D1074796

Clinical Practice

Principles and Practice of Ophthalmology

SECTION EDITORS

Eliot L. Berson, M.D.
Donald J. D'Amico, M.D.
Evangelos S. Gragoudas, M.D.
Charles L. Schepens, M.D.

Clinical Practice

Principles and Practice of Ophthalmology

Volume 2

DANIEL M. ALBERT, M.D.
Frederick A. Davis Professor and Chairman,
Department of Ophthalmology,
University of Wisconsin Medical School,
Madison, Wisconsin

FREDERICK A. JAKOBIEC, M.D., D.Sc.(Med.)
Henry Willard Williams Professor of Ophthalmology,
Professor of Pathology, and Chairman,
Department of Ophthalmology,
Harvard Medical School;
Chief, Department of Ophthalmology, and
Surgeon in Ophthalmology,
Massachusetts Eye and Ear Infirmary,
Boston, Massachusetts

NANCY L. ROBINSON, A.B.
Managing Editor

W.B. SAUNDERS COMPANY
A Division of Harcourt Brace & Company

Philadelphia   London   Toronto   Montreal   Sydney   Tokyo

W.B. SAUNDERS COMPANY
A Division of Harcourt Brace & Company

The Curtis Center
Independence Square West
Philadelphia, Pennsylvania 19106

Library of Congress Cataloging-in-Publication Data

Principles and practice of ophthalmology : clinical practice / [edited by]
Daniel M. Albert, Frederick A. Jakobiec.

    p.   cm.

ISBN 0–7216–3418–4 (5 v. set)

1. Ophthalmology.   I. Albert, Daniel M.   II. Jakobiec,
Frederick A.

[DNLM: 1. Eye Diseases.   2. Ophthalmology.   WW 140
P957 1994] RE46.P743 1994

617.7—dc20
DNLM/DLC   93–7247

PRINCIPLES AND PRACTICE OF OPHTHALMOLOGY: ISBN Volume 2 0–7216–6594–2
CLINICAL PRACTICE   5-Volume Set 0–7216–3418–4

Printed in the United States of America.

Last digit is the print number: 9   8   7   6   5   4   3   2   1

Contributors

Lloyd M. Aiello, MD
Associate Clinical Professor of Ophthalmology, Harvard Medical School; Director, Ophthalmology, and Active Staff, Joslin Diabetes Center; Chief, Section of Ophthalmology, and Active Staff, New England Deaconess Hospital; Associate Surgeon, Active Staff, Brigham and Women's Hospital; Associate Surgeon, Associate Staff, Massachusetts Eye and Ear Infirmity; Affiliate Staff, New England Baptist Hospital, Boston, Massachusetts

George K. Asdourian, MD
Professor of Ophthalmology, Department of Ophthalmology, University of Massachusetts Medical Center; Staff, University of Massachusetts Medical Center and The Medical Center of Central Massachusetts, Worcester, Massachusetts

Mark W. Balles, MD
Assistant Professor, Department of Ophthalmology, University of Minnesota Medical School; Director, Retina Service, University of Minnesota Hospital and Clinics, Minneapolis, Minnesota

Eliot L. Berson, MD
William F. Chatlos Professor of Ophthalmology and Director, Berman-Gund Laboratory for the Study of Retinal Degenerations, Harvard Medical School; Surgeon in Ophthalmology and Director, Electroretinography Service, Massachusetts Eye and Ear Infirmary, Boston, Massachusetts

Norman P. Blair, MD
Professor of Ophthalmology, University of Illinois at Chicago College of Medicine; Director, Vitreoretinal Service, University of Illinois at Chicago Eye and Ear Infirmary, Chicago, Illinois

Mark S. Blumenkranz, MD
Clinical Professor of Ophthalmology, Stanford University; Co-Director of Vitreoretinal Service, Stanford Medical Center, Stanford, California

Neil M. Bressler, MD
Associate Professor of Ophthalmology, Johns Hopkins University School of Medicine; Staff, Johns Hopkins Hospital and Francis Scott Key Medical Center; Consultant, Sinai Hospital, Baltimore, Maryland

Susan B. Bressler, MD
Associate Professor of Ophthalmology, Johns Hopkins University School of Medicine; Staff, Johns Hopkins Hospital and Francis Scott Key Medical Center; Consultant, Sinai Hospital, Baltimore, Maryland

Alfred Brini, MD
Professor Emeritus, Department of Ophthalmology, Université Louis Pasteur, Strasbourg, France

Norman E. Byer, MD
Clinical Professor of Ophthalmology, University of California, Los Angeles; Courtesy Staff, Torrance Memorial Hospital and Little Company of Mary Hospital, Torrance, California

Stanley Chang, MD
Associate Professor of Ophthalmology, Cornell University Medical College; Associate Attending, The New York Hospital and Memorial/Sloan-Kettering Medical Center, New York, New York

Nabil G. Chedid, MD
Research Fellow, Department of Ophthalmology, Harvard Medical School; Research Associate, Schepens Eye Research Institute; Clinical Fellow, Retina Associates, Boston, Massachusetts

Donald J. D'Amico, MD
Associate Professor of Ophthalmology, Harvard Medical School; Director, Diabetic Retinopathy Unit, and Associate Chief of Ophthalmology for Clinical Affairs, Massachusetts Eye and Ear Infirmary, Boston, Massachusetts

Monica A. De La Paz, MD
Clinical Fellow in Ophthalmology, Harvard Medical School; Retina Fellow, Massachusetts Eye and Ear Infirmary, Boston, Massachusetts

Maryanna Destro, MD
Clinical Instructor in Ophthalmology, Harvard Medical School; Assistant Clinical Professor, Tufts University School of Medicine; Assistant Surgeon, Massachusetts Eye and Ear Infirmary, Boston, Massachusetts

Jay S. Duker, MD
Associate Professor of Ophthalmology, Tufts University School of Medicine; Surgeon, New England Medical Center; Director, Vitreoretinal Service, New England Eye Center, Boston, Massachusetts

Bishara M. Faris, MD
Clinical Professor of Ophthalmology, Boston University School of Medicine; Lecturer on Ophthalmology, Harvard Medical School; Active Medical Staff, Boston University Medical Center and Boston City Hospital; Assistant in Ophthalmology, Massachusetts Eye and Ear Infirmary, Boston; Active Medical Staff, St. Vincent's Hospital, Worcester, Massachusetts

C. Stephen Foster, MD, FACS
Associate Professor of Ophthalmology, Harvard Medical School; Director, Immunology and Uveitis Service, Hilles Immunology Laboratory, and Rhoades Molecular Immunology Laboratory, Massachusetts Eye and Ear Infirmary, Boston, Massachusetts

Thomas R. Friberg, MS, MD
Professor of Ophthalmology, University of Pittsburgh School of Medicine and The Eye and Ear Institute; Staff, Eye and Ear Hospital, Veterans Administration Medical Center, Presbyterian-University Hospital, Pittsburgh, Pennsylvania

Ephraim Friedman, BA, MD
Professor of Ophthalmology, Harvard Medical School; Surgeon, Massachusetts Eye and Ear Infirmary, Boston, Massachusetts

Alexander R. Gaudio, MD
Clinical Instructor in Ophthalmology, Harvard Medical School; Senior Attending, Hartford Hospital; Associate Surgeon in Ophthalmology, Massachusetts Eye and Ear Infirmary, Boston, Massachusetts

Stephen C. Gieser, MD
Fellow, The Johns Hopkins School of Medicine; Senior Clinical Fellow, The Johns Hopkins Hospital, Baltimore, Maryland

Evangelos S. Gragoudas, MD
Associate Professor of Ophthalmology, Harvard Medical School; Director of Retina Service, Massachusetts Eye and Ear Infirmary, Boston, Massachusetts

David R. Guyer, MD
Staff, Retinal Service and Retinal Research Laboratory, Manhattan Eye, Ear, and Throat Hospital, New York, New York

Robert Haimovici, MD
Fellow, Retina Service, Harvard Medical School and Massachusetts Eye and Ear Infirmary, Boston, Massachusetts

Lawrence S. Halperin, MD
Attending, North Ridge Medical Center, Imperial Point Medical Center, and Boca Raton Community Hospital, Fort Lauderdale, Florida

Gary D. Haynie, MD
Clinical Fellow, Harvard Medical School; Fellow, Retina Service, Massachusetts Eye and Ear Infirmary, Boston, Massachusetts

Thomas R. Hedges III, MD
Associate Professor of Ophthalmology and Neurology, Tufts University School of Medicine; Ophthalmologist, New England Medical Center; Director of Neuro-ophthalmology, New England Eye Center, Boston, Massachusetts

Tatsuo Hirose, MD
Clinical Professor of Ophthalmology, Harvard Medical School; Associate Clinical Scientist, Schepens Eye Research Institute; Surgeon, Massachusetts Eye and Ear Infirmary, Boston, Massachusetts

David G. Hunter, MD, PhD
Staff, Pediatric Ophthalmology and Strabismus Service, The Wilmer Ophthalmological Institute, The Johns Hopkins Hospital, Baltimore, Maryland

Henry J. Kaplan, MD
Professor and Chairman, Department of Ophthalmology, Washington University School of Medicine; Attending, Barnes Hospital, St. Louis, Missouri

Shalom J. Kieval, MD
Associate Clinical Professor of Ophthalmology, Albany Medical College; Staff, Albany Medical Center Hospital, Albany Memorial Hospital, and Childs Hospital; Courtesy Staff, St. Peter's Hospital, Albany, New York

Sang H. Kim, MD
Visiting Associate Professor of Ophthalmology, University of Illinois at Chicago College of Medicine; Visiting Assistant Professor of Ophthalmology, University of Illinois at Chicago Eye and Ear Infirmary and Humana Michael Reese Health Plan, Chicago, Illinois

Arnold J. Kroll, MD
Clinical Professor of Ophthalmology, Tufts University School of Medicine and The New England Eye Center; Associate Surgeon of Ophthalmology, Massachusetts Eye and Ear Infirmary and The New England Eye Center, Boston, Massachusetts

Sara Krupsky, MD
Research Fellow, Massachusetts Eye and Ear Infirmary, Boston, Massachusetts

John S. Lean, MD, FRCS
Estelle Doheny Eye Hospital, Los Angeles, California

Carol M. Lee, MD
Clinical Assistant Professor, Department of Ophthalmology, New York University School of Medicine; Staff, Tisch Hospital, New York University Medical Center, New York, New York

Marc R. Levin, MD
Staff, Lutheran General Hospital, Park Ridge, Illinois

John I. Loewenstein, MD
Clinical Instructor in Ophthalmology, Harvard Medical School; Assistant in Ophthalmology, Massachusetts Eye and Ear Infirmary, Boston, Massachusetts

Peter L. Lou, MD
Clinical Instructor in Ophthalmology, Harvard Medical School; Assistant Surgeon in Ophthalmology, Massachusetts Eye and Ear Infirmary, Boston, Massachusetts

John C. Madigan, Jr., MD
Active Associate Staff, Hartford Hospital, Hartford, Connecticut

Raymond R. Margherio, MD
Senior Researcher and Clinical Professor of Biomedical Sciences (for Ophthalmology), Oakland University, Rochester; Chief, Department of Ophthalmology, William Beaumont Hospital, and Director, Beaumont Eye Institute, Detroit, Michigan

W. Wynn McMullen, MD
Assistant Clinical Professor of Ophthalmology, University of Texas Medical School at Houston; Active Staff, Hermann Hospital, Houston, Texas

Joan W. Miller, MD
Instructor in Ophthalmology, Harvard Medical School; Assistant Surgeon, Retina Service, Department of Ophthalmology, Massachusetts Eye and Ear Infirmary, Boston, Massachusetts

Jordi Monés, MD
Barcelona, Spain

Eric Mukai, BS
Medical Student, University of Vermont College of Medicine, Burlington, Vermont

Shizuo Mukai, MD
Assistant Professor of Ophthalmology, Harvard Medical School; Assistant in Ophthalmology, Massachusetts Eye and Ear Infirmary, Boston, Massachusetts

Robert P. Murphy, MD
Medical Staff, Department of Surgery, Division of Ophthalmology, Saint Joseph Hospital; Member, Greater Baltimore Medical Center Medical Staff with Consulting Privileges, Department of Ophthalmology; Consultant/Honorary Consultant, Medical Staff, Department of Ophthalmology, Sinai Hospital, Baltimore, Maryland

Don H. Nicholson, MD
Professor of Ophthalmology, Bascom Palmer Eye Institute, University of Miami School of Medicine; Peripatetic Staff, Anne Bates Leach Eye Hospital, Miami, Florida

Stuart W. Noorily, MD
Fellow, Department of Ophthalmology, The Johns Hopkins University School of Medicine; Assistant Instructor, Vitreoretinal Surgery Services, Wilmer Ophthalmological Institute, Baltimore, Maryland

R. Joseph Olk, MD
Associate Professor of Ophthalmology, Washington University School of Medicine; Attending Ophthalmologist, Barnes Hospital, St. Louis, Missouri

E. Mitchel Opremcak, MD
Assistant Professor of Ophthalmology, The Ohio State University College of Medicine; Staff, The University Hospitals and Columbus Children's Hospital, Columbus, Ohio

Andrew J. Packer, MD
Attending Staff, Hartford Hospital, Hartford, Connecticut

Samir C. Patel, MD
Assistant Professor of Ophthalmology and Director, Residency Program, University of Chicago, Department of Ophthalmology; Staff, University of Chicago Hospital and Weiss Memorial Hospital, Chicago, Illinois

Michael K. Pinnolis, MD
Instructor in Ophthalmology, Harvard Medical School; Assistant in Ophthalmology, Massachusetts Eye and Ear Infirmary; Affiliate Staff, Newton Wellesley Hospital, Boston, Massachusetts

Ronald C. Pruett, MD
Associate Clinical Professor of Ophthalmology, Harvard Medical School; Surgeon in Ophthalmology, Massachusetts Eye and Ear Infirmary, Boston, Massachusetts

Carmen A. Puliafito, MD
Professor and Chair, Department of Ophthalmology, Tufts University School of Medicine; Director, New England Eye Center; Full-time Staff, New England Medical Center, Boston, Massachusetts

Charles D. J. Regan, MD
Associate Professor of Ophthalmology, Harvard Medical School; Surgeon in Ophthalmology, Massachusetts Eye and Ear Infirmary, Boston, Massachusetts

Elias Reichel, MD
Instructor in Ophthalmology, Tufts University School of Medicine; Staff, New England Eye Center; New England Medical Center, Boston, Massachusetts

Steven J. Rose, MD
Clinical Assistant Professor of Ophthalmology, University of Rochester School of Medicine and Dentistry; Associate Attending Surgeon in Ophthalmology, Strong Memorial Hospital; St. Mary's Hospital; and Rochester General Hospital, Rochester, New York

Michael A. Sandberg, PhD
Associate Professor of Ophthalmology, Harvard Medical School; Research Associate, Massachusetts Eye and Ear Infirmary, Boston, Massachusetts

Charles L. Schepens, MD
Clinical Professor (Emeritus), Department of Ophthalmology, Harvard Medical School; Consulting Surgeon, Massachusetts Eye and Ear Infirmary, Boston, Massachusetts

Johanna M. Seddon, MD, MS
Associate Professor, Department of Ophthalmology, Harvard Medical School; Associate Surgeon in Ophthalmology, Massachusetts Eye and Ear Infirmary, Boston, Massachusetts

John A. Sorenson, MD
Attending Surgeon, Manhattan Eye, Ear, and Throat Hospital, New York, New York

Janet R. Sparrow, PhD
Assistant Professor of Anatomy in Ophthalmology and Assistant Professor of Cell Biology and Anatomy, Cornell University Medical College, New York, New York

Richard R. Tamesis, MD
Resident in Ophthalmology, University of Nebraska Eye Center, Omaha, Nebraska

David V. Weinberg, MD
Assistant Professor of Ophthalmology and Chief of Vitreoretinal Service, Northwestern University Medical School, Chicago, Illinois

Lawrence A. Yannuzzi, MD
Assistant Professor of Ophthalmology, Columbia-Presbyterian Medical Center; Vice Chairman and Director of Retinal Services, Manhattan Eye, Ear, and Throat Hospital, New York, New York

Lucy H. Y. Young, MD, PhD
Assistant Professor of Ophthalmology, Harvard Medical School; Assistant in Ophthalmology, Massachusetts Eye and Ear Infirmary, Boston, Massachusetts

To Ellie

D.M.A.

Preface

"INCIPIT." The medieval scribe would write this Latin word, meaning *so it begins,* to signal the start of the book he was transcribing. It was a dramatic word that conveyed promise of instruction and delight. In more modern times INCIPIT has been replaced by the PREFACE. It may be the first thing the reader sees, but it is, in fact, the last thing the author writes before the book goes to press. I appreciate the opportunity to make some personal comments regarding **Principles and Practice of Ophthalmology.**

One of the most exciting things about writing and editing a book in a learned field is that it puts the authors and editors in touch with those who have gone before. Each author shares with those who have labored in past years and in past centuries the tasks of assessing the knowledge that exists in his or her field, of determining what is important, and of trying to convey it to his or her peers. In the course of the work the author experiences the same anticipation, angst, and ennui of those who have gone before. He or she can well envision the various moments of triumph and despair that all authors and editors must feel as they organize, review, and revise the accumulating manuscripts and reassure, cajole, and make demands of their fellow editors, authors, and publisher.

This feeling of solidarity with early writers becomes even more profound when one is a collector and reviewer of books, and conversant with the history of one's field. In Ecclesiastes it is stated, "of the making of books, there is no end" (12:12). Indeed, there are more books than any other human artifact on earth. There is, however, a beginning to the "making of books" in any given field. The first ophthalmology book to be published was Benvenuto Grassi's *De Oculis* in Florence in 1474. Firmin Didot in his famous *Bibliographical Encyclopedia* wrote that Grassus, an Italian physician of the School of Solerno, lived in the 12th century and was the author of two books, *Ferrara Quarto* (1474) and the *Venetian Folio* (1497). Eye care in the 15th century was in the hands of itinerant barber-surgeons and quacks, and a treatise by a learned physician was a remarkable occurrence. The next book on the eye to appear was an anonymous pamphlet written for the layperson in 1538 and entitled *Ein Newes Hochnutzliches Büchlin von Erkantnus der Kranckheyten der Augen.* Like **Principles and Practice of Ophthalmology,** the *Büchlin* stated its intention to provide highly useful knowledge of eye diseases, the anatomy of the eye, and various remedies. It was illustrated with a full-page woodcut of the anatomy of the eye (Fig. 1). At the conclusion of the book, the publisher, Vogtherr, promised to bring more and better information to light shortly, and indeed, the next year he published a small book by Leonhart Fuchs (1501–1566) entitled *Alle Kranckheyt der Augen.*

Fuchs, a fervent Hippocratist, was Professor first of Philosophy and then of Medicine at Ingolstadt, Physician of the Margrave Georg of Brandenburg, and finally Professor at Tübingen for 31 years. Like the earlier *Büchlin,* his work begins with an anatomic woodcut (Fig. 2), then lists in tabular form various eye conditions, including strabismus, paralysis, amblyopia, and nictalops. The work uses a distinctly Greco-Roman terminology, presenting information on the parts of the eye and their affections, including conjunctivitis, ophthalmia, carcinoma, and "glaucoma." The book concludes with a remedy collection similar to that found in the *Büchlin.* Most significant in the association of Leonhart Fuchs with this book is the fact that a properly trained and

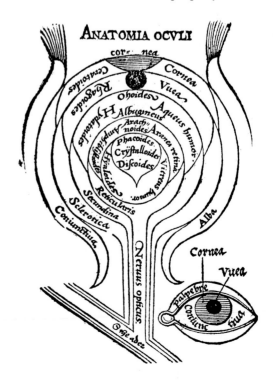

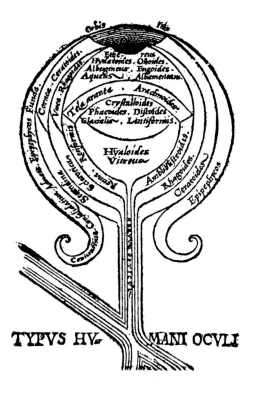

TYPVS HV-MANI OCVLI

well-recognized physician addressed the subject of ophthalmology.

Julius Hirschberg, the ophthalmic historian, noted that Fuch's *Alle Kranckheyt,* along with the anonymous *Büchlin,* apparently influenced Georg Bartisch in his writing of *Das ist Augendienst.* This latter work, published in 1583, marked the founding of modern ophthalmology. Bartisch (1535–1606) was an itinerant barber-surgeon but nonetheless a thoughtful and skillful surgeon, whose many innovations included the first procedure for extirpation of the globe for ocular cancer. Bartisch proposed standards for the individual who practices eye surgery, noting that rigorous training and concentration of effort were needed to practice this specialty successfully.

By the late 16th century, eye surgery and the treatment of eye disease began to move into the realm of the more formally trained and respected surgeon. This is evidenced by Jacques Guillemeau's *Traité des Maladies de l'Oeil,* published in 1585. Guillemeau (1550–1612) was a pupil of the surgical giant Ambroise Paré, and his book was an epitome of the existing knowledge on the subject.

The transition from couching of cataracts to the modern method of treating cataracts by extraction of the lens, as introduced by Jacques Daviel in 1753, further defined the skill and training necessary for the care of the eyes. The initiation of ophthalmology as a separate specialty within the realm of medicine and surgery was signaled by the publication of George Joseph Beer's two-volume *Lehre von den Augenkrankheiten* in 1813–1817. Beer (1763–1821) founded the first eye hospital in 1786 in Vienna, and his students became famous ophthalmic surgeons and professors throughout Europe.

In England, it was not only the demands of cataract surgery but also the great pandemic of trachoma following the Napoleonic wars that led to the establishment of ophthalmology as a recognized specialty. Benjamin Travers (1783–1858) published the earliest treatise in English on diseases of the eye, *A Synopsis of the Diseases of the Eye,* in 1820. In the United States, acceptance of ophthalmology as a specialty had to await the description of the ophthalmoscope by Helmholtz in 1851, and the additional need of special skills that using the early primitive "Augenspiegel" required.

As the complexity of ophthalmology increased and as subspecialization began to develop in the 19th century, multiauthored books began to appear. This culminated in the appearance in 1874 of the first volume of the Graefe-Saemisch *Handbuch.* The final volume of this great collective work, of which Alfred Carl Graefe (1830–1899) and Edwin Theodor Saemisch (1833–1909) were editors, appeared in 1880. The definitive second edition, which for more than a quarter of a century remained the most comprehensive and authoritative work in the field, appeared in 15 volumes between 1899 and 1918. The great French counterpart to the Graefe-Saemisch *Handbuch* was the *Encyclopédie Française d'Ophtalmologie,* which appeared in 9 volumes (1903–1910), edited by Octave Doin, and filled a similar role for the French-speaking ophthalmologist.

In 1896, the first of 4 volumes of Norris and Oliver's *System of Diseases of the Eye* was published in the United States. The senior editor, Dr. William Fisher Norris (1839–1901), was the first Clinical Professor of Diseases of the Eye at the University of Pennsylvania. Charles A. Oliver (1853–1911) was his student. Norris considered the *System* to be his monumental work. For each section he chose an outstanding authority in the field, having in the end more than 60 American, British, Dutch, French, and German ophthalmologists as contributors. Almost 6 years of combined labor on the part of the editors was needed for completion of the work. In 1913, Casey A. Wood (1856–1942) introduced the first of his 18 volumes of the *American Encyclopedia and Dictionary of Ophthalmology.* The final volume appeared in 1921. Drawn largely from the Graef-Saemisch *Handbuch* and the *Encyclopédie Française d'Ophtalmologie,* Wood's *Encyclopedia* provided information on the whole of ophthalmology through a strictly alphabetic sequence of subject headings.

The book from which the present work draws inspiration is Duke-Elder's *Textbook of Ophthalmology* (7 volumes; 1932) and particularly the second edition of this work entitled *System of Ophthalmology* (15 volumes, published between 1958 and 1976). The *System of Ophthalmology* was written by Sir Stewart Duke-Elder (1898–1978) in conjunction with his colleagues at the Institute of Ophthalmology in London. In 1976, when the last of his 15 volumes appeared, Duke-Elder wrote in the Preface:

> The writing of these two series, the *Textbook* and the *System,* has occupied all my available time for half a century. I cannot deny that its completion brings me relief on the recovery of my freedom, but at the same time it has left some sadness for I have enjoyed writing it. As

Edward Gibbon said on having written the last line of *The Decline and Fall of the Roman Empire:* "A sober melancholy has spread over my mind by the idea that I have taken everlasting leave of an old and agreeable companion."

Duke-Elder adds a final line that I hope will be more apropos to the present editors and contributors. "At the same time the prayer of Sir Francis Drake on the eve of the attack of the Spanish Armada is apposite: 'Give us to know that it is not the beginning but the continuing of the same until it is entirely finished which yieldeth the true glory.'" The void that developed as the Duke-Elder series became outdated has been partially filled by many fine books, notably Thomas Duane's excellent 5-volume *Clinical Ophthalmology.*

Inspiration to undertake a major work such as this is derived not only from the past books but from teachers and role models as well. For me, this includes Francis Heed Adler, Harold G. Scheie, William C. Frayer, David G. Cogan, Ludwig von Sallmann, Alan S. Rabson, Lorenz E. Zimmerman, Frederick C. Blodi, Claes H. Dohlman, and Matthew D. Davis.

Whereas the inspiration for the present text was derived from Duke-Elder's *Textbook* and *System* and from teachers and role models, learning how to write and organize a book came for me from Adler's *Textbook of Ophthalmology,* published by W. B. Saunders. This popular textbook for medical students and general practitioners was first produced by Dr. Sanford Gifford (1892–1945) in 1938. Francis Heed Adler (1895–1987), after writing the 6th edition, published in 1962, invited Harold G. Scheie (1909–1989); his successor as Chairman of Ophthalmology at the University of Pennsylvania, and myself to take over authorship. We completely rewrote this book and noted in the Preface to the 8th edition, published in 1969: "This book aims to provide the medical student and the practicing physician with a concise and profusely illustrated current text, organized in a convenient and useable manner, on the eye and its disorders. It is hoped that the beginning, or even practicing, ophthalmologist may find it of value."

In 1969 it was apparent that even for the intended audience, contributions by individuals expert in the subspecialties of ophthalmology were required. The book was published in Spanish and Chinese editions and was popular enough to warrant an updated 9th edition, which appeared in 1977. One of the high points of this work was interacting with John Dusseau, the Editor-in-Chief for the W. B. Saunders Company. As a 10th edition was contemplated, I became increasingly convinced that what was needed in current ophthalmology was a new, comprehensive, well-illustrated set of texts intended for the practicing ophthalmologist and written by outstanding authorities in the field. I envisioned a work that in one series of volumes would provide all of the basic clinical and scientific information required by practicing ophthalmologists in their everyday work. For more detailed or specialized information, this work should direct the practitioner to the pertinent journal articles or more specialized publications. As time pro-gressed, a plan for this work took shape and received support from the W. B. Saunders Company.

Memories of the formative stages of the **Principles and Practice of Ophthalmology** remain vivid: Proposing the project to Fred Jakobiec in the cafeteria of the Massachusetts Eye and Ear Infirmary in early 1989. Having dinner with Lew Reines, President and Chief Executive Officer, and Richard Zorab, Senior Medical Editor, at the Four Seasons Hotel in May 1989, where we agreed upon the scope of the work. My excitement as I walked across the Public Garden and down Charles Street back to the Infirmary, contemplating the work we were to undertake. Finalizing the outline for the book in Henry Allen's well-stocked "faculty lounge" in a dormitory at Colby College during the Lancaster Course. Meeting with members of the Harvard Faculty in the somber setting of the rare-book room to recruit the Section Editors. Persuading Nancy Robinson, my able assistant since 1969, to take on the job of Managing Editor. The receipt of our first manuscript from Dr. David Cogan.

We considered making this work a departmental undertaking, utilizing the faculty and alumni of various Harvard programs. However, the broad scope of the series required recruitment of outstanding authors from many institutions. Once the Section Editors were in place, there was never any doubt in my mind that this work would succeed. The Section Editors proved a hardworking and dedicated group, and their choice of authors reflects their good judgment and persuasive abilities. I believe that you will appreciate the scope of knowledge and the erudition.

The editorship of this book provided me not only with an insight into the knowledge and thinking of some of the finest minds in ophthalmology but also with an insight into their lives. What an overwhelmingly busy group of people! Work was completed not through intimidation with deadlines but by virtue of their love of ophthalmology and their desire to share their knowledge and experience. The talent, commitment, persistence, and good humor of the authors are truly what made this book a reality.

It was our intent to present a work that was at once scholarly and pragmatic, that dealt effectively with the complexities and subtleties of modern ophthalmology, but that did not overwhelm the reader. We have worked toward a series of volumes that contained the relevant basic science information to sustain and complement the clinical facts. We wanted a well-illustrated set that went beyond the illustrations in any textbook or system previously published, in terms of quantity and quality and usefulness of the pictures.

In specific terms, in editing the book we tried to identify and eliminate errors in accuracy. We worked to provide as uniform a literary style as is possible in light of the numerous contributors. We attempted to make as consistent as possible the level of detail presented in the many sections and chapters. Related to this, we sought to maintain the length according to our agreed-upon plan. We tried, as far as possible, to eliminate repetition and at the same time to prevent gaps in information. We worked to direct the location of information into a logical and convenient arrangement. We attempted to separate the basic science chapters to the major extent into the separate **Basic Sciences** volume, but at the same time to integrate basic science information with clinical detail in other sections as needed. These tasks were made challenging by the size of the work, the number of authors, and the limited options for change as material was received close to publishing deadlines. We believe that these efforts have succeeded in providing ophthalmologists and visual scientists with a useful resource in their practices. We shall know in succeeding years the level of this success and hope to have the opportunity to improve all these aspects as the book is updated and published in future editions. Bacon wrote: "Reading maketh a full man, conference a ready man, and writing an exact man." He should have added: *Editing maketh a humble man.*

I am personally grateful to a number of individuals for making this book a reality. Nancy Robinson leads the list. Her intelligent, gracious, and unceasing effort as Managing Editor was essential to its successful completion. Mr. Lewis Reines, President of the W. B. Saunders Company, has a profound knowledge of publishing and books that makes him a worthy successor to John Dusseau. Richard Zorab, the Senior Medical Editor, and Hazel N. Hacker, the Developmental Editor, are thoroughly professional and supportive individuals with whom it was a pleasure to work. Many of the black-and-white illustrations were drawn by Laurel Cook Lhowe and Marcia Williams; Kit Johnson provided many of the anterior segment photographs. Archival materials were retrieved with the aid of Richard Wolfe, Curator of Rare Books at the Francis A. Countway Library of Medicine, and Chris Nims and Kathleen Kennedy of the Howe Library at the Massachusetts Eye and Ear Infirmary.

The most exciting aspect of writing and editing a work of this type is that it puts one in touch with the present-day ophthalmologists and visual scientists as well as physicians training to be ophthalmologists in the future. We hope that this book will establish its own tradition of excellence and usefulness and that it will win it a place in the lives of ophthalmologists today and in the future.

"EXPLICIT," scribes wrote at the end of every book. EXPLICIT means *it has been unfolded.* Olmert notes in *The Smithsonian Book of Books,* "the unrolling or unfolding of knowledge is a powerful act because it shifts responsibility from writer to reader. . . . Great books endure because they help us interpret our lives. It's a personal quest, this grappling with the world and ourselves, and we need all the help we can get." We hope that this work will provide such help to the professional lives of ophthalmologists and visual scientists.

DANIEL M. ALBERT, M.D.
MADISON, WISCONSIN

To my beloved family, both living and elsewhere;
To my cherished teachers and trainees, both past and present;
To my incomparable patients, both cured and uncured;
And to my supportive colleagues and friends, all insufficiently
celebrated in my preface.

F.A.J.

Preface

Because of the pellucid beauty of the organ and tissues it studies, ophthalmology affords many pleasures and allurements. Although it might be more of a confessional than a verifiable statement, I have always believed that many individuals are also attracted to ophthalmology with the inchoate fantasy (later found to be erroneous) that it is an encapsulated and somewhat secessionist medical specialty one can totally master; this may indeed be an expression of the ophthalmic temperament's constitutive tropism toward control. Ophthalmology, furthermore, has long been a discipline that has generated exquisite teaching aids; most of the diseases and tissues we contend with are amenable to photographic documentation and elegant analysis by modern imaging and angiographic techniques. The quest for mastery in ophthalmology is marked by the periodic appearance of comprehensive textbooks, an example of which is the present enterprise.

If one person certainly could not do it today, is it possible for multiple authors to create a *Summa Ophthalmologica?* In my professional lifetime the most bruited effort was Duke-Elder's *System of Ophthalmology,* which encompassed 15 volumes, appearing ad seriatim from 1958 to 1976. As a resident-in-training, I remember anticipating the arrival of each new volume, and of devouring it from cover to cover because of the spectacular tour d'horizon that was provided. Early in my career, I was privileged to become involved with the orbit section of Duane's 5-volume *Clinical Ophthalmology* and subsequently with the anatomy, embryology, and teratology section of his 3-volume *Biomedical Foundations of Ophthalmology,* both of which were intended to supersede Duke-Elder. Now, having acquired more experience and maturity, I am aware that it is impossible for an ophthalmic diorama to rival the timelessness of Thomas Aquinas' *Summa Theologica,* Immanuel Kant's *Kritiken,* or Bertrand Russell's *Principia Mathematica,* all of which self-reflexively proceed from deductions based on a priori axioms. Ophthalmology is a contingent, empirical, and nonoracular discipline, and its intellectual artifacts necessarily reflect the imperfections and messiness of human inductive knowledge. At their best, the present and predecessor efforts to produce comprehensive ophthalmic textbooks are temporary codifications, inventories, and snapshots of an ever-unfolding field, much as sequential photograph albums reveal the fructifying growth and evolution of families over generations.

Why, then, was the present project undertaken, and what are its distinctive features? Dan Albert and I began jointly planning this work in early 1989, shortly after I arrived in Boston from New York City to become Chief of Ophthalmology at the Massachusetts Eye and Ear Infirmary and Chairman of the Department of Ophthalmology at the Harvard Medical School. We felt the time was right for a new gesamtwerk for ophthalmology, fraught as it might be with the limitations alluded to previously. We believed that the Harvard environment would be especially conducive to producing an outstanding work of scholarship. Initially the **Principles and Practice of Ophthalmology** textbook carried the subtitle "The Harvard System"; this was reflected in the contract signed with the publisher as well as in the stationery that was used throughout the project in correspondence with the contributors. Whereas it is true that all of the section editors and the vast majority of the 440 contributors are by design either present or past faculty or trainees of the Harvard Medical School, the Massachusetts Eye and Ear Infirmary, or the Schepens Eye Research Institute (now formally affiliated with the Harvard Department of Ophthalmology), it quickly became apparent that there was no single "Harvard" or systematic way of thinking about the various topics covered in these volumes. Even within the Harvard Department there are manifold approaches to basic science and clinical problems. Therefore, we were led to abandon the subtitle. Nonetheless, I personally am unabashedly proud that the high quality and erudition of the chapters derive from the intellectual formation that many contributors received from their association with the greater Harvard ophthalmic environment; well represented within this cadre are recent residents and fellows.

Of the 6 volumes, the longest **(Basic Sciences)** deals with the basic sciences of ophthalmology in ten sections. It is in this realm that one will expect the most rapid changes in subject matter in the immediate years ahead; on the other hand, this may be the most fecund and valuable of all the volumes, because there has not been a recent effort to synthesize the burgeoning of knowledge that has attended the revolutions in morphologic investigations, pharmacology, cell biology, immunology, and, lately, molecular genetics. Not every topic in the visual basic sciences could be covered: For example, an extensive and conventional repetition of the facts of embryology and anatomy has not been essayed, since there already exist serviceable references for these comparatively static subjects. The focus instead was on investigations that had been particularly rewarding and luminous over the past 10 years. My advice to readers is to approach each chapter in this volume as if it were an article in the *Scientific American* and to derive both knowledge and pleasure from these lapidary syntheses.

The 5 clinical volumes have been organized along the lines of standard anatomic and tissue-topographic demarcations. Additionally, there are systematic approaches to some established and newly emerging nodal points of knowledge: neuroophthalmology; the eye and systemic disease; pediatric ophthalmology; ocular oncology; ophthalmic pathology; trauma; diagnostic imaging; optical principles and applications; and psychological, social, and legal aspects of ophthalmology. Efforts were made to reduce unnecessary duplication from section to section in the coverage of various subjects; however, when it was felt that it would be profitable to have the same disease or topic covered from several perspectives, this was permitted. We are aware that, despite the length of our present undertaking, the end result is one of comprehensiveness but not exhaustiveness. It should be remembered that there already exist many published and revised multivolume treatises on subjects covered herein. What we have aimed for is to provide the generalist with a digestible up-to-date overview of ophthalmology and also to provide the superspecialist with readily accessible introductions to topics outside of his or her intensive areas of expertise.

Another distinctive feature of the present volumes is the prodigious number of illustrations, totaling well over 6000 if one includes tables, diagrams, and graphs. About half of these are in color, which enhances the aesthetic and teaching value of the entire project. The bibliographies are often daunting and will serve as pathfinders into the larger universe of their subjects. I would particularly like to thank Ms. Kit Johnson of the Infirmary for providing many of the color illustrations for diseases of the eyelids, conjunctiva, and anterior segment of the eye. For voluptuaries of ophthalmology, these and the fundus illustrations should provide a sumptuous feast.

It staggers the mind to contemplate the quotidian and oppressive amount of effort expended on this project—the incalculable atomistic acts of assemblage, the gently hectoring telephone calls, the background acquisition and scope of the basic science and clinical knowledge, the multiple textual revisions, the amassing of bibliographies and illustrations, and so on—and indeed the formidable cost of producing each of the individual chapters, much of which was borne by the authors themselves. Even as we are hopeful that these volumes will make a major positive impression on American and international ophthalmology, modesty in the face of our challenging task rather than arrogance has inspired the lofty goals that sustained the creation of the **Principles and Practice of Ophthalmology.** Still, I have no doubt that many of the chapters contained in these volumes are the most incandescent, scholarly, and useful summary presentations of their subjects that have been crafted up to now. In a many-authored textbook there

will be some unevenness, the result of the idiosyncrasies of the contributors as well as the state of development of their subject matter. My own criterion for the success of this enterprise is a simple one: that 50 percent or more of the chapters will have achieved the status of being the best overviews and introductions for their subjects. Regarding topics that should have been covered but were somehow missed or that were surveyed inadequately, the chief editors, the section editors, the authors, and the publisher will look forward to hearing from readers and reviewers about any constructive criticisms on how to improve the textbook in its next edition. We are also exploring various mechanisms for issuing supplemental chapters to rectify some of these perceived and real deficiencies before the next edition.

Based on my familiarity with ophthalmic texts, I think the present work is the largest ophthalmic publication ever to appear *all at once as a complete set.* The W. B. Saunders Company is consequently to be congratulated for having maintained the highest standards of production in terms of copy editing, printing, paper quality, indexing, and reproduction of color and black-and-white illustrations. Mr. Richard Zorab, Senior Medical Editor, was a tireless and relatively humane flogger of myself and the other contributors to meet realistic deadlines; Mrs. Hazel N. Hacker was our highly expert Developmental Editor, and Mrs. Linda R. Garber kept the movement of manuscripts and galleys on schedule with minimal breakage. Ms. Nancy Robinson was a compassionate, patient, and effective intradepartmental Managing Editor. I particularly applaud the ability of the publisher to keep the price of the 6 volumes, with all their color illustrations, at a respectable level so that they are within the reach of trainees, basic scientists, and clinicians in an era of highly competitive National Institutes of Health funding and when ophthalmic reimbursements are being ratcheted down.

It is my compressed personal philosophy that we live to feel, think, and act and that the highest emanations of these faculties are enthusiasm, creativity, and love. This textbook is a manifestation of all six of these capacities, served up in superabundance. May the response of the ophthalmic community be commensurate with the spiritual and intellectual largesse lavished by the contributors on these volumes. Finally, although I somewhat iconoclastically do not fully subscribe to the notion of role models (because I believe that each person should construct his or her unique identity and excellence by cultivating one's intrinsic gifts while at the same time selectively interiorizing the finest qualities of many exemplars), I would like to thank my many professional friends and colleagues who have played salutary roles in the parturition of my own career, and who have taught me and/or supported me to this point in my professional life so that I could participate in this magnificent and bracing academic adventure: Dean S. James Adelstein, Dr. Henry Allen, Dr. Myles Behrens, Mr. Alexander Bernhard, Dr. Frederick Blodi, Dr. Sheldon Buckler, Dr. Alston Callahan, Dr. Charles J. Campbell, Dr. H. Dwight Cavanaugh, Mr. Melville Chapin, Dr.

David Cogan, Dr. D. Jackson Coleman, Dr. Brian Curtin, Dr. Donald D'Amico, Dr. Arthur Gerard DeVoe, Dr. Jack Dodick, Dr. Claes Dohlman, Dr. Anthony Donn, Dr. Thomas Duane, Dr. Howard Eggers, Dr. Robert Ellsworth, Dr. Andrew Ferry, Dr. Ben Fine, Dr. Ramon L. Font, Dr. Max Forbes, Dr. Ephraim Friedman, Mr. J. Frank Gerrity, Dr. Gabriel Godman, Dr. Evangelos Gragoudas, Dr. W. Richard Green, Dr. Winston Harrison, the late Dr. Paul Henkind, Dr. George M. Howard, Dr. Takeo Iwamoto, Dr. Ira Snow Jones, Mrs. Diane Kaneb, Dr. Donald West King, Dr. Daniel M. Knowles, Dr. Raphael Lattes, Dr. Simmons Lessell, Dr. Harvey Lincoff, Mr. Martin Lipton, Dr. Richard Lisman, Mr. Richard MacKinnon, Dr. Ian McLean, Dr. Julian Manski, Dr. Norman Medow, Mr. August Meyer, Dr. George (Bud) Merriam, Jr., Dr. Karl Perzin, Dr. Kathryn Stein Pokorny, Dr. Elio Raviola, the late Dr. Algernon B. Reese, Mr. William Renchard, Dr. Rene Rodriguez-Sains, Dr. Evan Sacks, Dr. Charles Schepens, Dr. James Schutz, the late Dr. Sigmund Schutz, Dr. Jesse Sigelman, Mr. F. Curtis Smith, Dr. William Spencer, Ms. Cathleen Douglas Stone, Dr. R. David Sudarsky, Dr. Myron Tannenbaum, Dr. Elise Torczynski, Dean Daniel Tosteson, Dr. Arnold Turtz, Dr. Robert Uretz, the late Dr. Sigmund Wilens, Dr. Marianne Wolff, Dr. Myron Yanoff, and Dr. Lorenz E. Zimmerman.

I hope that this textbook will touch the lives of those who read it as much as these individuals have influenced my own.

Ad Astra Per Aspera!

FREDERICK A. JAKOBIEC, M.D., D.SC.(MED.)
BOSTON, MASSACHUSETTS

Contents

VOLUME 1

VOLUME 2

VOLUME 3

VOLUME 4

SECTION X

Ophthalmic Pathology, 2099
Edited by DANIEL M. ALBERT, THADDEUS P. DRYJA, and
FREDERICK A. JAKOBIEC

SECTION XI

Neuroophthalmology, 2387
Edited by JOSEPH F. RIZZO III and SIMMONS LESSELL

SECTION XII

Pediatric Ophthalmology, 2715
Edited by RICHARD M. ROBB and DAVID S. WALTON

VOLUME 5

SECTION IV

Retina and Vitreous

Edited by
EVANGELOS S. GRAGOUDAS and DONALD J. D'AMICO

Chapter 49

∎

Overview

EVANGELOS S. GRAGOUDAS and DONALD J. D'AMICO

Since the 1970s, there has been an unparalleled explosion of knowledge in the diagnosis and treatment of vitreoretinal disorders. Fluorescein angiography, laser photocoagulation, and vitrectomy were in their infancy in the early 1970s and now represent the most common diagnostic and therapeutic procedures for the vitreoretinal specialist. The major causes of blindness from retinal diseases include macular degeneration, diabetic retinopathy, and proliferative vitreoretinopathy, which were considered untreatable only a few years ago.

Major technologic advances and improvements in surgical techniques have led to the introduction of new or alternative therapies that have increased the effectiveness of the surgical procedures and diminished the number of inoperable cases. Modern vitrectomy machines, fine vitreous scissors and forceps, and endolasers, as well as the use of expansile gases, silicone oil, and liquid perfluorochemicals have improved the surgical success rate and saved numerous eyes from blindness.

Well-designed multicenter clinical trials have proved extremely helpful in defining the therapeutic approaches, as well as evaluating the results of treatment when compared with the natural history of the diseases studied. The Diabetic Retinopathy Study and the Macular Photocoagulation Study represent two of the most successful clinical trials in ophthalmology and in clinical medicine in general.

The treatment of endophthalmitis has been revolutionized, and many eyes that were uniformly lost only a few years ago can be now saved.

This section contains fresh information, numerous illustrations, and extensive references for a comprehensive vitreoretinal section.

Chapter 50 provides information on ophthalmoscopy and fundus biomicroscopy, which still represent the most important tools for a vitreoretinal examination. This is followed by Chapter 51 on fluorescein angiography and Chapter 52 on the newly applied indocyanine-green angiography. These most sophisticated imaging techniques have provided invaluable information in both the diagnosis and the management of retinal disorders.

A large number of chapters are devoted to the numerous disorders affecting the retinal vessels. Occlusion of arteries and retinal veins, diabetic retinopathy, and retinopathy of prematurity represent the more commonly observed vascular diseases, which are followed by Eales' disease, retinal macroaneurysms, retinal telangiectasia, familial exudative vitreoretinopathy, and Leber's idiopathic stellate neuroretinitis.

The macula can be affected by pathologic processes at the choroidal, retinal pigment epithelium, or neurosensory level and still represents one of the most challenging and difficult to treat areas of the fundus. Chapter 63 is devoted to central serous chorioretinopathy, which continues to puzzle the ophthalmologist regarding its pathogenesis, and Chapters 64 and 65 discuss age-related macular degeneration, which continues to be the major cause of blindness in the elderly population. The macula can be involved in several other disorders, such as angioid streaks, ocular histoplasmosis syndrome, degenerative myopia, macular holes, and cystoid macular edema after intraocular surgery. Disorders of unknown cause, such as acute posterior multifocal placoid pigment epitheliopathy, multiple evanescent white dot and related syndromes, and acute macular neuroretinopathy are discussed in detail. The retinochoroidal folds and epiretinal macular membranes many times can produce markedly decreased central vision from macular disturbance and are comprehensively reviewed. Retinal infections are currently diagnosed more accurately, and we have made considerable progress in their management. Toxoplasmosis, retinal manifestations of AIDS, acute retinal necrosis, viral infections, and ocular syphilis are extensively discussed. Subretinal fibrosis and uveitis syndrome, diffuse unilateral subacute neuroretinopathy, and frosted branch angiitis represent rather rare, but still very interesting, retinal disorders and have been addressed in separate chapters.

The retinal vasculature can be affected by several systemic disorders, and most of the systemic manifestations can be found in other sections of this book. In this section, the retinal findings of collagen disorders, retinopathy associated with blood anomalies, retinal lesions in sarcoidosis, hemoglobinopathies, and Behçet's disease have been discussed separately.

The retina can be injured in several ways, and separate chapters are devoted to photic maculopathy, radiation retinopathy, and retinal toxicity from systemic medications.

Peripheral retinal changes, such as lattice, retinal breaks, cystic retinal tufts, and retinoschisis continue to present controversial issues regarding management and have been addressed separately.

Vitreoretinal surgery is one of the most active subspecialties in ophthalmology and chapters on retinal detachment, scleral buckling surgery, proliferative vitreoretinopathy, vitreous surgery, vitreous substitutes, and intraocular foreign bodies have been devoted to these issues. Endophthalmitis has been surgically managed in many cases, and the state of the art in diagnosis and management has been addressed in a separate chapter.

The goal of this section is not to cover the whole vitreoretinal field as a subspecialty textbook but to provide an accurate guide that is detailed enough for the practicing ophthalmologist. We hope that our readers will enjoy it as much as we did in writing and editing this stimulating section. We would like to thank all the contributors for their efforts and hope that new research and better innovations will provide more effective diagnosis and management of retinal disorders in the next decade.

Chapter 50

■

Examination of the Retina: Ophthalmoscopy and Fundus Biomicroscopy

THOMAS R. FRIBERG

To thoroughly examine the ocular fundus, excellent powers of observation and clinical experience with ophthalmoscopy and biomicroscopy are necessary. Some individuals have almost a natural ability to use these specialized instruments to discover and document subtle retinal abnormalities. Most have considerably more difficulty, however. For instance, a novice might struggle and then finally see scattered retinal hemorrhages in the fundus of a patient's eye but then fail to note the location of the hemorrhages with respect to retinal landmarks. With practice, proper use of the instrumentation can be learned by almost anyone. Unfortunately, some clinicians never become good observers and remain unaware of the important distinction between seeing an abnormality and observing it.[1] Observation is a high-level activity, requiring mental processing and categorization of what is seen.

One method of improving observational skills is to use an examination routine whereby different regions of the fundus are evaluated in a specific sequence. For instance, an ophthalmologist might begin by examining the optic nerve; move on to the temporal vascular arcades, macula, and nasal retina; and finish by evaluating the equatorial and peripheral retina. By using an organized system of fundus evaluation, diagnostic oversights will be minimized.

PUPILLARY DILATATION

Examination of the fundus and especially the retinal periphery is greatly facilitated by a well-dilated pupil. Suggested mydriatic agents include 1 percent tropicamide (Mydriacyl) and 2.5 percent neosynephrine drops (Mydfrin), one drop of each in both eyes. Instillation of a topical anesthetic, such as 0.5 percent proparacaine hydrochloride, before instilling the dilating drops promotes more rapid mydriasis, as the anesthetic prevents reflex tearing and subsequent dilution of the mydriatic agent. Most patients' pupils dilate adequately after 20 to 30 min using this regimen. However, darkly pigmented irises dilate more slowly and remain dilated longer than do lightly colored irises, probably because the mydriatic agents are bound to the iris melanin and are released gradually.[2]

DIRECT OPHTHALMOSCOPE

To examine the ocular fundus, specialized instruments are necessary. The simplest is the direct ophthalmoscope, which is in essence a miniature flashlight held very close to the patient's eye and shined through the pupil (Fig. 50–1). The fundus is viewed monocularly through a small peephole located just above the illumination source of the instrument, producing an upright virtual image that magnifies the area of interest about 15 times.[3] This ophthalmoscope also has a dial containing neutralizing lenses, which is rotated to achieve the clearest retinal image.

Although magnification and resolution are quite good with the direct ophthalmoscope, difficulties inherent with its use include lack of stereopsis, inadequate illumination in the presence of media opacities, the necessity of placing the examiner's face in close proximity to the patient's face, a retinal image covering only about 8 degrees of the fundus,[3] and severe degradation of the image when significant lens opacities are present.[4, 5] It may be impossible to adequately examine eyes with a high degree of astigmatism or spherical ametropia using this instrument. Furthermore, the direct ophthalmoscope does not allow an undistorted view of the peripheral retina, limiting its use to visualizing the posterior retina only.

Largely because of its portability and simplicity, the direct ophthalmoscope is a useful screening device for

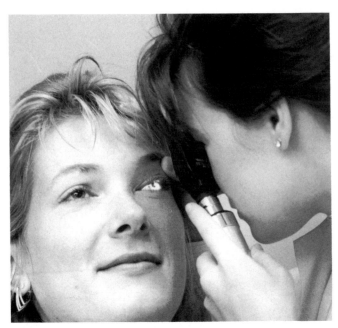

Figure 50–1. The direct ophthalmoscope is used like a flashlight to illuminate the patient's eye while the examiner looks through a small peephole. The left eye of the examiner is used to study the fundus of the patient's left eye. Conversely, the right eye is used to examine the patient's right eye.

the general practitioner who may wish to rule out papilledema, macular degeneration, or hypertensive or diabetic retinopathy. Many ophthalmologists have become facile with binocular slit-lamp biomicroscopes and specialized contact and noncontact fundus examination lenses, however, and observation of the ocular fundus with the direct ophthalmoscope is often redundant in the office setting.

BINOCULAR INDIRECT OPHTHALMOSCOPE

The binocular indirect ophthalmoscope, in conjunction with a high-quality aspherical hand-held lens, has become the indispensable standard for the proper examination of the fundus, especially when evaluating areas located outside the posterior pole (Fig. 50–2). Introduced by Schepens,[6] binocular indirect ophthalmoscopy offers a typical field of view of 25 degrees or more and excellent resolution of fundus details.[5] Stereopsis is enhanced, allowing the examiner to detect nuances of elevation and excavation of the retinal contour. The device is portable, permits evaluation of the retina with the patient in either the sitting or the supine position, and quickly gives a view of relatively large retinal areas. Furthermore, binocular indirect ophthalmoscopy has been incorporated into laser delivery systems, providing an important alternative to slit-lamp photocoagulation systems.[7]

Although an examination of the posterior fundus using the direct ophthalmoscope can be performed after a minimum of instruction, effective use of the indirect ophthalmoscope requires several hours of practice. The image formed by the indirect ophthalmoscope is physically located above the plane of the lens and, as with

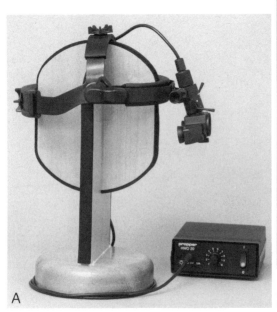
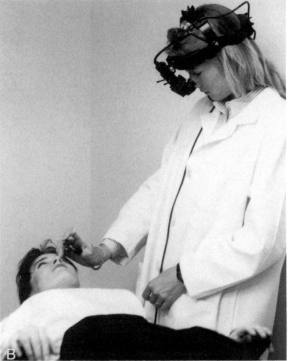

Figure 50–2. A, An example of a binocular indirect ophthalmoscope. The coronal and sagittal headbands and the interpupillary distance are adjustable. A transformer provides power for illumination. B, With the indirect ophthalmoscope adjusted and in place on the head, the examiner holds a lens over the patient's eye to form a retinal image.

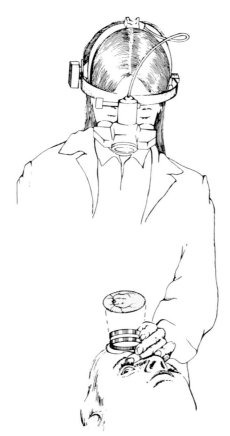

Figure 50–3. With indirect ophthalmoscopy, a real inverted image of the patient's fundus is formed in a plane located just above the hand-held lens.

all real images, is inverted (Fig. 50–3). This inversion creates considerable problems for the novice, especially when he or she tries to draw the observed abnormalities. In addition, the alignment of the indirect ophthalmoscope's illumination beam, the hand-held lens, the patient's pupil, and the ophthalmoscope oculars is crucial to obtaining a sharp image. Hence, prior to examining patients, it is beneficial to examine a model eye (Mira, Waltham, MA) manufactured for the purpose of practicing indirect ophthalmoscopy (Fig. 50–4).

EXAMINATION TECHNIQUE WITH THE INDIRECT OPHTHALMOSCOPE

To use the indirect ophthalmoscope, the examiner first adjusts the headbands so that the scope fits comfortably. A lightweight instrument is preferred. The illumination beam is turned on and the interpupillary distance of the eyepieces is adjusted so that both eyes can see the examiner's outstretched hand simultaneously. Next, the knob on the headset that controls the location of the illumination beam is rotated until the "footprint" of the light illuminates the superior portion of the outstretched hand. The head and body of the examiner should be positioned so that his or her viewing axis is in a line with the center of the patient's dilated

pupil. When this is done, a bright red reflex should appear through the oculars of the indirect ophthalmoscope.

Once a red reflex is visualized, the indirect hand-held lens is interposed along the imaginary line drawn between the examiner's pupil and the patient's pupil. The indirect lens should be held between the thumb and the forefinger of either hand and positioned a few centimeters from the patient's eye. The lens surface is oriented almost perpendicular to the illumination beam. To minimize problems with light reflections, the lens should be tilted very slightly, with the most convex side of the indirect lens facing the examiner (Fig. 50–5).

To steady the lens, the forth and fifth digits of the hand holding the lens should rest on the patient's face during the examination. The distance between the patient's eye and the lens should otherwise be as great as possible. To optimize the view, the lens is slowly moved toward or away from the patient's eye. When properly positioned, the image of the patient's fundus fills the lens and is in sharp focus. To examine different areas of the fundus, the viewing axis of the indirect ophthalmoscope, the center of the hand-held lens, and the patient's pupil must remain in alignment. A useful aid is to envision a solid rod representing the viewing axis of the indirect scope to which the center of the hand-held lens is fixed. This imaginary rod pivots at the center of the patient's pupil when examining the entire extent of the retina (Fig. 50–6). Indirect ophthalmoscopy is facilitated by having the patient in the supine position with the examiner standing, as this allows easy access to all retinal regions.

Many patients, especially those with light complexions, are photophobic when examined with bright light.

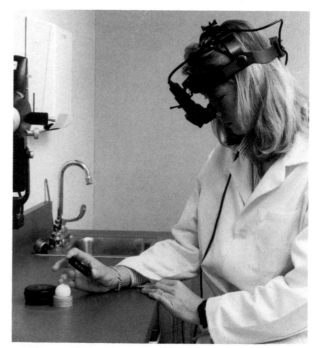

Figure 50–4. Pliable model eyes with realistic fundus details are valuable when learning binocular indirect ophthalmoscopy. They can also be indented to simulate scleral depression.

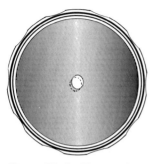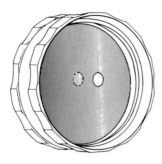

Figure 50–5. The most convex side of the hand-held lens is placed so that it faces the examiner. By tilting the lens very slightly, the bright light reflexes produced by the lens surfaces (*left*) do not enter the examiner's eye.

Hence, the illumination level of the ophthalmoscope must be low enough to allow examination of the fundus without causing patient discomfort and resultant squeezing of the eyelids. Conversely, the light must be sufficiently bright to allow observation of retinal details. For patient comfort, it is best to start with a dimmer light and increase its intensity as necessary.

The patient's eyelids should be held open with the examiner's fingers or with a lid speculum during indirect ophthalmoscopy. Either the hand holding the lens or the free hand can be used for this purpose, depending on whether scleral depression is being performed. Although a lid speculum potentially frees up one of the examiner's hands, an irrigating balanced salt solution such as BSS must be periodically instilled to prevent corneal drying when a speculum is used.

CHOICE OF HAND–HELD LENS

Numerous lenses are available for binocular indirect ophthalmoscopy. When selecting a lens, recall that angular magnification of fundus details is inversely proportional to the power of the hand-held lens. For example, a 20D lens will magnify the fundus details of an emmetropic eye about 2.3 times, whereas a 30D lens magnifies it about 1.5 times.[8] A high-quality 20D aspherical lens is widely used because it offers a good compromise between field of view and magnification. However, when viewing eyes with small pupils or eyes with hazy media, a 30D or 28D lens is often a better choice for the beginner. The field of view of the lens is generally directly proportional to the lens power, with a 20D aspherical lens providing about a 35-degree field.[3] Field of view is also a function of the diameter of the lens, with a larger field offered by a larger diameter lens. A comparison of field of view obtained when using a direct ophthalmoscope versus an indirect ophthalmoscope is shown in Figure 50–7.

SCLERAL DEPRESSION

To view the total extent of the peripheral fundus of the emmetropic eye, the wall of the eye must be depressed inward toward the visual axis. This examination technique, called *scleral depression*, should not be attempted until one is first accomplished at obtaining a sharp image of the posterior pole. If one cannot reliably image the posterior segment, attempting to view the retinal periphery with scleral depression is usually futile.

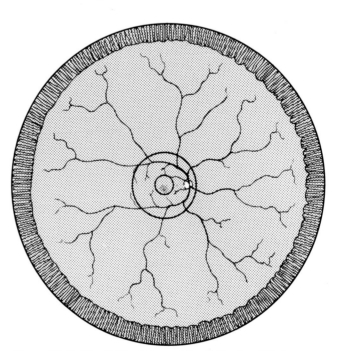

Figure 50–6. To view different regions of the fundus, the examiner moves his or her head and the hand-held lens as if there were an imaginary rod connecting the center of the patient's pupil, the center of the lens, and a point midway between the eyepieces of the indirect ophthalmoscope. The examiner then pivots around the central pupil to view the complete fundus.

Figure 50–7. The field of view of the indirect ophthalmoscope using a 20D lens (*outer circle*) is much larger than that provided by the direct ophthalmoscope (*inner circle*). However, the size of a given retinal lesion obtained using the direct ophthalmoscope appears commensurately bigger.

Several types of scleral depressors have been designed, and each has its advocates. The working end of most depressors consists of a metal shaft with an enlargement or crosspiece at the tip. Some depressors have a more elaborate construction with moving parts. Alternatively, one can simply use a cotton-tipped applicator pressed against the lids to accomplish the same goal, although some find the tip too bulky.

Pressure is exerted on the globe by pressing gently on the patient's partially opened eyelid until the peripheral retina is brought into view (Fig. 50–8). If excessive pressure is used, the patient will become uncomfortable, squeeze the eyelids shut, and prevent the examination from proceeding. With practice, patient discomfort should be minimal. Typically, scleral depression of the entire 360 degrees of the retinal periphery is easier to accomplish if the patient is in the supine position. The shaft of the depressor, the area of interest in the retinal periphery, and the central cornea should all be kept in the same plane during scleral depression.[9]

Scleral depression is not a static process whereby the peripheral retina is merely brought into view and observed. Gentle movement of the depressor in the vicinity of a suspicious area during observation may open up a previously unseen tear or demonstrate areas of vitreoretinal traction. Hence, to detect and diagnose subtle retinal abnormalities, dynamic scleral depression is required.

Topical anesthesia, such as a drop of 0.5 percent proparacaine hydrochloride may facilitate the examination with scleral depression. To limit patient discomfort, the complete examination should be performed without placing the depressor directly onto the conjunctival surface (Fig. 50–9). Occasionally, evaluation of some peripheral areas, particularly those at the 3 and 9 o'clock meridians, necessitates placement of the depressor directly on the globe.

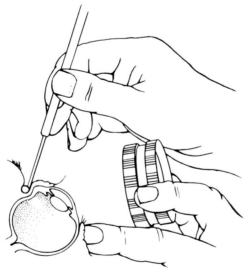

Figure 50–8. To perform scleral depression, light pressure is exerted on the globe through the patient's eyelids with the tip of the scleral depressor. The shaft of the depressor, the area of interest in the fundus, and the central cornea should all be in the same plane.

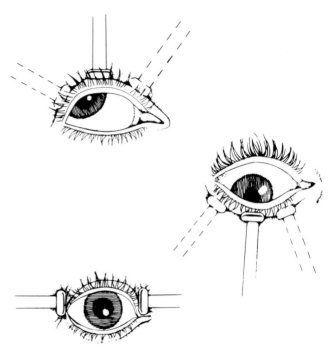

Figure 50–9. The scleral depressor is carefully repositioned along the upper and lower eyelids to completely examine all 360 degrees of the retinal periphery.

DOCUMENTING THE RETINAL FINDINGS

Detailed sketches of the fundus are made on durable drawing paper to document the retinal pathologic condition (Fig. 50–10). The location of a given lesion is drawn in reference to the major retinal veins, the meridional location of the lesion within the eye, and its relative peripheral location. The arteries are not typically drawn. By convention, the 12 o'clock meridian is placed at the top of the retinal drawing because it represents the uppermost part of the clock face. Keep in mind that mapping the retinal surface, which is spherical, on a flat piece of paper necessarily produces inaccuracies of scale in the finished drawing. For instance, the peripheral retina is disproportionally represented, just as the size of equatorial regions of the world are exaggerated in flat, polar maps generated by gnomonic projection.[10] Hence, a lesion of a given area will appear larger on the retinal drawing paper if it is located in the peripheral fundus than it would if it were located in the macula.

Because the retinal image is inverted during indirect ophthalmoscopy, beginners often make the mistake of assuming that the pathologic condition seen at the 6 o'clock position in the hand-held lens must be located at the 12 o'clock position in the eye. In fact, since only part of the fundus is imaged at a time, only the small fundus region that is being viewed is inverted (Fig. 50–11).[5] To avoid confusion, one can move the hand-held lens out of the way occasionally to observe which quadrant of the patient's eye the indirect ophthalmoscope is being directed toward.

When drawing the fundus, it is helpful to place the

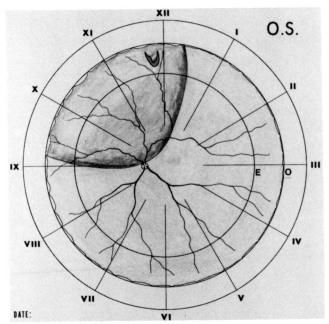

Figure 50–10. Drawing of a retinal detachment made on conventional retinal drawing paper. The center of the paper represents the fovea, the inner circle (E) represents the equator, and the outer circle (O) represents the ora serrata. The region defined by the two outermost circles represents the pars plana. On this paper, labeled O.S. for the left eye, the optic nerve is predrawn and located to the left of the fovea. Drawing paper labeled O.D. has the optic nerve drawn to the right of the fovea. Findings located on the drawing correspond to their clock hour location within the patient's eye, with 12 o'clock representing the superiormost portion of the globe. In this figure, a retinal detachment has been drawn extending from the 9:30 to the 12:30 positions. The retinal tear is drawn at the 11:45 position.

drawing paper on a clipboard and have the patient hold or support the clipboard on his or her chest. By orienting the paper so that its 12 o'clock meridian is directed inferiorly toward the patient's feet, the image fields can be visually translated directly onto the paper without

having to mentally invert them. Holding a pencil in one hand while holding the lens and the patient's eyelids open with the other hand greatly speeds up the process of generating an accurate retinal drawing (Fig. 50–12).

As retinal features are color-coded by convention (Table 50–1), color pencils are characteristically used for the retinal drawing.

LIMITATIONS OF THE INDIRECT OPHTHALMOSCOPE

Although the indirect ophthalmoscope is an invaluable instrument, it has limitations. A major drawback is that its magnification is insufficient to allow detection of small retinal abnormalities, particularly subtle macular lesions. For example, retinal microaneurysms, tiny areas of subretinal neovascularization, foveal cysts, and small round retinal breaks are often difficult to resolve with this instrument. For this reason, other ancillary devices are necessary to thoroughly evaluate the fundus.

BIOMICROSCOPY OF THE RETINA

The slit lamp is an essential instrument for fundus examination, particularly when a high degree of magnification is desired. It consists of a movable binocular biomicroscope mounted on a table and an intense illumination beam or slit beam of adjustable width that can be rotated 360 degrees in the vertical plane. Focusing is accomplished by moving a joystick located on the microscope platform. The slit lamp is used in conjunction with a diagnostic contact lens or hand-held lens to provide a high-quality magnified stereoscopic image of the fundus. Slit-lamp biomicroscopy of the fundus is particularly useful in determining whether the location of a hemorrhage is pre-, intra-, or subretinal; in detecting cystoid macular edema, and in diagnosing clinically significant macular thickening.

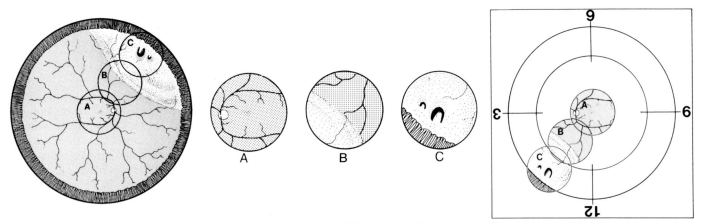

Figure 50–11. *Left,* Some fundus details located along the meridian at the 1:30 position on the clock are outlined by three circular areas, representing three areas to be viewed by indirect ophthalmoscopy. *Center,* The individual image fields of the fundus, as seen through the examiner's lens. Each field has been inverted by the optical system. *Right,* The salient details of each image field are drawn onto the fundus drawing paper. The paper is oriented with the 12 o'clock meridian directed toward the patient's feet. This allows the examiner to draw what he or she sees within each field as if it were being "pasted" directly on to the drawing paper. If the drawing paper were not inverted, the examiner would have to mentally invert the images before drawing them.

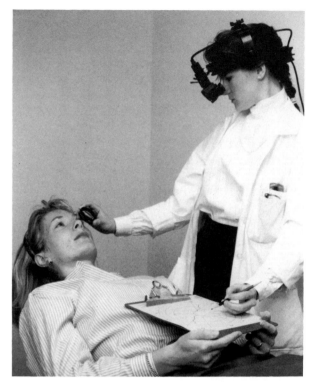

Figure 50–12. The patient's fundus findings can be documented rapidly if the lens is held in one hand while the examiner draws on the paper with a pencil held in the other hand. Again, the paper is purposely inverted.

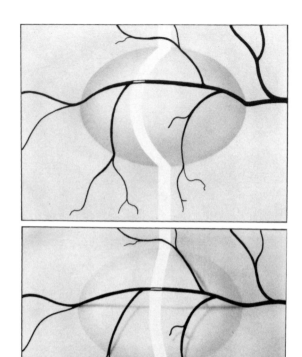

Figure 50–13. *Top,* A slit beam has been directed over a questionably elevated choroidal lesion. Bending of the beam is observed, indicating that the lesion is indeed elevated. *Bottom,* To detect a subtle elevation of the sensory retina, the area of suspicion is illuminated by the slit beam. Shadows of the retinal vessels are seen at the pigment epithelial level, indicating the presence of subretinal fluid and a shallow serous detachment of the sensory retina.

The slit lamp also provides optical sections of the vitreous body to allow detection of posterior vitreous detachments, abnormal vitreous surfaces, and vitreous floaters. Furthermore, the surface contours of a chorioretinal lesion are more apparent if a narrow beam of light is projected onto the lesion's surface. If an elevation or depression of a chorioretinal lesion is present, the slit beam on the retina will appear curved rather than straight (Fig. 50–13*A*). In some cases, when there is very little subretinal fluid, illumination of the retinal vessels with the slit beam produces shadows of the vessels at the level of the retinal pigment epithelium (Fig. 50–13*B*). Such shadows are further proof of retinal elevation.

If the slit beam of the biomicroscope is placed across an elevated retinal lesion, the behavior of the scattered light also provides important diagnostic clues. Often the borders of a small serous retinal or pigment epithelial detachment can be made to glow by positioning the slit beam across the elevation, making the lesion easier to demarcate. This technique is very useful in evaluating the posterior pole for the presence of a macular hole or for detecting cystic spaces within the fovea.

Slit-lamp examination methods can be separated into two major categories: (1) contact methods requiring the placement of a specialized contact lens onto the corneal surface to neutralize its power and (2) noncontact methods, which use the refractive power of the cornea and a special lens to form a fundus image. Noncontact fundus examinations are generally performed more rapidly, particularly if only the posterior pole requires evaluation. However, the patient may squeeze the eyelids shut during noncontact fundus evaluations. With diagnostic contact lenses, the eyelids cannot be closed, but corneal irritation may result if the examination is not performed gently. Furthermore, excessive pressure exerted on the eye during a contact lens evaluation may induce vasovagal reactions such as fainting and nausea. These side effects rarely occur if the examiner is experienced.

Table 50–1. COLOR CODING FOR RETINAL DRAWING

Color	Anatomic Feature
Red	Retinal arteries, retinal hemorrhage, attached retina, retinal neovascularization
Blue	Retinal veins, detached retina, retinal edema
Green	Media opacities, vitreous hemorrhage
Yellow	Retinal and choroidal exudates
Brown	Pigmented lesions, choroidal detachments
Red lined with blue	Retinal breaks

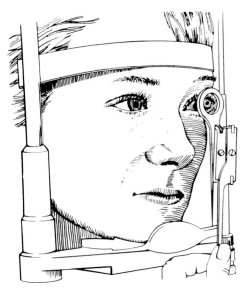

Figure 50–14. A high-power minus lens placed in front of the cornea forms a virtual image of the fundus. Moving a lever on the lens holder focuses the image, which is observed through the slit-lamp binoculars.

Noncontact Methods of Biomicroscopic Retinal Examination

PLANOCONCAVE LENSES

A planoconcave lens of high negative optical power, such as a Hruby lens, is incorporated into some slit-lamp biomicroscopes. To use this lens, a broad vertical slit beam is first rotated to illuminate the fundus from virtually a straight-on direction until the red reflex is clearly seen though the oculars. The lens is centered over the patient's cornea, positioned a few centimeters from the patient's eye, and focused via a lever until the fundus comes into view (Fig. 50–14). Some systems focus the lens more or less automatically. The image formed is upright and vertical, but the image quality is not uniformly good, especially near the edges of the field of view. This lens is used almost exclusively to view the posterior pole, as distortion seriously degrades the image if the fundus is viewed along any axis other than the approximate optical axis of the patient's eye.[11]

ASPHERICAL LENSES (60D, 78D, 90D) AND SLIT–LAMP INDIRECT OPHTHALMOSCOPY

A real image of the fundus is formed at the slit lamp several centimeters in front of the patient's eye when a high-powered plus lens is positioned in front of the cornea. This aerial image of the fundus is magnified by the slit-lamp optics. The resultant image is real, inverted, and of high quality if a superior high-power aspherical lens made for this purpose is used. Typically, indirect biomicroscopic lenses are positioned further away from the patient's eye than is the Hruby-type lens. With a lower power or longer focal length lens, the image is produced at a location farther in front of the patient's eye than with a higher power lens. Because some slit-lamp focusing tracks are limited in travel away from the patient, it may be impossible to obtain a clear fundus image with certain low-power indirect lenses.

Indirect ophthalmoscopy at the slit lamp is performed by placing the lens between the thumb and the forefinger, with the elbow supported by the slit-lamp table (Fig. 50–15). Because these lenses are of relatively high power, any movement of the examiner's hand induces sizable prism shift movements of the image. Some examiners prefer, therefore, to have the lens mounted on a small jointed holder affixed to the slit lamp (Volk Optical, Mentor, Ohio). As with indirect ophthalmoscopy, higher-power lenses provide wider fields of view at the expense of magnification.

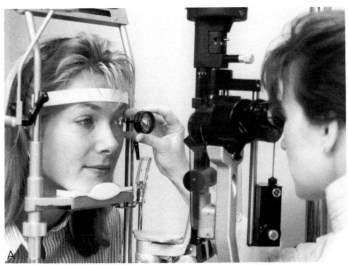
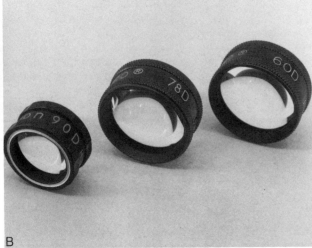

Figure 50–15. A, Binocular indirect ophthalmoscopy at the slit lamp is accomplished by holding a high-power plus lens in front of the cornea and focusing the slit lamp on the aerial image that forms anterior to the lens. B, Lenses of various powers provide the examiner with an array of magnification and field of view options.

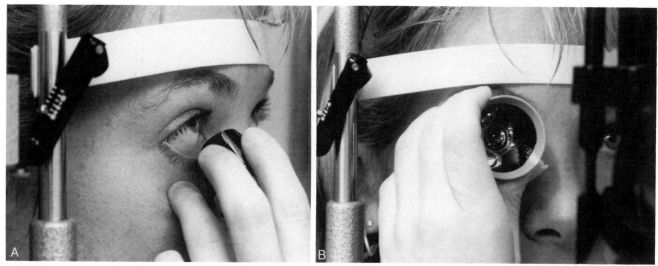

Figure 50–16. *A,* A diagnostic fundus contact lens containing an optical coupling fluid is placed on the anestheized cornea by holding the lids open while the patient looks up. *B,* The patient then gazes straight ahead to center the lens, which is held in place with very light pressure.

Although noncontact lenses are suitable for viewing the posterior pole, they do not by themselves provide an adequate view of the retinal periphery. Scleral depression can be attempted while viewing the fundus through these lenses, but this technique requires considerable practice and is technically difficult.

Contact Lens Methods of Biomicroscopic Retinal Examination

Prior to placing the diagnostic contact lens on the patient's cornea, a drop of a mild anesthetic agent such as 0.5 percent proparacaine hydrochloride is instilled. A viscous, clear liquid such as methylcellulose or hydroxypropyl methylcellulose (Goniosol) is placed in the concave portion of the lens to optically couple the lens to the cornea. With the patient looking up, the lids are held open and the lens is placed gently on the patient's cornea (Fig. 50–16). Small air bubbles are eliminated by exerting gentle pressure on the lens. When fundus photography is scheduled directly after removal of the diagnostic contact lens, any residual interface solutions remaining on the cornea can degrade the retinal image. Hence, many examiners prefer to use low-viscosity balanced salt solutions rather than thicker, more tenacious interface liquids. Unfortunately, balanced salt solutions are of such low viscosity that they will spill out of the fundus contact lens unless the lens is placed on the cornea in a smooth, rapid motion while the patient gazes ahead.

GOLDMANN THREE–MIRROR LENS

The three-mirror lens has a clear central portion for viewing the posterior pole, surrounded by three radially arranged mirrors (Fig. 50–17, *left*). Each mirror has a different inclination between its surface and the axis of the lens. Through the central posterior pole portion, the field of view is about 30 degrees for an emmetropic eye. The smallest mirror is used to view the anterior chamber angle and occasionally the far periphery of the fundus. The middle-sized mirror is configured to allow viewing of the retinal periphery anterior to the equator, and the largest mirror is chosen when the area of interest is within the equatorial and posterior equatorial region of the fundus (Fig. 50–18).[12]

The beam of the slit lamp should be projected along the radial axis of the mirror being used. This is achieved by rotating a collar or knob on the slit lamp, which, in turn, rotates the slit beam. With the patient gazing straight ahead, the best image is obtained when the front surface of the lens is kept perpendicular to the viewing axis of the slit lamp. By rotating the examination

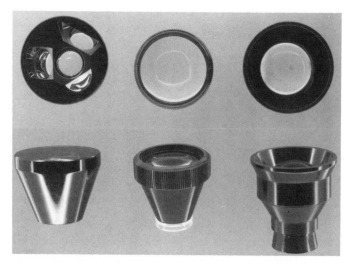

Figure 50–17. Specialized fundus contact examination lenses: *Left,* Goldmann's three-mirror contact lens; *center,* Mainster's biomicroscopic lens; *right,* Rodenstock's panfunduscopic lens. Each lens has specific attributes and shortcomings.

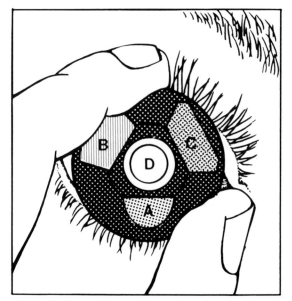
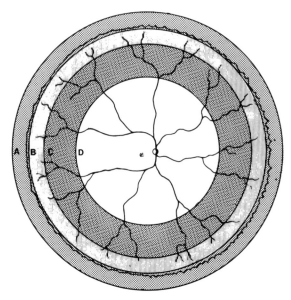

Figure 50–18. *Left,* The Goldmann three-mirror lens has a clear central zone (D) for examination of the posterior pole. The adjacent mirrors (A,B,C) are each inclined at different angles to the optical axis of the lens, providing visual access to different regions of the fundus as depicted (*right*).

mirror and readjusting the slit beam, all meridians of the retina can be evaluated.

Redirection of the patient's gaze facilitates viewing of more anteriorly or posteriorly located retinal regions positioned within a given mirror. If the patient moves her or his eye toward the mirror, a more posteriorly located portion of the fundus comes into view. If the eye is moved away from the mirror, more peripheral areas of the fundus are seen (Fig. 50–19). This change in image field with a change in the patient's gaze is especially important to note when photocoagulating a patient's eye through a mirror. The fovea may inadvertently appear within the treatment mirror of the lens on

extreme gaze. Failure to recognize the fovea in this situation can lead to its destruction by photocoagulation.

THREE–MIRROR LENS EXAMINATION COUPLED WITH SCLERAL DEPRESSION

A highly magnified view of the ora serrata and the most peripheral retina can be achieved by performing scleral depression during the three-mirror lens examination. This magnified examination of the retinal periphery is often easier to accomplish if the Goldmann lens is placed in a specialized conical holder, which, in turn, has a small depressor located along its circumference (Fig. 50–20). The middle-sized or smallest mirror should be inserted into the position opposite the depressor location. The lens holder is then held gently but firmly against the patient's eye, producing the desired scleral indentation. One type of lens holder incorporates an adjustable depressor that can be moved more pos-

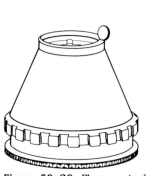

Figure 50–19. The patient's direction of gaze will influence the field being observed through each mirror of the Goldmann lens. If the patient looks toward the particular mirror being used for viewing, a more posteriorly located region of the fundus will be seen.

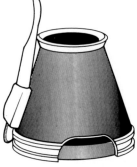

Figure 50–20. Placement of the Goldmann lens into a conical holder containing a scleral depressor at its periphery allows the examiner to perform scleral depression while using the slit-lamp biomicroscope. Two of these devices are illustrated.

teriorly along the sclera in any meridian.[13] Unfortunately, many patients find these scleral depression devices very uncomfortable, especially in inexperienced hands.

OTHER SPECIALIZED CONTACT LENSES

Goldmann's Posterior Fundus Contact Lens. If an examiner is primarily interested in studying the posterior retina, a small lightweight lens incorporating a peripheral flange at the point at which it touches the eyelids is often preferred over a larger, bulkier lens. The flange and smaller contact diameter make this lens more difficult to dislodge if the patient squeezes the eyelids.

Panfunduscopic Lens. The panfunduscopic lens (Rodenstock, Germany) (Fig. 50–17, *right*) consists of a meniscus lens coupled with a spherical lens located within the same lens holder housing. When the meniscus lens is placed on the cornea, the resultant image of the fundus is inverted, real, minified, and located well forward of the anterior lens surface. Magnification provided by the slit lamp counteracts the minification produced by the lens configuration. A wide-angle view of the fundus in an emmetropic eye, extending from the fovea to the equatorial region, is produced by such a panfunduscopic lens.[14] This device also facilitates the examination of the fundus through a poorly dilated pupil. However, panfunduscopic lenses are used more often during laser photocoagulation than for diagnostic purposes, primarily because the image of the retina is small and the view through the peripheral portions of this lens is not excellent.

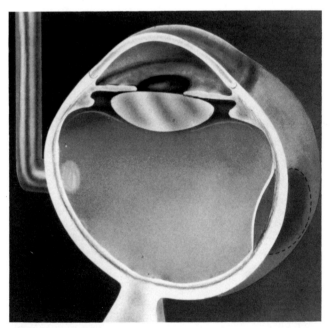

Figure 50–21. Transillumination. The globe is illuminated, through the sclera in this illustration, via a fiberoptic light source placed on the globe externally or on the cornea. In a darkened room, the sclera is observed, glowing yellow-orange. A dark choroidal lesion will block the transmission of light through the eye wall and will appear as a dark shadow surrounded by the red glow of the remainder of the sclera.

Mainster Lens. The Mainster lens (Ocular Instruments, Bellevue, Washington) (Fig. 50–17, *center*) provides a somewhat reduced field of view (45 degrees) compared with the panfunduscopic lens but also produces less minification.[15] Resolution with this lens is sufficient to detect retinal thickening from macular edema. The image size is comparable to that provided by the Goldmann lens, making the Mainster lens versatile for diagnostic as well as therapeutic purposes. The image plane is located quite anterior to the lens surface, however, making it difficult to view the fundi of patients with hyperopia or exophthalmos when using slit lamps with limited forward travel.

SPECIALIZED RETINAL EXAMINATION TECHNIQUES

If a fiberoptic probe or other suitable light source is placed against the sclera in a darkened room, the retina can be visualized using indirect ophthalmoscopy with the illuminating scope light turned off. This examination technique (transillumination ophthalmoscopy) requires that light be transmitted through the sclera and choroid. If an eye contains a solid pigmented mass, transillumination is useful in that the tumor will appear dark, whereas other choroidal lesions, such as a choroidal detachment, will be much more brightly illuminated.

Alternately, a transillumination light can be placed on the cornea so that it shines through the pupil. The examiner then observes the surface of the sclera, which should glow a uniformly orange color. A pigmented tumor or foreign body within the choroid will prevent the transillumination light from illuminating the sclera beneath it, and a dark shadow will be present within the affected scleral quadrant. In eyes that are lightly pigmented, a bright transilluminator may be directly applied to the sclera to achieve a similar effect (Fig. 50–21).

REFERENCES

1. Doyle AC: A scandal in Bohemia. *In* The Complete Works of Sherlock Holmes. Garden City, NY, Doubleday, 1892–1927, p 162.
2. Thompson HS: The pupil. *In* Moses RA, Hart WM (eds): Adler's Physiology of the Eye, Clinical Application. St Louis, CV Mosby, 1987, p 321.
3. Rubin ML: Magnification; Practical instruments: The indirect ophthalmoscope. *In* Optics for Clinicians, 2nd ed. Gainesville, FL, Triad, 1974, pp 235, 298.
4. Schepens CL: Methods of examination. *In* Retinal Detachment and Allied Diseases, vol. 1. Philadelphia, WB Saunders, 1983, pp 99–133.
5. Rosenthal ML, Fradin S: The technique of binocular indirect ophthalmoscopy. Highlights Ophthalmol 9:179–257, 1966.
6. Schepens CL: Progress in detachment surgery. Trans Am Acad Ophthalmol Otolaryngol 55:607–615, 1951.
7. Friberg TR: Clinical experience with a binocular indirect ophthalmoscope laser delivery system. Retina 7:28–31, 1987.
8. Rubin ML: The optics of indirect ophthalmoscopy. Sur Ophthalmol 9:449–464, 1964.
9. Chignell AH: Techniques of examination. *In* Retinal Detachment Surgery, 2nd ed, Berlin, Springer-Verlag, 1988, pp 14–25.
10. Kemp P (ed): The Oxford Companion to Ships and the Sea. London, Oxford University Press, 1976, p 346.

11. Tolentino FI, Schepens CL, Freeman HM: Instrumentation. *In* Vitreoretinal Disorders. Diagnosis and Management. Philadelphia, WB Saunders, 1976, pp 45–70.
12. Benson WE: Fundus examination and pre-operative management. *In* Retinal Detachment: Diagnosis and Management, 2nd ed. Philadelphia, JB Lippincott, 1988, pp 85–111.
13. Eisner G: Attachment for Goldmann three-mirror contact glass. For examination of the ora serrata and pars plana. Am J Ophthalmol 64:467–468, 1967.
14. Michels RG, Wilkinson CP, Rice TA: Pre-operative evaluation. *In* Michels RG (ed): Retinal Detachment. St Louis, CV Mosby, 1990, pp 325–378.
15. Mainster MA, Crossman JL, Erickson PJ, Heacock GL: Retinal laser lenses: Magnification, spot size, and field of view. Br J Ophthalmol 74:177–179, 1990.

Chapter 51

■

Examination of the Retina: Principles of Fluorescein Angiography

THOMAS R. FRIBERG

Although the fundus can be visualized using ophthalmoscopy and biomicroscopy, observation alone yields little information regarding blood flow through the retinal or choroidal vasculature, nor does it reveal subtle alterations in ocular physiology. Conversely, when an indicator dye such as sodium fluorescein is injected intravenously, the dye is confined within certain ocular tissues and freely leaks out of others. As the dye courses through the eye, photographic or video images of the fundus can demonstrate abnormalities within the sensory retina, pigment epithelium, sclera, choroid, and optic nerve. This powerful diagnostic study is known as *fluorescein angiography*.

HISTORY

During the 1950s and early 1960s, several investigators pioneered the use of intravenous fluorescein to evaluate the ocular circulation and chorioretinal disorders.[1] Fluorescein was first used clinically in the anterior segment, where fluorescent staining of corneal epithelial defects occurred when the topically placed dye was viewed with a blue light. MacLean and Maumenee performed angioscopy by injecting fluorescein intravenously into patients with choroidal tumors during ophthalmoscopy.[2] Flocks and coworkers[3] studied the retinal circulation in cats using various injectable dyes and cinephotography. Novotny and Alvis[4] perfected the use of sodium fluorescein as a dye for the photographic study of the human retinal circulation. Because they were the first to record on film the transit of fluorescein through the human retina, Novotny and Alvis are credited with producing the first fluorescein angiogram. Further innovations were made gradually, including the optimization of filters to improve the quality of the angiogram, development of improved fundus cameras, and stereoseparation to allow three-dimensional viewing.[5] Simultaneously, many clinicians studied ocular diseases with fluorescein angiography, establishing the intrinsic value of the technique.[6–8]

OVERVIEW

To perform fluorescein angiography, sodium fluorescein dye is injected into a peripheral vein. Up to 70 to 80 percent of the injected dye molecules are bound to serum albumin and other large protein molecules,[9] leaving an unbound portion that can diffuse through small intercellular spaces. As the dye enters the retinal and choroidal circulations, fluorescence is documented photographically using a special fundus camera and black and white film (Fig. 51–1). Ultimately, the dye is removed from the systemic circulation via the kidneys and liver.

With each exposure, the fundus is illuminated by light of a wavelength spectrum selected to excite sodium fluorescein molecules into a higher energy state. The excited molecules then release the incremental energy they just absorbed by fluorescing or giving off light at a wavelength higher than that of the excitation light. The wavelengths used to excite the fluorescein molecules are blue, peak between 465 and 490 nm, and are generated by placing a special filter in front of the illumination strobe lamp. The excited molecules produce yellow-green fluorescent light, the wavelength of which peaks between 520 and 530 nm. This light is detected by placing a barrier filter into the optical path between the fundus and the photographic film. Because the exciter and barrier filters transmit light of different wavelengths (Fig. 51–2), the exciter illumination is virtually invisible to the film. Hence, only substances capable of fluorescence are detected.

During fluorescein angiography, 20 to 30 individual

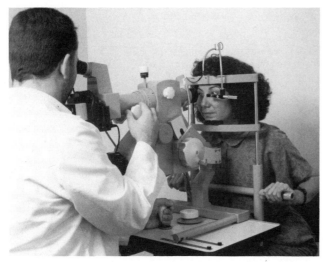

Figure 51–1. Fundus camera used for fluorescein angiography. Focusing is accomplished using a joystick (left hand) and is optimized via a focusing knob (right hand). Light from the strobe flash illuminates the fundus during the photographic exposure. Color transparencies are customarily obtained first, camera backs are changed, and the angiographic frames are recorded on black and white Kodak Tri-X film.

photographic frames of both the primary eye under evaluation and the fellow eye are exposed. The time elapsed since the intravenous injection is indicated on a timer and is recorded on each film frame. Characteristically, 5 ml of 10 percent sodium fluorescein are injected into a peripheral vein over a period of a few seconds. Angiograms are interpreted by evaluating the presence or lack of sodium fluorescein over time in various anatomic locations within the fundus. Stereophotography is preferred because stereoscopic viewing of the angiogram allows one to determine which retinal layers are involved when abnormalities are detected. The time required for vascular filling is also a useful parameter, especially in the diagnosis of ischemic and occlusive diseases.

INDICATIONS FOR ANGIOGRAPHY

There are few absolute rules regarding which patients should undergo fluorescein angiography. A reasonable guideline is to obtain a fluorescein angiogram if the results might alter the presumed diagnosis or the course of therapy or if a baseline study is required to document findings that could change over time. The study is essential when subretinal neovascularization near the fovea is suspected or if areas of macular edema need to be defined prior to laser treatment. Typically, diabetic patients with good vision who have only a few detectable microaneurysms and no macular edema on ophthalmoscopy are inappropriate candidates for study from a clinical standpoint. Furthermore, although fluorescein angiography complements the fundus examination, angiography and fundus photography cannot be used as substitutes for careful ophthalmoscopy. Various regions

of the fundus may be impossible to photograph, whereas other pathologic areas may simply be missed.

RISKS AND SIDE EFFECTS

For the most part, the risks of fluorescein angiography are limited.[10–12] Unavoidable side effects include temporary yellowing of the skin and conjunctivae and orange-yellow discoloration of the urine. The skin discoloration fades in 6 to 12 h, whereas urine fluorescence lasts from 24 to 36 h. A more unpleasant side effect is transient nausea lasting a few minutes, experienced by about 3 to 5 percent of patients. Concomitant vomiting is less frequent and can often be avoided by reassuring the patient that the nausea will pass quickly.[13]

If fluorescein dye extravasates into the skin during intravenous injection, local pain may be severe. Ice-cold compresses should be placed on the affected area for 5 to 10 min, and the patient should be reassessed over a period of hours or days if necessary until edema, pain, and redness resolve. Serious complications are more likely to occur when large amounts of dye extravasate. To avoid these problems, continual observation of the injection site during the course of the injection and monitoring the patient for pain are recommended.

Allergic reactions occur in less than 1 percent of patients undergoing fluorescein angiography.[12] Mild reactions such as pruritus or urticaria should be treated with antihistamines. However, any patient who experiences an allergic reaction must be observed carefully for

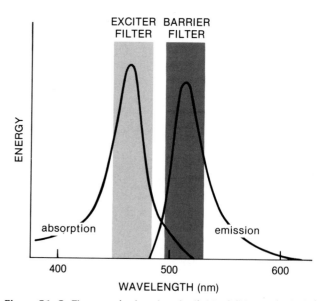

Figure 51–2. Fluorescein dye absorbs light, visible particularly in the blue spectrum as indicated by its absorption curve. It then fluoresces, producing green light with an emission spectrum similar to that shown on the right-hand curve. In the fundus camera, white light passes through an excitation filter to produce excitation wavelengths. A barrier filter, interposed in front of the film pack, only transmits light of longer wavelengths, so light simply reflected off the fundus is not detected. Overlap of the excitation and barrier filter wavelengths should be minimal (as shown with these "ideal" filters) to avoid pseudofluorescence.

the development of more severe sequelae such as bronchospasm or anaphylaxis. Although uncontrollable anaphylactic reactions to the dye leading to death are exceedingly rare, appropriate agents to treat severe reactions should be available on site. These include epinephrine for intravenous or intramuscular use, soluble corticosteroids, aminophylline for intravenous use, oxygen, and airway instrumentation.

Oral administration of sodium fluorescein is sometimes advocated for high-risk patients in lieu of intravenous injection. Unfortunately, the poor quality of the photographs after oral administration and the lack of normal filling phases limits the usefulness of this alternative. This method does provide interpretable late-phase photographs. Although fluorescein angiography may be performed safely during pregnancy with little apparent risk to either the woman or the fetus,[14] it is prudent to avoid this practice unless absolutely necessary.[15]

ANATOMIC CONSIDERATIONS

To properly interpret the fluorescein angiogram, knowledge of the normal anatomy of the posterior segment of the eye is germane (Fig. 51–3). The sensory retina is transparent, but the fovea appears yellow because of its high concentration of xanthophyll pigment. The retinal arterioles, capillaries, and veins are located in the superficial retinal layers. Tight junctions are present throughout the retinal vasculature, preventing molecules such as bound and unbound fluorescein dye from leaking out into the surrounding tissue.

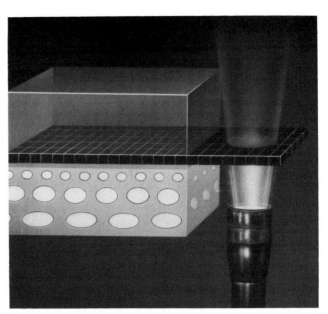

Figure 51–4. The pigment epithelial layer of the retina acts like an optical filter, attenuating the intensity of the underlying choroidal fluorescence, depicted here by the beam of a flashlight.

The pigment epithelium lies directly beneath the sensory retina and is composed of a unicellar layer of individual cells joined to one another at their apex by tight junctions. The pigment epithelial cells contain melanin, the concentration of which varies with the patient's pigmentation and race. In the central macula, the pigment epithelial cells are characteristically thicker and contain more pigment.

Beneath the pigment epithelium lie the choriocapillaris and choroid, which are separated from the retinal pigment epithelium (RPE) by Bruch's membrane. Vessels within the choriocapillaris have large fenestrations allowing free fluorescein molecules to quickly leak out into the surrounding choroidal tissue. Furthermore, since the choroid is made up of a relatively thick plexus of entangled capillaries and vessels, it is virtually impossible to resolve individual choroidal capillaries in the normal eye with fluorescein angiography. Bruch's membrane separates the retina from the choroid and is composed of a thin sandwich of elastic tissue surrounded on both sides by collagen layers and the basement membranes of the RPE cells and choriocapillaris. Bruch's membrane is not a barrier to the diffusion of sodium fluorescein molecules. However, fluorescein dye leaking from the choroidal tissue through Bruch's membrane is confined anteriorly by the tight intercellular junctions between the retinal pigment cells.[9] Therefore, the dye does not normally leak beneath or into the sensory retina.

Although fluorescein molecules are highly concentrated within the choroid, fluorescence from the choroidal layer is greatly attenuated by the pigment epithelial pigment granules. Hence, the RPE acts like an optical filter (Fig. 51–4). This attenuation effect is most prominent in the fovea in which the concentration of melanin is highest. Xanthophyll also blocks background choroi-

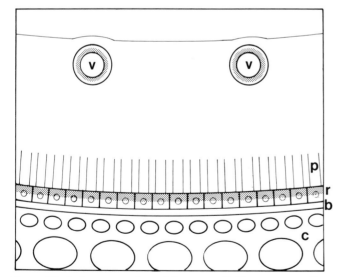

Figure 51–3. A cross section of the eye wall. The sensory retina contains vessels (v) located within its superficial layers, whereas the photoreceptors (p) are found in the deepest layer. The retinal pigment epithelial cells (r) lie directly adjacent to the photoreceptors and just above Bruch's membrane (b). The choroid (c), located beneath Bruch's membrane, provides nutrition to the other layers of the sensory retina. Normal barriers to fluorescein leakage are the tight junctions of both the retinal vasculature and the retinal pigment epithelium, as indicated by the shaded zones.

dal fluorescence, contributing to the darker angiographic appearance of the fovea.[9]

THE NORMAL FLUORESCEIN ANGIOGRAM

Exposure Sequence

Typically, angiographic frames are obtained 10 to 12 sec after fluorescein is injected into an antecubital vein. An initial exposure rate of one frame every few seconds documents the arteriolar and early venous filling phases of the study. Exposures are then made at less frequent intervals until about 20 to 25 frames are exposed. Late-phase photographs are taken after a pause of 10 to 30 min. These late-phase frames are essential to many studies, particularly when the extent of retinal and choroidal vascular leakage must be documented. The exact exposure sequencing routine of a fluorescein study will depend on the disease or disorder suspected. Many photographers use specific photographic protocols for the most common retinal diagnoses. Good communication between the physician ordering the study and the photographer is therefore essential.

Normal Findings

In the normal eye, the choriocapillaris quickly fills with dye about 10 to 15 sec after injection. If rapid-sequence photography is performed during this interval, a patchy, lobular choroidal pattern is observed as the retinal arteries begin to fill. This first phase is called the *early arterial phase* (Fig. 51–5A). Within seconds, the entire arterial side of the retinal vasculature is filled with fluorescein dye, marking the end of the arterial phase of the study (Fig. 51–5B). In the larger veins, thin

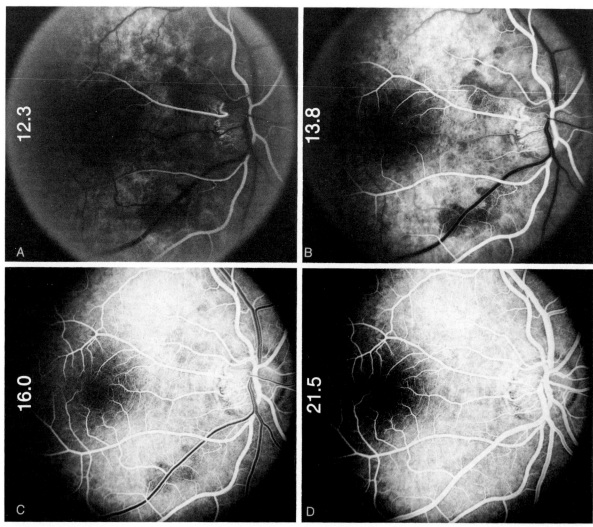

Figure 51–5. Normal fluorescein angiogram. Time after intravenous injection is indicated on each frame. The retinal arteries fill quickly in the arterial phase and the choroid simultaneously exhibits patchy filling of its lobules (A). The end of the arterial phase is characterized by complete filling of the arterioles with fluorescein dye (B). Shortly thereafter, dye begins to accumulate near the walls of the larger veins, marking the laminar flow or early arteriovenous phase (C). Gradually the concentration of dye in all vessels increases until it is maximal, indicating peak phase (D). During this phase, the foveal avascular zone is most apparent. By 30 sec after injection, the dye has begun to recirculate in the blood stream, decreasing its intensity in the eye.

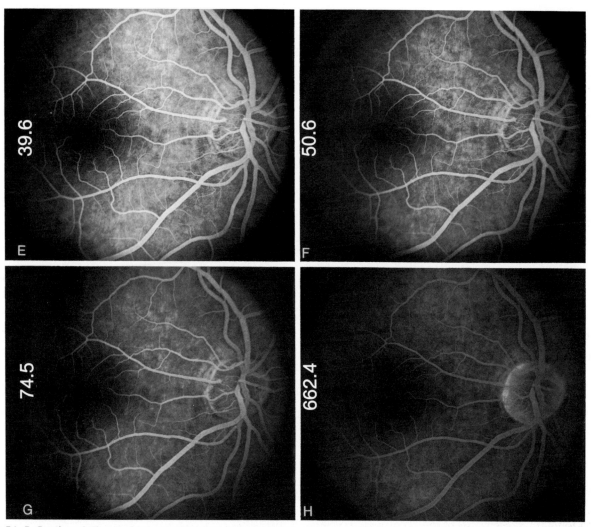

Figure 51–5 *Continued* The study thus enters the late arteriovenous phases (*E–G*). Ten minutes after injection and beyond, little fluorescein remains in the normal eye (*H*). These late-phase films are important, however, when evaluating an eye for macular edema and neovascularization. (*A–H*, Courtesy of Constantine Balouris, M.D.)

columns of fluorescein dye develop along the walls of the veins, indicating the beginning of the *arteriovenous phase* (Fig. 51–5C). These columns become wider within the next 5 to 15 sec until the entire lumen fills with dye. Filling progresses from the venous wall inward toward the central lumen because the velocity profile of venous blood flow is laminar, with little radial mixing of blood. The blood velocity is slowest near the wall and fastest at the center line.

Twenty to 25 sec after the injection of the dye bolus, the concentration of fluorescein within the choroid and retina is maximal. This point of the study, called the *peak phase,* is noteworthy because the foveal capillaries are best seen against the choroidal background at this time, often allowing the foveal avascular zone to be distinguished (Fig. 51–5D).

Thirty seconds after injection, the high concentration of dye within the retina and choroid begins to fade, decreasing both the retinal and the choroidal fluorescence. By this time, some of the injected fluorescein has returned to the heart and begins to recirculate (Fig. 51–5E).[4] Recirculation causes a continual reduction in retinal and choroidal fluorescence over the next few minutes (Fig. 51–5F and G) as the dye leaves the systemic blood stream.

The late phase begins about 10 min after injection, when the retinal and choroidal vessels stain only faintly (Fig. 51–5H). In the choroid, however, fluorescein has leaked out through fenestrations within the walls of the choroidal vessels and stains the tissue homogeneously. If the pigment epithelium contains much melanin, background fluorescence may be minimal in these late-phase frames. At 20 to 30 min after injection, little fluorescein is detectable unless abnormalities are present.[6]

To recapitulate, fluorescein is normally found first in the choroid and retinal arteries 10 to 15 sec after injection, and the dye intensity increases over the next 5 to 10 sec until peak fluorescence is reached and both the arteries and the veins are filled. The dye intensity then decreases gradually as fluorescein is distributed throughout the body until virtually no dye is seen in the retina about 15 to 20 min after injection. Fluorescein is contained within the retinal vasculature by the endothelial tight junctions and is confined beneath the pigment epithelial layer by the tight junctions located at the apical perimeter of each of the RPE cells.

INTERPRETATION OF THE FLUORESCEIN ANGIOGRAM

The fluorescein angiogram can be interpreted more accurately if the study includes color transparencies of the fundus. The negative 35-mm film strips, a positive transparency, or prints of the entire fluorescein study are reviewed concomitantly with the color slides. Both the slides and the fluorescein study are viewed stereoscopically on a viewbox using either a stereoscopic viewer or high-power magnifying lenses in a spectacle frame or by holding +10D lenses over each eye (Fig. 51–6).

To properly interpret the fluorescein angiogram, the reader must recognize when too much or too little fluorescein is present within a tissue at a given time compared with a normal study. Abnormalities are characterized using specific terminology. For example, too little fluorescence is called *hypofluorescence,* whereas excess fluorescence is termed *hyperfluorescence.* The sections that follow provide an introduction to normal and abnormal fluorescein findings.

Hypofluorescence

BLOCKED FLUORESCENCE

Excess melanin pigment within the RPE or choroid, such as found in hypertrophy of the RPE or in choroidal nevi, decreases the intensity of the background choroidal fluorescence. Melanin absorbs some of the blue excitation wavelengths and also attenuates the fluorescence

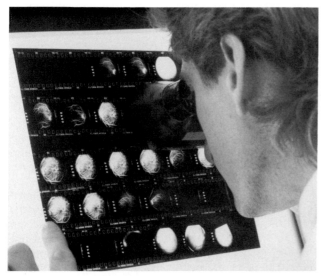

Figure 51–6. A positive transparency of the fluorescein study is interpreted at a light box. Adjacent frames that comprise stereo pairs are viewed stereoscopically using a suitable viewer.

occurring in the deeper choroidal layers. By convention, such hypofluorescence is called *blocked fluorescence.* Relatively opaque retinal abnormalities such as subretinal, intraretinal, or preretinal hemorrhage; cotton-wool spots; dense retinal exudates; and even vitreous opacities located very near the retina can cause hypofluorescence. Blocking defects are not characteristically time-dependent and are present throughout all phases in which background fluorescence is detectable. However, cotton-wool spots block more effectively in the early phases of the study, as dye eventually leaks out of the retinal capillaries in the region of the microinfarct. Examples of blocking defects are shown in Figure 51–7.

HYPOPERFUSION

If blood vessels fail to transport grossly normal amounts of fluorescein dye to a given area within the retina, choroid, or optic nerve, hypofluorescence from hypoperfusion is observed. Causes of hypoperfusion are numerous and include arteriolar and venous occlusions from emboli or thrombi, retinal ischemia related to systemic diseases such as diabetes mellitus, choroidal ischemia secondary to ophthalmic artery occlusion, focal loss of the choroidal vasculature from atrophy or scarring, and loss of perfusion of the optic nerve head from ischemia or atrophy. Hypoperfusion typically is most apparent during the arteriovenous phase of the fluorescein angiogram (Fig. 51–8). In later phases of the fluorescein study, the hypofluorescent defects often become less conspicuous, as partially occluded vessels may ultimately deliver adequate concentrations of dye to produce fluorescence.

Preinjection Fluorescence

AUTOFLUORESCENCE

Some chemical compounds that are present within the eye, such as vitamin A and lipofuscin, are capable of fluorescence. Compared with injected fluorescein dye, however, these substances are found in low concentrations and fluoresce inefficiently. However, drusen of the optic nerve head or large drusen of the pigment epithelium may contain enough fluorescent material to expose the photographic film prior to fluorescein injection. Such fluorescence occurring without the use of fluorescein dye is termed *autofluorescence.*

PSEUDOFLUORESCENCE

Excess fluorescence in a region during fluorescein transit has many possible causes. Rarely, the filters in the fundus camera are mismatched, erroneously indicating the presence of fluorescein when there is none. Hypofluorescence from this mismatch is called *pseudofluorescence.* Customarily, a preinjection photograph is taken of the fundus with the exciter and barrier filters in place. When these filters have been properly selected, virtually no fluorescence is seen prior to injection unless autofluorescence is present.

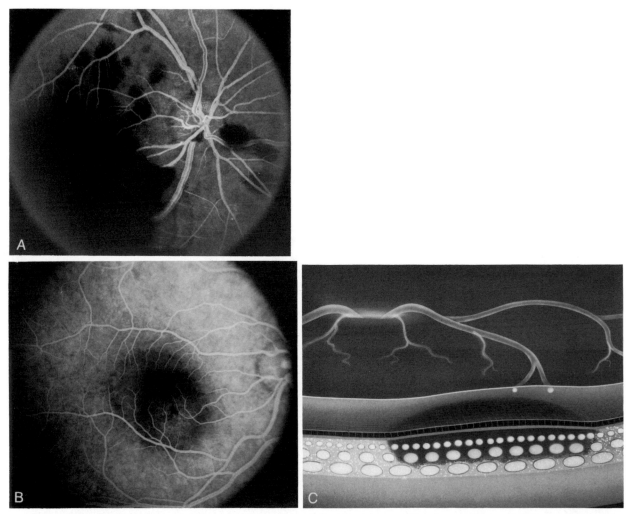

Figure 51–7. *A,* Hypofluorescence secondary to preretinal and intraretinal hemorrhage in a patient with Valsalva retinopathy. *B,* Hypofluorescence secondary to blocked choroidal fluorescence is shown in the area of the choroidal nevus located just inferonasal to the fovea. A few window defects (see Fig. 51–9) within the nevus exhibit hyperfluorescence. *C,* The mechanism of hypofluorescence is shown in cross section.

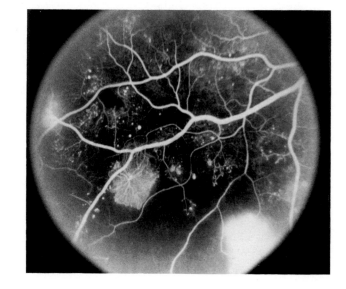

Figure 51–8. Hypoperfusion from retinal ischemia (in this case secondary to diabetes mellitus) causes hypofluorescence. The retinal capillary bed has been occluded, decreasing the concentration of intraretinal fluorescein that normally would be seen in this arteriovenous phase of the angiogram. The bright areas of hyperfluorescence are areas of retinal neovascularization that are typically found at the border between ischemic and nonischemic retina.

Hyperfluorescence

WINDOW DEFECT

The most common cause of excess fluorescence, called *hyperfluorescence,* is a focal loss of the pigment epithelial filter effect commonly referred to as a *window defect.* Even if only a few RPE cells lose their pigmentation because of atrophy or disease, fluorescein in the underlying choroid shines brightly through the defect. The brightness of a window defect depends on the concentration of fluorescein within the choroid. Window defects are thus seen early during the course of angiography, become brighter during the peak phase, and fade slowly as fluorescein leaves the eye (Fig. 51–9). Because the RPE tight junctions remain intact despite the depigmentation of the RPE, fluorescein does not leak out under the sensory retina at the window defect. Hence, the size of a window defect remains constant throughout the study.

LEAKAGE, STAINING, AND POOLING

Fluorescein is normally confined within the lumina of the retinal vessels by endothelial tight junctions. Furthermore, fluorescein is confined by the RPE layer of apical tight junctions present between adjacent cells. If the tight junctions of either the retina or the RPE are lacking or damaged, fluorescein can leak out into the surrounding tissues in which it is said to stain the tissue.

Staining may occur without abnormal leakage when there is defective filtering of fluorescence from the loss of pigment epithelium and choroidal melanin. An example is the staining of the sclera seen in an atrophic chorioretinal scar (Fig. 51–10). In this case, the source of the dye leakage is the normally leaky choroid surrounding the scar. Scleral staining is not seen in the angiogram until adequate amounts of dye have accumulated within the sclera. Hence, such staining is usually present in the late phases only.

Pooling is the accumulation of dye within an anatomic

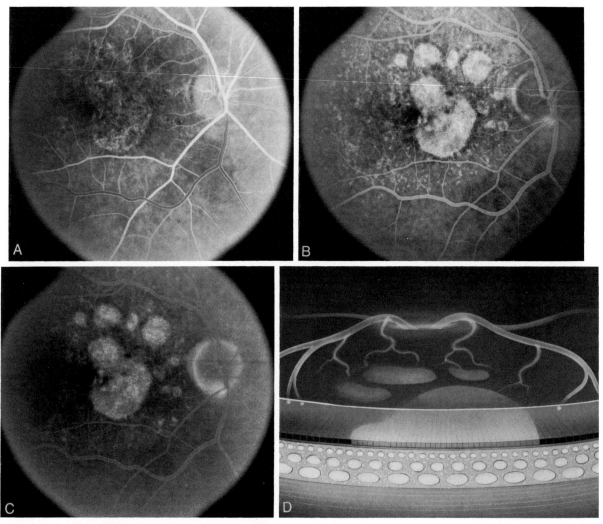

Figure 51–9. Loss of the normal attenuation effect of the retinal pigment epithelium creates a footprint-like pattern of hyperfluorescent window defects surrounding the fovea in this patient with age-related macular degeneration. Although the retinal pigment epithelium contains little pigment, its tight junctions are intact and prevent leakage of dye into the subretinal space. The defects increase in brightness through the peak phase (*A* and *B*) and slowly fade as fluorescein leaves the eye in the late phase (*C*). These defects do not change in size through the course of the study. *D,* The cause of the hyperfluorescent patches is shown schematically.

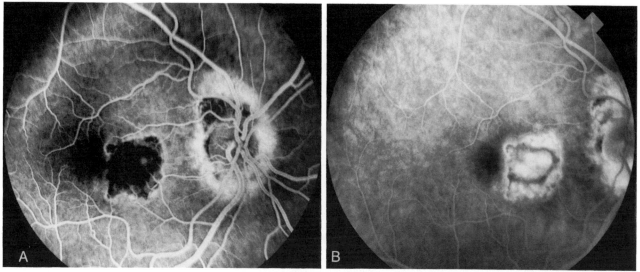

Figure 51–10. Atrophic chorioretinal scar (in this case secondary to laser photocoagulation) demonstrates staining of the sclera. This staining is not present early (A), as there is no overlying choroid, so accumulation of fluorescein in the sclera occurs slowly from the intact choroid surrounding the scar. B, Later phases show hyperfluorescence from scleral staining.

space and in the strictest sense can occur with or without abnormal leakage. Bright fluorescence develops in an area of pooling because many more photons of light are released per unit area when a deep pool of trapped fluorescein is illuminated by the excitation light (Fig. 51–11).

LEAKAGE FROM THE LOSS OF RETINAL TIGHT JUNCTIONS

Certain retinal disorders are associated with the breakdown of retinal endothelial tight junctions. In diabetic retinopathy, for instance, mural cells that nor-

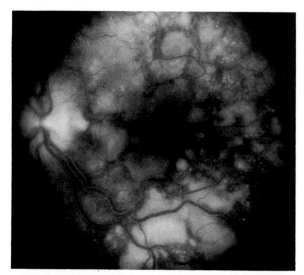

Figure 51–11. Fluorescein accumulating in a potential space is said to pool, and the high concentration of fluorescein molecules within this pool produces hyperfluorescence. In this patient with Harada's disease, considerable dye has leaked into several regions within the subretinal space, producing scattered pools of hyperfluorescence.

mally surround and support the retinal capillary endothelium are lost, causing microaneurysms to develop and allowing proteins and fluid to leak out between the capillary endothelial cells into the retinal tissue. On fluorescein angiography, this intraretinal leakage is seen as fluorescent staining (Fig. 51–12). Another example of retinal tight junction failure is aphakic cystoid macular edema in which the foveal capillaries become leaky and fluid accumulates in cystic spaces within the outer plexiform layer (Fig. 51–13). In both conditions, hyperfluorescence is more pronounced late in the study when more fluorescein has accumulated within the retina. Other causes of retinal vasculature damage that produces fluorescein leakage are central and branch retinal vein occlusion, ruptured retinal macroaneurysms, and retinal perivasculitis.

LEAKAGE FROM THE LOSS OF RPE TIGHT JUNCTIONS

The pigment epithelium normally is a barrier to movement of fluorescein from the choroidal tissue into the subretinal space. In central serous chorioretinopathy, for example, the RPE layer becomes defective, allowing fluorescein to leak out and pool beneath the sensory retina (Fig. 51–14).

LEAKAGE ACROSS BRUCH'S MEMBRANE

Fluorescein normally leaks across Bruch's membrane into the spaces between the pigment epithelium but not into the RPE cells themselves. The presence of tight junctions and an active transport mechanism confines the fluorescein beneath the pigment epithelial cell layer.

Abnormalities may develop along Bruch's membrane that allow dye to accumulate in high concentrations. For instance, in age-related macular degeneration and in some retinal dystrophies, multiple crystalline deposits

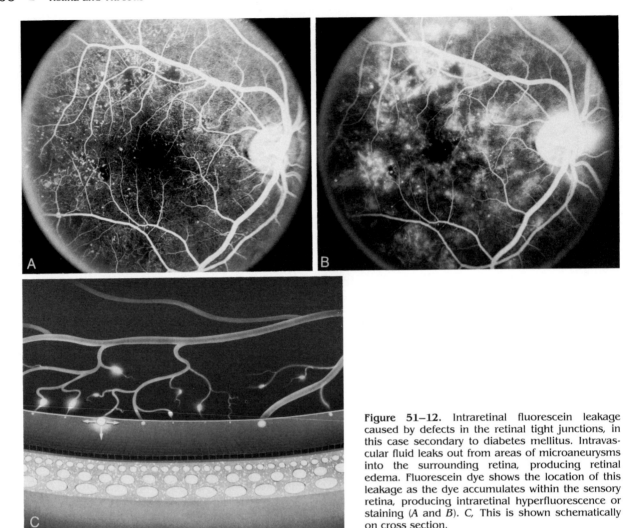

Figure 51–12. Intraretinal fluorescein leakage caused by defects in the retinal tight junctions, in this case secondary to diabetes mellitus. Intravascular fluid leaks out from areas of microaneurysms into the surrounding retina, producing retinal edema. Fluorescein dye shows the location of this leakage as the dye accumulates within the sensory retina, producing intraretinal hyperfluorescence or staining (A and B). C, This is shown schematically on cross section.

called *drusen* develop along the surface of Bruch's membrane. Furthermore, serous fluid may accumulate between Bruch's membrane and the RPE layers, a condition called *pigment epithelial detachment*. In these cases, the concentration of fluorescein is higher than normal, and fluorescence can be detected despite the presence of an intact pigment epithelial layer overlying the abnormalities. RPE detachments typically fluoresce early and become brighter as the study progresses, whereas the size of the hyperfluorescent area remains virtually constant (Fig. 51–15). Drusen typically exhibit progressive hyperfluorescence, with the margins of the drusen blurring somewhat in the later phases (Fig. 51–16).

LEAKAGE FROM THE LACK OF VASCULAR TIGHT JUNCTIONS

Leakage From Retinal Neovascularization

Retinal neovascularization, or the growth of new vessels from existing retinal or optic nerve head vessels, occurs in diabetic retinopathy, branch retinal vein occlusions, sickle cell disease, and almost any condition producing retinal ischemia. Regardless of the disease,

the new vessels lack tight junctions, allowing fluorescein to leak into the vitreous cavity throughout the course of the angiogram (Fig. 51–17). Hence, hyperfluorescence increases rapidly in the vicinity of the neovascularization, making angiography a sensitive method of detecting such a pathologic condition.

Leakage From Subretinal Neovascularization

The development of new vessels beneath the retina is called *subretinal neovascularization*. These vessels originate from the choriocapillaris and often grow through abnormalities in Bruch's membrane. Subretinal neovascularization occurs commonly in age-related macular degeneration, the presumed ocular histoplasmosis syndrome, and when Bruch's membrane is ruptured from trauma or disease. It is especially important to detect subretinal neovascularization in the macula because it may rapidly lead to retinal hemorrhage, scar formation, and permanent deterioration of central vision. The vessels in subretinal neovascularization appear considerably more leaky than normal vessels found within the inner layers of the choriocapillaris.

Text continued on page 711

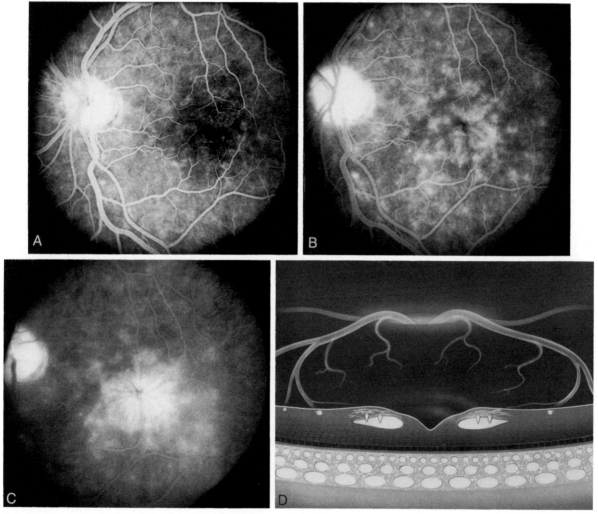

Figure 51–13. In an eye with aphakic cystoid macular edema, dye from the perifoveal retinal capillaries leaks into the outer plexiform layer and pools in cystic spaces (*A* and *B*). The petalloid pattern of fluorescence, which becomes most prominent in the late-phase films (*C*), is diagnostic of cystoid macular edema. Schematic cross section (*D*) depicts the source of the edema and the location of the cystic spaces in the perifoveal area.

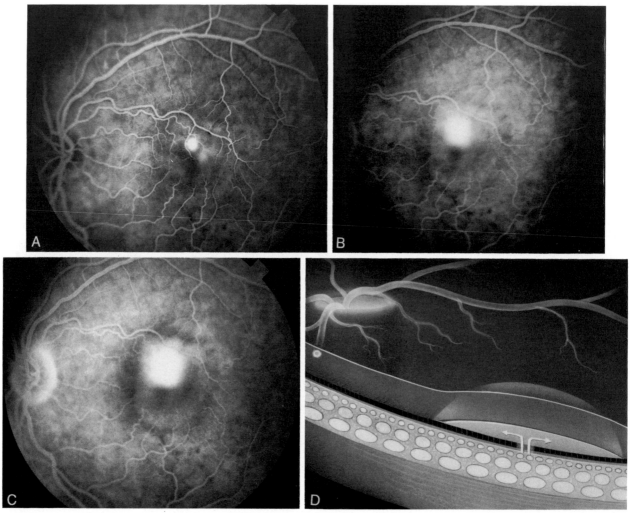

Figure 51–14. In this case of central serous chorioretinopathy, fluid from the choroid has leaked across defective tight junctions in the retinal pigment epithelium (*A*) and accumulates in the subretinal space. On fluorescein angiography, a small round area of hyperfluorescence is seen in the early-phase films and expands progressively as the dye is trapped (pools) within the subretinal space (*B* and *C*). *D*, Schematic representation of these fluorescein findings.

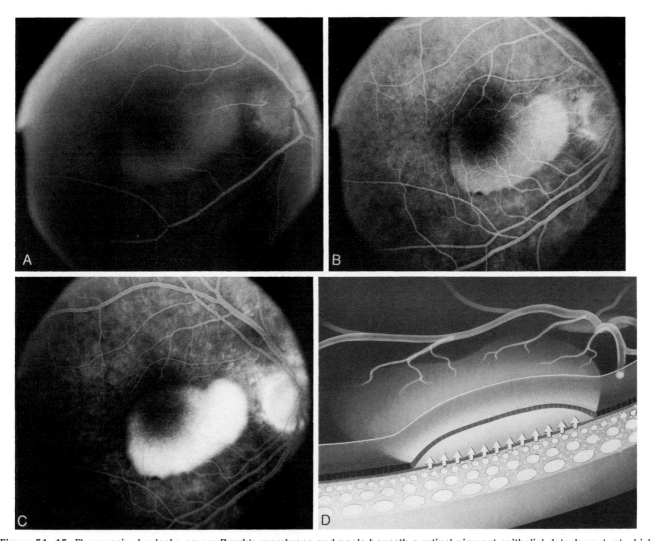

Figure 51–15. Fluorescein dye leaks across Bruch's membrane and pools beneath a retinal pigment epithelial detachment, at which point it is confined. Angiographically, progressive pooling is seen, but the extent of the hyperfluorescent area remains constant (A–C). D, Cross-sectional illustration depicts this course of events after fluorescein injection.

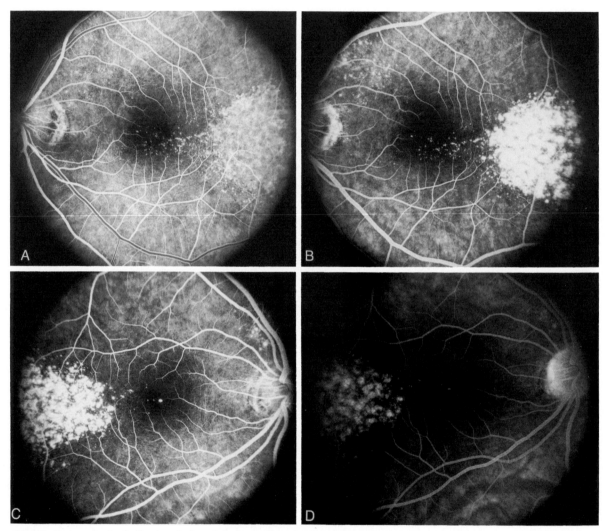

Figure 51–16. Drusen look similar to window defects on fluorescein angiography (*A*). Later in the study, however, the borders of drusen may become fuzzy (*B* and *C*). *D,* Arteriovenous late-phase photographs show staining of the drusen. (*A–D,* Courtesy of Roberta Wilson.)

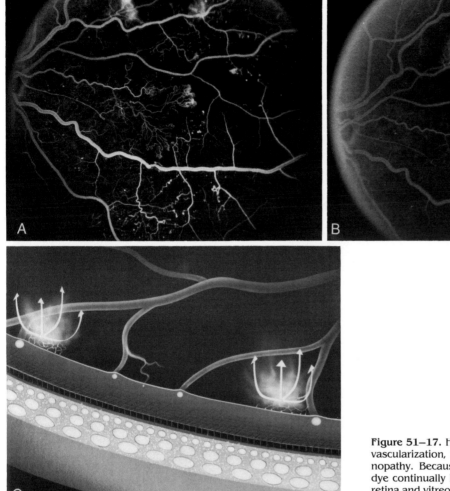

Figure 51–17. Hyperfluorescence caused by retinal neovascularization, in this case secondary to sickle cell retinopathy. Because the new vessels lack tight junctions, dye continually leaks out of the lumina (A), staining the retina and vitreous more intensely in the later phases (B). C, Illustration summarizes these events.

In the early phases, a subretinal neovascular net fills rapidly along with the choriocapillaris, glowing brightly as the peak phase is approached. Because the dye quickly leaks out of these new vessels, the area of leakage increases progressively with time. A dark hypofluorescent rim surrounding the new vessel membrane is often seen during the arteriovenous phase (Fig. 51–18).

One of the most frequent uses of fluorescein angiography is the detection of subretinal neovascularization. Laser photocoagulation has been shown to prevent visual loss in many patients with subretinal neovascular membranes.[16–18] Follow-up angiography is customarily performed about 3 wk after initial photocoagulation to make certain that no residual vessels remain. If vessels remain, additional laser treatment is often indicated.

Leakage From Retinal and Choroidal Tumor Vessels

Vessels within tumors of the retina and choroid characteristically lack tight junctions, allowing fluorescein dye to leak into and stain adjacent tissues. Examples of tumors associated with such vessels include combined hamartomas of the retina and pigment epithelium, cho-roidal hemangiomas, retinal angiomas (Fig. 51–19), choroidal melanomas, and astrocytic hamartomas.

INDOCYANINE GREEN ANGIOGRAPHY

When indocyanine green (ICG) dye is injected intravenously, it is confined almost completely by both the retinal and the choroidal vasculature, as ICG is highly bound to protein. This dye can be detected using infrared photography or video angiography.[19, 20] ICG fluoresces at a peak wavelength of 835 nm when illuminated by an infrared light having a peak wavelength of 805 nm.

With ICG angiography, subretinal neovascular membranes and other abnormalities of the choroidal vasculature are well demonstrated because the vascular patterns are not obscured by progressive leakage of dye from the choroidal vessels and because the pigment epithelium does not effectively block the choroidal fluorescence produced when infrared light illuminates the ICG dye. ICG is more highly confined to subretinal neovascular membranes when compared with sodium fluorescein, and fluorescence from ICG is better trans-

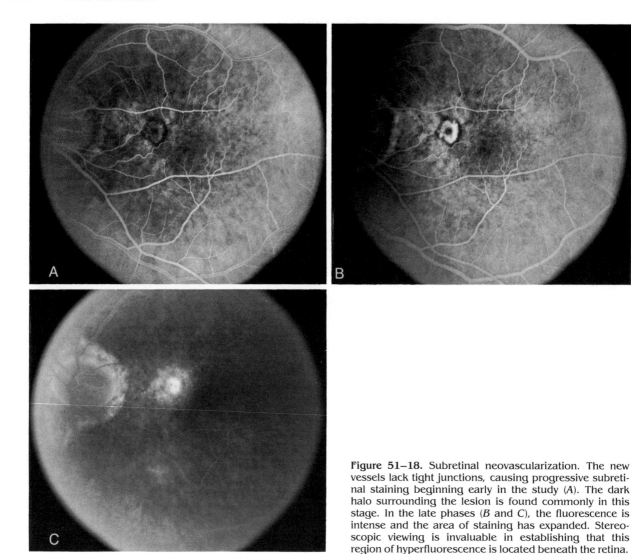

Figure 51–18. Subretinal neovascularization. The new vessels lack tight junctions, causing progressive subretinal staining beginning early in the study (A). The dark halo surrounding the lesion is found commonly in this stage. In the late phases (B and C), the fluorescence is intense and the area of staining has expanded. Stereoscopic viewing is invaluable in establishing that this region of hyperfluorescence is located beneath the retina.

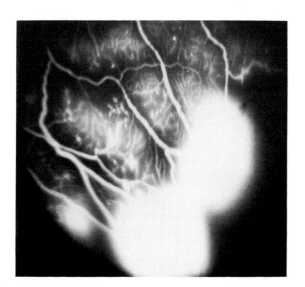

Figure 51–19. The retinal vessels in a patient with Coats' disease lack normal tight junctions, allowing fluorescein to leak out and progressively stain the adjacent vitreous.

mitted through blood, melanin, and exudate. Chorioretinal scars, which are hyperfluorescent on fluorescein angiography, are hypofluorescent on an ICG study. Thus, in regions of chorioretinal scarring, subretinal neovascularization is often more easily detectable when ICG, rather than fluorescein, angiography is used (Fig. 51–20).[20]

DIGITAL FLUORESCEIN ANGIOGRAPHY

Rather than use photographic film to record the fluorescein transit, fundus and fluorescein images can be documented electronically and stored on suitable storage media.[21, 22] A typical digital fundus imaging system (Fig. 51–21) consists of a high-resolution black and white video camera that replaces the camera back on the fundus camera. The fundus is imaged using only about a third of the light intensity required to expose photographic film. The resultant analog video image is

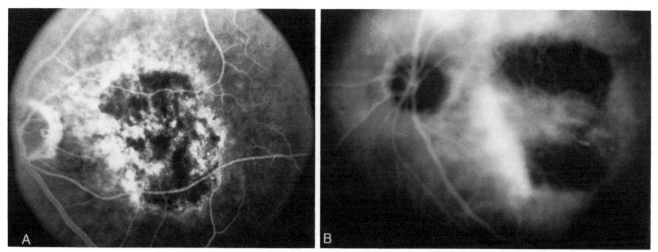

Figure 51–20. *A,* Fluorescein angiogram (arteriovenous phase) of the left eye in a patient with a large disciform area of chorioretinal atrophy centered at the fovea. A well-defined neovascular membrane cannot be discerned. *B,* Indocyanine green videoangiographic frame of the same eye demonstrates the presence of a large subretinal neovascular membrane beneath the fovea. (*A* and *B,* Courtesy of Maryanna Destro, M.D.)

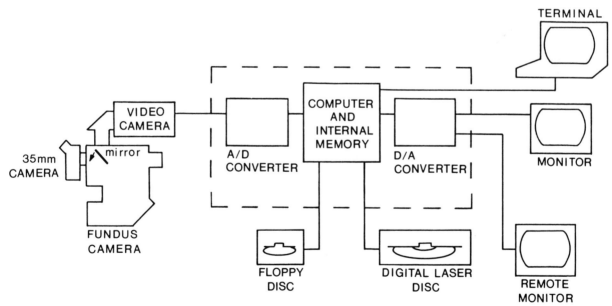

Figure 51–21. Schematic diagram of a typical digital acquisition system. Images are obtained using a fundus camera interfaced to a high-resolution video camera. The signal is digitized by an analog-to-digital convertor (A/D), and the image in digital form can then be manipulated by the image processor (*dotted lines*). Ultimately, the image is converted back to an analog signal (*D/A*) and viewed on a monitor. If desired, the images can be stored in computer storage devices such as an optical laser disc hard drive or floppy disc. High-quality transparencies can also be made using the digital image data. (From Friberg TR, Rehkopf PG, Warnicki JW, Eller AW: Use of directly acquired digital fundus and fluorescein angiographic images in the diagnosis of retinal disease. Retina 7:246–251, 1987.)

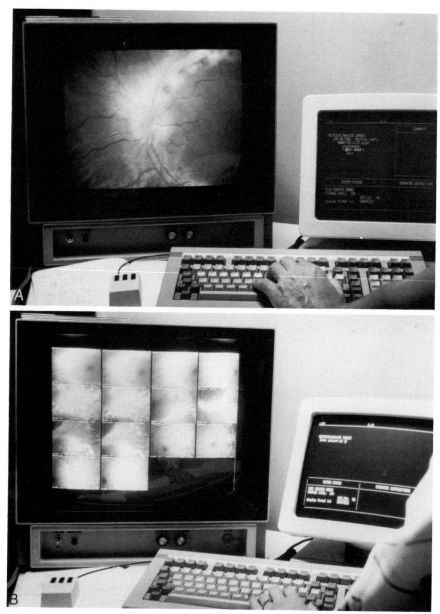

Figure 51–22. *A,* Electronic digital image of the fundus reassembled for viewing on a video monitor. *B,* Individual image may also be assembled into proof sheet form, allowing an overview of all the images in a study. (*A* and *B,* From Friberg TR, Rehkopf PG, Warnicki JW, Eller AW: Use of directly acquired digital fundus and fluorescein angiographic images in the diagnosis of retinal disease. Retina 7:246–251, 1987.)

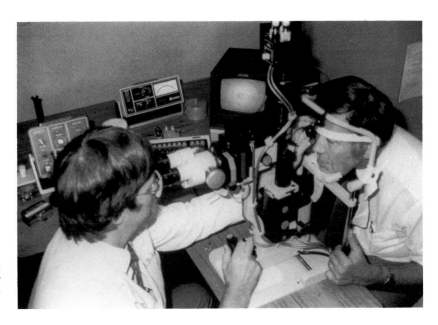

Figure 51–23. A video monitor placed on the laser console displays a bright digital image of high contrast that can serve as a guide to laser photocoagulation.

divided electronically into many tiny picture elements, or pixels, as the signal passes through an analog to digital convertor. Each pixel is assigned one of several hundred (usually 256) shades of color or gray, and the computer then stores the pixel information temporarily in its memory for display. These digital data may be permanently archived onto storage media such as a hard disc or an optical laser disc. By electronically reassembling the image, the fluorescein study or color images can be placed in a format and viewed on a high-resolution video monitor (Fig. 51–22).

Digital systems are particularly valuable in that they allow immediate assessment and treatment of chorioretinal diseases without the delay inherent in photographic film processing. In addition, images can be manipulated electronically to enhance or highlight subtle details or to facilitate analysis of a fundus pathologic condition.[23] Furthermore, the images can be enlarged and displayed on a television monitor. Placement of such a monitor adjacent to the laser delivery system console provides a guide for photocoagulation treatment of retinal lesions (Fig. 51–23).

A digital system with a pixel array of 1024 × 1024 elements yields excellent resolution of the fluorescein details and can be used in lieu of photographic techniques (Fig. 51–24). Systems using smaller numbers of pixels per frame yield clinically useful fluorescein results, but their lower resolution is noticeably inferior to the use of 35-mm film. If a hard-copy print is needed, the digital image can be printed via a high-quality laser printer either on a sheet of paper or in transparency form.

The relative advantages and disadvantages of on-line digital image acquisition systems when compared with film are summarized in Table 51–1. As the price of computer storage decreases and the speed of computers increases, use of such digital systems will predictably become more widespread. At present, the most serious disadvantages of digital imaging systems is the inability to economically obtain and store high-resolution color images and the inability to display high-quality fluorescein images stereoscopically in proof sheet form without first having to print the image.

SUMMARY

Although the basic principles of fluorescein angiography have been outlined in this chapter, proper interpretation of an angiographic study is a learned skill that must be refined by clinical experience. Several excellent and comprehensive texts are devoted entirely to the subject.[1, 8, 9] As an aid to recalling the physiologic basis of angiography, please refer to the flow charts for hyper- and hypofluorescence (Figs. 51–25 and 51–26), which are patterned after those developed by Schatz.[1, 13]

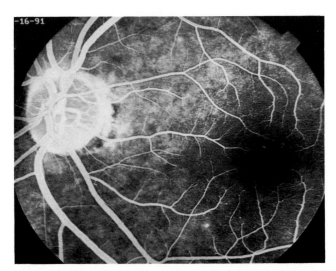

Figure 51–24. A fluorescein angiographic frame obtained digitally and composed of picture elements (pixels). The quality of this image compares well with the conventional photographic film. (Courtesy of Topcon.)

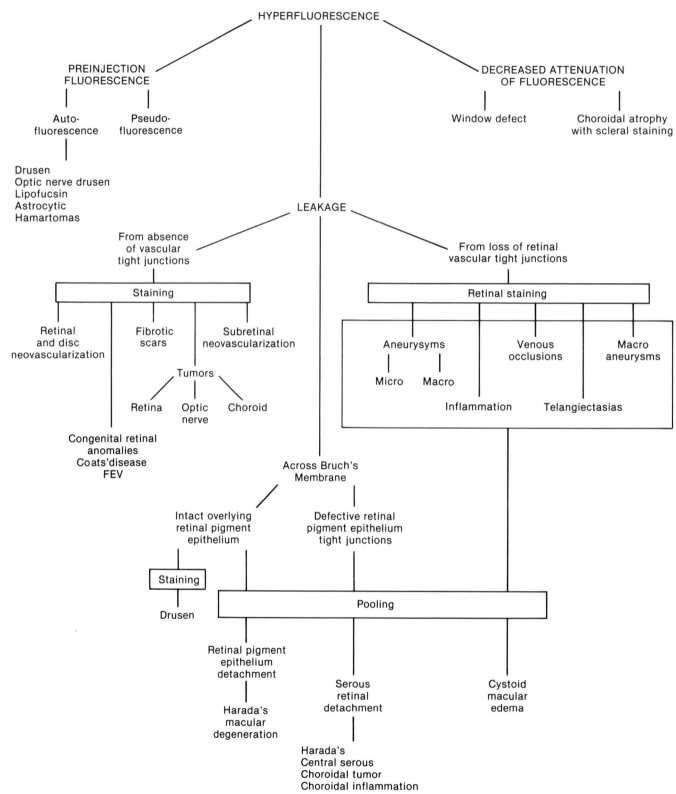

Figure 51–25. Flow chart for hyperfluorescence. Preinjection fluorescence has been placed on this chart for convenience. (FEV, familial exudative vitreoretinopathy.)

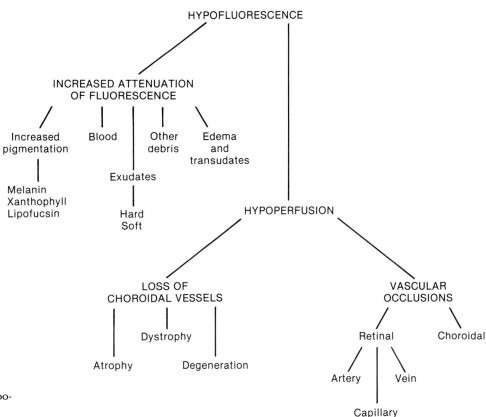

Figure 51–26. Flow chart for hypofluorescence.

Table 51–1. ON-LINE DIGITAL IMAGE ACQUISITION SYSTEMS

Advantages	Disadvantages
Instant fundus and fluorescein images	Less image resolution than film
Easy archiving of images onto storage media (optical discs and so on)	High-quality hard copy images require expensive digital printers
Image enhancement and analysis easily performed	System and files subject to computer malfunction and breakdown
Less light required to obtain images to conventional photography	Capital costs high for high-quality system
Images can be transmitted electronically to remote monitors	Systems do not yet allow economical use of high-quality color images; primarily for black and white imaging
Images seen with high contrast and can be easily magnified	
Elimination of film and development costs attendant with conventional photography	

REFERENCES

1. Schatz H, Burton TC, Yannuzzi LA, Rabb MF: History of fluorescein angiography. *In* Interpretation of Fundus Fluorescein Angiography. St Louis, CV Mosby, 1978, pp 3–9.
2. MacLean AL, Maumenee AE: Hemangioma of the choroid. Am J Ophthalmol 50:2–11, 1960.
3. Flocks M, Miller J, Chao P: Retinal circulation time with the aid of fundus cinephotography. Am J Ophthalmol 48:3–6, 1959.
4. Novotny HR, Alvis DL: A method of photographing fluorescein in circulating blood in the human retina. Circulation 24:82–86, 1961.
5. Allen L: Ocular fundus photography: Suggestions for achieving consistently good pictures and instructions for stereoscopic photography. Am J Ophthalmol 57:13–28, 1964.
6. Gass JDM: A fluorescein angiographic study of macular dysfunction secondary to retinal vascular diseases, Parts I to VI. Arch Ophthalmol 80:535–617, 1968.
7. Schatz H, George T, Liu JH, et al: Color fluorescein angiography: Its clinical role. Trans Am Acad Ophthalmol Otolaryngol 77:254–259, 1973.
8. Shikano S, Shimizu K: Atlas of Fluorescein Fundus Angiography. Philadelphia, WB Saunders, 1968.
9. Gass JDM: Pathophysiologic and histopathologic bases for interpretation of fluorescein angiography. *In* Stereoscopic Atlas of Macular Diseases. Diagnosis and Treatment, 3rd ed. St. Louis, CV Mosby, 1987, pp 19–41.
10. Amalric P, Piau C, Fenies MT: Incidents et accidents au cours de l'angiographie fluoresceinique. Bull Soc Ophthal Franc 68:968–973, 1968.
11. Pacirariu RI: Low incidence of side effects following intravenous fluorescein angiography. Ann Ophthalmol 14:32–36, 1982.
12. Butner RW, McPherson AR: Adverse reactions in intravenous fluorescein angiography. Ann Ophthalmol 15:1084–1086, 1983.
13. Berkow JW, Kelly JS, Orth DH: Fluorescein Angiography. A Guide to the Interpretation of Fluorescein Angiograms. American Academy of Ophthalmology Manual. San Francisco, 1984, pp 9–30.
14. Halperin LS, Olk J, Soubrane G, Coscas G: Safety of fluorescein angiography during pregnancy. Am J Ophthalmol 109:563–566, 1990.
15. Greenberg F, Lewis RA: Safety of fluorescein angiography during pregnancy. [Letter to the Editor with reply from Halperin LS, Olk J, Soubrane G, Coscas G] Am J Ophthalmol 110:323–325, 1990.

16. Macular Photocoagulation Study Group: Argon laser photocoagulation for senile macular degeneration: Results of a randomized clinical trial. Arch Ophthalmol 100:912–918, 1982.
17. Macular Photocoagulation Study Group: Argon laser photocoagulation for ocular histoplasmosis: Results of a randomized clinical trial. Arch Ophthalmol 101:1358–1361, 1983.
18. Macular Photocoagulation Study Group: Argon laser photocoagulation for idiopathic neovascularization: Results of a randomized clinical trial. Arch Ophthalmol 101:1358–1361, 1983.
19. Flowers RW, Hochheimer BF: Indocyanine green dye fluorescence and infrared absorption choroidal angiography performed simultaneously with fluorescein angiography. Johns Hopkins Med J 138:33–42, 1976.
20. Destro M, Puliafito CA: Indocyanine green videoangiography of choroidal neovascularizations. Ophthalmology 96:846–853, 1989.
21. Friberg TR, Rehkopf PG, Warnicki JW, Eller AW: Use of directly acquired digital fundus and fluorescein angiographic images in the diagnosis of retinal disease. Retina 7:246–251, 1987.
22. Friberg TR, Eller AW, Rehkopf P, Warnicki J: Use of digital fundus and fluorescein images in laser photocoagulation of the retina. In Gitter KA, Schatz H, Yannuzzi LA, McDonald HR (eds): Laser Photocoagulation of Retinal Disease. San Francisco, Pacifica Medical Press, 1988, pp 57–61.
23. Friberg TR, Campagna J: Central serous chorioretinopathy: An analysis of the clinical morphology using image-processing techniques. Graefes Arch Clin Exp Ophthalmol 227:201–205, 1989.

Chapter 52

■

Indocyanine Green Videoangiography

JORDI MONÉS, DAVID R. GUYER, SARA KRUPSKY,
EPHRAIM FRIEDMAN, and EVANGELOS S. GRAGOUDAS

Fluorescein angioscopy[1] and angiography[2] were important technologic advances in the study of retinal disorders. Although choroidal circulation patterns have been described with fluorescein angiography, the limitations of this technique for studying the choroid are well known.[3–6] The excitation and fluorescence of blue-green wavelengths (peak absorption 465 nm; peak fluorescence 525 nm) are absorbed and scattered by the pigment layers of the fundus, including the macular xanthophyll. Thus, the choroidal layers cannot be well visualized.[7–10] In addition, sodium fluorescein, which is 60 to 80 percent bound to plasma albumin,[11] rapidly leaks from the fenestrated choriocapillaris[4] and produces a diffuse background fluorescence, which further obscures the details of the choroidal vessels.[12] Finally, the intricate branching of the choroidal vascular system[13] is difficult to study with fluorescein angiography.[12]

Because the choroid is the major blood supply of the eye[14] and the outer retinal layers, a better method of studying this important tissue was needed. Near-infrared absorption angiography, using indocyanine green (ICG) as an absorbing dye, was first studied in the canine brain by Kogure and Choromokos in 1969.[15] This study led to the development of ICG choroidal angiography.

HISTORY OF ICG ANGIOGRAPHY

In 1969, a qualitative method of studying choroidal blood flow using reflective densitometry with ICG was reported.[16] After using infrared absorption ICG angiography to study the circulation of the dog cerebral surface,[15] Kogure and associates first demonstrated choroidal absorption angiography using intraarterial ICG injection and false-color infrared film in monkeys.[17] These investigators demonstrated filling of the smaller choroidal veins and occasional laminar filling of the larger choroidal veins. A choroidal arterial phase was not noted. David was the first to perform ICG absorption choroidal angiography in human patients in 1969.[18] These patients underwent intraarterial ICG injections during carotid angiography. He described diffuse choriocapillaris filling and choroidal veins draining toward the vortex veins. In 1971, Hochheimer[19] performed choroidal absorption angiography in cats using intravenous ICG injections and black-and-white infrared film. This study solved two major problems. The first was the use of intraarterial injections and the second was the inconsistency of the false-color infrared film.

Intravenous ICG absorption angiography was first successfully performed in humans by Flower and Hochheimer in 1972.[20, 21] With this method, the fundus is illuminated with infrared light and the reflected light exposes the photographic film. If larger vessels are filled with enough dye to absorb the incident light, the film will not be exposed.[21, 22] In 1973, Flower and Hochheimer described a method of ICG fluorescence angiography.[23] With this technique, direct fluorescence of the vessels occurred, the resolution improved, and the arterial and capillary dye phases were evident. In 1974, Flower developed a multispectral fundus camera.[12] Simultaneous ICG fluorescence and absorption angiography with fluorescein angiography was performed. This combination allowed comparison of the various types of angiograms. Clinical reports of ICG angiographic imaging of choroidal neovascular membranes, choroidal tumors, choroideremia, choroidal hemangiomas, and the presumed ocular histoplasmosis syndrome were published.[24–31] Further technologic improvements followed.[32–34] Visualization of the choriocapillaris filling pattern with ICG and study of the temporal differences of ICG and fluorescein choroidal filling were performed in monkeys.[33] Hyvärinen and Flower presented a case of a choroidal neovascular membrane in which the feeding choroidal artery was identified and photocoagulated.[35]

In 1985, Bischoff and Flower reported their 10 years of experience with ICG choroidal angiography.[36] This series included 180 angiograms of normal volunteers and 500 angiograms of patients with various fundus diseases. Hayashi and associates in 1986 performed ICG angiography in patients with central serous chorioretinopathy using an infrared-sensitive video camera.[37] Videoangiography has also been used by other investigators to study choroidal neovascular membranes[38–40] and choroidal blood flow.[41, 42] A digital computer system has also been used to study choroidal blood flow.[43, 44] Preliminary results with ICG videoangiography with the scanning laser ophthalmoscope were reported by Scheider and Schroedel in 1989,[45] and Scheider and coworkers recently described their experience with this technique and choroidal neovascularization.[46] More recently, a high-resolution digital imaging system has been adapted for diagnostic ICG angiography, which has been especially useful in imaging poorly defined choroidal neovascular membranes.[47, 48] Preliminary results have been presented on ICG dye-enhanced diode laser photocoagulation.[49, 50]

PHARMACOLOGY OF ICG

ICG was first used in 1957 to measure cardiac output.[51] It is a water-soluble tricarbocyanine dye, which is an anhydro-3,3,3′,3′-tetramethyl-1,1′-di-(4-sulfobutyl)-4,5,4′,5′-dibenzoindotricarbocyanine hydroxide sodium salt.

Its molecular weight is 775 daltons, and its empirical formula is $C_{43}H_{47}N_2O_6S_2Na$.[52] After intravenous injection, ICG is rapidly and almost completely bound to plasma proteins. It has been thought that ICG is bound to albumin in the blood.[53] However, 80 percent of ICG in human serum is actually bound to globulins, such as α-lipoproteins.[54]

The spectral absorption of ICG in aqueous solution with albumin is between 790 and 805 nm.[54–56] ICG is eliminated from the blood almost exclusively by the liver and is excreted into the bile. Reabsorption of ICG from the intestine does not occur.[55–58] ICG is not detected in the cerebrospinal fluid[58, 59] nor does it cross the placental barrier.[60]

TOXICITY OF ICG

ICG is not very toxic in animals.[61–65] Only a few side effects have been reported with clinical use.[53, 61, 66, 67] In 1978, 240,000 cases of ICG use were reviewed.[68] In the early years, when the presence of 5 percent iodide in Cardio-Green was not appreciated, there were some side effects in patients with iodide allergies. In addition, one patient had urticaria and three patients had anaphylactic reactions. One of these patients died. Among 43 patients who underwent chronic hemodialysis, 3 patients with nausea and 1 patient with a reversible anaphylactoid reaction to ICG were reported.[69]

No side effects have been reported in the ophthalmic literature. There were no complications after intravenous doses of 150 to 200 mg of ICG in one study.[70] During 700 procedures in another study, no side effects were reported.[36] Thus, ICG is relatively nontoxic and appears to be safer than fluorescein dye. Between 5 and 20 percent of patients receiving fluorescein dye suffer from nausea, headache, or dizziness, and 5 to 10 in 1000 patients have allergic reactions.[11] In 1986, a fluorescein angiography complication survey was published.[71] One in 63 patients had a moderate reaction (urticaria and syncope), and 1 in 1900 patients had a severe reaction (cardiopulmonary). The risk of death was estimated to be 1 in 222,000 patients.

Nevertheless, ICG may cause a severe anaphylactic reaction. ICG angiography should not be performed in patients who are allergic to iodide, in those who have a history of severe allergies, or in those who are uremic.[36] In addition, we would not recommend its use in patients with liver disease, as the dye is eliminated exclusively by this organ.

SPECIAL PROPERTIES OF ICG FOR CHOROIDAL ANGIOGRAPHY

ICG absorbs light in the near-infrared region of the spectrum (maximal absorption is approximately at 790 nm)[17] and also fluoresces in the near-infrared region (maximal emission is approximately at 835 nm).[72–74] Because of its activity at these longer wavelengths, ICG fluoresces through pigment and hemorrhage when it is excited by near-infrared light.

Approximately 98 percent of ICG is bound to plasma proteins,[53] and therefore, the dye probably does not leak from the choriocapillaris.[22] This property allows better visualization of the choroidal vessels because ICG remains in the choroidal vasculature longer than fluorescein does. However, some authors believe that ICG can pass through the fenestrations of the choriocapillaris.[37, 40] Bill stated that the choroidal blood vessels are permeable to substances with molecular weights of 17,000 to 156,000 daltons, such as myoglobin, albumin, and gamma globulin.[76] Thus, protein-bound ICG may pass through the fenestrations of the choriocapillaris to some extent.[36]

The liver rapidly removes ICG from the blood after intravenous injection.[53, 57, 77] Therefore, there is no significant ICG staining of normal ocular tissues.[17, 78]

Another advantage of ICG is that its peak absorption coincides with the emission spectrum of the diode laser. This property may allow selective ablation of chorioretinal lesions using ICG dye-enhanced diode laser photocoagulation when a target tissue containing ICG is exposed to the diode laser beam.[49, 50, 75]

TECHNIQUE OF ICG INJECTION

A dye concentration of 0.03 mg/ml is required for maximal fluorescence of ICG in the choroidal vessels. The dye is diluted 600 times before it enters the choroidal circulation. Thus, about 20 mg of ICG in 1 ml of aqueous solvent has to be rapidly injected intracubitally. We currently inject approximately 50 mg of ICG for diagnostic studies. Rapid injection is essential in order to delineate various choroidal filling phases because the majority of the dye bolus must be in the choroidal vessels before reaching the retinal vasculature.[79] This injection should be immediately followed by a flush of 5 ml of normal saline solution. The timing of photography should be determined by arm to retina time,[36] since the fundus cannot be observed. This transit time is approximately 10 sec in young patients and approximately 12 to 18 sec in older patients.[11]

CHARACTERISTICS OF INFRARED WAVELENGTHS

Near-infrared light is used to perform choroidal angiography because it can penetrate pigmented layers[7-9] better than the shorter wavelengths of visible light. The percentage of absorption in human retinal pigment epithelium and choroid for equal intensities is between 59 and 75 percent for 500 nm (blue-green visible light) and between 21 and 38 percent for 800 nm (near-infrared light).[10] Near-infrared light causes ICG to fluoresce. Patients note that infrared light appears as barely visible red light. Therefore, photophobic patients may tolerate this procedure better than fluorescein angiography.[20]

Since longer wavelengths are less scattered than shorter wavelengths, near-infrared angiography may be performed in patients with diffuse opacities in the ocular media, such as cataract or vitreous hemorrhage.[24] Infrared light is less harmful than shorter wavelength light to the retina; thus, a continuous light source may be used for high-speed angiography.[36] Thermal retinal damage, however, can be produced with the infrared light. With energies greater than 1 W/sq cm, the retinal temperature may rise 10°C, and acute retinal damage can occur. The safe time exposure must be calculated.[80] The risk of near-infrared–induced lens damage is minimal with choroidal angiography.[36]

MORPHOLOGIC FEATURES OF THE CHOROIDAL VASCULATURE

Normal Morphologic Choroidal Patterns

Most of the short posterior ciliary arteries enter the eye near the macula. These choroidal arteries travel radially to the equator. After they have perforated the sclera and have entered the choroid, they divide into smaller branches. Interarterial anastomoses are common in the choroid,[81] but they cannot be distinguished with ICG angiography. The choroidal arteries do not fill at the same time. The earliest detectable filling of the arteries is usually nasal to the fovea. This region is the area of highest blood perfusion pressure in the eye.[21] The individual vessels of the choriocapillaris cannot be distinguished. The choriocapillaris filling pattern produces a faint and diffuse homogeneous fluorescence that prevents a clear visualization of the deeper choroidal layers (Fig. 52–1).[79] Choroidal veins run parallel to the periphery and eventually form the vortex veins (Fig. 52–2). Venous anastomoses occur between large vessels.[81] Veins are larger and more fluorescent than arteries, but these changes cannot be used to differentiate them. A horizontal watershed area between the superior and the inferior vessels is sometimes present (Fig. 52–3).[36] Choroidal arteries fill between 0.5 and 1 sec earlier than does the central retinal artery. Different phases of the ICG angiogram have been described.[36, 82] The mean time values reported follow:

Choroidal artery to choroidal vein	1.8 sec
Central retinal artery to retinal vein (laminar)	2.0 sec
Central retinal artery to retinal vein (full)	6.2 sec
Choroidal artery to vortex vein (initial)	2.0 sec
Choroidal artery to vortex vein (maximal)	5.0 sec

ICG Angiography of Chorioretinal Disorders

AGE-RELATED MACULAR DEGENERATION

Macular disorders may occur secondary to specific choroidal vascular properties of this specialized area.[83]

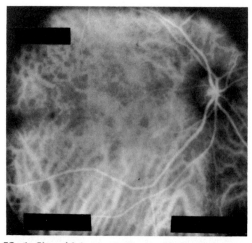

Figure 52–1. Choroidal venous phase of indocyanine green (ICG) angiography of a normal fundus. A diffuse, homogeneous fluorescence is noted in the macular area. Details of the deeper vessels in this area are not seen. Around the macular area, the choroidal veins are homogeneous in caliper and distributed uniformly to converge to form the vortex veins.

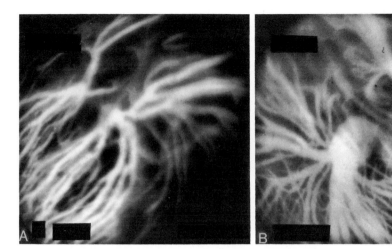

Figure 52–2. *A* and *B,* The choroidal veins converge to form the vortex veins, with a large variability of patterns.

Only short arteries and arterioles are present between the ciliary arteries and the choriocapillaris in the macula. This cluster of arterial branches is greater in the macula than in any other region. These findings may be responsible for the high pressure and rapid blood flow of the macula.[13, 21, 83] These pressure changes may cause choriocapillaris disease[83] and choroidal neovascularization.[84] The loss of contractility of the arterial wall that occurs with age may cause dilatation of the vessel.[85, 86] Watershed areas of both arterial and venous circulations may be present in the macular area.[87, 88] Hayashi and de Laey described a relationship between these choroidal "watershed zones" and macular lesions and showed evidence of abnormal choroidal vessels. They suggested that chronic choroidal insufficiency may cause choroidal neovascularization.[88]

Bischoff and Flower[36] reviewed 100 ICG angiograms of age-related macular degeneration and described four abnormal findings:

1. Delayed or irregular choroidal filling, or both. In some patients, the interval between choroidal arterial and choroidal venous filling was 3 to 4 sec. However, as these authors suggest, the significance of this finding is uncertain because the investigators did not study an age-matched control group.

2. Generalized arterial changes. These authors describe "wandering arteries" in some patients with age-related macular degeneration.

3. Localized arterial changes. Marked dilatation of macular choroidal arteries was observed in some patients. These arteries filled earlier than other vessels and often formed a loop close to the entrance site. These loops were anatomically related to overlying fundus lesions. The authors felt that a higher blood pressure in the choriocapillaris overlying vascular abnormalities may cause dilatation of the choriocapillaris and subsequent macular disease (Fig. 52–4).[84]

4. Choroidal neovascularization. This finding was observed by ICG angiography in only a small number of cases in Bischoff and Flower's series (Fig. 52–5). Only one case has been reported in which it was possible to identify and photocoagulate the feeding choroidal artery.[35]

Hayashi and colleagues reported that ICG angiography was particularly useful to detect occult choroidal neovascular membranes.[38] The same investigators showed that ICG leaks from choroidal neovascular

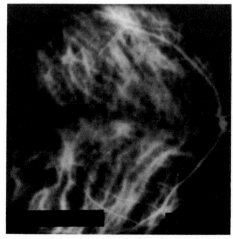

Figure 52–3. A horizontal watershed area between the superior and the inferior vessels is found in a minority of patients.

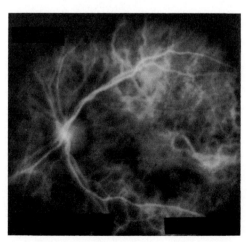

Figure 52–4. Choroidal midtransit phase of an ICG angiogram in a patient with age-related macular degeneration. Dilated tortuous arterial loops can be observed on the temporal side.

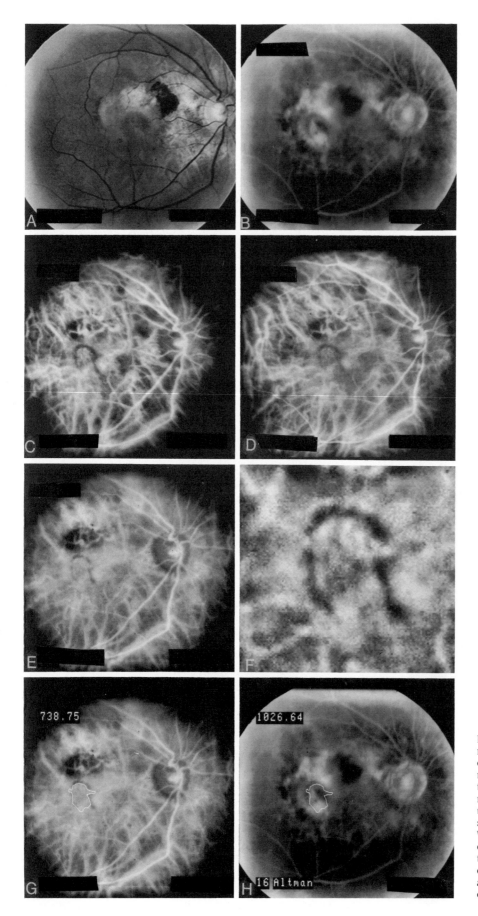

Figure 52–5. *A* and *B,* Red-free photography and the late phase of the fluorescein angiogram of a poorly defined choroidal neovascular membrane. *C–E,* In the ICG angiograms, the limits of the neovascular membrane can be better visualized. *F,* Increased magnification shows some feeding vessels. *G* and *H,* With computer analysis, the membrane observed in the ICG angiogram can be traced and superimposed on the fluorescein angiogram. In some instances, ICG angiography improves the definition of a choroidal neovascular membrane.

membranes into the subretinal space. However, the leakage is slower and of lesser magnitude than fluorescein leakage of choroidal neovascular membranes. This slow ICG leakage is sometimes useful in defining the borders of choroidal neovascular membranes and has delineated neovascularization not well-identified with fluorescein angiography.[40] Destro and Puliafito[39] also found this technique very useful to study occult choroidal neovascular membranes, particularly those with overlying hemorrhage or those that had recurred on the edge of previously treated areas. Choroidal neovascularization adjacent to chorioretinal scars showed greater contrast between the new vessels and the adjacent scar with ICG than with fluorescein angiography. Chorioretinal scars were hypofluorescent because of less ICG extravasation and the relative lack of choroidal vessels in those areas. ICG remained selectively in and around the choroidal neovascular membranes.[39] In addition, Scheider and coworkers described enhanced imaging of choroidal neovascularization by using the scanning laser ophthalmoscope with ICG angiography.[46]

High-resolution ICG images can now be produced by combining digital imaging systems and an ICG camera.[47, 48] This technologic advance now allows the theoretical advantage of ICG over fluorescein dye to finally be realized.

Yannuzzi and associates[48] showed that occult choroidal neovascularization could be converted into classic, well-defined choroidal neovascularization in 39 percent of the 129 patients in their series because of information obtained through digital ICG videoangiography. These authors found that digital ICG videoangiography is especially useful for patients with poorly defined choroidal neovascularization, pigment epithelial detachments, and recurrent choroidal neovascularization. In many cases, the late ICG images reveal a hyperfluorescent area corresponding to an area of subretinal neovascularization that cannot be detected by fluorescein angiography. The finding of a hyperfluorescent spot on the late ICG angiogram can separate the neovascularized portion from the serous portion of a pigment epithelial detachment.

DIABETIC RETINOPATHY

The choroidal angiography findings of 60 patients with diabetic retinopathy were reported by Bischoff and Flower.[36] Most of the patients with proliferative diabetic retinopathy showed irregular and delayed choroidal filling. Approximately 50 percent of patients with background diabetic retinopathy showed such changes.

CHOROIDAL TUMORS

Choroidal ICG absorption angiography and ICG fluorescence angiography have been used to study choroidal tumors.[24, 25, 27, 29, 36, 70, 90–93] This technique can visualize the vascularization and filling patterns of nonpigmented and lightly pigmented tumors. The near-infrared light is absorbed by melanin of heavily pigmented tumors, such as choroidal melanomas, and thus blocks ICG fluorescence (Fig. 52–6). Nevertheless, the borders of the

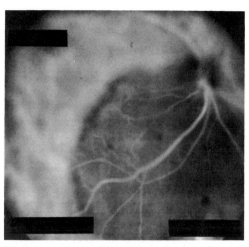

Figure 52–6. Late phase of the ICG angiogram of a patient with a juxtapapillary choroidal melanoma. No intratumoral vessels can be noted because the heavy pigmentation of the tumor absorbs the near-infrared wavelengths.

pigmented tumors may be better delineated by ICG angiography than by fluorescein angiography, and therefore ICG angiography may serve as a more accurate tool for assessment of tumor growth.[24, 25, 36] Bischoff and Flower reported that in some lightly pigmented tumors ICG angiography was able to resolve some of the larger vessels of the tumor with staining of their walls and leakage into the mass.[36]

In contrast to pigmented choroidal melanomas, choroidal hemangiomas show progressive hyperfluorescence because they are composed of vascular channels;[29, 90, 91] thus, ICG angiography may be useful in distinguishing choroidal hemangiomas from some choroidal melanomas. Choroidal metastasis originating from different primary tumors will show different angiographic characteristics, depending on the vascularity and pigmentation of the mass: Metastasis of breast carcinoma blocks choroidal fluorescence,[93] whereas metastasis of thyroid carcinoma[70] and metastatic bronchial carcinoid tumors[93] are hyperfluorescent on ICG angiography. However, intense late hyperfluorescence may be more characteristically observed with choroidal hemangiomas than with choroidal metastasis.

CHOROIDITIS

In patients with birdshot choroiditis, ICG angiography was found to be superior to fluorescein angiography in defining the typical patches. Multiple hypofluorescent lesions radiating to the periphery are observed between the choroidal veins.[93] These lesions are consistent with choriocapillary drop-out and sometimes are more evident on later stages of the angiogram (Fig. 52–7). In patients with serpiginous choroiditis, actively inflamed areas within the lesion block choroidal fluorescence (Fig. 52–8).[92] With resolution, the choroidal vessels' fluorescence can be seen in the previously hypofluorescent areas. Late hyperfluorescence can be seen at sites at which a choroidal neovascular membrane has evolved. Overt leakage from choroidal vessels was observed on

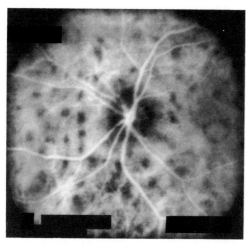

Figure 52–7. Multiple hypofluorescent lesions straddle the choroidal veins in birdshot choroiditis.

ICG angiography in a patient with acute choroiditis.[93] Complete clinical and angiographic resolution was noted following treatment.

OTHER CONDITIONS

Choroidal involvement in the presumed ocular histoplasmosis syndrome has been described with ICG angiography.[31, 36] Bischoff and Flower reported no significant abnormality in ICG angiograms of patients with

Best's disease.[36] In these eyes, it is our experience that a hypofluorescent lesion in the macula can be found, which most likely corresponds to a blocking effect of the abnormal material, although choroidal nonperfusion at that area cannot be ruled out.

ICG choroidal angiography has also been used to study central serous chorioretinopathy.[37, 94] Hayashi and associates[37] have reported 30 such cases. They noted that ICG leaked from the choriocapillaris through a defect in the retinal pigment epithelium into the subretinal space and that hyperfluorescent areas were present near the leakage point. They suggested that the hyperfluorescent area may represent retinal pigment epithelial degeneration, since it did not correspond to a choroidal vascular pattern and no accompanying choroidal vasculature abnormalities were present. Delayed choroidal filling was noted in 5 of 21 eyes with hyperfluorescent areas.[37]

Reduced filling of the choriocapillaris in cases of myopia has been noted with ICG angiography.[36] ICG angiography is also particularly useful in patients with mild vitreous hemorrhage, which prevents evaluation by fluorescein angiography.[36]

CHOROIDAL BLOOD FLOW STUDIES

ICG angiography has also been used to investigate ocular hemodynamics. This technique is enhanced by

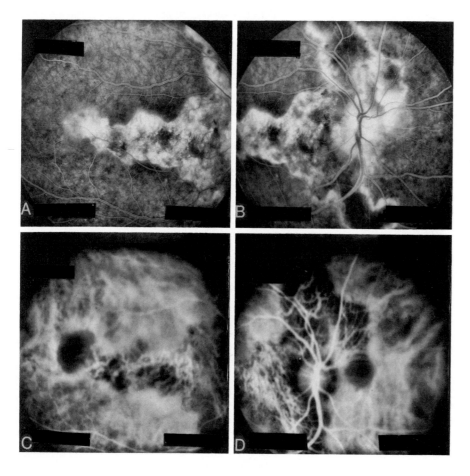

Figure 52–8. *A* and *B*, Late phases of a fluorescein angiogram of an eye with a recurrence of serpiginous choroidopathy. *C* and *D*, Late phase of the ICG angiogram shows marked hypofluorescence in the areas of active inflammation.

the low affinity of ICG to ocular tissue structures as shown with ^{123}I ICG measurements.[78] Flower, Bischoff, Prünte and their associates[41-44] have used choroidal filling times to assess the velocity of the choroidal circulation with some success. These techniques have yet to demonstrate clinical usefulness. Ernest and Goldstick in 1979 estimated choroidal blood flow in monkeys by determining the rate of clearance of ICG from the choroidal circulation.[95] Several authors have attempted to quantify morphologic and dynamic parameters in the choroidal circulation. Quantification of effective nutrient choroidal blood flow is difficult, however. Fluorescence is a superficial phenomenon, it is not proportional to the quantity of dye in the blood vessel,[79, 96] and it depends on multiple variables such as vessel size, the cardiovascular system, and the injection technique.[97]

ICG–ENHANCED DIODE LASER PHOTOCOAGULATION

Since the emission and absorption peaks of the diode laser and ICG are similar, ICG dye-enhanced diode laser photocoagulation may allow selective ablation of the ICG-containing choroidal neovascular membrane and relative sparing of the normal neighboring retina. This experimental technique may be especially useful in treating subfoveal choroidal neovascular membranes by potentially allowing highly selective membrane closure.[49, 50] In addition, we have successfully treated one patient with peripheral retinal telangiectasia and vitreous hemorrhage with this technique. It should be emphasized that this technique is experimental at present. Further investigation is necessary to determine the role, if any, for this treatment.

REFERENCES

1. MacLean AL, Maumenee AE: Hemangioma of the choroid. Trans Am Ophthalmol Soc 57:171, 1959.
2. Novotny HR, Alvis DL: A method of photographing fluorescence in circulating blood of the human eye. Am J Ophthalmol 50:176, 1960.
3. Maumenee AE: Fluorescein angiography in the diagnosis and treatment of lesions of the ocular fundus. (The 1968 Doyne Lecture.) Trans Ophthalmol Soc UK 88:529, 1968.
4. Hyvärinen L, Maumenee AE, George T, et al: Fluorescein angiography of the choriocapillaris. Am J Ophthalmol 67:653, 1969.
5. Archer D, Krill AF, Newell FW: Fluorescein studies of normal choroidal circulation. Am J Ophthalmol 69:543, 1970.
6. Archer DB, Krill AE, Ernest JT: Choroidal vascular aspects of degenerations of the retinal pigment epithelium. Trans Ophthalmol Soc UK 92:187, 1972.
7. Wald G: The photochemistry of vision. Doc Ophthalmol 3:94, 1949.
8. Geeraets WJ, Williams RC, Chang G, et al: The loss of light energy in retina and choroid. Arch Ophthalmol 64:606, 1960.
9. Behrendt T, Wilson LA: Spectral reflectance photography of the retina. Am J Ophthalmol 59:1079, 1965.
10. Geeraets WJ, Berry ER: Ocular spectral characteristics as related to hazards from lasers and other light sources. Am J Ophthalmol 66:15, 1968.
11. Bloome MA: Fluorescein angiography: Risks. Vision Res 20:1083, 1980.
12. Flower RW: Choroidal angiography using indocyanine green: A review and progress report. Ophthalmol Dig 36:18, 1974.
13. Ring HG, Fujino T: Observations on the anatomy and pathology of the choroidal vasculature. Arch Ophthalmol 78:431, 1967.
14. Friedman E, Kopald HH, Smith TR, et al: Retinal and choroidal blood flow determined with krypton-85 anesthetized animals. Invest Ophthalmol 3:539, 1964.
15. Kogure K, Choromokos E: Infrared absorption angiography. J Appl Physiol 26:154, 1969.
16. Collela ME, Pilkerton AR: Determination of choroidal blood flow in man. Invest Ophthalmol 8:460, 1969.
17. Kogure K, David NJ, Yamanouchi U, et al: Infrared absorption angiography of the fundus circulation. Arch Ophthalmol 83:209, 1970.
18. David NJ: Infrared absorption fundus angiography. In Proceedings International Symposium Fluorescein Angiography, Albi 1969. Basel, Karger, 1971, p 189.
19. Hochheimer BF: Angiography of the retina with indocyanine green. Arch Ophthalmol 86:564, 1971.
20. Flower RW, Hochheimer BF: Clinical infrared absorption angiography of the choroid. Am J Ophthalmol 73:458, 1972.
21. Flower RW: Infrared absorption angiography of the choroid and some observations on the effects of high intraocular pressures. Am J Ophthalmol 74:600, 1972.
22. Brown N, Strong R: Infrared fundus angiography. Br J Ophthalmol 57:797, 1973.
23. Flower RW, Hochheimer BF: A clinical technique and apparatus for simultaneous angiography of the separate retinal and choroidal circulations. Invest Ophthalmol 12:248, 1973.
24. Patz A, Flower RW, Klein ML, et al: Clinical application of indocyanine green angiography. Doc Ophthalmol Proc Ser 9:245, 1976.
25. Orth DH, Patz A, Flower RW: Potential clinical applications of indocyanine green choroidal angiography. Preliminary report. Eye Ear Nose Throat Monthly 55:15, 1976.
26. Craandijk A, Van Beek CA: Indocyanine green fluorescence angiography of the choroid. Br J Ophthalmol 60:377, 1976.
27. Chopdar A, Turk AM, Hill DW: Fluorescent infra-red angiography of the fundus oculi using indocyanine green dye. Trans Ophthalmol Soc UK 98:142, 1978.
28. Forsius H, Hyvärinen L, Nieminen H, et al: Fluorescein and indocyanine green fluorescence angiography in study of affected males and in female carriers with choroideremia. A preliminary report. Acta Ophthalmol 55:459, 1977.
29. Bonnet M, Habozit F, Magnard G: Valeur de l'angiographie en infra-rouge au vert d'indocyanine dans le diagnostic clinique des angiomes de la choroide. Bull Soc Ophthalmol Fr 76:713, 1976.
30. Bacin F, Buffet JM: Un diagnostic difficile: L'angiome choroidien isole. J Fr Ophthalmol 1:197, 1978.
31. Saari M: Disciform detachment of the macula. II. Fluorescein and indocyanine green fluorescence angiographic findings in juvenile haemorrhagic macular choroidopathy. Acta Ophthalmol 55:530, 1977.
32. Flower RW: Simple adaptors for fast conversion of a fundus camera for rapid-sequence ICG fluorescence choroidal angiography. J Biol Photogr Assoc 45:43, 1977.
33. Flower RW: Choroidal fluorescent dye filling patterns. A comparison of high-speed indocyanine green and fluorescein angiograms. Int Ophthalmol 2:143, 1980.
34. Hayashi K, Nakase Y, Nishiyama A, et al: Indocyanine green fluorescence angiography, Report 2. Studies of new interference filters. Acta Soc Ophthalmol Jpn 86:1532, 1982.
35. Hyvärinen L, Flower RW: Indocyanine green fluorescence angiography. Acta Ophthalmol 58:528, 1980.
36. Bischoff PM, Flower RW: Ten years' experience with choroidal angiography using indocyanine green dye: A new routine examination or an epilogue? Doc Ophthalmol 60:235, 1985.
37. Hayashi K, Hasegawa Y, Tokoro T: Indocyanine green angiography of central serous chorioretinopathy. Int Ophthalmol 9:37, 1986.
38. Hayashi K, Hasegawa Y, Tokoro T, et al: Value of indocyanine green angiography in the diagnosis of occult choroidal neovascular membrane. Jpn J Clin Ophthalmol 42:827, 1988.
39. Destro M, Puliafito CA: Indocyanine green videoangiography of choroidal neovascularization. Ophthalmology 96:846, 1989.
40. Hayashi K, Hasegawa Y, Tazawa Y, et al: Clinical application of indocyanine angiography to choroidal neovascularization. Jpn J Ophthalmol 33:57, 1989.

41. Prünte P, Niesel P: Quantification of choroidal blood-flow parameters using indocyanine green video-fluorescence angiography and statistical picture analysis. Ophthalmologica 226:55, 1988.

42. Bischoff P: Quantitative Untersuchung der normalen Aderhautzirkulation. Fortschr Ophthalmol 86:107, 1989.

43. Flower RW, Klein GJ: Pulsatile flow in the choroidal circulation: A preliminary investigation. Eye 4:310, 1990.

44. Klein GJ, Baumgartner R, Flower RW: An image processing approach to characterizing choroidal blood flow. Invest Ophthalmol Vis Sci 31:629, 1990.

45. Scheider A, Schroedel C: High resolution indocyanine green angiography with scanning laser ophthalmoscope. Am J Ophthalmol 108:458, 1989.

46. Scheider A, Kaboth A, Neuhauser L: Detection of subretinal neovascular membranes with indocyanine green and infrared scanning laser ophthalmoscope. Am J Ophthalmol 113:45, 1992.

47. Guyer DR, Puliafito CA, Monés JM, et al: Indocyanine-green digital angiography and choroidal neovascularization. Ophthalmology 92:287, 1992.

48. Yannuzzi LA, Slakter JS, Sorenson J, et al: Digital indocyanine green videoangiography and choroidal neovascularization. Retina 12:191, 1992.

49. Puliafito CA, Guyer DR, Monés JM, et al: Indocyanine-green digital angiography and dye-enhanced diode laser photocoagulation of choroidal neovascularization. Invest Ophthalmol Vis Sci 32(Suppl):712, 1991.

50. Balles MW, Puliafito CA, Kliman GH, et al: Indocyanine green dye–enhanced diode laser photocoagulation of subretinal neovascular membranes. Invest Ophthalmol Vis Sci 31(Suppl):882, 1990.

51. Fox IJ, Wodd EH: Applications of dilution curves recorded from the right side or venous circulation with the aid of a new indicator dye. Proc Mayo Clin 32:541, 1957.

52. Paumgartner G: The handling of indocyanine green by the liver. Schweiz Med Wochenschr 105(17 Suppl):1, 1975.

53. Cherrick GR, Stein SW, Leevy CM, et al: Indocyanine green: Observations on its physical properties, plasma decay, and hepatic extraction. J Clin Invest 39:592, 1960.

54. Baker KJ: Binding of sulfobromophthalein (BSP) sodium and indocyanine green (ICG) by plasma α1-lipoproteins. Proc Soc Exp Biol Med 122:957, 1966.

55. Leevy CM, Bender J, Silverberg M, et al: Physiology of dye extraction by the liver: Comparative studies of sulfobromophthalein and indocyanine green. Ann NY Acad Sci 111:161, 1963.

56. Goresky CA: Initial distribution and rate of uptake of sulfobromophthalein in the liver. Am J Physiol 207:13, 1964.

57. Wheeler HO, Cranston WI, Mettzer JI: Hepatic uptake and biliary excretion of indocyanine green in the dog. Proc Soc Exp Biol Med 99:11, 1958.

58. Ketterer SG, Wiegand BD: Hepatic clearance of indocyanine green. Clin Res 7:289, 1959.

59. Ketterer SG, Wiegand BD: The excretion of indocyanine green and its use in the estimation of hepatic blood flow. Clin Res 7:71, 1959.

60. Probst P, Paumgartner G, Caucig H, et al: Studies on clearance and placental transfer of indocyanine green during labor. Clin Chim Acta 29:157, 1970.

61. Fox IJ, Wodd EH: Indocyanine green: Physical and physiologic properties. Mayo Clin Proc 35:732, 1960.

62. Warner GS: Laboratory animal toxicity studies on cardiogreen. Documentation of Hynson, Wescott & Dunning, Baltimore, 1971.

63. Tokoro T, Hayashi K, Muto M, et al: Studies on choroidal circulation. Report I: Fundamental studies on the infrared absorption angiography. Jpn J Ophthalmol 30:173, 1976.

64. Lutty GA: The acute intravenous toxicity of biological stains, dyes, and other fluorescent substances. Toxicol Appl Pharmacol 44:225, 1978.

65. Lutty GA: An intraperitoneal survey of biological stains, dyes, and other fluorescent substances. Bull Nippon Kanhoh-Shihiso Kenkyusho 50:25, 1979.

66. Leevy CM, Smith F, Kierman T: Liver function test. In Bochus HL (ed): Gastroenterology, 3rd ed, vol. 3. Philadelphia, WB Saunders, 1976, p 68.

67. Shabetai R, Adolph RJ: Principles of cardiac catheterization. In Fowler NO (ed): Cardiac Diagnosis and Treatment, 3rd ed. Hagerstown, MD, Harper & Row, 1980, p 117.

68. Carski TR, Staller BJ, Hepner G: Adverse reactions after administration of indocyanine green. JAMA 240:635, 1978.

69. Iseki K, Onoyama K, Fujimi S: Shock caused by indocyanine green dye in chronic hemodialysis patients. [Letter] Clin Nephrol 14:210, 1980.

70. Bacin F, Buffet JM, Mutel N: Angiographie par absorption, en infrarouge, au vert d'indocyanine. Aspects chez le sujet normal et dans les tumeurs choroidiennes. Bull Soc Ophthalmol Fr 81:315, 1981.

71. Yannuzzi LA, Rohrer KT, Tindel LJ, et al: Fluorescein angiography complication survey. Ophthalmology 93:611, 1986.

72. Flower RW: High-speed human choroidal angiography using indocyanine green dye and a continous light source. Doc Ophthalmol Proc Ser 9:59, 1976.

73. Flower RW, Hochheimer BF: Indocyanine green dye fluorescence and infrared absorption choroidal angiography performed simultaneously with fluorescein angiography. Johns Hopkins Med J 138:33, 1976.

74. Benson RC, Kues HA: Fluorescence properties of indocyanine green as related to angiography. Phys Med Biol 23:159, 1978.

75. Puliafito CA, Destro M, To K, et al: Dye enhanced photocoagulation of choroidal neovascularization. ARVO Abstracts. Invest Ophthalmol Vis Sci 29(Suppl):414, 1988.

76. Bill A: Capillary permeability to and extravascular dynamics of myoglobin, albumin and gammaglobulin in the uvea. Acta Physiol Scand 73:204, 1968.

77. Ketterer SG, Wiegard BD, Rapaport E: Hepatic uptake and biliary excretion of indocyanine green and its use in estimation of hepatic blood flow in dogs. Am J Physiol 199:481, 1960.

78. Ansari A, Lambrecht RM, Packer S, et al: Note on the distribution of iodine 123–labeled indocyanine green in the eye. XVIII. Invest Ophthalmol 14:780, 1975.

79. Flower RW: Injection technique for indocyanine green and sodium fluorescein dye angiography of the eye. Invest Ophthalmol 12:881, 1973.

80. American National Standards Institute (ANSI): Safe use of lasers, Standard Z-136.1. New York, ANSI, 1976.

81. Shimizu K, Ujiie K (eds): In The Structure of the Ocular Vessels. Tokyo, New York, Ikagu-Shoin, 1978, p 51.

82. Bischoff PM, Speiser P: Angiographic study of the vortex vein circulation. Graefes Arch Clin Exp Ophthalmol 224:122, 1986.

83. Potts AM: An hypothesis on macular disease. Trans Am Acad Ophthalmol Otolaryngol 70:1058, 1966.

84. Bischoff PM, Flower RW: High blood pressure in choroidal arteries as a possible pathogenetic mechanism in senile macular degeneration. [Letter] Am J Ophthalmol 96:398, 1983.

85. Green WR, Key SN: Senile macular degeneration. A histopathologic study. Trans Am Ophthalmol Soc 75:180, 1977.

86. Garner A: Vascular disorders. In Garner A, Klintworth GK (eds): Pathobiology of Ocular Disease, Part B. New York, Marcel Dekker, 1982, p 1479.

87. Hayreh SS: Recent advances in fluorescein fundus angiography. Br J Ophthalmol 58:391, 1974.

88. Hayashi K, de Laey JJ: Indocyanine green angiography of choroidal neovascular membranes. Ophthalmologica 190:30, 1985.

89. François P, Turut P, Delannoy C: L'angiofluorographie choroidienne a l'indocyanine. Bull Soc Ophthalmol Fr 77:971, 1977.

90. Bonnet M, Francoz-Taillanter N: Hemangiomes caverneux de la choroide (revue clinique de 10 cas). Bull Soc Ophthalmol Fr 81:455, 1981.

91. Quentel G, Coscas G: Angiographie en fluorescence infrarouge au vert d'indocyanine. Bull Soc Ophthalmol Fr 84:559, 1984.

92. Bischoff P: Badeutung der Infrarotangiographie fur die Differentialdiagnostik der Aderhauttumoren. Klin Monatsbl Augenheilkd 186:187, 1985.

93. Krupsky S, Friedman E, Foster CS, et al: Indocyanine green angiography in choroidal diseases. Invest Ophthalmol Vis Sci 33:723, 1992.

94. Speiser P, Bischoff P: Die sogenannte Chorioretinopathia centralis serosa im Lichte der Aderhautangiographie. Klin Monatsbl Augenheilkd 185:378, 1984.

95. Ernest JT, Goldstick TK: Choroidal blood flow measurement in the monkey by clearance of indocyanine green dye. Exp Eye Res 29:7, 1979.

96. Miszalok V: Video-Angiographie: Methode und Nomenklatur. Klin Monatsbl Augenheilkd 190:217, 1987.

97. Flower RW, Hochheimer BF: Quantification of indicator dye concentration in ocular blood. Exp Eye Res 25:103, 1977.

Chapter 53

■

Arterial Occlusions

MARYANNA DESTRO and EVANGELOS S. GRAGOUDAS

The retina normally derives its blood supply from the internal carotid artery via the ophthalmic artery, from which branch the central retinal artery and the ciliary arteries. The central retinal artery enters the eye within the optic nerve sheath and then branches to supply blood to the inner layers of the retina, extending from the inner aspect of the inner nuclear layer to the nerve fiber layer. Branches of the ciliary arteries provide blood to the choriocapillaris, which, in turn, supplies blood to the outer layers of the retina, extending from the outer aspect of the inner nuclear layer to the retinal pigment epithelium.[1] Compromise of the retinal perfusion may occur secondary to occlusion anywhere along this arterial system and may present clinically with changes ranging from focal occlusion of small retinal arterioles (cotton-wool spots) to global ischemia from ophthalmic artery occlusion.

The causes of retinal occlusive disease are multiple and include partial or complete obstruction of blood flow secondary to (1) luminal obstruction by emboli; (2) luminal narrowing from atherosclerosis with thrombosis, arteriosclerosis, vasospasm, vasculitis, or external compression; and (3) retinal hypoperfusion from systemic hypotension, ocular hypertension, or blood dyscrasias.[1]

COTTON-WOOL SPOTS

Cotton-wool spots are transient, small, whitish opacities with feathery edges located within the superficial retina and represent microinfarctions of small retinal arterioles. They are most frequently seen in the peripapillary and posterior retina, and they may cause symptoms of small scotomas of acute onset. In the majority of cases, these cotton-wool spots are an indication of a systemic vascular disease, the most common of which is diabetes mellitus. Excluding diabetes, Brown and associates noted that a general systemic evaluation yielded an underlying cause in 95 percent of patients presenting with retinal cotton-wool spots (Table 53–1).[2]

Retinal ischemia occurs in arteriolar occlusion, with disruption of normal retinal cellular metabolism and transport and accumulation of cellular debris from disrupted axoplasmic flow. This axoplasmic debris is thought to produce the characteristic whitish color of the cotton-wool spot. Light microscopy reveals characteristic cytoid bodies within the nerve fiber layer, which by electron micrographic studies have been shown to be composed largely of degenerated mitochondria and other intracellular debris.[3] Fluorescein angiography of cotton-wool spots may reveal hypofluorescence, which is secondary to both blocked fluorescence by this cellular debris and arteriolar nonperfusion. Adjacent fluorescein

Table 53–1. DISEASES ASSOCIATED WITH RETINAL COTTON-WOOL SPOTS

Trauma
  Amniotic fluid emboli
  Carbon monoxide poisoning
  Cardiac surgery
  Carotid artery ligation
  Fat emboli
  Purtscher's disease
  Radiation retinopathy

Infection
  AIDS
  Leber's stellate neuroretinitis
  Pneumonia
  Rheumatic fever
  Rift Valley fever
  Rocky Mountain spotted fever
  Subacute bacterial endocarditis
  Typhus

Neoplasm
  Atrial myxoma
  Carcinomatous cachexia
  Hodgkin's lymphoma
  Leukemia
  Multiple myeloma
  Pheochromocytoma

Congenital
  Congenital arteriole prepapillary loops
  Disc drusen

Hematologic
  Anemia
  Dysproteinemia
  Leukopenia
  Thrombocytopenia

Endocrine/Gastrointestinal
  Acute pancreatitis
  Cirrhosis with anemia
  Diabetic retinopathy
  Gastric ulcer syndrome

Collagen Vascular Disease
  Behçet's disease
  Dermatomyositis
  Rheumatoid arthritis
  Scleroderma
  Systemic lupus erythematosus
  Polyarteritis nodosa
  Temporal arteritis

Vascular Disease
  Aortic arch syndrome
  Carotid occlusion disease
  Hypotension
  Hypovolemia
  Ischemic optic neuropathy
  Malignant hypertension
  Renal vascular disease
  Toxemia of pregnancy
  Atherosclerosis
  Arteriosclerosis

Idiopathic/Other
  Idiopathic recurrent branch retinal artery occlusion
  Primary amyloidosis

leakage from associated microaneurysms may also be noted, along with capillary irregularity and remodeling. After clinical resolution of the cotton-wool spot, fluorescein angiography may reveal reperfusion or ingrowth of new capillaries within the previously infarcted area.[4] The appearance of cotton-wool spots is nonspecific and similar in many of the previously mentioned vascular diseases, and the spots tend to disappear over a period of weeks to several months.[5, 6] In some diseases, such as AIDS, the presence and number of cotton-wool spots have been noted to indicate a poor systemic prognosis and may be useful in monitoring the severity of systemic disease (Fig. 53–1).[7]

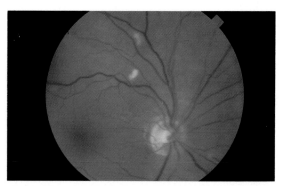

Figure 53–1. Cotton-wool spots in a patient with AIDS.

BRANCH RETINAL ARTERY OCCLUSION

Patients with acute branch retinal artery occlusion typically present in the seventh decade of life with the sudden onset of unilateral, painless partial visual loss associated with a corresponding visual field deficit. They may give a history of fleeting episodes of similar visual loss (amaurosis fugax) or relate a history of previous neurologic loss (transient ischemic attacks or strokes). In up to three quarters of patients, carotid occlusive disease or systemic hypertension may be present.[8, 9] Much less frequently, patients are younger (less than 30 yr old) and have associated cardiac disease or other vasculopathies.[10]

On ophthalmoscopy, acute occlusion of one or more branches of the central retinal artery presents with a discrete zone of retinal whitening within the distribution of the occluded arteriole distal to the site of obstruction (Fig. 53–2). This site of obstruction often occurs at a bifurcation of the vessel and is often caused by the presence of an embolus that has traveled downstream to become lodged at this bifurcation. In a study of 201 eyes with branch retinal artery occlusion, Ros and colleagues found that the temporal branches of the central retinal artery were involved in 98 percent of their cases and that emboli were visible in 62 percent of eyes.[11] In other eyes, perivascular sheathing at the site of a previous embolus may be seen.

Less frequently, branch retinal arteriole occlusions may occur secondary to (1) thrombosis, often in association with atherosclerosis;[12] (2) vasculitis, which may

be localized to the eye (e.g., toxoplasmosis retinitis) (Fig. 53–3),[13] may be systemic (temporal arteritis),[14] may be associated with leukoemboli[15] (e.g., collagen vascular diseases),[16] or may be secondary to traumatic insult (e.g., x-ray irradiation);[17] (3) vasospasm, such as may occur in association with migraine;[18] (4) compressive lesions, such as have been reported in association with optic nerve drusen[19] or swelling of the optic nerve from papillitis, papilledema, anterior ischemic optic neuropathy, retrobulbar injection, intrasheath hemorrhage, central retinal vein occlusion, or neoplasm;[20–23] or (5) blood dyscrasias, such as seen in association with sickle cell disease.[24] In addition, a syndrome of recurrent idiopathic branch retinal arterial occlusions has also been described.[25]

Acutely, fluorescein angiography reveals delayed or no filling of the occluded branch retinal artery, which is associated with hypofluorescence of the surrounding ischemic retina (see Fig. 53–2B). This hypofluorescence may be due to both the lack of normal perfusion and blockage of underlying fluorescence by intracellular edema and axoplasmic debris. In some cases, vessels distal to the site of occlusion will fill via retrograde flow from the adjacent capillary bed of perfused retinal vessels. Fluorescein staining of the occlusion site and the vessel's wall may be seen in the late-phase angiogram. After dissolution of the obstruction, retinal blood flow is usually restored, although the previously occluded vessel may remain narrowed or may become sclerotic. In addition, artery-to-artery anastomoses may occasionally be seen and are highly suggestive of previous branch retinal artery occlusion.[9]

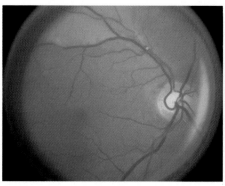

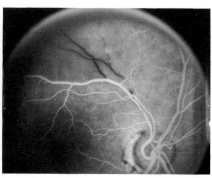

A   B

Figure 53–2. Superotemporal branch retinal artery occlusion. Note acute retinal whitening in the distribution of the occluded arteriole distal to the embolus *(A),* with lack of fluorescein filling on the corresponding angiogram *(B).*

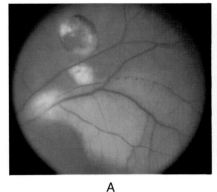
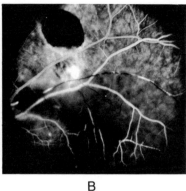

Figure 53–3. *A* and *B*, Superotemporal branch retinal artery occlusion secondary to acute toxoplasmic retinochoroiditis. Note acute retinal whitening associated with retinal arteriole occlusion distal to the focus of retinochoroiditis. Note also the prevalence of old toxoplasmic chorioretinal scars superior to the occlusion.

A   B

Histologic evaluation within a week after an acute branch retinal artery occlusion reveals swelling of the inner retinal layers with intracellular edema and cellular autolysis. After a period of a month or more, this inner retinal tissue extending from the nerve fiber layer outward to the inner nuclear layer reveals extensive cell loss with associated gliosis.[4]

When the branch retinal artery occlusion is caused by retinal emboli, most frequently they are composed of endogenous platelet-fibrin plugs, which are dull, whitish gray, and often elongated.[26, 27] In addition, they are readily friable and often fragment into numerous smaller emboli, which may be seen along a single vessel or may become lodged in multiple smaller distal retinal branches. These platelet-fibrin emboli most frequently originate from ulcerated atheromatous plaques located along the walls of the common or internal carotid artery.[28, 29] Cholesterol emboli (Hollenhorst's plaques) are also frequently seen lodged at arteriole bifurcations in these patients.[30–32] However, these emboli are iridescent, orangish, and often appear as thin crystalline plates, which may become more visible with induced arterial pulsation from mild digital ocular compression by the examiner. Cholesterol emboli alone are not usually thought to be sufficient to significantly obstruct blood flow, as some portion of the blood frequently passes around them. However, if they are large or combined with platelet-fibrin plugs, they may occasionally cause significant arterial obstruction.[33]

A third type of endogenous embolus, the calcific embolus, is most frequently seen within the large retinal arterioles overlying or adjacent to the optic disc (Fig. 53–4). The calcific emboli are typically single, large, and dull, dirty white and frequently originate from diseased cardiac valves.[34] Although they are seen less frequently than either platelet-fibrin or cholesterol emboli, when present they often cause arterial occlusion.[27, 33]

Less frequent causes of endogenous emboli leading to retinal arterial occlusion include leukoemboli,[15] as may occur in association with vasculitis, Purtcher's retinopathy (Fig. 53–5), and septic endocarditis; fat emboli, as may occur following traumatic long bone fractures;[35] amniotic fluid emboli, as may occur as a complication of pregnancy;[36] and tumor emboli, as may occur in association with atrial myxoma.[37]

A large variety of exogenous retinal emboli have also been reported to cause retinal branch artery occlusion.

Many of these substances, such as talc, are impurities introduced into the blood stream by intravenous drug abusers (Fig. 53–6).[38, 39] Other substances, such as corticosteroid emboli, are inadvertently injected into the arterial system during intralesional steroid treatment for various head and neck lesions.[40] Still others, including air emboli and small pieces of synthetic materials from intravascular cannulae and cardiac and vascular prostheses, may also enter the blood stream following trauma or surgery (Table 53–2).[33]

Clinically, after several weeks normal retinal transparency returns and visual acuity begins to improve. In nearly 90 percent of patients without other ocular disease, acuity may return to 20/40 or better; however, in most cases some degree of permanent visual loss persists.[11] In addition, persistent narrowing of the vessels or optic atrophy may occur. Rarely, secondary complications of retinal neovascularization and, very rarely, rubeosis may develop.[9]

Treatment of acute branch retinal artery occlusion is of questionable benefit because most patients regain good vision, and they appear to have a similar outcome with or without treatment.[11] However, in cases affecting the foveal circulation, treatment similar to that for central retinal artery occlusion (as described further on) may be attempted.

As previously noted, patients who present with evidence of retinal arterial occlusive disease should undergo a thorough general physical examination, with particular attention being directed toward the cardiovascular and cerebrovascular systems. The majority of patients older

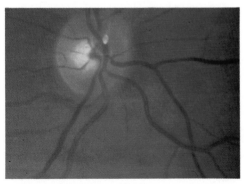

Figure 53–4. Calcific embolus overlying the optic disc in a patient with cardiac valvular disease.

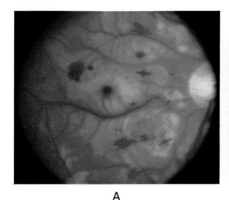
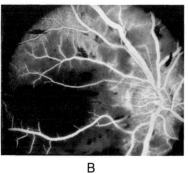

A   B

Figure 53–5. *A* and *B*, Presumed Purtscher's retinopathy in a patient following severe chest compression injury.

than 40 yr of age with arterial occlusion have been found to have significant carotid occlusive disease, hypertension, or cardiac disease, or a combination, and younger patients frequently have been noted to suffer from cardiac disease or vasculopathy. Furthermore, a number of studies have reported decreased survival rates in these patients in comparison with age-matched controls.[41–43]

CILIORETINAL ARTERY OCCLUSION

In up to 32 percent of eyes, a cilioretinal artery is present, which may contribute in part to the papillomacular retinal circulation.[44] As such, it may also become occluded, either alone or in combination with central retinal vein occlusion or anterior ischemic optic neuropathy. As in branch retinal artery occlusion, isolated cilioretinal artery occlusion usually presents with the sudden onset of a visual scotoma, with acute whitening of the retinal tissue within the vessel's distribution (Fig. 53–7). Also, similar to branch retinal artery occlusion, the visual prognosis for most patients with isolated cilioretinal artery occlusion is good, unless significant foveal involvement occurs. The causes and evaluation of cilioretinal artery occlusion are similar to those of branch and central retinal artery occlusions.

CENTRAL RETINAL ARTERY OCCLUSION

Patients with acute central retinal artery occlusion usually present with the sudden onset of profound, unilateral, painless visual loss, often in the range of counting fingers to light perception vision. As in branch retinal artery occlusion, patients may relate previous episodes of amaurosis fugax. Acutely, ophthalmoscopy reveals diffuse retinal arteriole constriction, often with visible emboli or segmentation ("boxcarring") of blood flow. The ischemic retinal tissue becomes diffusely pale within hours of the onset of occlusion, with the exception of the fovea, which retains a reddish hue (Fig. 53–8 *A*). This diffuse pallor is due to the loss of retinal transparency as intracellular edema, cellular necrosis, and accumulation of cellular debris develop, similar to that seen in branch retinal artery occlusion. The foveal cherry-red spot occurs because the retina in the foveal region is very thin, allowing visibility of the underlying patent choroidal circulation.

Acutely, fluorescein angiography reveals filling of the choroid and ciliary branches perfusing the optic nerve head while displaying delayed retinal arterial filling with a prolongation of the arteriovenous circulation time (Fig. 53–8*B*). Some filling of the proximal branches of

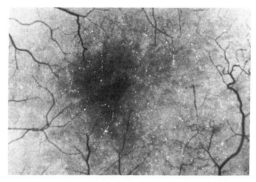

Figure 53–6. Multiple talc retinal emboli in an intravenous drug abuser. (From Friberg TR, Gragoudas ES, Regan CDJ: Talc emboli and macular ischemia in intravenous drug abuse. Arch Ophthalmol 97:1089–1091, 1979. Copyright 1979, American Medical Association.)

Table 53–2. CAUSES OF RETINAL EMBOLI

Endogenous Sources
  Atrial myxoma
  Atheromatosis plaque–carotid disease
  Amniotic fluid emboli
  Cardiac valvular disease
  Disseminated intravascular coagulation
  Erythrocyte aggregation (sickle cell disease)
  Fat emboli
  Leukoemboli
  Metastatic tumors (malignant melanoma, breast
    adenocarcinoma)
  Septic emboli

Exogenous Sources
  Air
  Artificial valves, catheters, prostheses
  Cornstarch
  Mercury
  Silicone
  Steroids
  Talc

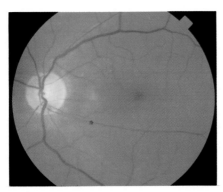

Figure 53–7. Acute retinal whitening within the distribution of an occluded cilioretinal artery.

Table 53–3. SYSTEMIC DISEASES ASSOCIATED WITH CENTRAL RETINAL ARTERY OCCLUSION

Atheromatous vascular disease
Arteriosclerotic vascular disease
Blood dyscrasias
Cardiac valvular disease
Carotid occlusive disease
Compressive vascular disease
Diabetes mellitus
Embolic disease
Hypertension
Vasculitis
Vasospasm

the central retinal artery and vein usually occurs via collaterals from the peripapillary ciliary vessels. In the late-phase angiogram, staining of the disc and occasionally the retinal vessels may be seen.[45]

The patient's age and underlying causes of central retinal artery occlusion are similar to those in branch retinal artery occlusion. In approximately 20 percent of cases, retinal emboli can be seen, within either the central retinal artery or its branches.[46] Other causes of central retinal artery occlusion include thrombosis or hemorrhage into an atheromatous plaque, as well as vasculitis (including temporal arteritis), vasospasm, compression, and blood dyscrasias, as seen in branch retinal artery occlusion (Fig. 53–9). Two thirds of all patients are reported to have associated hypertension, and up to one quarter of patients have carotid occlusive disease, diabetes, or cardiac valvular disease, or a combination,[46, 47] which significantly contributes to their poor survival compared with that of the general population (Table 53–3).

Histologically, the occlusion of the central retinal artery usually occurs at the level of the lamina cribrosa or at its posterior aspect, although occlusion anterior to this level may also occur.[4] Similar to branch retinal artery occlusion, intracellular edema and cellular necrosis with pyknotic nuclei of the inner retinal cell layers are seen within the first week. Chronically, diffuse inner retinal atrophy and gliosis are noted involving the inner two thirds of the inner nuclear layer, as well as the inner plexiform, ganglion cell, and nerve fiber layers.[4]

The natural history of central retinal artery occlusion is generally one of persistent severe visual loss in the range of counting fingers to light perception, although some patients regain useful vision.[48] Up to one tenth of patients may be more fortunate in retaining their central visual acuity because of the presence of a patent cilioretinal artery perfusing the fovea (Fig. 53–10).[2] After several weeks, the acute retinal opacification fades and circulation is restored. However, diffusely narrowed retinal arterioles usually persist, and optic atrophy develops with time. An afferent pupillary defect also usually persists. The development of secondary complications, including rubeosis and retinal and disc neovascularization, has generally been thought to be rare; however, recent studies have indicated that the incidence of rubeosis following central retinal artery occlusion may be as high as 20 percent.[50] Fortunately, bilateral involvement is rare, and when present it is highly suggestive of arteritic disease.[14]

The retina is particularly susceptible to hypoxic injury because of its high rate of oxygen consumption. Hayreh and associates reported irreversible cell injury following 90 min of total central retinal artery occlusion in their primate model.[51] Thus, acute central retinal artery occlusion is one of the true therapeutic emergencies in ophthalmology, as time is of the essence if vision is to be successfully restored. Many patients unfortunately present for evaluation and treatment after this critical period has already passed. Nevertheless, most authorities recommend attempting treatment during the first 24 hr following acute visual loss. Currently, this treatment consists of attempts to improve perfusion by lowering

Figure 53–8. *A* and *B,* Acute central retinal artery occlusion with a foveal "cherry-red spot." Note delayed retinal arteriole filling with prolonged arteriole venous circulation time on the corresponding fluorescein angiogram *(B)*.

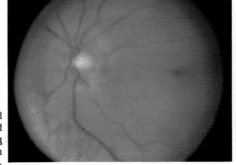

A

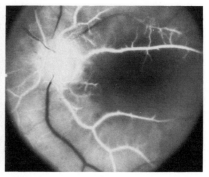

B

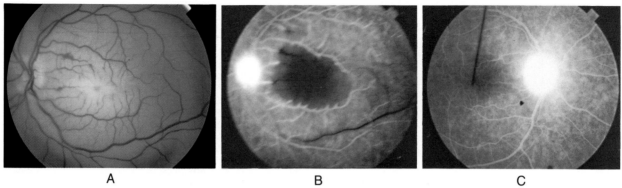

Figure 53–9. *A–C,* Acute central retinal artery occlusion in a patient with AIDS and bilateral papillitis. Note delayed retinal perfusion in the left eye as well as bilateral optic disc staining.

the intraocular pressure—medically by administration of acetazolamide and other ocular hypotensive agents and surgically via anterior chamber paracentesis. In addition, ocular massage may help to lower the intraocular pressure and possibly dislodge an offending embolus, and inhalation of a 95 percent oxygen–5 percent carbon dioxide mixture may also assist in increasing oxygenation while inducing vasodilatation.[48, 52] In addition, in a small number of patients, the central retinal artery occlusion occurs secondary to temporal arteritis, and it is important to obtain an erythrocyte sedimentation rate and initiate prompt systemic corticosteroid therapy in these patients, particularly because their visual loss can quickly become bilateral.[14]

Despite these maneuvers, however, significant visual loss persists in the majority of patients with central artery occlusion. Prompted by the lack of an effective treatment, a number of other therapeutic interventions have been attempted with limited success to date. They include the systemic and retrobulbar administration of vasodilatory drugs, hyperbaric oxygen, and antifibrinolytic drugs, as well as surgical attempts to remove the intravascular embolus and direct injection of antifibrinolytic drugs into the supraorbital artery.[52–55]

Recently, attention has been turned toward a different therapeutic approach aimed more at protecting the retinal tissue from the damaging effects of hypoxia rather than at attempting to acutely restore circulation itself. In fact, it has been found that much of the cellular injury following a hypoxic event occurs during the time of reperfusion. These therapeutic maneuvers have been extrapolated from studies investigating central nervous system injury such as occurs in stroke and spinal cord trauma. From these studies, it has become apparent that much of the cellular injury and death in the hypoxic and ischemic states appear to be due not to the lack of oxygen per se but to the release of toxic by-products and chemical mediators of cellular injury.[56] These toxic by-products and chemical mediators include compounds leading to intracellular acidosis, as well as to the release or production of excitotoxins (neurosynaptic compounds that can produce cell death when released in ischemic states), and free radicals (unstable oxygen compounds with unpaired outer electrons that can cause extensive cell injury when unchecked).[56, 58] Discovery of these toxic compounds has led to the use of hypothermia and barbiturate-induced coma in an attempt to lower the rate of cellular metabolism and thus protect against the development of acidosis and the production of these toxic metabolic by-products,[59] and to the use of excitotoxin blocking agents[57] and antioxidants and free radical scavengers in an attempt to block the damaging effects of the released chemical mediators of ischemic cell injury.[58] Such attempts may hold exciting new possibilities in developing an effective method of treatment for retinal occlusive disease.

CAROTID ARTERY OCCLUSION

Severe carotid artery stenosis of greater than or equal to 90 percent may lead to a chronic global compromise

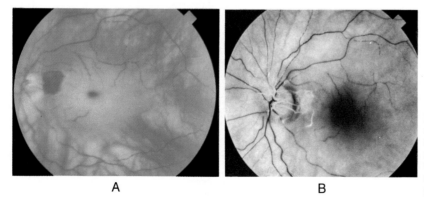

Figure 53–10. *A* and *B,* Acute central retinal artery occlusion in a patient with a patent cilioretinal artery. Unfortunately, this cilioretinal artery did not perfuse the fovea. Note filling of the cilioretinal artery and lack of filling of the retinal arterioles on the corresponding fluorescein angiogram *(B).*

of ocular perfusion known as the ocular ischemic syndrome.[60] This syndrome occurs most frequently in one eye of older men, with visual loss and ocular pain being the most frequent presenting ocular complaints. The degree of visual loss is variable, with visual acuity ranging from 20/20 to no light perception, and the ocular pain is characteristically described as a dull periocular ache, which is thought to be due either to ischemia itself or to associated secondary neovascular glaucoma. Ophthalmic examination often reveals dot-blot retinal hemorrhages, which occur primarily in the midperiphery and may extend into the posterior pole, as well as narrowed retinal arterioles and dilatation of the retinal veins without significant tortuosity (Fig. 53–11A). In addition, decreased ocular perfusion pressure may be demonstrated by ophthalmodynamometry. Rubeosis may be present in two thirds of eyes (Fig. 53–11B). Of those eyes with rubeosis, approximately one half will develop neovascular glaucoma. Other eyes may be normotensive despite a closed filtration angle, secondary to concomitant ciliary body hypoperfusion with decreased aqueous production.

Fluorescein angiography demonstrates increased arteriovenous circulation in 95 percent of patients (Fig. 53–11C), retinal vascular staining (primarily arteriole) in 85 percent of patients, and prolonged patchy choroidal filling in 60 percent of patients.[60]

Similar to central retinal artery occlusion, systemic diseases most often associated with ocular ischemic syndrome include hypertension, atherosclerotic cardiovascular disease, diabetic mellitus, cerebrovascular disease, and peripheral vascular disease. The 5-yr mortality rate has been reported to be approximately 40 percent.[61]

The differential diagnosis in eyes with ocular ischemic syndrome includes mild nonischemic central retinal vein occlusion, diabetes mellitus, chronic ophthalmic artery occlusion, and causes of the aortic arch syndrome, including syphilis, dissecting aneurysms, and Takayasu's disease.[9] Clinical features that may be helpful in differentiating ocular ischemic syndrome from mild central retinal vein occlusion include decreased ophthalmodynamometry readings and delayed fluorescein choroidal filling, which are features not typically seen in central retinal vein occlusion. In ocular ischemic syndrome, the retinal veins are typically dilated but not tortuous, in contrast to the venous tortuosity commonly seen in central retinal vein occlusion. Furthermore, on fluorescein angiography, retinal vascular staining in ocular ischemic syndrome is primarily arterial, whereas staining in central retinal vein occlusion is primarily venous.[60] Likewise, the retinal hemorrhages seen in diabetes mellitus are more frequently bilateral and associated with hard exudate and normal fluorescein filling times, which are features not typical of ocular ischemic syndrome.[60]

The visual prognosis in ocular ischemic syndrome is generally poor, particularly in the presence of rubeosis.[61] Attempts to treat the associated neovascular glaucoma may include panretinal laser photocoagulation if the anterior chamber filtration angle is still open or filtration procedures and cyclodestructive photocoagulation or cryopexy if the angle is closed.[62] Some reports of visual improvement following surgical resolution of carotid occlusion have been published;[63] however, other investigators have been unable to confirm them.[62]

OPHTHALMIC ARTERY OCCLUSION

When acute obstruction occurs at the level of the ophthalmic artery, both the ciliary (and thus choroidal) and the retinal circulations are affected, and the extent of the ischemic injury and visual loss is even more severe, with patients often presenting with bare light perception or no light perception in the affected eye.[64] On examination, the eye may be hypotonous, and the retinal vessels are markedly constricted. A foveal cherry-red spot may or may not be visible. Fluorescein angiography in the acute phase demonstrates poor choroidal and papillary filling, as well as blocked retinal artery filling. Obstruction at this level may be due to an embolus, particularly from atheromatous carotid disease, or to other entities, such as vasculitis. In most cases, the severe visual loss is permanent and chronic ocular signs develop, including narrowed retinal vessels, optic atrophy, and a diffuse pigmentary disturbance secondary to choroidal injury.

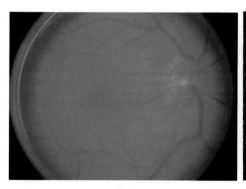
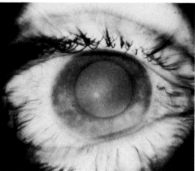
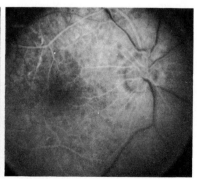

A   B   C

Figure 53–11. Ocular ischemic syndrome in a patient with carotid occlusive disease. Note the retinal arteriolar narrowing and retinal venous dilatation without tortuosity (A), fluorescein leakage from associated iris neovascularization (B), and delayed retinal perfusion on fluorescein angiography (C).

In contrast to central retinal artery occlusion, in which only the b-wave (corresponding to inner retinal ischemia) of the electroretinogram is diminished,[65] both the b-wave and the a-wave are usually diminished or lacking in ophthalmic artery occlusions, reflecting the global degree of ocular ischemia.[66]

COMBINED CENTRAL RETINAL ARTERY AND VEIN OCCLUSION

Occasionally, patients present with acute severe visual loss secondary to occlusion of both the central retinal artery and the central retinal vein. Ophthalmoscopically, whitening of the posterior pole, with or without a cherry-red spot, and dilated retinal veins, optic disc edema, and intraretinal hemorrhages are seen. Fluorescein angiography typically demonstrates normal choroidal filling with severe retinal occlusion, and a high percentage of these eyes develop rubeosis and neovascular glaucoma.[67] According to Brown, almost one third of these cases occur secondary to traumatic retrobulbar injection, with either direct injury to the vessels themselves or indirect injury secondary to injection within the optic nerve sheath.[9] In such cases, localized retinal detachment may also be seen.[21] Other causes may include vasculitis, neoplastic infiltration of the optic nerve, and other systemic conditions associated with central retinal artery occlusion.[67]

Visual loss is generally severe and permanent, and treatment is generally ineffective, although panretinal photocoagulation may be helpful in preventing secondary neovascular glaucoma.

REFERENCES

1. Appen RE, Ray SH, Cogan DG: Central retinal artery occlusion. Am J Ophthalmol 79:374–381, 1975.
2. Brown GC, Brown MM, Hiller T, et al: Cotton wool spots. Retina 5:206–214, 1985.
3. McLeod D, Marshall J, Kohner EM, et al: The role of axoplasmic transport in the pathogenesis of retinal cotton wool spots. Br J Ophthalmol 61:177–191, 1977.
4. Green WR: Retina. In Spencer WH (ed): Ophthalmic Pathology; An Atlas and Textbook, 3rd ed, vol. 2. Philadelphia, WB Saunders, 1985, pp 624–631.
5. Kohner EM, Doller YCT, Bulpitt CJ: Cotton wool spots in diabetic retinopathy. Diabetes 18:691–704, 1969.
6. Freeman WR, Lerner CW, Mines JA, et al: A prospective study of the ophthalmologic findings in the acquired immunodeficiency syndrome. Am J Ophthalmol 97:133, 1984.
7. Brezin A, Girard B, Rosenheim M, et al: Cotton wool spots and AIDS-related complex. Int Ophthalmol 14:37–41, 1990.
8. Kollarits CR, Lubow M, Hissong SL: Retinal Strokes. I. Incidence of carotid atheromata. JAMA 222:1273, 1972.
9. Brown GC: Arterial obstruction disease and the eye. Int Ophthalmol Clin North Am 3:373–392, 1990.
10. Brown GC, Magargal CE, Shields JA, et al: Retinal arterial obstruction in children and young adults. Ophthalmology 88:18, 1981.
11. Ros MA, Magargal LE, Uram M: Branch retinal artery occlusion: A review of 201 eyes. Ann Ophthalmol 3:103–107, 1989.
12. Brownstein S, Font RL, Alper MG: Atheromatous plaques of the retinal blood vessels: Histologic confirmation of ophthalmoscopically visible lesions. Arch Ophthalmol 90:49, 1973.
13. Williamson TH, Meyer PA: Branch retinal artery occlusion in Toxoplasma retinochoroiditis. Br J Ophthalmol 4:253, 1991.
14. Mohan K, Gupta A, Jain IS, et al: Bilateral central retinal artery occlusion in occult temporal arteritis. J Clin Neuro Ophthalmol 4:270–272, 1989.
15. Shapiro I, Jacob HS: Leukoembolization in ocular vascular occlusion. Am J Ophthalmol 14:60, 1982.
16. Fitzpatrick EP, Chesen N, Rahn EK: The lupus anticoagulant and retinal vaso-occlusive disease. Am J Ophthalmol 4:148–152, 1990.
17. Irvin AR, Alvarado JA, Wara MM, et al: Radiation retinopathy: An experimental model for the ischemia-proliferative retinopathies. Trans Am Ophthalmol Soc 79:103, 1981.
18. Wolter JR, Burchfield NJ: Ocular migraine in a young man resulting in unilateral transient blindness and retinal edema. J Pediatr Ophthalmol 8:173, 1971.
19. Neuman NJ, Lessell S, Brandt EM: Bilateral central retinal artery occlusion, disc drusen, and migraine. Am J Ophthalmol 3:235–240, 1989.
20. Gupta A, Jalali S, Bansal RK, et al: Anterior ischemia optic neuropathy and branch retinal artery occlusion in cavernous sinus thrombosis. J Clin Neuroophthalmol 3:193–196, 1990.
21. Mieler WF, Bennett SR, Platt LW, et al: Localized retinal detachment with combined central retinal artery and vein occlusion after retrobulbar anesthesia. Retina 4:278–283, 1990.
22. Duker JS, Cohen MS, Bonon GC, et al: Combined branch retinal artery and central retinal vein occlusion. Retina 2:105–112, 1990.
23. Baker RS, Buncio JR: Sudden visual loss in pseudotumor cerebri due to central retinal artery occlusion. Arch Neurol 41:1274, 1984.
24. Shaw HE Jr, Osher RH, Smith JL: Amaurosis fugax associated with SC hemogliobinopathy and lupus erythematosus. Am J Ophthalmol 87:281, 1979.
25. Capone A Jr, Meredith TA: Profound central visual loss and ocular neovascularization in idiopathic recurrent branch retina artery occlusion. Retina 4:265–268, 1990.
26. Millifisher CM: Observations of the fundus ocular in transient monocular blindness. Neurology 9:333–347, 1959.
27. Arruga J, Sanders M: Ophthalmologic findings in 70 patients with evidence of retinal embolism. Ophthalmology 89:1336–1347, 1982.
28. McBrine DJ, Bradley RD, Ashton N: The nature of retinal emboli in stenosis of the internal carotid artery. Lancet 1:697–699, 1963.
29. Ross Russell RW: The source of retinal emboli. Lancet 2:789–792, 1968.
30. Witmer R, Schmid A: Cholesterinekristall Als Retinaler Arteriellar Embolus. Ophthalomolgica 135:432–433, 1958.
31. David NJ, Klintworth GK, Friedberg SJ, et al: Fatal atheromatous cerebral embolism associated with bright plaques in the retinal arterioles. Report of a Case. Neurology 13:708–713, 1963.
32. Hollenhorst RW: Vascular status of patients who have cholesterol emboli in the retina. Am J Ophthalmol 61:1159–1165, 1966.
33. Young BR: The significance of retinal emboli. J Clin Neuro Ophthalmol 3:190–194, 1989.
34. Holley KE, Bahn C, McGoon DC, et al: Calcific embolization associated with valvotomy for cardiac aortic stenosis. Circulation 28:175–181, 1963.
35. Chuang EC, Miller FS III, Kalina RE: Retinal lesions following long bone fractures. Ophthalmology 92:370, 1985.
36. Change M, Herbert WNP: Retinal arteriolar occlusions following amniotic fluid embolism. Ophthalmology 91:1634–1637, 1984.
37. Yasuma F, Tsuzuki M, Yasuma T: Retinal embolism from left atrial myxoma. Jpn Heart J 4:527–532, 1989.
38. Friberg TR, Gragoudas ES, Regan CDJ: Talc emboli and macular ischemia in intravenous drug abuse. Arch Ophthalmol 97:1089–1091, 1979.
39. Schatz H, Drake M: Self-injected retinal emboli. Ophthalmology 86:468, 1979.
40. Whiteman DW, Rosen DA, Pinkerton RMH: Retinal and choroidal embolism after intranasal corticosteroid injection. Am J Ophthalmol 89:851, 1980.
41. Pfaffenbach DR, Hollenhorst RW: Morbidity and survivorship of patients with embolic cholesterol and crystals in the ocular fundus. Am J Ophthalmol 75:66, 1973.
42. Savino PJ, Laser JS, Cassady J: Retinal strokes: Is the patient at risk? Arch Ophthalmol 95:1185–1189, 1977.
43. Lotentzen SE: Occlusion of the central retinal artery: A follow-up. Arch Ophthalmol 47:690–703, 1969.

44. Justice J Jr, Lehmann RP: Cilioretinal arteries: A study based on review of steroid fundus photographs and fluorescein angiographic findings. Arch Ophthalmol 4:1355–1358, 1976.
45. Schatz H: Essential Fluorescein Angiography. San Francisco, Pacific Medical Press, 1983, pp 17–19.
46. Brown GC, Margargal LE: Central retinal artery obstruction and visual acuity. Ophthalmology 89:14–19, 1982.
47. Shah HG, Brown GC, Goldberg RE: Digital subtraction carotid angiography and retinal arteriole obstruction. Ophthalmology 92:68–72, 1985.
48. Augsburger JJ, Magargal LE: Visual prognosis following treatment of acute central retinal artery occlusion, Br J Ophthalmol 64:913–917, 1980.
49. Brown GC, Shields JA: Cilioretinal arteries and retinal arteriole occlusion. Arch Ophthalmol 97:84–92, 1979.
50. Duker JS, Siralingam A, Brown GC, et al: A prospective study of acute retinal artery obstruction: The incidence of secondary neovascularization. Arch Ophthalmol 3:339–342, 1991.
51. Hayreh SS, Kolder HF, Neingeist TA: Central retinal artery occlusion and retinal tolerance time. Ophthalmology 87:75–78, 1980.
52. Ffytche TJ: A rationalization of treatment of central retinal artery occlusion. Trans Ophthalmol Soc UK 94:468–479, 1974.
53. Gold D: Retinal arterial occlusion. Trans Am Acad Ophthalmol Otolaryngol 83:397–408, 1977.
54. Watson PG: The treatment of acute retinal arterial occlusion. In Cant JS (ed): The Ocular Circulation in Health and Disease. St Louis, CV Mosby, 1969, pp 234–245.
55. Peyman GA, Gremillion CM Jr: Surgical removal of a branch retinal artery embolus. A case report. Int Ophthalmol 4:295–298, 1990.
56. Bresnick GH: Excitotoxins: Possible new mechanisms for pathogenesis of ischemic retinal damage. Arch Ophthalmol 107:339, 1989.
57. Yoon YH, Marmor MF: Dextromethorphan protects the retina against ischemic injury in vivo. Arch Ophthalmol 107:409–411, 1989.
58. Hall ED, Pazara BA, Braughbor JM: 21-Aminosteroid lipid peroxidation inhibitor U74006F protects against cerebroischemia in gerbils. Stroke 19:997–1002, 1988.
59. Pulido JS, Fukuda M, Howe CA, et al: Barbiturates protect retinal cells from hypoxia in cell culture. Arch Ophthalmol 107:1809–1812, 1989.
60. Brown GC, Magargal LE: The ocular ischemia syndrome. Clinical fluorescein angiographic and carotid angiographic features. Int Ophthalmol 11:239–251, 1988.
61. Sivalingam A, Brown GC, Magargal LE: The ocular ischemia syndrome. II. Mortality and systemic morbidity. Int Ophthalmol 13:187–191, 1989.
62. Sivalingam A, Brown GC, Magargal LE: The ocular ischemic syndrome. III. Visual prognosis on the effect of treatment. Int Ophthalmol 15:15–20, 1991.
63. Neupert JR, Brubaker RT, Kearns TP, et al: Rapid resolution of venous stasis retinopathy after carotid endarterectomy. Am J Ophthalmol 81:600–602, 1976.
64. Brown CG, Magargal LE, Sergott R: Obstruction of the retinal and choroidal circulation. Ophthalmology 93:1373–1382, 1986.
65. Nillson SEG: Human retinal vascular obstructions. Acta Ophthalmol 49:111, 1971.
66. Fugino T, Hamasaki DI: The effect of occluding the retinal and choroidal circulations on the electroretinogram of monkeys. J Physiol 180:837, 1965.
67. Richard RD: Simultaneous occlusion of the central retinal artery and vein. Trans Am Ophthalmol Soc 77:191–209, 1979.

Chapter 54

■

Venous Occlusive Diseases of the Retina

DAVID V. WEINBERG and JOHANNA M. SEDDON

Venous occlusive diseases are among the most common retinal diseases seen in clinical practice. In a large population-based study from Israel, the 4-yr incidence of retinal vein occlusion for patients aged 40 yr and older was 2.14/1000. For patients older than 64 yr of age, the 4-yr incidence was 5.36/1000.[1] Branch retinal vein occlusion (BRVO) alone was second only to diabetes as a cause of retinal vascular disease in patients referred to the Retina Vascular Center at the Wilmer Institute.[2] Recognition of these diseases is of particular importance because their complications are a cause of significant visual morbidity. Timely intervention can substantially reduce the incidence and severity of these complications. Improved understanding of medical conditions associated with these diseases may have implications for the patient's general well-being.

The two anatomic categories of venous occlusive disease are BRVO and central retinal vein occlusion (CVRO). Hemicentral retinal vein occlusion (HCRVO) pathologically is a variant of CRVO, but because of an anatomic variation it affects only half of the retina.

The list of potential complications of all venous occlusive diseases is the same; however, the relative frequency of occurrence of these complications differs from one anatomic category to another. The pathologic forces at work as a result of venous occlusion are probably the same in all cases. The risk of the development of any particular complication can be attributed to the location of the injury, the extent and severity of the damage, and the adequacy of compensatory mechanisms.

CRVO

There are few entities in ophthalmology as distinctive and dramatic as the appearance of a fresh CVRO. In its classic appearance there is edema of the optic disc and retina, marked dilatation and tortuosity of the retinal veins, and extensive superficial and deep retinal hemorrhages radiating outward from the optic disc and extending into the periphery in all quadrants (Fig. 54–1). In this form, there is rarely any diagnostic confusion. In less severe instances or late in the course of disease, the diagnosis may be less obvious.

In the mildest form of the disease, there may be only vascular dilatation and tortuosity, disc hyperemia, and a few retinal hemorrhages (Fig. 54–2). In this form, the condition is likely to resolve without sequelae. At the other extreme, there may be nearly confluent hemorrhages, cotton-wool spots, massive retinal and macular edema, and extensive capillary nonperfusion. In these cases one can expect to see severe visual impairment and a marked tendency for the development of rubeosis iridis and neovascular glaucoma.

The clinical course following CRVO is highly variable. In some cases, the signs of occlusion disappear in a few months, leaving little if any permanent injury. Intermediate cases may leave persistent hemorrhage, macular edema, and microvascular abnormalities such as microaneurysms. In ischemic disease, complications may develop, such as rubeosis iridis, neovascular glaucoma, retinal or disc neovascularization, and vitreous hemorrhage.

Pathophysiology

Full understanding of the pathophysiology of CRVO has been obscured, largely because of the lack of a satisfactory animal model. Hayreh, using evidence from clinical and animal data, argued that nonischemic CRVO was due to simple occlusion of the retinal venous system and that ischemic CRVO was due to a combined occlusion of the arterial and venous circulations.[3–5] In his monkey experiments, he and his coworkers occluded the central retinal vessels at the site of entry into the optic nerve. The clinical picture of ischemic CRVO with hemorrhage was reproduced only by occlusion of the central retinal vein with temporary occlusion of the central retinal artery.

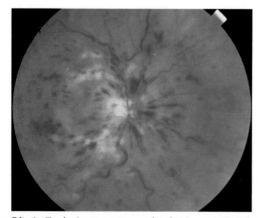

Figure 54–1. Typical appearance of a fresh central retinal vein occlusion, with disc edema, venous dilatation and tortuosity, cotton-wool spots, and retinal hemorrhages in all quadrants.

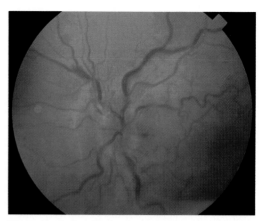

Figure 54–2. Central retinal vein occlusion demonstrating disc hyperemia and venous dilatation and tortuosity, with mild retinal hemorrhages.

Other experimental and pathologic studies have contradicted Hayreh's assertions. Fujino and coworkers found that more anterior obstruction of the central retinal vein alone produced a picture similar to the clinical appearance of an ischemic CRVO.[6]

Klein and Olwin divided CRVO into three subsets: (1) those resulting from external compression of the vein; (2) those resulting from primary disease of the veins, such as vasculitis; and (3) those resulting from thrombosis.[7, 8] In the largest histopathologic series to date, Green and coinvestigators supported the hypothesis that thrombus formation is the primary event in CRVO.[9] They found fresh or recanalized thrombus in the region of the lamina cribrosa in 29 of 29 enucleated eyes following CRVO. Endothelial proliferation and inflammation were commonly associated findings, but both were believed to be secondary to thrombus formation rather than to primary events. Most of the eyes reported in this study had chronic, ischemic CRVO and had been enucleated for neovascular glaucoma. The few eyes with fresh occlusions occurred in patients in the terminal stages of severe systemic disease. Eyes with fresh and nonischemic CRVOs were underrepresented in this series.

The reason that thrombus formation tends to occur in the region of the lamina cribrosa is unknown. The close anatomic association of the central retinal artery and the central retinal vein in this region, as well as the narrowing of the central retinal vessels as they pass through the lamina cribrosa, may contribute to turbulent flow and thrombus formation.[10]

Associated Conditions

The average age of patients presenting with CRVO is the early to mid 60s. Ninety percent of patients with CRVO are older than 50 yr of age.[11] There is a slight male preponderance.[12–14]

Some authors have considered CRVO in young individuals as a distinct entity. A presumed inflammatory cause led to the use of terms such as *papillophlebitis* and *benign retinal vasculitis*. The eyes described in these categories resemble nonischemic CRVO, with a tendency toward exaggerated disc edema and a relatively benign clinical course, usually with complete or nearly complete recovery.[15–17] Other than the younger age of the patients, there is little reason to distinguish these cases from other examples of nonischemic CRVO. One uncontrolled series reported a higher than expected incidence of collagen vascular disease in young CRVO patients.[14] The importance of inflammation in the pathogenesis of CRVO remains to be proved.[18]

Many ocular and systemic conditions have been associated with CRVO. In uncontrolled studies, 40 percent or more of patients with CRVO had preexisting open-angle glaucoma, or this condition developed during follow-up.[19, 20] A high prevalence of systemic hypertension has consistently been associated with CRVO—about 60 percent of cases in several large series.[14, 21–25] Other conditions associated with CRVO in numerous series include diabetes and cardiovascular and peripheral vascular disease. In younger patients with CRVO, one series reported a higher than expected incidence of cardiovascular death,[26] and another reported a high prevalence of collagen vascular disease.[14]

The previously described data linking CRVO with other ocular and systemic diseases are chiefly from series of CRVO patients without control groups. Elman and coworkers compared rates of hypertension, diabetes, cardiovascular disease, cerebrovascular disease, and mortality among white CRVO patients and a control group from the Wilmer Ophthalmological Institute and to another control group based on a national survey.[27] The prevalence of hypertension was significantly higher in the CRVO group than in either control group. Diabetes was significantly more prevalent when compared with the national survey controls but not when compared with the Wilmer controls. Rates of cardiovascular disease, cerebrovascular disease, and mortality did not differ significantly among the groups. Rath and associates compared patients with vein occlusions (CRVO, BRVO, and HCRVO) with patients from a general ophthalmology patient population. Male gender, systemic hypertension, and open-angle glaucoma were significantly more common in the patients with vein occlusions.[120] The ongoing multicenter Eye Disorder Case Control Study should provide additional epidemiologic information about this important subject.

Several hematologic factors have been implicated as risk factors for venous occlusive disease, including elevated lipid and cholesterol levels.[25, 28] Elevated serum viscosity may be a contributing factor in both BRVO and CRVO, particularly in predisposing to the ischemic forms of these diseases.[29, 30] Systemic diseases that result in increased hyperviscosity syndromes such as polycythemia and Waldenstrom's macroglobulinemia can cause a clinical picture of bilateral CRVO.[31, 32] In these cases of severe secondary hyperviscosity, normalization of the viscosity may cause dramatic improvement of the retinal abnormalities.

Lupus anticoagulant factor is a circulating immunoglobulin that may cause mild prolongation of coagulation studies, especially partial thromboplastin time, but paradoxically is associated with thrombosis. This factor occurs in a subset of patients with lupus but can also occur in patients without lupus. Patients with this factor frequently test positive for antiphospholipid antibodies, including anticardiolipin, and may demonstrate a false-positive result on the Venereal Disease Research Laboratory (VDRL) test. In addition to systemic thrombosis and spontaneous abortion, patients may demonstrate occlusions of the retinal arterial, retinal venous, and choroidal circulations.[33–37]

Classification

It has long been recognized that some CRVOs follow a relatively benign clinical course, whereas in others severe complications and visual loss develops. Since photocoagulation therapy appears to be beneficial in preventing these complications, it is valuable for clinicians to be able to identify those patients at high risk. Hayreh advocated the notion that the disease CRVO was actually two distinct entities. *Hemorrhagic retinopathy* was his term for the more severe form of CRVO, with a high attendant risk for the development of neovascular complications. *Venous stasis retinopathy* was the term used to describe the milder form of the disease, which had a relatively benign course.[38] *Venous stasis retinopathy* had previously been coined by Kearns and Hollenhorst to describe a similar-appearing retinopathy resulting from chronic retinal ischemia due to carotid artery disease.[39] The use of this term to describe two similar-appearing entities has led to considerable ambiguity and confusion, and its application should probably be abandoned. Other terms used to distinguish mild from severe CRVO include *partial* and *complete* and *nonischemic* and *ischemic*. The choice of terminology is less important than an understanding of factors that are useful in distinguishing eyes at risk for neovascular complications. Parameters to be considered in the evaluation of a CRVO include visual acuity, degree of afferent pupillary defect, ophthalmoscopic findings, fluorescein angiographic findings, and electroretinographic abnormalities.

The common factor that correlates each of the predictors with the risk of neovascularization is retinal ischemia. Magargal and associates classified CRVOs based on the proportion of nonperfused retina (ischemic index).[40] They found a bimodal distribution, with 42 percent well-perfused eyes, 43 percent very ischemic eyes (defined as an ischemic index of 50 percent or greater), and 15 percent in intermediate categories. The risk of neovascularization was proportional to the degree of ischemia.[40] Although no standard criteria have been established, one practical working definition defined ischemia as five or more disc areas of retinal nonperfusion.[14] Based on several large series, approximately two thirds of all CRVOs can be roughly categorized as nonischemic, and one third can be classified as ischemic.[12, 14, 41] The cases of CRVO with the greatest degree of ischemia should be watched closely because two thirds or more of these will develop neovascular complications, most commonly and most ominously rubeosis iridis.[12, 13, 22, 40] Rubeosis rarely develops in truly nonischemic CRVO. Classification of ischemia is imperfect, and it is well documented that approximately 1 in 10 initially nonischemic CRVOs can become ischemic and assume the risks of the latter form,[12, 14, 22, 42] so vigilance is warranted in all cases. Any CRVO for which the perfusion cannot be assessed should be followed very closely until its status can be ascertained.

Methods of Evaluation

Visual Acuity. In acute CRVO, visual acuity ranges from normal to just the ability to see hand motions.[14] The long-term visual prognosis ranges from full recovery to absolute blindness. Most patients with ischemic CRVO have visual acuity of 20/100 or worse. Patients with nonischemic CRVO tend to have better visual acuity, but vision may be very poor because of macular edema or other nonischemic complications.[12, 14, 21] Among all CRVO patients, there is a strong correlation between initial and final visual acuity,[43] with acuity remaining within three lines of the initial acuity in half of affected eyes. In eyes in which the visual acuity changes three or more lines, there is more often a loss than a gain.[14]

Afferent Pupillary Defect. A quantitative measurement of relative afferent pupil defect in eyes with CRVO has been shown to correlate well with retinal ischemia and to be a good predictor of eyes at risk for neovascular complications. Ninety percent of eyes designated nonischemic by other criteria had relative afferent defects of 0.3 log units or less. Ninety-one percent of eyes with ischemic CRVOs had relative afferent defects of 1.2 log units or more.[44]

Intraocular Pressure. The association between elevated intraocular pressure and CRVO has already been discussed. Immediately following CRVO, the intraocular pressure is typically slightly lower in the affected eye than in the fellow eye. This relative pressure difference diminishes with time, and symmetry returns over the ensuing weeks to months.[20, 45, 46]

Visual Fields. Central and peripheral visual field abnormalities are more common in ischemic than in nonischemic CRVO.[38]

Fundus Findings. The clinical picture of acute CRVO has already been described. Cotton-wool spots are indicators of ischemia. The presence of 10 or more cotton-wool spots was found to be a risk factor for the development of rubeosis iridis.[22]

The resolution of fundus findings is quite variable and unpredictable. The retinal hemorrhages tend to decrease in number over many months and may disappear entirely; however, some may persist for years, particularly in the periphery. The dilatation and tortuosity of the involved retinal veins typically diminishes over time, and marked sheathing of the retinal veins may develop. Disc edema regresses, and in ischemic cases disc pallor may develop. Collateral vessels at the optic disc may develop in mild or severe occlusions (Fig. 54–3). Evi-

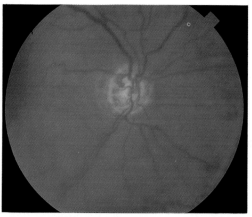

Figure 54–3. Typical, tortuous appearance of disc collaterals following a central retinal vein occlusion.

dence of retinal microvascular injury may persist in the form of microaneuerysms, persistent macular edema, and macular pigment irregularity. In ischemic CRVO, neovascularization of the disc or retina may appear weeks or months after the acute event.

Fluorescein Angiography. The characteristic fluorescein angiographic findings in CRVO are the result of changes in vascular caliber, abnormal vascular permeability, and closure of the retinal capillaries.[41, 47, 48] Fluorescein angiography is helpful in making the diagnosis of CRVO, identifying complications, and selecting patients for treatment.

The appearance of fluorescein in the retinal arteries following its injection is normal to slightly delayed. The arteriovenous transit time is typically prolonged (Fig. 54–4).[48] Prolongation beyond 20 sec is associated with a greater risk of rubeosis iridis.[22] Staining of the walls of the retinal veins has also been shown to be an indicator of ischemia.[22]

Fluorescein angiographic assessment of capillary closure may be hindered by hemorrhages obscuring the retinal capillaries. Standard angiographic views of the posterior pole may neglect areas of more peripheral ischemia. Also, intraobserver and interobserver repro-

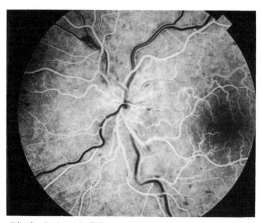

Figure 54–4. Delayed filling of the retinal venous system in a central retinal vein occlusion. This frame, taken 14 sec after the appearance of fluorescein in the retinal arteries, shows minimal filling of the retinal venous system.

ducibility in grading nonperfusion is imperfect.[49] Despite these limitations, fluorescein angiography has been the most widely used method for the evaluation of retinal perfusion and the prediction of eyes at risk for the neovascular complications of CRVO. Most reports have divided eyes into only two or three categories of ischemia and have shown a clearly increased risk of neovascularization among eyes with severe ischemia.[12–14, 21, 22] Small areas of nonperfusion may not put the eye at risk for neovascularization but can be visually significant if located near the fovea. An intact perifoveal capillary net is usually required for good final visual acuity.[47]

Retinal edema results from abnormal permeability of the retinal vessels. It may be distributed throughout the retina but tends to be most severe in the macula in which it may take on a diffuse pattern or the typical petaloid pattern of cystoid macular edema. Edema occurs in both ischemic and nonischemic forms of CRVO but tends to be more diffuse and severe in the ischemic form.

Electroretinography. Several studies have shown that electroretinographic abnormalities correlate well with other indices of ischemia and identify eyes at risk for neovascularization. The parameters most often cited as indicators of ischemia are reduced b-wave amplitude, a reduced b:a wave ratio, and prolonged b-wave implicit time.[51–55]

Complications

Macular Edema. Macular edema may occur in mild or severe cases and is one of the leading causes of visual loss in central vein occlusion. It results from leakage of the perifoveal small vessels secondary to hydrostatic stress and ischemia. The edema typically takes on the clinical and fluorescein angiographic appearance of cystoid macular edema and may be transient or persistent.

Hemorrhage. The presence of retinal hemorrhage is practically essential for the diagnosis of acute CRVO; however, the amount of hemorrhage is highly variable. If hemorrhage occurs in the fovea, visual acuity will be affected. Extensive hemorrhage makes the fluorescein angiographic evaluation of ischemia difficult by blocking the fluorescence of retinal capillaries, and it may interfere with photocoagulation. Occasionally, acute CRVO may lead to vitreous hemorrhage, which if severe enough may obscure the fundus and the diagnosis. Vitreous hemorrhage may also occur as a later complication caused by disc or retinal neovascularization.

Ischemia. Ischemia is responsible both directly and indirectly for visual morbidity in CRVO. Ischemia refers to closure of the retinal capillaries and is described angiographically as *capillary dropout* or *"capillary nonperfusion."* If ischemia affects the capillaries surrounding the foveal avascular zone, vision is usually irreversibly impaired. Ischemia is believed to be the factor that, by an unknown mechanism, stimulates neovascularization. In general, the greater the extent and severity of ischemia, the greater the risk of neovascularization. As previously mentioned, in several large series about two thirds of CRVOs were classified as nonischemic. When

ischemia was defined as five or more disc areas of capillary nonperfusion, leakage or staining of a venule wall, or retinal or anterior segment neovascularization, 64 percent of cases were classified as nonischemic and 36 percent were classified as ischemic.[14]

Neovascularization. The proliferation of new blood vessels is a complication of many ischemic processes affecting the retina. Retinal ischemia may lead to neovascularization, which may take place on the optic disc, on the retina, in the angle, and on the iris (rubeosis iridis). Neovascularization of the disc and of the retina following CRVO is less common than neovascularization of the iris.[56] Iris and angle neovascularization are the most dreaded complications of CRVO because they may progress swiftly, leading to intractable neovascular glaucoma, pain, and blindness. The risk of rubeosis iridis is greatest in the early months after a CRVO but may occur later. The overall incidence of rubeosis among all CRVOs is about 20 percent.[12, 22, 40] Among the ischemic eyes, rubeosis with or without neovascular glaucoma occurs in 45 to 80 percent of eyes. In nonischemic eyes, the rate of iris neovascularization has generally been reported to be less than 5 percent.[12, 13, 22, 40] Neovascularization of the optic disc or retina is usually considered a rare complication but was reported in 24 percent of ischemic CRVOs.[14]

Retinal Detachment. Rhegmatogenous retinal detachment has been described coincidental with or following CRVO.[57, 58] Other than a temporal association with CRVO, these detachments did not differ from other retinal detachments caused by peripheral retinal breaks. Exudative retinal detachment—with turbid subretinal fluid, subretinal exudate, and retinal ischemia—may also occur as a late complication of CRVO.[59]

Other Vascular Complications. Microaneurysms, similar in appearance to those seen in diabetic retinopathy, typically develop in the retina following venous occlusion. A less frequent occurrence is the formation of large aneurysms of the retina that look similar to arterial macroaneurysms but appear to arise from the capillary circulation (Fig. 54–5).[60]

Collateral channels between the retinal and the ciliary circulations (sometimes called *optociliary* vessels) de-

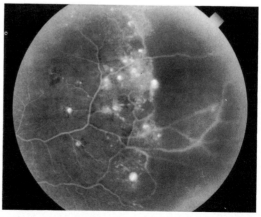

Figure 54–5. Large capillary aneurysms that occurred following a central retinal vein occlusion. Peripheral to the aneurysms is a large area of nonperfusion.

velop in about 50 percent of cases. They appear as tortuous vascular loops on or adjacent to the optic disc (see Fig. 54–3). They may be confused with disc neovascularization but can usually be distinguished by their larger caliber and lack of leakage on fluorescein angiography. Some studies have suggested that development of collaterals is associated with an improved visual prognosis,[26, 61] whereas others have refuted this assertion.[14]

The occlusion of one or more cilioretinal arteries is sometimes found concurrently with CRVO. Cilioretinal arteries have a lower perfusion pressure than does the retinal arterial circulation and presumably appear occluded because they cannot overcome the increased vascular resistance resulting from CRVO.[62–64]

Hard exudate is an infrequent complication of CRVO. When large amounts of hard exudate occur, there appears to be an association with increased ischemia and poor visual acuity[59, 65] as well as elevated serum triglyceride levels.[65]

Treatment

Photocoagulation. Panretinal photocoagulation using a xenon arc[41, 46] or an argon laser[66] has been shown to virtually eliminate the risk of neovascular glaucoma in CRVO. Although definite guidelines have not been established, common clinical practice is the application of prophylactic photocoagulation to eyes considered ischemic. Some eyes, particularly those with extensive retinal hemorrhage, cannot be clearly categorized at the initial evaluation. Eyes in this "indeterminate" category must be followed closely until their perfusion status can be determined. Eyes initially classified as nonischemic are not immune from neovascular complications and may subsequently be classified as ischemic. These eyes must also be watched carefully and considered for treatment if signs of ischemia develop.

The efficacy of laser photocoagulation for the treatment of macular edema secondary to CRVO has never been subjected to a randomized clinical trial. The proven benefit of photocoagulation for macular edema following BRVO and clinical experience suggest that this treatment may be worthwhile in patients with chronic macular edema following CRVO.[67] An ongoing multicenter trial should help define the benefits of panretinal photocoagulation and macular photocoagulation for complications of CRVO.

Medical Therapy. The use of anticoagulants was recommended by some investigators based on the experience of uncontrolled trials in the 1940s and 1950s.[8, 68–71] A randomized clinical trial of intravenous streptokinase in CRVO suggested a reduction in the rate of neovascular glaucoma in treated patients, but there was an unacceptable risk of vitreous hemorrhage shortly after the institution of therapy.[72] The use of systemic anticoagulation carries significant morbidity and cannot be recommended unless a randomized clinical trial can prove benefits that outweigh its substantial risks.

BRVO

In BRVO, the fundus abnormalities are similar to CRVO except that only a portion of the retina is involved. BRVOs occur at arteriovenous intersections, and the area of retina drained by the occluded vein is principally affected. This usually defines an arcuate wedge of retina with its apex at the site of obstruction (Fig. 54–6). The area of retina involved depends on the size and location of the involved vein. In general, the nearer the occlusion occurs to the optic disc, the greater the extent of the affected retina and the more serious the complications.[73, 74] The visual impact of a BRVO is partly related to the site and size of the occlusion, but even very tiny occlusions can be visually significant if the fovea is affected (Fig. 54–7).[75]

The involved retina demonstrates variable degrees of venous dilatation and tortuosity, superficial and deep retinal hemorrhage, cotton-wool spots, and retinal edema. The clinical course following BRVO is variable, with the potential for minimal to severe permanent anatomic and functional damage.

Pathophysiology

BRVOs occur almost exclusively at arteriovenous intersections. Manifestations of hypertensive retinopathy in the form of venous "nicking" or Gunn's sign is frequently observed in eyes with BRVO. At arteriovenous intersections, the crossing artery and vein share a common adventitial sheath, and the vascular walls are fused. Despite the clinical appearance, Seitz demonstrated histologically that the retinal vein is not compressed by the artery at intersections at which nicking is observed.[76] The physiologic importance of arteriovenous crossings in BRVO is still poorly understood. In normal eyes, retinal arteries cross over (innermost to) retinal veins at 70 to 75 percent of all arteriovenous intersections, and veins cross over arteries at 25 to 30

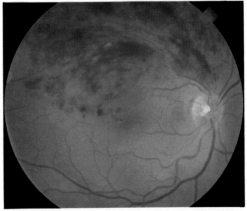

Figure 54–6. Large superotemporal branch retinal vein occlusion occurring at an arteriorvenous intersection near the superior margin of the disc.

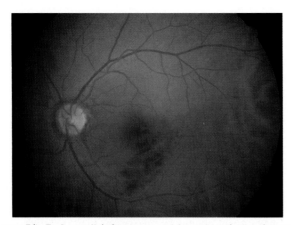

Figure 54–7. A small inferotemporal branch retinal vein occlusion. Although the area of affected retina is small, the hemorrhage and edema extend into the fovea and have reduced vision.

percent of intersections.[77, 78] For reasons that are unclear, BRVOs occur almost exclusively at arterial overcrossings.[78, 79]

The precise "event" responsible for the constellation of findings in BRVO has been the subject of some controversy. Some authors have suggested that BRVO is actually a result of arterial insufficiency.[24, 80] Experimental studies have demonstrated that most of the manifestations of BRVO in humans, including nonperfusion and secondary changes in the retinal arteries, can be reproduced by experimental occlusion of the retinal veins in animals.[81–86]

Frangieh and associates in a histopathologic study of nine cases of BRVO found fresh or recanalized venous thrombus at the site of occlusion in all cases and concluded that thrombus of the branch vein was probably the primary event, and the other vascular changes occurred secondarily.[87]

Associated Conditions

BRVO tends to be a disease of older adults, most commonly 60 to 70 yr.[73, 88, 89] Systemic hypertension and its characteristic retinal vascular changes have long been associated with BRVO based mostly on clinical observation and uncontrolled series.[2, 90] One half to two thirds of patients in large series have been reported to also have systemic hypertension.[73–75, 89, 91, 92] One case control study found male gender, hypertension, and hyperopia to be more common among BRVO patients than among age-matched controls. Diabetes mellitus and open-angle glaucoma occurred more frequently among BRVO patients than among controls, but the differences were not statistically significant.[88] The possible importance of serum lipids, viscosity, and other circulating factors was discussed in CRVO. The results of the Eye Disorder Case Control Study are expected to improve our knowledge of the epidemiologic associations of BRVO.

Methods of Evaluation

Visual Acuity. If visual acuity is acutely affected in BRVO, it is because the macula has been affected by hemorrhage, edema, or ischemia. Later in the course of the disease, these complications, as well as others, such as vitreous hemorrhage or retinal detachment, may impair vision. The visual acuity in acute BRVO may be unaffected to severely impaired. Overall, the visual prognosis is good, with 50 to 60 percent of untreated patients having a final visual acuity of 20/40 or better. About 20 to 25 percent of patients are left with 20/200 or worse, and the remainder have visual acuity from 20/50 to 20/100. A final acuity of the patient only being able to see hand motions or worse occurs rarely.[73, 74, 89, 93, 94]

Fundus Findings. The classic appearance of a fresh BRVO has been described and illustrated and is rarely mistaken. Small macular BRVOs are less dramatic in appearance and may not be recognized (Fig. 54–7).[75] In long-standing cases, after the characteristic pattern of hemorrhage is resolved, the sequelae of BRVO may be mistaken for other vasculopathies such as diabetic retinopathy. The typical distribution of the microvascular abnormalities and the presence of intraretinal collaterals draining across the median raphe are clues to the presence of an old BRVO. In more ischemic cases, sclerosis and sheathing of the retinal veins and arteries in the distribution of the occlusion may develop.[48, 95]

Fluorescein Angiography. As with CRVO, the angiographic findings reflect changes in the permeability, caliber, and patency of the retinal vessels. Venous filling in the area of the occlusion is delayed relative to the unaffected retina,[73, 96] and in most cases the fluorescein column is narrowed at the site of occlusion.[96] In some cases, a small area of early hyperfluorescence occurs just proximal to the site of occlusion.[89, 96] Fluorescein angiography is useful in evaluating ischemia, which is important in determining eyes at risk for neovascular complications, or determining if macular ischemia may be contributing to visual impairment (Fig. 54–8). Retinal hemorrhages block fluorescence and may make assessment of perfusion difficult.

Retinal edema is common within and surrounding the distribution of the occluded vein. Macular edema is the most common visually significant complication of BRVO. The petaloid pattern of cystoid macular edema may involve all or only part of the macula.

Complications

The same pathologic forces are at work in BRVO and CRVO. The resultant complications are similar but occur at different frequencies in the two diseases. In BRVO, variations in the size of the affected retina, the severity of the damage to the area, and the location of the affected area all influence the outcome. BRVOs occurring away from the fovea and without neovascular complications are often asymptomatic.

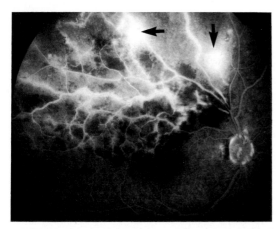

Figure 54–8. Fluorescein angiogram of an ischemic branch retinal vein occlusion demonstrating widespread capillary nonperfusion and staining of the retinal veins. The two areas of intense hyperfluorescence *(arrows)* are due to retinal neovascularization.

Edema. Macular edema is the most common complication of BRVO and the leading cause of visual loss.[73, 97] In one series, macular edema was initially found in 100 percent of cases and persisted in 62 percent of untreated patients.[89]

Hemorrhage. Retinal hemorrhage is one of the hallmarks of acute BRVO. Hemorrhages within the fovea may be responsible for early visual loss. Hemorrhage usually resolves weeks or months after the acute occlusion but may persist much longer. The presence of severe hemorrhage makes interpretation of fluorescein angiography more difficult and may interfere with the delivery of photocoagulation. Vitreous hemorrhage may rarely occur as a complication of acute BRVO,[47] but more frequently it occurs later in the course as a result of retinal and disc neovascularization.

Ischemia. Ischemia contributes directly and indirectly to the visual morbidity in BRVO. As with CRVO, ischemia involving the fovea limits the potential for visual improvement following BRVO. Retinal ischemia is associated with an increased risk of neovascular complications.[91] Some BRVOs originally classified as nonischemic may progress to become ischemic.[94, 95, 98]

Neovascularization. The most common site of neovascularization following BRVO is the retina. Retinal neovascularization usually occurs at the border of perfused and nonperfused retina (Fig. 54–9) but can rarely occur away from the territory of the BRVO.[99] Neovascularization of the optic disc is much less common, and when it occurs, it tends to be concurrent with retinal neovascularization.[91] Iris neovascularization is very rare following BRVO. Hayreh and coworkers reported a 28.8 percent incidence of neovascular complications following "major" BRVO.[12] Most of these cases were retinal or retinal and disc neovascularization. Only 1.6 percent developed iris neovascularization. Other studies have reported an incidence of retinal neovascularization of 22 to 24 percent.[73, 89, 94]

In the Branch Vein Occlusion Study, neovascularization developed in 22 percent of eyes with BRVO without regard to degree of nonperfusion. The incidence of neovascularization was 36 percent in eyes with five disc diameters or more of retinal nonperfusion.[94] Shilling and Kohner found an incidence of 62 percent among eyes with greater than four disc diameters of nonperfusion, and 0 percent among eyes without this degree of nonperfusion.[91]

Several studies have shown that the majority of untreated eyes with retinal or disc neovascularization will develop vitreous hemorrhage.[73, 74, 91, 94]

Other Vascular Complications. Microvascular abnormalities are common sequelae to BRVO. Dilated capillaries and microaneurysms develop in the territory of the vein occlusion. Chronic leakage by these abnormal vessels can contribute to macular edema and cause the deposition of lipid (hard exudates) in the retina. Large capillary or venous macroaneurysms may develop within the territory of the occlusion in BRVO as well as in CRVO.[60, 100, 101] Sheathing of the retinal arteries and veins often develops in the territory of the occlusion (Fig. 54–10).

Collateral vessels that develop following BRVO are different from those occurring after CRVO. Collateral channels may form and pass from the territory of the occlusion to a point proximal to the site of occlusion or to an uninvolved vein. The most characteristic type of collaterals are small, tortuous venous channels that cross the horizontal raphe (usually temporal to the fovea) and drain into the venous circulation of the uninvolved quadrant (Fig. 54–11).

Retinal Detachment. Retinal breaks occurring as a result of BRVO may lead to rhegmatogenous retinal detachments. This is a rare complication of BRVO, but when breaks occur they tend to be located posterior to the equator and result from traction exerted by fibrovascular proliferation.[102–105] Other rhegmatogenous detachments following BRVO have been attributed to traction unrelated to neovascularization and to ischemic retinal degeneration with hole formation.[58, 105–107]

Exudative retinal detachment may occur as a complication of BRVO. These detachments occur within the territory affected by the occlusion, are associated with ischemia, and seem to resolve when treated with photocoagulation.[104, 108, 109]

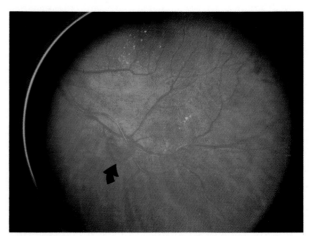

Figure 54–9. A tuft of retinal neovascularization *(arrow)* along the vascular arcade in a long-standing inferotemporal branch retinal vein occlusion.

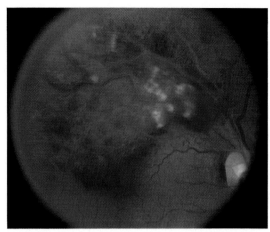

Figure 54–10. Branch retinal vein occlusion with hemorrhage, cotton-wool spots, and sheathing of the retinal veins.

Other. Sequelae of BRVO that may be visually significant when the macula is involved include epiretinal membrane, retinal pigment epithelial irregularity, subretinal scarring, and a macular hole.[73, 89, 110]

Treatment

We are fortunate to have the results of a randomized clinical study that demonstrated the effectiveness of photocoagulation in reducing the morbidity of the two major complications of BRVO: macular edema and retinal neovascularization. Prior to the branch vein occlusion study, there were numerous uncontrolled studies suggesting the benefit of photocoagulation in treating macular edema resulting from BRVO.[67, 74, 111–114] In 1984, the Branch Retinal Vein Occlusion Study reported the results of a randomized trial of no treatment versus laser photocoagulation for a selected group of eyes with BRVO.[93] Eligible eyes had a BRVO with a duration of 3 to 18 mo and a visual acuity of 20/40 or worse attributable to macular edema. A group of randomly

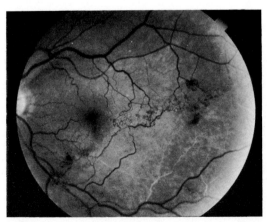

Figure 54–11. Appearance of venous collaterals following a branch retinal vein occlusion. The channels cross the median raphe temporal to the fovea and drain from the affected to the nonaffected quadrant.

selected patients received a grid pattern of argon laser photocoagulation applied to the area of macular capillary leakage. Using 100-μ spots, spaced approximately one burn width apart, treatment was allowed to extend no closer to the fovea than the avascular zone and no further peripherally than the major vascular arcades.[115] After 3 yr, treated eyes were more likely to have an improvement in vision, were more likely to have a final visual acuity of 20/40 or better, and had an average visual acuity better than that of untreated eyes.[93]

The other aspect of the BRVO study addressed the efficacy of scatter laser photocoagulation for the prevention of retinal neovascularization and vitreous hemorrhage following BRVO. Eyes with BRVO involving at least a 5-disc diameter area of retina were randomized to photocoagulation treatment versus observation. Treatment consisted of medium-intensity 200- to 500-μ argon laser burns spaced one burn width apart, covering the entire area of involved retina, except within two disc diameters of the fovea. Twenty-four percent of the untreated eyes developed neovascularization versus 12 percent of the treated eyes. Of eyes developing neovascularization, all initially had five disc diameters or more of nonperfusion, or they developed this degree of nonperfusion during follow-up.[94]

Eyes with neovascularization at the time of entry into the study were randomized to the same treatment versus nontreatment protocol. Sixty-one percent of the untreated eyes developed vitreous hemorrhage versus 29 percent of the treated eyes.

The study was not designed to determine whether nonperfused eyes should be prophylactically treated or observed and treated only if neovascularization develops; however, analysis of the available data led the authors to conclude ". . . there may be no advantage to treating before the development of neovascularization."[94]

HCRVO

In some eyes, the veins that drain the superior and inferior halves of the retina do not merge into a common central retinal vein until they unite proximal to the lamina cribrosa. This configuration has been observed in approximately one in five eyes.[116] In these eyes, the pathologic events that typically cause a CRVO may affect only one of these veins, creating a picture of a retinal vein occlusion affecting only the superior or inferior half of the retina (Fig. 54–12).[117, 118] The pathogenesis of HCRVO is more like CRVO than it is like BRVO. This has been supported by a study showing that the risk factors for HCRVO are more similar to CRVO than to BRVO.[119]

The clinical findings and complications of HCRVO are somewhat of a hybrid of CRVO and BRVO. The typical manifestations of venous occlusion are principally limited to the superior or inferior retinal hemisphere; however, there may be some spillover into the opposite hemisphere. Macular edema is common. For neovascular complications, Hayreh and colleagues divided HCRVOs into *venous stasis* and *hemorrhagic* as they

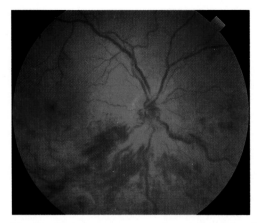

Figure 54–12. Typical appearance of an inferior hemicentral retinal vein occlusion. Findings are similar to central retinal vein occlusion but affect only half of the retina.

did with CRVOs. Roughly two thirds of HCRVOs were classified as venous stasis, and one third were classified as hemorrhagic. Neovascular complications were not found in any of the hemivenous stasis retinopathy group. Among the hemihemorrhagic group, 13 percent developed iris neovascularization, 29 percent developed disc neovascularization, and 42 percent developed retinal neovascularization.[12] Thus, for ischemic HCRVO, the risk of iris neovascularization is greater than for BRVO but less than for ischemic CRVO. The risk of disc or retinal neovascularization appears to be greater in HCRVO than in either BRVO or ischemic CRVO. Collateral channels may form at the disc (as in CRVO) as well as across the median raphe (as in BRVO).[117]

The utility of photocoagulation for the prevention and treatment of complications in HCRVO has not been investigated. Since the rate of neovascular complications is relatively high following ischemic HCRVO, the prophylactic application of scatter photocoagulation in the affected retinal hemisphere may be considered. For the treatment of chronic macular edema following HCRVO, it is probably reasonable to extrapolate the guidelines established by the BRVO study.[94]

REFERENCES

1. David R, Zangwill L, Badarna M, et al: Epidemiology of retinal vein occlusion and its association with glaucoma and increased intraocular pressure. Ophthalmologica 197:69, 1988.
2. Orth DH, Patz A: Retinal branch vein occlusion. Surv Ophthalmol 22:357, 1978.
3. Hayreh SS: So-called "central retinal vein occlusion" I. Pathogenesis, terminology, clinical features. Ophthalmologica 17:1, 1976.
4. Hayreh SS: Occlusion of the central retinal vessels. Br J Ophthalmol 49:626, 1965.
5. Hayreh SS: Pathogenesis of occlusion of the central retinal vessels. Am J Ophthalmol 72:998, 1971.
6. Fujino T, Curtin VT, Norton EWD: Experimental central retinal vein occlusion. A comparison of intraocular and extraocular occlusion. Arch Ophthalmol 81:395, 1969.
7. Klein BA: Sidelights on retinal venous occlusion. Am J Ophthalmol 61:25, 1966.
8. Klein BA, Olwin JH: A survey of the pathogenesis of retinal venous occlusion. Emphasis upon choice of therapy and analysis of the therapeutic results in fifty-three patients. AMA Arch Ophthalmol 56:207, 1956.
9. Green WR, Chan CC, Hutchins GM, et al: Central retinal vein occlusions: A prospective histopathologic study of 29 eyes in 28 cases. Retina 1:27, 1981.
10. Green WR: Retina. In Spencer WH, (ed): Ophthalmic Pathology, An Atlas and Textbook, 3rd ed. Philadelphia, WB Saunders, 1985, p 589.
11. Gutman FA: Evaluation of a patient with central retinal vein occlusion. Ophthalmology 90:481, 1990.
12. Hayreh SS, Rojas P, Podhajsky P, et al: Ocular neovascularization with retinal vascular occlusion III. Incidence of ocular neovascularization with retinal vein occlusion. Ophthalmology 90:488, 1983.
13. Magargal LE, Brown GC, Augsburger JJ, et al: Neovascular glaucoma following central retinal vein obstruction. Ophthalmology 88:1095, 1981.
14. Quinlan PM, Elman MJ, Kaur Bhatt A, et al: The natural course of central retinal vein occlusion. Am J Ophthalmol 110:118, 1990.
15. Lyle TK, Wybar K: Retinal vasculitis. Br J Ophthalmol 45:778, 1961.
16. Lonn LI, Hoyt WF: Papillophlebitis: A cause of protracted yet benign optic disc edema. Eye, Ear, Nose, Throat Monthly 45:62, 1966.
17. Hart CD, Sanders MD, Miller SJH: Benign retinal vasculitis. Clinical and fluorescein angiographic study. Br J Ophthalmol 55:721, 1971.
18. Walters RF, Spalton DJ: Central retinal vein occlusion in people aged 40 years or less: A review of 17 patients. Br J Ophthalmol 74:30, 1990.
19. Dreyden RM: Central retinal vein occlusion and chronic simple glaucoma. Arch Ophthalmol 73:659, 1965.
20. Bertelsen TI: The relationship between primary thrombosis in the retinal veins and primary glaucoma. Acta Ophthalmol 39:603, 1961.
21. Zegarra H, Gutman FA, Conforto J: The natural course of central retinal vein occlusion. Ophthalmology 86:1931, 1979.
22. Sinclair SH, Gragoudas ES: Prognosis for rubeosis iridis following central retinal vein occlusion. Br J Ophthalmol 63:735, 1979.
23. Zegarra H, Gutman FA, Zarkov N, et al: Partial occlusion of the central retinal vein. Am J Ophthalmol 96:330, 1983.
24. Paton A, Rubenstein K, Smith VH: Arterial insufficiency in retinal venous occlusion. Trans Ophthalmol Soc UK 84:559, 1964.
25. McGrath MA, Wechler F, Hunyor ABL, et al: Systemic factors contributory to retinal vein occlusion. Arch Intern Med 138:216, 1978.
26. Priluck IA, Robertson DM, Hollenhorst RW: Long-term follow-up of occlusion of the central retinal vein in young adults. Am J Ophthalmol 90:190, 1980.
27. Elman MJ, Kaur Bhatt A, Quinlan PM, et al: The risk of systemic vascular disease and mortality in patients with central retinal vein occlusion. Ophthalmology 97:1543, 1990.
28. Dodson PM, Galton DJ, Hamilton AM, et al: Retinal vein occlusion and the prevalence of lipoprotein abnormalities. Br J Ophthalmol 66:161, 1982.
29. Ring CP, Pearson TC, Sanders MD, et al: Viscosity and retinal vein thrombosis. Br J Ophthalmol 60:397, 1976.
30. Trope GE, Lowe GDO, McArdle BM, et al: Abnormal blood viscosity and haemostasis in long-standing retinal vein occlusion. Br J Ophthalmol 67:137, 1983.
31. Spalter HF: Abnormal serum proteins and retinal vein thrombosis. AMA Arch Ophthalmol 62:868, 1959.
32. Luxenberg MN, Mausolf FA: Retinal circulation in the hyperviscosity syndrome. Am J Ophthalmol 70:588, 1970.
33. Levine SR, Crofts JW, Lesser GR, et al: Visual symptoms associated with the presence of a lupus anticoagulant. Ophthalmology 95:686, 1988.
34. Pulido JS, Ward LM, Fishman GA, et al: Antiphospholipid antibodies associated with retinal vascular disease. Retina 7:215, 1987.
35. Asherson RA, Merry P, Acheson JF, et al: Antiphospholipid antibodies: A risk factor for occlusive ocular vascular disease in systemic lupus erythematosus and the "primary" antiphospholipid syndrome. Ann Rheum Dis 48:358, 1989.

36. Kleiner RC, Najarian LV, Schatten S, et al: Vaso-occlusive retinopathy associated with antiphospholipid antibodies (lupus anticoagulant retinopathy). Ophthalmology 96:896, 1989.
37. Snyers B, Lambert M, Hardy JP: Retinal and choroidal vaso-occlusive disease in systemic lupus erythematosus associated with antiphospholipid antibodies. Retina 10:255, 1991.
38. Hayreh SS: Classification of central retinal vein occlusion. Ophthalmology 90:458, 1983.
39. Kearns TP, Hollenhorst RW: Venous-stasis retinopathy of occlusive disease of the carotid artery. Proc Staff Mtg Mayo Clin 38:304, 1963.
40. Magargal LE, Donoso LA, Sanborn GE: Retinal ischemia and risk of neovascularization following central retinal vein obstruction. Ophthalmology 89:1241, 1982.
41. Laatikainen L, Kohner EM, Khoury D, et al: Panretinal photocoagulation in central retinal vein occlusion: A randomized controlled clinical study. Br J Ophthalmol 61:741, 1977.
42. Miturn J, Brown GC: Progression of nonischemic central retinal vein obstruction to the ischemic variant. Ophthalmology 93:1158, 1986.
43. Ebert EM, Seddon JM, Egan KM, et al: Visual outcome following diagnosis of retinal vein occlusion. Invest Ophthalmol Vis Sci 32(Suppl):1143, 1991.
44. Servais GE, Thompson HS, Hayreh SS: Relative afferent pupillary defect in central retinal vein occlusion. Ophthalmology 93:301, 1986.
45. Moore RF: Some observations on the intraocular tension in cases of thrombosis of the retinal veins. Trans Ophthalmol Soc UK 42:115, 1922.
46. May DR, Klein ML, Peyman GA, et al: Xenon arc panretinal photocoagulation for central retinal vein occlusion: A randomized prospective study. Br J Ophthalmol 63:725, 1979.
47. Laatikainen L, Kohner EM: Fluorescein angiography and its prognostic significance in central retinal vein occlusion. Br J Ophthalmol 60:411, 1976.
48. Gass JDM: A fluorescein angiographic study of macular dysfunction secondary to retinal vascular disease. II. Retinal vein obstruction. Arch Ophthalmol 80:550, 1968.
49. Welch JC, Augsburger JJ: Assessment of angiographic retinal capillary nonperfusion in central retinal vein occlusion. Am J Ophthalmol 103:761, 1987.
50. Sabates R, Hirose T, McMeel JW: Electroretinography in the prognosis and classification of central retinal vein occlusion. Arch Ophthalmol 101:232, 1983.
51. Hayreh SS, Klugman MR, Podhajsky P, et al: Electroretinography in central retinal vein occlusion. Correlation of electroretinographic changes with pupillary abnormalities. Graefes Arch Clin Exp Ophthalmol 227:549, 1989.
52. Breton ME, Quinn GE, Keene SS, et al: Electroretinogram parameters at presentation as predictors of rubeosis in central retinal vein occlusion patients. Ophthalmology 96:1343, 1989.
53. Johnson MA, Marcus S, Elman MJ, et al: Neovascularization in central retinal vein occlusion: Electroretinographic findings. Arch Ophthalmol 106:348, 1988.
54. Kay SB, Harding SP: Early electroretinography in unilateral central retinal vein occlusion as a predictor of rubeosis iridis. Arch Ophthalmol 106:353, 1988.
55. Bresnick GH: Following up patients with central retinal vein occlusion. Arch Ophthalmol 106:324, 1988.
56. Chan C, Little HL: Infrequency of retinal neovascularization following central retinal vein occlusion. Ophthalmology 86:256, 1979.
57. Lembach RG, Davidorf FH: Acute onset of central retinal vein occlusion and retinal detachment. Ann Ophthalmol 7:983, 1975.
58. Zauberman H: Retinopathy of retinal detachment after major vascular occlusions. Br J Ophthalmol 52:117, 1968.
59. Weinberg D, Jampol LM, Schatz H, et al: Exudative retinal detachment following central and hemicentral retinal vein occlusion. Arch Ophthalmol 108:271, 1990.
60. Schulman J, Jampol LM, Goldberg MF: Large capillary aneurysms secondary to retinal venous obstruction. Br J Ophthalmol 65:36, 1981.
61. Blinder KJ, Khan JA, Giangiacomo J, et al: Optociliary veins and visual prognosis after central retinal vein occlusion. Ann Ophthalmol 21:192, 1989.
62. McCleod D, Ring CP: Cilio-retinal infarction after retinal vein occlusion. Br J Ophthalmol 60:419, 1976.
63. Brown GC, Moffat K, Cruess A, et al: Cilioretinal artery obstruction. Retina 3:182, 1983.
64. Schatz H, Fong ACO, McDonald HR, et al: Cilioretinal artery occlusion in young adults with central retinal vein occlusion. Ophthalmology 98:594, 1991.
65. Brown GC: Central retinal vein obstruction with lipid exudate. Arch Ophthalmol 107:1001, 1989.
66. Magargal LE, Brown GC, Augsburger JJ, et al: Efficacy of panretinal photocoagulation in preventing neovascular glaucoma following ischemic central retinal vein obstruction. Ophthalmology 89:780, 1982.
67. Gutman FA, Zegarra H: Macular edema secondary to occlusion of the retinal veins. Surv Opthalmol 28:462, 1984.
68. Vannas S, Orma H: Experience of treating retinal venous occlusion with anticoagulant and antisclerosis therapy. AMA Arch Ophthalmol 58:812, 1957.
69. Duff IF, Falls HF, Linman JW: Anticoagulant therapy in occlusive vascular disease of the retina. AMA Arch Ophthalmol 46:601, 1951.
70. Klein BA: Prevention of retinal venous occlusion with special reference to ambulatory dicumarol therapy. Am J Ophthalmol 33:175, 1950.
71. Van Loon JA: The causes and therapy of thrombosis of the retinal veins. Ophthalmologica 141:467, 1961.
72. Kohner EM, Pettit JE, Hamilton AM, et al: Streptokinase in central retinal vein occlusion: A controlled clinical trial. Br Med J 1:550, 1976.
73. Gutman FA, Zegarra H: The natural course of temporal retinal branch vein occlusion. Trans Am Acad Ophthalmol Otolaryngol 78:OP178, 1974.
74. Blankenship GW, Okun E: Retinal tributary vein occlusion. Arch Ophthalmol 89:363, 1973.
75. Joffe L, Goldberg RE, Magargal LE, et al: Macular branch vein occlusion. Ophthalmology 87:91, 1980.
76. Seitz R (Blodi FC, translator): The crossing phenomenon. In The Retinal Vessels. St Louis, CV Mosby, 1964, pp 20–74.
77. Jensen VA: Clinical studies of tributary thrombosis in the central retinal vein. Acta Ophthalmol Suppl 10:1, 1936.
78. Weinberg D, Dodwell DG, Fern SA: Anatomy of arteriovenous crossings in branch retinal vein occlusion. Am J Ophthalmol 109:298, 1990.
79. Duker JS, Brown GC: Anterior location of the crossing artery in branch retinal vein occlusion. Arch Ophthalmol 107:998, 1989.
80. Rabinowicz IM, Litman S, Michaelson IC: Branch venous thrombosis—A pathological report. Trans Ophthalmol Soc UK 88:191, 1968.
81. Kohner EM, Dollery CT, Shakib M, et al: Experimental retinal branch vein occlusion. Am J Ophthalmol 69:778, 1970.
82. Hamilton AM, Marshall J, Kohner EM, et al: Retinal new vessel formation following experimental vein occlusion. Exp Eye Res 20:493, 1975.
83. Hamilton AM, Kohner EM, Rosen D, et al: Experimental retinal branch vein occlusion in rhesus monkeys. I. Clinical appearances. Br J Ophthalmol 63:377, 1979.
84. Hockley DJ, Tripathi RC, Ashton N: Experimental retinal branch vein occlusion in the monkey. Histopathological and ultrastructural studies. Trans Ophthalmol Soc UK 96:202, 1976.
85. Hockley DJ, Tripathi RC, Ashton N: Experimental retinal branch vein occlusion in rhesus monkeys. III. Histopathological and electron microscopical studies. Br J Ophthalmol 63:393, 1979.
86. Rosen DA, Marshall J, Kohner EM, et al: Experimental retinal branch vein occlusion in rhesus monkeys. II. Retinal blood flow studies. Br J Ophthalmol 63:388 1979.
87. Frangieh GT, Green WR, Barraquer-Somers E, et al: Histopathologic study of nine branch retinal vein occlusions. Arch Ophthalmol 100:1132, 1982.
88. Johnston RL, Brucker AJ, Steinmann W, et al: Risk factors of branch retinal vein occlusion. Arch Ophthalmol 103:1831, 1985.
89. Michels RG, Gass JDM: The natural course of retinal branch vein obstruction. Trans Am Acad Ophthalmol Otolaryngol 78:OP166, 1974.

90. Leber T: Die Krankheite der Netzhaut und des Sehnerven. *In* Graefe A, Saemich T (eds): Handbuch der Gesammten Augeheilkunde, Pathologie und Therapie. Leipzig, Verlag Von Wilhelm Engelmann, 1877, p 521.
91. Shilling JS, Kohner EM: New vessel formation in retinal branch vein occlusion. Br J Ophthalmol 60:810, 1976.
92. Appiah AP, Trempe CL: Risk factors associated with branch vs. central retinal vein occlusion. Ann Ophthalmol 21:153, 1989.
93. The Branch Vein Occlusion Study Group: Argon laser photocoagulation for macular edema in branch vein occlusion. Am J Ophthalmol 98:271, 1984.
94. The Branch Vein Occlusion Study Group: Argon laser scatter photocoagulation for prevention of neovascularization and vitreous hemorrhage in branch vein occlusion. Arch Ophthalmol 104:34, 1986.
95. Shilling JS: Vascular changes after retinal branch vein occlusion. Trans Ophthalmol Soc UK 96:193, 1976.
96. Clemett RS: Retinal branch vein occlusion. Changes at the site of obstruction. Br J Ophthalmol 58:548, 1974.
97. Gutman FA: Macular edema in branch retinal vein occlusion: Prognosis and management. Trans Am Acad Opthalmol Otolaryngol 83:OP488, 1977.
98. Brown GC, Kimmel AS, Magargal LE, et al: Progressive capillary nonperfusion in temporal branch retinal vein occlusion. Ann Ophthalmol 21:290, 1989.
99. Finkelstein D, Clarkson J, Diddie K, et al: Branch vein occlusion. Retinal neovascularization outside the involved segment. Ophthalmology 89:1357, 1982.
100. Magargal LE, Augsburger JJ, Hyman D, et al: Venous macroaneurysm following branch retinal vein obstruction. Ann Ophthalmol 12:685, 1980.
101. Sanborn GE, Magargal LE: Venous macroaneurysm associated with branch retinal vein obstruction. Ann Ophthalmol 16:464, 1984.
102. Joondeph HC, Joondeph BC: Posterior traction retinal breaks complicating branch retinal vein occlusion. Retina 8:136, 1988.
103. Joondeph HC, Goldberg MF: Rhegmatogenous retinal detachments after tributary retinal vein occlusion. Am J Ophthalmol 80:253, 1975.
104. Gutman FA, Zegarra H: Retinal detachment secondary to retinal branch vein occlusions. Trans Am Acad Ophthalmol Otolaryngol 81:OP491, 1976.
105. Regenbogen L, Godel V, Feiler-Ofrey V, et al: Retinal breaks secondary to vascular accidents. Am J Ophthalmol 84:187, 1977.
106. Ramos-Umpierre A, Berrocal JA: Retinal detachment following branch vein occlusion: Case report. Ann Ophthalmol 9:339, 1977.
107. Chess J, Eichen A: Rhegmatogenous retinal detachment associated with branch vein occlusion.
108. Schatz H, Yannuzzi L, Stransky TJ: Retinal detachment secondary to branch vein occlusion. Part I. Ann Ophthalmol 8:1437, 1976.
109. Schatz H, Yannuzzi L, Stransky TJ: Retinal detachment secondary to branch vein occlusion. Part II. Ann Ophthalmol 8:1461, 1976.
110. Wise GN, Wangvivat Y: The exaggerated macular response to retinal disease. Am J Ophthalmol 61:1359, 1966.
111. Flindall RJ: Photocoagulation in chronic cystoid macular edema secondary to branch vein occlusion. Can J Ophthalmol 7:395, 1972.
112. Gitter KA, Cohen G, Baber BW: Photocoagulation in venous occlusive disease. Am J Ophthalmol 79:578, 1975.
113. Campbell CJ, Wise GN: Photocoagulation therapy of branch vein obstructions. Am J Ophthalmol 75:28, 1973.
114. Wetzig PC: The treatment of acute branch retinal vein occlusion by photocoagulation. Am J Ophthalmol 87:65, 1979.
115. The Branch Vein Occlusion Study Group: Argon laser photocoagulation for macular edema in branch vein occlusion. Am J Ophthalmol 99:219, 1985.
116. Chopdar A: Dual trunk central retinal vein incidence in clinical practice. Arch Ophthalmol 102:85, 1984.
117. Hayreh SS, Hayreh MS: Hemi-central retinal vein occlusion. Pathogenesis, clinical features, and natural history. Arch Ophthalmol 98:1600, 1980.
118. Chopdar A: Hemi-central retinal vein occlusion. Pathogenesis, clinical features, natural history and incidence of dual trunk central retinal vein. Trans Ophthalmol Soc UK 102:241, 1982.
119. Appiah AP, Trempe CL: Differences in contributory factors among hemicentral, central, and branch retinal vein occlusions. Ophthalmology 96:364, 1989.
120. Rath EZ, Frank RN, Shin DH, et al: Risk factors for renal vein occlusions. A case-control study. Ophthalmology 99:509, 1992.

■

Chapter 55

Diagnosis, Management, and Treatment of Nonproliferative Diabetic Retinopathy and Macular Edema*

LLOYD M. AIELLO

SIGNIFICANCE OF APPROACHING AND REACHING HIGH-RISK PROLIFERATIVE DIABETIC RETINOPATHY AND CLINICALLY SIGNIFICANT MACULAR EDEMA

In 1967, the first evidence of the effectiveness of scatter (panretinal) laser photocoagulation surgery to treat diabetic retinopathy was promulgated in the ophthalmic and medical communities.[1] Since these promising beginnings, dramatic strides in controlling diabetic retinopathy and macular edema have been made through the effective use of scatter (panretinal) laser and other surgical techniques, a fact strongly supported by the findings of three major nationwide randomized controlled clinical trials—the Diabetic Retinopathy Study (DRS),[2–15] the Early Treatment Diabetic Retinopathy Study (ETDRS),[16–28] and the Diabetic Retinopathy Vitrectomy Study (DRVS).[29–33] Scientists can now offer the hope that proper diagnosis and treatment can virtually eliminate the 5-yr risk of severe visual loss from proliferative diabetic retinopathy (PDR) by the year 2000 for the 7 million Americans who have been diagnosed with diabetes mellitus.

Nevertheless, diabetic retinopathy remains a leading cause of blindness in the United States for citizens between the ages of 20 and 74 yr. This blindness usually results from nonresolving vitreous hemorrhage, traction retinal detachment, or diabetic macular edema. However, the 5-yr risk of *severe visual loss* (SVL)† can be reduced to less than 5 percent if a person with diabetic retinopathy approaching or just reaching high-risk proliferative retinopathy (as defined further on), undergoes scatter (panretinal) laser photocoagulation surgery. Furthermore, people with *clinically significant diabetic macular edema* (CSME) can have the risk of *moderate visual loss* (MVL) reduced to approximately 12 percent or less if they undergo appropriate focal laser surgery. Since

diabetic retinopathy is often asymptomatic in its most treatable stages, its early detection through regularly scheduled ocular examinations becomes critical.

This chapter reviews the prognostic implications of the lesions of diabetic retinopathy and the risks of progression, with particular emphasis on identifying patients at risk of visual loss and in need of laser surgery. The laser treatment techniques are only generally described in this chapter but are carefully detailed in ETDRS Reports Nos. 3 and 4.[18, 19]

EPIDEMIOLOGY OF DIABETIC RETINOPATHY

An estimated 14 million Americans have diabetes mellitus, but only half of these cases have been diagnosed.[34, 35] Ten to 15 percent of the diabetic population has insulin-dependent diabetes mellitus (IDDM; type I), which is usually diagnosed before the age of 40 yr. The majority of diabetic patients, however, have non–insulin-dependent diabetes mellitus (NIDDM; type II), which is usually diagnosed after the age of 40 yr. These patients may or may not be treated with insulin. Al-

Table 55–1. ABBREVIATIONS AND DEFINITIONS

PDR	Proliferative diabetic retinopathy
NPDR	Nonproliferative diabetic retinopathy
H/Ma	Hemorrhages or microaneurysms, or both
HE	Hard exudates
SE (CWS)	Soft exudates (cotton-wool spots)
VB	Venous beading
IRMA	Intraretinal microvascular abnormality
NVD	New vessels on or witihin 1 disc diameter of disc margin
NVE	New vessels elsewhere in the retina outside of disc and 1 disc diameter from disc margin
FPD	Fibrous proliferations on or within 1 disc diameter of disc margin
FPE	Fibrous proliferations elsewhere, not FPD
SVL	Severe visual loss: Visual acuity ≤5/200 at two consecutive completed 4-mo follow-up visits
MVL	Moderate visual loss: A doubling of the visual angle (e.g., 20/40 to 20/80 at two consecutive completed 4-mo follow-up visits)
CSME	Clinically significant macular edema

---

*The Early Treatment Diabetic Retinopathy Study (ETDRS) Reports[16–28] form the basis of this chapter, are widely quoted and paraphrased, and set the standards of care for patients with diabetic retinopathy.

†Italicized terms and abbreviations are defined in Tables 55–1 and 55–7.

though those with type I diabetes mellitus experience a high incidence of severe ocular complications and are more likely to have significant ocular problems during their lifetimes, those with type II diabetes mellitus make up the majority of clinical cases with diabetic eye disease because of their overall larger numbers.

Diabetic retinopathy is a highly specific vascular complication of both type I and type II diabetes mellitus, and the duration of diabetes is a significant risk factor for the development of retinopathy. After 20 yr of diabetes, nearly all patients with IDDM, and more than 60 percent of patients with NIDDM, have some degree of retinopathy. Although at present there is no known cure for diabetic retinopathy and diabetic macular edema, and no known means to prevent these conditions from occurring, laser surgery and other surgical modalities help minimize the risk of MVL and SVL from these conditions and, in some cases, restore useful vision for those who have suffered visual loss. These surgical modalities, particularly laser treatment, are most effective when initiated at the time a person *approaches* or just reaches *high-risk PDR* or before visual acuity is lost from diabetic macular edema.[24]

The 5-yr risk of SVL from high-risk PDR may be as high as 60 percent, and the risk of MVL from CSME may be as high as 25 to 30 percent. Since PDR and CSME may cause no ocular or visual symptoms when the retinal lesions are most amenable to treatment, the responsibility is to identify eyes at risk of visual loss and ensure that the patients receive referral for laser surgery at the most appropriate time. Even minor errors in diagnosing the level of retinopathy (see Table 55–8) can result in a significant increase in a person's risk of visual loss.

Furthermore, collateral health and medical problems present a significant risk for the development and progression of diabetic retinopathy (Table 55–2). These factors include pregnancy,[36–38] chronic hyperglycemia,[39–42] hypertension,[43] renal disease,[41] and hyperlipidemia.[44] Patients with these conditions require careful medical evaluation and follow-up for the progression of diabetic retinopathy.

CLINICAL TRIALS

Three nationwide randomized clinical trials have largely determined the strategies for appropriate clinical management of patients with diabetic retinopathy.

The DRS (Table 55–3) conclusively demonstrated that scatter (panretinal) photocoagulation significantly reduces the risk of SVL from PDR, particularly when high-risk PDR is present.

The ETDRS provided valuable information concerning the timing of scatter (panretinal) laser surgery for advancing diabetic retinopathy and conclusively demonstrated that focal photocoagulation for CSME reduces the risk of MVL by 50 percent or more (Table 55–4).

Furthermore, the ETDRS demonstrated that both early scatter (panretinal) laser surgery (before the onset of high-risk PDR) and deferral of treatment "until and

Table 55–2. MEDICAL COMPLICATIONS

Condition	Comment
Risk Indicators of Diabetic Retinopathy	
Joint contractures	Association of retinopathy and contractures has been established. Eye examination is indicated. Care of joint contractures is important.
Neuropathy	Peripheral neuropathy may result in difficulty handling contact lenses. Neuropathy in lower extremities may alter mobility in such a way that restoration and maintenance of as much vision as possible is important.
Conditions That May Affect the Course of Diabetic Retinopathy	
Hypertension	Appropriate medical treatment is indicated for prevention of cardiovascular disease, stroke, and death. Hypertension itself may result in hypertensive retinopathy superimposed on diabetic retinopathy.
Elevated triglycerides and lipids	Appropriate management to normalize is important. Proper diet and reduced levels may result in less retinal vessel leakage.
Proteinuria; elevated creatinine	Aggressive management of renal disease is indicated to avoid renal retinopathy, which may increase risk of progression of diabetic retinopathy.
Cardiovascular disease	Increased risk of cardiac disease, particularly coronary vascular disease, is often associated with an increase in the attenuation and arteriosclerotic closure of the arterial system of the retina. A decreased risk of hemorrhage into the vitreous may result, but there also may be a decrease in retinal function with associated decrease in vision. Management of cardiovascular disease may help relieve some of the ischemic process in the retina. Aggressive cardiovascular management is important.
Clinical trials	There are no clinical trials that have specifically shown that control of systemic conditions that may affect the eyes (the four previous entries) prevents the progression of diabetic retinopathy. However, clinical experience suggests an association with the systemic benefits of appropriate treatment of these problems.

as soon as high-risk PDR developed are effective in reducing the risk of SVL." Scatter laser surgery, therefore, should be considered as an eye approaches the high-risk stage and "usually should not be delayed if the eye has reached the high-risk proliferative stage."[24]

The DRVS provided guidelines for the most opportune time to consider vitrectomy surgery for patients with type I and type II diabetes mellitus and vitreous hemorrhage (Table 55–5)[29, 30, 33] or severe PDR in eyes with useful vision (Table 55–5).[31, 32] Early vitrectomy

Table 55–3. DIABETIC RETINOPATHY STUDY

Major Eligibility Criteria
1. Visual acuity ≥20/100 in each eye.
2. PDR in at least one eye or severe NPDR in both.
3. Both eyes suitable for photocoagulation.

Major Design Features
1. One eye of each patient was assigned randomly to photocoagulation (scatter [panretinal], local [direct confluent treatment of surface new vessels], and focal [for macular edema] as appropriate). The other eye was assigned to follow-up without photocoagulation.
2. The eye assigned to treatment was then randomly assigned to argon laser or xenon arc photocoagulation.

Major Conclusions
1. Photocoagulation reduced risk of severe visual loss by 50% or more. (SVL = VA* <5/200 at two consecutively completed 4-mo follow-up visits.)
2. Modest risks of decrease in visual acuity (usually only 1 line) and visual field (risks greater with xenon than argon photocoagulation).
3. Treatment benefit outweighs risks for eyes with high-risk PDR (50% 5-yr rate of SVL in such eyes without treatment was reduced to 20% by treatment).

Prepared by M. Davis, M.D., and the ETDRS Research Group for the American Academy of Ophthalmology Diabetes 2000 Program.
*VA, visual acuity.

for eyes with recent severe vitreous hemorrhage and visual acuity less than 5/200 was beneficial, especially for patients with type I diabetes mellitus. Furthermore, the chance of achieving visual acuity of 10/20 or better increased when early vitrectomy was performed in eyes with severe new vessels, again, especially for patients with type I diabetes mellitus.

Table 55–4. EARLY TREATMENT DIABETIC RETINOPATHY STUDY

Major Eligibility Criteria
1. Visual acuity ≥20/40 (≥20/400 if reduction caused by macular edema).
2. Mild NPDR to non–high-risk PDR, with or without macular edema.
3. Both eyes suitable for photocoagulation.

Major Design Features
1. One eye of each patient assigned randomly to early photocoagulation and the other to deferral (careful follow-up and photocoagulation if high-risk PDR develops).
2. Patients assigned randomly to aspirin or placebo.

Major Conclusions
1. Focal photocoagulation (direct laser for focal leaks and grid laser for diffuse leaks) reduced the risk of moderate visual loss (doubling of the visual angle) by 50% or more and increased the chance of a small improvement in visual acuity.
2. Both early scatter with or without focal photocoagulation and deferral were followed by low rates of severe visual loss (5-yr rates in deferral subgroups were 2–10%; in early photocoagulation groups these rates were 2–6%).
3. Focal photocoagulation should be considered for eyes with CSME.
4. Scatter photocoagulation is not indicated for mild to moderate NPDR but should be considered as retinopathy approaches the high-risk stage and usually should not be delayed when the high-risk stage is present.

Prepared by M. Davis, M.D., and the ETDRS Research Group for the American Academy of Ophthalmology Diabetes 2000 Program.

Table 55–5. DIABETIC RETINOPATHY VITRECTOMY STUDY

Group H—Recent Severe Vitreous Hemorrhage

Major Eligibility Criteria
1. VA* ≤ 5/200.
2. VH† consistent with VA, duration 1–6 mo.
3. Macula attached by ultrasound.

Major Design Features
1. In most patients, only one eye is eligible.
2. Eligible eye or eyes assigned randomly to early vitrectomy or conventional management (vitrectomy if center of macula detaches or if VH persists for 1 yr, photocoagulation as needed and as possible).

Major Conclusions
1. Chance of recovery of VA ≥10/20 increased by early vitrectomy, at least in patients with type 1 diabetes, who were younger and had more severe PDR (in most severe PDR group, ≥10/20 at 4 yr in 50% of early vitrectomy group versus 12% in conventional management group).

Group NR—Very Severe PDR With Useful Vision

Major Eligibility Criteria
1. VA ≥10/200.
2. Center of macula attached.
3. Extensive, active, neovascular, or fibrovascular proliferations.

Major Design Features
1. Same as group H (except conventional management included vitrectomy after a 6-mo waiting period in eyes that developed severe VH).

Major Conclusions
1. Chance of VA ≥10/20 increased by early vitrectomy, at least for eyes with very severe new vessels.

Prepared by M. Davis, M.D., and the ETDRS Research Group for American Academy of Ophthalmology Diabetes 2000 Program.
*VA, visual acuity.
†VH, vitreous hemorrhage.

DIAGNOSIS, CLASSIFICATION, AND MANAGEMENT OF DIABETIC RETINOPATHY

Retinal Lesions

Various retinal lesions identify the risk of progression of retinopathy and visual loss (Table 55–6).

The first clinical signs of diabetic retinopathy are *microaneurysms*, which are saccular outpouchings of retinal capillaries (Fig. 55–1). Ruptured microaneurysms, decompensated capillaries, and intraretinal microvascular abnormalities result in *intraretinal hemorrhages*. The clinical appearance of these hemorrhages reflects the retinal architecture of the retinal level at which the hemorrhage occurs. Hemorrhages in the nerve fiber layer assume a more flame-shaped appearance, coinciding with the structure of the nerve fiber layer that runs parallel to the retinal surface. Hemorrhages deeper in the retina, at which point the arrangement of cells is more or less perpendicular to the surface of the retina, assume a pinpoint or dot shape.

Intraretinal microvascular abnormalities (IRMAs) (Fig. 55–2) represent either new vessel growth within the retina or, more likely, preexisting vessels with endothelial cell proliferation that become "shunts" through

Table 55–6. PDR AT 1-YR VISIT BY SEVERITY OF INDIVIDUAL LESION

Lesion	Grade	PDR in 1 Yr (%)
HMA	Present in 2–5 fields	9
	Very severe	57
IRMA	None	9
	Moderate in 2–5 fields	57
VB	Lacking	15
	Present in 2–5 fields	59

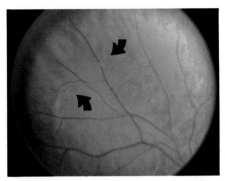

Figure 55–2. Standard photograph No. 8A of the Modified Airlee House Classification of Diabetic Retinopathy demonstrating intraretinal microvascular abnormalities (IRMAs) *(arrows)*. (Courtesy of the ETDRS.)

areas of nonperfusion. IRMAs may be seen adjacent to cotton-wool spots. Multiple IRMAs mark a severe stage of nonproliferative retinopathy, and frank neovascularization is likely to appear on the surface of the retina or optic disc within a short time.

Venous caliber abnormalities (Fig. 55–3) are indicators of severe retinal hypoxia. These abnormalities can be venous dilatation, venous beading, or loop formation. There are large areas of nonperfusion adjacent to the veins. Treatment with scatter (panretinal) photocoagulation may cause these abnormal veins to become less dilated and more regular.

Proliferative retinopathy (Fig. 55–4) is marked by proliferating endothelial cell tubules. The rate of growth of these new vessels is variable. They grow either at or near the optic disc *(neovascularization of the disc [NVD])* or elsewhere in the retina *(neovascularization elsewhere [NVE])*. Translucent fibrous tissue often appears adjacent to the new vessels. This fibroglial tissue appears opaque and becomes adherent to the adjacent vitreous.

Patients with *high-risk PDR* require immediate scatter laser photocoagulation. High-risk PDR is characterized by one or more of the following lesions:

- NVD that is approximately one-quarter to one-third disc area or more in size (i.e., greater than or equal to NVD in standard photograph No. 10A) (Fig. 55–4);
- NVD less than one-quarter disc area in size if fresh vitreous or preretinal hemorrhage is present;

- NVE greater than or equal to one-half disc area in size if fresh vitreous or preretinal hemorrhage is present (Fig. 55–5).

Therefore, attention must be paid to the presence or lack of new vessels, the location of new vessels, the severity of new vessels, and the presence or lack of preretinal or vitreous hemorrhages.[4]

Levels of Diabetic Retinopathy: Nonproliferative Diabetic Retinopathy and Early PDR

It is crucial to consider scatter (panretinal) laser surgery as retinopathy approaches or reaches the high-risk stage of proliferative retinopathy. An eye is considered to be *approaching the high-risk stage* when there are retinal signs of severe or very severe nonproliferative diabetic retinopathy (NPDR), with or without new vessels, or extensive new vessels, not quite fulfilling the definition of high-risk retinopathy associated with any level of NPDR. The baseline level of retinopathy indicates the risk of progression from the NPDR stage to early PDR and to high-risk PDR (Tables 55–7 to 55–9).

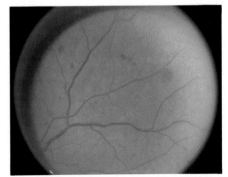

Figure 55–1. Standard photograph No. 2A of the Modified Airlee House Classification of Diabetic Retinopathy demonstrating a moderate degree of hemorrhage or microaneurysms, or both. (Courtesy of the Early Treatment Diabetic Retinopathy Study [ETDRS].)

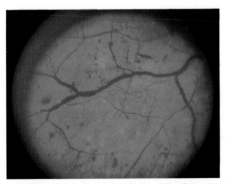

Figure 55–3. Standard photograph No. 6B of the Modified Airlee House Classification of Diabetic Retinopathy demonstrating venous beading. (Courtesy of the ETDRS.)

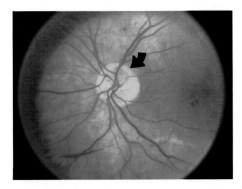

Figure 55–4. Standard photograph No. 10A of the Modified Airlee House Classification of Diabetic Retinopathy demonstrating neovascularization of the optic disc (NVD) *(arrows)*, covering approximately one quarter to one third of the disc area. (Courtesy of the ETDRS.)

NPDR LEVELS

Diabetic retinopathy is broadly classified as NPDR and PDR. Diabetic macular edema can occur with either NPDR or PDR and is discussed separately. Accurate diagnosis of a patient's "diabetic retinopathy level" is critical because there is a varying risk of progression to PDR and high-risk PDR depending on the specific NPDR level (Fig. 55–6; see also Table 55–8).

Mild NPDR is marked by at least one retinal microaneurysm, but hemorrhages and microaneurysms are less than those in ETDRS standard photograph No. 2A (see Fig. 55–1 and Table 55–7). No other retinal lesion or abnormality associated with diabetes is present. Those with mild NPDR have a 5 percent risk of progression to PDR within 1 yr and a 15 percent risk of progression to high-risk PDR within 5 yr (see Table 55–8).

Moderate NPDR (see Table 55–7) is characterized by hemorrhages or microaneurysms, or both (H/Ma), greater than those pictured in ETDRS standard photograph No. 2A. Soft exudates, venous beading, and IRMAs are definitely present to a mild degree. The risk of progression to PDR within 1 yr is 12 to 27 percent, and the risk of progression to high-risk PDR within 5 yr is 33 percent (see Table 55–8).

Table 55–7. LEVELS OF RETINOPATHY

NPDR

A. Mild NPDR
   At least one microaneurysm
   Definition not met for B, C, D, E, F
B. Moderate NPDR
   > standard photograph No. 2A (Fig. 55–1)
   Soft exudates, VB, and IRMAs definitely present
   Definition not met for C, D, E. F
C. Severe NPDR
   H/Ma > standard photograph No. 2A (Fig. 55–1) in all 4 quadrants
   VB in 2 or more quadrants (Fig. 55–3)
   IRMA > standard photograph No. 8A in at least 1 quadrant (Fig. 55–2)
D. Very Severe NPDR
   Any two or more of C.
   Definition not met for E, F.

PDR

(Composed of: [1] NVD or NVE, [2] preretinal or vitreous hemorrhage, [3] fibrous tissue proliferation)

E. Early PDR
   New vessels
   Definition not met for F
F. High-risk PDR
   NVD ≥1/3–1/2 disc area (Fig. 55–4) *or*
   NVD and vitreous or preretinal hemorrhage *or*
   NVE ≥1/2 disc area and preretinal or vitreous hemorrhage (Fig. 55–5)

CSME

1. Thickening of the retina located ≤500 μ from the center of the macula *or*
2. Hard exudates with thickening of the adjacent retina located ≤500 μ from the center of the macula *or*
3. A zone of retinal thickening, 1 disc area or larger in size located ≤1 disc diameter from the center of the macula.

Patients with mild or moderate NPDR generally are not candidates for scatter (panretinal) laser surgery and can be followed safely at 6- to 12-mo intervals as determined by the examiner. The presence of macular edema, even with mild or moderate degrees of NPDR, requires follow-up in a shorter period, and if CSME is

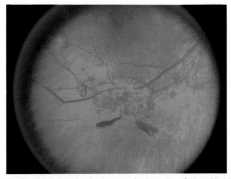

Figure 55–5. Standard photograph No. 7 of the Modified Airlie House Classification of Diabetic Retinopathy demonstrating neovascularization elsewhere (NVE) in the retina greater than one half disc diameter with a fresh hemorrhage present. (Courtesy of the ETDRS.)

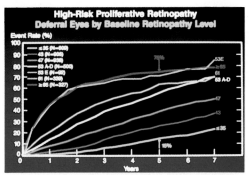

Figure 55–6. Life table cumulative event rates of high-risk proliferative retinopathy by level of retinopathy severity scale at baseline in eyes assigned to deferral of photocoagulation in the ETDRS. Level ≤35, mild nonproliferative diabetic retinopathy (NPDR); level 43, moderate NPDR; level 47, moderate to severe NPDR; level 53A–D, severe NPDR; level 53E, very severe NPDR; level 61, early proliferative diabetic retinopathy (PDR); level 65, PDR < high-risk PDR.[27] (Courtesy of the ETDRS.)

Table 55–8. GENERAL MANAGEMENT RECOMMENDATIONS

	Natural Course		Evaluation		Treatment Strategies		
	Rate of Progression to:		Color Fundus				Follow-up
Level of Retinopathy	PDR 1 Yr	HRC* 5 Yr	Photograph	FA†	PRP‡	Focal	(mos)
Mild NPDR	5%	15%					
No macular edema			No	No	No	No	12
Macular edema			Yes	Occasionally	No	No	4–6
CSME			Yes	Yes	No	Yes	2–4
Moderate NPDR	12–27%	33%					
No macular edema			Yes	No	No	No	6–8
Macular edema (not CSME)			Yes	Occasionally	No	No	4–6
CSME			Yes	Yes	No	Yes	2–4
Severe NPDR	52%	60%					
No macular edema			Yes	No	Rarely	No	3–4
Macular edema (not CSME)			Yes	Occasionally	Occasionally after focal	Occasionally	2–3
CSME			Yes	Yes	Occasionally after focal	Yes	2–3
Very severe NPDR	75%	75%					
No macular edema			Yes	No	Occasionally	No	2–3
Macular edema (not CSME)			Yes	Occasionally	Occasionally after focal	Occasionally	2–3
CSME			Yes	Yes	Occasionally after focal	Yes	2–3
Non–high-risk PDR		75%					
No macular edema			Yes	No	Occasionally	No	2–3
Macular edema (not CSME)			Yes	Occasionally	Occasionally after focal	Occasionally	2–3
CSME			Yes	Yes	Occasionally after focal	Yes	2–3
High-risk PDR							
No macular edema			Yes	No	Yes	No	2–3
Macular edema			Yes	Yes	Yes	Usually	1–2
CSME			Yes	Yes	Yes	Yes	1–2

*HRC, high-risk characteristic proliferative retinopathy.
†FA, fluorescein angiography.
‡PRP, proliferative retinopathy photocoagulation.

present, focal laser treatment is advisable (see Table 55–8). Coincident medical problems or pregnancy will influence the period of reevaluation.

Severe NPDR, based on the severity of H/Ma, IRMAs, and venous beading, is characterized by any one of the following lesions (see Table 55–7):

- H/Ma > standard photograph No. 2A (see Fig. 55–1) in four quadrants *or*
- Venous beading (see Fig. 55–3) in two or more quadrants *or*
- IRMAs > standard photograph No. 8A (see Fig. 55–2) in at least one quadrant

Eyes with severe NPDR have a 52 percent risk of developing PDR within 1 yr and a 60 percent risk of developing high-risk PDR within 5 yr. These patients require follow-up evaluation in 2 to 4 mo. Treatment of CSME is strongly indicated because of the risk of the development of PDR and high-risk PDR, and some eyes with macular edema, even if not clinically significant, may require focal treatment in preparation for impending scatter (panretinal) laser surgery, which may also be indicated as determined by the clinical judgment of the retinal specialist (see Table 55–8).

Eyes with *very severe NPDR* (see Table 55–7) have two or more lesions of severe NPDR but no frank neovascularization. There is a 75 percent risk of developing PDR within 1 yr. Patients with very severe NPDR may be candidates for scatter (panretinal) laser surgery, and macular edema, if present, may require treatment. Very close follow-up evaluation at 2- to 3-mo intervals is important (see Table 55–8).

EARLY PDR LEVEL

Diabetic retinopathy marked by new vessel growth on the optic disc (NVD) or elsewhere (NVE) on the retina

Table 55–9. COMPLICATIONS AND SIDE EFFECTS OF SCATTER (PANRETINAL) LASER PHOTOCOAGULATION

Field constriction and nyctalopia
  Depends upon extent and intensity of scatter laser burns
Foveal burn
  Identify landmarks prior to treatment
Macular edema
  May result in permanent decrease in visual acuity
Foveal traction
  Do not treat over blood
  Avoid puncture of Bruch's membrane
Serous or choroidal detachment
  Acute angle-closure glaucoma is possible
Anterior segment
  Posterior synechiae
  Cornea and lens burns
  Internal ophthalmoplegia
  Less frequent with multiple sessions and light to moderately
    intense burns
Pain
  Peripheral retina—more painful
  Use retrobulbar anesthesia as needed
  Reassurance
Retrobulbar hemorrhage
  Continue with treatment
  Watch central retinal artery
  Retrobulbar anesthesia required infrequently
Hypoglycemia
  Anxiety, pain, upright → shock, seizure
Loss of follow-up may result from
  Pain
  Retrobulbar hemorrhage
  Intercurrent illness
  Lack of caring explanation
  Lack of persistent rescheduling

or by fibrous tissue proliferation is designated PDR. *Early PDR* does not meet the definition of high-risk PDR (see Table 55–7). Eyes with early PDR (less than high-risk PDR) have a 75 percent risk of developing high-risk PDR within a 5-yr period. These eyes may require scatter (panretinal) laser surgery, and macular edema, even if not clinically significant, may benefit from focal treatment before scatter treatment is initiated (see Table 55–8).

Patients with *severe* and *very severe NPDR* and *early PDR* (less than high-risk PDR) should be considered for early scatter (panretinal) laser surgery, particularly if there are new vessels in the presence of severe or very severe NPDR, elevated new vessels, or NVD. In the presence of macular edema, patients with severe NPDR or worse should be considered for focal treatment of macular edema, whether the macular edema is clinically significant or not, in preparation for the impending need of scatter laser photocoagulation (see Table 55–8).

Role of Clinical Fluorescein Angiography in the Management of Diabetic Retinopathy

Fluorescein angiography of the macula in the presence of CSME is fundamental for the detection of treatable lesions, as described further on. However, its use to identify lesions such as NVE or feeder vessels on NVD

is not necessary because scatter (panretinal) laser surgery is the method of choice for the treatment of diabetic retinopathy as it approaches or reaches the high-risk stage.

Angiographic risk factors for progression of NPDR to PDR have been identified.[26, 28] Analysis of data from the untreated (deferred) eyes in the ETDRS indicates that the following lesions are independently related to outcome: (1) fluorescein leakage, (2) capillary loss on fluorescein angiography, (3) capillary dilatation on fluorescein angiography, and (4) these color fundus photographic risk factors: IRMAs, venous beading, and H/Ma. Hard and soft exudates have an inverse relationship to progression. It is widely accepted that capillary loss as documented on fluoroscein angiography is a risk factor for progression of NPDR to PDR.[26, 28, 45–47] However, capillary dilatation on fluorescein angiography, fluorescein leakage, and capillary loss on fluorescein angiography, and the ETDRS color fundus photographic retinopathy severity levels are all closely correlated. Although the fluorescein angiography abnormalities provide additional prognostic information, the color fundus photographic gradings of retinopathy levels of both eyes give the same prognostic results.[27, 28] Therefore, the increase in power to predict progression from NPDR to PDR by fluorescein angiography is "not of significant clinical importance to warrant routine FA."[28]

Periodic follow-up retinal examinations, however, are necessary. The appropriate interval can be determined by skillful grading of seven standard field stereo color fundus photographs or by retinal examination by an ophthalmologist experienced in the management of diabetic eye disease. Because the retinal level of diabetic retinopathy derived from color fundus photography is predictive enough to establish frequency of follow-up, because fluorescein angiography classification cannot identify all cases destined to progress, and because initiation of scatter (panretinal) laser photocoagulation should be considered as diabetic retinopathy approaches (before or just as it reaches) the high-risk stage, "periodic follow-up of all patients with diabetic retinopathy continues to be of fundamental clinical importance."[28]

Diabetic Macular Edema

Diabetic macular edema may be present at any level of retinopathy (see Table 55–8) and alters the structure of the macula in any of these manners, significantly affecting its function:

- Macular edema, i.e., a collection of intraretinal fluid in the macula with or without lipid exudates and with or without cystoid changes;
- Nonperfusion of parafoveal capillaries with or without intraretinal fluid;
- Traction in the macula by fibrous tissue proliferation causing dragging of the retinal tissue, surface wrinkling, or detachment of the macula;
- Intraretinal or preretinal hemorrhage in the macula;
- Lamellar or full-thickness retinal hole formation;
- Any combination of the preceding.

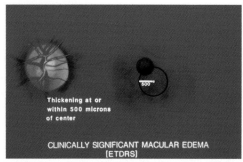

Figure 55–7. Schematic representation of clinically significant macular edema (CSME), with thickening of the macula less than 500 μ from the center of the macula. (Courtesy of Robert Murphy, M.D.)

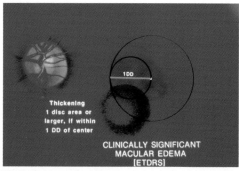

Figure 55–9. Schematic representation of area of thickening, 1 disc diameter in size, part of which is within 1 disc diameter of the center of the macula. (Courtesy of Robert Murphy, M.D.)

Clinically, *macular edema* is retinal thickening within 2 disc diameters of the center of the macula (*not* fluorescein leakage without thickening). Retinal thickening or hard exudates with adjacent retinal thickening that threatens or involves the center of the macula is considered to be clinically significant. CSME as defined by the ETDRS includes any *one* of these lesions (see Table 55–7):

- Retinal thickening at or within 500 μ of the center of the macula (Fig. 55–7); *or*
- Hard exudates at or within 500 μ of the center of the macula, if there is thickening of the adjacent retina (Fig. 55–8); *or*

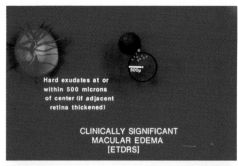

A

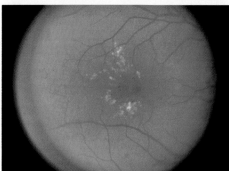

B

Figure 55–8. *A,* Schematic representation of CSME with hard exudates at or within 500 μ of the center of the macula, with thickening of the retina adjacent to the exudates. (Courtesy of Robert Murphy, M.D.) *B,* Clinical appearance of hard exudates less than 500 μ from the center of the macula. There is thickening of the adjacent retina, which is not appreciated without stereoscopic observation. (Courtesy of the ETDRS.)

- An area or areas of retinal thickening at least 1 disc area in size, at least part of which is within 1 disc diameter of the center of the macula (Figs. 55–9 and 55–10).

There are particular retinal lesions identified on fluorescein angiography that are amenable to treatment. The "treatable lesions" associated with macular edema include:

- Focal leaks >500 μ from the center of the macula thought to be causing retinal thickening or hard exudates (Fig. 55–11);
- Focal leaks 300 to 500 μ from the center of the macula thought to be causing retinal thickening or hard exudates if the treating ophthalmologist does not believe that treatment is likely to destroy the remaining perifoveal capillary network (Fig. 55–11);
- Areas of diffuse leakage that have not been treated previously (Fig. 55–12); *or*
- Avascular zones, other than the normal foveal avascular zone, not previously treated (Fig. 55–12*B*)

Focal laser surgery for CSME consists of either direct laser treatment, grid laser treatment, or a combination of direct focal laser and grid laser treatment. These treatment methods are described in detail elsewhere.[17, 19]

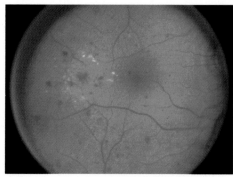

Figure 55–10. Clinical photograph showing macular edema greater than 500 μ from the center of the macula (the edema is not appreciated without stereoscopic evaluation). (Courtesy of the ETDRS.)

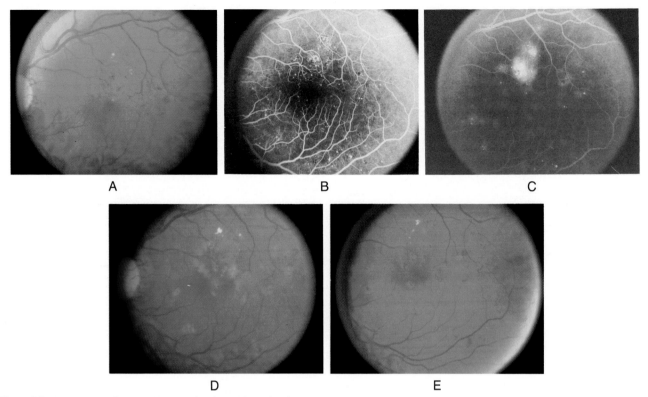

Figure 55–11. *A,* There is a small area of retinal thickening just above the center of the macula (poorly appreciated without stereopsis), which is detectable monocularly because of blurring of the choroidal pattern. Several microaneurysms are visible within the thickened area. There is a little hard exudate around the edges of the edematous patch, some of which extends almost to the center of the macula. Thickening extends to within 500 μ of the center of the macula (clinically significant macular edema). Visual acuity is 20/15. *B,* In the 17- to 18-sec phase of the fluorescein angiogram, microaneurysms and slightly dilated capillaries are visible in the area of thickening. *C,* The 7-min phase of the angiogram shows leakage into the retina from the two groups of microaneurysms noted in *B. D,* Treatment has been applied to most of the microaneurysms. *E,* Four months later, the appearance of the retina is satisfactory: The center of the macula is flat and most of the thickening noted before treatment has disappeared. Visual acuity remains at 20/15. (*A–E,* Courtesy of the ETDRS.)

Table 55–8 summarizes the management recommendations for CSME at the various retinopathy levels.

LASER PHOTOCOAGULATION

Timing of Photocoagulation

The 3-yr risk of MVL from macular edema in the ETDRS without focal laser treatment was 30 percent. Focal laser surgery for CSME reduced this risk to 15 percent,[16] amounting to a reduction in the risk of moderate visual loss of approximately 50 percent. Focal treatment also increased the chance of improvement in visual acuity of 1 line or more. Conversely, scatter (panretinal) laser surgery was not effective in managing diabetic macular edema and in some cases may have had a deleterious effect on the progression of macular edema.

Eyes with CSME and retinopathy that is approaching high-risk PDR are best treated first with focal photocoagulation for the macular edema 6 to 8 wk before initiating scatter (panretinal) laser surgery. Eyes with mild or moderate NPDR and CSME respond best to prompt focal photocoagulation, with scatter treatment delayed unless very severe NPDR or high-risk PDR occurs. Delaying scatter photocoagulation while focal treatment is being completed is unlikely to increase the risk of SVL provided that the retinopathy is not progressing rapidly and careful follow-up can be maintained. Delaying scatter photocoagulation while focal treatment is completed in eyes with high-risk PDR usually is not advisable.

Focal treatment is not attended by adverse effects on central visual field or color vision when eyes so treated were compared with eyes assigned to deferral of focal treatment.[17] Any harmful effects of early photocoagulation reflected by constriction of the peripheral visual fields seem to be mostly due to scatter photocoagulation. Because the principal benefit of treatment is to prevent a further decrease in visual acuity, focal laser surgery should be considered in all eyes with CSME, especially if the center of the macula is threatened or involved, even if normal visual acuity is present.

The DRS had demonstrated in 1976 that scatter (panretinal) photocoagulation was effective in reducing the risk of severe visual loss from high-risk PDR. One question of concern for the ETDRS was whether earlier

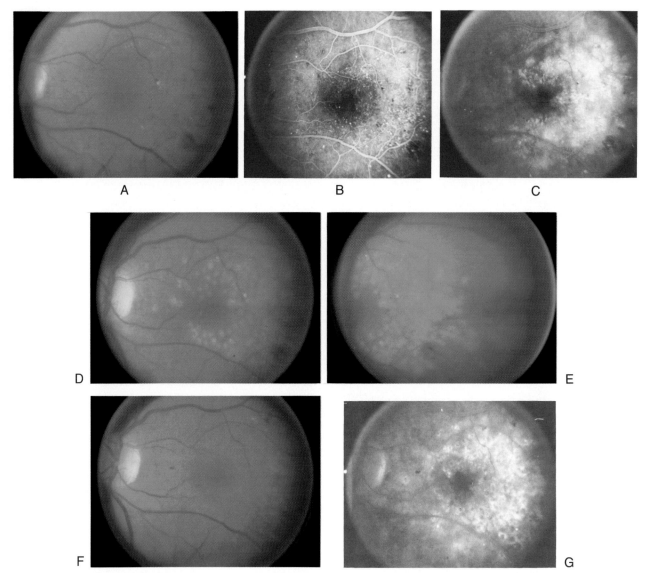

Figure 55–12. *A,* Clinical photograph showing retinal thickening temporal to the center of the macula extending just to the center. Visual acuity is 20/40+3. *B,* Early phase of the angiogram shows capillary loss adjacent to the foveal avascular zone, capillary dilatation, and scattered microaneurysms. *C,* The 7-min phase of the angiogram shows extensive small cystoid spaces temporal to the center of the macula and above and below it. The center appears uninvolved. *D,* The microaneurysms have been treated focally. In addition, laser burns have been applied in a grid pattern to the areas of diffuse leakage. *E,* The temporal extent of the grid laser treatment. *F,* Four months later, hemorrhages and hard exudates have decreased, and the retinal thickening can no longer be detected. Visual acuity is 20/25. *G,* The 7-min phase of the angiogram showing disappearance of most of the cystoid spaces visible in *C.* (*A–G,* Courtesy of the ETDRS.)

scatter photocoagulation, before the development of high-risk PDR, justified the side effects and risks of laser surgery (see Table 55–9), since the DRS did not provide a clear choice between prompt treatment and deferral of treatment unless there was progression to high-risk PDR.

In the ETDRS, early treatment, compared with deferral of photocoagulation until high-risk PDR develops,[22] was associated with a small reduction in the incidence of SVL, but 5-yr rates of SVL were low for both the early treatment group and the group assigned to deferral of treatment (2.6 percent and 3.7 percent, respectively). Provided careful follow-up can be maintained, scatter laser surgery is *not* recommended for

eyes with mild or moderate NPDR.[24] When retinopathy is more severe (i.e., severe or very severe NPDR and early PDR), scatter photocoagulation should be "considered and usually should not be delayed if the eye has reached the high-risk proliferative stage."[24]

As retinopathy approaches the high-risk stage (very severe NPDR or early PDR), the benefits and risks of early photocoagulation may be roughly balanced; the benefit of a reduction of the risk of SVL from early photocoagulation may be more important in an eye that has almost a 50 percent risk of reaching a high-risk stage within 1 yr. Initiating scatter photocoagulation early in at least one eye seems particularly appropriate when both eyes are approaching the high-risk stage, because optimal timing of photocoagulation may be difficult if both eyes need photocoagulation simultaneously. Also, prompt scatter photocoagulation should be considered for eyes with neovascularization in the anterior chamber angle, whether or not high-risk proliferative retinopathy is present.

Treatment Program

Table 55–8 presents the treatment program for diabetic retinopathy, which consists of:

- Initial scatter laser photocoagulation treatment as the diabetic retinopathy approaches or reaches the high-risk stage or initial focal laser photocoagulation in the presence of clinically significant macular edema;
- Careful follow-up at 4-mo intervals following the treatment;
- Retreatment of persistent or recurrent treatable lesions.

As high-risk PDR is reached, the major threat for SVL is traction retinal detachment; a lesser threat is vitreous hemorrhage. The primary goal of the scatter laser surgery is the prevention of traction retinal detachment, particularly involving the macula.

Scatter laser photocoagulation involves placement of multiple argon blue-green or green or krypton red laser burns in the midperipheral retina in two or more sessions, consisting of a total of 1200 to 1600 laser burns of moderate intensity and 500-μ-diameter spot size spaced one-half burn width apart. Focal photocoagulation for macular edema uses an argon green–only laser to treat focal lesions (such as microaneurysms that fill or leak during fluorescein angiography) and other treatable lesions (see earlier discussion) located between 500 and 3000 μ from the center of the macula. The response to laser treatment varies, but the goal of scatter treatment is to prevent the onset or induce the regression of neovascularization without vitreous hemorrhage or fibrovascular proliferation.

Various strategies are involved in follow-up treatment. The ocular lesions to be considered for follow-up photocoagulation include new, flat neovascularization or elevated neovascularization, new, persistent or recurrent CSME, and rarely, feeder vessels to NVD. The treatment methods include additional scatter laser treatment, local laser to NVE, focal laser for CSME, pars plana vitrectomy for recurrent hemorrhages with fibrovascular proliferation causing traction, or perhaps merely continued observation. Further scatter treatment may be placed between previously placed laser scars as long as these scars do not become confluent and the extent of the scatter treatment is not such as to totally destroy retinal function.

Although laser surgery is often considered painless, some pain may be associated with the treatment in younger patients. There also may be some pain when the peripheral retina is treated. Complications and side effects of laser photocoagulation are summarized in Table 55–9.

In summary, scatter treatment significantly reduces the risk of SVL from PDR. Both early scatter treatment prior to development of high-risk PDR and deferral of treatment until high-risk PDR develops reduce the risk of severe visual loss. The rates of SVL are low for each group. Consequently, it is recommended that scatter laser treatment *not* be used for mild to moderate NPDR. For severe NPDR and early PDR, scatter treatment is appropriate when close follow-up is unlikely or the disease process is progressing rapidly.

FUTURE HORIZONS

Present strategies for dealing with diabetic retinopathy address retinopathy that is already established. The Diabetes Control and Complications Trial (DCCT), a nationwide clinical trial testing very tight control of blood glucose levels versus standard control of blood glucose levels, is investigating the effect of tight control on the development of retinopathy itself. The DCCT will determine whether the efforts and risks of very tight control of blood glucose levels are justifiable by reduction in renal and retinal complications of diabetes. Although most practitioners believe it is prudent to maintain blood glucose levels under as strict control as possible in order to minimize the complications of diabetes mellitus, the results of the DCCT should firmly establish any benefit of very tight control.

Another multicentered clinical trial, the Sorbinil Retinopathy Trial (Table 55–10), tested whether a daily dose of sorbinil, an aldose reductase inhibitor (ARI), reduces the complications of diabetic retinopathy.

Over a 3-yr period, the drug had no clinically important effect on the course of diabetic retinopathy in adults with IDDM of moderate duration.[48] The group taking sorbinil, however, did show a slightly slower progression rate in microaneurysm count. Forthcoming reports will address the effect of sorbinil on diabetic neuropathy and diabetic nephropathy.

Table 55–10. SORBINIL RETINOPATHY STUDY (SRT)

SRT Evaluating
Effect on onset and progression of diabetic retinopathy
Effect on neuropathy and nephropathy
Safety and tolerance of sorbinil

SRT Design Features
Type I for 1–15 yr
Random sorbinil or placebo
Follow-up for 3 yr
250 mg daily

SRT Results (250 mg)
No effect on onset of diabetic retinopathy
No effect on progression of diabetic retinopathy
Hypersensitivity in 7% of subjects
Slightly fewer microaneurysms
No effect on blood pressure, hemoglobin A_{1C}

Limitations of SRT
Diabetic retinopathy not early enough
Duration of SRT too short
Dosage (250 mg) too small
Unknown effect on retina

There were complications from the use of the drug in the study population. Nearly 7 percent of the initial 202 participants had adverse reactions, including toxic epidermal necrolysis, erythema multiforme, and the Stevens-Johnson syndrome. It is unlikely that sorbinil will achieve prophylactic usage because of the hypersensitivity reactions and outcome similarities between the group treated with sorbinil and the control group in the study. Other aldose reductase inhibitors, notably tolrestat, which has a different chemical structure than sorbinil, are currently under investigation in the United States and Canada. Although the Sorbinil Retinopathy Trial research group reports discouraging results, there is hope, based on animal studies and study protocol, that successful intervention with aldose reductase inhibitors in the future will prevent or retard the progression of diabetic retinopathy.

Other research is addressing mechanisms contributing to altered retinal blood flow and retinal vascular complications in diabetes.[49, 50] Various metabolic and hormonal factors are suspected in the initiation and progression of retinal vascular abnormalities. Retinal blood flow is decreased in patients who have had diabetes less than 5 yr. Furthermore, a direct relationship between decreased retinal blood flow and the activation of protein kinase C in the rat model has been shown. Identifying these biochemical alterations associated with hyperglycemia with functional changes in retinal circulation may provide methods of preventing the development of diabetic retinopathy.

Other studies address the modulation of retinal blood flow by vasoactive agents such as angiotensin II, histamine, and oxygen. Inhibition of angiotensin II, histamine, and aldose reductase with insulin therapy or islet cell transplants may normalize retinal blood flow in diabetes. The prevalence of antipericyte antibodies, a reflection of pericyte degeneration, may be related to early development of diabetic retinopathy.

GUIDELINES

Until modalities are in place to prevent or cure diabetic retinopathy, the emphasis must be on identification, careful follow-up, and timely laser photocoagulation in patients with diabetic retinopathy. Proper care will result in reduction of personal suffering for those involved, as well as a substantial cost savings for the involved individuals and their families and the United States as a whole.[51] Therefore, strict guidelines have been established for the ocular care of people with diabetes (Table 55–11; see also Table 55–8).

All diabetic patients should be informed of the possibility of the development of retinopathy with or without symptoms and the associated threat of visual loss. The natural course and treatment of diabetic retinopathy should be discussed and the importance of routine examination stressed. Patients should be informed of the possible relationship between the level of control of diabetes and the subsequent development of ocular and other medical complications as the rationale for their

Table 55–11. EYE EXAMINATION SCHEDULE

Type of Diabetes Mellitus	Recommendation Time of First Examination	Routine Minimal Follow-up*
Type I; IDDM	5 yr after onset or	Yearly
Type II; NIDDM	At time of diagnosis	Yearly
During pregnancy	Prior to pregnancy for counseling Early in first trimester Each trimester or more frequently as indicated	3–6 months post partum

*Abnormal findings will dictate more frequent follow-up examinations (see Table 55–8).

partnership with the health care team. Patients should be informed that diabetic nephropathy, as manifested by proteinuria, requires aggressive early treatment to avoid superimposed renal retinopathy (and the possible associated risk of neovascular glaucoma). The association of joint contractures, hypertension, cardiovascular disease, elevated lipid levels, and neuropathy with onset and progression of diabetic retinopathy should be discussed.

Diabetic women contemplating pregnancy should have a complete eye examination prior to conception. Pregnant women with diabetes should have their eyes examined early in each trimester of pregnancy and should have a postpartum examination 3 to 6 mo following delivery. Since pregnancy may exacerbate existing retinopathy and may be associated with hypertension, careful medical and ocular observation is crucial during pregnancy. Retinopathy status may have an impact on the type of delivery, and close communication among the various members of the health care team is essential.

Patients with diabetic retinopathy, even in its mildest form, must be informed of the availability and benefits of early and timely laser photocoagulation therapy in reducing the risk of visual loss. The management program outlined in Table 55–8 is fundamental. Furthermore, patients with visual impairment of any degree, legal blindness, or total blindness should be informed of the availability of visual, vocational, and psychosocial rehabilitation programs. Information concerning these programs should be made available to each patient as indicated by his or her medical and visual condition.

CONCLUSIONS

In its earliest stages, diabetic retinopathy usually causes no symptoms. Visual acuity may be excellent, and upon evaluation and diagnosis, a patient may deny the presence of retinopathy. It is crucial at this stage for a patient's physician to initiate a careful program of education and follow-up of any ocular condition.

If retinal disease progresses, visual acuity may be compromised by macular edema or episodes of vitreous hemorrhage. Difficulty in the work or home environment may result. Although denial may continue, anger may result. Fear of blindness and other complications of diabetes, including death, may also occur. If visual acuity drops to 20/200 or worse, a patient may remain in a state of uncertainty until the retinopathy is in quiescence secondary to laser treatment, vitreoretinal surgery, or the natural history of the disease process. Anger and fear continue. Once the retinopathy is in remission and the vision is stable, a patient is in a position to accept the situation and make the appropriate psychologic and social adjustments. At this time, visual and vocational rehabilitation may be successful.

Communication among all members of a patient's health care team is of paramount importance in dealing with the physical and psychologic stresses of visual loss from diabetes. Faced with the inability to prevent or cure diabetic retinopathy, the main concern of all doctors must now focus on its early detection. Patient access, careful follow-up, and timely laser photocoagulation are fundamental to the successful elimination of blindness by the year 2000—the goal of the American Academy of Ophthalmology Diabetes 2000 program.

Acknowledgment

Special thanks to Rita Botti and Ann Kopple in preparing this manuscript and to Jerry Cavallerano, O.D., Ph.D., for his linguistic and organizational skills.

REFERENCES

1. Aiello LM, Beetham WP, Balodimos MC, et al: Ruby laser photocoagulation in treatment of diabetic proliferating retinopathy: Preliminary report. *In* Goldberg MF, Fine S (eds): Symposium on the Treatment of Diabetic Retinopathy. Public Health Service Publication No. 1890. Washington, DC, US Government Printing Office, 1969, pp 437–463.
2. Diabetic Retinopathy Study Report Number 1: Preliminary report on effects of photocoagulation therapy. Am J Ophthalmol 81:1–14, 1976.
3. Diabetic Retinopathy Study Report Number 2: Photocoagulation of proliferative diabetic retinopathy. Ophthalmology 85:82, 1978.
4. Diabetic Retinopathy Study Report Number 3: Four risk factors for severe visual loss in diabetic retinopathy. Arch Ophthalmol 97:658, 1979.
5. Diabetic Retinopathy Study Report Number 4: A short report of long-range results. Proceedings of the 10th Congress of International Diabetes Federation. New York, Excerpta Medica, 1980.
6. Diabetic Retinopathy Study Report Number 5: Photocoagulation treatment of proliferative diabetic retinopathy. Relationship of adverse treatment effects to retinopathy severity. Dev Ophthalmol 2:1–15, 1981.
7. Diabetic Retinopathy Study Report Number 6: Design, methods, and baseline results. Invest Ophthalmol Vis Sci 21:149–209, 1981.
8. Diabetic Retinopathy Study Report Number 7: A modification of the Airlie House Classification of Diabetic Retinopathy. Invest Ophthalmol Vis Sci 21:210–226, 1981.
9. Diabetic Retinopathy Study Report Number 8: Photocoagulation treatment of proliferative diabetic retinopathy. Clinical application of Diabetic Retinopathy Study (DRS) Findings. Ophthalmology 88:583–600, 1981.
10. Diabetic Retinopathy Study Report Number 9: Assessing possible late treatment effects in stopping clinical trials early: A case study by F. Ederer, MJ Podgor. Controlled Clin Trials 5:373–381, 1984.
11. Diabetic Retinopathy Study Report Number 10: Factors influencing the development of visual loss in advanced diabetic retinopathy. Invest Ophthalmol Vis Sci 26:983–991, 1985.
12. Diabetic Retinopathy Study Report Number 11: Intraocular pressure following panretinal photocoagulation for diabetic retinopathy. Arch Ophthalmol 105:807–809, 1987.
13. Diabetic Retinopathy Study Report Number 12: Macular edema in Diabetic Retinopathy Study patients. Ophthalmology 94:754–760, 1987.
14. Diabetic Retinopathy Study Report Number 13: Factors associated with visual outcome after photocoagulation for diabetic retinopathy. Invest Ophthalmol Vis Sci 30:23–28, 1989.
15. Diabetic Retinopathy Study Report Number 14: Indications for photocoagulation treatment of diabetic retinopathy. Int Ophthalmol Clin 27:239–253, 1987.
16. Early Treatment Diabetic Retinopathy Study Report Number 1: Photocoagulation for diabetic macular edema. Arch Ophthalmol 103:1796–1806, 1985.
17. Early Treatment Diabetic Retinopathy Study Report Number 2: Treatment techniques and clinical guidelines for photocoagulation of diabetic macular edema. Ophthalmology 94:761–774, 1987.
18. Early Treatment Diabetic Retinopathy Study Report Number 3: Techniques for scatter and local photocoagulation treatment of diabetic retinopathy. Int Ophthalmol Clin 27:254–264, 1987.
19. Early Treatment Diabetic Retinopathy Study Report Number 4: Photocoagulation for diabetic macular edema. Int Ophthalmol Clin 27:265–272, 1987.
20. Early Treatment Diabetic Retinopathy Study Case Reports Numbers 3 and 4: Case reports to accompany Early Treatment Diabetic Retinopathy Study Reports Numbers 3 and 4. Int Ophthalmol Clin 27:273–333, 1987.
21. Early Treatment Diabetic Retinopathy Study Report Number 5: Detection of diabetic macular edema. Ophthalmoscopy versus photography. Ophthalmology 96:746–751, 1989.
22. Early Treatment Diabetic Retinopathy Study Report Number 7: Early Treatment Diabetic Retinopathy Study design and baseline patient characteristics. Ophthalmology 98:741–756, 1991.
23. Early Treatment Diabetic Retinopathy Study Report Number 8: Effects of aspirin treatment on diabetic retinopathy. Ophthalmology 98:757–765, 1991.
24. Early Treatment Diabetic Retinopathy Study Report Number 9: Early photocoagulation for diabetic retinopathy. Ophthalmology 98:766–785, 1991.
25. Early Treatment Diabetic Retinopathy Study Report Number 10: Grading diabetic retinopathy from stereoscopic color fundus photographs—An extension of the modified Airlie House Classification. Ophthalmology 98:786–806, 1991.
26. Early Treatment Diabetic Retinopathy Study Report Number 11: Classification of diabetic retinopathy from fluorescein angiograms. Ophthalmology 98:807–822, 1991.
27. Early Treatment Diabetic Retinopathy Study Report Number 12: Fundus photographic risk factors for progression of diabetic retinopathy. Ophthalmology 98:823, 833, 1991.
28. Early Treatment Diabetic Retinopathy Study Report Number 13: Fluorescein angiographic risk factors for progression of diabetic retinopathy. Ophthalmology 98:834–840, 1991.
29. Diabetic Retinopathy Vitrectomy Study Report Number 1: Two-year course of visual acuity in severe proliferative diabetic retinopathy with conventional management. Ophthalmology 92:492–502, 1985.
30. Diabetic Retinopathy Vitrectomy Study Report Number 2: Early vitrectomy for severe vitreous hemorrhage in diabetic retinopathy. Two-year results of a randomized trial. Arch Ophthalmol 103:1644–1652, 1985.
31. Diabetic Retinopathy Vitrectomy Study Report Number 3: Early vitrectomy for severe proliferative diabetic retinopathy in eyes with useful vision. Results of a randomized trial. Ophthalmology 95:1307–1320, 1988.
32. Diabetic Retinopathy Vitrectomy Study Report Number 4: Early vitrectomy for severe proliferative diabetic retinopathy in eyes with useful vision. Clinical application of results of a randomized trial. Ophthalmology 95:1331–1334, 1988.
33. Diabetic Retinopathy Vitrectomy Study Report Number 5: Early vitrectomy for severe vitreous hemorrhage in diabetic retinopathy. Four-year results of a randomized trial. Arch Ophthalmol 108:958–964, 1990.
34. Klein R, Klein BEK, Moss SE, et al: The Wisconsin Epidemiologic Study of Diabetic Retinopathy. II. Prevalence and risk of diabetic retinopathy when age at diagnosis is less than 30 years. Arch Ophthalmol 102:520–526, 1984.

35. Klein R, Klein BEK, Moss SE, et al: The Wisconsin Epidemiologic Study of Diabetic Retinopathy. III. Prevalence and risk of diabetic retinopathy when age at diagnosis is 30 or more years. Arch Ophthalmol 102:527–532, 1984.
36. Moloney JBM, Drury MI: The effect of pregnancy on the natural course of diabetic retinopathy. Am J Ophthalmol 93:745–756, 1982.
37. Serup L: Influence of pregnancy on diabetic retinopathy. Acta Endocrinol 277:122–124, 1986.
38. Phelps RL, Sakol P, Metzger BE, et al: Changes in diabetic retinopathy during pregnancy: Correlations with regulation of hyperglycemia. Arch Ophthalmol 104:1806–1810, 1986.
39. The Kroc Collaborative Study Group: Blood glucose control and the evolution of diabetic retinopathy and albuminuria. N Engl J Med 311:365–372, 1984.
40. Grunwald JE, Riva CE, Martin DB, et al: Effect of insulin-induced decrease in blood glucose on the human diabetic retinal circulation. Ophthalmology 94:1614–1620, 1987.
41. Chase HP, Jackson WE, Hoops SL, et al: Glucose control in the renal and retinal complications of insulin-dependent diabetes. JAMA 261:1155–1160, 1989.
42. Brinchmann-Hansen O, Dahl-Jorgensen K, Hanssen KF, et al: Effects of intensified insulin treatment on various lesions of diabetic retinopathy. Am J Ophthalmol 100:644–653, 1985.
43. Krolewski AS, Canessa M, Warram JH, et al: Predisposition to hypertension and susceptibility to renal disease in insulin-dependent diabetes mellitus. N Engl J Med 318:140–145, 1988.
44. Stern MP, Patterson JK, Haffner SM, et al: Lack of awareness and treatment of hyperlipidemia in type II diabetes in a community survey. JAMA 262:360–364, 1989.
45. Bresnick GH: Background diabetic retinopathy. In Ryan SJ (ed): Retina, vol. 2. Medical Retina. St Louis, CV Mosby, 1989, pp 327–366.
46. Shimizu K, Kobayashi Y, Muraoka K: Midperipheral fundus involvement in diabetic retinopathy. Ophthalmology 88:601–612, 1981.
47. Takashi N, Muroka K, Shimizu K: Distribution of capillary nonperfusion in early-stage diabetic retinopathy. Ophthalmology 91:1431–1439, 1984.
48. The Sorbinil Retinopathy Trial Research Group: A randomized trial of sorbinil, an aldose reductase inhibitor in diabetic retinopathy. Arch Ophthalmol 108:1234–1244, 1990.
49. de la Rubia Sanchez G, Oliver-Pozo J, Shiba T, King GL: Modulation of endothelin-1 (ET-1) receptor on retinal pericytes by elevated glucose levels. Invest Ophthalmol Vis Sci 32:3110, 1991.
50. Shiba T, Bursell S-E, Clermont A, et al: Protein kinase C (PKC) activation is a causal factor for the alteration of retinal blood flow in diabetes of short duration. Invest Ophthalmol Vis Sci 32:785, 1991.
51. Javitt JC, Aiello LP, Bassi LJ, et al: Detecting and treating retinopathy in patients with type I diabetes mellitus. Savings associated with improved implementation of current guidelines. Ophthalmology 98:1565–1574, 1991.

Chapter 56

■

Proliferative Diabetic Retinopathy

JOAN W. MILLER and DONALD J. D'AMICO

HISTORY AND DEFINITION

With the introduction of insulin in the 1930s, diabetes mellitus ceased to be a rapidly fatal disease of young individuals, and coma as a cause of death fell from 60 to 4 percent.[1] The medical care of diabetics instead shifted to the management of vascular complications, including cardiac disease, renal failure, and diabetic retinopathy. In the 1970s, it was well demonstrated that laser photocoagulation could substantially reduce visual loss and blindness from diabetic retinopathy.[2, 3] Advances in vitreoretinal surgery have further made an impact on severe proliferative retinopathy. Even so, diabetic eye disease remains a severe medical and social problem afflicting individuals during their productive years. Diabetic retinopathy is responsible for at least 12 percent of the new cases of blindness each year in the United States. In 1985, the public welfare expense and lost income was estimated to be approximately $75 million annually.[4]

Proliferative diabetic retinopathy (PDR) is characterized by new vessels arising from the surface of the retina. New vessels may grow from the vessels on the surface of the optic disc directly into the vitreous cavity (neovascularization at the disc; NVD). They may also originate from the retinal circulation elsewhere (neovascularization elsewhere in the retina; NVE) and grow along the partially detached posterior hyaloid, also termed the *posterior vitreous face* (Fig. 56–1). Fibroblasts and glial elements accompany the new vessels, and proliferation of this fibroglial tissue can become the predominant feature of the retinopathy. PDR also includes rubeosis iridis or new vessels on the surface of the iris or in the anterior chamber angle.

PATHOGENESIS

The exact pathogenesis of retinal neovascularization remains unclear. Observations implicate substances released from ischemic retina that stimulate new vessel growth from susceptible vessels both locally and at distant locations in the eye (Fig. 56–2). Neovascularization is not a response limited to diabetes but is probably a programmed response to retinal ischemia. Ashton, Kohner, and others remarked on the associa-

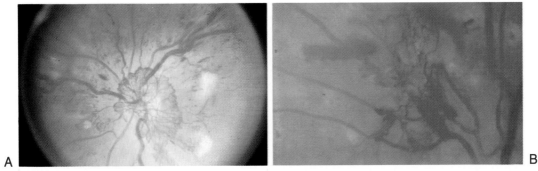

Figure 56–1. Proliferative diabetic retinopathy. *A,* Neovascularization at the disc (NVD). *B,* Neovascularization elsewhere (NVE).

tion of retinal capillary nonperfusion and adjacent retinal neovascularization.[5, 6] In other diseases, such as venous occlusive disease, sickle cell retinopathy, and retrolental fibroplasia, the appearance of retinal neovascularization coincides with the appearance of significant areas of capillary closure. The causes of capillary closure may differ in different disease states.

In diabetes, there are early functional changes that have been observed, including alterations in retinal blood flow and a breakdown in the blood-retinal barrier that is demonstrated by increased leakage from retinal blood vessels measured by vitreous fluorophotometry.[7–9] Morphologic changes include microaneurysms, dot hemorrhages, cotton-wool spots, venous caliber abnormalities, and intraretinal microvascular abnormalities. Microaneurysms appear in clusters and surround areas of capillary closure; they probably represent a response to capillary closure. Intraretinal microvascular abnormalities (IRMAs) are also found adjacent to areas of capillary drop-out. Controversy exists as to whether these

abnormalities represent dilated and abnormal retinal capillaries or early intraretinal neovascularization.[8]

With more extensive areas of capillary and arteriolar occlusion, neovascularization appears. NVE develops from retinal vessels and tends to appear adjacent to regions of nonperfusion. NVD originates from vessels on the disc and appears coincident with significant areas of nonperfusion in the midperiphery. Investigators have postulated the existence of and attempted to find a diffusible factor or factors that stimulate new vessel growth.

Factors capable of modulating angiogenesis are typically examined in vitro by measuring their effect on cultured endothelial cells and in various in vivo models such as the chick chorioallantoic membrane (CAM) model.[10, 11] Using these techniques, Glaser and associates were able to demonstrate angiogenic activity from human, bovine, and rabbit retina, which was not present in other tissues, including bovine skeletal muscle, heart, or liver.[12–14] They also found that human vitreous from

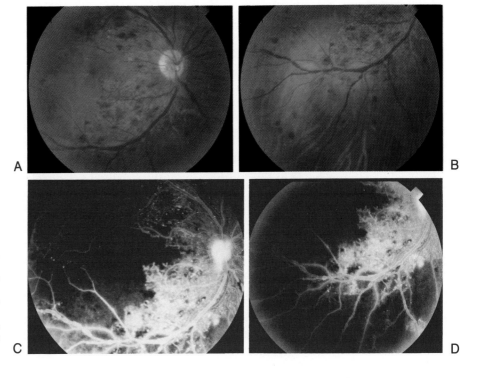

Figure 56–2. Severe retinal ischemia with rubeosis. *A,* Photograph of the right eye of a 27-year-old diabetic man who presented with rubeosis and neovascular glaucoma in each eye. There is NVD, and visual acuity is 20/200. *B,* View of inferotemporal arcade with numerous intraretinal hemorrhages and subtle intraretinal whitening. *C,* Fluorescein angiogram documenting severe capillary nonperfusion of the entire temporal macula and beyond; there is also hyperfluorescence indicating NVD. *D,* Inferior view showing nearly complete lack of capillary perfusion outside the peripapillary area.

patients with PDR stimulated endothelial cell growth in vitro.[15] However, no one has yet isolated and identified the factor or factors responsible for intraocular angiogenesis.

Factors that modulate angiogenesis have been isolated from other systems. One important group is the heparin-binding fibroblast growth factors, so named because their purification is facilitated by heparin affinity chromatography.[11] The fibroblast growth factors are potent stimulators of angiogenesis in the chick CAM model, although the endothelial cell may not be the only target cell. These factors appear to be incorporated into the basal lamina of endothelial cells and may normally serve an intracellular function. However, they may be released into the extracellular environment with cell damage and facilitate the repair process.[16, 17] Basic fibroblast growth factor has been shown to bind to basement membranes, including the lens capsule and inner limiting membrane of the retina, Descemet's membrane, and the basement membrane of vascular endothelium.[15, 18] Basic fibroblast growth factor also binds with high affinity to endothelial cells.

Other growth factors that are being investigated include transforming growth factors-α and -β.[11, 15] These factors were named for their ability to transform fibroblasts, namely, to make their growth in vitro anchorage-independent. However, they have both been shown more recently to be angiogenic in vivo. Transforming growth factor-β may be a bifunctional modulator of angiogenesis. In vivo it demonstrates angiogenic capability, whereas in vitro it inhibits the proliferation of vascular endothelial cells. This paradox may be partly explained by the fact that transforming growth factor-β is strongly chemotactic for macrophages, which may secondarily promote angiogenesis in vivo. This underscores the complexity of interpreting the modulation of angiogenesis in vivo, in which the interplay of factors depends on the external milieu or tone of the whole control system. Certain prostaglandins are angiogenic, possibly through the mediation of macrophages.[10] Platelet factor 4, which is released from platelets during aggregation, inhibits angiogenesis in in vivo models and prevents the proliferation of endothelial cells in vitro.[19] Retinal pigment epithelial cells grown in culture have been demonstrated to release substances that inhibit angiogenesis in the in vivo chick CAM model.[20] However, the retinal pigment epithelium (RPE) is also known to have a trophic effect on the choriocapillaris, as destruction of the RPE, which can be accomplished in the iodate model, leads to atrophy of the choriocapillaris.[15]

The control of angiogenesis has been likened by Folkman and Klagsbrun to the control of blood coagulation. The system is maintained for long periods in a state of readiness, without capillary growth and with a variety of interplaying controls. However, with the proper stimulus, the system is able to respond with rapid capillary growth, responding either to a physiologic demand or to a pathologic condition such as a wound, ischemia, or tumor.[11]

The vitreous appears to have at least a mechanical effect on the development of proliferative tissue. Ret-rospective studies have shown that although a complete posterior vitreous detachment (PVD) occurs in diabetes as a function of aging, partial PVD is seen in diabetics with proliferative retinopathy far more commonly than in individuals without diabetes or in diabetics with background retinopathy.[21] The posterior vitreous face remains attached to the retinal vessels at the sites of proliferation and provides a scaffold along which the new vessels and fibrous tissue can grow. The resulting tractional forces can lead to the development of traction retinal detachment. Precocious PVD, occurring prior to the development of proliferative retinopathy, appears to protect patients from traction retinal detachments.[22]

EPIDEMIOLOGY

Epidemiologic studies are important in elucidating the systemic, ocular, and genetic factors associated with the development and progression of diabetic retinopathy. Understanding these factors gives insight into the pathophysiology of the disease, as well as indicates the direction treatment should take in individual patients and in the health care system as a whole.

The Wisconsin Epidemiologic Study of Diabetic Retinopathy (WESDR) was a large population-based study of 2366 subjects divided into two groups: the younger-onset group or those diagnosed with diabetes before age 30 yr and the older-onset group or those diagnosed with diabetes after age 30 yr.[23, 24] The older-onset group was subdivided into those who took insulin and those who did not. In the younger-onset group, the prevalence of any retinopathy was closely related to the duration of diabetes, ranging from 2 percent in subjects with diabetes for less than 2 yr, to 98 percent in subjects with diabetes for 15 yr or more.[23] The severity of retinopathy in this group also increased with the duration of diabetes: The prevalence of PDR ranged from 0 percent in subjects with diabetes for less than 5 yr to 25 percent in subjects with diabetes for 15 yr, and 56 percent in subjects with diabetes for 20 yr or more. In the younger-onset group macular edema is rare before diabetes has been present 10 yr, but its prevalence reaches 21 percent after 20 or more yr of disease. In a population examined at the Joslin Clinic, macular edema was more common in the older-onset group, and in patients younger than the age of 50 yr, it was associated with preproliferative or proliferative retinopathy.[25]

In contrast to the younger-onset group, the older-onset group was more likely to have retinopathy at the time diabetes was diagnosed. The prevalence of any retinopathy in this group in the WESDR was 30 percent in insulin-taking subjects and 23 percent in those not taking insulin who had had diabetes for less than 2 yr.[24] This increased to 85 percent in the insulin-taking group and 58 percent in the group not taking insulin after 15 yr or more of diabetes. Proliferative retinopathy was also found in this group. After 15 yr or more of diabetes, the prevalence of PDR was 20 percent in those taking insulin, and 4 percent in those not taking insulin.

Incidence and progression of retinopathy was also studied in the WESDR. The younger-onset group had the highest 4-yr incidence of any retinopathy (59 percent), as well as progression (41 percent), and progression to PDR (10.5 percent).[23] Older-onset patients taking insulin had a 47 percent 4-yr incidence of any retinopathy, 34 percent incidence of progression, and 7 percent incidence of progression to PDR.[24] In those not using insulin, these numbers were all lower, with only a 34 percent incidence of any retinopathy. The incidence of legal blindness was 3 percent over 4 yr in the older-onset group on insulin versus 1.5 percent in the younger-onset group.

Various investigators have attempted to determine the characteristics associated with the severity or progression of retinopathy. As already evidenced, the duration of diabetes is important in all patients. The WESDR also found that elevated glycosylated hemoglobin levels were associated with more severe retinopathy in all groups. Proteinuria was associated with severe retinopathy in younger-onset subjects who had diabetes for 10 yr or more, as well as in the older-onset group. Elevated diastolic blood pressure and male sex was associated with more severe retinopathy in the younger-onset group and with elevated systolic blood pressure in the older-onset group.[23, 24]

A prospective study was carried out at the Joslin Clinic in 153 patients with long-standing diabetes, 90 percent of whom were in the early-onset category.[26] The risk of progression to preproliferative or proliferative retinopathy increased in the presence of background retinopathy, even if it was slight. The risk of progression increased exponentially with increasing hemoglobin A1c. Diastolic blood pressure less than 70 mmHg and increasing age were protective factors. Since the study involved patients with long-standing diabetes (duration 16 to 60 yr), the results may not apply to patients in the early course of the disease.

Genetic factors have been investigated, particularly the histocompatibility antigens (HLA) with varying findings.[27] Baker and Rand and associates reported that patients with HLA-DR phenotypes 4/0, 3/0, and X/X (neither 3 nor 4) had three to four times the risk of proliferative retinopathy than that found in patients with the HLA-DR phenotypes usually associated with diabetes (HLA-DR 3/4, 3/X, 4/X). In patients with myopia (2 D or greater) this risk was not evident.[27, 28]

Several studies have reported significant mortality associated with PDR. In a cohort study at the Joslin Center, Rand and colleagues demonstrated that the risk of death was not attributable to PDR itself.[29] The increased risk of death was found only in PDR patients with diabetic nephropathy as evidenced by persistent proteinuria.

OCULAR CONSEQUENCES OF NEOVASCULAR PROLIFERATION

Diagnosis and Fluorescein Evaluation

Neovascularization occurs most frequently in the posterior pole or within 45 degrees of the optic disc.[30] It is very commonly observed on the disc itself. New vessels on the disc can be easily overlooked in their early stages, beginning as fine loops or networks of vessels. The vessels gradually increase in caliber to one eighth to one quarter the diameter of a retinal vein at the optic disc. The vessels often form a cartwheel configuration with vessels radiating out from the center to a circumferential peripheral vessel (see Fig. 56–1A). Occasionally, new vessels will appear like normal retinal vessels, having a large caliber and extending across the retina without forming networks. However, these vessels can be distinguished because they will cross both arterioles and venules. Disc neovascularization is best identified using a magnified stereoscopic view, by either contact or precorneal lens, or with stereoscopic photography.

NVE is best detected by a thorough fundus examination, with binocular indirect ophthalmoscopy combined with biomicroscopy using a lens. Fundus photographs are also helpful in detecting early NVE. Neovascularization typically occurs adjacent to areas of capillary closure, marked by cotton-wool spots and hemorrhagic microaneurysms (see Fig. 56–1B). Intraretinal microvascular abnormalities (IRMA) may be difficult to differentiate from early NVE. *IRMA* is the term used to describe irregular, segmental dilatation of retinal capillaries, representing early neovascular changes or shunt vessels. On fluorescein angiography, IRMA typically do not leak as profusely as do new vessels (Fig. 56–3). However, angiography is not rou-

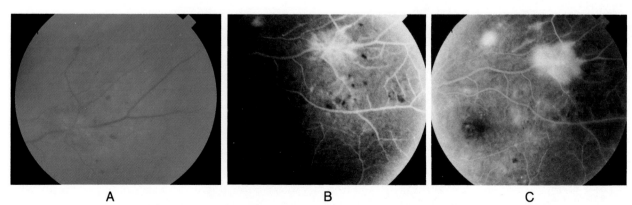

Figure 56–3. Fluorescein angiography of neovascularization. *A,* NVE along the vascular arcade. *B,* Early fluorescein transit defines NVE. *C,* Late transit showing continued leakage from NVE.

tinely required to screen for neovascularization. Borderline lesions will be revealed with careful follow-up.

Vitreous and Preretinal Hemorrhage

While the posterior hyaloid remains attached, neovascular proliferations appear to be on or slightly anterior to the retina and are usually asymptomatic. Small hemorrhages may occur near the growing tips of the vessels, but they usually remain subhyaloid. As the posterior hyaloid detaches, hemorrhages become less confined and symptoms appear (Fig. 56–4). Vitreous detachment usually begins in the posterior pole on either side of the vascular arcades, over the fovea, or temporal to the macula. Progression of vitreous detachment is halted whenever a tuft of neovascularization or a particularly strong attachment to a retinal vessel is encountered. The tuft may be pulled forward as the vitreous contracts, with or without detachment of the underlying retina. The vitreous detachment will continue to the periphery, at which point the vitreous is permanently attached to the vitreous base. The vitreous usually remains attached at the disc if there are fibrovascular proliferations present.

This process leads to a variety of complicated patterns of partial vitreous detachment, unified by the pathophysiology favoring attachment of the vitreous to neovascularization, major retinal vessels, the disc, and obligatorily, the peripheral vitreous base. The outer contour of the partially detached vitreous has been termed the *vitreous cone,* with the widest aspect of the cone anteriorly and a variable stem of the cone oriented at the posterior pole. The posterior vitreous face and its attachments in a given eye are critical to the understand-

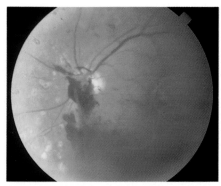

Figure 56–4. A complication of neovascularization. Vitreous hemorrhage from NVD.

ing of the surgical approaches in PDR (Fig. 56–5). The posterior vitreous face serves as a surface that may loculate hemorrhage. In addition, it may also have perforations that at times may cause it to be confused with an epiretinal membrane or even a macular hole.

Vitreous hemorrhage may occur as a result of vitreous traction on new vessels. Contraction of the vitreous or fibrovascular proliferation can lead to avulsion of a retinal vessel, usually a vein, and vitreous hemorrhage. Hemorrhage may also be associated with Valsalva maneuvers related to coughing or vomiting, or it is occasionally associated with insulin reactions.[31] Most of the time, it occurs during sleep and is unrelated to any obvious factor. Results of the Early Treatment of Diabetic Retinopathy Study indicate that aspirin use does not increase the risk of vitreous hemorrhage.[32]

Blood in the fluid vitreous behind the detached posterior vitreous face remains red until it is absorbed, which usually occurs over weeks to months. Hemorrhage

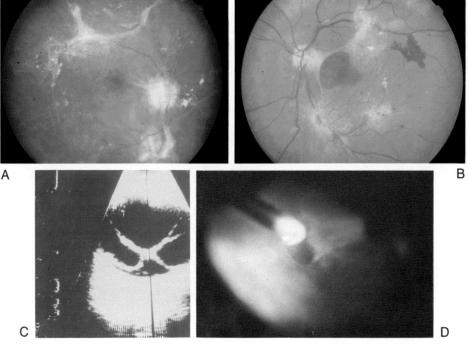

Figure 56–5. Posterior hyaloid (posterior vitreous face) configurations in proliferative diabetic retinopathy. *A,* The posterior hyaloid is attached across the macula, at the disc, and just beyond each arcade; outside of these areas, the vitreous is detached. In this eye, the posterior hyaloid is fibrotic and slightly separated from the surface of the macula, rendering it visible. The underlying retina is totally attached, and the visual acuity is 20/30. *B,* Posterior hyaloid with large hole centrally, simulating an epiretinal membrane with hole. The residual attachment points of the posterior hyaloid at the disc in superior, inferior, and inferotemporal locations may be seen. The retina is attached, and visual acuity is 20/30. *C,* Ultrasound demonstrating traction retinal detachment and vitreous attachments (vitreous cone). *D,* Intraoperative view of vitreous surgery with creation of an opening in the detached peripheral vitreous with the vitrectomy instrument; the membranous character of this tissue is shown.

into the formed vitreous tends to turn white over time and may require months to clear.

Vitreous Traction and Fibrous Proliferation

Early in the course of neovascularization, the new vessels appear bare, but as they develop, delicate white fibrous tissue can be seen adjacent to the vessels. This tissue increases as the vessels develop and may subsequently contract. Distortion and disruption of the normal retinal tissue may result in conjunction with the process of vitreous detachment (Fig. 56–6).

Contraction of the posterior vitreous face and fibrovascular proliferation may lead to traction retinal detachment. Since fibrous proliferation usually progresses along the temporal arcades, the retina along the temporal arcades is usually the first to detach. Progression of the detachment can then extend centrally and peripherally. The rate of progression required for an extramacular traction detachment to involve the macula may be as low as 15 percent in a single year.[33] In contrast to rhegmatogenous retinal detachments, traction detachments are typically concave and localized and do not extend to the ora serrata. Traction retinal detachments, in PDR have many configurations, depending on the location, number, and severity of attachments of the posterior vitreous face to neovascularization and its associated fibrovascular tissue; the activity of the neovascularization also plays a role. The configurations may range from an isolated traction detachment outside the arcades associated with an area of NVE that has regressed to a traction detachment of the entire posterior

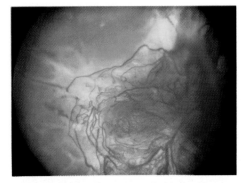

Figure 56–6. Very severe neovascularization with vascular overgrowth obscuring the retina and traction retinal detachment.

retina with extensive contact of the retina, neovascular tissue, and the posterior vitreous face. The varying configurations have implications for the indications for surgical intervention and for the prognosis for successful reattachment. Traction retinal detachments may also develop retinal breaks, either atrophic or tractional. The resulting combined traction–rhegmatogenous detachment typically progresses, although in some cases the detachment may remain stable despite the break, particularly in an eye that has undergone extensive panretinal photocoagulation (Fig. 56–7). Detachments involving the fovea have obvious impact on vision. However, in other cases, the fibrovascular tissue may overgrow and obscure the fovea, reducing vision without actual foveal detachment. Contraction of fibrovascular tissue can also lead to distortion or horizontal displacement of the macula (tangential traction). Visual acuity may be reduced in this condition because of striae in the macula, and surgery may result in visual improvement.[34]

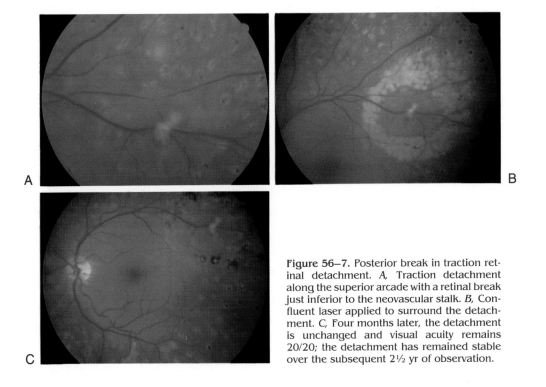

Figure 56–7. Posterior break in traction retinal detachment. *A,* Traction detachment along the superior arcade with a retinal break just inferior to the neovascular stalk. *B,* Confluent laser applied to surround the detachment. *C,* Four months later, the detachment is unchanged and visual acuity remains 20/20; the detachment has remained stable over the subsequent 2½ yr of observation.

Rubeosis

Iris neovascularization or rubeosis is a complication of proliferative retinopathy. Rubeosis is characterized by networks of branching vessels over the surface of the iris, with vessels crossing the scleral spur on gonioscopy. Usually the new vessels are apparent on clinical examination, but fluorescein angiography is occasionally helpful in demonstrating leakage from the new vessels. Rubeosis is observed in the setting of proliferative changes and retinal ischemia and also in long-standing retinal detachment related to diabetic retinopathy. It is most dramatically evident in eyes with retinal detachment following unsuccessful vitrectomy. In this setting, rubeosis will develop in almost all cases and will progress rapidly if the underlying detachment is not repaired.

Involutional PDR

All diabetic retinopathy eventually reaches an involutional stage. The visual outcome is variable and depends on the degree of structural alteration in the posterior pole. Vitreous detachment is completed, except in areas in which fibrovascular proliferations prevent complete separation, and fibrovascular proliferation ceases. Usually there is some element of traction detachment by the time this phase is reached, and it typically involves the macula. The optic nerve develops some pallor, and the retinal arterioles become attenuated. Retinal hemorrhages and microaneurysms are rare, and pigmentary changes in the RPE may be seen. Fibrous tissue may be thinner and translucent, with the appearance of vitreous veils in contact with diaphanous retina. Visual loss at the involutional phase may relate to macular detachment, macular ischemia, long-standing macular edema, or optic nerve disease (Fig. 56–8).

TREATMENT OF PDR

Beetham's Observations Leading to Rationale for Laser Therapy

Early investigators observed that certain ocular conditions seemed to prevent severe diabetic retinopathy. Eyes with chorioretinal scarring, optic atrophy, retinitis pigmentosa, and high myopia were protected from severe proliferative retinopathy.[35] Beetham, studying patients at the Joslin Clinic, described spontaneous resolution of PDR in approximately 10 percent of patients.[36] The fundus picture in these patients consisted of lacy, reticulated proliferative tissue; attenuated arterioles; and obliterated vessels appearing as white lines. The fundus picture resembled that of the ocular conditions described earlier, as well as the fundus picture that develops after successful hypophysectomy for PDR. It was recognized that this appearance could be achieved with photocoagulation.

Early Laser Trials (Direct Ablation)

Meyer-Schwickerath and Schott first used light photocoagulation to treat diabetic retinopathy in 1955.[37] The xenon arc they used produced white light emitting multiple wavelengths. Lesions of moderate therapeutic intensity were full-thickness retinal burns histologically, with destruction of inner retina, explaining the frequent occurrence of visual field defects. With the xenon arc, one could obliterate vessels directly, treating flat neovascular patches, dilated retinal capillaries, microaneurysms, and edematous retina. Treating elevated vessels required increased power and resulted in extensive retinal destruction. The best results were obtained by Meyer-Schwickerath and Schott in patients with nonproliferative retinopathy and early PDR.[37] Several months to years following treatment with the xenon arc, flat neovascular patches remained scarred and atrophic; there was a decrease in exudates, retinal edema, and venous dilatation. New retinal vessels disappeared even if not treated directly. Atrophic changes progressed over 4 to 8 yr. Of 73 patients with nonproliferative diabetic retinopathy treated with the xenon arc and followed for 1 to 9 yr, only 1 patient developed PDR. However, diffuse treatments of the retina resulted in large visual field defects, hemorrhage, and fibrous proliferation and traction.

Aiello and colleagues postulated that in order to reproduce the involutional fundus picture, one needed to be able to produce multiple small, "harmless" chorioretinal scars in the posterior pole.[38] Clearly, this was not possible with the xenon arc. However, with the development of the ruby laser, this treatment approach became possible. The ruby laser emits monochromatic energy at 694.3 nm, a wavelength transmitted through ocular media and absorbed well by the RPE and choroid. It transmits fairly well through blood, permitting treatment through mild vitreous hemorrhage but also making the laser less effective in treating vessels directly. The laser emits energy for less than 1 msec. In experimental studies by Campbell and coworkers, the thermal changes were smaller and more narrowly confined than those found with xenon arc use. In 1965, Campbell and coworkers reported the results of treating 220 patients for a variety of conditions, including retinal tears, retinoschisis, retinal detachment, angiomas, and chorioretinitis.[39]

Beetham and associates began using the ruby laser to treat patients with diabetic retinopathy in 1967. By 1969, they had treated 329 patients with various degrees of proliferating retinopathy, treating one eye and using the second eye as a control, in patients in whom the degree of retinopathy was approximately the same.[35] Most of the patients treated had flat neovascularization of the retina, or early NVD plus or minus NVE. Patients were medically evaluated and followed by complete ocular examinations, including refraction, field examination, fundus photography, and fluorescein angiography. The ruby laser was used at a 2.5-degree aperture to produce 750 individual chorioretinal lesions of grade 1 or 2

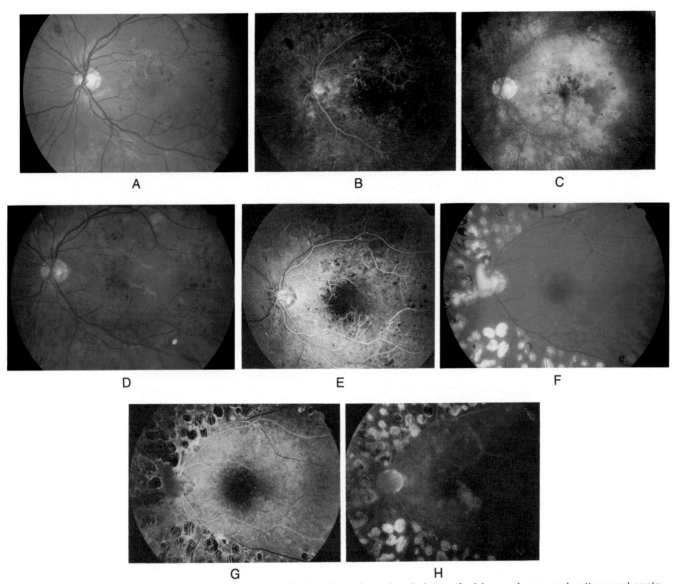

Figure 56–8. Macular ischemia in a 21-year-old man with diabetic retinopathy. *A,* Intraretinal hemorrhages and cotton-wool spots; visual acuity is 20/30. *B,* Fluorescein angiogram demonstrates macular capillary nonperfusion and early disc neovascularization. *C,* Late phase of the angiogram showing continued ischemia with diffuse leakage in the macula. *D,* Six months later, cotton-wool spots have increased and visual acuity is 20/50. *E,* Fluorescein angiogram now displays extensive capillary nonperfusion, most prominent in the temporal macula. NVD has increased, and visual acuity is 20/50. *F,* Eight years later, after extensive panretinal photocoagulation as well as a vitrectomy for vitreous hemorrhage, regressed proliferative changes are noted. Sclerotic vessels are seen temporally, and visual acuity is 20/80. *G,* Fluorescein angiogram shows delayed filling of temporal vessels and a greatly increased foveal avascular zone. *H,* Late phase of the angiogram shows continued ischemia, vascular wall leakage in the temporal vessels, and macular edema resulting from intraretinal vascular abnormalities.

intensity. Applications were placed in all areas of the posterior pole, avoiding the disc, macula, and papillomacular bundle.

With 1 to 2 yr of follow-up, there was regression of neovascularization in the treated eyes, which was statistically significant.[35] Eighty percent of the treated eyes showed some regression, and 54 percent had complete disappearance of neovascularization, with the control eyes remaining unchanged or worsening. Aiello and colleagues also noted a decrease in the diffuse angiopathy of the posterior pole, even in the untreated area

of the papillomacular bundle.[38] Results in patients with more severe proliferative retinopathy were more disappointing, although with fewer patients falling into these groups, statistical comparisons could not be made. Of seven patients with elevated disc neovascularization who were treated with ruby laser, two patients showed improvement, three patients suffered severe vitreous hemorrhage, with one experiencing severe fibrous proliferans after the hemorrhage, and two patients remained stable. None of the treated patients in any group experienced sector visual field defects, and there was no related vitreous traction, iritis, cataracts, or elevated intraocular pressure.

In summary, Aiello and Beetham and associates noted the following results after treatment: Neovascular nets disappeared or became nonfilling, diffuse angiopathy improved, dot-blot hemorrhages decreased, retinal edema decreased, the disc became paler, there was no change in fibrous proliferation, and the retinal veins were noted to be less "leaky" by fluorescein angiography.[35, 38] The pathophysiologic mechanism by which the laser treatment worked was unclear, possibly involving the reduction in metabolic demand by destroying functioning retinal tissue or altering the hemodynamic status of the retinal-choroid layer. More than 20 yr later it is still unclear, although alterations in the levels of various modulators of angiogenesis are felt to play a role. Aiello and Beetham and associates felt that a "green" laser might be useful to directly treat elevated vessels prone to hemorrhage, as there would be greater absorption by the blood column. They also believed that their results warranted a large, long-term, controlled study.

Pituitary Ablation

Pituitary ablation remains a controversial and infrequently used method of treating PDR. Houssay first noted that hypophysectomy reduced the severity of diabetes in pancreatectomized dogs in 1930.[40] Interest was further generated by a report by Poulsen in 1953 of remission of diabetic retinopathy in a woman with Sheehan's syndrome, or postpartum anterior pituitary insufficiency.[42] Luft and coworkers introduced the technique in humans in the 1950s.[41] Various techniques of pituitary ablation were tried, including surgical hypophysectomy, transsphenoidal hypophysectomy, yttrium-90 implantation, x-irradiation, proton beam irradiation, and stereotactic hypophysectomy using radiofrequency coagulation.

Both short- and long-term follow-up of patients undergoing pituitary ablation demonstrated a stabilization of visual acuity in survivors, an improvement in both disc and peripheral neovascularization, and a reduction in exudates, microaneurysms, and hemorrhages.[9, 42, 43] However, the complications of treatment were frequent and significant. As reported by Sharp and associates they included debilitating postural hypotension and asymptomatic hypoglycemia, with several related deaths. Osteoporosis and avascular necrosis of the hip were reported and were related to steroid replacement. Sterility led to episodes of severe depression in several patients and suicide in at least one case. In the group from London treated with yttrium-90, the 5-yr mortality rate was 18 percent, and the 10-yr rate was 51 percent.[43]

With the advent of photocoagulation and vitrectomy, both of which are effective and associated with fewer risks and complications, pituitary ablation for PDR is no longer performed.

Diabetic Retinopathy Study and Modern Panretinal Photocoagulation

INDICATIONS

The early studies of Beetham and Aiello and associates suggested a beneficial effect of laser photocoagulation in controlling PDR. The Diabetic Retinopathy Study (DRS) was a multicenter randomized prospective study designed to determine whether laser treatment in diabetics prevented severe visual loss. It proved very quickly that severe visual loss (visual acuity < 5/200) occurred about 60 percent less frequently in eyes treated with photocoagulation than in eyes assigned to no treatment.[2, 3] The study was also able to identify certain high-risk characteristics in subgroups of patients that led to poor outcome without treatment and in which treatment clearly was of benefit.[44] After 4 yr, the study was changed to allow treatment of previously untreated eyes that developed these high-risk characteristics.

The high-risk characteristics demonstrated by the DRS follow:

- Moderate to severe neovascularization of the disc (greater than standard photograph 10A)
- Any neovascularization of the disc with vitreous or preretinal hemorrhage
- Moderate to severe NVE with vitreous or preretinal hemorrhage

Other indications, although not clearly demonstrated by the study, are also widely employed, and are summarized in Table 56–1. They include widespread capillary drop-out, moderate to severe NVE alone, and rubeosis with or without neovascular glaucoma. Special consideration should also be given to the history, compliance, medical complications precluding follow-up, and other clinical aspects seen in the patient. For instance, it may be argued that a juvenile diabetic with visual loss caused by severe proliferative retinopathy in one eye should be treated in the second eye when any degree of proliferative retinopathy, preproliferative retinopathy, or increasing retinal ischemia is documented. Similarly, a pregnant woman with proliferative changes may be treated sooner because of the possibility of rapid progression of the retinopathy, particularly if tight metabolic control is instituted.

TECHNIQUE

Laser photocoagulation has effectively replaced the xenon arc photocoagulator as the instrument of choice. Multiple wavelengths and instruments are available and effective. Argon green (514 nm) is most commonly employed, and the energy is well absorbed by blood-filled vessels and by pigment in the RPE. Argon blue-green (488 nm) is rarely used, although it was the standard of therapy for the DRS: It is more widely scattered by media and may lead to long-term retinal toxicity in the treating physician. Dye yellow (577 nm)

Table 56–1. INDICATIONS FOR PANRETINAL PHOTOCOAGULATION FOR PROLIFERATIVE DIABETIC RETINOPATHY

DRS High-risk Characteristics
NVD of moderate to severe degree (greater than standard photo 10A)
NVD of any degree if associated with preretinal or vitreous hemorrhage
NVE of moderate to severe degree if associated with preretinal or vitreous hemorrhage

Additional Indications Widely Employed
Rubeosis with or without neovascular glaucoma
Moderate to severe NVE alone, particularly in juvenile diabetic patients
Widespread retinal ischemia and capillary drop-out on fluorescein angiography

Special Situations for Consideration of Panretinal Photocoagulation
PDR developing in pregnancy, particularly with the institution of tight metabolic control
Preproliferative retinopathy in the second eye of a juvenile diabetic patient with severe proliferative retinopathy in the other eye

Key: DRS, Diabetic Retinopathy Study; NVD, neovascularization at the disc; NVE, neovascularization elsewhere in the retina; PDR, proliferative diabetic retinopathy.

is well absorbed by blood and may permit direct treatment of new vessels in certain instances, such as NVE persisting after panretinal photocoagulation. Krypton red (647 nm) offers better penetration through nuclear sclerotic cataracts and, to a lesser extent, vitreous hemorrhage than does the argon green wavelength. Improved penetration in the choroid may make this wavelength more painful to the patient. More recently, solid-state diode lasers emitting wavelengths between 780 and 850 nm have become available for medical use. They offer the advantage of small size and portability, as well as low power requirements. The longer wavelengths can penetrate media opacity but require more power to produce equivalent retinal lesions and may be associated with more patient discomfort.

Laser photocoagulation can be delivered through a slit-lamp system, an indirect ophthalmoscope, or an endolaser probe. Transpupillary slit-lamp delivery is the most common delivery system for the treatment of adults. The indirect ophthalmoscope laser is available with argon or diode lasers and permits panretinal photocoagulation in patients under general anesthesia or in a recumbent position. The endolaser, either argon or diode, is restricted to use at vitrectomy.

Topical anesthesia is usually adequate, although retrobulbar anesthesia may be needed for retreatments, treatment with longer wavelengths, or indirect ophthalmoscope delivery. Oral diazepam supplementation can also be useful in a patient who is very nervous. The lenses used for slit-lamp delivery include the Rodenstock panfundoscopic lens, the Volk quadraspheric lens, and the Goldmann three-mirror lens. The Rodenstock and Volk lenses allow one to view a large area of the fundus during treatment and are increasingly popular for the performance of panretinal photocoagulation. With these lenses, the image is inverted, and far-peripheral burns are more difficult to place than with the Goldmann lens. The Rodenstock and Volk lenses magnify the spot size, and relatively more power is required for these lenses. The Goldmann lens allows placement of far-peripheral burns but provides a view of only a small area of the retina.

Spot size depends on the lens selected, usually 500 μ for the Goldmann lens and 200 μ for the Rodenstock lens, to achieve a 500-μ burn. Occasionally, larger lesions are employed for heavy therapy (e.g., when treating rubeosis). The duration is typically 0.1 to 0.2 sec. Longer durations can be used in patients with media opacity, as well as for treatment with longer wavelengths. The power should be titrated to produce a gray-white burn. Treatment should begin at 100 mW with the Goldmann lens or 150 mW with the Rodenstock or Volk lens, although a heavily pigmented fundus in an aphakic or pseudophakic eye suggests an even lower initial setting. The number of spots is less critical than is the response to therapy and follow-up. The DRS protocol specified 800 to 1600 spots 500 μ in size, but typical therapy with a Rodenstock or Volk lens is 600 to 1000 200-μ spots (500-μ spot at the retina). The burns should be placed 1 to 1½ burn widths apart, with focal confluent bombardment of the NVE. If possible, the treatment inferiorly should be heavier than the treatment superiorly to preserve downgaze field. In treating the temporal raphe, a barrier line should be placed 2.5 disc diameters temporal to the center of the macula, with treatment extending distal to the barrier. Panretinal treatments are usually divided over two to three sessions but may be given in a single session if required. One study found no significant long-term differences in single-session versus multiple-session treatment, but fewer transient choroidal and exudative retinal detachments were observed in the multiple-session group.[45]

RESULTS

The DRS clearly demonstrated that photocoagulation in selected diabetics reduced the risk of severe visual loss. Eligible patients for the DRS had proliferative retinopathy in at least one eye or severe nonproliferative retinopathy in two eyes and visual acuity of 20/100 or better in each eye. One eye was randomly assigned to treatment, and treatment was randomized between argon laser and xenon arc photocoagulation. The rate of severe visual loss (visual acuity <5/200) was reduced by treatment from 16 percent in nontreated eyes over 2 yr to 6 percent in treated eyes, a reduction of 57 percent.[2, 3, 46] The DRS identified certain subgroups, based on the severity of retinopathy, for which the treatment effect outweighed any harmful effect. These retinopathy gradings (called high-risk characteristics and discussed earlier) and severe visual loss in these patients fell from 26 percent in nontreated eyes to 11 percent in treated eyes.[2, 44, 46] Harmful effects of treatment were also identified and were somewhat greater in the xenon-treated group of the DRS. Estimates of persistent visual acuity loss attributable to treatment in the xenon-treated eyes were 19 percent with loss of 1 line of visual acuity and 11 percent with loss of 2 lines.[46, 47] In the argon-treated group, these numbers were 11 percent and 3 percent, respectively. Twenty-five percent of the xenon-treated eyes demonstrated a modest loss of visual field, and an additional 25 percent had more severe loss of visual field. Five percent of patients in the argon group showed some constriction in visual field. It was felt that some adverse treatment effects were related to focal treatment of NVD and elevated NVE, and this aspect of treatment was abandoned.[46] Other studies comparing the use of xenon arc and laser photocoagulation failed to demonstrate any significant difference in the two modalities, either in effectiveness or in the rate of visual loss related to treatment.[48, 49] However, they did confirm the greater risk of field loss occurring after xenon arc treatment, which probably correlates with the inner retinal damage from a xenon arc burn that is evident on histopathologic examination.[48]

Regression of neovascularization occurs in 30 to 55 percent of eyes after laser photocoagulation using various treatment approaches and may correlate with visual prognosis (Fig. 56–9). The DRS found complete regression of disc neovascularization in 29.8 percent of cases and partial regression in 24.5 percent of eyes 12 mo after treatment.[3] Blankenship compared central and peripheral photocoagulation and found a trend toward decreased visual loss (related to treatment) in the peripheral distribution group and a slightly smaller loss of visual field. Regression of disc neovascularization was similar in both groups, with 47 percent complete regression in the peripheral distribution group versus 40 percent in the central distribution group. In both groups, 33 percent of patients had partial regression of disc neovascularization following photocoagulation.[50] Regression of neovascularization should be assessed several weeks after photocoagulation as a prognostic indicator and to determine whether additional treatment is necessary. Doft and Blankenship have shown that regression of neovascularization 3 wk after treatment is a good indicator of longer-term visual results.[51] Vine suggests that eyes be assessed 6 to 8 wk after laser treatment, and treatment augmented if high-risk characteristics persist.[52] He described a group of "nonresponders" who continued to have high-risk characteristics despite augmented panretinal photocoagulation averaging 3000 Goldmann burns. Approximately 50 percent of these "nonresponders" did respond to additional low-intensity, but extensive, photocoagulation, reaching an average of 7550 Goldmann burns, with preservation of visual acuity.

Although the DRS used blue-green argon wavelengths or xenon arc for photocoagulation, other wavelengths are employed by treating ophthalmologists. Argon green has replaced argon blue-green to avoid long-term retinal toxicity in the treating physician. Dye yellow, krypton red, and diodes emitting in the near-infrared spectrum have all been used for panretinal photocoagulation. Studies have compared the effectiveness of certain wavelengths but not all. Krypton red photocoagulation was demonstrated to be as effective as argon blue-green for the treatment of PDR, comparing visual outcome, regression of vessels, and incidence of complications.[53]

There is some controversy regarding photocoagulation in the presence of traction retinal detachment. Certainly if the traction retinal detachment involves the fovea, vitrectomy is indicated. However, concerns are often expressed that photocoagulation in patients with extrafoveal traction detachments will lead to worsening of the detachment and involvement of the fovea. The DRS found that harmful treatment effects, including decreased visual acuity, were associated with preexisting fibrous proliferations and localized retinal detachments, particularly in the xenon-treated group.[47] However, the report also confirmed that those patients with severe proliferative retinopathy still benefitted from argon laser treatment. Some authors have suggested "prophylactic vitrectomy" for traction retinal detachments "threatening" the macula.[54] This approach may unnecessarily subject some patients to the risks of vitrectomy surgery. One study investigating argon laser photocoagulation in patients with severe proliferative retinopathy and posterior extrafoveal traction detachments found that after treatment, detachments rarely progress to involve the fovea.[55] In this study, the area of detachment was avoided with otherwise standard photocoagulation techniques and without any effort to wall off the detachment.[55] Panretinal photocoagulation with careful follow-up should be the first line of therapy in patients with proliferative retinopathy and traction retinal detachments not involving the fovea.

The DRS found that eyes with high-risk characteristics have a 2-yr risk of severe visual loss of 25 percent. Scatter photocoagulation reduces the risk of severe visual loss by 50 percent or more. Eyes with severe nonproliferative retinopathy or proliferative retinopathy without high-risk characteristics have a 2-yr risk of

Figure 56–9. Progression of proliferative diabetic retinopathy despite panretinal photocoagulation. A, A 29-year-old man with preproliferative changes in the right eye. Vascular dilatation, cotton-wool spots, and intraretinal hemorrhages are seen. Visual acuity is 20/25. B, Superior retina with similar preproliferative changes. C, Fluorescein angiogram with numerous microaneurysms with leakage and an enlarged foveal avascular zone. D, Superior retina with capillary nonperfusion and leakage into the vascular walls. E, Patient was lost to follow-up for 1½ yr and now presents with severe NVD; visual acuity is 20/25. F, Fluorescein angiogram shows marked progression of ischemic changes in association with prominent leakage from NVD. G, Angiogram of superior retina shows greatly increased ischemia compared with previous angiogram. H, Angiogram of nasal retina documents almost total closure of capillary bed in association with areas of neovascularization. I, Six months later, NVD progresses despite extensive and repeated panretinal photocoagulation. J, After an additional 10 mo, a traction retinal detachment involving the fovea develops. The retina is obscured by neovascular tissue, and visual acuity is at the counting fingers level at 1 ft. K, One year after vitrectomy and endolaser treatment, the retina is attached but displays vascular and optic atrophy, and visual acuity is 20/200.

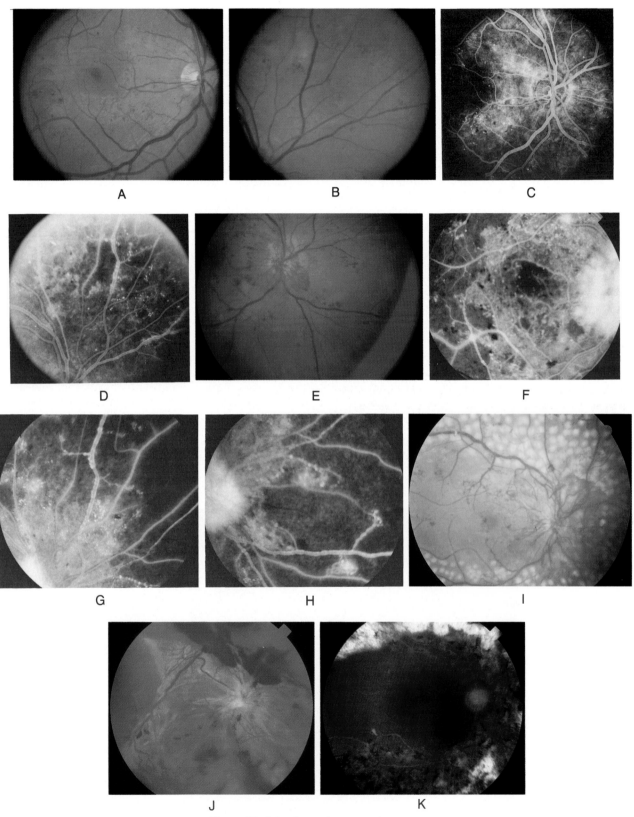

Figure 56–9 *See legend on opposite page*

severe visual loss of 3 to 7 percent. Thus the risk of visual acuity loss relating to treatment assumes greater relative importance.[46] The DRS was unable to determine whether deferral of treatment with observation in this group was better than early treatment. The Early Treatment of Diabetic Retinopathy Study was designed in part to determine the optimal timing of photocoagulation. Early treatment for nonproliferative retinopathy was compared with deferral of photocoagulation until high-risk characteristics developed. There was a small reduction in the rate of severe visual loss with early treatment, but the rates of severe visual loss were low in both groups (2.6 percent for the early treatment group and 3.7 percent for the deferral group).[56] Therefore, as long as careful follow-up can be provided for the patient, scatter laser photocoagulation is not recommended for eyes with mild or moderate nonproliferative retinopathy. The physician must, of course, incorporate some clinical judgment, including assessment of the fellow eye, progression of lens opacities, and other conditions.

COMPLICATIONS

Laser photocoagulation is clearly an effective treatment but can result in complications (Table 56–2). These complications may occur during treatment or in the immediate postoperative period or may present as long-term problems (Fig. 56–10). Pain during treatment is usually transient but may require retrobulbar anesthesia for completion of the session. Increased intraocular pressure can occur, particularly after heavy treatment, as a result of choroidal swelling and angle shallowing, but it usually resolves after 48 hr.[57] It can usually be avoided with divided sessions or lighter treatment. The

Table 56–2. COMPLICATIONS OF PANRETINAL PHOTOCOAGULATION

Foveal burn	Pain during treatment
Optic disc damage	Increased intraocular pressure
Macular edema	Corneal abrasion
Choroidal hemorrhage	Mydriasis–paresis of
Choroidal neovascularization	accommodation
Choroidal detachment	Loss of visual field
Exudative retinal detachment	Loss of dark adaptation
Vitreous hemorrhage	Lens opacities
	Increase in traction detachments

cornea in diabetic patients is very sensitive to contact lens trauma, and corneal abrasion during treatment may result in a persistent epithelial defect. The cornea should be inspected after treatment and any abrasions treated appropriately. Mydriasis is the result of laser damage to nerves in the uveal tract and is permanent; paralysis of accommodation can occur but is usually transient.[58]

Macular edema and a loss of visual acuity of 1 to 3 lines can occur and is more common in patients with perifoveal capillary nonperfusion. Recovery usually occurs over 2 to 4 wk, but visual loss may be permanent. Visual field loss secondary to photocoagulation was documented in the DRS and is related to the extent of treatment;[46] loss of dark adaptation can also occur after panretinal photocoagulation.[59] Choroidal detachment and exudative retinal detachment are usually the result of very heavy panretinal photocoagulation and usually resolve spontaneously.[60] Choroidal hemorrhage can occur with a very heavy burn, particularly with longer wavelengths, but is usually limited and resolves spontaneously. Subretinal neovascularization has been reported and should be treated if it is macular.[61] Foveal

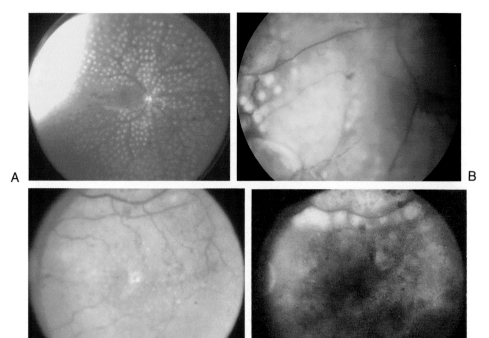

Figure 56–10. Panretinal photocoagulation and complications. A, Wide-angle photograph of a typical panretinal photocoagulation pattern. B, Choroidal and exudative retinal detachment following extensive photocoagulation for rubeosis. C, Macular edema 2 wk after panretinal photocoagulation; visual acuity is at the counting fingers level at 2 ft, and visual acuity is 20/30. D, Fluorescein angiogram documents cystoid edema; edema resolved in 1 mo with visual recovery.

burns are caused by the surgeon's disorientation or by unfortunate ocular movement and result in permanent loss of central acuity, but there may be some improvement after the initial loss. Vision loss has also been reported in association with peripapillary treatment.[62] Vitreous hemorrhage can result from rupture of neovascular vessels during treatment (rarely) or from shrinkage and regression of neovascular tissue after treatment (commonly). Hemorrhage that occurs after panretinal photocoagulation usually resolves with time but may occasionally require vitrectomy. Direct treatment of neovascularization with green (514 nm) or yellow (577 nm) wavelengths has a limited role and is restricted to eyes with recurrent vitreous hemorrhage and persistent neovascularization despite complete panretinal photocoagulation.

Lens opacities can occur with high energy and misfocusing, particularly with the panfundus-style lenses, and are usually permanent but nonprogressive.[63, 64] Vascular occlusion can result from placement of burns over a vessel. Frequently the vessel will again become patent. Although heavy treatment with the xenon arc photocoagulator in eyes with active vitreoretinal traction can lead to progression of an extrafoveal traction retinal detachment into the fovea in certain cases, data indicate that argon laser therapy may be safely performed in these eyes.[55] Care should be taken to avoid heavy treatment near areas of vitreoretinal traction.

The Role of Vitrectomy for PDR

INDICATIONS

Laser photocoagulation allows effective treatment of moderate to severe PDR. However, although treatment substantially reduces the risk of severe visual loss, PDR in a certain number of eyes progresses to traction retinal detachment and vision loss. Standard laser cannot be performed in eyes with vitreous hemorrhage precluding visualization of the retina. Vitrectomy was first introduced by Machemer in the 1970s as a method of removing nonclearing vitreous hemorrhage.[65] As techniques and instrumentation have improved, its indications have broadened (Table 56–3).[66, 67]

Removing dense, nonclearing vitreous hemorrhage

Table 56–3. INDICATIONS FOR VITRECTOMY IN PROLIFERATIVE DIABETIC RETINOPATHY

Vitreous hemorrhage
  Nonclearing, based on duration and visual need
  To permit photocoagulation of active retinopathy
Traction retinal detachment involving the fovea
Visual loss due to macular striae or distortion (tangential traction)
Combined traction–rhegmatogenous retinal detachment
Rubeosis with media opacity precluding panretinal photocoagulation
Visual loss due to epiretinal membrane or opacified posterior vitreous face
Progressive neovascularization unresponsive to retinal ablation

remains an important indication for vitrectomy in diabetics. The Diabetic Vitrectomy Study Group studied the timing of vitrectomy and its effect on visual outcome and complications.[68, 69] They included patients with severe vitreous hemorrhage (visual acuity <5/200) and compared early vitrectomy (after 1 mo) with deferred vitrectomy (after 1 yr). In patients with type I diabetes, early vitrectomy offered a greater chance of visual recovery. In type II diabetes and mixed type diabetes, the visual results were essentially the same whether vitrectomy was performed early or after 1 yr. However, the study was performed without standardized photocoagulation management in the deferred vitrectomy group and without the use of endolaser photocoagulation in diabetic vitrectomy in either group, and the validity of its conclusions may be questioned. Nevertheless, early vitrectomy offers the chance for prompt recovery of vision, which is of greatest importance to patients who do not have useful vision in the fellow eye.[67]

Progressive fibrovascular proliferation in diabetes can lead to traction retinal detachment. Posterior traction detachments not involving the fovea may remain stable and should be observed.[33, 55, 67] However, once the fovea is involved, vitrectomy is indicated. Surgery should be performed promptly, as degenerative changes in the detached retina will prevent visual recovery after reattachment (Fig. 56–11). The combination of vitreous traction and membrane contraction can lead to retinal holes and combined traction-rhegmatogenous retinal detachments, which need to be approached via pars plana vitrectomy.

Some patients present with cataract and proliferative disease. If adequate panretinal photocoagulation cannot be performed because of media opacity, there are several management options. Cataract surgery can be performed using extracapsular or phacoemulsification techniques, with panretinal photocoagulation performed within a few days of surgery. It should be kept in mind that proliferation may progress rapidly after cataract extraction. Alternatively, pars plana vitrectomy and the endolaser can be used in conjunction with lensectomy (via the pars plana or limbal approach) with intraocular lens placement.[33, 67]

Iris neovascularization, with or without angle involvement, and glaucoma are conventionally treated with panretinal photocoagulation. Vitrectomy with endolaser use is indicated in patients with media opacities, such as cataract or vitreous hemorrhage, or when retinal reattachment is necessary.[67, 70]

Epiretinal membranes develop in diabetes after premacular hemorrhages or after extensive photocoagulation. Vitrectomy is indicated when the patient's vision is compromised enough to warrant surgery.

TECHNIQUE

The details of vitrectomy surgery are discussed in Chapter 100 and are not repeated here. The goals of vitrectomy in diabetic retinopathy are simple in concept. One major objective is to remove media opacities, either

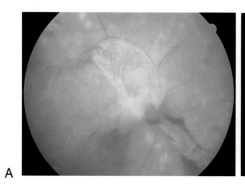
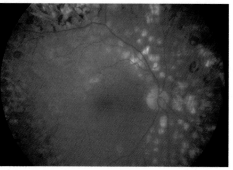

A   B

Figure 56–11. Traction retinal detachment involving the fovea. A, Preoperative photograph illustrating extensive neovascularization emanating from the disc with traction detachment; visual acuity is 20/400. B, Postoperative photograph after vitrectomy showing retinal reattachment and removal of neovascular tissue; visual acuity is 20/40.

vitreous hemorrhage or cataract. The second objective is to relieve vitreous traction causing detachment, distortion, or displacement of the fovea, either transvitreal traction from anterior vitreous to posterior attachments or tangential traction from proliferative tissue adherent to the retinal surface. As dissection is performed, it is important to obtain hemostasis to preserve visualization and allow for effective endophotocoagulation. The final goal is to perform retinal ablation, usually by laser, to prevent subsequent neovascular proliferation.[67]

Two major differences in the technical approach to diabetic vitrectomy are (1) the segmentation technique and (2) the delamination and en bloc resection techniques. In all approaches, the anterior vitreous is removed to permit visualization and to create a fluid space posterior to the lens. In segmentation, an opening is made in the mid-peripheral detached vitreous where it is typically separated from the underlying retina.[65, 67] This opening is extended 360 degrees at the equator and eliminates anteroposterior traction. This "truncation of the vitreous cone" separates the posterior vitreous face with its attachments to the retina from the vitreous base anteriorly. Segmentation then proceeds with dissection of the posterior vitreous face with vertical scissors cuts around each neovascular attachment of the posterior vitreous face to the underlying retina.[33, 67] The end result is the segmentation of the posterior vitreous face into small islands of residual neovascular attachments, and this segmentation relieves contraction between these points and permits reattachment of the retina. These islands can then be trimmed with the vitrectomy instrument.

In delamination and en bloc resection techniques, the anteroposterior traction is not relieved initially but is used to facilitate dissection of the posterior vitreous face in a horizontal fashion. In the delamination technique, an opening is created in the posterior vitreous face over the macula, gaining access to the surgical plane between the posterior vitreous face and the retina. Horizontal scissors transection across the neovascular attachments above the disc and major vascular arcades is performed radiating outward from the posterior pole, ultimately freeing the retina from the posterior vitreous face entirely.[33] In the conceptually similar en bloc technique, access to this same surgical plane is accomplished by creating an opening in the peripheral detached vitreous and then proceeding with horizontal scissors transection across the posterior pole.[71] In both techniques, the

dissection is concluded by using the vitrectomy instrument to remove the now freed posterior vitreous face as it hangs supported by the remaining attachments to the anterior vitreous base.

It should be emphasized that each of the previously mentioned techniques has adherents and detractors. The segmentation technique is criticized for the incomplete removal of proliferative tissue from the retina with possible recurrent hemorrhage or membrane proliferation, and the horizontal dissection techniques are criticized because there is a greater frequency of retinal breaks and a possibility of increased intraocular hemorrhage from transection across the neovascular stalks. These differences remain largely theoretical at the present time, and a combination of surgical approaches is frequently required in a given eye.

Diathermy is used as needed to obtain hemostasis, but most hemorrhages can be controlled by elevation of the infusion fluid height.[67] Air-fluid exchange with internal drainage of subretinal fluid is used in cases of retinal detachment with posterior retinal break, as described in Chapter 97. Panretinal endophotocoagulation is performed when there is active neovascularization or preoperative iris neovascularization or if panretinal photocoagulation has not been performed prior to surgery.[33, 70] Endophotocoagulation is also used to treat iatrogenic retinal breaks. Transscleral cryopexy remains a useful tool when extensive retinal ablation is required or the fundus view is lost. Intraocular tamponade with air, long-acting gas, or silicone oil is used in cases of retinal detachment.

RESULTS

The results of vitrectomy for PDR have improved steadily over the past 2 decades because of increasing vitreoretinal surgical sophistication in general and the introduction of the endolaser and the continuing development of intraocular tamponades in particular. Surgical results in patients with vitreous hemorrhage alone suggest that 71 to 78 percent of patients will have improved vision 6 mo after vitrectomy[72–74] and that 76 percent of patients will have visual acuity of 5/200 or better. For patients with traction retinal detachment involving the fovea, 57 to 75 percent of patients will have improved visual acuity,[75–80] with 20/200 or greater acuity at 6 mo in 40 to 54 percent of patients (Fig. 56–12).[77, 79, 80] Anatomic reattachment of the macula can now be ob-

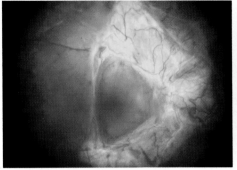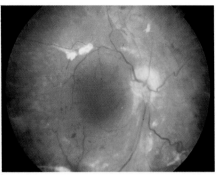

Figure 56–12. Traction retinal detachment involving the fovea. *A,* Preoperative photograph showing severe neovascularization with detachment of the fovea. Visual acuity is 20/400. *B,* Postoperative appearance after vitrectomy showing retinal reattachment with continued inferior distortion of the macula; visual acuity is 20/200.

A

B

tained intraoperatively in the great majority of cases,[76, 77] but recurrent macular detachment (resulting from recurrent epiretinal tissue or rhegmatogenous detachment) occurs in 5 to 23 percent of cases.[76, 79, 80] For patients with combined traction-rhegmatogenous retinal detachment who require vitrectomy for management, long-term macular reattachment is obtained in 64 percent of cases, and improved visual acuity is observed in 53 percent of cases, with 55 percent of these patients having postoperative visual acuity greater than 5/200.[81] These results are an improvement over earlier series in which scleral buckling alone was available for repair; in these series, the retina was reattached in 46 percent of cases and 43 percent of subjects had improved visual acuity.[82] For patients with distortion of the macula from contraction of proliferative tissue (tangential traction syndrome), visual acuity was improved in four of four patients in one report (Fig. 56–13).[34] In large series, preoperative factors associated with a negative prognostic value for visual recovery include iris neovascularization, cataract, visual acuity less than 5/200, and retinal detachment.[83] Long-term studies indicate the stability of visual and anatomic results of vitreoretinal surgery for PDR.[84] However, postoperative complications such as rubeosis (with or without neovascular glaucoma), retinal detachment, recurrent vitreous hemorrhage, and anterior hyaloid fibrovascular proliferation are the chief causes of irreparable visual loss in these patients.[72–81, 85, 86]

COMPLICATIONS

A comprehensive discussion of the complications of vitrectomy is found in Chapter 100; complications of particular relevance to diabetic vitrectomy are briefly highlighted here. Postoperative complications following vitrectomy can be early (within the first week) or late (weeks to months later). Early complications are frequent but can usually be treated successfully. The cornea of the diabetic individual is susceptible to injury at surgery, and epithelial defects may be difficult to heal, requiring pressure patching and occasionally bandage contact lens for resolution.[67] Cataract formation may occur from direct lens trauma at the time of vitrectomy or from exposure to intraocular gas postoperatively.[33, 67] Lens removal should be performed if visually significant, after the posterior segment is stable or sooner if significant complications arise from lens-induced glaucoma or inflammation.

Postoperative hemorrhage usually resolves spontaneously over several weeks. If the fundus is obscured, ultrasound should be performed periodically to exclude retinal detachment.[33, 67] If the blood does not clear within several weeks or if there is a concurrent retinal detachment, reoperation is indicated. Ghost cell glaucoma is an infrequent complication but usually requires a washout procedure to control the intraocular pressure.[33] Retinal detachment after vitrectomy may result from unrecognized retinal holes or traction and requires

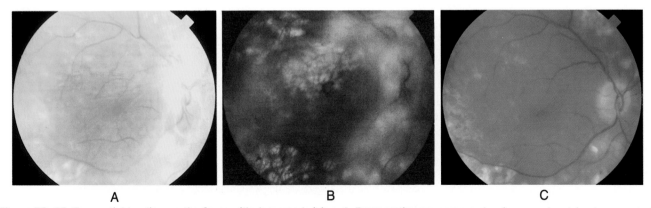

A

B

C

Figure 56–13. Tangential traction on the fovea with decreased vision. *A,* Preoperative appearance showing macular striae to regressed neovascular tissue to the disc. Visual acuity is 20/80. *B,* Fluorescein angiogram documents extensive cystoid edema, primarily affecting the area of traction. *C,* Postoperative photograph 2 mo after vitrectomy and removal of posterior vitreous face; traction is relieved and visual acuity is 20/70.

reoperation.[33, 67] Endophthalmitis is rare and should be diagnosed and treated emergently. Glial recurrence occurs rarely; the glial tissue proliferates directly on the retinal surface and is managed surgically with a segmentation-delamination approach.[33]

Iris and angle neovascularization may develop after vitrectomy; it is usually related to rhegmatogenous retinal detachment or extensive retinal ischemia (Fig. 56–14A).[33, 67] Surgery for the retinal detachment, with extensive panretinal photocoagulation, is indicated. Anterior hyaloid fibrovascular proliferation is a serious complication of diabetic vitrectomy and is most commonly observed in juvenile diabetic patients with severe retinal ischemia undergoing vitrectomy without lens removal.[85, 86] In this situation, extensive neovascularization develops posterior to the lens and along the anterior hyaloid (Fig. 56–14B). Unless surgical intervention, including lensectomy and extensive peripheral retinal ablation, is performed promptly, these eyes are invariably lost.

OCULAR AND SYSTEMIC INTERACTIONS

Ocular Surgery

Cataracts occur commonly in diabetic patients and may require surgical intervention both for visual rehabilitation and for visualization of the fundus. Cataract surgery in diabetics may be more complicated than in the general population, however, with poorer postoperative results, including an increased incidence of cystoid macular edema, an increased risk of progression of the retinopathy, and an increased risk of anterior segment neovascularization.[87, 88]

Cheng and Franklin studied 28 eyes in 21 patients with diabetes who were undergoing cataract extraction but did not have retinopathy preoperatively.[87] Although most patients had extracapsular surgery with posterior chamber lens implantation, four patients with anterior chamber intraocular lenses or iris clip lenses were included. Although two patients acquired background

diabetic retinopathy postoperatively, the corrected visual acuities were 20/40 or better in 88 percent of the patients 12 mo postoperatively. These results compare favorably with those of nondiabetic individuals. Conversely, in 18 eyes of 15 patients with retinopathy preoperatively there was a poorer outcome, with one third of the patients having postoperative visual acuities of less than 20/200. Eight of 18 eyes developed cystoid macular edema. Jaffe described eight patients who progressed from background diabetic retinopathy to severe exudative maculopathy after extracapsular cataract extraction, with diffuse retinal thickening and fluorescein leakage.[89] Six of eight patients received photocoagulation treatment, and postoperative visual acuity was worse in 6 of the eight patients.

Sebestyen studied 74 patients with either no background diabetic retinopathy or mild background retinopathy who were undergoing cataract extraction and lens implantation. He found a similar risk of progression between the operated and the unoperated eyes.[90] Alpar prospectively studied the risk of progression of retinopathy in patients undergoing either extracapsular or intracapsular surgery.[91] He found the lowest incidence of progression of retinopathy in the group undergoing extracapsular extraction but did not differentiate on the basis of preoperative retinopathy, which appears from other studies to be an important factor. It is speculated, however, that an intact lens capsule or anterior hyaloid face acting as a semipermeable barrier between the anterior and the posterior chambers may reduce the risk of postoperative complications, both neovascular and inflammatory.

Aiello and coworkers retrospectively studied 154 diabetic patients who had undergone routine intracapsular cataract extraction in one eye only.[88] The second eye served as a control, and neither eye received laser photocoagulation before surgery or during the first year after surgery. Although most of the eyes had either no diabetic retinopathy or background retinopathy, eyes were included with both quiescent PDR and active PDR. In all of the patients, regardless of the degree of preoperative retinopathy, there was a statistically significant increased risk of rubeosis iridis and neovascular glau-

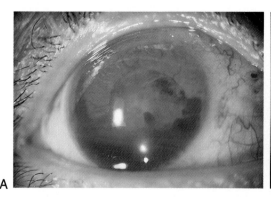 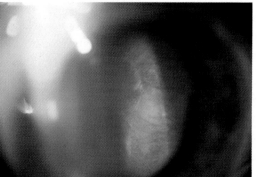

Figure 56–14. Complications of vitrectomy. *A,* Rubeosis, hyphema, neovascular glaucoma, and recurrent detachment following failed vitrectomy for traction retinal detachment involving the fovea; visual acuity is at the no–light perception level. *B,* Anterior hyaloid fibrovascular proliferation in a 22-year-old man after phakic diabetic vitrectomy. Visual acuity is at the seeing hand motions level, and the eye was lost despite repeat surgery.

coma (8 versus 0 percent). In patients with active PDR preoperatively, the risk was even higher (40 versus 0 percent). There was also an increased risk of vitreous hemorrhage after surgery, but this was significant only for the group with no background retinopathy or mild background retinopathy preoperatively and not for those with proliferative retinopathy, probably because of the small number of patients in this group.

Given the increased risks associated with cataract surgery in patients with diabetic retinopathy, special consideration should be made both preoperatively and postoperatively. The preoperative assessment of the visual impairment caused by cataract may be more difficult in the diabetic patient, and use of the blue field entoptoscope and potential acuity meter may be helpful.[92] Even in cases in which the retina appears unremarkable, patients should be cautioned that there may be progression of diabetic changes postoperatively, with resultant poorer visual acuity. When a cataract is developing in a diabetic patient, effort should be made to perform indicated laser photocoagulation, particularly panretinal photocoagulation for active PDR, before the density of the cataract precludes treatment.

Surgery should be directed toward maintaining an adequate aperture for viewing (and possibly treating) the fundus, and an extracapsular technique with "in the bag" placement of an intraocular lens is probably preferred. Because of the increased rate of macular edema postoperatively in diabetic patients, it may be worth considering topical or oral nonsteroidal antiinflammatory agents as well as topical or depot steroids. Wounds should be sutured well to allow laser photocoagulation with a contact lens within 2 to 3 wk of surgery if this proves necessary. If yttrium-aluminum-garnet (YAG) capsulotomy is indicated postoperatively, again the aperture should allow visualization of the retina to the equator. Close follow-up postoperatively is essential, with examination of the iris for neovascularization and a dilated examination of the fundus for macular edema or progression of retinopathy, with consideration of focal or scatter photocoagulation as indicated.

Glucose Control

With the introduction of insulin arose the question, as yet unanswered, Is there a level of glycemic control that would prevent the secondary complications of diabetes? If there is such a level, at what point in the course of the disease must the intervention be made? Most clinical studies have shown an association between poor control of blood glucose levels and increased severity of retinopathy.[23, 24, 26, 28, 93] In the WESDR, an elevated glycosylated hemoglobin level was associated with more severe retinopathy in the younger-onset and older-onset diabetics.[23, 24] In a series at the Joslin Clinic, the risk of PDR in long-standing diabetes was related to elevated glycosylated hemoglobin levels.[26, 28] Several prospective studies have begun placing diabetic patients on continuous subcutaneous insulin infusion (CSII) systems or multidose (three to four doses/day) insulin treatment regimens with home glucose monitoring.[94–96]

The Kroc collaborative study involved 70 patients with diabetes and nonproliferative retinopathy who were randomized to CSII or conventional injection treatment.[94] Over 8 mo, glycosylated hemoglobin and blood glucose levels reached near-normal levels in the treatment group. The level of retinopathy progressed in both groups but was worse in the treatment group, with increased cotton-wool spots and IRMAs. After 2 yr of follow-up, however, little difference was found in the rates of progression between the two groups.[26, 28] The Oslo group, studying 45 patients randomized to CSII, multidose insulin, or conventional insulin therapy, also reported an initial worsening of retinopathy, with microaneurysms and IRMAs.[95] One patient experienced severe preproliferative retinopathy in both eyes after 3 mo of CSII and was followed without laser intervention but continued on CSII with regression of the retinopathy after several months.[97] After 2 yr of follow-up, patients receiving CSII or multiple injections had a lower rate of progression of retinopathy, as measured by the number of microaneurysms and hemorrhages, than did the conventionally treated group. Both studies, as well as other case reports,[98] suggest that rapid achievement of good glycemic control in diabetics with previously poor metabolic control may be detrimental, particularly in patients with preproliferative or proliferative retinopathy.

These trials are limited because of their small study population, short duration, and patient make-up, with varying duration of diabetes and varying degrees of retinopathy. The Diabetes Control and Complications Trial is a large randomized controlled trial, involving 1400 insulin-dependent subjects, designed to study both primary prevention and secondary intervention.[96, 99] Patients are randomized to standard therapy or intensive therapy of multidose insulin injections or CSII. The primary prevention study involves 728 subjects who have had diabetes for 1 to 5 yr and who have no retinopathy or evidence of renal disease. The secondary intervention study involves 715 subjects who have had diabetes for 1 to 15 yr, with minimal background diabetic retinopathy and minimal diabetic nephropathy. The trial has been estimated to have sufficient statistical power to detect a 30 percent reduction in the risk for the development and progression of diabetic retinopathy.

Pregnancy

The role of pregnancy in the progression of diabetic retinopathy remains somewhat controversial. In his 1950 report, Beetham found that disease in pregnant diabetic patients without retinopathy did not progress during the pregnancy.[100] However, patients with evidence of proliferative retinopathy at the onset of pregnancy did so poorly that he recommended that they not undertake pregnancy. In a study by Rodman and associates in 1979, it was found that 8 percent of 201 pregnant diabetic women with no background retinopathy or mild background retinopathy at the onset of pregnancy had the retinopathy progress during pregnancy.[101] In 127 women with proliferative disease, 25 percent had the retinopathy progress during pregnancy. Laatikainen and colleagues prospectively studied 73 consecutive pregnant patients and noted no significant progression of retinopathy in patients who lacked or had minimal retinopathy at the beginning of pregnancy.[102] However, 13 of 20 patients (65 percent) with frank retinopathy in the first trimester were observed to have progressive disease during pregnancy.

Klein and coworkers reported on a prospective case-control study comparing pregnant and nonpregnant insulin-taking diabetic women.[103] Risk factors that were evaluated for the progression of retinopathy included glycosylated hemoglobin, duration of diabetes, current age, diastolic blood pressure, number of past pregnancies, and current pregnancy. Women with evidence of proliferative retinopathy or evidence of previous panretinal photocoagulation were not considered to be at risk for progression, and their data were not included in evaluating risk factors for progression. After correcting for glycosylated hemoglobin level, current pregnancy was found to be significantly associated with progression, with an adjusted odds ratio of 2.3. Diastolic blood pressure had a smaller effect on progression. Pregnant women were significantly more likely to have a decrease in visual acuity, although this was only a mean difference of less than 1 Snellen letter poorer. Klein and coworkers noted that the metabolic control of the pregnant group was markedly better than that of the nonpregnant group.[103] This is probably because of the current obstetric practice of attempting tighter metabolic control during pregnancy. It has been postulated that progression of retinopathy during pregnancy may be at least partly related to the rapid tightening of metabolic control. Laatikainen and associates studied 40 pregnant patients randomized at the end of their first trimester to conventional insulin therapy and CSII.[104] They found that the risk of progression of retinopathy was the same. However, 2 of the patients in the CSII group progressed from background to proliferative retinopathy. Both patients had a rapid decrease in their glycosylated hemoglobin level as they entered CSII treatment. None of the patients in the conventional therapy group developed proliferative changes.

Diabetic retinopathy may also be a predictor of pregnancy outcome. Diabetic patients taking insulin are known to be at increased risk of an adverse pregnancy outcome, including abortion, perinatal death, and severe congenital anomalies. Klein and associates evaluated various risk factors as predictors for adverse outcome and found that the severity of retinopathy was the only variable to significantly predict an adverse outcome.[105]

Pregnancy in diabetic patients is a crucial time for coordinated care by ophthalmologists, obstetricians, and internists. Guidelines for patient care should be understood by all members of the team. Pregnant diabetic patients should be seen during the first month of pregnancy. If no retinopathy is found, follow-up each trimester is sufficient unless the patient becomes symptomatic. An exception is made if the patient is being brought under tighter metabolic control, which could increase the risk of progression of the retinopathy. Improvement in metabolic control should be gradual. Patients with

preproliferative or proliferative disease should be followed every 1 to 2 mo. Laser photocoagulation should be considered earlier in pregnant diabetics than in nonpregnant diabetics when there is evidence of early proliferative or active preproliferative retinopathy. These findings will be revealed by careful ophthalmoscopic and biomicroscopic examination, and fluorescein angiography can usually be avoided in the assessment of the pregnant diabetic patient. Although there are no firm data on the risk of vitreous hemorrhage in patients with proliferative retinopathy, PDR is not an indication for cesarean section.

Hypertension

The relationship between hypertension and the development of diabetic retinopathy is not clear. In the WESDR, the presence and severity of retinopathy were associated with elevated diastolic blood pressure in younger-onset diabetics after 10 yr or more of diabetes and with elevated systolic blood pressure in the older-onset diabetics.[23, 24] In a case-control study at the Joslin Clinic, Rand and associates found that hypertension was associated with proliferative retinopathy in patients who had had diabetes for 15 yr or more.[28] This association remained significant even if cases with renal disease were excluded. In a prospective study at the Joslin Clinic, Janka and coworkers found different rates of progression of severe retinopathy in patients with diastolic blood pressures less than or greater than 70 mmHg.[26, 106] Chase and colleagues also found that elevated diastolic blood pressure, even just to high-normal values, carried an increased risk of retinopathy in young diabetics.[107] Since hypertension is a known risk factor for stroke and myocardial infarction, it is important that elevated blood pressure be treated in the diabetic patient, regardless of its effect on retinopathy.

Renal Disease

Approximately one third of juvenile-onset insulin-dependent diabetics experience diabetic nephropathy, with the highest risk in the second decade of diabetes.[108] Several risk factors may be involved in the development of diabetic nephropathy, including genetic predisposition, hypertension, and poor glycemic control. Severe retinopathy is more likely to be found in patients with renal insufficiency. In the WESDR, proteinuria was strongly associated with severe retinopathy in the younger-onset diabetics with 10 yr or more of diabetes.[23] Older-onset diabetics with proteinuria were also more likely to have proliferative retinopathy.[24] Renal retinopathy will overlie diabetic retinopathy in uremic patients and consists of a hypertensive component and a uremic component.[9] The hypertensive changes include nerve fiber layer hemorrhages, cotton-wool spots, and a narrowing and irregular caliber of the retinal arterioles. The uremic changes include disc edema and diffuse retinal edema, which may lead to massive macular edema. Treatment of the renal failure, including with diuretics, dialysis, or renal transplantation, may result in decreased retinal and macular edema. Laser photocoagulation is not very effective in this group of patients; it is important to consider laser photocoagulation treatment for preproliferative retinopathy or early proliferative changes in the diabetic patient experiencing renal failure.

The treatment of renal failure may result in a different set of ocular problems. Patients on hemodialysis are at increased risk of elevated intraocular pressure, particularly in eyes that have undergone vitrectomy. Renal transplant patients are at an increased risk of acquiring cataract from chronic corticosteroid treatment or cytomegalovirus retinitis from chronic immunosuppression.[109]

Pancreas Transplantation

Pancreas transplantation, alone or in combination with renal transplantation, is a relatively new and risky procedure performed on diabetic patients with advanced diabetic nephropathy in conjunction with renal transplantation. Several investigators have begun to examine the effect of transplantation on diabetic retinopathy, although all the studies to date have been limited by low numbers and short follow-up. Petersen and Vine reported on eight patients who underwent combined pancreas and renal transplantation from cadaver donors.[110] Four patients successfully retained functioning pancreas transplants for at least 12 mo, whereas four patients with failed pancreas transplants but functioning renal transplants served as the controls. Successful pancreas transplantation led to a euglycemic state, with normal fasting blood glucose and glycosylated hemoglobin levels. However, the progression of retinopathy appeared unaffected. Three of the study group eyes had an increase in capillary closure versus no increase in the control eyes. Four of the study group eyes versus two of the control eyes had an increase in preretinal gliosis. One eye in each group had worsening of proliferative retinopathy. Comparing the variables of visual acuity, macular edema, capillary closure, disc neovascularization, preretinal neovascularization, preretinal gliosis, and severity of retinopathy, no statistically significant difference between the two groups was seen.

Ramsay and associates reported on the ophthalmic outcomes of pancreas transplant recipients, again comparing successful and unsuccessful transplantations.[111] Twenty-two patients were in the successful transplantation group and 16 patients were in the control group, with follow-up averaging 24 mo. Although the investigators noted no substantial difference in the progression of retinopathy in the two groups after 2 yr, they observed a trend toward less progression of retinopathy in the treated group after 3 yr. In order to adequately study the ophthalmic outcomes of pancreas transplantation recipients, it will probably be necessary to pool the patients in transplantation centers across the United States under a common protocol.

Pancreas transplantation still carries significant morbidity and mortality and requires chronic immunosuppression. As a result, the procedure has been limited to patients with end-stage nephropathy, which is a group with a high incidence of advanced retinopathy, many of whom have already received panretinal photocoagulation. It may be difficult to show an effect of pancreas transplantation and normoglycemia on this advanced and already treated eye disease. Furthermore, it does not clarify the issue of whether normoglycemia induced in a diabetic soon after diagnosis could prevent or reduce the incidence of secondary complications.

GUIDELINES FOR EYE CARE OF PATIENTS WITH DIABETES MELLITUS

Optimal eye care for the diabetic patient should reflect coordinated effort from the primary physician, ophthalmologist, and patient. It is essential that the primary physician understand the indications for examination by a qualified ophthalmologist. The following guidelines have been adapted from the Joslin Diabetes Center.[9]

1. All patients with diabetes should be informed that sight-threatening eye disease is a common complication of diabetes. Diabetic eye disease can be present with good vision, and early detection and treatment improves the prognosis.

2. Patients with juvenile-onset diabetes should have a complete ophthalmic examination including history of visual symptoms, measurement of visual acuity and intraocular pressure, and ophthalmoscopic examination through dilated pupils.

3. Individuals with older-onset diabetes should have the preceding ophthalmic examination at the time of diagnosis of the diabetes.

4. After the initial ophthalmic examination, patients with diabetes should be examined yearly, unless more frequent examinations are indicated by their eye disease.

5. Any woman with diabetes who becomes pregnant should be examined for retinopathy early in the first trimester and thereafter as indicated by any abnormality.

6. Any woman with diabetes planning pregnancy should be examined and followed for retinopathy.

7. Patients should be under the care of a retina specialist or ophthalmologist experienced in the care of diabetic retinopathy when their eye findings indicate severe background retinopathy, proliferative retinopathy, or macular edema.

8. Patients with functionally decreased vision should undergo low-vision evaluation and appropriate visual, vocational, and psychosocial rehabilitation.

REFERENCES

1. Waite JH, Beetham WP: The visual mechanism in diabetes mellitus: Comparative study of 2002 diabetics and 457 non-diabetics for control. N Engl J Med 212:367, 429, 1935.
2. The Diabetic Retinopathy Study Research Group: Preliminary report on effects of photocoagulation therapy. Am J Ophthalmol 81:1, 1976.
3. The Diabetic Retinopathy Study Research Group: Photocoagulation treatment of proliferative diabetic retinopathy: The second report of diabetic retinopathy study findings. Ophthalmology 85:82, 1978.

4. Klein R, Klein BE: Vision disorders in diabetes. *In* Harris MI, Hamman RF (eds): Diabetes Data Compiled 1984. Washington, DC, US Government Printing Office, 1985, p XIII.

5. Ashton N: Retinal vascularization in health and disease. Proctor Award Lecture of the Association for Research in Ophthalmology. Am J Ophthalmol 44:7, 1957.

6. Kohner EM, Schilling JS, Hamilton AM: The role of avascular retina in new vessel formation. Metab Ophthalmol 1:15, 1976.

7. Plehwe WE, Sleightholm MA, Kohner EM, et al: Does vitreous fluorophotometry reflect severity of early diabetic retinopathy? Br J Ophthalmol 73:255, 1989.

8. Frank RN: Diabetic retinopathy: Current concepts of evaluation and treatment. Clin Endocrinol Metab 15:933, 1986.

9. Aiello LM, Rand LI, Sebestyen JG, et al: The eyes and diabetes. *In* Marble A (ed): Joslin's Diabetes Mellitus, 12th ed. Philadelphia, Lea & Febiger, 1985.

10. Folkman J: Angiogenesis and its inhibitors. *In* DeVita VT Jr, Hellman S, Rosenberg SA (eds): Important Advances in Oncology, part I. Philadelphia, JB Lippincott, 1985, p 42.

11. Folkman J, Klagsbrun M: Angiogenic factors. Science 235:442, 1987.

12. Glaser BM, D'Amore PA, Michels RG, et al: Demonstration of vasoproliferative activity from mammalian retina. J Cell Biol 84:298, 1980.

13. Glaser BM, D'Amore PA, Michels RG, et al: The demonstration of angiogenic activity from ocular tissues. Preliminary report. Ophthalmology 87:440, 1980.

14. D'Amore PA, Glaser BM, Brunson SK, et al: Angiogenic activity from bovine retina: Partial purification and characterization. Proc Natl Acad Sci USA 78:3068, 1981.

15. Glaser BM: Extracellular modulating factors and the control of intraocular neovascularization. Arch Ophthalmol 106:603, 1988.

16. Folkman J, Klagsbrun M, Sasse J, et al: A heparin-binding angiogenic protein—basic fibroblast growth factor—is stored within basement membrane. Am J Pathol 130:393, 1988.

17. Vlodavsky I, Folkman J, Sullivan R, et al: Endothelial cell–derived basic fibroblast growth factor: Synthesis and deposition into subendothelial extracellular matrix. Proc Natl Acad Sci USA 84:2292, 1987.

18. Soubrane G, Jerdan J, Karpouzas I, et al: Binding of basic fibroblast growth factor to normal and neovascularized rabbit cornea. Invest Ophthalmol Vis Sci 31:323, 1990.

19. Maione TE, Gray GS, Petro J, et al: Inhibition of angiogenesis by recombinant human platelet factor-4 and related peptides. Science 247:77, 1990.

20. Glaser BM, Campochiaro PA, Davis JL Jr, et al: Retinal pigment epithelial cells release an inhibitor of neovascularization. Arch Ophthalmol 103:1870, 1985.

21. Tagawa H, McMeel JW, Furukawa H, et al: Role of the vitreous in diabetic retinopathy. I. Vitreous changes in diabetic retinopathy and in physiologic aging. Ophthalmology 93:596, 1986.

22. Foos RY, Kreiger AE, Forsythe AB, et al: Posterior vitreous detachment in diabetic subjects. Ophthalmology 87:122, 1980.

23. Klein R, Klein BEK, Moss SE, et al: Diabetic Retinopathy. II. Prevalence and risk of diabetic retinopathy when age at diagnosis is less than 30 years. Arch Ophthalmol 102:520, 1984.

24. Klein R, Klein BEK, Moss SE, et al: The Wisconsin Epidemiologic Study of Diabetic Retinopathy. III. Prevalence and risk of diabetic retinopathy when age at diagnosis is 30 or more years. Arch Ophthalmol 102:527, 1984.

25. Aiello LM, Rand LI, Briones JC, et al: Diabetic retinopathy in Joslin Clinic patients with adult-onset diabetes. Ophthalmology 88:619, 1981.

26. Janka JU, Warram JH, Rand LI, et al: Risk factors for progression of background retinopathy in long-standing IDDM. Diabetes 38:460, 1989.

27. Baker RS, Rand LI, Krolewski AS, et al: Influence of JLA-DR phenotype and myopia on the risk of nonproliferative and proliferative diabetic retinopathy. Am J Ophthalmol 102:693, 1986.

28. Rand LI, Krolewski AS, Aiello LM, et al: Multiple factors in the prediction of risk of proliferative diabetic retinopathy. N Engl J Med 3113:1433, 1985.

29. Rand LI, Krolewski AS, Warram JH: Late complications: The critical period. *In* Friedman EA, L'Esperance A (eds): Diabetic Renal-Retinal Syndrome, vol. 3. New York, Grune & Stratton, 1986.

30. Diabetic Retinopathy Study Research Group: Report 6: Design, methods, and baseline results. Invest Ophthalmol Vis Sci 21:149, 1981.

31. Davis MD: Proliferative diabetic retinopathy. *In* Ryan SJ (ed): Retina. St Louis, CV Mosby, 1989.

32. Early Treatment of Diabetic Retinopathy Study Group: Effects of aspirin treatment on diabetic retinopathy. ETDRS Report No. 8. Ophthalmology 98:757, 1991.

33. Charles S: Vitreous Microsurgery. Baltimore, Williams & Wilkins, 1981.

34. Packer AJ: Vitrectomy for progressive macular traction associated with proliferative diabetic retinopathy. Arch Ophthalmol 105:1679, 1987.

35. Beetham WP, Aiello LM, Balodimos MC, et al: Ruby laser photocoagulation of early diabetic neovascular retinopathy. Arch Ophthalmol 83:261, 1970.

36. Beetham WP: Visual prognosis of proliferating diabetic retinopathy. Br J Ophthalmol 47:611, 1963.

37. Meyer-Schwickerath GRE, Schott K: Diabetic retinopathy and photocoagulation. Am J Ophthalmol 66:597, 1968.

38. Aiello LM, Beetham WP, Balodimos MC, et al: Ruby laser photocoagulation in treatment of diabetic proliferating retinopathy: Preliminary report. *In* Goldberg MF, Fine SL (eds): Symposium on the Treatment of Diabetic Retinopathy, Bulletin 1890. Washington, DC, Public Health Service, 1969, p 437.

39. Campbell CJ, Koester CJ, Curtice V, et al: Clinical studies in laser photocoagulation. Arch Ophthalmol 74:57, 1965.

40. Poulsen JE: Diabetes and anterior pituitary insufficiency. Final course and postmortem study of a diabetic patient with Sheehan's syndrome. Diabetes 15:73, 1966.

41. Luft R, Olivecrona H, Ikkos D, et al: Hypophysectomy in man: Further experiences in severe diabetes mellitus. Br Med J 2:752, 1955.

42. Poulsen JE: Recovery from retinopathy in a case of diabetes with Simmonds' disease. Diabetes 2:7, 1953.

43. Sharp PS, Fallon TJ, Brazier OJ, et al: Long-term follow-up of patients who underwent yttrium-90 pituitary implantation for treatment of proliferative diabetic retinopathy. Diabetologia 30:199, 1987.

44. The Diabetic Retinopathy Study Research Group: Four risk factors for severe visual loss in diabetic retinopathy. The third report from the DRS. Arch Ophthalmol 97:654, 1979.

45. Doft BH, Blankenship GW: Single versus multiple treatment sessions of argon laser panretinal photocoagulation for proliferative diabetic retinopathy. Ophthalmology 89:772, 1982.

46. The Diabetic Retinopathy Study Research Group: Photocoagulation treatment of proliferative diabetic retinopathy. Clinical applications of DRS findings. DRS Report No. 8. Ophthalmology 88:583, 1981.

47. The Diabetic Retinopathy Study Research Group: Photocoagulation treatment of proliferative diabetic retinopathy: Relationship of adverse treatment effects to retinopathy severity. DRS Report No. 5. Dev Ophthalmol 2:248, 1981.

48. Plumb AP, Swan AV, Chignell AH, et al: A comparative trial of xenon arc and argon laser photocoagulation in the treatment of proliferative diabetic retinopathy. Br J Ophthalmol 66:213, 1982.

49. Okun E, Johnston GP, Boniuk I, et al: Xenon arc photocoagulation of proliferative diabetic retinopathy. A review of 2688 consecutive eyes in the format of the Diabetic Retinopathy Study. Ophthalmology 91:1458 1984.

50. Blankenship GW: A clinical comparison of central and peripheral argon laser panretinal photocoagulation for proliferative diabetic retinopathy. Ophthalmology 95:170, 1988.

51. Doft BH, Blankenship G: Retinopathy risk factor regression after laser panretinal photocoagulation for proliferative diabetic retinopathy. Ophthalmology 91:1453, 1984.

52. Vine AK: The efficacy of additional argon laser photocoagulation for persistent, severe proliferative diabetic retinopathy. Ophthalmology 92:1532, 1985.

53. Blankenship GW: Red krypton and blue-green argon panretinal

laser photocoagulation for proliferative diabetic retinopathy: A laboratory and clinical comparison. Trans Am Ophthalmol Soc 134:967, 1986.

54. Shea M: Early vitrectomy in proliferative diabetic retinopathy. Arch Ophthalmol 101:1204, 1983.

55. D'Amico DJ: Diabetic traction retinal detachments threatening the fovea and panretinal argon laser photocoagulation. Semin Ophthalmol 6:11, 1991.

56. Early Treatment Diabetic Retinopathy Study Group: Early photocoagulation for diabetic retinopathy. ETDRS No. 9. Ophthalmology 98:766, 1991.

57. Blondeau P, Pavan PR, Phelps CD: Acute pressure elevation following panretinal photocoagulation. Arch Ophthalmol 99:1239, 1981.

58. Lobes LA, Bourgon P: Pupillary abnormalities induced by argon laser photocoagulation. Ophthalmology 92:234, 1985.

59. Pender PM, Benson WE, Compton H, et al: The effects of panretinal photocoagulation on dark adaptation in diabetics with proliferative retinopathy. Ophthalmology 88:635, 1981.

60. Kleiner RC, Elman MJ, Murphy RP, et al: Transient severe visual loss after panretinal photocoagulation. Am J Ophthalmol 106:298, 1988.

61. Wallow I, Johns K, Barry P, et al: Chorioretinal and choriovitreal neovascularization after photocoagulation for proliferative diabetic retinopathy. A clinicopathologic correlation. Ophthalmology 92:523, 1985.

62. Swartz M, Apple DJ, Creel D: Sudden severe visual loss associated with peripapillary burns during panretinal argon photocoagulation. Br J Ophthalmol 67:517, 1983.

63. McCanna R, Chandra SR, Stevens TS, et al: Argon laser–induced cataract as a complication of retinal photocoagulation. Arch Ophthalmol 100:1071, 1982.

64. Lakhanpal V, Schocket SS, Rchards RD, et al: Photocoagulation-induced lens opacity. Arch Ophthalmol 100:1068, 1982.

65. Machemer R: Vitrectomy: A Pars Plana Approach. New York, Grune & Stratton, 1975.

66. Aaberg TM, Abrams GW: Changing indications and techniques for vitrectomy in management of complications of diabetic retinopathy. Ophthalmology 94:775, 1987.

67. Michels RG: Proliferative diabetic retinopathy. Pathophysiology of extraretinal complications and principles of vitreous surgery. Retina 1:1, 1981.

68. The Diabetic Retinopathy Vitrectomy Study Research Group: Early vitrectomy for severe vitreous hemorrhage in diabetic retinopathy. Arch Ophthalmol 103:1644, 1985.

69. The Diabetic Retinopathy Vitrectomy Study Group: Two-year course of visual acuity in severe proliferative diabetic retinopathy with conventional management. Diabetic Retinopathy Vitrectomy Study (DRVS) Report #1. Ophthalmology 92:492, 1985.

70. McCuen BW, Rinkoff JS: Silicone oil for progressive anterior ocular neovascularization after failed diabetic vitrectomy. Arch Ophthalmol 197:677, 1989.

71. Abrams GW, Williams GA: "En bloc" excision of diabetic membranes. Am J Ophthalmol 103:302, 1987.

72. Mandelcorn MS, Blankenship G, Machemer R: Pars plana vitrectomy for the management of severe diabetic retinopathy. Am J Ophthalmol 81:561, 1976.

73. Michels RG, Rice TA, Rice EF: Vitrectomy for diabetic vitreous hemorrhage. Am J Ophthalmol 95:12, 1983.

74. Peyman GA, Raichand M, Huamonte FU, et al: Vitrectomy in 125 eyes with diabetic vitreous hemorrhage. Br J Ophthalmol 60:752, 1976.

75. Barrie T, Feretis E, Leaver P, McLeod D: Closed microsurgery for diabetic traction macular detachment. Br J Ophthalmol 66:754, 1982.

76. Williams DF, Williams GA, Hartz A, et al: Results of vitrectomy for diabetic traction retinal detachments using the en bloc excision technique. Ophthalmology 96:752, 1989.

77. Aaberg TM: Clinical results in vitrectomy for diabetic traction retinal detachment. Am J Ophthalmol 88:246, 1979.

78. Hutton WL, Bernstein I, Fuller D: Diabetic traction retinal detachment: Factors influencing final visual acuity. Ophthalmology 87:1071, 1980.

79. Tolentino FI, Freeman HM, Tolentino FL: Closed vitrectomy in the management of diabetic traction retinal detachment. Ophthalmology 87:1078, 1980.

80. Rice TA, Michels RG, Rice EF: Vitrectomy for diabetic traction retinal detachment involving the macula. Am J Ophthalmol 95:22, 1983.

81. Rice TA, Michels RG, Rice EF: Vitrectomy for diabetic rhegmatogenous retinal detachment. Am J Ophthalmol 95:34, 1983.

82. Miller SA, Shafrin F, Bresnick GH, et al: Scleral buckling for diabetic retinal detachments secondary to proliferative diabetic retinopathy. Am J Ophthalmol 89:103, 1980.

83. Thompson JT, Auer CL, de Bustros S, et al: Prognostic indicators of success and failure in vitrectomy for diabetic retinopathy. Ophthalmology 93:290, 1986.

84. Blankenship G, Machemer R: Long-term diabetic vitrectomy results: Report of 10-year follow-up. Ophthalmology 92:503, 1985.

85. Lewis H, Abrams GW, Williams GA: Anterior hyaloidal fibrovascular proliferation after diabetic vitrectomy. Am J Ophthalmol 104:607, 1987.

86. Lewis H, Abrams GW, Foos RY: Clinicopathologic findings in anterior hyaloidal fibrovascular proliferation after diabetic vitrectomy. Am J Ophthalmol 104:614, 1987.

87. Cheng H, Franklin SL: Treatment of cataract in diabetics with and without retinopathy. Eye 2:607, 1988.

88. Aiello LM, Wand M, Liang G: Neovascular glaucoma and vitreous hemorrhage following cataract surgery in patients with diabetes mellitus. Ophthalmology 90:814, 1983.

89. Jaffe GJ, Burton TC: Progression of nonproliferative diabetic retinopathy following cataract extraction. Arch Ophthalmol 106:745, 1988.

90. Sebestyen JG: Intraocular lenses and diabetes mellitus. Am J Ophthalmol 101:425, 1986.

91. Alpar JJ: Diabetes: Cataract extraction and intraocular lenses. J Cataract Refract Surg 13:43, 1987.

92. Lischwe TD, Ide CH: Predicting visual acuity after cataract surgery using the blue field entoptoscope and projected slides. Ophthalmology 95:256, 1988.

93. Orchard TJ, Dorman JS, Maser RE, et al: Factors associated with avoidance of severe complications after 25 yr of IDDM: Pittsburgh Epidemiology of Diabetes Complications Study 1. Diabetes Care 13:741, 1990.

94. Kroc Collaborative Study Group: Blood glucose control and the evolution of diabetic retinopathy and albuminuria: A preliminary multicenter trial. N Engl J Med 311:365, 1984.

95. Dahl-Jorgensen K, Brinchmann-Hanses O, Hanssen KF, et al: Effect of near normoglycemia for two years on progression of early diabetic retinopathy, nephropathy, and neuropathy: The Oslo study. Br Med J 293:1195, 1986.

96. The DCCT Research Group: Diabetes Control and Complications Trial (DCCT): Results of feasibility study. Diabetes Care 10:1, 1987.

97. Rosenlund EF, Haakens K, Brinchmann-Hanses O, et al: Transient proliferative diabetic retinopathy during intensified insulin treatment. Am J Ophthalmol 105:618, 1988.

98. Dandona P, Bolger JP, Boag F, et al: Rapid development and progression of proliferative retinopathy after strict diabetic control. Br Med J 290:895, 1985.

99. Zinman B: The physiologic replacement of insulin, an elusive goal. N Engl J Med 321:363, 1989.

100. Beetham WP: Diabetic retinopathy in pregnancy. Trans Am Ophthalmol Soc 48:205, 1950.

101. Rodman HM, Singerman LJ, Aiello LM, et al: Diabetic retinopathy and its relationship to pregnancy. In Merkaty TR, Adams PAJ (eds): The Diabetic Pregnancy, a Perinatal Perspective. New York, Grune & Stratton, 1979.

102. Laatikainen L, Larinkari J, Teramo K, et al: Occurrence and prognostic significance of retinopathy in diabetic pregnancy. Metab Pediatr Ophthalmol 4:191, 1980.

103. Klein BEK, Moss SE, Klein R: Effect of pregnancy on progression of diabetic retinopathy. Diabetes Care 13:34, 1990.

104. Laatikainen L, Teramo K, Hieta-Heikeraninen, et al: A controlled study of the influence of continuous subcutaneous insulin infusion treatment on diabetic retinopathy during pregnancy. Acta Med Scand 221:367, 1987.

105. Klein BEK, Klein R, Meur ST, et al: Does the severity of diabetic retinopathy predict pregnancy outcome? J Diabetic Compl 2:179, 1988.
106. Janka HU, Ziegler AG, Valsania P, et al: Impact of blood pressure on diabetic retinopathy. Diabetic Metab 15:333, 1989.
107. Chase HP, Garg SK, Jackson WE, et al: Blood pressure and retinopathy in type I diabetes. Ophthalmology 97:155, 1990.
108. Krolewski AS, Canessa M, Warram JH, et al: Predisposition to hypertension and susceptibility to renal disease in insulin-dependent diabetes mellitus. N Engl J Med 318:140, 1988.
109. Klein R: Recent developments in the understanding and management of diabetic retinopathy. Med Clin North Am 72:1415, 1988.
110. Petersen MR, Vine A: The University of Michigan Pancreas Transplant Evaluation Committee: Progression of diabetic retinopathy after pancreas transplantation. Ophthalmology 97:496, 1990.
111. Ramsay RC, Goetz FC, Sutherland DER, et al: Progression of diabetic retinopathy after pancreas transplantation for insulin-dependent diabetes mellitus. N Engl J Med 318:208, 1988.

Chapter 57

■

Advanced Retinopathy of Prematurity

DAVID G. HUNTER, SHIZUO MUKAI, and TATSUO HIROSE

Retinopathy of prematurity (ROP)—the proliferation of abnormal retinal blood vessels that occurs in newborn infants—has been an important cause of childhood blindness since it was first recognized by Terry in 1942.[1] A near-epidemic of ROP occurred in the decade following its discovery. After Patz and associates[2] confirmed a link between ROP and high oxygen concentrations, oxygen supplementation was curtailed and the incidence decreased. Unfortunately, the decreased incidence of ROP was met with an increase of cerebral palsy and hyaline membrane disease.[3] Since then, the minimal level of oxygen has been given to preserve life and keep neurologic systems intact. Advances in neonatology have led to an increase in the survival of very young premature infants since the 1970s, with a corresponding resurgence of ROP. This chapter focuses on the surgical therapy of advanced ROP and discusses the correlation of surgical success with advances in the understanding of disease pathogenesis. New therapeutic maneuvers are also addressed.

CLINICAL FEATURES[4-14]

Forms of ROP

Prior to the development of indirect ophthalmoscopy, the vascular proliferation of ROP typically was not recognized until a fibroblastic mass was seen behind the lens (retrolental fibroplasia). The earliest stages of acute ROP are now recognized 6 to 8 wk after delivery. Acute ROP typically develops gradually and can regress spontaneously at any stage. After regression of the acute process, scarring or cicatricial disease persists throughout life.[15-17]

Mild Acute ROP. The first clinically apparent manifestation of acute ROP is the development of a demarcation line between vascular and avascular retina. The demarcation line remains within the plane of the retina. It is thin, white, and flat. Avascular retina is present anterior to the line, whereas numerous abnormally branched and tortuous vessels are present posterior to the line.

The demarcation line develops into the "ridge" as ROP progresses. The ridge (also known as the shunt or mesenchymal shunt) is a thickened white or pink structure that extends out of the plane of the retina. Vessels leave the posterior retinal surface to enter the ridge but do not extend into the vitreous. Mild forms of acute ROP usually regress without additional sequelae.

Severe Acute ROP. With further progression, the proliferative vessels may extend upward into the vitreous. Fibrovascular proliferation gives the posterior surface of the ridge a ragged appearance. The retinal vessels near the ridge become dilated and tortuous. If ROP continues to progress, myofibroblasts migrate into the vitreous from the ridge and form a fibrovascular mass that contracts and leads to tractional retinal detachment. Fluid from abnormal neovascular tufts accumulates in the subretinal space.

In some cases, the veins in the posterior pole become quite dilated and the arteries become tortuous ("plus" disease), which is often associated with iris vascular engorgement. Retinal hemorrhage and vitreous haze are other signs of advancing disease.[18] When "plus" disease occurs in the posterior part of the eye, progression of ROP may be very rapid. This unusually aggressive form of ROP has been called "rush" disease by some.[19, 20] In "rush" disease, ROP develops in patients with extremely low birth weight (less than 1000g) by age 3 to 5 wk. The course of disease in some of these patients progresses rapidly to severe ROP and retinal detachment.

Scarring. Significant permanent changes from ROP result from the vitreoretinal traction exerted by fibrous tissue in the vitreous. The severity of disability depends on the location and extent of this fibrous tissue formation. With mild traction, the posterior retinal vessels are straightened somewhat. With more extensive traction, the posterior vessels and the macula are dragged toward the periphery. In more severe cases, all retinal vessels are drawn into a fold that runs radially from the disc. When the scarring is most severe, proliferative tissue extends around the entire circumference of the eye, with a totally detached retina drawn behind the lens.

Classification

The International Classification of ROP was developed in 1984 to standardize the clinical assessment of acute ROP.[21, 22] This classification is based on three clinical parameters: stage of vascular proliferation (Table 57–1), location of disease (proximity to optic disc), and extent of involvement (in clock hours). The International Classification is discussed in more detail in the Pediatric Ophthalmology section, in a later volume of this work.

Diagnosis

Examination Technique. Dilating drops must be used with caution in premature infants.[23] Phenylephrine, 10 percent, can cause tachycardia and hypertension, and concentrations of cyclopentolate greater than 1 percent can cause vomiting or ileus. Phenylephrine, 2.5 percent, tropicamide, 0.5 percent, and cyclopentolate, 1 percent, are generally safe. Oculocardiac reactions do occur, sometimes requiring resuscitative measures. Corneal clouding, transient cataract, postpartum intraretinal hemorrhage, and the tunica vasculosa lentis can interfere with retinal visualization in the youngest premature infants.

Screening.[6, 24, 25] All infants with a birth weight of less than 1250 to 1500 g should be screened. Larger premature infants who have had more than 50 days of supplemental oxygen should also be examined. Eye examina-

Table 57–1. STAGES OF ROP AS DEFINED BY THE INTERNATIONAL CLASSIFICATION OF ROP

Stage	Characteristics
1	Demarcation line
2	Ridge
3	Ridge with extraretinal fibrovascular proliferation
4	Subtotal retinal detachment
	A. Extrafoveal
	B. Including fovea
5	Total retinal detachment

Funnel:	Anterior	Posterior
	Open	Open
	Narrow	Narrow
	Open	Narrow
	Narrow	Open

From Hunter DG, Mukai S: Retinopathy of prematurity: Pathogenesis, diagnosis, and treatment. Int Ophthalmol Clin 32:163–184, 1992.

tions should begin by 4 to 5 wk of age. It is important to note the extent of avascular retina. When the avascular zone is wide (zone 1 or posterior zone 2), the chances of ROP progression are high.[26–28] Once disease is detected, weekly examinations are required to identify eyes that cross the threshold for treatment. Twice/wk examinations may be necessary in extremely severe cases such as zone 1+ disease. Examinations should continue until vascularization has extended to the extreme periphery near the ora serrata. If there is no disease, the timing of follow-up examinations depends on individual risk factors.

SURGICAL TREATMENT

Peripheral Retinal Ablation

The major cause of blindness in ROP is tractional retinal detachment or tractional retinal folds resulting from contraction of fibrovascular proliferative tissues that develop on the surface of the retina and within the vitreous cavity. The development of fibrovascular proliferation is always preceded by neovascularization at the junction of vascular and avascular retina. Neovascularization is presumably induced by secretion of angiogenic factors in the avascular retina. In ROP, the severity of the vasoproliferative response appears to correlate positively with the extent of avascular retina.[26, 27] Thus, treatment of acute ROP might best be directed toward eliminating the source of the vasoproliferative response. Ablation of the peripheral retina by photocoagulation or cryotherapy, which has been used successfully for many years,[29–32] can help achieve this goal.

Photocoagulation. Nagata[33] began to treat acute ROP with xenon photocoagulation in the late 1960s. Initially he treated the neovascular tufts but soon found that coagulation of the avascular zone anterior to the ridge was effective, whereas treatment of neovascular tissue or vascular retina posterior to the ridge was harmful rather than helpful. Photocoagulation continued to be practiced, mainly in Japan, for acute ROP until it was replaced by cryotherapy. With cryotherapy, it was relatively easier to treat the peripheral retina, with a better view of the fundus through the indirect ophthalmoscope. In addition, photocoagulation was generally performed in the operating room, whereas cryotherapy could be performed in the nursery.

The introduction of indirect ophthalmoscope–mounted lasers has led to renewed interest in photocoagulation of the peripheral retina for ROP.[34] A prospective, randomized clinical trial of indirect ophthalmoscopic laser photocoagulation has been performed by McNamara and associates.[35] In that study, argon green laser was used to treat infants with threshold ROP. The outcome of laser-treated infants was statistically indistinguishable from a cryotherapy-treated control group. There was a trend toward more favorable outcomes in the laser-treated group, although the difference was not statistically significant in this group of

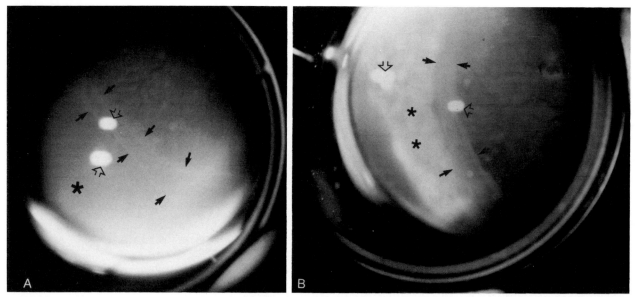

Figure 57–1. *A,* Fundus photograph of stage 3 moderate retinopathy of prematurity (ROP). The *solid arrows* show a large ridge with extraretinal fibrovascular proliferation. Peripheral to this ridge is a large area of avascular retina indicated by an *asterisk.* Two *open arrows* indicate light reflected from the condensing lens. *B,* Fundus photograph of the same eye immediately after ablation of the avascular retina anterior to the ridge by diode laser coagulation. The *solid arrows* show a ridge with extraretinal fibrovascular proliferation. The treated area of avascular retina shows extensive coagulation marks *(asterisk).* In this case, laser coagulation was applied in three to four contiguous rows anterior to the ridge without treating all the way up to the ora serrata. Treatment was as effective as cryotherapy. Two *open arrows* indicate light reflected from the condensing lens.

28 eyes. The authors felt that laser treatment was preferable to cryotherapy, as it was easier to place discrete scars, with less perceived infant discomfort.

There are other advantages of indirect laser photocoagulation over cryotherapy. Indirect laser treatment does not require as much manipulation of the globe. It is particularly promising for treatment of disease located in zone 1 or posterior zone 2, in which cryotherapy is technically difficult and requires conjunctival incision. A disadvantage of the blue-green argon laser is in the treatment of eyes with a persistent tunica vasculosa lentis. In these eyes, patent blood vessels cross the anterior surface of the lens. When blue-green laser is delivered through the pupil, these vessels are coagulated, which induces miosis and opacifies the media.

In our experience, the diode laser, which operates in infrared wavelengths, appears to be as effective as the argon laser for peripheral retinal ablation in acute ROP (Fig. 57–1). An advantage of the diode laser over the argon laser is that its longer wavelength allows treatment through a persistent tunica vasculosa lentis without coagulation of the anterior vessels.

Cryotherapy. Acute ROP has been treated with cryotherapy nearly as long as it has been treated with photocoagulation, with Yamashita[32] first reporting on its efficacy in 1972. Although many specialists subsequently reported a beneficial effect of cryotherapy, conflicting reports led to continued controversy over its usefulness. Widespread acceptance of cryotherapy was initially limited by the lack of a controlled study conclusively demonstrating efficacy. Furthermore, complications such as bleeding following treatment of the ridge (shunt) and late retinal detachment have been reported.[36] To

determine the efficacy of cryotherapy, a multicenter double-blind controlled study (the "cryo-ROP" study) was conducted.[28] Table 57–2 describes the definitions of threshold and prethreshold for the development of blinding consequences of ROP in this study. Threshold eyes were eligible for treatment, whereas prethreshold eyes were observed. In eyes with symmetric disease, one eye was treated and the other observed. With asymmetric disease, individual eyes were randomized for treatment or observation. Treatment was applied to a contiguous expanse of the entire avascular retina. The ridge itself was not treated. Treatment was repeated if "plus" disease persisted. Any eye with retinal detachment, posterior retinal fold, or retrolental tissue obscuring the posterior pole was considered to have an unfavorable outcome. At 12 months, 47 percent of control eyes had an unfavorable outcome, compared with 26 percent of treated eyes. Thus treatment is now recommended in at least one eye of nearly all patients with threshold ROP. However, because of uncertainty about the long-term sequelae of cryotherapy, the authors of

Table 57–2. THRESHOLD AND PRETHRESHOLD ROP AS DEFINED FOR THE CRYO-ROP STUDY

	Stage	Zone	Extent
Prethreshold	< 2 +	1	Any
	2 +, or 3	2	Any
Threshold	3+	1 or 2	5 contiguous or 8 cumulative

From Hunter DG, Mukai S: Retinopathy of prematurity: Pathogenesis, diagnosis, and treatment. Int Ophthalmol Clin 32:163–184, 1992.

the study refrained from advocating treatment of both eyes in every case, except in cases of bilateral stage 3 +, zone 1 retinopathy. They suggested that each patient with symmetric threshold disease be considered on an individual basis.

It is difficult to draw conclusions about treatment of zone 1 ROP from the cryo-ROP study. Only 12 eyes (8 percent) in the study had zone 1 disease. Eyes with zone 1 disease are more difficult to treat, but the outcome data of this group were combined with those of the eyes with zone 2 disease. The study did not address the timing of cryotherapy except to state that it should commence within 72 hr of the recognition of threshold disease. Timing of treatment may have a substantial influence on the success of treatment, especially in eyes with zone 1 disease.

The cryotherapy study design and recommendations may be conservative.[38, 39] Hindle[38] states that control eyes were released for treatment too late to prevent visual disability. Kretzer and colleagues recommend a second ring of treatment to the ridge in any patient with stage 3b (moderate) or greater ROP.[40, 41] This treatment should be performed after the initial therapy in order to allow the engorged vessels in the ridge time to regress. Their recommendations are based on ultrastructural studies, which indicate that myofibroblasts emerge from the ridge in eyes with stage 3b disease. The myofibroblasts migrate into the vitreous and contract, leading to retinal detachment even after the avascular retina has been destroyed. Thus, Kretzer and Hittner[37] predict that retinal detachments will develop in some of the early successes of the cryo-ROP study because of the lack of treatment to this area. Cryotherapy at threshold may be too late in infants with zone 1 disease, as the disease can progress rapidly to retinal detachment.

The decision to treat both eyes in patients who have bilateral stage 3 + disease ultimately depends on the risk that unrecognized late complications of cryotherapy will emerge.[42, 43] Thus far, there is little evidence of such complications. Greven and Tasman[44] described three cases of rhegmatogenous retinal detachment occurring at the junction of treated and untreated areas 1 to 4 yr following cryotherapy. Topilow and Ackerman saw only one case of retinal detachment in 25 treated infants followed for an average of 2 yr.[45] Ben-Sira and associates[46] followed patients for 8 yr after treatment and found only a higher incidence of myopia. Seiberth and colleagues[47] found no evidence of increased refractive errors 2 to 7 yr after cryotherapy.

Even when cryotherapy fails and retinal detachment ensues, subsequent surgical intervention may be technically less difficult in an eye that has been treated preoperatively. The induced shrinkage of neovascular tufts may decrease the bleeding, fibrin production, and scarring that follow vitrectomy.[48]

Cryotherapy is generally performed in the operating room with continuous monitoring by an anesthesiologist or neonatologist.[49, 50] General anesthesia is used in most published protocols, although local anesthesia is also acceptable. Treatment is administered transconjunctivally if possible. In cases of posterior disease, a small limbal peritomy is performed to permit subconjunctival treatment. The entire avascular retina peripheral to the ridge is ablated (Fig. 57–2). Contiguous transretinal cryotherapy marks are placed. To avoid vitreous hemorrhage, applications must be delicately placed, with sufficient time between treatments to allow the ice ball to melt. The cryoprobe should be removed at intervals of 5 min to avoid prolonged ocular hypertension with central retinal artery compromise. The response to therapy is usually observable within a few days. Retreatment may be required in patients in whom untreated areas persist in the setting of "plus" disease, especially if there is a shallow segmental retinal detachment or progression

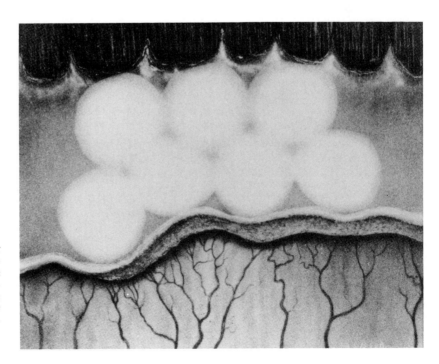

Figure 57–2. Fundus drawing of the avascular retina immediately after five spots of cryoapplications shown as white spots anterior to the fibrovascular ridge. (From Cryotherapy for Retinopathy of Prematurity Cooperative Group: Multicenter trial of cryotherapy for retinopathy of prematurity: Preliminary results. Arch Ophthalmol 106:471–479, 1988. Copyright 1988, American Medical Association.)

of extraretinal fibrovascular proliferation contiguous with a skipped area.

Retinal Detachment Surgery[17, 51–53]

Once retinal detachment occurs, it can progress rapidly. Peripheral detachments posterior to the ridge can proceed to total retinal detachment within a day, and total detachments can become closed funnels within a week. In acute ROP, tractional detachment is most commonly observed. Tractional detachments originate at the ridge, at which point myofibroblasts pull in a "purse string" configuration. Less commonly, when plasma leaks from abnormal neovascular tufts, subretinal fluid collects. Shallow exudative detachments of avascular retina anterior to the ridge do not normally require surgical intervention.[54]

Rhegmatogenous detachments are only rarely seen in acute ROP and are usually iatrogenic at this age. In contrast, they are the most common retinal detachment seen in older children and adults with cicatricial ROP. Many of these cases are long-standing, unnoticed by the patient until subretinal fluid expands into a large enough area to be visually symptomatic. The detached retina is thin, with multiple small equatorial breaks hidden by a vitreous membrane. Tractional detachments are also seen as late sequelae.

Scleral Buckling. Scleral buckling can be used to treat milder forms of retinal detachment in acute ROP.[27, 55] Greven and Tasman[56] reported success with scleral buckling in 13 of 22 eyes with stages 4b and 5 (open-open configuration) ROP. More than 50 percent of patients had satisfactory anatomic results in most other studies.[54, 57, 58] Scleral buckling is an accepted treatment for ROP patients with rhegmatogenous detachment.[59]

The timing of scleral buckling in the management of nonrhegmatogenous stage 4a detachment is controversial, as partial nonrhegmatogenous detachments often reattach spontaneously. However, the duration of retinal detachment influences prognosis, as the retina becomes dysplastic after relatively brief periods of detachment.[58] Thus, scleral buckling should be considered in early posterior tractional detachments and in large exudative detachments. There is less agreement about surgery in tractional detachments that do not involve the posterior pole. Until a randomized, controlled trial of surgery for advanced ROP is performed, the decision to undertake surgery in these controversial cases must be determined on an individual basis.

Cryotherapy is often performed at the time of retinal detachment surgery, especially in tractional or exudative cases with continued active neovascularization. However, cryotherapy is much less effective in shrinking neovascularization once the retina is detached to the extent that surgery is required. If cryotherapy has already been performed, the buckling procedure should be performed without additional retinal ablation. A silicone band is used to encircle the globe at the site of ridge elevation. External drainage of subretinal fluid is necessary if the retina is highly elevated. Greven and

Tasman[56] recommend scleral dissection in some patients and fluid drainage in nearly all patients.

The silicone band may cause globe constriction as ocular growth proceeds in such small eyes. Machemer and deJuan[57] do not routinely remove the band unless there is clinically apparent retardation of ocular growth. Greven and Tasman[56] also leave the band in place in most cases. McPherson and coworkers[58] and Orellana[54] state that the band ideally should be transected 3 to 6 mo postoperatively to permit normal ocular growth.

Prophylactic Scleral Buckle. The uniform loss of macular vision in infants who have undergone therapeutic scleral buckling for zone 1 stage 4b or 5 (macula detached) ROP has been noted by Hittner and Kretzer.[60] They proposed two reasons for the poor outcome in these infants. First, explosive ocular growth occurs following development of ROP in these infants, whereas the area of vascularized retina does not increase. The distance between the temporal optic disc and the center of the macula remains precisely 4 mm from preterm to adulthood. Thus, tractional factors are exaggerated with ocular growth. Second, the retinal interaction with pigment epithelium is critical to normal retinal development. An interruption of the normal configuration for even a few days may result in irreversible dysmorphic changes. These considerations led to the proposal that these extremely low birth weight infants be treated with a prophylactic scleral buckle at the time of cryotherapy for threshold ROP. Macular detachment or ectopia has not yet developed in 80 percent of eyes in these infants with zone 1 disease who were treated with a prophylactic scleral buckle.

Vitrectomy. Vitrectomy may be considered when scleral buckling fails, a high retinal detachment is present, media opacification by vitreous strands occurs, or a fibroblastic membrane is observed behind the lens. With advances in surgical approaches to ROP, the retina can be reattached in an apparently unsalvageable eye (Fig. 57–3). This is achieved by meticulous removal of proliferative membranes, sometimes combined with scleral buckling, during vitrectomy surgery.[58, 61–65]

There are two major approaches to vitrectomy in advanced ROP: closed and "open sky." Each technique has its advocates. Charles,[61, 66] Machemer and deJuan,[57, 62] and Trese[67] have all used the closed technique for management of ROP. The small size of the eye and extensive proliferation necessitated several modifications of the standard closed-vitrectomy approach used in adults. Sewn-in infusion cannulas cannot be used; instead, a bent 20-gauge blunt cannula is necessary. When the retina is pulled so far anteriorly that it abuts the lens, the cannula must be inserted through the iris root or anterior ciliary body to avoid entering the subretinal space; thus, a sector iridectomy is often required. Machemer and deJuan[57] recommend the corneal limbal approach to avoid tearing of the anteriorly pulled retina by the instrument as it is inserted through the pars plicata. Following lensectomy, the epiretinal-retrolental membrane is dissected by scissors delamination and removed with the vitrectomy instrument. Hyaluronic acid is used in closed vitrectomy by Trese[67] and

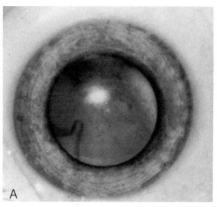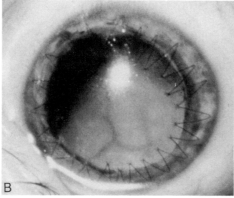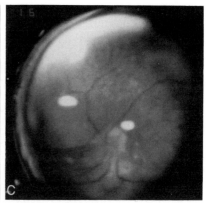

Figure 57–3. Photograph of the eye of a 16-month-old boy with stage 5 ROP. The retina is totally detached and pulled forward toward the lens. The vessels of the detached retina are seen through the thin retrolental fibrous membrane. B, Photograph of the same eye 1½ mo after open-sky vitrectomy. C, Fundus photograph of the same eye. The retina is attached with retinal vessels drawn into the broad dry fold inferiorly.

others. Blacharski and Charles[68] advocate intraoperative thrombin infusion to minimize bleeding. Charles does not normally use encircling bands following vitrectomy. He reports an anatomic success rate of 46 percent (Table 57–3).[61]

The open-sky technique was developed by Schepens in 1981.[64] In this technique, the cornea is removed with a 7- to 8-mm trephine and stored in culture medium during surgery.[17] A Flieringa ring is used to preserve the shape of the eye during surgery. The eye is irrigated with chilled balanced salt solution during the procedure to minimize fibrin formation. Iridotomies are made at the 12 and the 6 o'clock positions, and the lens is removed with a cryoprobe. This allows direct visualization of the transparent anterior hyaloid and the fibrous white retrolental membrane. The strongly adherent retrolental membrane and the fibrous mass filling the funnel of detached retina are cut and removed as a block. Hyaluronic acid is used to expand the funnel of detachment and to identify the location of the adhesion of the fibrous tissues to the detached retina to facilitate dissection of these tissues. The iridotomies are closed with 10–0 polypropylene sutures, and the corneal button

is replaced with 10–0 nylon sutures. Scleral buckling is performed by Hirose and coworkers[52] 4 to 8 wk later if the retina shows no sign of reattachment. They report a 39-percent anatomic success rate using this technique (Table 57–3). Eyes with the closed-closed configuration had a 29-percent reattachment rate; all other eyes had reattachment rates of greater than 60 percent. McPherson and associates[69] had a 22-percent anatomic success rate with open funnels and an 11-percent success rate with closed funnels using the open-sky technique, whereas Tasman and colleagues[70] had a 35-percent anatomic success rate (Table 57–3).

Time will tell which technique gives superior results. The results depend in part on the selection of cases. The advantage of the closed technique is the avoidance of removal and replacement of the corneal button. The disadvantages include the need for a pars plicata or iris root entry site because of the extreme anterior displacement of the retina and the difficulty maneuvering vitrectomy instruments within the small closed space of the premature infant eye. Incomplete removal of residual peripheral membranes results in only "partial" reattachment (Table 57–3). Reported disadvantages of the open-

Table 57–3. RESULTS OF VITRECTOMY FOR STAGE 5 ROP

Study	Yr	No. of Patients	Anatomic Success (%)	Functional Success* (%)	Technique
Trese[67]	1984	40	40	28	Closed
Charles[61]	1986	586	46	35–45	Closed
Trese[48]†	1987	10	80	30‡	Closed
Zilis et al[65]	1990	121	9–40§	11	Closed
McPherson et al[69]	1986	47	13	4	Open sky
Tasman et al[70]	1987	23	35	4	Open sky
Hirose et al[52]‖	1974–1989	524	39	46¶	Open sky
Hirose et al[52]	1984–1989	123	67	41¶**	Open sky
Cryo-ROP[75]	1991	71	28	3	Either

*Functional success is "fixation and following" unless otherwise noted.
†Preoperative cryotherapy.
‡"Grasp brightly colored objects 2.5 cm in diameter."
§9 percent complete, 31 percent partial reattachments.
‖94 percent of patients had leukocoria.
¶Ambulatory vision.
**62 percent had recordable pattern visual-evoked response.

sky technique include increased complexity of postoperative management because of the need for a corneal graft, prolonged hypotony, and a longer operating time. In experienced hands, however, operative time is less than 2 h.[52] Choroidal detachments are rare, and corneal endothelial cell density changes little.[71] The advantage of the open-sky technique is the excellent visualization of the pathologic process and the direct access to the retrolental membrane. This makes more complete removal of peripheral membranes possible; thus, the retina is subjected to less stretch when it is reattached at the posterior pole. Some cases that would be inoperable by the closed technique can be repaired using the open-sky method. The main drawback of open-sky vitrectomy is the difficulty exposing the posterior pole in eyes with a narrow funnel. The use of additional hyaluronic acid is helpful in these situations.

The optimal timing of vitrectomy remains to be determined. In patients with stage 5 ROP, a session of cryotherapy before surgery may promote quiescence of the vasoproliferative process, allowing earlier repair of the detachment.[48] Chong and colleagues[72] recommend operating as soon as "plus" disease has regressed. At this stage, the detachment is typically still an open funnel; however, adhesion of the membrane to the retina is very strong, and complete removal of the fibrous tissues from the retina is extremely difficult, with an increased chance of reproliferation. Thus, the potential functional advantage of operating early must be weighed against the increased difficulty of extracting adherent membranes and the increased postoperative fibrin production (with development of secondary membranes) if vitrectomy is performed too soon. The optimal time for surgery may be after 6 mo of age but before the patient is 1 yr old. One may operate earlier if the eye has been treated with cryotherapy or photocoagulation and the fundus is dry with no sign of active vasoproliferation. Even when surgery is delayed for years, it may be worth attempting repair in some cases, as ambulatory acuity has been obtained postoperatively in patients with long-standing retinal detachment up to 3 yr of age.[52]

Iatrogenic retinal breaks produced during vitrectomy surgery are extremely difficult to close. Peripheral breaks may be closed by scleral buckling, but breaks formed in the posterior pole in infants with ROP are impossible to close either with scleral buckling or with air-fluid exchange and internal drainage of subretinal fluid. Other factors that can make ROP surgery more difficult include the presence of a persistent hyaloid artery,[73] intraocular bleeding, multiple circular retinal folds, and tilting of the funnel toward one quadrant.[52]

Although anatomic reattachment can be achieved in eyes with severe disease using either technique, vision has been disappointingly poor.[72, 74] Machemer and de-Juan reported an anatomic success rate of 64 percent and a functional success rate of 43 percent in stage 4 cases.[57] Patients with stage 5 ROP do not fare as well (see Table 57–3). Stage 5 cases with the open-open configuration have the best prognosis; the closed-closed configuration is least likely to result in recovery of useful vision.[65]

In the cryo-ROP study, the visual outcome of infants who progressed to stage 5 retinal detachment was studied retrospectively.[75] Surgery was performed by several different surgeons using different techniques. There were no standardized preoperative criteria for undertaking vitrectomy, and patients were not randomized. The configuration of detachment (open versus closed funnel) was not specified. The anatomic success rate was 28 percent in operated eyes, with a functional success rate of 3 percent. Although data were not specified for all eyes that did not undergo vitrectomy, 1 of the 10 eyes described had spontaneous resolution of the retinal detachment. Eyes that underwent vitrectomy had a lower incidence of glaucoma and shallow anterior chamber compared with unoperated eyes. The rates of corneal opacity, hypotony, and vitreous hemorrhage were similar in the two groups. Thus, although surgical approaches to ROP are meeting with improved rates of retinal reattachment in ROP, the visual outcomes to date indicate that the emphasis must remain on prevention of retinal detachment.[75]

THEORETICAL BASIS OF THERAPEUTIC APPROACHES

Retinal Vascular Development[37, 76]

At a gestational age of 6 wk, the hyaloid artery enters the eye and begins to fill the vitreous cavity with vessels. The retina remains avascular until 16 wk of gestational age, when mesenchymal spindle cells arise from the adventitia of the hyaloid artery and migrate peripherally through cystoid spaces as the outer plexiform layer differentiates. The migrating spindle cells form a circumferential apron that advances peripherally toward the ora serrata. Spindle cells behind the advancing apron form solid cords that canalize and metamorphose into capillary endothelial cells. Although spindle cells reach the temporal ora serrata by 29 wk of gestational age, fully formed inner retinal vessels do not reach the ora serrata until term. The entire process of retinal vascular development occurs in the hypoxic in utero environment.

Early Models of ROP Pathogenesis

Experimental models of kitten and puppy retinal neovascularization led Ashton and Patz and their colleagues[12, 77] to propose that elevated oxygen levels lead to retinal vasoconstriction, which can cause permanent vessel obliteration. According to this once widely accepted theory, endothelial cell proliferation adjacent to closed capillaries followed return to room air, leading to new vessel growth.

The kitten retinal vasculature studied by Ashton and associates was almost completely obliterated by elevated oxygen. Kretzer and coworkers[78] performed electron microscopic studies of eyes from preterm infants at high risk for the development of ROP in an attempt to confirm this model in humans. None of the eyes examined demonstrated retinal vasoobliteration or endothelial cell destruction, nor was there any evidence of inner retinal hypoxia or ischemia.

The observation that ROP can develop in infants exposed to minimal supplemental oxygen also suggests that human ROP may not be caused by oxygen-induced vasoconstriction. In addition, the vasoobliteration hypothesis cannot explain the efficacy of cryotherapy of the avascular peripheral retina. This theory was based on analysis of animal models of retinal vascularization that do not develop via spindle cells and on experimental models of retinopathy that do not progress to retinal detachment.

Spindle Cell Model of ROP Pathogenesis

Kretzer and associates[78, 79] have proposed that the spindle cells in the periphery of the immature retina are critical to the pathogenesis of ROP. According to this theory, developing spindle cells are bombarded with oxygen free radicals when they are removed from the hypoxic in utero environment at birth. The reduced free radical scavenging capability of preterm infants allows extensive plasma membrane lipid peroxidation to occur. Spindle cell plasma membranes form extensive intercellular linkages via gap junctions in response to this injury. Once linked by gap junctions, spindle cells are no longer able to migrate or canalize normally. Instead, they begin active protein synthesis. These "activated" spindle cells probably secrete an angiogenic factor that promotes vasoproliferation at the border between vascular and avascular retina.[40]

Two months after the initial insult, usually after stage 3+ disease has developed, myofibroblasts differentiate from a stem cell line in the shunt. These cells form a contractile sheet that invades the vitreous, inducing traction that leads to retinal detachment. Existing tractional forces are accentuated by the rapid ocular growth that occurs between 24 and 40 wk.[37] Contraction of the shunt with retinal stretching, contraction of proliferative tissue with retinal elevation, and intravitreal proliferation ultimately cause detachment of the retina. The location of proliferative tissue is in part determined by the detached retinal configuration.[80]

Targets of Therapy

Many of the clinical features of ROP can be explained by the spindle cell hypothesis. Undifferentiated spindle cells are not normally present in the eye at term, and immaturity is central to the development of ROP. More immature infants have larger expanses of spindle cells, which makes them more susceptible to the development of ROP. The observation that ROP can develop without the presence of high oxygen tension is supported by evidence that cell damage, environmental stress, low pH, and lipid peroxidation can all induce gap junction formation. According to the spindle cell model of pathogenesis, disease progression should be slowed or prevented by delivery of adequate levels of antioxidants to the retina.[81]

Cryotherapy is a logical treatment option because it destroys spindle cells, the probable source of angiogenic factor. Most of the spindle cells in the avascular inner retina must be destroyed for cryotherapy to induce regression of ROP. In the smallest preterm infants, additional spindle cells emerge from the hyaloid artery adventitia and vascularized retina as development continues; thus, multiple sessions of cryotherapy may be necessary. Ideally, the myofibroblasts at the retina-vitreous interface should also be obliterated by transretinal cryotherapy. To destroy the sheets of myofibroblasts before they have migrated from the shunt into the vitreous, Kretzer and Hittner[37] advocate a second session of cryotherapy directly to the shunt 3 to 7 days after the initial treatment. During the second cryotherapy treatment, any extraretinal fibrovascular proliferation should be destroyed to prevent contraction of myofibroblasts in this area. This extensive chorioretinal scar from cryotherapy functions as a new ora serrata at the periphery of vascularized retina, which eliminates transmission of tractional forces to functioning retina.

Ultrastructural observations of eyes with retinal detachments of less than 8 wk duration demonstrate a grossly disorganized retina, with atrophic nuclear layers and a distorted inner layer.[82] Disorganization and death may occur earlier than is seen in mature retinas because of the extraordinary dependence of the developing retina (the macula in particular) on interactions with surrounding tissues. This may explain why such poor functional results are obtained in many patients despite anatomic reattachment—a dysmorphic retina has little visual potential whether attached or not.

SUMMARY

Interest in ROP has grown along with the increasing incidence of the disease. During the 1980s, a widely accepted classification of the disease process was agreed upon, new approaches to its prevention and treatment were developed, and advances in our understanding of the risk factors and pathogenesis of the disease emerged. Despite these advances, the incidence of ROP continues to increase. The increasing use of surfactant in the neonatal intensive care unit[83] may result in increased survival of infants weighing less than 600 g, with an additional surge of cases of ROP.

Treatments of advanced stages of acute ROP have also been refined, with properly timed cryotherapy or laser photocoagulation preventing retinal detachment, and meticulous vitrectomy techniques successfully removing tractional forces. The improved anatomic success rates of vitreoretinal surgery have been confounded by disappointingly poor visual function. Still, surgery should be pursued when indicated, as even attaining hand motion visual acuity allows many patients to remain ambulatory. Further modifications of treatment protocols, with an emphasis on preventing retinal detachment, will be necessary before significantly better acuity can be retained in eyes with severe stages of this devastating disease.

REFERENCES

1. Terry TL: Extreme prematurity and fibroblastic overgrowth of persistent vascular sheath behind each crystalline lens. I. Preliminary report. Am J Ophthalmol 25:203, 1942.
2. Patz A, Hoeck LE, DeLaCruz E: Studies on the effect of high oxygen administration in retrolental fibroplasia. Nursery observations. Am J Ophthalmol 35:1248–1253, 1952.
3. McDonald AD: Neurological and ophthalmic disorders in children of very low birth weight. Br Med J 1:895, 1962.
4. Archambault P, Gomolin JE: Incidence of retinopathy of prematurity among infants weighing 2000 g or less at birth. Can J Ophthalmol 22:218–220, 1987.
5. Cats BP, Tan KE: Retinopathy of prematurity: Review of a four-year period. Br J Ophthalmol 69:500–503, 1985.
6. Clemett RS, Darlow BA, Hidajat RR, Tarr KH: Retinopathy of prematurity: Review of a five-year period, examination techniques and recommendations for screening. Aust NZ J Ophthalmol 14:121–125, 1986.
7. Gibson DL, Sheps SB, Schechter MT, et al: Retinopathy of prematurity: A new epidemic? Pediatrics 83:486–492, 1989.
8. Harden AF: Retinopathy of prematurity—A long-term follow-up. Trans Ophthalmol Soc UK 105:717–719, 1986.
9. Hoon AH, Jan JE, Whitfield MF, et al: Changing pattern of retinopathy of prematurity: A 37-year clinic experience. Pediatrics 82:344–349, 1988.
10. Keith CG, Doyle LW, Kitchen WH, Murton LJ: Retinopathy of prematurity in infants of 24–30 weeks' gestational age. Med J Aust 150:293–296, 1989.
11. Ng YK, Fielder AR, Shaw DE, Levene MI: Epidemiology of retinopathy of prematurity. Lancet 2:1235–1238, 1988.
12. Payne JW, Patz A: Current status of retrolental fibroplasia: The retinopathy of prematurity. Ann Clin Res 11:205, 1979.
13. Schulenburg WE, Prendiville A, Ohri R: Natural history of retinopathy of prematurity. Br J Ophthalmol 71:837–843, 1987.
14. Valentine PH, Jackson JC, Kalina RE, Woodrum DE: Increased survival of low birth weight infants: Impact on the incidence of retinopathy of prematurity. Pediatrics 84:442–445, 1989.
15. Ben-Sira I, Nissenkorn I, Kremer I: Retinopathy of prematurity. Surv Ophthalmol 33:1–16, 1988.
16. Biglan AW, Cheng KP, Brown DR: Update on retinopathy of prematurity. Int Ophthalmol Clin 29:2–9, 1989.
17. Hirose T, Lou PL: Retinopathy of prematurity. Int Ophthalmol Clin 26:1–23, 1986.
18. Bachynski BN, Kincaid MC, Nussbaum J, Green WR: A hemorrhagic form of zone 1 retinopathy of prematurity. J Pediatr Ophthalmol Strabismus 26:56–60, 1989.
19. Majima A: Studies on retinopathy of prematurity. 1. Statistical analysis of factors related to occurrence and progression in active phase. Jpn J Ophthalmol 21:404–420, 1977.
20. Nissenkorn I, Kremer I, Gilad E, et al: "Rush" type retinopathy of prematurity: Report of three cases. Br J Ophthalmol 71:559–562, 1987.
21. Committee for the Classification of ROP: An international classification of ROP. Arch Ophthalmol 102:1130–1134, 1984.
22. Committee for the Classification of ROP: An international classification of retinopathy of prematurity. II. The classification of retinal detachment. Arch Ophthalmol 105:906–912, 1987.
23. Bates JH, Burnstine RA: Consequences of retinopathy of prematurity examinations. Case report. Arch Ophthalmol 105:618–619, 1987.
24. Stannard KP, Mushin AS, Gamsu HR: Screening for retinopathy of prematurity in a regional neonatal intensive care unit. Eye 3:371–378, 1989.
25. Tan KE, Cats BP: Timely incidence of retinopathy of prematurity and its consequences for the screening strategy. Am J Perinatol 6:337–340, 1989.
26. Yoshizumi M, Toyotuku H, Tanoue F, et al: Prognosis and avascular area in active stages of retinopathy of prematurity. Folia Ophthal Jpn 27:861–866, 1976.
27. Topilow HM, Ackerman AL, Wang FM: The treatment of advanced retinopathy of prematurity with cryotherapy and scleral buckling procedure. Ophthalmology 92:379–387, 1985.
28. Cryotherapy for Retinopathy of Prematurity Cooperative Group: Multicenter trial of cryotherapy for retinopathy of prematurity. One year outcome—Structure and function. Arch Ophthalmol 108:1408–1416, 1990.
29. Ben-Sira I, Nissenkorn I, Gurnwald E, et al: Treatment of acute retrolental fibroplasia by cryopexy. Br J Ophthalmol 64:758–762, 1980.
30. Hindle NW: Cryotherapy for retinopathy of prematurity to prevent retrolental fibroplasia. Can J Ophthalmol 17:207–212, 1982.
31. Tasman W, Brown GC, Naidoff M, et al: Cryotherapy for active retinopathy of prematurity. Graefes Arch Clin Exp Ophthalmol 225:3–4, 1987.
32. Yamashita Y: Studies on retinopathy of prematurity. III. Cryocautery for retinopathy of prematurity. Jpn J Clin Ophthalmol 26:385–393, 1972.
33. Nagata M: The possibility of treatment for the retinopathy of prematurity by photocoagulation. Ophthalmology (Japan) 10:719–727, 1968.
34. Landers MB, Semple HC, Ruben JB, Serdahl C: Argon laser photocoagulation for advanced retinopathy of prematurity. Am J Ophthalmol 110:429–431, 1990.
35. McNamara JA, Tasman W, Brown GC, Federman JL: Laser photocoagulation for stage 3 + retinopathy of prematurity. Ophthalmology 98:576–580, 1991.
36. Brown GC, Tasman WS, Naidoff M, et al: Systemic complications associated with retinal cryoablation for retinopathy of prematurity. Ophthalmology 97:855–858, 1990.
37. Kretzer FL, Hittner HM: Retinopathy of prematurity: Clinical implications of retinal development. Arch Dis Child 63:1151–1167, 1988.
38. Hindle NW: Cryotherapy for retinopathy of prematurity. [Letter] Surv Ophthalmol 33:134–135, 1988.
39. Hindle NW: Cryotherapy for retinopathy of prematurity, [Letter] Arch Ophthalmol 108:1375, 1990.
40. Kretzer FL, Hittner HM: Spindle cells and retinopathy of prematurity: Interpretations and predictions. Birth Defects 24:147–168, 1988.
41. Kretzer FL, McPherson AR, Hittner HM: An interpretation of retinopathy of prematurity in terms of spindle cells: Relationship to vitamin E prophylaxis and cryotherapy. Graefes Arch Ophthalmol Clin Exp Ophthalmol 224:205–214, 1986.
42. Phelps DL, Phelps CE: Cryotherapy in infants with retinopathy of prematurity. A decision model for treating one or both eyes. JAMA 261:1751–1756, 1989.
43. Teller J, Nissenkorn I, Ben-Sira I, Abraham FA: Ocular dimensions following cryotherapy for active stage of retinopathy of prematurity. Metab Pediatr Syst Ophthalmol 11:81–82, 1988.
44. Greven CM, Tasman W: Rhegmatogenous retinal detachment following cryotherapy in retinopathy of prematurity. Arch Ophthalmol 107:1017–1018, 1989.
45. Topilow HW, Ackerman AL: Cryotherapy for stage 3 + retinopathy of prematurity: Visual and anatomic results. Ophthalmol Surg 20:864–871, 1989.
46. Ben-Sira I, Nissenkorn I, Weinberger D, et al: Long-term results of cryotherapy for active stages of retinopathy of prematurity. Ophthalmology 93:1423–1428, 1986.
47. Seiberth V, Knorz MC, Trinkmann R: Refractive errors after cryotherapy in retinopathy of prematurity. Ophthalmologica 201:5–8, 1990.
48. Trese MT: Surgical therapy for stage V retinopathy of prematurity. A two-step approach. Graefes Arch Clin Exp Ophthalmol 225:266–268, 1987.
49. Cryotherapy for Retinopathy of Prematurity Cooperative Group: Multicenter trial of cryotherapy for retinopathy of prematurity: Preliminary results. Arch Ophthalmol 106:471–479, 1988.
50. McPherson AR, Hittner HM, Kretzer FL: Treatment of acute retinopathy of prematurity with cryotherapy. In McPherson AR, Hittner HM, Kretzer FL (eds): Retinopathy of Prematurity—Current Concepts and Controversies. Toronto, BC Decker, 1986, pp 161–178.

51. Hirose T, Schepens CL: Open-sky vitrectomy in total retinal detachment in cicatricial retinopathy of prematurity. Ophthalmology 91(Suppl):73, 1984.
52. Hirose T, Schepens CL, Katsumi O, Mehta MC: Open-sky vitrectomy for severe retinal detachment caused by advanced retinopathy of prematurity. *In* Flynn J (ed): Retinopathy of Prematurity. New York, Springer-Verlag, 1992, pp 95–114.
53. Tasman W: Surgical approaches to retinal detachment in retinopathy of prematurity. Birth Defects 24:265–274, 1988.
54. Orellana J: Scleral buckling in acute retinopathy of prematurity stages 4 and 5. *In* Eichenbaum JW, Mamelok AE, Mittl RN, Orellana J (eds): Treatment of Retinopathy of Prematurity. Chicago, Yearbook Medical, 1991, pp 194–213.
55. McPherson AR, Hittner HM: Scleral buckling in 2½ to 11-month-old premature infants with retinal detachment associated with acute retrolental fibroplasia. Ophthalmology 86:819–835, 1979.
56. Greven C, Tasman W: Scleral buckling in stages 4B and 5 retinopathy of prematurity. Ophthalmology 97:817–820, 1990.
57. Machemer R, deJuan E: Retinopathy of prematurity: Approaches to surgical therepy. Aust NZ J Ophthalmol 18:47–45, 1990.
58. McPherson AR, Hittner HM, Kretzer FL: Treatment of acute retinopathy of prematurity by scleral buckling. *In* McPherson AR, Hittner HM, Kretzer FL (eds): Retinopathy of Prematurity—Current Concepts and Controversies. Toronto, BC Decker, 1986, pp 179–192.
59. Sneed SR, Pulido JS, Blodi CF, et al: Surgical management of late-onset retinal detachments associated with regressed retinopathy of prematurity. Ophthalmology 97:179–183, 1990.
60. Mintz-Hittner HA, Kretzer FL: The rationale for cryotherapy with a prophylactic scleral buckle for zone 1 threshold retinopathy of prematurity. Doc Ophthalmol 74:263–268, 1990.
61. Charles S: Vitrectomy with ciliary body entry for retrolental fibroplasia. *In* McPherson AR, Hittner HM, Kretzer FL (eds): Retinopathy of Prematurity—Current Concepts and Controversies. Toronto, BC Decker, 1986, pp 225–234.
62. deJuan E Jr, Machemer R: Retinopathy of prematurity. Surgical technique. Retina 7:63–69, 1987.
63. Jabbour NM, Eller AE, Hirose T, et al: Stage 5 retinopathy of prematurity. Prognostic value of morphologic findings. Ophthalmology 94:1640–1646, 1987.
64. Schepens CL: Clinical and research aspects of subtotal open-sky vitrectomy. Am J Ophthalmol 91:143, 1981.
65. Zilis JD, deJuan E, Machemer R: Advanced retinopathy of prematurity. The anatomic and visual results of vitreous surgery. Ophthalmology 97:821–826, 1990.
66. Charles S: Vitreoretinal surgery for retinopathy of prematurity. Birth Defects 24:287–293, 1988.
67. Trese MT: Surgical results of stage V retrolental fibroplasia and timing of surgical repair. Ophthalmology 91:461–466, 1984.
68. Blacharski PA, Charles S: Thrombin infusion to control bleeding during vitrectomy for stage V retinopathy of prematurity. Arch Ophthalmol 105:203–205, 1987.
69. McPherson AR, Hittner HM, Moura RA, Kretzer FL: Treatment of retrolental fibroplasia with open-sky vitrectomy. *In* McPherson AR, Hittner HM, Kretzer FL (eds): Retinopathy of Prematurity—Current Concepts and Controversies. Toronto, BC, Decker, 1986, pp 225–234.
70. Tasman W, Borrone RN, Bolling J: Open-sky vitrectomy for total retinal detachment in retinopathy of prematurity. Ophthalmology 94:449–452, 1987.
71. Sawa M, Hirose T, Kenyon KR: Endothelial specular microscopy in children with retrolental fibroplasia undergoing open-sky vitrectomy. Jpn J Ophthalmol 34:1–14, 1990.
72. Chong LP, Machemer R, de Juan E: Vitrectomy for advanced stages of retinopathy of prematurity. Am J Ophthalmol 102:710–716, 1986.
73. Eller AW, Jabbour NM, Hirose T, Schepens CL: Retinopathy of prematurity. The association of a persistent hyaloid artery. Ophthalmology 94:444–448, 1987.
74. Topilow HW, Ackerman AL, Wang FM, Strome RR: Successful treatment of advanced retinopathy of prematurity. Ophthalmic Surg 19:781–785, 1988.
75. Quinn GE, Dobson V, Barr CC, et al: Visual acuity in infants after vitrectomy for severe retinopathy of prematurity. Ophthalmology 98:5–13, 1991.
76. Fielder AR, Moseley MJ, Ng YK: The immature visual system and premature birth. Br Med Bull 44:1093–1118, 1988.
77. Ashton N, Ward B, Serpell G: Effect of oxygen on developing retinal vessels with particular reference to the problem of retrolental fibroplasia. Br J Ophthalmol 38:397–432, 1954.
78. Kretzer FL, Mehta RS, Johnson AT, et al: Vitamin E protects against retinopathy of prematurity through action on spindle cells. Nature 309(5971):793–795, 1984.
79. Kretzer FL, Hunter DG, Mehta RS, et al: Spindle cells as vasoformative elements in the developing human retina: Vitamin E modulation. *In* Coates PW, Markwald RR, Kenney AD (eds): Developing and Regenerating Vertebrate Nervous Systems. New York, Alan R Liss, 1983, pp 199–210.
80. Machemer R: Description and pathogenesis of late stages of retinopathy of prematurity. Birth Defects 24:275–280, 1988.
81. Hittner HM, Godio LB, Rudolph AJ, et al: Retrolental fibroplasia: Efficacy of vitamin E in a double-blind clinical study of preterm infants. N Engl J Med 305:1365–1371, 1981.
82. Kretzer FL, Mehta RS, Brown ES, Mintz-Hittner HA: The pathogenesis of retinopathy of prematurity as it relates to surgical treatment. Doc Ophthalmol 74:205–211, 1990.
83. Kendig JW, Notter RH, Cox C, et al: A comparison of surfactant as immediate prophylaxis and as rescue therapy in newborns of less than 30 weeks' gestation. N Engl J Med 324:865–871, 1991.

Chapter 58

■

Eales Disease

STEPHEN C. GIESER and ROBERT P. MURPHY

Eales disease is an idiopathic obliterative vasculopathy that primarily affects the peripheral retina. Although previously considered to afflict healthy young adults, it is seen in persons of all ages and is usually bilateral. Vascular sheathing and focal occlusion of peripheral retinal vessels occur early in the course of the disease. With progression, large areas of nonperfusion can develop, extending posteriorly. Neovascularization can occur at the junction of the perfused and nonperfused retina, frequently resulting in recurrent vitreous hemorrhages. Retinal neovascularization in Eales disease appears to respond well to laser treatment.

HISTORY

The disease is named after Henry Eales, an ophthalmologist who in 1880 described a syndrome of recurrent vitreous hemorrhages in young men with epistaxis and constipation.[1] He termed this new entity *primary recurrent retinal hemorrhage*. Using the newly developed direct ophthalmoscope, Eales documented abnormal retinal veins and zones in the peripheral retina that were free of capillaries.[2]

In spite of these astute early observations, the entity he described differs considerably from the disease that now bears his name. He did not observe any new vessels or inflammation preceding or accompanying the hemorrhages. Eales erroneously felt that this disease was associated with epistaxis, and he attributed the hemorrhages to increased venous pressure caused by constipation.

In 1887, Wadsworth described associated inflammation and neovascularization with this disease.[3] Since then, numerous authors have grouped periphlebitis retinae and idiopathic recurrent vitreous hemorrhages with or without retinal perivasculitis under the term *Eales disease.*

Not all authors have felt that Eales disease is a specific entity. Duke-Elder felt that Eales disease represented the clinical manifestation of many diseases.[4] Since then, refined diagnostic tests have demonstrated that many of the so-called idiopathic hemorrhages are the result of diseases with known causes, such as sarcoidosis, systemic lupus erythematosus, diabetes mellitus, sickle cell disease, and collagen vascular disease.

However, after elimination of these causes, there remains a group of patients with idiopathic peripheral nonperfusion and perivasculitis of the retina. Many investigators now agree that Eales disease is a distinct entity comprising characteristic funduscopic and fluorescein angiographic features.[5] Although this disease has been called *periphlebitis retinae*,[6] emphasizing the abnormalities of retinal venules, evidence suggests that the inflammation in this disease affects both arterioles and venules.[7]

EPIDEMIOLOGY

Eales disease is uncommon in North America; however, this disorder is responsible for widespread visual loss in India, Pakistan, and Afghanistan. It typically affects healthy young adults. The average age at onset is 20 to 30 yr. Patients usually present with symptoms of vitreous hemorrhage, such as floaters or decreased vision. The majority of patients experience bilateral, although often asymmetric, involvement.

Most reports, including Eales' original description, indicate a male predominance. However, Murphy and coworkers found an equal prevalence of men and women in their study of 55 patients.[7]

CLINICAL FEATURES

Inflammation

Signs of ocular inflammation are commonly encountered in Eales disease, especially early in its course. Vascular sheathing is seen in most patients (Fig. 58–1). The degree of sheathing ranges from fine white lines on both sides of the blood column to thick exudative sheathing. The thin white lines tend to be continuous, whereas the heavy, exudative sheathing is often segmental.

Areas of vascular sheathing frequently demonstrate hyperfluorescence in fluorescein angiography (Fig. 58–2). However, there is no direct correlation between the regions of sheathing and staining. The intensity of the hyperfluorescence seen on the fluorescein angiograms does not correlate with the intensity of inflammation.

In the century since Eales' observation of altered retinal veins, many investigators have described Eales disease as a primary disease of altered retinal veins. Elliot and Harris suggested the term *periphlebitis retinae* for this disorder.[6] However, more recent studies have reported equal involvement of arteriolar and venular sheathing.[7] Because of the evidence of arteriolar involvement (Fig. 58–1B), this disease should be considered a retinal vasculitis or vasculopathy.

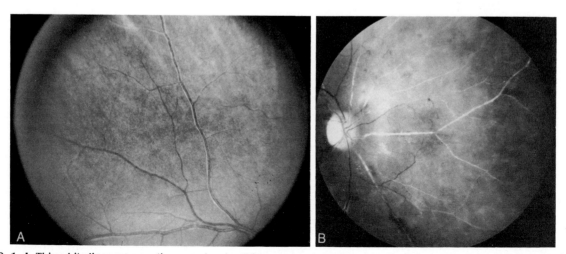

Figure 58–1. *A,* Thin white lines representing vascular sheathing surround a retinal venule. (From Gieser SC, Murphy RP, Eales disease. *In* Ryan S [ed]: Retina, St Louis, CV Mosby, 1989.) *B,* Extensive arteriolar sheathing with retinal vascular nonperfusion nasal to disc.

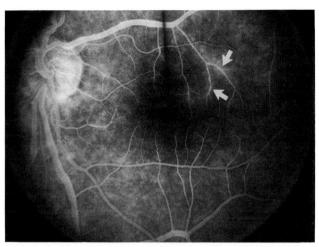

Figure 58–2. Fluorescein angiogram demonstrates abnormal staining of a small retinal venule *(arrows)* in a patient with Eales disease. There was venous sheathing in this area.

Keratic precipitates, anterior chamber cell and flare, and vitreous cells have been observed in patients with Eales disease.[7] Cystoid macular edema occurs in eyes with extensive sheathing. Although the exact cause of the macular edema is unknown, it may be associated with low-grade inflammation.

Nonperfusion

Peripheral retinal nonperfusion is present in all patients with this disease. The extent of the perfusion ranges from small areas in the far periphery to massive nonperfusion extending into the posterior pole (Fig. 58–3). The nonperfusion is generally confluent and sharply demarcated from the posterior perfused retina. The temporal retina is most commonly affected.

The microvascular abnormalities may be so severe that the fundus resembles Coats' disease. Fine white

lines representing the remains of obliterated large vessels (ghost vessels) are often seen in the area of nonperfusion.

Elliot[8] and Spitznas[9] have documented the vascular abnormalities at the junction of the anteroperipheral nonperfused retina and the posterior perfused retina. Intraretinal hemorrhages often first appear in the affected area, followed by an increase in vascular tortuosity with frequent collateral formation around occluded vessels (see Fig. 58–3). Microaneurysms, arteriovenous shunts, and venous beading are commonly seen at the junction (Fig. 58–4). Fluorescein angiography enhances these abnormalities and often demonstrates staining at the stumps of obliterated vessels.

Patients with Eales disease can also experience branch vein occlusion (BVO). The BVO can be either single or multiple. Unlike patients with primary BVO, in whom the pathologic condition is confined to one quadrant, patients with Eales disease have more extensive involvement of the peripheral retina that does not respect the horizontal midline.

Neovascularization

The retinal nonperfusion leads to the eventual development of new vessels. The neovascularization can form either on the disc or elsewhere in the retina. Neovascularization of the iris has also been described. These abnormal blood vessels frequently bleed and are the major cause of visual loss in this disease.

Many investigators have proposed that an ischemic retina produces a diffusible substance that stimulates neovascularization. In Eales disease, the ischemia is predominantly peripheral, and thus the development of peripheral neovascularization is not surprising.

The neovascularization often occurs along the junction of perfused and nonperfused retina, similar to the appearance of sickle cell retinopathy. The neovascularization frequently has a prominent fibrous component. Occasionally, patients have extensive retinal and vitreal proliferation of avascular sheets and strands of fibrous

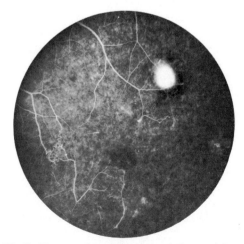

Figure 58–3. Fluorescein angiogram of the peripheral retina demonstrating the junction of normally perfused retinal vessels adjacent to an area of nonperfused retina. Note the vascular abnormalities and the small area of neovascularization at the junctional zone.

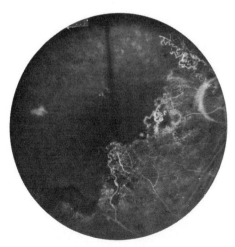

Figure 58–4. Fluorescein angiogram demonstrates severe nonperfusion of retinal vasculature involving the macula.

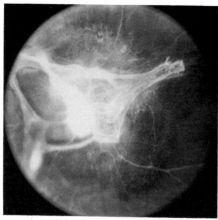

Figure 58–5. Hypovascular fibroproliferation emanating from the disc of a patient with advanced Eales disease.

scar tissue (Fig. 58–5). The anteroposterior traction resulting from the fibrovascular membrane places these eyes at risk of developing retinal detachment.

VISUAL PROGNOSIS

The natural course of this disease is variable. Although the visual acuity in patients with Eales disease ranges from normal to no light perception, most eyes retain good acuity. In spite of extensive anteroperipheral nonperfusion, the macula is usually spared, preserving central vision. Murphy and coworkers reported that 67 percent of their patients had final visual acuity in the better eye that ranged from 20/15 to 20/40. Twenty-four percent had visual acuity that ranged from 20/50 to 20/200, and 9 percent had visual acuity worse than 20/200.[7]

Vitreous hemorrhage is the most frequent cause of visual loss. Usually the hemorrhage settles to the lower portion of the vitreous and is gradually reabsorbed within several weeks or months, with the return of normal central vision.

Severe, permanent visual loss usually results from complications associated with neovascularization, such as persistent vitreous hemorrhage, retinal detachment, and neovascular glaucoma. Occasionally, loss of vision is caused by cystoid macular edema, macular holes, retinal telangiectasia, or epiretinal membrane. In some patients, relentless nonperfusion progresses across the macula (see Fig. 58–4); visual acuity in these eyes is usually less than 20/400.

TREATMENT

Eales offered his patients a mixture of laxative, digitalis, and belladonna.[1] Other remedies have included vitamin C, thyroid extract, and high-dose steroids. None of these treatments has been conclusively beneficial.

Although no prospective, controlled clinical trial has been performed on patients with this disease, investigators generally agree that peripheral scatter photocoagulation of an ischemic retina is the treatment of choice for the neovascularization of Eales disease (Fig. 58–6).[10, 11] The treatment is similar to that used for other vasoproliferative diseases of the retina, such as diabetic and sickle cell retinopathies. Several investigators have demonstrated favorable results with light-intensity, full-scatter argon laser photocoagulation to the nonperfused retina and to the junction of perfusion and nonperfusion.[11] Others have used a combination of cryotherapy and laser photocoagulation.[12] Because nonperfused retina is more fragile than perfused retina, caution should be exercised when treating these patients.

Vitrectomy can be employed for removing persistent vitreous hemorrhages and fibrosis, often with good results.[13] No treatment is known to prevent or reverse the nonperfusion or capillary drop-out.

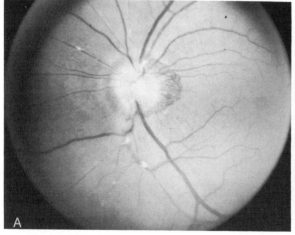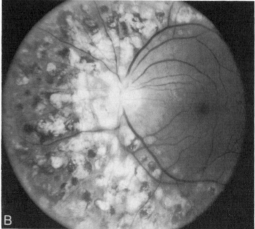

Figure 58–6. *A,* Neovascularization of the disc. Note the segmental exudative arteriolar sheathing. *B,* Same patient as in Figure 58–6*A,* 2.5 yr later. The patient has had total regression of the neovascularization after treatment with scatter photocoagulation of all areas of nonperfused retina. Note that the former areas of arteriolar sheathing have resolved. (*A* and *B,* From Gieser SC, Murphy RP: Eales disease. *In* Ryan S [ed]: Retina. St Louis, CV Mosby, 1989.)

ETIOLOGY

As an idiopathic entity, Eales disease must first be differentiated from retinal vasculopathies with known causes. Systemic diseases such as diabetes mellitus, sickle cell hemoglobinopathies, sarcoidosis, and systemic lupus erythematosus can manifest retinal inflammation, nonperfusion, and neovascularization. However, one can rule out these conditions with a careful history and appropriate laboratory tests.

Many investigators have emphasized a relationship between Eales disease and tuberculosis.[8, 9] Although there is a higher than normal incidence of positive reaction to the tuberculin protein, no one has demonstrated any evidence that the ocular changes are related to infection of the eye or retina by tuberculin bacteria. Renie and colleagues noted in their group of 32 patients that 48 percent had either tuberculosis or a history of exposure to tuberculosis.[14]

Electrophoretic study of serum proteins in patients with Eales disease has shown a rise in α-globulins and reduced albumin levels.[15] Isoelectric focusing of the serum samples has revealed several unique proteins in these patients.[16] It is possible that altered immune reactivity to an extraneous agent may play a role in the pathogenesis of Eales disease.

Some patients with Eales disease have a concomitant vestibuloauditory dysfunction. Renie and colleagues discovered sensorineural hearing loss in 24 percent of their 35 patients with this disease and vestibuloauditory dysfunction in 50 percent of their patients.[14] The concomitant vestibuloauditory abnormalities suggest that the pathologic features of this disease are not limited to the eye.

There are multiple case reports of diseases of the central nervous system in patients with Eales disease, including multiple sclerosis, cerebellar ataxia, myelopathy, and hemiplegia. Additionally, several investigators have noted an increased prevalence of immunologic disorders.[17]

Eales disease is a long-recognized, but poorly understood, disorder. Until we understand more about the cause and pathogenesis of Eales disease, we will continue to be able to treat only the secondary complications of this disorder.

REFERENCES

1. Eales H: Causes of retinal hemorrhage associated with epistaxis and constipation. Birm Med Rev 9:262, 1880.
2. Eales H: Primary retinal hemorrhages in young men. Ophthalmol Rev 1:41, 1882.
3. Wadsworth OF: Recurrent retinal hemorrhage, followed by the development of blood vessels in the vitreous. Ophthalmol Rev 6:289–299, 1887.
4. Duke-Elder WS: Diseases of the retina. *In* Duke-Elder WS (ed): System of Ophthalmology, vol. 10. St Louis, CV Mosby, 1967.
5. Gieser SC, Murphy RP: Eales disease. *In* Ryan S (ed): Retinal Disease. St Louis, CV Mosby, 1989.
6. Elliot AJ, Harris GS: The present status of the diagnosis and treatment of periphlebitis retinae (Eales disease). Can J Ophthalmol 4:117, 1969.
7. Murphy RP, Gieser SC, Fine SL, Patz A: Retinal and vitreous findings in Eales disease. Invest Ophthalmol Vis Sci 27:121, 1986.
8. Elliot AJ: Thirty-year observation of patients with Eales disease. Am J Ophthalmol 80:404, 1975.
9. Spitznas M, Meyer-Schwickerath G, Stephan B: The clinical picture of Eales disease. Graefes Arch Clin Exp Ophthalmol 194:73, 1975.
10. Spitznas M, Meyer-Schwickerath G, Stephan B: Treatment of Eales disease with photocoagulation. Graefes Arch Clin Exp Ophthalmol 194:73, 1975.
11. Magargal LE, Walsh AW, Magargal HO, Robb-Doyle E: Treatment of Eales disease with scatter photocoagulation. Ann Ophthalmol 21:300, 1989.
12. Das T, Namperumalsamy P: Combined photocoagulation and cryotherapy in treatment of Eales retinopathy. Indian J Ophthalmol 35:108, 1987.
13. Smiddy WE, Isernhagen RD, Michels RG, Glaser BM: Vitrectomy for nondiabetic vitreous hemorrhage. Retina 8:88, 1988.
14. Renie WA, Murphy RP, Anderson KC, et al: The evaluation of patients with Eales disease. Retina 3:243, 1983.
15. Rengarajan K, Muthukkaruppan VR, Namperumalsamy P: Biochemical analysis of serum proteins from Eales patients. Curr Eye Res 8:1259, 1989.
16. Pratap VB, Mehra MK, Gupta RK: Electrophoretic pattern of serum proteins in Eales disease. Indian J Ophthalmol 23:14, 1976.
17. Muthukkaruppan V, Rengarajan K, Chakkalath HR, Namperumalsamy P: Immunological status of patients of Eales disease. Indian J Med Res 90:351, 1989.

Chapter 59

∎

Retinal Arterial Macroaneurysms

MARC R. LEVIN and EVANGELOS S. GRAGOUDAS

Aneurysmal alterations of the retinal vasculature are a common occurrence in clinical ophthalmic practice. These changes most commonly involve the retinal veins or capillaries and are usually seen as a sequel to diabetes mellitus, venous occlusive disease, sickle cell disease, or radiation retinopathy. Less commonly, larger aneurysms arise directly from the major retinal arteries. Although they were described sporadically in the earlier literature,[1, 2] the first systematic study of large arterial aneurysms was published in 1973 by Robertson,[2] in which he formally established the distinct clinical entity currently known as *retinal arterial macroaneurysms*.

DEFINITION AND DESCRIPTION

Retinal arterial macroaneurysms may be defined as fusiform or saccular dilatations of the retinal arteries, usually arising within the first three orders of bifurcation. Their diameter exceeds 100 μ (arbitrarily the upper limit of typical microaneurysms) but typically is not greater than about 250 μ. Multiple aneurysms are common, occurring in approximately 20 percent of affected eyes. They usually involve different arteries in the same eye, although 10 percent of patients have bilateral disease. Patients may present with multiple aneurysms along the same artery. The most common involvement is along the superotemporal or inferotemporal arcades, with the nasal vessels more rarely involved. This pattern may be more apparent than real because patients with aneurysms confined to the nasal circulation have less chance of experiencing symptomatic macular involvement and, subsequently, probably do not seek medical attention. Rarely, macroaneurysms can occur directly on the optic nerve head[3] or arise from a cilioretinal artery.[4] They often occur at bifurcation sites and at arteriovenous crossings and have been seen to develop in vessels with a documented history of embolic damage.[5] Approximately 10 percent of macroaneurysms are pulsatile on initial presentation, but the literature is discordant as to whether this is a sign of impending rupture.[6-8]

DEMOGRAPHICS

The typical patient presenting with a macroaneurysm is usually an older woman, greater than 60 yr of age, with an established history of systemic hypertension. The female preponderance is on the order of 3:1.[2, 6, 7] Approximately 75 percent of patients have a history of hypertension. Hypertension and arteriosclerotic vascular disease are the only consistent disease associations in patients harboring macroaneurysms.

FUNDUS APPEARANCE

The presentation of a patient with a macroaneurysm is variable. Retinal arterial macroaneurysms can be found on routine examination in asymptomatic patients. Sudden, severe visual loss may result from rupture of the aneurysm and resultant hemorrhage into the subretinal space, the subinternal limiting membrane space, the retrohyaloid space, or the vitreous (Fig. 59–1). Hemorrhage can also occur intraretinally. Often a typical

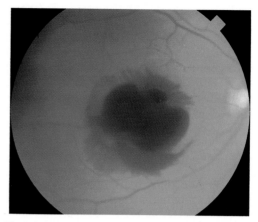

Figure 59–1. Large hemorrhage obscuring the macroaneurysm.

"hourglass hemorrhage" occurs, consisting of simultaneous subretinal and preretinal collections of blood. Serous fluid can collect intraretinally, producing diffuse, focal, or cystoid macular edema, or it can accumulate subretinally, detaching the macula and producing a gradual diminution in visual acuity. Lipid exudates can also cause a gradual decrease in vision by migrating into the macula (Fig. 59–2).

Secondary epiretinal membranes may form as subhyaloid or subinternal limiting membrane hemorrhage resorbs and can cause persistent decreased visual acuity even after the macroaneurysm itself and bleeding attributed to it have resolved. If the macroaneurysm is large and occurs at an arteriovenous crossing, a branch retinal vein occlusion may be produced secondarily, and symptoms may result from manifestations of the vein occlusion or the macroaneurysm, or both.

ANGIOGRAPHIC FINDINGS

The most common fluorescein angiographic appearance of a macroaneurysm is immediate uniform filling. Partial filling may also occur if the aneurysm is spontaneously involuting or partially thrombosed (Fig. 59–3). Leakage from the macroaneurysm is common. The involved artery is typically patent but may be narrowed proximal and distal to the macroaneurysm, although obliteration of the distal portion of the artery has been

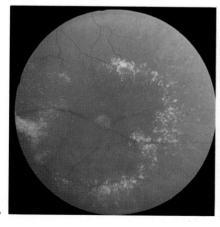
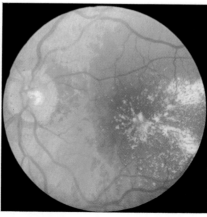

Figure 59–2. A and B, Peripherally located aneurysm with lipid exudate involving the fovea.

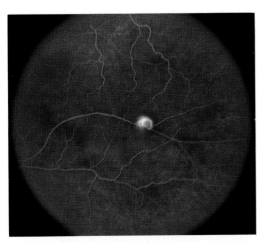

Figure 59–3. Fluorescein angiogram showing rapid, incomplete filling of macroaneurysm, which is consistent with partial thrombosis.

reported.[9] The area surrounding the macroaneurysm often shows capillary microaneurysms and nonprofusion, intraretinal microvascular abnormalities, telangiectasis, and fluorescein dye leakage. Occasionally, all evidence of the macroaneurysm is hidden from view by overlying hemorrhage, and only a high index of suspicion combined with serial examinations and angiography as the hemorrhage clears will result in an accurate diagnosis. Cystoid or diffuse macular edema, may be seen in delayed views. Distortion of the retinal vascular architecture may be noted in cases in which epiretinal membranes have formed.

PATHOGENESIS AND PATHOLOGIC APPEARANCE

The exact pathogenetic mechanism of macroaneurysm formation is uncertain. However, several observations and associations have led investigators to at least three hypotheses.

Lewis and colleagues[5] observed a patient in whom a macroaneurysm developed at the site of a documented incomplete embolic occlusion of a retinal artery. These authors postulate that embolic injury results in focal damage to blood vessel walls, causing weakening of the walls and subsequent aneurysm formation.

Retinal arterial macroaneurysms have been noted to be similar to intracerebral miliary aneurysms seen in elderly hypertensive patients, especially women.[2, 7] Since hypertension is commonly associated with retinal arterial macroaneurysms, it is thought that chronic vascular wall damage caused by hypertension and associated arteriosclerotic changes predispose the vessels to focal dilatation in the presence of continued increased intraluminal pressure.

Lavin and associates[7] have noted that at the point of arteriovenous crossing, there is no adventitia, and the two blood vessels share a common coat. The arterial wall thus has less support at these locations, and with increased intraluminal pressure in the hypertensive patient, ectasia of the arterial wall results.

After development of the macroaneurysm, symptoms are produced from leakage from the macroaneurysm as well as from the surrounding microvascular alterations that are usually present. Histopathologically, actual aneurysmal sites show thickening of the arterial walls secondary to a fibrin laminated clot accompanied by hypertrophy of the muscular layer. A thrombus will often partially or entirely fill the macroaneurysm. Thickened, hyalinized arterial walls are common in adjacent arterioles. The areas surrounding the macroaneurysm, clinically noted to show microvascular changes such as capillary loss, telangiectasias, and products of vascular leakage, typically show corroborating histologic findings including dilatation of the capillary bed, hemorrhage, lipid, edema, and photoreceptor degeneration.[10]

NATURAL HISTORY

The natural history of macroaneurysms varies and is dependent on the clinical presentation.

Abdel-Khalek and Richardson[6] reported the natural history of macroaneurysms, segregating them by clinical presentation into acute and chronic decompensation. Acute decompensation was typified by hemorrhage into the retina, subretinal space, subhyaloid space, or vitreous, and it produced sudden visual loss. Chronic decompensation was characterized by more gradual visual loss from the accumulation of macular edema and lipid exudate.

Following presumed aneurysmal rupture associated with the acute decompensation category, several pathways were followed. In some subjects, the arterial perforation closed, leaving an intact aneurysm that could rebleed or continue to leak fluid and exudate. Other aneurysms spontaneously closed, forming Z-shaped kinks at the former aneurysm site (Fig. 59–4). Subjects with only an intraretinal hemorrhage often experienced a yellow-gray, saddle-shaped plaque centered on the macroaneurysm, with surrounding exudate. The involved arteriole often became heavily sheathed.

In the group of patients with chronic decompensation, several macroaneurysms were treated with photocoagulation because edema and lipid exudate had already involved the central macular area and caused decreased visual acuity. In five subjects in whom macular function was not threatened, no treatment was undertaken. None of these cases ever progressed to involve the macula, although only one spontaneously closed during the study.

Following closure of these chronically decompensating aneurysms, either spontaneously or as a result of photocoagulation, kinking occurred at the aneurysmal site. Arteriolar constriction also occurred, usually proximal but occasionally distal to the macroaneurysm site. Arterial sheathing distal to the macroaneurysm was commonly seen, but distal arterial closure is rare, even after therapy.

These authors reported a better visual prognosis with macroaneurysms presenting with acute hemorrhage, as have other investigators.[7, 8] Of the eight patients in this category, only two patients had a final visual acuity of 6/18 or less. The remaining six patients had visual acuity of 6/12 or better. Of the patients with chronic aneurys-

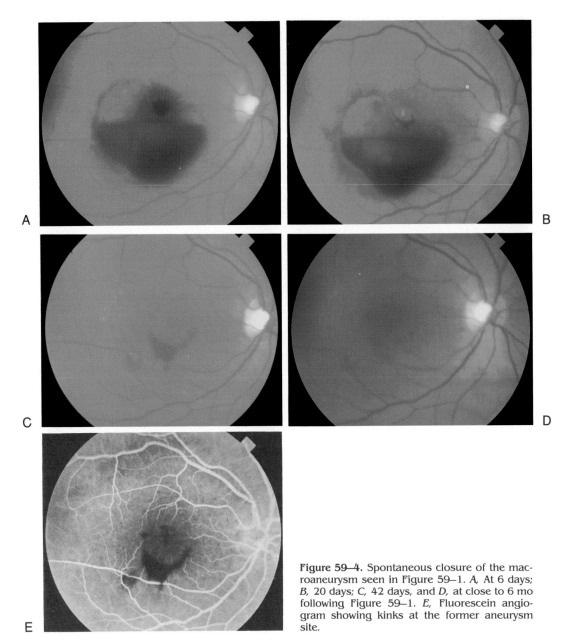

Figure 59–4. Spontaneous closure of the macroaneurysm seen in Figure 59–1. *A,* At 6 days; *B,* 20 days; *C,* 42 days, and *D,* at close to 6 mo following Figure 59–1. *E,* Fluorescein angiogram showing kinks at the former aneurysm site.

mal decompensation, one patient had visual acuity of 6/60, two patients had visual acuity of 6/36, and one patient had visual acuity of 6/18, with only six patients arriving at visual acuity of 6/12 or better. These authors concluded that acute hemorrhage infrequently leads to marked decreases in visual acuity, whereas macular edema and exudate commonly lead to a poorer visual outcome.

Palestine and associates[8] investigated the natural course of macroaneurysms using a similar strategy. They divided their patients into three groups. Group A included eyes with hemorrhage, exudate, edema, or the macroaneurysm within the vascular arcades, accompanied by decreased visual acuity. Group B included eyes with hemorrhage, exudate, edema, or the macroaneurysm within the arcades but without an effect on visual acuity. Group C included eyes in which all the pathologic features were peripheral to the vascular arcades. These investigators concluded that eyes in group A could do poorly and that the prognosis was variable. Eyes in

group B did better but needed to be observed periodically to be certain they did not convert to the group A type of eyes. Group C eyes typically did well without therapy. These investigators, as did Abdel-Khalek and Richardson,[6] also noted that eyes presenting with acute vitreous or subinternal limiting membrane hemorrhage tended to do well.

Cleary and associates[9] reviewed the natural history of macroaneurysms in 20 patients. They observed that the macroaneurysms almost always closed spontaneously after acute hemorrhage, whereas they rarely did so when macular edema was the presenting pathologic condition. They again concluded that the prognosis was good in patients presenting with hemorrhage and was poorer in those presenting with macular edema. Both the degree of chronicity and the severity of the macular edema affected the prognosis.

As already noted, a question has been raised in the literature regarding the significance of pulsation of the macroaneurysm. Some investigators[6] believe that this is a sign of imminent rupture, although most believe that it has no relationship to eventual rupture and that there are no reliable signs of impending rupture.[7]

DIFFERENTIAL DIAGNOSIS

In cases uncomplicated by a poor view of the fundus, the diagnosis of retinal arterial macroaneurysm is straightforward. Often, however, the true nature of the pathologic condition is obscured by hemorrhage, whether in the vitreous, intraretinally, or preretinally. A typical "hourglass" type of hemorrhage should alert the clinician to the possibility of a macroaneurysm. In addition, several entities closely resemble retinal arterial macroaneurysms and are not always easily distinguishable. Spalter[11] has even gone so far as to call retinal arterial macroaneurysms another "masquerade" syndrome.

Microaneurysms such as those that occur secondary to diabetes mellitus, radiation retinopathy, sickle cell disease, and branch retinal vein occlusion are usually not confused with retinal arterial macroaneurysms. They are smaller, and the nature of the underlying disease is often well established.

Schulman and colleagues[12] described large capillary macroaneurysms occurring secondary to retinal venous obstructive disease. They were similar in size to macroaneurysms but originated from the venous side of the capillary bed. They caused decreased visual acuity as a result of macular edema and exudate as well as serous elevation of the macula, mechanisms shared in common with retinal arterial macroaneurysms.

Venous macroaneurysms have been reported following branch retinal vein occlusion.[13] Decreased visual acuity in this situation was caused by chronic cystoid macular edema. Cousins and associates[14] reviewed the photographs and fluorescein angiograms of patients who participated in the Collaborative Branch Vein Occlusion Study through the Bascom Palmer Eye Institute. They noted that four types of macroaneurysms could be seen following branch retinal vein occlusion. Typical retinal arterial macroaneurysms, indistinguishable from the idiopathic variety, were common and occurred within the zone of the branch retinal vein occlusion. Venous macroaneurysms were similar in size but slower to fill angiographically because they occurred along the obstructed vein. Capillary aneurysms were also seen, similar to those reported by Schulman and colleagues.[12] Finally, they described a new type of macroaneurysm that they called the *collateral-associated* macroaneurysm. These were associated with clearly identifiable dilated collateral vessels on fluorescein angiography. All four types of these macroaneurysms were associated with intraretinal lipid or hemorrhagic exudation, often involving the macula. On fluorescein angiography, the macroaneurysms were typically found to be present in areas of capillary nonperfusion. Eighty-four percent of these eyes were classified as having severe nonperfusion for purposes of the Branch Vein Occlusion Study.

Branch retinal vein occlusions have been reported to masquerade as retinal arterial macroaneurysms; this is known as the *Bonnet sign*[15] The classic Bonnet sign consists of intraretinal hemorrhage at an arteriovenous crossing simulating a macroaneurysm.

There is one report of a retinal arterial macroaneurysm presenting as a mass lesion of the optic nerve; only with serial follow-up was the proper diagnosis ultimately made.[3] There has been one case report of Valsalva retinopathy occurring as the result of a ruptured retinal arterial macroaneurysm.[16]

Before retinal arterial macroaneurysms became a familiar clinical entity, they were commonly confused with retinal telangiectasis, Leber's miliary aneurysms, or Coats' disease. These patients have unilateral disease consisting of multiple telangiectatic vessels in the midperiphery, predominantly on the venous side of the circulation and are usually present in childhood, often with massive exudation including exudative retinal detachment.

Von Hippel's angiomatosis usually shows a distinct genetic component. When small, the angiomas may be confused with macroaneurysms, but when well developed, they are typically much larger and accompanied by large, tortuous feeder and draining vessels. Similar-sized retinal angiomas may occur unassociated with von Hippel's disease; they do not have large feeder and drainage vessels unless the tumors become quite large.

A common presenting situation is that of an elderly patient with an acute subretinal hemorrhage in the macula. There is often a surrounding area of subretinal lipid exudate, and the appearance can closely mimic exudative age-related macular degeneration. The macroaneurysm may be obscured by the retinal hemorrhage. In these cases, only a high index of suspicion coupled with fluorescein angiography, which may be repeated after the hemorrhage has resolved, will lead to the proper diagnosis.

Since approximately 10 percent of retinal arterial macroaneurysms present with vitreous hemorrhage, this diagnosis must be borne in mind when no retinal detachment, retinal tear, or avulsed retinal vessel is found after the vitreous hemorrhage clears. The retinal arterial macroaneurysm may involute prior to adequate fundus viewing and leave only subtle telltale signs of its presence as the cause of the vitreous hemorrhage.

If massive subretinal or subretinal pigment epithelial hemorrhage occurs, rarely this presentation may be mistaken for a choroidal melanoma.

MANAGEMENT

Although there have been no prospective, controlled, randomized clinical studies involving laser photocoagulation treatment of retinal arterial macroaneurysms, empirical treatment guidelines have been established by numerous investigators. The major controversies with respect to treatment involve whether or not to treat and having elected to treat whether to do so by direct or indirect photocoagulation and with which wavelength.

Most authorities agree that a quiet macroaneurysm that is asymptomatic without visible leakage should not be treated but should continue to be monitored until spontaneous fibrosis occurs. Ghost macroaneurysms (i.e., those that are already spontaneously fibrosed and show the kinked vessel Z-sign or the saddle-shaped plaque) also should not be treated, as they have run their natural course and will remain quiescent. Similarly, macroaneurysms that have ruptured and bled acutely rarely rebleed,[17] so observation is adequate in these cases. Aneurysms that leak fluid or exudate, or both, and threaten to involve or already involve the central macula should be considered for therapy. Treatment has been shown to shorten the duration of macroaneurysm patency.[7] The duration of the hemorrhage and exudate as well as its severity will determine the ultimate visual outcome.

Abdel-Khalek and Richardson[6] treated macroaneurysms with direct photocoagulation using the argon laser and xenon arc. Two of these patients also received perianeurysmal treatment preceding the direct treatment. No bleeding or other complications occurred from the direct therapy. The macroaneurysms were closed in all cases. The indications for treatment included recurrent bleeding or the threat of such, though the investigators do not provide a definition of threat. Other investigators have found that recurrent bleeding is rare and that treatment is not necessary in these cases.[7, 8] They also advocate treatment in cases in which macular edema and exudate are present. This should be undertaken early in the course of the disease because the longer the exudate and edema are present, the less the chance of improving the visual acuity and preventing permanent macular damage. Closure of the macroaneurysm has been shown to enhance the rate of resorption of retinal exudate,[5] although the exudate may initially appear to worsen or increase because of more rapid and selective resorption of retinal edema fluid, which may cause further precipitation of lipid exudate.

Palestine and associates[8] treated several eyes with macroaneurysms that had produced macular edema and exudate. They specifically advised against treating the aneurysm or the artery directly because of the possibility of rupture of the aneurysm, although they acknowledged that this complication had not been reported. These investigators, as did Lewis and colleagues,[5] treated the area of the microvascular changes surrounding the aneurysm and found that this predictably produced involution of the aneurysm. They also noted an early increase in lipid exudation, as less protein-rich fluid was initially resorbed. Complete resolution of the exudate took several months.

Lavin and associates[7] treated hemorrhagic and exudative macroaneurysms when the macula was involved, with a combination of direct and perianeurysmal techniques using the argon laser. They achieved closure of the macroaneurysms without complications and again noted that the visual prognosis depended on the degree of intraretinal hemorrhage and exudate in the central macula.

Joondeph and colleagues[8] treated macroaneurysms using the yellow dye laser. They used a technique of partially overlapping burns applied to just the peripheral margin of the macroaneurysm, sparing the feeding and draining arterioles. They successfully closed all the macroaneurysms in one treatment and reported no complications of therapy.

Mainster and Whitacre[19] also used the yellow dye

laser with a similar technique to successfully close five macroaneurysms. They also reported no complications. However, Russell and Folk,[20] after having successfully treated 15 macroaneurysms with the argon laser, used the yellow dye laser on one patient and immediately produced a branch retinal artery occlusion after applying only four burns to the macroaneurysm. Their treatment technique was not well described but appeared to involve a more direct treatment to the macroaneurysm than did either of the previous two reports involving the yellow dye laser.

These aforementioned treatment techniques are routinely used for managing the vision-threatening consequences of macroaneurysms. Ancillary techniques have been reported. Tassignon and coworkers used a Q-switched neodymium-yttrium-aluminum-garnet laser to release a retrohyaloid hemorrhage resulting from a ruptured macroaneurysm, thus facilitating more rapid resorption of the blood than would have occurred spontaneously.

Our recommendation is to treat, either directly or indirectly or with a combination technique, those macroaneurysms that produce decreased visual acuity as a result of leakage of blood, exudate or fluid into the macula or via the production of a serous macular detachment (Fig. 59–5). *Threatening the fovea* may be defined as progression of exudate toward the fovea, especially when the pathologic condition is located within the vascular arcades. Treatment should be undertaken early if the visual acuity is already compromised because a temporal threshold for permanent macular damage is not well established and may, indeed, vary from patient to patient. The macroaneurysms may be treated with either the argon or the yellow dye laser, although the yellow dye laser may be inherently more dangerous, and direct treatment with this mode of therapy probably should be avoided. Although the yellow dye and argon lasers have not been compared in a single study, all investigators have reported predictable, reliable closure of macroaneurysms, usually with a single argon laser treatment, before the advent of the dye laser. Despite prompt closure of the macroaneurysm, visual acuity may not improve dramatically if permanent macular damage has already occurred.

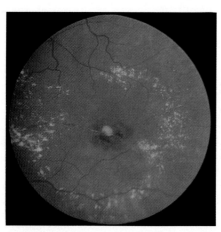

Figure 59–5. Appearance of macroaneurysm 3 mo after argon-green laser photocoagulation.

SUMMARY

Retinal arterial macroaneurysms are a well-defined retinal vascular disorder consisting of saccular or fusiform dilatations of the major retinal arterioles, usually within the first three orders of bifurcation. They usually occur in older, hypertensive women. Diagnosis can sometimes be difficult, and a high index of suspicion is required. Their natural history is often benign, with many progressing to spontaneous fibrosis and involution with retention of good visual acuity. The visual acuity is decreased as the result of macular involvement with hemorrhage, exudate, edema, or serous detachment or from vitreous or preretinal hemorrhage. Selected patients may be successfully treated using any of several different photocoagulation techniques, but the visual prognosis cannot be reliably predicted in individual cases.

REFERENCES

1. Rabb MF, Gagliano DA, Teske MP: Retinal arterial macroaneurysms. Surv Ophthalmol 33:73, 1988.
2. Robertson DM: Macroaneurysms of the retinal arteries. Trans Am Acad Ophthalmol Otolaryngol 77:OP55, 1973.
3. Brown GC, Weinstock F: Arterial macroaneurysm on the optic disc presenting as a mass lesion. Ann Ophthalmol 17:519, 1985.
4. Giuffre G, Montalto FP, Amodei G: Development of an isolated retinal macroaneurysm of the cilioretinal artery. Br J Ophthalmol 71:445, 1987.
5. Lewis RA, Norton MH, Wise GN: Acquired arterial macroaneurysms of the retina. Br J Ophthalmol 60:21, 1976.
6. Abdel-Khalek MN, Richardson J: Retinal macroaneurysm: Natural history and guidelines for treatment. Br J Ophthalmol 70:2, 1986.
7. Lavin MJ, Marsh RJ, Peart S, et al: Retinal arterial macroaneurysms: A retrospective study of 40 patients. Br J Ophthalmol 71:817, 1987.
8. Palestine AG, Robertson DM, Goldstein BG: Macroaneurysms of the retinal arteries. Am J Ophthalmol 93:164, 1982.
9. Cleary PE, Kohner EM, Hamilton AM, et al: Retinal macroaneurysms. Br J Ophthalmol 59:355, 1975.
10. Fichte C, Streeten BW, Friedman AH: A histopathologic study of retinal arterial aneurysms. Am J Ophthalmol 85:509, 1978.
11. Spalter HF: Retinal macroaneurysms: A new masquerade syndrome. Trans Am Ophthalmol Soc 80:113, 1982.
12. Schulman J, Jampol LM, Goldberg MF: Large capillary aneurysms secondary to retinal venous obstruction. Br J Ophthalmol 65:36, 1981.
13. Sanborn GE, Magargal LE: Venous macroaneurysm associated with branch retinal vein obstruction. Ann Ophthalmol 16:464, 1984.
14. Cousins SW, Flynn HW, Clarkson JG: Macroaneurysms associated with retinal branch vein occlusion. Am J Ophthalmol 109:567, 1990.
15. Kimmel AS, Magargal LE, Morrison DL, et al: Temporal branch retinal vein obstruction masquerading as a retinal arterial macroaneurysm: The Bonnet sign. Ann Ophthalmol 21:251, 1989.
16. Avins LR, Krummenacher TK: Valsalva maculopathy due to a retinal arterial macroaneurysm. Ann Ophthalmol 15:421, 1983.
17. Nadel AJ, Gupta KK: Macroaneurysms of the retinal arteries. Arch Ophthalmol 94:1092, 1976.
18. Joondeph BC, Joondeph HC, Blair NP: Retinal macroaneurysms treated with the yellow dye laser. Retina 9:187, 1989.
19. Mainster MA, Whitacre MM: Dye yellow photocoagulation of retinal arterial macroaneurysms. Am J Ophthalmol 105:97, 1988.
20. Russell SR, Folk JR: Branch retinal artery occlusion after dye yellow photocoagulation of an arterial macroaneurysm. Am J Ophthalmol 104:186, 1987.
21. Tassignon MJ, Stempels N, Van Mulders L: Retrohyaloid premacular hemorrhage treated by q-switched Nd-YAG laser. Graefe's Arch Clin Exp Ophthalmol 227:440, 1989.

Chapter 60

■

Coats' Disease and Retinal Telangiectasia

MARYANNA DESTRO and EVANGELOS S. GRAGOUDAS

PRIMARY OR CONGENITAL RETINAL TELANGIECTASIA (COATS' DISEASE, LEBER'S MILIARY ANEURYSMS)

Coats' disease (congenital retinal telangiectasia, Leber's miliary aneurysms) is a developmental retinal vascular anomaly consisting of leaking telangiectatic and aneurysmal retinal vessels with associated lipid exudation, which most frequently occurs in one eye of otherwise healthy, juvenile boys.[1] Initially described as separate entities, the milder (Leber's miliary aneurysms)[2] and more severe (Coats' disease)[3, 4] forms of this retinal vascular anomaly are now considered by most authorities to be variable expressions of the same disease and are therefore currently grouped under the common name of *Coats' disease.*[1, 5]

Demographics

Coats' disease has reportedly occurred in patients ranging from 4 mos of age[6] to those in the seventh decade of life;[7] however, the majority of cases occur by 20 yr of age, with the peak incidence occurring toward

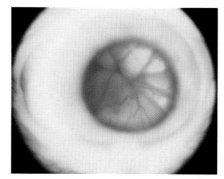

Figure 60–1. Leukocoria secondary to total exudative retinal detachment in a child with Coats' disease.

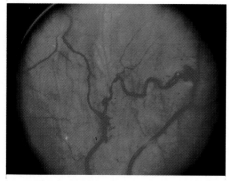

Figure 60–2. Asymptomatic localized focus of a retinal telangiectasis in a patient with mild Coats' disease.

the end of the first decade of life.[7] Greater than two thirds of cases occur in males, with 90 percent occurring in one eye of otherwise healthy patients.[8] Most are diagnosed after parents note leukocoria or strabismus or after a school vision screening is failed (Fig. 60–1). Milder cases may be detected at the time of routine ophthalmic examination.[9]

Etiology

The cause of Coats' disease is unknown, and there does not appear to be any genetic, familial, racial, or ethnic predisposition. However, isolated cases of a Coats type of eye disease and various genetic disorders have been reported, including one patient with a pericentric inversion on chromosome 3[10] and another patient with a deletion on chromosome 13 (initially causing a misdiagnosis of retinoblastoma).[11] In addition, retinal vascular changes similar to those in Coats' disease have been noted in patients with fasciocapsulohumeral muscular dystrophy,[12] Turner's syndrome,[13] Senior-Loken syndrome,[14] and one variant of the epidermal nevus syndrome.[15] In addition, changes similar to those in Coats' disease have been noted in up to 3.6 percent of patients with retinitis pigmentosa.[16]

Clinical Presentation

In mild cases, one or more localized foci of retinal telangiectasis are noted within the retinal capillary bed, primarily in the temporal quadrants (Fig. 60–2). One or more quadrants may be involved, and there may be variable amounts of associated retinal edema and lipid exudate within and beneath the retina, which may partially or totally obscure visualization of the telangiectatic vessels.[1] Microaneurysms, areas of capillary nonperfusion, and saccular outpouchings of retinal venules (so-called light bulb dilatations) may also be seen.[17] Vision usually becomes affected when hard exudate accumulates beneath the fovea or when cystoid macular edema or exudative macular detachment occurs (Fig. 60–3). Long-standing subfoveal hard exudate may organize into a fibrous disciform scar and may be associated with subretinal choroidal neovascularization (Fig. 60–4).[7]

Natural History

Although the extent and rate of development of these findings are variable, the disease is usually progressive.[7] With further accumulation of lipid-laden exudate, a

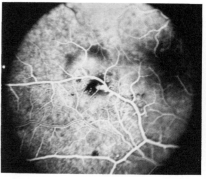 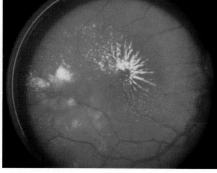 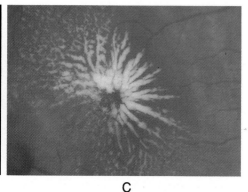

A   B   C

Figure 60–3. Retinal telangiectasis in a patient with Coats' disease resulting in decreased visual acuity secondary to macular edema and lipid exudation. Note the area of retinal telangiectasis temporal to the fovea visualized on fluorescein angiography (A), as well as the macular star formation secondary to lipid exudation (B and C). B denotes the appearance following recent laser photocoagulation to the region of telangiectasis.

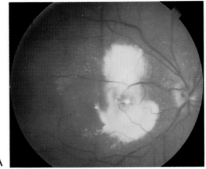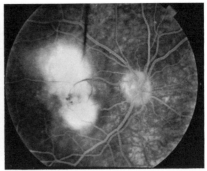

Figure 60–4. *A* and *B*, Subretinal choroidal neovascularization with organized fibrotic disciform scar following long-standing subfoveal lipid exudate in a patient with Coats' disease.

yellow or greenish-yellow subretinal mass may develop in association with localized exudative retinal detachment (Fig. 60–5). This subretinal lipid may coalesce into crystalline bodies, and multiple subretinal masses may occur (Fig. 60–6A). With further progression, total exudative retinal detachment may develop, which when chronic, may lead to rubeosis, neovascular glaucoma, cataract, uveitis, and phthisis.[7] In addition, retinal and vitreous hemorrhage, neovascularization of the disc and retina, and proliferative vitreoretinopathy may occur (Fig. 60–6B).[7]

Classification

Coats initially divided this entity into three varieties: Type I included cases of abnormal exudation without apparent vascular changes, type II included cases with both exudation and abnormal vessels (hemorrhage and telangiectasia), and type III included cases with exudation surrounding a large retinal angioma.[3, 4] With the advent of fluorescein angiography, it became apparent that abnormal retinal vessels were present in both types I and II, which varied only in the degree of vessel obscuration, depending on whether the exudate was deposited deep within the retinal or subretinal space or within the superficial layers of the retina. Type III was subsequently determined to be synonymous with Von Hippel's angiomatosis retinae.[7]

In 1917, Leber described the condition of "Leber's

miliary retinal aneurysms," in which telangiectatic retinal vessels were noted without lipid exudation.[2] In his later report in 1915, he concluded that his described syndrome was most likely a milder variant of Coats' disease,[5] and this opinion was further supported by Reese, who described two cases of typical "Leber's disease" progressing to typical Coats' disease.[1]

Gomez Morales described a classification of staging that was based on the severity of the clinical findings.[7] In stage 1, isolated focal exudates alone were noted. In stage 2, massive exudation was seen. These stages were followed by stage 3, in which a partial exudative retinal detachment was noted; stage 4, in which the retina was totally detached; and stage 5, in which secondary complications of chronic retinal detachment were seen. Sigelman described a similar classification, differing only in stages 1 and 2, which he described as consisting of telangiectasis only and focal intraretinal exudates, respectively.[18]

In addition, some authors have classified Coats' disease into the juvenile (<30 yr) form and the much less common adult (>30 yr) form, which has been reported to be associated with hypercholesterolemia.[19]

Differential Diagnosis

In children, the differential diagnosis of Coats' disease includes other entities causing intraocular mass lesions, leukocoria, or strabismus. They include retinoblastoma, toxocariasis, persistent hyperplastic primary vitreous, retinopathy of prematurity, familial exudative vitreoretinopathy, congenital cataract, retinal angiomatosis, incontinentia pigmenti, endophthalmitis, and pars planitis (Table 60–1).[20]

In both children and adults, other retinal telangiectatic and retinal diseases may also mimic Coats' disease, including branch retinal vein occlusion,[21] diabetic retinopathy,[22] radiation retinopathy,[23] juxtafoveal telangiectasia (see further on), Eales disease,[24] and various causes of vasculitis.[25]

In cases in which a subretinal mass is present, the differential diagnosis includes retinoblastoma, malignant melanoma, choroidal metastasis, choroidal hemangioma, eccentric disciform age-related macular degeneration, and exophytic retinal capillary hemangioma.[26] Besides the patient's history, several features may be

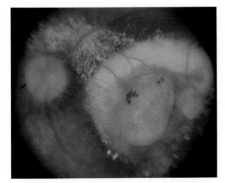

Figure 60–5. Subretinal mass with associated localized exudative retinal detachment secondary to progressive accumulation of subretinal lipid exudate in a patient with Coats' disease.

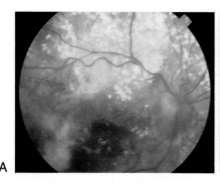

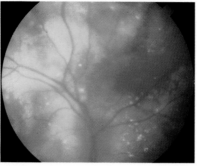

A

B

Figure 60–6. *A* and *B,* Subretinal choles-terol-rich "crystalline bodies" and associated hemorrhage in a patient with Coats' disease.

helpful in distinguishing these diseases from Coats' disease. In children, retinopathy of prematurity, familial exudative vitreoretinopathy, and pars planitis are often bilateral and occur in either sex, whereas Coats' disease most frequently occurs unilaterally in boys. In addition, in persistent hyperplastic primary vitreous, the eye is often microphthalmic and prominent ciliary processes may be seen, findings that are not typical of Coats' disease.[27] High levels of·serum antibodies to *Toxocara canis* aid in distinguishing cases of ocular toxocariasis.[28] In addition, in contrast to retinoblastoma, the masses in Coats' disease are usually yellow rather than white and are rarely calcified. Also, the overlying telangiectatic vessels in Coats' disease do not typically occur in retinoblastoma.[29]

In some cases of Coats' disease, the telangiectatic vessels may form small retinal angiomas, which may be confused with angiomatosis retinae. However, these lesions do not typically grow to larger than 0.5 disc diameter and do not display large feeder vessels, in contrast to angiomatosis retinae (Von Hippel's disease) (Fig. 60–7).[30]

At all ages, ancillary diagnostic tests, including fluorescein angiography, ultrasonography, computed axial tomography, and more recently, magnetic resonance

Table 60–1. DIFFERENTIAL DIAGNOSIS OF COATS' DISEASE

Retinoblastoma
Familial exudative vitreoretinopathy
Retinopathy of prematurity
Retinal toxocariasis
Persistent hyperplastic primary vitreous
Retinal angiomatosis
Incontinentia pigmenti
Pars planitis
Congenital cataract
Malignant melanoma
Choroidal metastasis
Choroidal hemangioma
Eccentric disciform age-related macular degeneration
Exophytic retinal capillary hemangioma
Branch retinal vein occlusion
Idiopathic acquired juxtafoveal telangiectasia
Other causes of acquired juxtafoveal telangiectasia
   (see Table 60–2)

imaging may all be helpful in establishing the correct diagnosis.[31]

Fluorescein Angiography

At the time Coats originally described this disease, he did not have the advantage of fluorescein angiography, which demonstrates typical retinal vascular changes, including areas of capillary nonperfusion, saccular and beadlike "light bulb" dilatations of retinal vessels (which may be both arterial and venous), and associated general dilatation of the adjacent capillary bed.[32] These abnormal retinal vessels typically leak fluorescein, which may pool within the intraretinal spaces of associated cystoid macular edema or within the subretinal space (Fig. 60–8).[8, 32]

Pathologic Features

The pathogenic mechanism underlying Coats' disease is thought to be an abnormal permeability of the vascular endothelial cells. This has been supported by Mc-Gettrick and Loeffler, who demonstrated ultrastructural evidence of endothelial cell fenestrations and interendothelial cell separation.[33] This results in breakdown of the blood-retinal barrier with subsequent leakage of blood components into the retinal tissue and subretinal space. In some areas, PAS-positive thickening of the capillary wall (resulting from a deposition of basement membrane–type material and blood components), with a relatively normal luminal diameter and intact endothelium, is seen, whereas in other areas, the capillary wall is markedly thinned, with irregular enlargement of the luminal size and total lack of the endothelial layer.[18] Necrosis of abnormal endothelial cells is thought to lead to the development of irregular dilatation and telangiectasis of the vessel walls, with formation of microaneurysms and areas of capillary closure.[18] With breakdown of the blood-retinal barrier, massive outpouring of lipid-rich exudate into the subretinal and retinal space occurs. Cholesterol crystals and cholesterol-laden macrophages (ghost cells) are frequently seen within the subretinal space, and aspiration of this material has been proposed by some to be a useful diagnostic procedure in selected patients with subretinal masses (Fig. 60–9).[34]

Figure 60–7. A and B, Peripheral angiomatous mass in a patient with Coats' disease. Fluorescein angiography aids in distinguishing this lesion from angiomatosis retinae. Note the typical retinal vascular changes of Coats' disease, including capillary nonperfusion, saccular and beadlike "light bulb" dilatations of the retinal vessels, and associated dilatation of the adjacent capillary bed.

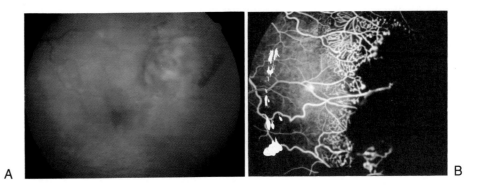

Figure 60–8. A and B, Typical "light bulb" dilatation demonstrating fluorescein leakage in the late-phase angiogram in a patient with Coats' disease.

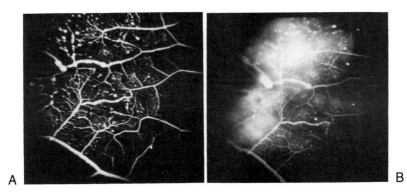

Figure 60–9. Cholesterol crystals of subretinal fluid aspirate in a patient with Coats' disease as visualized with H & E staining (A) and polarized microscopy (B).

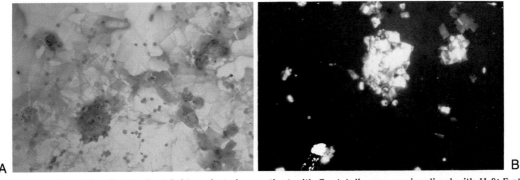

Figure 60–10. A and B, Laser photocoagulation of localized retinal telangiectasis in a patient with Coats' disease. Multiple treatment sessions may be necessary to assure complete vascular closure, and careful follow-up is required to document regression of the abnormal vessels, as well as to detect new areas of telangiectasis.

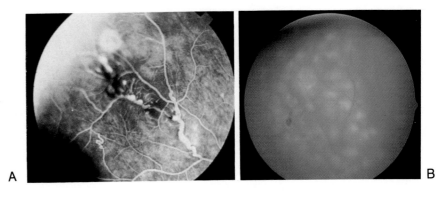

Treatment

Since most cases of Coats' disease tend to be progressive with associated visual loss, surgical intervention is generally recommended in all except the most mild and the most severe cases.[18, 35] The primary goal of treatment is to obliterate the abnormal leaking retinal vessels in order to allow subsequent absorption of the lipid exudate. In mild cases, obliteration of these vessels may be accomplished with laser photocoagulation, or transscleral cryopexy (Fig. 60–10). It is important to treat the entire area of abnormal vessels; fluorescein angiography or angioscopy may aid in visualizing the full extent of vascular disease. In addition, the recent availability of indirect laser photocoagulation may facilitate treatment, particularly in children requiring general anesthesia and supine positioning.[36]

In areas of thick exudation, there may be inadequate absorption of laser energy; in such areas, the triple freeze-thaw method of transscleral retinal cryopexy may be more effective.[18] Multiple treatment sessions may be necessary to assure complete vascular closure, and careful follow-up is required to document regression of the abnormal vessels, as well as to detect new areas of telangiectasis, which have been reported to occur as late as 5 yr following the initial treatment.[30]

In more advanced cases associated with exudative retinal detachment, surgical drainage of subretinal fluid and exudate may be necessary to allow treatment of abnormal retinal vessels with either photocoagulation or cyropexy.[18, 30, 37] This may be attempted externally, with or without placement of a scleral buckle, or internally in conjunction with pars plana vitrectomy (Fig. 60–11). Although visual function may be severely limited, particularly in cases of total retinal detachment, such surgical maneuvers may successfully reattach the retina and cause regression of the exudative retinopathy, thereby stabilizing the eye and preventing the subsequent development of phthisis, painful neovascular glaucoma, and the need for enucleation.[38] However, in end-stage cases of total blindness and organized retinal detachment, surgical attempts other than for palliation are probably not warranted, since there is little likelihood of anatomic or functional success.

Egerer and coworkers reported regression of disease in 15 of 18 eyes without retinal detachment, using xenon arc photocoagulation and transscleral cryopexy.[37] Those patients who did not respond were more likely to have had three or more quadrants of retinal vascular involvement. In 4 cases associated with retinal detachment, surgical reattachment with drainage of subretinal fluid and exudate followed by diathermy successfully resulted in resorption of the abnormal exudate.

More recently, Pauleikhoff and associates reported an overall treatment success rate of 52.1 percent in a large retrospective study of 197 treated eyes.[39] In cases with no associated retinal detachment, treatment was successful in accomplishing complete vascular closure and exudate absorption in 67.3 percent of patients, whereas in cases with exudative detachment, the rate of treatment success decreased to 23.8 percent. Their treatment strategies included photocoagulation or cryopexy (80.1 percent), diathermy (13.6 percent), and retinal detachment surgery (6.3 percent). Final visual acuities, with a mean follow-up period of 68.2 mos, were 20/25 or greater in 15.3 percent of patients, between 20/30 and 20/200 in 39.4 percent of patients, and less than 20/400 in 45.3 percent of patients. Four percent of treated eyes required enucleation. The reported complications of treatment have included worsening exudative detachment or inflammation, or both, macular pucker, proliferative vitreoretinopathy, and retinal and vitreous hemorrhage.[7, 18, 35, 37]

JUXTAFOVEAL RETINAL TELANGIECTASIA

Retinal telangiectasia localized to the foveal region alone in one or both eyes is termed *juxtafoveal telangiectasia*. Such a change may be congenital, and thus a mild variant of Coats' disease, or may be acquired and seen as an isolated finding in middle-aged or older patients.[40] These idiopathic forms of telangiectasia must be distinguished from secondary telangiectasia caused by other retinal vascular diseases (Table 60–2).

Gass has classified these patients into several groups based on clinical findings and natural history.

Group IA: Unilateral Congenital Parafoveolar Telangiectasia

Patients with group IA disease most likely have a localized, very mild form of primary, congenital retinal telangiectasia (Coats' disease). Most typically these find-

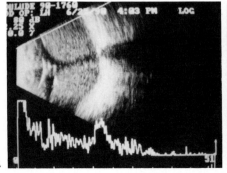
A

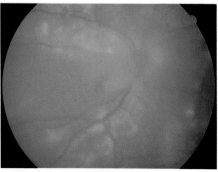
B

Figure 60–11. *A,* B-scan ultrasound depicting total exudative retinal detachment in a patient with Coats' disease. *B,* This patient's retina was successfully reattached via pars plana vitrectomy with internal drainage of subretinal fluid and endolaser photocoagulation.

Table 60–2. DIFFERENTIAL DIAGNOSIS OF IDIOPATHIC TELANGIECTASIA

Diabetic retinopathy
Branch retinal vein occlusion/central retinal vein occlusion
Radiation retinopathy
Tapetoretinal dystrophy
Inflammatory retinopathy/Irvine-Gass syndrome
Coats' disease
Eales disease
Adult-onset pseudovitelliform foveal macular dystrophy
Best's disease
Age-related macular degeneration
Choroiditis
Sickle cell retinopathy
Polycythemia vera retinopathy
Canthaxanthine crystalline retinopathy
Other crystalline retinopathies
Localized retinal capillary hemangioma
Hypertensive retinopathy
Ocular ischemic syndrome/carotid artery obstruction

ings occur in one eye of middle-aged men who present with mild blurring of central vision, with visual acuity in the range of 20/25 to 20/40. Telangiectatic capillaries are noted within 2 disc diameters of the center of the fovea, occurring primarily along the temporal parafoveal region and often associated with yellow lipid exudate (Fig. 60–12). Fluorescein angiography confirms these telangiectatic capillaries, which may also be associated with localized serous retinal detachment. In some patients, laser photocoagulation may be helpful in preserving central visual acuity. However, visual loss in this group of patients tends to be mild, and reports of spontaneous resolution may occur.

Group IB: Unilateral, Idiopathic Parafoveolar Telangiectasia

The cause of this subtype of juxtafoveal telangiectasia is unknown. It may be an acquired retinal vascular change or possibly a very mild form of congenital telangiectasia (Coats' disease). This form of telangiectasia occurs most often in middle-aged men who present with mild visual blurring and metamorphopsia in one eye. However, visual acuity is most frequently 20/25 or better, and serous exudation is limited to a very focal area of telangiectasia usually less than 1 clock hour in size along the edge of the foveal avascular zone, with or without associated lipid deposition. Fluorescein angiography reveals this very discrete area of capillary telangiectasia with minimal staining. Typically, good visual acuity is maintained, and laser therapy is usually not advised because of the good visual prognosis and the proximity of the telangiectatic changes to the center of the fovea.

Group II: Bilateral Idiopathic Acquired Parafoveolar Telangiectasia

This is the most common form of juxtafoveal telangiectasia, and it occurs in both sexes, most frequently in the fifth and sixth decades of life. In addition, there may be a familial component in this disease. Patients typically present with mild blurring of vision in one or both eyes, and blunting of the foveal reflex with a mild grayish appearance of the parafoveal retina is noted on slit-lamp biomicroscopy. These findings are typically bilateral, symmetric, associated with minimal serous exudation and no lipid deposition, and confined to an area 1 disc diameter or smaller in size. Most frequently, these telangiectatic areas are noted in the temporal parafoveolar region, although the parafoveolar capillary network for 360 degrees may be involved. In addition, glistening white or yellowish-white dots may be noted in the superficial parafoveal retina (Fig. 60–13). Fluorescein angiography initially reveals mild dilatation and intraretinal staining within the parafoveal region. Most patients experience a slowly progressive loss of central visual acuity with clinical evidence of central foveal atrophy. In some patients, small, yellow lesions, 0.33 disc diameter in size, develop within the foveal avascular zone and may be confused with adult-onset pseudovitelliform foveal macular dystrophy or Best's disease. Not infrequently, patients experience medium-sized right-angle retinal venules, which appear to drain the areas of parafoveolar telangiectasis and may be associ-

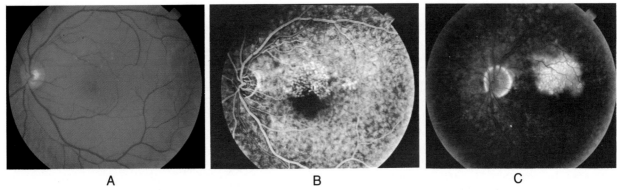

| A | B | C |

Figure 60–12. A–C, Unilateral congenital parafoveolar telangiectasia (group IA). Note the telangiectatic capillaries within the superior parafoveolar region associated with yellow lipid exudate and fluorescein leakage.

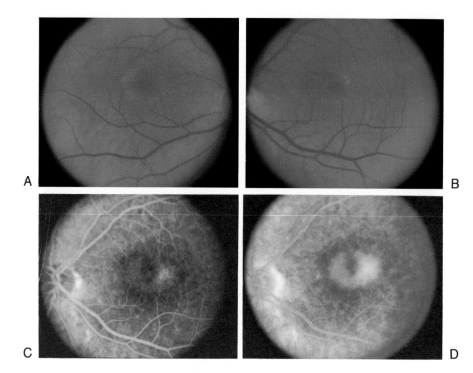

Figure 60–13. A–D, Bilateral idiopathic acquired parafoveolar telangiectasia (group II). Note the bilateral grayish parafoveolar appearance, as well as yellowish superficial retinal dots noted on the color photographs and parafoveolar leakage on fluorescein angiography.

ated with the development of stellate plaques of retinal pigment epithelial hyperplasia, as well as the development of retinochoroidal anastomosis and choroidal neovascularization.[8, 40] When such choroidal neovascularization occurs, there may be rapid loss of central visual acuity. These stellate plaques of retinal pigment epithelial hypertrophy and choroidal neovascularization may lead to the misdiagnosis of age-related macular degeneration or chorioretinal scarring secondary to focal macular choroiditis. The pathogenesis of this form of retinal juxtafoveal telangiectasia is unknown. Gass has suggested that the right-angle draining venules may suggest a chronic venous obstructive disorder.[8] Other authors have suggested a possible relationship with diabetes mellitus because of a significant incidence of abnormal glucose tolerance test results in their group of patients.[41] Histopathologic light and electron microscopic evaluation of one patient by Green and colleagues revealed thickening of retinal vessel walls secondary to marked proliferation of basement membrane, as well as degeneration of endothelial cells and pericytes, findings not unlike those seen in diabetic retinopathy.[42] It is of interest that in this case the authors noted minimal evidence of actual capillary telangiectasia.

Laser photocoagulation is not generally recommended for the majority of these patients because the abnormal vessels are close to the center of the fovea and the visual acuity remains relatively good. In selected cases, however, macular grid photocoagulation with either krypton red or dye yellow laser within the areas of telangiectasia may be helpful in the management of chronic macular edema, and in some patients macular laser photocoagulation of choroidal neovascular membranes may stabilize central visual acuity.[9]

Group III: Bilateral Idiopathic Perifoveolar Telangiectasia and Capillary Occlusion

Gass has reported two patients with this seemingly rare form of juxtafoveal telangiectasia.[8] These patients both presented in the fifth decade of life with progressive bilateral central visual loss associated with telangiectasia and progressive obliteration of the perifoveolar capillary network. Prominent aneurysmal dilatation of the tips of these capillaries, as well as the lack of fluorescein leakage, helps to distinguish these cases from other types of juxtafoveal telangiectasia. In both of these patients, optic disc pallor and hyperactive deep tendon reflexes were noted. In addition, Gass reported similar findings in one patient with polycythemia vera, as well as in patients with sickle cell retinopathy.[8]

REFERENCES

1. Reese AB: Telangiectasis of the retina and Coats' disease. Am J Ophthalmol 42:1–8, 1956.
2. Leber TH: Verber ein durch Yorkommen miltipler Miliaraneurisi men Characterisierte Form von Retinal -degeneration. Graefes Arch Clin Exp Ophthalmol 81:1–14, 1912.
3. Coats G: Forms of retinal disease with massive exudation. R Lond Ophthalmic Hosp Rep 17:440–525, 1908.
4. Coats G: Ueber Retinitis exudativa (retinitis hemorrhagiga externa). Graefes Arch Clin Exp Ophthalmol 81:275–327, 1912.
5. Leber TH: Retinitis exudativa (Coats), Retinitis und Chorioretinitis Serofibrinosa Degeraus. Graefe Saemisch Augenheikld 7:1267–1319, 1915.
6. Dow DS: Coats' disease: occurrence in a four-month-old infant. South Med J 66:836–838, 1973.
7. Gomez Morales A: Coats' disease. Am J Ophthalmol 60:855–864, 1965.

8. Gass JDM: Stereoscopic Atlas of Macular Diseases: Diagnosis and Treatment, 3rd ed. St Louis, CV Mosby, 1987, pp 384–397.
9. Brucker A, Robinson F: Primary retinal vascular abnormalities. In Yannuzzi LA (ed): Laser Photocoagulation of the Macula. Philadelphia, JB Lippincott, 1989, pp 115–133.
10. Skuta GL, France TD, Stevens TS, et al: Apparent Coats' disease and pericentric inversion of chromosome 3. Am J Ophthalmol 104:84–86, 1987.
11. Genkova P, Toncheva D, Tzoneva M: Deletion of 13q 12.1 in a child with Coats' disease. Acta Paediatr Hung 27:141–143, 1986.
12. Fitzsimons RB, Gurwin ED, Bird AC: Retinal vascular abnormalities in facioscapulohumeral muscular dystrophy. A general association with genetic and therapeutic implications. Brain 110:631–648, 1987.
13. Asdourian G: Vascular anomalies of the retina. In Peyman GA, Sanders DR, Goldberg MF (eds): Principles and Practice of Ophthalmology, Philadelphia, WB Saunders, 1980.
14. Schuman JS, Lieberman KV, Friedman AH, et al: Senior-Loken syndrome (familial renal-retinal dystrophy) and Coats' disease. Am J Ophthalmol 100:822–827, 1985.
15. Burch JV, Leveille AS, Morse PH: Ichthyosis hystrix epidermal nevus syndrome and Coats' disease. Am J Ophthalmol 89:25–30, 1980.
16. Khan JA, Ide CH, Strickland MP: Coats'-type retinitis pigmentosa. Surv Ophthalmol 32:317–332, 1988.
17. Green WR: Retina. In Spencer WH (ed): Ophthalmic Pathology, 3rd ed. Philadelphia, WB Saunders, 1985, pp 624–643.
18. Sigelman J: Retinal diseases: Pathogenesis, laser therapy, and surgery. Boston, Little, Brown, 1984, pp 331–349.
19. Woods AC, Duke J: Coats' disease I. Review of the literature, diagnostic criteria, clinical findings, and plasma lipid studies. Br J Ophthalmol 47:385–412, 1963.
20. Chang M, McLean IW, Merritt JC: Coats' disease: A study of 62 histologically confirmed cases. J Pediatr Ophthalmol Strabismus 21:163–168, 1984.
21. Scimeca G, Magargal LE, Augsburger JJ: Chronic exudative ischemic superior temporal branch retinal vein obstruction simulating Coats' disease. Ann Ophthalmol 18:118–120, 1986.
22. Ashton N: Studies of the retinal capillaries in relation to diabetic and other retinopathies. Am J Ophthalmol 90:203, 1980.
23. Hayreh SS: Post-radiation retinopathy: A fluorescence fundus angiographic study. Br J Ophthalmol 54:705, 1970.
24. Recine WA, Murphy RP, Anderson K, et al: The evaluation of patients with Eales' disease. Retina 3:243, 1983.
25. Ffytche TJ: Retinal vasculitis: A review of the clinical signs. Trans Ophthalmol Soc UK 97:457, 1977.
26. Gass JDM: Differential Diagnosis of Intraocular Tumors: A Stereoscopic Presentation, St Louis, CV Mosby, 1974.
27. Spencer WH: Vitreous. In Spencer WH (ed): Ophthalmic Pathology, 3rd ed. Philadelphia, WB Saunders, 1985.
28. Poloard ZF, Jarrett WH, Hagler WS, et al: ELISA for diagnosis of ocular toxocariasis. Ophthalmology 86:743, 1979.
29. Shields CL, Shields JA, Shah P: Retinal blastoma in older children. Ophthalmology 98:395–399, 1991.
30. Chisolm IA, Foulds WS, Christison D: Investigation and therapy of Coats' disease. Trans Ophthalmol Soc UK 94:335, 1974.
31. Mafee MF, Goldberg MF, Cohen SB, et al: Magnetic resonance imaging versus computed tomography of leukocoric eyes and use of in-vitro proton magnetic resonance spectroscopy of retinal blastoma. Ophthalmology 96:965–975, 1989.
32. Schatz H: Essential Fluorescein Angiography. San Anselmo, CA, Pacific Medical, 1983.
33. McGettrick PM, Loeffler KU: Bilateral Coats' disease in an infant (a clinical, angiographic, light and electron microscopic study). Eye 1:136–145, 1987.
34. Kremer I, Nissenhorn I, Ben-Sira I: Cytologic and biochemical examination of the subretinal fluid in the diagnosis of Coats' disease. Acta Ophthalmol (Copenh) 67:342–346, 1989.
35. Ridley ME, Shields JA, Brown GL, et al: Coats' disease: Evaluation of management. Ophthalmology 89:1381–1387, 1982.
36. Sneed SK, Blodi CF, Pulido JS: Treatment of Coats' disease with the binocular indirect argon laser photocoagulator. [Letter] Arch Ophthalmol 107:789–790, 1989.
37. Egerer I, Tasman W, Tomer TO: Coats' disease. Arch Ophthalmol 97:109–112, 1974.
38. Silodor SW, Augsburger JJ, Shields JA: Natural history and management of advanced Coats' disease. Ophthalmic Surg 19:89–93, 1988.
39. Pauleikhoff D, Kruger K, Heinrich T, et al: Epidemiologic features and therapeutic results in Coats' disease. Invest Ophthalmol 29(Suppl):335, 1988.
40. Gass JDM, Oyakawa RT: Idiopathic juxtafoveolar retinal telangiectasis. Arch Ophthalmol 100:769, 1982.
41. Millay RH, Klein ML, Handelman IL, et al: Abnormal glucose metabolism and parafoveal telangiectasia. Am J Ophthalmol 102:363–370, 1986.
42. Green WR, Quigley HA, DeLaCruz Z, et al: Parafoveal retinal telangiectasis: Light and electron microscopic studies. Trans Ophthalmol Soc UK 100:162, 1980.

Chapter 61

■

Leber's Idiopathic Stellate Neuroretinitis

DAVID R. GUYER and DONALD J. D'AMICO

HISTORICAL PERSPECTIVE

In 1916, Leber[1] first described idiopathic stellate neuroretinitis as a disorder of unilateral vision loss associated with optic disc edema and macular star formation. He observed that this idiopathic disease was a self-limited, benign condition and distinguished it from other secondary forms of stellate retinopathy. The latter types of stellate retinopathy were often observed secondary to hypertension, albuminuria, or nephritis. Ricci[2] reviewed the literature in 1961. Additional idiopathic cases were reported by Francois and associates[3] in 1969 (two cases), Papastratigakis and coworkers[4] in 1981 (one case), and Carroll and Franklin[5] in 1982 (three cases). The classic paper on Leber's idiopathic stellate neuroretinitis (LISN) is a study of 27 patients by Dreyer and colleagues[6] in 1984. These authors stated that this condition is not a maculopathy but rather a primary disease of the optic nerve, involving leaking optic disc capillaries.[6, 7] They suggested that neuroretinitis and stellate maculopathy are, respectively, generalized and inappropriate names for the condition. Instead, they commented that patients with optic disc edema, a macular star, and no other ocular or systemic associations, except for a viral prodome, represent a specific entity. Dreyer and colleagues[6] suggested the name LISN for such patients. They stated that multiple hematogenous infectious agents, including those that cause leptospirosis and cat-scratch fever, may be responsible for at least some cases of LISN.

Maitland and Miller[8] reported 12 additional patients and concluded that this condition was a self-limited, benign, systemic inflammatory disorder. In this chapter, we discuss the clinical characteristics, fluorescein angiographic findings, natural history, pathophysiology, differential diagnosis, and treatment of this rare condition.

CLINICAL CHARACTERISTICS

Demographics

Patients with LISN are usually between 8 and 55 yr old (average, 22 to 30 yr).[6, 8] Men and women are affected equally.[6, 8] Bilaterality is noted in 7 to 33 percent of cases.[6, 8]

Systemic Associations

A viral prodrome is present in 42 to 63 percent of LISN cases.[6, 8] Upper respiratory, gastrointestinal, and genitourinary system symptoms, with or without headache, are common. The following have all been reported to occur in association with LISN: leptospirosis,[6] cat-scratch fever,[6, 9] peripheral idiopathic seventh nerve palsy (Bell's palsy),[5] chickenpox,[8] influenza,[3, 5] mumps,[8] exanthematous viral illness,[8] and trauma.[8] No association between LISN and multiple sclerosis has been reported.[6, 8]

Ocular Symptoms

LISN patients complain of decreased and blurred vision. Rarely, retrobulbar pain or pain on eye movement may be present.[6]

Ophthalmic Findings
(Figs. 61–1 to 61–3 and Table 61–1)

Visual acuity initially can range from 20/20 to light perception vision.[6, 8] However, initial visual acuity is usually 20/50 to 20/200.[10] Approximately 75 percent of patients will have an afferent pupillary defect.[6] Cecocentral and central scotomas are the most commonly observed visual field defects, but arcuate defects may also be present.[6, 8]

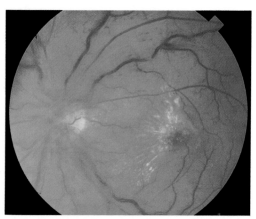

Figure 61–1. Ophthalmoscopic appearance of Leber's idiopathic stellate neuroretinitis (LISN) with optic disc edema and macular star exudate. The patient was a 25-year-old woman with a 1-mo history of scotoma and decreased vision in the left eye. The patient had numerous cats at home and was otherwise healthy. Visual acuity was 20/40; serologic test results for syphilis were negative, and the neurologic examination was otherwise normal.

In a few patients, anterior chamber cell and flare may be noted.[6] Posterior vitreous cells are observed in 87 percent of cases. The following findings may be present on ophthalmoscopic examination.[6, 8–10]

1. *Optic disc edema*: Optic disc swelling is the earliest sign of LISN. The swelling can be mild or severe, with secondary edema of the peripapillary retina. In very severe cases, juxtapapillary splinter hemorrhages may be present. The edema is usually diffuse but can rarely be segmental. The optic disc swelling starts to resolve in approximately 2 wk but can take 8 to 12 wk to totally disappear.[6]

2. *Optic disc atrophy*: In unusual cases, optic disc pallor may occur. In the series of Dreyer and colleagues,[6] 5 of 29 eyes (17 percent) experienced optic disc atrophy. In 2 of these cases, the optic disc pallor was associated with large afferent pupillary defects, optic disc–related visual field changes, and a poor visual

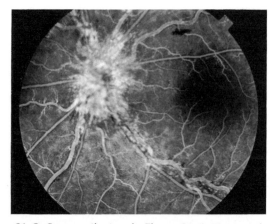

Figure 61–2. Same patient as in Figure 61–1. Fluorescein angiography documents leakage from peripapillary capillaries and secondary venous engorgement, but there is no leakage from the perifoveal capillaries.

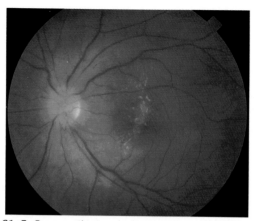

Figure 61–3. Same patient as in Figures 61–1 and 61–2. Seven weeks later, the visual acuity has improved to 20/30 + 2, and partial resolution of the optic disc edema and macular exudates is observed.

outcome. Thus, this constellation of findings may represent a subgroup of patients with a poor prognosis.

3. *Macular star*: The optic disc swelling leads to an exudative peripapillary retinal detachment. Finally, a macular star develops approximately 9 to 12 days after the onset of decreased vision.[6] The macular star usually starts to disappear after 1 mo, but it can take 6 to 12 mo until it totally resolves.[6]

4. *Residual retinal pigment epithelial defects*: Occasionally small retinal pigment epithelial defects can occur after resolution of the macular star.[6] These defects correspond to regions of previous heavy lipid accumulation and usually have no effect on visual acuity.

5. *Chorioretinitis*: Small, slightly elevated yellow-white spots at the level of deep retina or Bruch's membrane and the choriocapillaris have rarely been reported.[5, 6, 8] These spots disappear slowly and become chorioretinal scars. In the series of Dreyer and colleagues[6] three such cases were reported. In one case, *Leptospira* was cultured from the cerebrospinal fluid. In the second case, a finger abscess was present, and in the third case, a history of cat-exposure and a viral illness was noted. Thus, a septic retinitis is presumably present in such cases.

6. *Inflammatory sheathing of the peripapillary veins*: Two cases of LISN with inflammatory sheathing of the peripapillary veins have been reported.[6]

Table 61–1. CLINICAL FINDINGS

Decreased vision
Afferent pupillary defect
Visual field defects
Cell and flare
Vitritis
Optic disc edema
Optic disc atrophy
Macular star
Retinal pigment epithelium defects
Chorioretinitis
Vascular sheathing

Laboratory Findings

In the series of Dreyer and colleagues,[6] only a limited laboratory work-up was performed in most patients. The erythrocyte sedimentation rate was elevated in four of six patients tested (67 percent), and the white blood cell count was elevated with a normal differential in three of six individuals tested (50 percent). Antinuclear antibodies, rheumatoid factor, and syphilis test results were normal in all patients tested. Cerebrospinal fluid findings can include an increased white blood cell count and lymphocyte pleocytosis, increased or normal protein content, and increased opening pressure.[6, 8] In addition, *Leptospira* was isolated from cerebrospinal fluid culture in one case.[6]

FLUORESCEIN ANGIOGRAPHIC FINDINGS

Hyperpermeability of the deep optic disc capillaries is demonstrated by fluorescein angiography.[6, 7] The optic nerve hyperfluorescence is usually diffuse but can be segmental. On occasion, optic disc hyperfluorescence can be noted in asymptomatic fellow eyes. In four such patients in the series of Dreyer and colleagues,[6] none of the fellow eyes had LISN during follow-up examination. It should be emphasized that fluorescein angiography reveals no perifoveal capillary leakage or macular abnormalities in this disorder. We have studied one patient with LISN with digital indocyanine green videoangiography. The choroidal vasculature was normal in this case.

NATURAL HISTORY

During the first week of this condition, decreased vision, vitreous cells, and optic disc swelling are present. A peripapillary exudative retinal detachment occurs secondary to the optic disc edema. After the first week, the optic disc edema and peripapillary retinal detachment begin to resolve. Total resolution of the disc edema takes 8 to 12 wk.[6] The macular star forms after the first week and begins to disappear after 1 mo.[6] However, it may take 6 to 12 mo to observe total resolution of the exudates.[6] Long-term sequelae, such as retinal pigment epithelial changes and optic disc atrophy, occur on occasion.[6, 8] The former do not lead to permanent vision loss, whereas the latter may cause permanent decreased visual acuity.[6, 8]

In the series of Dreyer and colleagues,[6] visual acuity at follow-up examination (median, 14 mo; range, 3 wk to 10 yr) was 20/20 or better in 66 percent of cases, 20/20 to 20/40 in 31 percent of cases, and 20/400 in 3 percent of cases. Vision returned to 20/40 or better in 28 of 29 cases (97 percent) by 6 to 8 wk. Maitland and Miller[8] also reported that LISN patients have an excellent prognosis. In their series, 13 of 16 eyes (81 percent) had a visual acuity of 20/50 or better at follow-up examination (range, 1 mo to 2 yr).

However, a small subset (3 to 19 percent) of LISN patients have a poor prognosis.[6, 8] In these cases, optic disc atrophy occurs. Large optic disc–related visual field defects and afferent pupillary defects are often observed in these patients. It has been suggested that a viral vasculitis may destroy prelaminar arterioles in these cases and cause an anterior ischemic optic neuropathy.[6]

Involvement of the fellow eye may on occasion occur months to years later.[10] Dreyer and colleagues[6] reported one patient in their series who experienced LISN in the fellow eye 3 yr after the initial episode.

PATHOPHYSIOLOGY

This disorder is caused either by a direct viral invasion or by a systemic virally induced autoimmune mechanism.[8, 11, 12] The latter hypothesis is favored because culture results are often negative, visual recovery usually occurs, and vision loss often occurs after a viral prodrome.[8] The capillaries of the optic disc are primarily affected, causing the edema and exudation.[6, 7] Protein and lipid exudation from the deep optic disc capillaries spreads into the subretinal space and outer plexiform layer.[6, 7] The serous material reabsorbs, and the lipid that precipitates in the outer plexiform layer is engulfed by macrophages. A fine stellate macular star is thus formed. Wolter and associates[13] have suggested a mechanism of macular star formation. Deposition of fat-containing phagocytic cells and free lipids from degenerated neurons occurs in the outer plexiform and inner nuclear layers. The stellate pattern results from the radial and loose configuration of the outer plexiform layer in the macula.

A hematogenously spread infection is probably the causative agent. Several findings support this hypothesis. First, a viral prodrome is present in 42 to 63 percent of cases.[6–8] Second, the condition can be bilateral. Third, segmental disc hyperfluorescence can occur, and the prelaminar vasculature is segmental in nature. Finally, several infectious agents, including those causing leptospirosis and cat-scratch fever, have been implicated as causative in this disorder.[6, 8–10]

Histopathologic material has not been available for study in this condition.

DIFFERENTIAL DIAGNOSIS

(Table 61–2)

The differential diagnosis of LISN includes conditions that can produce a macular star or neuroretinitis, or both. These disorders include the following:

1. *Anterior ischemic optic neuropathy (AION):* On rare occasions, AION can produce optic disc swelling and a macular star. Dreyer and colleagues[6] described three such cases with presumed atherosclerosis. Visual recovery does not usually occur with AION but commonly occurs with LISN. In addition, AION patients are usually elderly, whereas LISN patients are often

Table 61–2. DIFFERENTIAL DIAGNOSIS

Anterior ischemic optic neuropathy
Branch retinal vein occlusion
Systemic hypertension, diabetes mellitus, and nephritis
Syphilis
Diffuse unilateral subacute neuroretinitis
Nonspecific uveitis
Papillophlebitis
Trauma
Toxoplasmosis of the optic nerve head
Juxtapapillary angiomas
Severe disc swelling of any cause
Hemifacial atrophy
Sarcoidosis
Septic optic neuritis
Tuberculosis
Toxocaral granuloma
Acute solar maculopathy

young. An afferent pupillary defect may occur with either condition. Cecocentral and central visual field defects are more common with LISN, and altitudinal visual field defects are more characteristic of AION. However, AION can also produce central field deficits.

2. *Branch retinal vein occlusion (BRVO):* BRVO is a rare cause of a macular star.[6] The classic fundus picture of BRVO, which includes retinal hemorrhages, should distinguish it from LISN in most cases.

3. *Systemic hypertension, diabetes mellitus and nephritis:* In Leber's original report[1] he distinguished LISN from neuroretinitis secondary to these systemic conditions. Bilaterality and progression without intervention are characteristic of neuroretinitis secondary to systemic diseases. In addition, characteristic fundus changes caused by these systemic conditions, such as background diabetic retinopathy, can distinguish these disorders from LISN.

4. *Syphilis:* This disease can produce a clinical picture indistinguishable from LISN,[6] often during the early asymptomatic neurosyphilitic period.[14] Serologic studies should be performed on all patients suspected of having LISN.[8]

5. *Diffuse unilateral subacute neuroretinitis (DUSN):* DUSN infrequently causes a macular star; however, DUSN can appear similar to early LISN cases without macular star formation.[6, 10] A nematode should be searched for in such cases.

6. *Nonspecific uveitis:* Dreyer and colleagues[6] described five patients with neuroretinitis and nonspecific uveitis.

7. *Papillophlebitis:* This condition is probably a mild central retinal vein occlusion, with optic disc swelling, which occurs in young patients. It can rarely cause a macular star and be confused with LISN.[6]

8. *Other conditions:* A macular star can infrequently be caused by or associated with trauma, presumed toxoplasmosis of the optic nerve, juxtapapillary angiomas, severe disc swelling of any cause, hemifacial atrophy, and sarcoid or septic optic neuritis.[6, 8, 10] Neuroretinitis can also rarely be caused by tuberculosis and a toxocaral granuloma within the optic nerve head.[15, 16] Children may experience an anterior optic neuritis and

papillitis, which may resemble neuroretinitis. Multiple sclerosis may develop in such patients.[6] Finally, the residual retinal pigment epithelial defects, which may occur after resolution of the macular star, may be confused with acute solar maculopathy.[6] A history of sun gazing can differentiate these conditions.

MANAGEMENT

Syphilis serologic tests (Venereal Disease Research Laboratory [VDRL] and fluorescent treponemal antibody absorption test [FTA-ABS]) should be performed on all patients to detect early asymptomatic neurosyphilis.[8] In typical cases, blood pressure measurements and routine blood tests should also be performed.[8] In atypical presentations, other measures such as cerebrospinal fluid examination may be necessary.[8] Dreyer and colleagues[6] treated 13 patients with oral or periocular steroids and followed an additional 13 patients. They stated that their sample size was too small to detect any possible beneficial effect of treatment. However, these authors did not note any obvious difference in final visual acuity between treated and untreated groups.

REFERENCES

1. Leber T: Die psuedonephritischen Netzhauterkrankungen, die Retinitis stellata: Die Purtschersche Netzhautaffektion nach schwerer Schadelverletzung. In Graefe AC, Saemische T (eds): Graefe-Saemisch Handbuch der der Augerheilkunde, 2nd ed, Vol 7, pt 2, Chap. 10. Leipzig, East Germany, Englemann, 1916, p 1319.
2. Ricci A: La retinite pseudo-albuminurigue de Leber (retinitis stellata). Ann Ocul 194:1038–1047, 1961.
3. Francois J, Verriest G, De Laey JJ: Leber's idiopathic stellate retinopathy. Am J Ophthalmol 68:340–345, 1969.
4. Papastratigakis B, Stavrakas E, Phanouriakis C, et al: Leber's idiopathic stellate maculopathy. Ophthalmologica 183:68–71, 1981.
5. Carroll DM, Franklin RM: Leber's idiopathic stellate retinopathy. Am J Ophthalmol 93:96–101, 1982.
6. Dreyer RF, Hopen G, Gass JDM, Smith JL: Leber's idiopathic stellate neuroretinitis. Arch Ophthalmol 102:1140–1145, 1984.
7. Gass JDM: Diseases of the optic nerve that may simulate macular disease. Trans Am Acad Ophthalmol Otolaryngol 83: 766–769, 1977.
8. Maitland CG, Miller NR: Neuroretinitis. Arch Ophthalmol 102:1146–1150, 1984.
9. Bar S, Segal M, Shapira R, Savir H: Neuroretinitis associated with cat-scratch disease. Am J Ophthalmol 110:703–705, 1990.
10. Gass JDM: Stereoscopic Atlas of Macular Diseases, 3rd ed. St Louis, CV Mosby, 1987, pp 746–751.
11. Johnson BL, Wisotzkey HM: Neuroretinitis associated with herpes simplex encephalitis in an adult. Am J Ophthalmol 83:481–489, 1977.
12. Selbst RG, Selhorst JB, Harbison JW, et al: Parainfectious optic neuritis: Report and review following varicella. Arch Neurol 40:347–350, 1983.
13. Wolter JR, Philips RL, Butler GR: The star-figure of the macular area. Arch Ophthalmol 60:49–59, 1958.
14. Folk JC, Weingeist TA, Corbett JJ, et al: Syphilitic neuroretinitis. Am J Ophthalmol 95:480–486, 1983.
15. Duke-Elder S, Dobree JH: Diseases of the retina. In Duke-Elder S (ed): System of Ophthalmology, vol. 10. St Louis, CV Mosby, 1967, pp 246–248.
16. Bird AC, Smith JL, Curtin VT: Nematode optic neuritis. Am J Ophthalmol 69:72–77, 1970.

Chapter 62

■

Familial Exudative Vitreoretinopathy

SHIZUO MUKAI, ERIC MUKAI, and CARMEN A. PULIAFITO

In 1969, Criswick and Schepens[1] reported on six patients with abnormalities of the retina and vitreous that were clinically similar to retinopathy of prematurity but without a history of prematurity or oxygen supplementation. Two of the patients were related by blood, and the other four patients were members of another family and were related by blood. Criswick and Schepens called this entity *familial exudative vitreoretinopathy* (FEVR, which is also known as the Criswick-Schepens syndrome) because of the familial and exudative nature of the disease. Both FEVR and retinopathy of prematurity are characterized by avascularity of the peripheral retina, which is especially evident on fluorescein angiography. In both diseases reactive fibrovascular proliferations develop that may lead to cicatricial changes and retinal traction in the temporal periphery, resulting in dragged discs, ectopic maculas, retinal detachments, and falciform retinal folds. Visual loss is primarily due to retinal detachment.[2]

FEVR is a rare disorder that is slowly progressive.[3] Gow and Oliver[4] identified the inheritance of FEVR as autosomal dominant, and similar observations have been made by others.[2, 3, 5–15] Because of this, some have suggested the terms *dominant exudative vitreoretinopathy*,[5, 6] *autosomal dominant exudative vitreoretinopathy*,[3, 7] or *hereditary exudative vitreoretinopathy*,[8] to describe these kindreds. The cause of FEVR is not known.

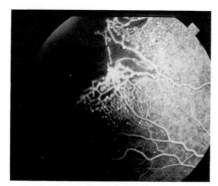

Figure 62–1. Fluorescein angiogram demonstrating the peripheral avascular zone, vascular engorgement and telangiectasia, microaneurysms, and shunt vessels in stage 1 disease.

CLINICAL CHARACTERISTICS

FEVR is a vitreoretinal disorder that is clinically similar to retinopathy of prematurity, except that there is a positive family history, usually in an autosomal dominant pattern, and there is no history of prematurity or oxygen supplementation. The disease is often asymptomatic in the early stages and progresses very slowly. Based on fundoscopic and fluorescein angiographic observations, Canny and Oliver have developed a useful staging scheme.[9] The three stages describe mild, moderate, and severe forms of FEVR, and each stage can be seen at any age.

Stage 1 describes the mild form of FEVR. Fundus examination during this stage reveals vitreoretinal changes in the periphery between the equator and the ora serrata, including the white-with-pressure and white-without-pressure signs, peripheral cystoid degeneration, and vitreous bands. There is a peripheral avascular zone that is difficult to see clinically. Exudation, neovascularization, and fibrovascular proliferation are not present at this initial stage. Fluorescein angiography demonstrates the peripheral avascular zone clearly (Fig. 62–1). Vascular engorgement and telangiectasia, capillary microaneurysms, arteriovenous shunts, and straightened vessels are present in the temporal periphery and can leak fluorescein. There is abnormal arborization of the vessels in the periphery, and these vessels terminate along a scalloped or curvilinear border with the avascular zone. In cases in which there are wider zones of peripheral avascularity, a wedge-shaped area of avascularization may be seen in the temporal meridian. Chorioretinal atrophy is often associated with this V-shaped zone of avascularization.[16] In many individuals, the peripheral avascular zone persists into adult life without regression or progression to proliferation.[8] This is in contrast to retinopathy of prematurity in which the peripheral retina subsequently vascularizes.

It is not known why the peripheral retina does not vascularize completely in FEVR. Whether this disease is a primary disorder affecting retinal vessel development[4, 10] rather than a true vitreoretinopathy, as originally suggested by Criswick and Schepens,[1] is still to be determined. Although congenital nonvascularization of the retinal periphery is the most common characteristic of the mildest phenotypes, vitreal changes are also noted in these patients. It also remains uncertain whether a secondary vasoocclusive process (e.g., associated with hematologic disease) is a factor in the pathogenesis of FEVR. Laqua[10] performed extensive hematologic examinations in one of his patients with FEVR and did not find any evidence of a hematologic disorder. Platelet dysfunction may play a role in FEVR, but this is still not fully determined.[17–19]

Stage 2 FEVR is the moderate form of the disease and represents the proliferative and exudative stage of this disease. In addition to the stage 1 findings already described, neovascularization, fibrovascular proliferation, and subretinal and intraretinal exudation are seen, especially in the temporal periphery (Figs. 62–2 and 62–3). A localized traction retinal detachment may also be present. The fibrovascular lesion contracts and exerts traction on the retina, producing an ectopic macula and a dragged disc (Fig. 62–4).[9] A fluorescein angiogram shows neovascularization, often in a sea fan pattern, developing from the retinal vessels at the vascular-

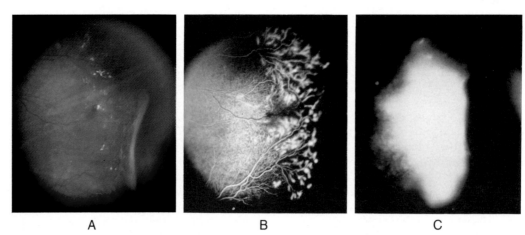

A   B   C

Figure 62–2. A, The temporal periphery in stage 2 familial exudative vitreoretinopathy (FEVR). Fibrovascular ridge and retinal exudation are seen. B, Early fluorescein angiogram of the same area showing neovascularization at the vascular-avascular border. C, Late fluorescein angiogram of the same area showing extensive leakage of the fluorescein dye. (A–C, Courtesy of Tatsuo Hirose, M.D.)

avascular border and growing anteriorly into the avascular retina. The temporal region of the retina is again the most common area for neovascularization. There is abrupt cessation of the retinal capillary network at the scalloped edge posterior to the fibrovascular mass. These terminal capillaries also leak fluorescein. Fibrovascular masses stain with fluorescein, and large feeder vessels may also be seen.[5, 16]

Stage 3 represents the advanced stage of FEVR. A cicatricial lesion in the temporal periphery pulls the retina and causes traction retinal detachments, falciform retinal folds, and rhegmatogenous retinal detachments. Massive intraretinal and subretinal exudation is present and can result in an exudative retinal detachment (Fig. 62–5). The exudative component of the disease may resemble Coats' disease and is different from retinopathy of prematurity. The degree of exudation is usually less than that found in Coats' disease, and exudative retinal detachments are rare. Anterior segment changes, including cataracts, iris atrophy, rubeosis iridis, and neovascular glaucoma, as well as band keratopathy, can also occur.[9]

Retinal detachments are relatively common in FEVR and constitute the major cause of visual loss in these patients. The incidence of retinal detachment ranges between 20 and 32 percent.[2, 13, 20] The rhegmatogenous form is the most common form of retinal detachment, and between 25 and 63 percent of all retinal detachments in FEVR are of this type. A variety of retinal breaks have been observed, including round holes, horseshoe tears, and giant tears. Rhegmatogenous retinal detachments usually occur in the second and third decades of life. At least in the Japanese population, rhegmatogenous retinal detachments from FEVR appear to constitute a significant proportion of all rhegmatogenous retinal detachments. Hashimoto and associates showed that in 576 consecutive cases of all rhegmatogenous retinal detachments, 5 percent were in FEVR patients. When he looked at all rhegmatogenous retinal detachments in patients less than 30 yr of age, a surprising 12 percent were in patients with FEVR.[20]

Retinal breaks in FEVR are thought to be caused by a combination of vitreoretinal traction and retinal atrophy. Vitreous bands and adhesions are seen even in the

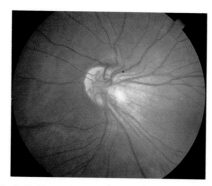

Figure 62–4. Patient with stage 2 FEVR with a dragged disc.

early stages of FEVR. Neovascularization and fibrovascular proliferation produce additional traction. The peripheral retina in patients with FEVR is also avascular and atrophic. Atrophic holes are seen in the periphery in many cases. The combination of vitreoretinal traction and atrophic retina makes these eyes more susceptible to retinal tears.[2, 21] The rhegmatogenous retinal detachments tend to be difficult cases that often lead to proliferative vitreoretinopathy and require multiple procedures.[2, 22] There is also one reported case of significant postoperative uveitis.[23] Vitreous hemorrhage in patients with FEVR is rare but may be an ominous sign; two cases described by van Nouhuys resulted in rapid progression to closed-funnel retinal detachments.[2]

Falciform retinal folds are also relatively common and are found in 15 to 39 percent of eyes with FEVR.[2, 14] The folds usually extend from the optic nerve head to the temporal or inferotemporal periphery, at which point there are cicatricial connections to the mass of fibrous tissue at the peripheral retina and lens equator.[24, 25] The distance between the peripheral retina and the lens equator is very short in the neonatal eye, and this accounts for the anterior adhesions. The folds appear to be caused by severe traction of the retina resulting from the organization of peripheral neovascularization and fibrovascular mass. The folds usually occur in the first decade of life and do not show progression.

Traction retinal detachments are less common and occur at a rate of 6 to 10 percent in eyes with FEVR.[2, 20] They usually occur before the age of 10 yr and show very little progression. Exudation does not play a major

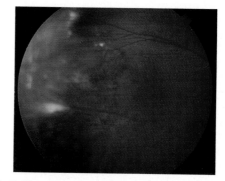

Figure 62–3. The temporal periphery in stage 2 disease demonstrating intraretinal and subretinal exudation, pigmentary changes, and straightening of retinal vessels.

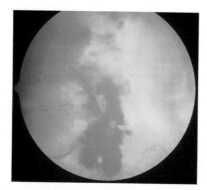

Figure 62–5. Stage 3 FEVR in a patient with retinal hemorrhage and severe exudative retinal detachment.

role in causing retinal detachments, and significant exudative retinal detachments are rare.[2]

DIFFERENTIAL DIAGNOSIS

FEVR is characterized by nonvascularization of the peripheral retina, familial occurrence (usually autosomal dominant), dragged disc and macula, retinal exudation, retinal detachment, and retinal folds. The clinical features are most similar to retinopathy of prematurity and include peripheral nonvascularization, reactive fibrovascular proliferations, and cicatricial changes with severe traction on the retina. Important differentiating features are a family history of the disorder and no history of prematurity or oxygen supplementation. The peripheral avascular retina does not vascularize in FEVR as it typically does in retinopathy of prematurity, and exudation, which is common in FEVR, is very rare in retinopathy of prematurity.[10]

In addition to retinopathy of prematurity, possible alternative differential diagnoses of patients having peripheral retinal nonvascularization with neovascular proliferation include sickle cell trait and disease and other hemoglobinopathies, Eales disease, incontinentia pigmenti, and autosomal dominant neovascularization as described by Gitter and coworkers.[26] Diseases causing dragged discs, ectopic maculas, and falciform retinal folds also need to be considered, especially hereditary falciform retinal folds, persistent hyperplastic primary vitreous, *Toxocara canis* infection, Norrie's disease, and incontinentia pigmenti.[6, 14] Causes of peripheral retinal fibrous or exudative mass lesions include Coats' disease, angiomatosis retinae, *Toxocara canis* infection, and pars planitis.[10, 21]

GENETICS

FEVR is inherited as an autosomal dominant trait in most families.[2, 3, 5–15] Penetrance is close to 100 percent, and there is significant phenotypic variability, as previously described. McKusick's catalog of inherited diseases lists FEVR under autosomal dominant phenotypes, No. 13378.[27] Although it is less common, an X-linked form of FEVR appears to exist; two four-generation kindreds of this type were described by Trese and colleagues.[28] Interestingly, in one of the original families described by Criswick and Schepens,[1] three brothers and a maternal uncle were affected, and a distant male relative related through females was blind. This kindred shows inheritance consistent with that of an X-linked recessive trait. Sporadic cases of FEVR also exist[13, 29] and may represent somatic or new germinal mutations. Genetic counseling should be given after careful examination of each family.

The exact nature of the genetic defect in this disease is not known. With the identification of many large families with this disease, especially in the Netherlands[2, 5, 6, 24] and Japan,[13–16, 20, 22, 23, 30–35] it is our hope that modern molecular genetic techniques can be applied, possibly by candidate gene analysis or by linkage analysis, to identify the mutations that cause FEVR. Understanding the genetic defect will help elucidate the cause of disease and may help in the study of related diseases.

PATHOLOGIC FEATURES

Histopathologic studies of six eyes enucleated for end-stage FEVR have been reported.[11, 24, 36, 37] These eyes were enucleated for phthisis, neovascular glaucoma, acute angle closure, and possible retinoblastoma (in a 6-week-old infant). Many of the histopathologic findings are those typically associated with chronic retinal detachments, neovascular glaucoma, and phthisis bulbi. This discussion concentrates on the findings unique to FEVR. No pathologic findings in either stage 1 or stage 2 disease are available.

Retinal detachment and prominent preretinal and vitreal membrane formation are seen in all cases. Brockhurst and associates[36] observed a thick, acellular preretinal membrane consisting of amorphous material. This membrane is seen just posterior to the ora serrata and extends posteriorly. Multiple adhesions to the retina cause large retinal folds. A cellular fibrous membrane with pigment is also seen in the vitreous. van Nouhuys'[24] case of the 6-week-old infant with possible retinoblastoma shows the preretinal membrane to extend much more anteriorly and attach to the lens capsule. Intraretinal and subretinal exudation is also seen, but the degree of exudation and the extent of telangiectatic vessels are less than those usually seen in Coats' disease.[37] Nicholson and Galvis[11] observed areas of necrosis and acute inflammation surrounding the fibrovascular tissue in the temporal periphery of the retina.

PREVENTION AND TREATMENT

The major cause of visual loss in cases of FEVR is retinal detachment. When retinal detachments occur in eyes with FEVR, they tend to be complicated and difficult to repair, often requiring multiple surgical procedures.[2, 20] Some of the detachments are similar to those seen in retinopathy of prematurity. Retinal detachments are more difficult and have the worst prognosis in younger children; rhegmatogenous retinal detachment in an adolescent patient with FEVR has a high likelihood of progressing to proliferative vitreoretinopathy and redetachment. The key to retinal detachment repair in patients with FEVR is to release the peripheral vitreoretinal traction using meticulous membrane dissection and scleral buckling.[22]

As in retinopathy of prematurity, the goal, then, is to try to prevent the retinal detachment seen in stage 3 FEVR. Early examination (including dilated fundus examination with scleral depression) of children who have a positive family history is mandatory in identifying those with early proliferative changes. The neovascular and fibrovascular process can then be treated by prophylactic photocoagulation or cryotherapy. There are very few descriptions of FEVR in neonates and infants, and early examination will also give us a better understanding of how FEVR presents in this population. The application of a retinoablative procedure to the avascular retina alone or together with the neovascular frond appears to be effective in aborting the proliferative process.[2, 38] The destruction of the proliferative process is thought to diminish the subsequent cicatricial process that leads to retinal detachment. A randomized study to test the effectiveness of prophylactic cryotherapy or photocoagulation would be difficult to carry out because of the rarity and slow progression of the disease. It is not currently clear whether we can prevent the retinal detachments that present quite early in life, since stage 3 FEVR can already be present in very young patients.[39]

The cicatricial process makes the direct detection of subtle retinal detachments difficult. Vitreous cells and haze, poor mydriasis, aqueous cells and flare, and posterior synechiae are all signs of retinal detachment in a patient with FEVR. Ultrasonography is important in the diagnosis of retinal detachments in eyes with media opacities. An increase in angle kappa is evidence of increasing peripheral traction.[2] The role of electrophysiologic testing is uncertain.[34]

REFERENCES

1. Criswick VG, Schepens CL: Familial exudative vitreoretinopathy. Am J Ophthalmol 68:578–594, 1969.
2. van Nouhuys CE: Juvenile retinal detachment as a complication of familial exudative vitreoretinopathy. Fortschr Ophthalmol 86:221–223, 1989.
3. Ober RR, Bird AC, Hamilton AM, Sehmi K: Autosomal dominant exudative vitreoretinopathy. Br J Ophthalmol 64:112–120, 1980.
4. Gow J, Oliver GL: Familial exudative vitreoretinopathy: An expanded view. Arch Ophthalmol 86:150–155, 1971.
5. Nijhuis FA, Deutman AF, Aan de Kerk AL: Fluorescein angiography in mild stages of dominant exudative vitreoretinopathy. Mod Probl Ophthalmol 20:107–114, 1979.
6. van Nouhuys CE: Congenital retinal fold as a sign of dominant exudative vitreoretinopathy. Graefes Arch Clin Exp Ophthalmol 217:55–67, 1981.
7. Feldman EL, Norris JL, Cleasby GW: Autosomal dominant exudative vitreoretinopathy. Arch Ophthalmol 101:1532–1535, 1983.
8. Tasman W, Augsburger JJ, Shields JA, et al: Familial exudative vitreoretinopathy. Trans Am Ophthalmol Soc 79:211–226, 1981.
9. Canny CLB, Oliver GL: Fluorescein angiographic findings in familial exudative vitreoretinopathy. Arch Ophthalmol 94:1114–1120, 1976.
10. Laqua H: Familial exudative vitreoretinopathy. Graefes Arch Clin Exp Ophthalmol 213:121–133, 1980.
11. Nicholson DH, Galvis V: Criswick-Schepens syndrome (familial exudative vitreoretinopathy): Study of a Colombian kindred. Arch Ophthalmol 102:1519–1522, 1984.
12. Saraux H, Laroche L, Koenig F: Retinopathie exudative a transmission dominante. Presentation d'un nouveau pedigree. J Fr Ophthalmol 8:155–158, 1985.
13. Miyakubo H, Inohara N, Hashimoto K: Retinal involvement in familial exudative vitreoretinopathy. Ophthalmologica 185:125–135, 1982.
14. Nishimura M, Yamana T, Sugino M, et al: Falciform retinal fold as sign of familial exudative vitreoretinopathy. Jpn J Ophthalmol 27:40–53, 1983.
15. Oshio K, Oshima K: A family of vitreoretinopathy with developmental anomaly of retinal vessels. Folia Ophthalmol Jpn 27:138–144, 1976.
16. Miyakubo H, Hashimoto K, Miyakubo S: Retinal vascular pattern in familial exudative vitreoretinopathy. Ophthalmology 91:1524–1530, 1984.
17. Chaudhuri PR, Rosenthal AR, Goulstine DB, et al: Familial exudative vitreoretinopathy associated with familial thrombocytopathy. Br J Ophthalmol 67:755–758, 1983.
18. Friedrich CA, Francis KA, Kim HC: Familial exudative vitreoretinopathy (FEVR) and platelet dysfunction. Br J Ophthalmol 73:477–478, 1989.
19. Gole GA, Goodall K, James MJ: Familial exudative vitreoretinopathy. Br J Ophthalmol 69:76, 1985.
20. Hashimoto K, Miyakubo H, Inohara N, Tada H: Juvenile retinal detachment and familial exudative vitreoretinopathy. Jpn J Clin Ophthalmol 37:797–803, 1983.
21. Dudgeon J: Familial exudative vitreo-retinopathy. Trans Ophthalmol Soc UK 99:45–49, 1979.
22. Tano Y, Ikeda T: Treatment of familial exudative vitreoretinopathy with pars plana vitrectomy. Ophthalmology 97(Suppl):152, 1990.
23. Okubo Y, Okubo A, Kubono T, Shimizu H: Familial exudative vitreoretinopathy, rhegmatogenous retinal detachment and postoperative uveitis with massive subretinal exudation. Nippon Ganka Gakkai Zasshi 88:1151–1156, 1984.
24. van Nouhuys CE: Dominant exudative vitreoretinopathy and other vascular developmental disorders of the peripheral retina. Doc Ophthalmol 54:1–414, 1982.
25. Campo RV: Similarity of familial exudative vitreoretinopathy and retinopathy of prematurity. Arch Ophthalmol 101:821, 1983.
26. Gitter KA, Rothchild H, Waltman DD, et al: Dominantly inherited peripheral retinal neovascularization. Arch Ophthalmol 96:1601–1605, 1978.
27. McKusick VA: Mendelian Inheritance in Man: Catalog of Autosomal Dominant, Autosomal Recessive, and X-linked Phenotypes, 9th ed. Baltimore, The Johns Hopkins University Press, 1990, p 244.
28. Trese MT, Hartzer MR, Shastry BS: X-Chromosome–Linked Familial Exudative Vitreoretinopathy. Presented at 8th International Congress of Human Genetics, Washington, DC, 1991.
29. Schulman J, Jampol LM, Schwartz H: Peripheral proliferative retinopathy without oxygen therapy in a full-term infant. Am J Ophthalmol 90:509–514, 1980.
30. Kosaka A, Arimoto H, Kubota N: A case of vitreo-retinal dystrophy. Jpn J Clin Ophthalmol 36:105–108, 1982.
31. Nishimura M, Yamana T, Minei M, Ueda K: Vitreoretinal involvements in mild stages of familial exudative vitreoretinopathy. Nippon Ganka Gakkai Zasshi 86:1213–1223, 1982.
32. Nishimura M, Yamana T, Ueda K, et al: Family studies of retinopathy of prematurity in full-term infants. Nippon Ganka Gakkai Zasshi 86:702–710, 1982.
33. Nishimura M, Kohno T, Sanui H, et al: Familial angiodysplastic vitreoretinopathy. Folia Ophthalmol Jpn 30:1560–1570, 1979.
34. Ohkubo H, Tanino T: Electrophysiological findings in familial exudative vitreoretinopathy. Doc Ophthalmol 65:461–469, 1987.
35. Yoshitake H, Uchida S, Nishimura T: Fundus changes similar to those of retinopathy of prematurity in full-term infants. Folia Ophthalmol Jpn 32:2016–2022, 1981.
36. Brockhurst RJ, Albert DM, Zakov ZN: Pathologic findings in familial exudative vitreoretinopathy. Arch Ophthalmol 99:2143–2146, 1981.
37. Boldrey EE, Egbert P, Gass JDM, Friberg T: The histopathology of familial exudative vitreoretinopathy: A report of two cases. Arch Ophthalmol 103:238–241, 1985.
38. Bergen RL, Glassman R: Familial exudative vitreoretinopathy. Ann Ophthalmol 15:275–276, 1983.
39. Slusher MM, Hutton WE: Familial exudative vitreoretinopathy. Am J Ophthalmol 87:152–156, 1979.

Chapter 63

■

Central Serous Chorioretinopathy

DAVID R. GUYER and EVANGELOS S. GRAGOUDAS

HISTORICAL PERSPECTIVE

Central serous chorioretinopathy (CSC) or idiopathic macular serous detachment was first described in 1866 by Von Graefe[1] and termed *recurrent central retinitis.* Since then this condition has been described under various names, reflecting the lack of a precise clinical definition for this disorder in the past and the uncertainty over which tissue site was primarily disturbed. In 1916, Fuchs[2] reported additional cases, and in 1927, Horniker[3] named the condition *central angiospastic retinitis.* In the mid to late 1930s, this disorder was termed *idiopathic flat detachment of the macula* by Walsh and Sloane[4] and *central angiospastic retinopathy* by Gifford and Marquardt.[5] These latter authors believed that the disease was due to an angioneurotic diathesis. In 1953, Klien[6] divided these cases into three groups: central angiospastic retinopathy, central angiospastic chorioretinopathy, and central angioneurotic chorioretinopathy. This author attributed the condition to autonomic nervous system dysfunction. In the mid to late 1950s, Bennett[7] and Maumenee[8] stated that CSC belonged in the spectrum of macular disciform degeneration. The name *central serous retinopathy* was applied to this condition by Bennett in 1955.[7] Peripheral retinal changes associated with CSC were subsequently described.[9]

Maumenee[10] and Gass[11] provided great insight into our current understanding of CSC in the mid 1960s. Maumenee[10] described the unique fluorescein angiographic appearance of CSC—a leak through the retinal pigment epithelium (RPE). Then in 1967 Gass[11] provided the classic description of the disease and reported on the fluorescein angiographic findings in 15 additional patients. He also suggested that the disorder be termed *central serous choroidopathy.*

CLINICAL CHARACTERISTICS

Demographics

CSC occurs in young to middle-aged individuals, usually about 20 to 45 yr of age.[1, 7, 11–21] The diagnosis must be questioned in patients older than 50 yr, as these individuals are often found later to have age-related macular degeneration and choroidal neovascularization. Although CSC in a 7-year-old girl has been reported, this patient may actually have had posterior scleritis.[22, 23]

There is a male predominance of 8 to 10:1.[7, 21, 24–27] The condition is uncommon in blacks but is common in whites, Hispanics, and probably Asians, especially those of Japanese origin.[28–30] The severe form of CSC may occur more frequently in individuals from Southeast Asia or those of Latin origin.[12] Mild hyperopia is often noted in CSC patients.[28, 31]

Systemic Associations

Patients with CSC may occasionally complain of a migraine-like headache.[11] In addition, these patients often are noted to have various personality traits, including a type A personality, hypochondria, hysteria, and conversional neurosis. Werry and Arends,[32] using the Minnesota Multiphasic Personality Inventory Test, showed that CSC patients are more likely to show hypochondria or hysteria and have a conversional neurosis than are controls. Yannuzzi,[28] using the Jenkins Activity Survey, has reported that, when compared with controls, CSC patients are more likely to exhibit type A personality.

Ocular Symptoms

Patients with CSC complain of decreased or blurred vision, metamorphopsia, micropsia, paracentral scotomas, and chromatopsia.

Ophthalmic Findings

Visual acuity in the acute state of this disorder can range from 20/20 to 20/200 or better.[21] In one series, 52 percent of patients had visual acuity of 20/30 or better at presentation.[21] With a small hyperopic correction, vision can usually be improved. The anterior segment and vitreous are normal.

The following findings may be present on fundus examination (Table 63–1):[11, 12, 21]

1. *Serous retinal detachment*: A round to oval, well-delineated shallow serous retinal detachment is present in the macula (Fig. 63–1). This mildly darkened area is surrounded by a halo of light reflex and has an average size of two disc diameters. The normal foveal reflex is not apparent.

2. *Serous detachment of the RPE*: One or more discrete yellow to yellow-gray, round to oval, well-demarcated areas of detached RPE may be observed. These

Table 63–1. OPHTHALMIC FINDINGS

Serous retinal detachment
Serous detachment of the retinal pigment epithelium (RPE)
Subretinal precipitates
Extramacular RPE atrophic tracts
Multiple bullous serous retinal and RPE detachments
RPE atrophic changes

areas are often present under the superior half of the macular detachment but sometimes may be present above the macular detachment when gravity forces the subretinal fluid inferiorly.[11] These detachments are often less than one quarter of a disc diameter in size and have a grayish halo around them. Pigment changes may be present on the detachment's surface and occasionally can be seen only with fluorescein angiography.

3. *Subretinal precipitates*: Multiple, variably sized yellow dotlike precipitates probably caused by subretinal fluid turbidity may be noticed at the level of the RPE (Fig. 63–2).[11] Diffuse gray-white subretinal deposits, which may represent fibrin, are occasionally present (Fig. 63–3).[12] In the fovea, a small, yellow, round spot may be seen, which may be caused by increased xanthophyll visibility.

4. *Extramacular RPE atrophic tracts*: Yannuzzi and coworkers[9] described 25 patients with extramacular inferior hemispheric RPE atrophic tracts related to an antecedent retinal detachment. Five of these patients actually had a peripheral retinal detachment. Other findings that were reported in this subset of CSC patients included retinal capillary telangiectasia, retinal capillary leakage, cystoid macular edema, lipid deposition, choriocapillaris atrophy, choroidal neovascularization, and disciform scar formation. These patients often had a poor visual prognosis, and thus these authors suggest that CSC may not always be a benign condition. Extramacular RPE atrophic tracts have also previously been reported by others.[33, 34] Gass[34] describes this as a pseudoretinitis pigmentosa–like atypical CSC presentation with prolonged and recurrent serous retinal detachment. He states that it is more frequent in patients of Latin or Asian ancestry and that bone spicules may be present. He also notes that frequent recurrences, permanent vision loss, and significant superior field vision loss are common.

5. *Multiple bullous serous retinal and RPE detachments*: An atypical presentation of CSC is that of multiple bullous serous retinal detachments, usually seen in healthy middle-aged men.[12, 17, 35, 36] These posterior pole or midperipheral detachments are often associated with subretinal fibrinous exudate and multiple serous RPE detachments with areas of shifting subretinal fluid.

6. *RPE atrophic changes*: RPE changes corresponding to previous CSC episodes may be present in either or both eyes.

FLUORESCEIN ANGIOGRAPHIC CHARACTERISTICS

Maumenee[10] first described the classic RPE leak noted on fluorescein angiography. Gass[11] then described 15

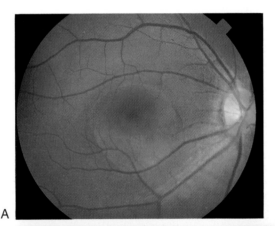

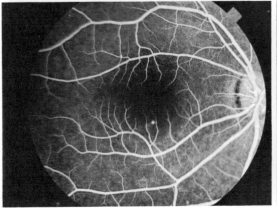

Figure 63–1. *A*, A serous macular detachment consistent with central serous chorioretinopathy. Fluorescein angiography reveals a typical smokestack configuration. *B*, Early phase. *C*, Late phase.

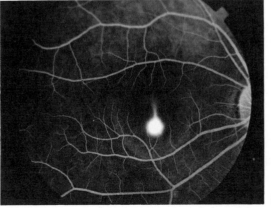

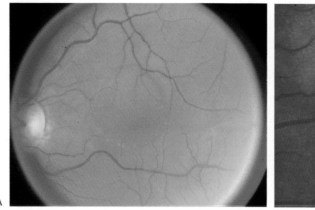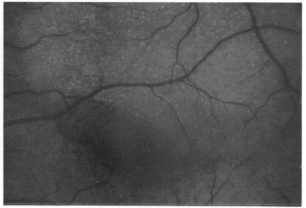

Figure 63–2. A and B, Subretinal precipitates can be observed in some cases of central serous chorioretinopathy.

additional cases. Early in the angiogram, there is a focal dotlike hyperfluorescence representing the leakage of dye from the choroid through the RPE. Later, dye accumulates beneath the sensory retinal detachment but does not extend outside the borders of the detachment. Two types of leakage may occur. The classic or smoke-stack-type leakage, first described by Shimizu and Tobari in 1971,[37] occurs in 7 to 20 percent of cases (see Fig. 63–1).[25, 26, 37, 38] The leakage first ascends superiorly, like a smokestack, and then spreads laterally. This type of leakage is thought to occur secondary to convection currents and a pressure gradient between the subretinal fluid and the dye entering the detachment. There is speculation that this gradient exists because of different protein concentrations. In up to 93 percent of CSC cases, however, the smokestack-type leakage is not seen.[38] Instead, a leakage point with uniform dye filling is appreciated.

Spitznas and Huke[38] have studied the number, shape, and topography of leakage points in 430 eyes with CSC. One leakage point was present in 71.6 percent of cases, two points were present in 17 percent of cases, three points were present in 5.1 percent of cases, four points were present in 4 percent of cases, five points were present in 1.6 percent of cases, six points were present in 0.5 percent of cases, and seven points were present in 0.2 percent of cases. The most common location for

a leakage point was in the upper nasal quadrant (33.2 percent). This finding is confirmed by other studies.[27, 37, 39] The leakage point was found in the lower nasal quadrant in 21.2 percent of cases and in the upper temporal quadrant in 19 percent of cases.[38] The lower temporal quadrant was the least likely area to contain a leakage point (14.8 percent).

Most leakage points are within a 1-mm area around the fovea, but they can occur in an area greater than 3 mm from the foveal avascular zone in 11.8 percent of cases.[38] In less than 10 percent of cases, the leakage point is found in the fovea,[31] and in 10 to 30 percent of cases, the leakage point is found in the papillomacular bundle.[7, 27, 37, 38] In recurrent cases, the leakage point is within 1 mm of the initial leakage point in 80 percent of patients.[25, 38]

Friberg and Campagna[40] have studied the leakage points using digital image processing in 53 cases of CSC. They found that there is a nonrandom distribution of leaks near the center of the detachments and that a detachment associated with a smokestack-type leak is larger than that from a less active pinpoint leak.

Other rare CSC leakage patterns include diffuse leakage without an obvious leakage point, a healed CSC scar that still leaks, and a pinpoint RPE detachment leak.[25] Other common associated fluorescein angiographic findings include RPE changes secondary to old CSC episodes and areas of hyperfluorescence corresponding to RPE detachments.

If a leakage point is not observed on fluorescein angiography, the extramacular and, especially, superior areas should be studied. Gravity may have caused the leakage point to remain outside the detached area. In some cases, a leakage point will not be found because the leak has healed. In these cases, the detachment will usually resolve in days to weeks. Finally, several other conditions may mimic CSC clinically, and thus in these cases, a leakage point will not be found (see Differential Diagnosis).

NATURAL HISTORY

The visual prognosis for CSC patients is relatively good.[21, 24] In the series of Klein and associates,[21] reso-

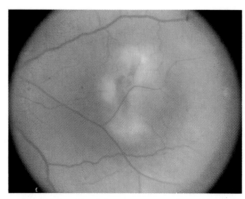

Figure 63–3. Fibrin deposition is present in this patient with central serous chorioretinopathy.

lution was noted in all 34 eyes studied prospectively without any treatment. The average resolution time was 3 mos. All patients had visual acuity of 20/40 or better, and 94 percent of the eyes had visual acuity of 20/30 or better at follow-up examination (average, 23 mos). These authors concluded that CSC was a benign and self-limiting condition, which seldom required laser photocoagulation therapy. In the study by Gilbert and coworkers,[25] approximately 75 percent of their patients had 20/20 vision at last follow-up examination. If the patient initially had a visual acuity of worse than 20/30, he or she usually gained two to three lines of vision. However, even after resolution of the serous detachment, patients with CSC may still have minor visual complaints, including decreased color vision, relative scotomas, micropsia, metamorphopsia, decreased contrast sensitivity, and nyctalopia.[21, 41, 42]

Resolution of the detachment occurs by 3 to 4 mo;[11] however, improvement in visual acuity can occur up to 12 mo following resolution of the detachment.[21] RPE abnormalities occur at and around the previous areas of leakage. In addition, focal yellow deposits, precipitates, and cystic changes may be present.[11]

In a small number of cases, the visual outcome may not be as favorable. Levine and associates[33] suggest that the visual prognosis of CSC patients is not as benign as previously thought. In a long-term study of 14 eyes by fluorescein angiography, these authors concluded that CSC may be a diffuse, progressive RPE disorder. Nonleaking RPE defects were present inside the previously detached areas in all cases and were also present outside these areas in 43 percent of cases. In the fellow eye, 42 percent had new RPE window defects. Two lines of visual acuity were lost in 29 percent of the eyes with CSC and in 8 percent of the fellow eyes. These authors suggest that CSC is a progressive bilateral asymmetric disease with diffuse RPE abnormalities outside the area of previous detachment. However, the demographics of their population is not typical of CSC; 23 percent of their patients were black, and the average age was older than usual. Thus, they may have studied an unusual subset of patients with this condition.

Yannuzzi and coworkers[9] have also suggested that for a subset of CSC patients, the visual prognosis may not be so benign. In their series of a subset of 32 CSC eyes with peripheral RPE atrophic tracts, 25 percent of patients had a final visual acuity of 20/200 or worse.

Recurrences are an additional problem in patients with CSC. Klein and associates[21] reported recurrences by observation or history in 45 percent of the patients in their series. Gilbert and coworkers[25] reported that 51 percent of their untreated patients had a single resolving CSC episode based on previous historical episodes, clinically observed recurrences, and probable persistent detachments. Recurrences can occur many years later. The recurrent leakage point is within 1 mm of the initial leakage point in 80 percent of patients.[25, 38]

Thus, although the visual prognosis of CSC patients is usually very good, a small subset of patients may have a poor visual outcome. Uncommon complications of the disease, such as peripheral tracts and detachments, macular edema, choroidal neovascularization, and RPE atrophy may occur.

PATHOPHYSIOLOGY

The pathophysiology of CSC is highly controversial.[11, 16, 43–47] The debate centers not only on the underlying cause of the condition but also on whether it is primarily a disease of the choroid or the RPE. Numerous causes have been proposed for CSC.[28] They include syphilis,[1, 2] tuberculosis,[48] malnutrition,[49] vitreous traction,[50] hypotony,[49] allergy,[51, 52] toxicity,[14, 53] infection,[1, 2, 48, 54] vessel spasm,[3, 5, 6, 55] episcleritis,[22] familial causes,[12, 13] increased venous pressure with vortex vein stasis and eosinophilia,[56] relationship to hemorrhagic disciform macular degeneration,[7, 8] and psychogenic behavior.[5, 11, 28, 32, 57]

Spitznas[47] suggests that the RPE is damaged via an immunologic, infectious, circulatory, or neuronal mechanism, which causes the RPE to secrete ions in a chorioretinal direction (toward the retina). Neighboring RPE cells pump the fluid back in a retinochoroidal direction (toward the choroid).

Others[44, 46] state that a passive RPE leak could not overwhelm the RPE pump of the neighboring normal RPE, and therefore dysfunction of the neighboring RPE must also occur. Thus, they suggest that CSC has more diffuse RPE abnormalities. However, increased choroidal permeability and fluid pressure may be great enough to overwhelm even neighboring RPE cells.

Yannuzzi[28] suggests that CSC may have a multifactorial cause consisting of genetic, environmental, and behavioral factors. Experimental animal CSC models[58–64] defend the hypothesis that elevated catecholamine levels may be important in the pathogenesis of this disorder. Horniker,[3] in 1927, first suggested the psychogenic-related hypothesis of CSC. He believed that these patients had a constitutional angioneurosis, which led to angiospasm and exudation. Since then, other authors have suggested a psychogenic component to this disease.[5, 11, 28, 32, 57] Associated personality traits include hypochondria, hysterics, neuroses, and type A behavior.[28, 32]

Several investigators[58–61] have shown that intravenous epinephrine can create a CSC-like picture in rabbits. Yoshioka and associates[62–64] reported that repeated intravenous epinephrine injections in monkeys also can produce an animal model of CSC. Thus, from the personality traits of patients with CSC and experimental animal studies, it seems possible that an adrenergic reaction may cause damage to the choriocapillaris. This insult may cause choriocapillaris hyperpermeability, which leads to RPE cell degeneration. Pregnancy also may induce CSC, perhaps through hormonal and psychogenic mechanisms.[65–68] In addition, dialysis or organ transplantation, or both, may cause CSC.[69, 70] Friberg and Eller[69] reported two patients who acquired CSC within 9 mo after cardiac transplantation and one patient in whom bilateral CSC developed within 6 mos after renal transplantation. Each of these three patients had an elevated blood urea nitrogen level at the time of presentation.

It appears that CSC is a multifactorial disease in which stress is one of many risk factors. CSC probably results primarily from increased choriocapillaris permeability, which causes secondary RPE changes. A primary role of the RPE in this condition, however, cannot be totally discounted. One report[71] of indocyanine green angiography in a patient with CSC suggests choroidal hyperpermeability at the area of leakage. We are currently conducting an investigation of CSC patients with digital indocyanine green angiography to learn more about the possible choroidal circulatory abnormalities in this perplexing disorder.

Several electrophysiologic studies have been performed on CSC patients. Nagata and Honda[72] studied focal electroretinograms (ERG) in 28 patients. They found an initially diminished macular response (b waves) in approximately 90 percent of patients. Only two patients showed a normal focal ERG at follow-up examination. Miyake and associates[73] reported significantly reduced local macula responses on ERG in 24 patients. Oscillatory potentials and b waves were affected more than a waves. At resolution, 18 patients were studied and showed recovery of the b waves and shortened implicit times. However, oscillatory potentials did not recover, suggesting a middle to inner retinal layer abnormality. Foveal densitometry studies[74] revealed abnormal two-way densities of pigment in 12 of 14 CSC patients, with slow regeneration. Chuang and associates[75] noted a loss in sensitivity of 3 log units in patients with acute CSC using psychophysical and photochemical methods to study visual depression and rod dysfunction.

HISTOPATHOLOGY

Limited histopathologic material exists on CSC. Three reports describe serous macular detachments without defects or detachments in the RPE.[56, 76, 77] However, some of these cases were not confirmed to be CSC by fluorescein angiography or were not typical CSC cases, or both. Two additional cases[12, 78] have been reported. No choriocapillaris abnormalities were noted in either case. One eye had an RPE detachment, and examination of the other eye revealed a gray-white exudate composed of fibrin.

Yoshioka and Katsume[64] have described the ultrastructural findings in the intravenous epinephrine–induced monkey model of CSC. These authors found a focal area of degenerated RPE with adjacent damaged choriocapillaris endothelial cells. These endothelial abnormalities were sealed by platelet-fibrin clots. Histopathologic studies of acute cases are necessary to further elucidate the pathogenesis of this disease.

DIFFERENTIAL DIAGNOSIS

Although the clinical and fluorescein angiographic features of CSC are often classic, several entities should be considered in the differential diagnosis, including the following (Table 63–2).

1. *Tumors*: Choroidal melanoma, choroidal hemangioma, choroidal metastasis, leukemia, choroidal infiltrates, and choroidal osteoma can occasionally present

Table 63–2. DIFFERENTIAL DIAGNOSIS

Tumors
Presumed ocular histoplasmosis syndrome
Posterior scleritis
Harada's disease
Sympathetic ophthalmia
Benign reactive lymphoid hyperplasia of the uvea
Collagen vascular disorders
Sarcoidosis
Idiopathic uveal effusion syndrome
Malignant hypertension
Toxemia of pregnancy
Disseminated intravascular coagulopathy
Age-related macular degeneration
Retinal hole
Optic nerve pit with serous macular detachment
Trauma
Following surgery

diagnostic difficulties, especially in patients with a large RPE detachment and a small retinal detachment.

2. *Infectious and inflammatory disorders*: Several infectious and inflammatory conditions should be considered in the differential diagnosis. The presumed ocular histoplasmosis syndrome can present with a serous macular detachment. However, peripapillar atrophy, histoplasmosis spots, and choroidal neovascularization distinguish this disease from CSC. Posterior scleritis can produce a retinal detachment like CSC, but it can be differentiated from CSC by the scleral involvement, intraocular inflammation, and a subretinal mass. A serous retinal detachment is also observed in patients with Harada's disease who, unlike CSC patients, may have systemic symptoms, optic disc swelling, a thickened choroid on ultrasonography, and multiple pinpoint leaks on fluorescein angiography. Patients with serous retinal detachment secondary to sympathetic ophthalmia will have a past history of ocular trauma or surgery and inflammation in both eyes. CSC can be confused with benign reactive lymphoid hyperplasia of the uvea, which can also cause a serous macular detachment. This latter disease can produce diffuse uveal thickening, a yellow to gray fundus color change, RPE changes, acute angle-closure glaucoma, extensive retinal detachment, and inflammation. Collagen vascular disorders can lead to serous macular detachments, with or without involvement of the retinal vasculature, and should be considered in the differential diagnosis of CSC. Sarcoidosis can be distinguished from CSC by the presence of a choroidal granuloma, retinal vasculature changes, and optic nerve involvement. Patients with the idiopathic uveal effusion syndrome may present with a serous macular detachment. However, they usually have choroidal and ciliary body detachments.

3. *Vascular disorders*: Malignant hypertension can produce a serous retinal detachment. The presence of systemic hypertension, Elschnig's spots, shifting fluid, and choroidal or retinal vasculature changes, or both, can distinguish it from CSC. Serous retinal detachment can occur in toxemia of pregnancy. The systemic findings of hypertension, proteinuria, and edema will separate this condition from CSC seen in pregnant women. Disseminated intravascular coagulopathy also should be

considered in the differential diagnosis of serous retinal detachment and can be distinguished by its systemic findings.

4. *Age-related macular degeneration*: Choroidal neovascularization secondary to age-related macular degeneration may be difficult to distinguish from CSC in patients older than 50 yr of age. Often the choroidal neovascularization may be small or poorly defined, and a focal leakage point may suggest the diagnosis of CSC. Thus, because CSC usually occurs in young to middle-aged patients, one must be very cautious in diagnosing CSC in a patient more than 50 yr of age. Repeating the fluorescein angiogram 2 to 3 wk later is often helpful because choroidal neovascularization may become apparent with time.

RPE detachments caused by age-related macular degeneration can also be confused with CSC. This condition usually occurs in patients with drusen, in which large RPE detachments are present with associated small serous retinal detachments. In these cases, a discrete leakage point, as seen in CSC, is not apparent on fluorescein angiography, and early diffuse hyperfluorescence occurs. Choroidal neovascularization may be associated with these RPE detachments and must be searched for carefully with fluorescein and indocyanine green angiography.

5. *Retinal hole*: A peripheral retinal hole, usually found superiorly, should be searched for in cases of retinal detachment without a focal leakage point on fluorescein angiography. In addition, macular holes in patients with high myopia can cause posterior pole detachments.

6. *Optic nerve pit with serous macular detachment*: Optic nerve pits with serous macular detachments can mimic cases of CSC. Pits should be looked for in all patients with CSC, but especially when focal leakage points are not present on fluorescein angiography.

7. *Trauma and surgery*: Ocular contusion and associated macular detachment can on occasion mimic CSC. Rarely, in the early postoperative period or after scleral buckling surgery or pneumatic retinopexy,[79] a CSC-like picture of exudative retinal detachment can occur.

8. *Rare macular disorders*: Best's dystrophy and retinal pigment epitheliitis can, on rare occasions, be confused with CSC. The latter disorder does not cause a macular detachment, but the RPE changes can sometimes be confused with resolved cases of CSC.

TREATMENT

Medical Treatment

No medical therapy has been shown to be effective for patients with CSC. Tranquilizers, sedatives, and barbiturates have been advocated to decrease the psychogenic component of this disorder, but their efficacy has not been demonstrated. It has been suggested that β-blockers might be a reasonable pharmacologic intervention to investigate, especially if these patients are found to have abnormal serum epinephrine levels.[28] The rationale for investigating β-blocker intervention is based on the personality trait surveys[28, 32] and the intravenous epinephrine–induced animal CSC models[58–64] discussed previously.

Acetazolamide has also been suggested as possibly beneficial for patients with CSC. This drug may be able to cause earlier resolution of the detachment either by increasing the RPE pump or perhaps by altering choroidal hemodyamics.[80]

Laser Photocoagulation Treatment

There has been great controversy in the literature regarding the use of laser photocoagulation for CSC patients.

In a prospective study of 34 untreated CSC cases, Klein and associates[21] reported that all cases resolved and that 94 percent of the eyes had visual acuity of 20/30 or better at follow-up examination (average, 23 mos).

Laser photocoagulation to the leakage site also has been suggested for CSC patients. In 1967, Gass[11] described five treated cases and stated that the use of laser photocoagulation was encouraging. In 1974, Watzke and associates[81] showed that ruby laser photocoagulation could shorten the duration of disease by 2 mo but that it had no effect on final visual acuity or recurrence rate. Spitznas[31] reported on a nonrandomized study of 139 untreated and 109 xenon arc–treated cases of CSC. Treatment was applied in either a direct (to the leakage point) or an indirect (the detachment's edge was treated but not the leakage point) fashion. The final visual acuity (median 20/25) was identical in all three groups. The duration of CSC was 80 days in the untreated group and only 10 days in both treated groups. Recurrences were noted in 45 percent of untreated patients, 38 percent of indirectly coagulated patients, and only 8.8 percent of directly treated patients. He concluded that directly treated patients had a shortened duration of disease and a recurrence rate that was five times lower. He suggested that the xenon arc's large spot size destroys not only the abnormal hypersecreting RPE cells but also the neighboring RPE cells that could be responsible for future recurrences. Robertson and Ilstrup,[82] in a prospective randomized trial of argon laser photocoagulation, concluded that direct treatment shortened the duration of the disease by 2 mo. Gilbert and coworkers[25] did not find a difference in final visual acuity or recurrence rate in argon laser–treated and untreated patients in their series.

Indirect treatment has also been advocated for CSC patients. However, Robertson and Ilstrup,[82] in a prospective randomized trial of argon laser photocoagulation, concluded that indirect treatment is ineffective. Watzke and colleagues[83] also showed that indirect argon laser treatment was inferior to direct treatment. Finally, in the study of Spitznas,[31] the duration of disease was less in indirectly treated patients than in untreated individuals, but the recurrence rate was lower only for directly treated patients.

The xenon arc, ruby laser, and argon laser have all been used to treat CSC. Slusher[84] showed that krypton laser photocoagulation may be beneficial and suggests that this wavelength may be more tissue-selective.

The consensus from the preceding studies and others is that direct laser treatment to the leakage site shortens the course of disease[81–88] but does not affect the final visual acuity or recurrence rate.[21, 25, 34]

When should one treat CSC with laser photocoagulation? First, it should be understood by the physician and patient that treatment only shortens the duration of the disease and does not affect the final visual acuity or recurrence rate. Therefore, photocoagulation should be performed only for occupational reasons or when the well-informed patient prefers treatment to shorten the duration of the disease. Second, the leakage point must be well defined. When it is unclear if a patient has CSC or choroidal neovascularization, follow-up and repetition of fluorescein angiography every 2 to 3 wk is advisable.[85] Choroidal neovascularization may become more apparent with time. In addition, the leakage point should be at least 500 μ from the center of the foveal avascular zone; if it is not, treatment probably should not be performed.

Several authors[12, 85] provide guidelines for treatment. Laser photocoagulation should be performed to the leakage site with low-intensity energy. We suggest using three to five 100 to 200 micron–sized spots of 0.1 or 0.2 sec duration, with low (100 to 200 mW) energy. Spot sizes less than 100 μ should be avoided because of the risk of choroidal neovascularization.[85] Treatment should produce a minimal white color change, unlike the heavy treatment used to photocoagulate choroidal neovascularization. Careful follow-up of these patients for recurrences or laser-induced complications is essential.

Laser photocoagulation is not a benign procedure. Besides the potential for foveal damage, laser treatment for CSC may also cause traction lines and iatrogenic choroidal neovascularization. Schatz and coworkers[89] described 27 cases of choroidal neovascularization following laser photocoagulation. These authors state that some of the choroidal neovascularization was iatrogenically produced, whereas some cases may have been choroidal neovascularization masquerading as CSC. Gass[34] states that 2 to 5 percent of treated patients will acquire choroidal neovascularization. However, choroidal neovascularization complications have not been reported in other large series of treated CSC cases.[25, 31]

REFERENCES

1. von Graefe A: Ueber centrale recidivierende Retinitis. Graefes Arch Clin Exp Ophthalmol 12:211–215, 1866.
2. Fuchs E: Ein Fall zentraler, Rezidivierender Syphilitischer Netzhaut-entzundung. Centralbl f Prakt Augenh 40:105–108, 1916.
3. Horniker E: Su di una forma retinite centrale di origine vasoneurotica (retinite central capillaro-spastica). Ann Ottal 55:578–600, 1927.
4. Walsh FB, Sloan LL: Idiopathic flat detachment of the macula. Am J Ophthalmol 19:195–228, 1936.
5. Gifford SR, Marquardt G: Central angiospastic retinopathy. Arch Ophthalmol 21:211–228, 1939.
6. Klien BA: Macular lesions of vascular origin. II. Functional vascular conditions leading to damage of the macula lutea. Am J Ophthalmol 36:1–13, 1953.
7. Bennett G: Central serous retinopathy. Br J Ophthalmol 39:605–618, 1955.
8. Maumenee AE: Serous and hemorrhagic disciform detachment of the macula. Trans Pacific Coast Oto-Ophthalmol Soc 40:139–160, 1959.
9. Yannuzzi LA, Shakin J, Fisher Y, et al: Peripheral retinal detachment and retinal pigment epithelial atrophic tracts secondary to central serous pigment epitheliopathy. Ophthalmology 91:1554–1572, 1984.
10. Maumenee AE: Symposium: Macular diseases, clinical manifestations. Trans Am Acad Ophthalmol Otolaryngol 69:605–613, 1965.
11. Gass JDM: Pathogenesis of disciform detachment of the neuroepithelium. II. Idiopathic central serous choroidopathy. Am J Ophthalmol 63:587–615, 1967.
12. Gass JDM: Stereoscopic Atlas of Macular Diseases. St. Louis, CV Mosby, 1987, pp 46–59.
13. Gragoudas ES: Unpublished data.
14. Burton TC: Central serous retinopathy. In Blodi FC (ed): Current Concepts in Ophthalmology, vol 3. St Louis, CV Mosby, 1972, pp 1–28.
15. Edwards TS, Priestley BS: Central angiospastic retinopathy. Am J Ophthalmol 57:988–996, 1964.
16. Gass JD, Norton EWD, Justice J: Serous detachment of the retinal pigment epithelium. Trans Am Acad Ophthalmol Otolaryngol 70:990–1015, 1966.
17. Gass JDM: Bullous retinal detachment: An unusual manifestation of idiopathic central serous choroidopathy. Am J Ophthalmol 75:810–821, 1973.
18. Klein BA: Symposium: Macular diseases, clinical manifestations. I. Central serous retinopathy and chorioretinopathy. Trans Am Acad Ophthalmol Otolaryngol 69:614–620, 1965.
19. Mitsui Y, Sakanishi R: Central angiospastic retinopathy. Am J Ophthalmol 41:105–114, 1956.
20. Straatsma BR, Allen RA, Pettit TH: Central serous retinopathy. Trans Pacific Coast Oto-Ophthalmol Soc 47:107–127, 1966.
21. Klein ML, van Buskirk EM, Friedman E, et al: Experience with nontreatment of central serous choroidopathy. Arch Ophthalmol 91:247–250, 1974.
22. Fine SL, Owens SL: Central serous retinopathy in a 7-year-old girl. Am J Ophthalmol 90:871–873, 1980.
23. Fine SL: Personal communication, 1989.
24. Cohen D, Gaudric A, Coscas G, et al: Epitheliopathie retinienne diffuse et chorioretinopathie sereuse centrale, J Fr Ophthalmol 6:339–349, 1983.
25. Gilbert CM, Owens SL, Smith PD, Fine SL: Long-term follow-up of central serous chorioretinopathy. Br J Ophthalmol 68:815–820, 1984.
26. Spitznas M: Central serous chorioretinopathy. Ophthalmology 87(8S):88, 1980.
27. Wessing A: Grundsatzliches zum diagnostoschen Fortschritt durch die Fluoreszenzangiographie. Ber Dtsch Ophthalmol Ges 73:566–568, 1973.
28. Yannuzzi LA: Type A behavior and central serous chorioretinopathy. Trans Am Ophthalmol Soc 84:799–845, 1986.
29. Hirose I: Therapy of central serous retinopathy. Folia Ophthalmol Jpn 20:1003–1034, 1969.
30. Fukunaga K: Central chorioretinopathy with disharmony of the autonomic nervous system. Acta Soc Ophthalmol Jpn 73:1468–1477, 1969.
31. Spitznas M: Central serous retinopathy. In Ryan SJ (ed): Retina. St Louis, CV Mosby, 1989, pp 217–227.
32. Werry H, Arends C: Untersuchung zur Objektivierung von Personlichkeitsmerkmalen bei Patienten mit Retinopathia centralis serosa. Klin Monatsbl Augenheilkd 172:363–370, 1978.
33. Levine R, Brucker AJ, Robinson F: Long-term follow-up of idiopathic central serous chorioretinopathy by fluorescein angiography. Ophthalmology 96:854–859, 1989.
34. Gass JDM: Photocoagulation treatment of idiopathic central serous choroidopathy. Trans Am Acad Ophthalmol Otolaryngol 83:456–463, 1977.
35. Mazzuca DE, Benson WE: Central serous retinopathy: Variants. Surv Ophthalmol 31:170–174, 1986.
36. Benson WE, Shields JA, Annesley WH, Tasman W: Central

serous chorioretinopathy with bullous retinal detachment. Ann Ophthalmol 12:920–924, 1980.

37. Shimizu K, Tobari I: Central serous retinopathy dynamics of subretinal fluid. Mod Probl Ophthalmol 9:152–157, 1971.

38. Spitznas M, Huke J: Number, shape, and topography of leakage points in acute type I central serous retinopathy. Graefes Arch Clin Exp Ophthalmol 225:437–440, 1987.

39. Bonamour G, Bonnet M, Grange JD, et al: Topographische Studien uber angiographisch beobachtete Lasionen bei Retinitis centralis serosa. Klin Monatsbl Augenheikd 171:862–866, 1977.

40. Friberg TR, Campagna J: Central serous chorioretinopathy: An analysis of the clinical morphology using image-processing techniques. Graefes Arch Ophthalmol 227:201–205, 1989.

41. Folk JC, Thompson HS, Han DP, Brown CK: Visual function abnormalities in central serous retinopathy. Arch Ophthalmol 102:1299–1302, 1984.

42. Tsuneoka H, Kabayama T, Fukada J, Narazaki S: Night visual acuity in patients with idiopathic central serous choroidopathy. Jpn J Ophthalmol 24:178–187, 1980.

43. Piccolino FC: Central serous retinopathy: Some considerations on the pathogenesis. Ophthalmologica 182:204–210, 1981.

44. Marmor MF: Control of subretinal fluid: Experimental and clinical studies. Eye 4:340–344, 1990.

45. Nadel AJ, Turan MI, Coles RS: Central serous retinopathy: A generalized disease of the pigment epithelium. Mod Probl Ophthalmol 20:76–88, 1979.

46. Negi A, Marmor MF: Experimental serous retinal detachment and focal pigment epithelium damage. Arch Ophthalmol 102:445–449, 1984.

47. Spitznas M: Pathogenesis of central serous retinopathy: A new working hypothesis. Graefes Arch Clin Exp Ophthalmol 224:321–324, 1986.

48. Kitahara S: Ueber klinische Beobachtungen bei der in Japan haufig vorkommenden Chorioretinitis centralsi serosa. Klin Monatsbl Augenheilkd 97:345–362, 1936.

49. Duke-Elder WS: System of Ophthalmology: Diseases of the Retina, vol 10. St. Louis, CV Mosby, 1967, pp 121–137.

50. Tolentinto FI, Freeman HM, Schepens CC: Vitreoretinal traction in serous and hemorrhagic macular retinopathy. Arch Ophthalmol 78:23–20, 1967.

51. Bettman JW: Allergic retinosis. Am J Ophthalmol 28:1323–1328, 1945.

52. Berens S, Sayad WY, Girard LJ: Symposium on ocular allergy. The uveal tract and retina: Consideration of certain experimental and clinical concepts. Trans Am Acad Ophthalmol Otolaryngol 56:220–241, 1952.

53. Redman SI: A review of solar retinitis as it may pertain to macular lesions seen in persons of the armed forces. Am J Ophthalmol 28:1155–1165, 1945.

54. Sie-Boen-Lian: The etiologic agent of serous central chorioretinitis. Ophthalmologica 148:263–270, 1964.

55. Henry F: Angiospastic retinopathy. Am J Ophthalmol 35:1509–1510, 1952.

56. Klien BA: Macular and extramacular serous chorioretinopathy. Am J Ophthalmol 51:231–242, 1961.

57. Lipowski ZJ, Kiriakos RZ: Psychosomatic aspects of central serous retinopathy: A review and case report. Psychosomatics 12:398–401, 1971.

58. Ikeda I, Komi T, Nakaji K, et al: Chorioretinitis central serous. Acta Soc Ophthalmol Jpn 60:1261–1266, 1956.

59. Nagayoski K: Experimental study of chorioretinopathy by intravenous injection of adrenaline. Acta Soc Ophthalmol Jpn 75:1720–1727, 1971.

60. Miki T, Sunada I, Higaki T: Studies on chorioretinitis induced in rabbits by stress (repeated administration of epinephrine). Acta Soc Ophthalmol Jpn 75:1037–1045, 1972.

61. Yasuzumi T, Miki T, Sugimoto K: Electron microscopic studies of epinephrine choroiditis in rabbits. I. Pigment epithelium and Bruch's membrane in the healed stage. Acta Soc Ophthalmol Jpn 78:588–598, 1974.

62. Yoshioka H, Sugita T, Nagayoski K: Fluorescein angiography findings in experimental retinopathy produced by intravenous adrenaline injection. Folia Ophthalmol Jpn 21:648–652, 1970.

63. Yoshioka H, Katsume Y, Akune H: Experimental central serous chorioretinopathy in monkey eyes. II. Fluorescein angiographic findings. Ophthalmologica 185:168–178, 1982.

64. Yoshioka H, Katsume Y: Experimental central serous chorioretinopathy. III. Ultrastructural findings. Jpn J Ophthalmol 26:397–409, 1982.

65. Bedrossian RH: Central serous retinopathy and pregnancy. Am J Ophthalmol 78:152, 1974.

66. Chumbley LC, Frank RN: Central serous retinopathy and pregnancy. Am J Ophthalmol 77:158–160, 1974.

67. Cruysberg JRM, Deutman AF: Visual disturbances during pregnancy caused by central serous choroidopathy. Br J Ophthalmol 66:240–241, 1982.

68. Fastenberg DM, Ober RR: Central serous choroidopathy in pregnancy. Arch Ophthalmol 101:1055–1058, 1983.

69. Friberg TR, Eller AW: Serous retinal detachment resembling central serous chorioretinopathy following organ transplantation. Graefes Arch Clin Exp Ophthalmol 228:305–309, 1990.

70. Gragoudas ES: Unpublished data.

71. Kazuhiko H, Hasegawa Y, Tokoro T: Indocyanine green angiography of central serous chorioretinopathy. Int Ophthalmol 9:37–41, 1986.

72. Nagata M, Honda Y: Macular ERG in central serous retinopathy. Jpn J Ophthalmol 15:9–16, 1971.

73. Miyake Y, Shiroyama N, Ota I, Horiguchi M: Local macular electroretinographic responses in idiopathic central serous chorioretinopathy. Am J Ophthalmol 106:546–550, 1988.

74. van Meel GJ, Smith VC, Pokorny J, van Norren D: Foveal densitometry in central serous choroidopathy. Am J Ophthalmol 98:359–368, 1984.

75. Chuang EL, Sharp DM, Fitzke FW, et al: Retinal dysfunction in central serous retinopathy. Eye 1:120–125, 1987.

76. Fry WE, Spaeth EB: Subacute circumscribed macular retinochoroiditis simulating intraocular tumor. Trans Am Acad Ophthalmol 59:346–355, 1955.

77. Ikui H: Histopathological examination of central serous retinopathy. Folia Ophthalmol Jpn 20:1035–1043, 1969.

78. de Venecia G: Fluorescein angiographic smoke stack. Case presentation at Verhoeff Society Meeting. Washington DC, April 24–25, 1982.

79. Ambler JS, Zagarra H, Myers SM: Chronic macular detachment following pneumatic retinopexy. Retina 10:125–130, 1990.

80. Cox SN, Hay E, Bird AC: Treatment of chronic macular edema with acetazolamide. Arch Ophthalmol 106:1190–1195, 1988.

81. Watzke RC, Burton TC, Leverton PE: Ruby laser photocoagulation therapy of central serous retinopathy. I. A controlled clinical trial. II. Factors affecting prognosis. Trans Am Acad Ophthalmol Otolaryngol 78:205–211, 1974.

82. Robertson DM, Ilstrup D: Direct, indirect, and sham laser photocoagulation in the management of central serous chorioretinopathy. Am J Ophthalmol 95:457–466, 1983.

83. Watzke RC, Burton TC, Woolson RF: Direct and indirect laser photocoagulation of central serous choroidopathy. Am J Ophthalmol 88:914–918, 1979.

84. Slusher MM: Krypton red laser photocoagulation in selected cases of central serous chorioretinopathy. Retina 6:81–84, 1986.

85. Robertson DM: Argon laser photocoagulation treatment in central serous chorioretinopathy. Ophthalmology 93:972–974, 1986.

86. Landers MB III, Shaw HE Jr, Anderson WB Jr, Sinyai AJ: Argon laser treatment of central serous chorioretinopathy. Ann Ophthalmol 9:1567–1572, 1977.

87. Leaver P, Williams C: Argon laser photocoagulation in the treatment of central serous chorioretinopathy. Br J Ophthalmol 63:674–677, 1979.

88. Theodossiadis G, Tongos D: Treatment of central serous chorioretinopathy: A comparative study with and without light coagulation. Ophthalmologica 169:416–431, 1974.

89. Schatz H, Yannuzzi LA, Gitter KA: Subretinal neovascularization following argon laser photocoagulation treatment for central serous chorioretinopathy: Complication or misdiagnosis? Trans Am Acad Ophthalmol Otoloaryngol 83:OP893–906, 1977.

Chapter 64

Age-related Macular Degeneration: Drusen and Geographic Atrophy

SUSAN B. BRESSLER, NEIL M. BRESSLER, and
EVANGELOS S. GRAGOUDAS

Age-related macular degeneration (AMD) may be classified into a neovascular (exudative) form (discussed in Chapter 65) and a nonneovascular (nonexudative) form. The nonneovascular form features drusen and abnormalities of the retinal pigment epithelium (RPE), such as geographic atrophy, nongeographic areas of atrophy, and focal areas of hyperpigmentation within the macula. The clinical features, clinicopathologic correlation, differential diagnosis, natural course, and treatment of the nonneovascular form of AMD are reviewed in this chapter. (The epidemiology of AMD is discussed in *Principles and Practice of Ophthalmology: Basic Sciences,* Chap. 109.)

CLINICAL FEATURES AND CLINICOPATHOLOGIC CORRELATION

Drusen

Multiple small, yellow-white lesions at the level of the RPE within the macula, commonly found in patients older than 50 yr, are called *drusen*. The term *drusen* is derived from the German word *druse,* which means gland, indicating that these yellow-white deposits reminded early investigators of glandular structures.[1]

The relationship of drusen to AMD is somewhat confusing because there are several types of yellow-white lesions that may be seen at the level of the RPE within the macula. These lesions may be conveniently categorized into (1) small, hard drusen; (2) large, soft drusen; and (3) cuticular (basal laminar) drusen. Large, soft drusen are the form of drusen most commonly considered to be a feature of AMD.

Small, Hard Drusen (Fig. 64–1). Small drusen have been defined in most studies as being less than 50 μ in length[2, 3] or less than 63 μ in diameter.[4] The borders of small drusen are almost always[2, 3] distinct and well defined, contributing to the designation of hard drusen. Small, hard drusen are not believed to be a feature of AMD for the following reasons: (1) the presence of at least one small druse in the macula is nearly ubiquitous on fundus photographs[2] and postmortem examination[5] in individuals older than 40 yr; (2) the presence of small, hard drusen is not age-related;[2] (3) their presence is not associated with an increased risk of the development of

the neovascular form of AMD when compared with large, soft drusen;[3] and (4) clinicopathologic correlation demonstrates that these small lesions represent either a lipidization of a few RPE cells[6] or a *localized* accumulation (nodule) of hyaline material in the inner and outer collagenous zones of Bruch's membrane,[7] which can be totally normal on either side of this nodule. The presence of these localized accumulations in an otherwise normal Bruch's membrane makes it unlikely that these small, hard drusen are a feature of a diffusely dysfunctioning RPE–Bruch's membrane–choriocapillaris complex.

Large, Soft Drusen. Large drusen have been defined in most studies as greater than or equal to 63 μ in diameter.[4] The borders of large drusen may be poorly demarcated, without sharp edges,[2, 4] contributing to the designation of *soft* drusen (Fig. 64–2). Histologically, these large, soft drusen correspond to either (1) diffuse thickening of the inner aspect of Bruch's membrane in which overlying areas of hypopigmentation of the RPE correspond to the drusen seen clinically or (2) amorphous material located between a detached, thickened inner aspect of Bruch's membrane and the remainder of Bruch's membrane (Fig. 64–2*B*). Clinically, one cannot

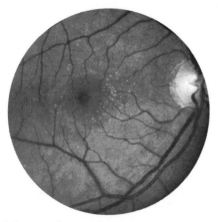

Figure 64–1. Hard drusen usually appear clinically as small yellow punctate lesions at the level of the retinal pigment epithelium (RPE) with sharp discrete borders. These changes have been shown to correspond to lipoid degeneration of a few discrete retinal pigment epithelial cells without evidence of diffuse thickening of the inner aspect of Bruch's membrane throughout the macula.

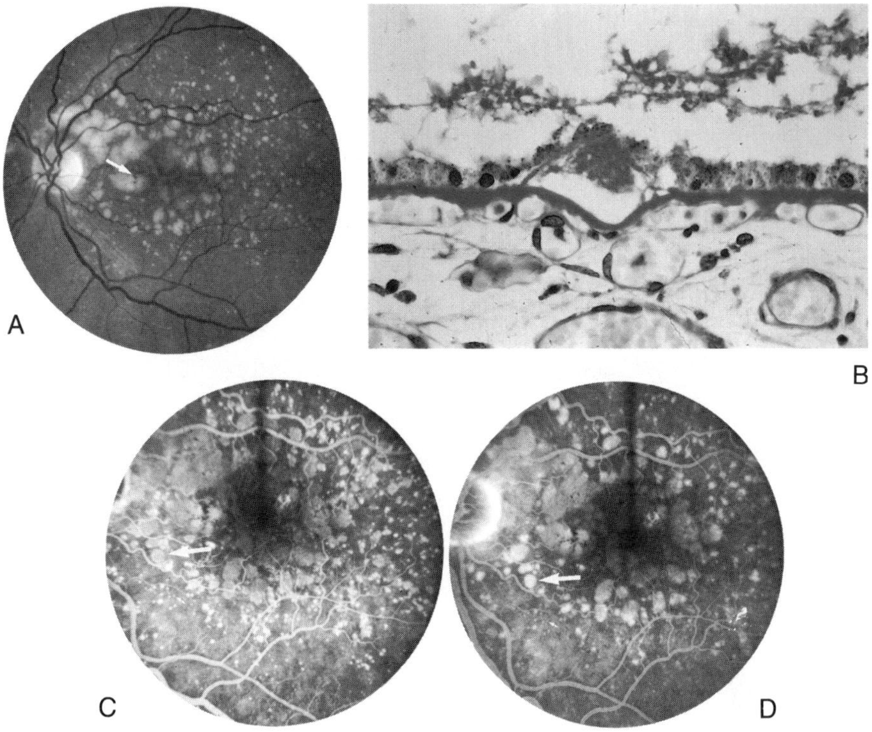

Figure 64–2. Soft drusen are seen clinically as large yellow lesions with amorphous, ill-defined borders (arrow) at the level of the RPE (A). It is suspected that the soft drusen noted clinically usually correspond to areas of diffuse thickening of the inner aspect of Bruch's membrane at the point at which focal areas of RPE hypopigmentation have developed in areas overlying this diffuse thickening or at the point at which fracturing of the diffusely thickened inner aspect of Bruch's membrane has separated from the remaining outer aspect of Bruch's membrane (B). It is suspected that drusen may stain more intensely (arrow) in the late phases of the angiogram (C and D) when this fracturing is present, presumably because the fluorescein molecules collect between the detached inner aspect and the remainder of Bruch's membrane.

detect the diffuse thickening of the inner aspect of Bruch's membrane; however, when there are areas of RPE hypopigmentation overlying this diffusely thickened Bruch's membrane or when this diffuse thickening weakens the inner aspect of Bruch's membrane and predisposes it to separation, or both, one recognizes these areas clinically as soft drusen.

The term *soft drusen* for *clinical* descriptive purposes[2] is slightly different from the term *soft drusen* for *pathologic* descriptions.[7] Pathologically, soft drusen refers to amorphous material located between a thickened, detached inner aspect of Bruch's membrane and the remainder of this membrane (see Fig. 64–2B). Thus, not all drusen identified as soft clinically correspond to soft drusen pathologically. On clinical examination, some of these soft drusen will correspond only to areas of hypopigmented RPE overlying a diffusely thickened aspect of Bruch's membrane, whereas other soft drusen will correspond to soft drusen pathologically, with detachment of a diffusely thickened inner aspect of Bruch's membrane (see Fig. 64–2B).

Clinically, soft drusen are believed to be an early feature of AMD for the following reasons: (1) the presence of soft drusen is age-related;[2] (2) their presence is associated with an increased risk of the development of the neovascular form of AMD when compared with small, hard drusen;[3] (3) clinicopathologic correlation demonstrates that the presence of soft drusen represents *diffuse* thickening of the inner aspect of Bruch's membrane throughout the macula;[7, 8] and (4) with the neovascular form of AMD (see Chap. 65), pathologic features, including choroidal neovascularization or disciform scarring are usually noted in eyes that also have diffuse thickening of the inner aspect of Bruch's membrane throughout the macular region.[7–10]

On angiography, staining of drusen (see Fig. 64–2D) may be noted in areas in which overlying RPE hypopigmentation allows increased visualization of choroidal fluorescence and/or in areas in which fracturing of this diffuse thickening provides a space for fluorescein molecules to pool (see Fig. 64–2B). Some investigators have suggested that the hydrophobic or hydrophilic properties of drusen, determined by their lipid composition, may account for hypo- or hyperfluorescence, respectively.[11] However, this latter theory does not as yet have direct fluoroangiographic-pathologic correlation.

Abnormalities of the RPE

The development of diffuse thickening of the inner aspect of Bruch's membrane associated with the clinical recognition of soft drusen also may be accompanied by abnormalities of the RPE. These abnormalities include geographic atrophy of the RPE, nongeographic atrophy of the RPE, focal hyperpigmentation, and dystrophic calcification of Bruch's membrane.

Geographic Atrophy of the RPE. Geographic atrophy of the RPE (also called areolar atrophy) consists of one to several areas of well-demarcated depigmentation in which the underlying larger choroidal vessels may be seen and the overlying sensory retina may appear thinned (Fig. 64–3A). Clinically, two patterns have been suggested to lead to geographic atrophy in eyes that are presumed to have AMD. In one scenario, areas of large, soft, confluent drusen progress to geographic atrophy in multifocal areas corresponding to the location of the large, confluent drusen. In the second scenario, the central macula contains tiny areas of reticulated hypo-

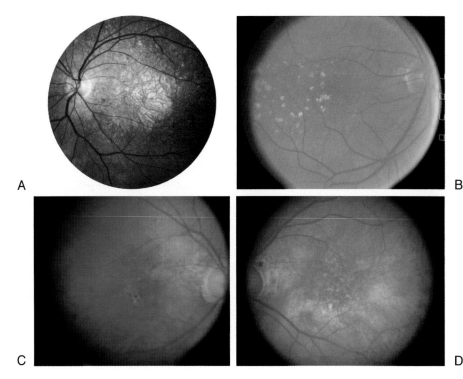

A

B

C

D

Figure 64–3. Abnormalities of the RPE secondary to age-related macular degeneration. *A,* An area of geographic atrophy, with well-demarcated loss of pigmentation of the RPE and overlying thinning of the sensory retina with more apparent underlying choroidal vasculature. *B,* Calcified drusen that correspond histologically to dystrophic calcification at the level of the outer retina. *C,* Focal hyperpigmentation or pigment clumps correspond to clumps of pigment at the level of the RPE or within the outer aspects of the sensory retina. *D,* Nongeographic atrophy refers to a finding of tiny mottled areas of hypo- and hyperpigmentation that may show some thinning of the overlying sensory retina.

and hyperpigmentation, which progress to one large area of geographic atrophy that spreads fairly contiguously in a horseshoe pattern around the fovea, eventually completely surrounding it (lending to a bull's-eye maculopathy). Only after many years, does it finally spread to include the fovea within the area of geographic atrophy. Clinicopathologic correlation of these changes has shown replacement of soft drusen with fibrous tissue or dystrophic calcification.[12] The RPE overlying these areas ultimately disappears, producing small areas of geographic atrophy. The underlying choriocapillaris may be sclerosed, with thickening of the intercapillary septae.[7] The areas of geographic atrophy are usually accompanied by loss of overlying photoreceptors, accounting for the visual loss that is noted when the geographic atrophy extends through the center of the macula. Dystrophic calcification may accompany geographic atrophy and appears clinically as glistening bright yellow specks within drusen that are undergoing atrophy (Fig. 64–3*B*), contributing to the term *calcified drusen.*[7]

Angiography of geographic atrophy demonstrates early hyperfluorescence of atrophic areas, presumably resulting from increased transmission of choroidal fluorescence because of hypopigmentation, attenuation, or lack of RPE. In the late frames, persistent staining of the areas of geographic atrophy will be noted, probably because of increased visibility of the fluorescein staining of the choroidal and scleral tissue through the atrophic RPE.

Focal Hyperpigmentation. Focal hyperpigmentation of the RPE consists of areas of increased pigmentation at the level of the outer retina (Fig. 64–3*C*). Clinical studies have shown that focal clumps of hyperpigmentation identified on color fundus photographs are asso-

ciated with an increased risk of the development of choroidal neovascularization.[3, 13] Some investigators have hypothesized that areas of focal hyperpigmentation on color fundus photographs may be associated with an increased risk of choroidal neovascularization because the areas of hyperpigmentation represent disturbances of the RPE overlying occult choroidal neovascularization.[14] However, clinicopathologic correlation has shown that these areas can correlate with areas of intraretinal pigment migration to the level of the photoreceptor nuclei with no evidence of choroidal neovascularization.[7]

Nongeographic Atrophy. Nongeographic atrophy consists of areas of stippled, punctate hypopigmentation in which the underlying choroidal vessels are not more readily apparent than in areas without nongeographic atrophy, but in which the overlying sensory retina appears to be thinned on stereoscopic examination (Fig. 64–3*D*).[2] Nongeographic atrophy has been reported to identify a subgroup of patients who are at an increased risk of the development of recurrent choroidal neovascularization following previously successful laser treatment.[4] Clinicopathologic correlation (unpublished data) depicted on color fundus photography has shown that these areas appear to correlate to mottled areas of relative hypopigmentation of the RPE overlying a diffusely thickened inner aspect of Bruch's membrane. These areas are similar to the pathologic correlate of large, soft drusen identified clinically, except the areas of nongeographic atrophy have minute foci of hypopigmentation often interspersed with clumps of hyperpigmentation, whereas clinically apparent soft drusen have broader areas of RPE hypopigmentation, but often do not have clumps of hyperpigmentation within the drusen.

DIFFERENTIAL DIAGNOSIS

A variety of maculopathies might be confused with the nonneovascular features of AMD and they should be differentiated from drusen or abnormalities of the RPE. These other conditions often have a different prognosis from the nonneovascular features of AMD. A variety of factors, including demographics, morphologic features, and distribution of the fundus and angiographic changes, will help to differentiate these conditions from AMD.

Cuticular (Basal Laminar) Drusen. Innumerable small, uniformly sized, discretely round, slightly raised, yellow subretinal lesions (Fig. 64–4A) that are best seen with angiography (Fig. 64–4B) and usually present in middle-age (40s to 60s) are called *cuticular (basal laminar) drusen.*[15-17] They may be differentiated from more typical soft drusen in that retroillumination biomicroscopically demonstrates semitranslucency of innumerable similar-sized basal laminar drusen, as opposed to variably sized, more typical soft drusen that appear opaquely yellow and are not semitranslucent. On angiography, cuticular drusen will demonstrate early, bright, uniform hyperfluorescence compared with the variable, less bright hyperfluorescence of more typical soft drusen and the lack of bright hyperfluorescence of small, hard drusen.

The term *basal laminar drusen* should not be confused with the term *basal laminar deposits*, which refers to the wide-spaced collagen located between the plasma membrane and the basement membrane of the RPE, or the term *basal linear deposits*, which refers to the granular, electron-dense, lipid-rich material seen ultrastructurally *external* to the basement membrane of the RPE. In fact, the term *basal linear deposits* corresponds to the diffuse thickening of the inner aspect of Bruch's membrane, which was described previously as *diffuse drusen*. Clinicopathologic correlation has shown that cuticular drusen consist of an extremely thick inner aspect of Bruch's membrane with overlying nodular excrescences, all beneath the RPE. Since no cuticle exists, and to avoid the use of the confusing terms *basal laminar* and *basal linear* deposits, it has been proposed that the clinical features depicted in Figure 64–4 be called *diffuse drusen with overlying nodular excrescences* to more accurately describe what they are.

Patients with this unusual form of drusen may experience pseudovitelliform detachments consisting of yellowish material at the level of the outer retina. The material appears to obscure details of the RPE, suggesting that it is present between the sensory retina and the RPE. On angiography, these detachments show early hypofluorescence (see Fig. 64–4B), presumably because of the ability of the yellowish material to block the underlying fluorescence of the choriocapillaris. Progressive staining of the yellowish material becomes apparent in the middle- and late-transit phases of the angiogram (see Fig. 64–4C), presumably because of the incompetence of the RPE's zonula occludens, which fails to keep fluorescein from diffusing from the choriocapillaris to the subsensory retinal space, with subsequent staining of the yellowish material.

Since this hyperfluorescence may mimic choroidal neovascularization, one must recognize its appearance in order to avoid unnecessary photocoagulation of a pseudovitelliform detachment. The natural course of these detachments can be spontaneous clearing (see Fig. 64–4D) with extremely slow development of atrophy or clearing associated with marked geographic atrophy.

These pseudovitelliform detachments should be differentiated from true vitelliform detachments seen in Best's disease (in which the electrooculogram will be

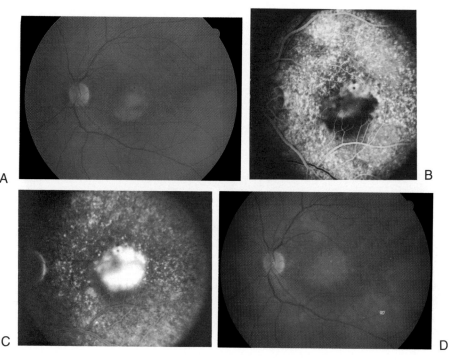

Figure 64–4. Basal laminar or cuticular drusen. *A,* Color photograph showing innumerable small, uniformly sized, discretely round, and slightly raised yellow subretinal lesions and dull yellow material in the central macula referred to as a *pseudovitelliform detachment. B,* Angiogram helps highlight basal laminar drusen. In addition, hypofluorescence, presumably from the associated pseudovitelliform detachment, blocks the underlying fluorescence of the choriocapillaris. *C,* Progressive staining of the pseudovitelliform detachment material becomes apparent in the middle- and late-transit phases of the angiogram. *D,* With time, the pseudovitelliform detachment can clear spontaneously. Geographic atrophy will sometimes develop with clearing.

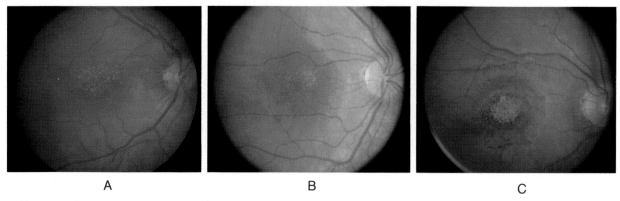

A   B   C

Figure 64–5. Dominant drusen. A, A young woman in her 20s demonstrates typical large drusen, some of which have discrete boundaries. Similar findings are noted in her 9-year-old son (B) and her 6-year-old son (C).

abnormal) and from pattern dystrophies of the RPE that may show pseudovitelliform-like detachments (see further on).

Patients with basal laminar or cuticular drusen have a diseased Bruch's membrane and are at risk of the development of choroidal neovascularization. Therefore, careful scrutiny of any bright hyperfluorescence that appears to leak in these patients must determine whether the features are due to the presence of choroidal neovascularization or progressive staining of the pseudovitelliform detachment. Sometimes this differentiation is extremely difficult to make.

Dominant Drusen in Young Individuals. Patients in their teens or 20s may present with large (greater than 63 μ), discrete nodular drusen, often in a very symmetric distribution (such as temporal to the fovea or nasal to the optic nerve). Even children of these patients who are less than 10 yr may have discrete drusen (Fig. 64–5). In the experience of the authors, these patients may go years without choroidal neovascularization or atrophy developing and therefore suffer no significant visual loss. When these lesions are in the macula, they could presumably cause focal disturbances of Bruch's membrane and may increase the risk of the development of choroidal neovascularization.

Pattern Dystrophy of the RPE (Adult Vitelliform, Adult-onset Foveal Pigment Epithelial Dystrophy, Butterfly-shaped Pigment Dystrophy, Reticular Dystrophy of the Pigment Epithelium). Patients with pattern dystrophy of the RPE will show a reticulated pattern of pigmentation, usually fairly symmetric between the two eyes and often without the presence of more typical soft drusen (Fig. 64–6).[18] These dystrophies may have a yellowish deposition at the level of the outer retina, often with a central area of greenish hyperpigmentation (sometimes best seen with transillumination of the yellowish material) and occasionally surrounded by a petaloid pattern of hyperpigmentation, which is more obvious on angiography (Fig. 64–6B).

Clinicopathologic correlation of pattern dystrophies of the RPE has shown a thick layer of slightly granular, eosinophilic, PAS-positive material lying between a thinned atrophic RPE and Bruch's membrane, with central pigment clumping from large pigment-laden cells and extracellular melanin pigment lying between the sensory retina and Bruch's membrane.[19] These lesions have been observed both within families and sporadically. Although they are often located in the center of the macula, they may present eccentrically (Fig. 64–7), accounting for the variety of appearances on presentation. The pseudovitelliform detachments will not show disruption or layering of the yellow pigment dependently, as is seen in the vitelliform lesions of Best's disease. The disturbance of Bruch's membrane histologically presumably places these patients at increased risk of the development of choroidal neovascularization through breaks in the outer aspect of Bruch's membrane.

Bull's-eye Maculopathy. A variety of conditions may produce a bull's-eye maculopathy (usually referring to

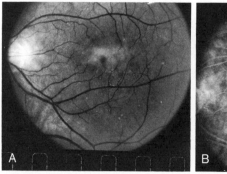
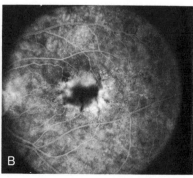

Figure 64–6. Pattern dystrophy of the RPE. A, Typical pattern dystrophy in which blocked fluorescence on angiography corresponds to pigment clumping or greenish discoloration seen at the level of the RPE, surrounded by hyperfluorescence corresponding to dull yellowish material that has sometimes been termed a *pseudovitelliform detachment.* B, The angiogram highlights not only the blocked fluorescence but also very prominent staining with persistent bright hyperfluorescence in the late phase of the angiogram, but no leakage. The absence of leakage helps confirm the absence of choroidal neovascularization.

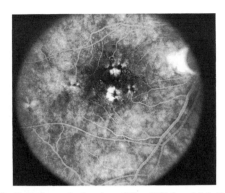

Figure 64–7. Pattern dystrophy of the RPE in which the blocked fluorescence and hyperfluorescence occur in a multifocal distribution outside of the foveal center.

an area of central pigmentation of the retina surrounded circumferentially by an area of relative hypopigmentation and sometimes surrounded once again circumferentially by an area of increased pigmentation). This condition may progress to geographic atrophy of the RPE, which typically is similar to the geographic atrophy seen in AMD.[20] These conditions usually can be differentiated from geographic atrophy associated with AMD. The bull's-eye maculopathies result in a central area of geographic atrophy with no associated soft drusen, whereas geographic atrophy in AMD is usually multifocal, with preservation of the fovea until the very late stages. In addition, the bull's-eye maculopathies occur in early or midlife, whereas geographic atrophy is seen most often in patients in their late 70s and 80s, with increasing prevalence into the 90s. The causes of some of these maculopathies include central areolar choroidal–RPE dystrophy, the Bardet-Biedl syndrome, concentric annular macular dystrophy, chloroquine retinopathy, cone dystrophy, fenestrated sheen macular dystrophy, the Hallervorden-Spatz syndrome, and fundus flavimaculatus.

NATURAL COURSE

Drusen

The natural course of an eye with drusen depends on whether the fellow eye has drusen with no evidence of neovascular AMD or whether the eye with drusen is the fellow eye of a patient whose other eye has already developed the neovascular form of AMD.

The most accurate information on the natural course of fellow eyes with neovascular AMD is provided from the 5-yr prospective follow-up in the Macular Photocoagulation Study. In this investigation, macular characteristics were graded in a masked fashion without knowledge of the subsequent course or treatment of either eye using a standardized classification scheme.[3] Eyes with no large drusen and no focal hyperpigmentation were at a 10 percent risk of developing choroidal neovascularization within 5 yr. Eyes with large drusen or focal hyperpigmentation had a 30 percent risk of devel-

oping choroidal neovascularization within 5 yr. Eyes with both large drusen and focal hyperpigmentation had about a 60 percent risk of acquiring choroidal neovascularization within 5 yr.[3]

The development of significant severe visual loss occurred almost exclusively in eyes in which choroidal neovascularization developed. Overall, 30 of 127 eyes developed choroidal neovascularization during the follow-up period. Of the remaining 97 eyes in which choroidal neovascularization did not develop, the average visual acuity loss over 5 yr was only 0.4 line.

Very small retrospective studies in patients in whom both eyes have drusen with no evidence of neovascular AMD in either eye suggest that in 8.5 to 18 percent of eyes, visual acuity deteriorates to 20/200 or worse in at least one eye. The deterioration was almost always due to the development of choroidal neovascularization.[13, 22] These studies may be biased given that the patients were referred to centers specializing in retinal diseases and may not represent the general population. More accurate information may come from the Baltimore Longitudinal Study on Aging, a prospective follow-up of healthy volunteers over a 10-yr period; from follow-up of the Framingham Eye Study; from follow-up in the Chesapeake Bay Watermen Study; and from follow-up in the Age-Related Eye Disease Study.

Geographic Atrophy

In a study of 208 patients who presented with geographic atrophy,[23] the geographic atrophy had a tendency to start outside of the foveal center. By the time the atrophy encroached within 750 μ of the foveal center, it approached 1 disc diameter. Even after progression, a small part of the fovea tended to be spared for a long time, and eyes with 100 percent involvement of the fovea showed atrophy of more than 7 disc diameters. Visual acuity was related to the percentage of fovea affected but varied widely within each group. It was rather difficult to predict the visual acuity within a narrow margin of certainty from the anatomic appearance of the atrophy alone. Nevertheless, central fixation tended to be lost when atrophy occupied 85 percent or more of the fovea. The condition was very symmetric, with one half of the patients presenting with geographic atrophy bilaterally and an additional 25 percent having evidence of prior choroidal neovascularization in the fellow eye.[23]

In the same study,[23] the progression of atrophy was documented retrospectively in 61 patients who were followed for an average of 29 mo. Sarks and Sarks noted that geographic atrophy involved areas affected by incipient atrophy, defined as areas of diffuse stippled RPE hyperpigmentation and stippled atrophy, as shown in Figure 64–3. Seven of the 61 patients (11 percent) experienced choroidal neovascularization during follow-up. Only one of these 7 patients had advanced atrophy; the remaining 6 patients had atrophy that averaged 1 disc diameter. Perhaps widespread areas of atrophy are associated with a decreased risk of the development of choroidal neovascularization, whereas small areas of atrophy, in the presence of a diffuse macular pathologic condition and thickening of the inner aspect of Bruch's membrane, have a moderate risk of the development of choroidal neovascularization. Histologic studies have shown that almost 35 percent of individuals with choroidal neovascularization also have areas of geographic atrophy.[8] Large areas of atrophy may not be associated with the development of choroidal neovascularization based on monkey models of experimentally produced choroidal neovascularization[24] in which the RPE was selectively destroyed by the administration of ornithine or sodium iodide prior to the attempt to produce choroidal neovascularization. The presence of some RPE was necessary in experimentally induced choroidal neovascularization following creation of a break in Bruch's membrane using laser. Nevertheless, even widespread areas of atrophy in conditions such as choroideremia[25] or gyrate atrophy[26] have been associated with the development of choroidal neovascularization, although their incidence is so low that they have only been reported as single case reports.

The development of subretinal hemorrhage in eyes with geographic atrophy does not necessarily imply the presence of choroidal neovascularization. Nasrallah and associates[27] have reported on eight patients in whom small subretinal hemorrhages spontaneously cleared over a 15-mo period without evidence of choroidal neovascularization at the time of the hemorrhage nor evidence of choroidal neovascularization or disciform scarring with clearing of the hemorrhage. These subretinal hemorrhages may reflect rupture of normal choriocapillaris, as it is seen in subretinal hemorrhages occurring in myopic patients with lacquer cracks in which choroidal neovascularization is not growing through the lacquer crack.[28]

MANAGEMENT

Since the risk of visual loss in eyes with drusen results predominantly from the development of choroidal neovascularization, the ideal treatment should be directed toward the prevention of choroidal neovascularization. No known treatment exists at this time.

In a small pilot trial[29] oral zinc administration was associated with a small decrease in the frequency of progressive visual loss in patients with drusen and atrophic changes. However, there are several reasons to withhold any recommendation on using oral zinc in patients with macular degeneration at this time. The natural history studies from the Macular Photocoagulation Study suggest that patients who do not experience choroidal neovascularization have a loss of visual acuity of 0.4 line over a 5-yr period without any treatment; even in this small pilot study,[29] zinc has not been shown to prevent the development of choroidal neovascularization. The difference in visual acuity between zinc-treated and placebo-treated patients was only 0.8 line in patients followed for 18 mo and only 0.6 line in patients followed for 19 to 24 mo. There was no correlation between initial visual acuity and baseline serum zinc levels among the patients in this study. Finally, the systemic toxicity associated with zinc, and particularly anemia, even if not found in this small pilot study, might be a problem in a larger scale study in which many patients remain on zinc for a long time.

There are no data to suggest that ultraviolet light is associated with the development of AMD,[30] although a small correlation has been seen between increased exposures of visible light over a 20-yr period and the development of geographic atrophy or disciform scarring.[31] Since the use of sunglasses that block out some visible light is relatively inexpensive and without side effects, this should certainly not be discouraged.

The most important aspect of management in patients with drusen at the present time is education. These patients are at increased risk of acquiring choroidal neovascularization, especially if one eye has already been affected, and data suggest that diagnosis at the earliest onset of the choroidal neovascularization provides the greatest chance of being successful.[32, 33] Therefore, patients should monitor their central vision every day in each eye at risk for the development of choroidal neovascularization, and they should contact their ophthalmologist promptly if they notice any metamorphopsia or scotoma, which may suggest the onset of choroidal neovascularization. Evaluation by an ophthalmologist should include careful contact lens biomicroscopy for the presence of subretinal fluid or hemorrhage and, if necessary, fluorescein angiography to determine whether or not choroidal neovascularization is present.

Unfortunately, some patients may experience choroidal neovascularization asymptomatically,[34] and many ophthalmologists recommend that patients who have drusen be followed every 6 mo in the hope of detecting asymptomatic choroidal neovascularization that might still be amenable to treatment.[35]

Geographic Atrophy of the RPE

Management of eyes with geographic atrophy is similar to that described for choroidal neovascularization. In addition, since extension of geographic atrophy through the foveal center can result in severe visual loss even without the development of disciform scarring from choroidal neovascularization, patients who have lost central vision in both eyes from geographic atrophy may benefit from low-vision aids (see Chap. 294).

CONCLUSIONS AND FUTURE RESEARCH

Although fairly uniform descriptions of the nonneovascular features of AMD have been presented, there still is little information on the cause or progression of these changes. Hopefully, current and future epidemiologic studies will lead to better understanding of the pathogenesis of these changes. Interventional trials may allow us to understand what can be done to prevent the development of these changes in the first place or prevent progression to the visually disabling stage of atrophy or choroidal neovascularization.

REFERENCES

1. Donders FC: Beitrage zur pathogischen Anatomie des Auges. Graefes Arch Ophthalmol 1:106, 1855.
2. Bressler NM, Bressler SB, West SK, et al: The grading and prevalence of macular degeneration in Chesapeake Bay watermen. Arch Ophthalmol 107:847–852, 1989.
3. Bressler SB, Maguire MG, Bressler NM, Fine SL: The Macular Photocoagulation Study Group: Relationship of drusen and abnormalities of the retinal pigment epithelium to the prognosis of neovascular macular degeneration. Arch Ophthalmol 108:1442–1447, 1990.
4. Macular Photocoagulation Study Group: Persistent and recurrent neovascularization after krypton laser photocoagulation for neovascular lesions of age-related macular degeneration. Arch Ophthalmol 108:825–831, 1990.
5. Coffey AJH, Brownstein S: The prevalence of macular drusen in postmortem eyes. Am J Ophthalmol 102:164–171, 1986.
6. El Baba F, Green WR, Fleischmann J, et al: Clinicopathologic correlation of lipidization and detachment of the retinal pigment epithelium. Am J Ophthalmol 101:576, 1986.
7. Green WR, McDonnell PH, Yeo JH: Pathologic features of senile macular degeneration. Ophthalmology 92:615–627, 1985.
8. Green WR, Key SN: Senile macular degeneration: A histopathologic study. Trans Am Ophthalmol Soc 75:180–254, 1977.
9. Sarks SH: Drusen and their relationship to senile macular degeneration. Aust J Ophthalmol 8:117–130, 1980.
10. Sarks SH: Ageing and degeneration in the macular region: A clinicopathologic study. Br J Ophthalmol 60:324–341, 1976.
11. Pouleikhoff D, Barondes MJ, Minassian D, et al: Drusen as risk factors in age-related macular degeneration. Am J Ophthalmol 109:38–43, 1990.
12. Sarks JP, Sarks SH, Killingsworth MC: Evolution of geographic atrophy of the retinal pigment epithelium. Eye 2:552–577, 1988.
13. Smiddy WE, Fine SL: Prognosis of patients with bilateral macular drusen. Ophthalmology 91:271–277, 1984.
14. Jampol LM: Discussion of prognosis of patients with bilateral macular drusen. Ophthalmology 91:276–277, 1984.
15. Gass JDM, Jallow S, Davis B: Adult vitelliform macular detachment occurring in patients with basal laminar drusen. Am J Ophthalmol 99:445–459, 1985.
16. Kenyon KR, Maumenee AE, Ryan SJ, et al: Diffuse drusen and associated complications. Am J Ophthalmol 100:119–128, 1985.
17. Bressler NM, Bressler SB, Fine SL: Age-related macular degeneration. Surv Ophthalmol 32:375–413, 1988.
18. Gass JDM: A clinicopathologic study of a peculiar foveomacular dystrophy. Trans Am Ophthalmol Soc 72:139, 1974.
19. Todd K, Schatz H, Crawford JB: Pathologic findings in pseudo-vitelliform macular degeneration. Invest Ophthalmol Vis Sci 27:198, 1986.
20. Gass JDM: Stereoscopic Atlas of Macular Diseases: Diagnosis and Treatment, 3rd ed, vol. 1. St Louis, CV Mosby, 1987, p 264.
21. Wilkinson CP, Bressler NM, Burgess D, et al: Five-year changes in visual acuity of fellow eyes of patients with extrafoveal choroidal neovascularization in age-related macular degeneration. Invest Ophthalmol Vis Sci 232:712, 1991.
22. Gass JDM: Drusen and disciform macular detachment and degeneration. Arch Ophthalmol 90:206–217, 1973.
23. Sarks SH, Sarks JP: Age-related macular degeneration: Atrophic form. In Ryan SJ, Schachat AP, Murphy RP, Patz A (eds): Retina. St Louis, CV Mosby, 1989, pp 149–173.
24. Itagaki T, Ohkuma H, Yamagishi K, et al: Studies on experimental subretinal neovascularization, relationship between new vessels and retinal pigment epithelium. Ther Res 5:665–670, 1986.
25. Robinson D, Tiedman J: Choroideremia associated with a subretinal neovascular membrane: Case report. Retina 7:70–74, 1987.
26. Giovanni A, Amato GP, Pazzaglia A, et al: Sub-retinal neovascularisations of uncommon origin. In BenEzra D, Ryan SJ, Glaser BM, Murphy RP (eds): Ocular Circulation and Neovascularisation. Dordrecht, The Netherlands, Martinus Nijhoff/Dr W Junk, 1987, pp 313–317.
27. Nasrallah F, Jalkh AE, Trempe CL, et al: Subretinal hemorrhage in atrophic age-related macular degeneration. Am J Ophthalmol 107:38–41, 1989.
28. Klein RM, Green S: The development of lacquer cracks in pathologic myopia. Am J Ophthalmol 106:282–285, 1988.
29. Newsome DA, Swartz M, Leone NC, et al: Oral zinc in macular degeneration. Arch Ophthalmol 106:192–198, 1988.
30. West SK, Rosenthal FS, Bressler NM, et al: Exposure to sunlight and other risk factors for age-related macular degeneration. Arch Ophthalmol 107:875–879, 1989.
31. Taylor HR, Munoz B, West SK, et al: Visible light and risk of age-related macular degeneration. Trans Am Ophthalmol Soc 88:163–178, 1990.
32. Bird AC: Treatment of senile macular degeneration by photocoagulation. Br J Ophthalmol 58:367–376, 1974.
33. Macular Photocoagulation Study Group: Laser photocoagulation of subfoveal neovascular lesions in age-related macular degeneration. Results of a randomized clinical trial. Arch Ophthalmol 109:1219–1231, 1991.
34. Moisseiev J, Bressler NM: Asymptomatic neovascular membranes in the second eye of patients with visual loss from age-related macular degeneration (AMD). Invest Ophthalmol Vis Sci 31:462, 1990.
35. American Academy of Ophthalmology Quality of Care Committee Retina Panel: Macular Degeneration. American Academy of Ophthalmology Preferred Practice Pattern. San Francisco, American Academy of Ophthalmology, 1990.

Chapter 65

Age-related Macular Degeneration: Choroidal Neovascularization

NEIL M. BRESSLER, SUSAN B. BRESSLER, and
EVANGELOS S. GRAGOUDAS

Although most patients with age-related macular degeneration (AMD) manifest only drusen or abnormalities of the retinal pigment epithelium (RPE), the majority of patients who experience severe visual loss from AMD do so because of the development of choroidal neovascularization (CNV) and related manifestations such as serous or hemorrhagic detachment of the RPE and fibrovascular disciform scarring. The pathogenesis, clinical features, differential diagnosis, natural course, and treatment of the neovascular form of AMD are reviewed in this chapter. (The nonneovascular form of AMD, including drusen and abnormalities of the RPE such as geographic atrophy, is reviewed in Chapter 64.)

PATHOGENESIS

The pathogenesis of the development of CNV is largely unknown. In part, clinical[1-4] and histologic reports[5,6] suggest that the presence of diffuse thickening of the inner aspect of Bruch's membrane (associated with large, soft drusen clinically) predisposes Bruch's membrane to develop cracks through which ingrowth of new vessels from the choriocapillaris can occur. This hypothesis is supported by the finding of CNV in other pathologic entities in which breaks in Bruch's membrane occur, such as pathologic myopia[7] and angioid streaks.[8] However, it is unlikely that a break in Bruch's membrane alone necessarily predisposes to the development of CNV. Histologic studies have shown that in eyes with AMD, breaks in Bruch's membrane can be identified not only in areas of CNV but also in areas in which no new vessels can be identified.[5]

Experimental studies have also suggested that other cellular processes may have a role in the development of the CNV beyond merely a disturbance in Bruch's membrane. Laboratory studies have shown that endothelial cells can elaborate enzymes necessary for the digestion of a basement membrane such as Bruch's membrane.[9] This finding would support the concept that endothelial cells from the choriocapillaris could produce a break in Bruch's membrane, rather than presuming that CNV only grows through preexisting breaks in Bruch's membrane. Other reports have suggested that a granulomatous inflammatory response to degenerated Bruch's membrane may be an important factor in the

development of CNV. In histologic studies, eyes with AMD had an increased prevalence of lymphocytes, macrophages, and fibroblasts within Bruch's membrane when compared with control eyes without AMD.[10-12] These findings would suggest that a low-grade chronic inflammatory response may be involved in the development of AMD. Although these inflammatory cells have been shown histologically to be *associated* with the presence of the nonneovascular and neovascular stages of AMD, the studies have not shown that inflammatory cells necessarily lead to the development of CNV. Therefore, these studies cannot determine whether these inflammatory cells represent a response to existing degenerative changes within Bruch's membrane or whether the inflammatory cells act as essential mediators of degeneration, with subsequent development of CNV.

Experimentally produced CNV developing around retinal laser burns in the monkey eye have also shown the presence of macrophages at the site of developing CNV.[13,14] Again, it is not known whether these macrophages represent a response to damaged retina from a laser burn or whether they act as mediators of CNV. Also, this model of CNV differs from CNV in AMD in that experimentally produced CNV proliferates internal to the RPE (between the sensory retina and the RPE),[13] whereas CNV associated with AMD initially proliferates external to the RPE (within the thickened inner aspect of Bruch's membrane).[5,6]

A relationship of scleral rigidity with choroidal neovascular disease in AMD has been suggested in a pilot study in which increased scleral rigidity was found to be associated with the presence of AMD.[15] The possibility of compromised blood flow in the vortex veins by progressively increased scleral rigidity was hypothesized to account for these findings, but further investigation is required.

Recent results from a case control study (personal communication, E. S. Gragoudas, 1991) also demonstrated that the risk of CNV is associated with low blood levels of micronutrients with antioxidant potential, cigarette smoking, higher levels of serum cholesterol, and parity greater than zero. Decreased risk was associated with higher levels of carotenoids and use of postmenopausal exogenous estrogens in women. The associations with estrogens, cigarette smoking, and serum cholesterol are intriguing because sphingomyelins and cholesterol esters similar to those found in arteriosclerotic plaques are found in aging sclera.[16] Perhaps these factors may in some way account for increased scleral rigidity.

Regardless of the pathogenesis of CNV in AMD, clinicopathologic correlative studies[5, 6, 17] and natural history studies[2, 18–22] have shown that CNV is often accompanied by the ingrowth of fibrous scar tissue, eventually resulting in a disciform scar. This CNV-scar complex may have a variety of complex clinical and angiographic appearances. An understanding of these features is critical in the identification, proper management, and treatment of the choroidal neovascular form of AMD.

CLINICAL FEATURES

Symptoms of CNV

CNV should be suspected in any patient (usually older than 65 yr with large, soft drusen) who complains of metamorphopsia, central or paracentral scotoma, or any sudden, nonspecific change in central vision.[23, 24] Any of these symptoms should alert the ophthalmologist to look for signs of CNV, which are outlined further on. However, not all patients with CNV will be symptomatic[25] or will note changes of metamorphopsia on home-testing with an Amsler grid.[26] Therefore, even *asymptomatic* patients older than 65 yr with large, soft drusen on clinical examination probably should be scrutinized for signs of CNV on periodic examination.

Signs of CNV

In the early stages of the neovascular form of AMD, before disciform scarring has developed clinically, biomicroscopic clues to the presence of CNV may include any or all of the following: the presence of subretinal or intraretinal lipids, elevation of the RPE, cystic changes in the sensory retina, or visualization of the choroidal neovascular vessels themselves. The vessels may be seen as a yellow-green discoloration frequently surrounded by a pigmented ring and are often visualized best with transillumination of the RPE with a thin slit beam on biomicroscopy. The presence of subretinal or sub-RPE blood may be so extensive as to obscure all other signs of CNV; often though, this blood, if present, will be along the periphery of the CNV (Fig. 65–1). Other causes of subretinal or sub-RPE hemorrhage should be ruled out, including macroaneurysms, lacquer cracks in pathologic myopia, traumatic choroidal rupture, choroidal tumors, or subretinal hemorrhage within areas of geographic atrophy when no CNV is seen on angiography. (Presumably, the subretinal hemorrhage within areas of geographic atrophy without CNV on angiography is from disruption of the choriocapillaris in association with the geographic atrophy.[27])

Although CNV secondary to AMD has classically been described in association with subretinal hemorrhage, many cases may present with little or no hemorrhage, the predominant sign being the more subtle finding of subretinal fluid. Often, one needs a contact lens examination with biomicroscopy and a thin slit beam to detect this subretinal fluid. The anterior portion of the beam will bow forward convexly and there will be an increased distance between the surface of the slit beam, which is visualized on the surface of the sensory retina, and the posterior portion of the beam, which is visualized on the surface of the RPE. As subretinal fluid is absorbed at the periphery of the CNV, subretinal lipid may precipitate in a circumferential pattern around the CNV and thereby help to alert the ophthalmologist to the presence of CNV. Other biomicroscopic signs of CNV, as already mentioned, include the elevation of the RPE, presumably caused by the presence of CNV and fibrovascular proliferation beneath the RPE,[17, 28] pigment proliferation overlying the CNV,[29] or the actual choroidal neovascular vessels themselves (occasionally seen when the overlying RPE pigmentation is markedly attenuated).

If CNV secondary to AMD is suspected from symptoms or signs, fluorescein angiography is indicated for the following reasons: (1) to confirm the diagnosis of CNV, (2) to determine if treatment is indicated (as discussed further on), and (3) if treatment is indicated, to serve as a guide as to treatment location.

Fluorescein Angiographic Features of CNV

A set of photographs to facilitate the identification of the variety of appearances of CNV secondary to AMD includes (1) a black-and-white stereo pair of the macula obtained with green (monochromatic) filter; (2) rapid-sequence photographs of the macula taken during the

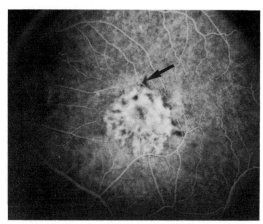

Figure 65–1. Subfoveal choroidal neovascularization (CNV) with contiguous blood *(arrow)*. The boundaries of the entire lesion (the CNV and blood) are well demarcated; the entire lesion is less than 3.5 disc areas; the lesion would meet the eligibility criteria of the Macular Photocoagulation Study (MPS). (From Macular Photocoagulation Study Group: Laser photocoagulation of subfoveal neovascular lesions in age-related macular degeneration. Results of a randomized clinical trial. Arch Ophthalmol 109:1220–1231, 1991. Copyright 1991, American Medical Association.)

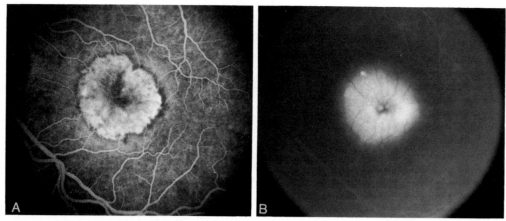

Figure 65–2. Classic CNV. *A,* Early phase of fluorescein angiogram of classic CNV in which boundaries of the neovascular lesion are well demarcated. *B,* Late phase of angiogram showing pooling of dye in subsensory retinal space, obscuring boundaries of CNV demarcated in earlier phase of angiogram. *(A and B,* From Macular Photocoagulation Study Group: Subfoveal neovascular lesions in age-related macular degeneration. Guidelines for evaluation and treatment in the Macular Photocoagulation Study. Arch Ophthalmol 109:1242–1257, 1991. Copyright 1991, American Medical Association.)

dye transit, including at least one stereo pair; (3) stereo pairs of the macula taken at approximately 30, 40, 60, 90, 120, and 180 sec after dye injection; (4) late stereo pairs of the macula taken at 5 and 10 min after dye injection; and (5) stereoscopic color fundus photographs of the macula.[30] Since CNV growth can be a continuous process,[31, 32] the size of the CNV and the area of retina to be treated can change within a short time. Therefore, a fluorescein angiogram should ideally be obtained on the same day as any contemplated treatment and probably no more than 96 hr prior to treatment.

Two basic angiographic patterns of CNV, recognized in the Macular Photocoagulation Studies[30, 33, 34] and described by independent investigators,[17, 20, 23, 24, 35–37] include classic and occult CNV.

Classic CNV. This condition is characterized by well-demarcated boundaries of hyperfluorescence that can be

discerned in the early phase of the angiogram (Fig. 65–2 *A*) with progressive dye leakage pooling in the overlying subsensory retinal space (Fig. 65–2 *B*). Only occasionally will fluorescein angiography identify the actual capillary network of the CNV secondary to AMD. This latter observation is contrary to the widely held view that CNV presents angiographically as a lacy network of vessels. This lacy pattern may be seen commonly in CNV secondary to other pathologic entities, such as the ocular histoplasmosis syndrome, but is unusual in AMD.

Occult CNV. This condition encompasses a variety of fluorescein angiographic appearances that do not conform with the classic description of CNV. The occult forms may be categorized into fibrovascular pigment epithelial detachments (PEDs) and late leakage of undetermined source. In fibrovascular PEDs (Fig. 65–3),

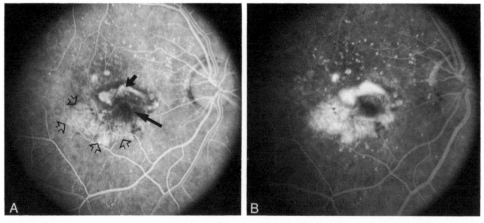

Figure 65–3. Recurrent classic and occult CNV (with fibrovascular pigment epithelial detachment). *A,* Early phase of fluorescein angiogram showing areas of classic CNV *(small solid arrow),* scar from prior laser treatment *(large solid arrow),* and irregular elevation of retinal pigment epithelium (RPE) with stippled hyperfluorescence *(open arrows)* representing fibrovascular pigment epithelial detachment (PED) inferotemporal to scar. *B,* One minute after fluorescein injection fluorescein leakage is apparent from the classic CNV, and increased intensity of stippled hyperfluorescence corresponding to fibrovascular PED is noted. The boundaries of the fibrovascular PED remain well demarcated. At each clock hour, the boundary of the lesion is clearly demarcated and would meet eligibility criteria in the MPS trials. *(A and B,* From Macular Photocoagulation Study Group: Subfoveal neovascular lesions in age-related macular degeneration. Guidelines for evaluation and treatment in the Macular Photocoagulation Study. Arch Ophthalmol 109:1242–1257, 1991. Copyright 1991, American Medical Association.)

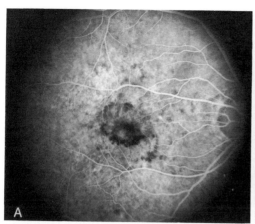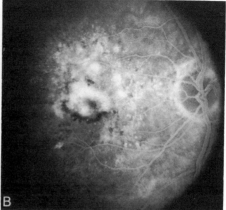

Figure 65–4. Occult CNV with late leakage of undetermined source. *A,* Early phase of angiogram. *B,* Middle phase of angiogram shows pinpoints of speckled hyperfluorescence and larger areas of hyperfluorescence with accumulation of fluorescein leakage in overlying subsensory retinal space. The source of the leakage cannot be discerned from earlier phases of the angiogram. The lesion does not meet the MPS eligibility criteria that the boundaries of neovascularization be well demarcated; therefore, treatment is not considered for this lesion. (*A* and *B,* From Macular Photocoagulation Study Group: Subfoveal neovascular lesions in age-related macular degeneration. Guidelines for evaluation and treatment in the Macular Photocoagulation Study. Arch Ophthalmol 109:1242–1257, 1991. Copyright 1991, American Medical Association.)

areas of irregular elevation of the RPE are often most easily detectable on *stereoscopic* fluorescein angiography. These areas usually are not as discrete or bright as areas of classic CNV in pictures taken during the transit; by 1 to 2 min after fluorescein injection, an area of stippled hyperfluorescence becomes apparent (Fig. 65–3*B*). By 10 min, there is persistence of fluorescein staining or leakage within a sensory retinal detachment overlying this area.

Late leakage of undetermined source consists of areas of late choroidal fluorescein leakage, often appearing as speckled hyperfluorescence, with pooling of dye in the overlying subsensory retinal space, in which there is no discernible, discrete, well-demarcated area of hyperfluorescence that might be considered the source of leakage from earlier photography (Fig. 65–4).

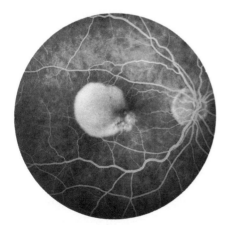

Figure 65–5. Early-phase fluorescein angiogram of a serous detachment of the RPE. A uniform elevation of the RPE, with uniform pooling of fluorescein dye, and a smooth contour to the surface of the elevated RPE, with well-demarcated borders in the early phase of the angiogram, are noted. Persistent bright hyperfluorescence continued within these well-demarcated boundaries in the late phase of this angiogram (not shown).

Angiographic Features That Obscure the Boundaries of CNV

Three features can obscure the boundaries of CNV and are important to recognize when attempting to delineate the boundaries of the choroidal neovascular lesion. Two of these features *block* the angiographic view of choroidal fluorescence. They include (1) blood contiguous with the CNV that is thick enough to obscure the normal choroidal fluorescence; (2) elevated areas of blocked fluorescence due to hyperplastic pigment or fibrous tissue; and (3) a serous detachment of the RPE (Fig. 65–5). The bright, reasonably uniform early hyperfluorescence associated with a serous detachment of the RPE may obscure hyperfluorescence from the CNV and interfere with the ability to judge how far CNV extends under the area of the serous detachment.

Other Clinical and Angiographic Features of CNV Secondary to AMD

Fading CNV. CNV occasionally may be recognized in the early- or middle-transit phase of the angiogram with *fading* in the late phase, so that no leakage can be discerned in the area that was presumed to harbor CNV (Fig. 65–6).[30] Most ophthalmologists are reluctant to treat areas of CNV that fade. These areas usually are not associated with overlying subretinal fluid (in conjunction with the lack of fluorescein leakage on angiography), so one can only presume that this region may go on to disciform scarring. Perhaps these areas represent CNV histologically, but without evidence of subretinal fluid or late leakage, one cannot be sure that this pattern definitively represents CNV, and laser destruction of this area may obliterate retina unnecessarily.

Feeder Vessels. These vessels may be identified as

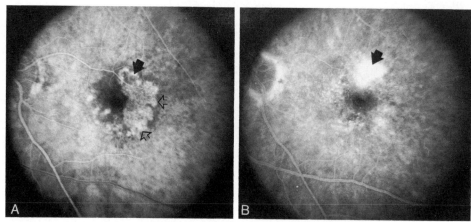

Figure 65–6. Fading fluorescence of CNV. *A,* Early phase of angiogram shows classic CNV *(solid arrows)* with contiguous areas of slightly elevated hyperfluorescent RPE *(open arrows)*, presumably representing a fibrovascular pigment epithelial detachment, and other less well-demarcated areas of hyperfluorescence nasal to fovea. *B,* Later phase of angiogram shows fluorescein leakage from classic CNV *(arrow)*. However, areas of elevated hyperfluorescent RPE noted on early phase of angiogram begin to fade in later phase. Faded areas are not considered a lesion component to be treated in 1991 by MPS treatment protocol because hyperfluorescence does not have enough leakage or staining in the late phase of the angiogram to be considered occult CNV. Before 1988, most ophthalmologists would have considered treatment of the classic CNV with late leakage *(arrow)*. By current interpretations, treatment of area of classic CNV still might be contemplated, but ophthalmologists would be concerned about untreated areas of presumed occult CNV that fade in the late phase of the angiogram, even though most ophthalmologists would not consider treatment of this presumed occult CNV that fades in the late phase. *(A and B,* From Macular Photocoagulation Study Group: Subfoveal neovascular lesions in age-related macular degeneration. Guidelines for evaluation and treatment in the Macular Photocoagulation Study. Arch Ophthalmol 109:1242–1257, 1991. Copyright 1991, American Medical Association.)

choroidal vessels apparent during the transit phase of the angiogram connected unequivocally to leaking choroidal capillaries (Fig. 65–7). Although feeder vessels have been described as extending from a laser scar to recurrent CNV across the perimeter of the laser scar,[23, 30, 38] feeder vessels also may be seen in untreated eyes. In the latter situation, peripheral untreated areas of CNV may be connected by feeder vessels to more central areas of CNV that are evolving toward natural scar formation.[30]

Loculated Fluid. This fluid consists of a well-demar-

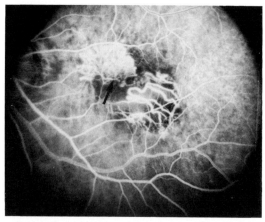

Figure 65–7. Recurrent CNV with feeder vessel *(arrow),* as well as larger choroidal vessels seen within central portion of scar from previous laser treatment. (From Macular Photocoagulation Study Group: Subfoveal neovascular lesions in age-related macular degeneration. Guidelines for evaluation and treatment in the Macular Photocoagulation Study. Arch Ophthalmol 109:1242–1257, 1991. Copyright 1991, American Medical Association.)

cated area of hyperfluorescence that appears to represent pooling of fluorescein in a compartmentalized space anterior to the choroidal neovascular leakage.[39] Although the loculated fluid may conform to a pattern of typical cystoid macular edema, it can also pool within an area deep to the sensory retina in a shape that does not bear any resemblance to cystoid macular edema (Fig. 65–8).[39]

Tears or Rips of the RPE. An acute tear or rip of the RPE may occur spontaneously (Fig. 65–9) or during laser photocoagulation of a choroidal neovascular lesion.[40–45] Visual acuity may fall precipitously, especially when associated CNV has an opportunity to destroy foveal photoreceptors. When there is no CNV, RPE tears through the fovea may be associated with preservation of good central visual acuity provided that the *torn area,* and not the scrolled-up RPE, underlies the foveal center.[46] Angiography demonstrates early, bright, sharply demarcated hyperfluorescence within the torn region. Blocked fluorescence corresponding to heaped-up RPE will be noted at one side of the lesion. The bright hyperfluorescence presumably corresponds to fluorescein dye within the choriocapillaris that quickly leaks into the choroidal and scleral tissues and is not blocked by pigment that is normally otherwise present within the overlying RPE. No leakage of dye is seen if no overlying sensory retinal detachment is present. The lack of a sensory retinal detachment over a tear of the RPE may be due to the higher osmotic pressure of the choroid compared with the subretinal space, which allows fluid to be removed from the subretinal space at a rapid rate when the tight junctions of the RPE are lacking and unable to prevent free movement of fluid.[47]

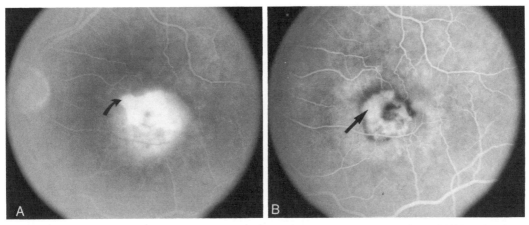

Figure 65–8. Example of an eye in which the borders of loculated fluid extend beyond the borders of CNV. In late-transit frames *(A)*, the area of loculated fluid *(arrow)* extends beyond the area of the borders of the CNV as defined in the early-transit phase of the angiogram *(B, arrow)*. (A and B, From Bressler NM, Bressler SB, Alexander J, et al: Loculated fluid: A previously undescribed fluorescein angiographic finding in choroidal neovascularization associated with macular degeneration. Arch Ophthalmol 109:211–215, 1991. Copyright 1991, American Medical Association.)

Disciform Scar. The term *disciform scar* is used to describe the yellow-white fibrous tissue that often accompanies CNV. The lesion may also contain brown or black pigment, depending on the degree of pigment proliferation from the RPE within the scar. The disciform scarring may have a variety of appearances depending on its location within the retina (sub-RPE or subretinal), the degree of associated CNV with the scarring, the presence of chorioretinal anastomosis within the scar, or the amount of RPE atrophy accompanying the scar (Fig. 65–10). The natural course of most choroidal neovascular lesions secondary to AMD consists of scarring within the central portion of the

lesion with continued signs of active CNV at the periphery of the lesion (including subretinal fluid, hemorrhage, or lipid). Therefore, most disciform scars secondary to AMD could be termed *CNV-scar* when they include both a fibrous component noted on biomicroscopy and a neovascular component represented by subretinal fluid–hemorrhage–lipid on biomicroscopy and accompanied by leakage from CNV on angiography (Fig. 65–10B). Occasionally, these disciform scars may develop anterior to the posterior pole. These peripheral disciform scars may become quite large with irregular shapes or they may be accompanied by hemorrhage, leading to the suspicion of a tumor such as a melanoma, until they are evaluated with ultrasound (see further on).

Vitreous Hemorrhage. Occasionally, hemorrhage from CNV or CNV-scarring extends into the vitreous space.[48, 49] Any patient with a massive vitreous hemorrhage in one eye and features of AMD in the fellow eye should be suspected of harboring CNV in the eye with vitreous hemorrhage. Ultrasonography should be performed to rule out a rhegmatogenous retinal tear or detachment, choroidal melanoma, and other less common causes of vitreous hemorrhage. Sonographically, the posterior pole or peripheral lesion is relatively flat and broad-based, with a fairly homogeneous pattern and without signs of choroidal excavation. The vitreous hemorrhage clears in approximately 75 percent of patients. If the hemorrhage does not clear, consideration of a vitrectomy to restore peripheral vision should be considered, taking into account how restoration of that peripheral vision will improve the patient's quality of life, given the unlikelihood of restoration of central vision.

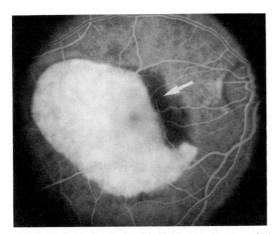

Figure 65–9. Retinal pigment epithelial tear seen on early-transit phase of fluorescein angiogram demonstrating extremely sharp, well-demarcated hyperfluorescence. Continued intense staining was seen in the late phase of the angiogram with no leakage. An early blocked fluorescence *(arrow)* presumably corresponds to the redundant, folded, torn pigment epithelium. (From Bressler NM, Finkelstein D, Sunness JS, et al: Retinal pigment epithelial tears through the fovea with preservation of good visual acuity. Arch Ophthalmol 108:1694–1697, 1990. Copyright 1990, American Medical Association.)

RPE Detachments in AMD

Various changes in AMD may result in elevation or detachment of the RPE as seen on stereoscopic biomi-

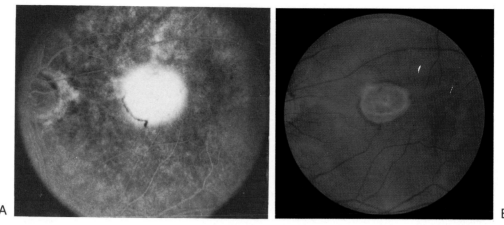

Figure 65–10. CNV-disciform scarring. *A,* Subretinal and sub-RPE fibrosis, as well as subretinal fluid and hemorrhage, is seen on color photograph. The latter presumably are indicative of persistent vascular tissue within the fibrosis. *B,* Fluorescein angiography of CNV-scarring demonstrating some blocked fluorescence corresponding to the fibrotic tissue as well as leakage toward the periphery of the lesion, presumably from CNV associated with the scarring. (*A* and *B,* From Macular Photocoagulation Study Group: Subfoveal neovascular lesions in age-related macular degeneration. Guidelines for evaluation and treatment in the Macular Photocoagulation Study. Arch Ophthalmol 109:1242–1257, 1991. Copyright 1991, American Medical Association.)

croscopic or angiographic evaluation. The term *RPE detachment* secondary to AMD in the ophthalmic literature remains confusing because various RPE detachments may have quite different prognoses and managements, and yet several series may have included some or all of these RPE detachments in their reports. RPE detachments secondary to AMD that may be readily recognized and probably should be differentiated include the following: (1) *fibrovascular PEDs* which are a subset of occult CNV (see Fig. 65–3); (2) *elevated areas of RPE that block fluorescence* because of hyperplastic pigment or fibrous tissue (see Fig. 65–3); (3) *serous detachments of the RPE* (see Fig. 65–5); (4) *hemorrhagic detachments of the RPE,* in which blood from a choroidal neovascular lesion is noted beneath or exterior to the RPE; and (5) *drusenoid RPE detachments,* in which large areas of confluent, soft drusen are noted.[50]

Elevated blocked fluorescence may be differentiated from fibrovascular PEDs and serous detachments of the RPE in that blocked fluorescence is noted within the area of elevated RPE throughout the angiogram. One of the more difficult differentiations is between fibrovascular PEDs and serous detachment of the RPE. Although they probably have been lumped together in several series that have examined RPE detachments,[51–56] some of these clinical reports have attempted to identify certain features that might distinguish between serous detachments of the RPE and areas of elevation of the RPE that may harbor occult CNV.[53] Using descriptions from the Macular Photocoagulation Study (MPS), fibrovascular PEDs (as a subset of occult CNV) have been distinguished from classic serous detachments of the RPE in that the former have slow filling with a stippled appearance to the surface of the RPE by the middle phase of the angiogram and may show pooling of dye in the overlying subsensory retinal space in the late phase, whereas the latter show uniform, bright hyperfluorescence in the early phase with a smooth contour to the RPE by the middle phase and

little, if any, leakage into the overlying sensory retinal space by the late phase.

A hemorrhagic detachment of the RPE will block choroidal fluorescence just as blocked fluorescence from hyperplastic pigment or fibrous tissue does. However, in hemorrhagic detachments of the RPE, the dark appearance on biomicroscopy caused by the moundlike collection of blood beneath the RPE will help to differentiate it from areas of elevated blocked fluorescence caused by hyperplastic pigment or fibrous tissue as discussed previously. Occasionally, a hemorrhagic detachment of the RPE may be mistaken for a choroidal melanoma, but usually hemorrhagic detachments of the RPE will not demonstrate low internal reflectivity, as is seen characteristically in choroidal melanomas.

The final feature of AMD that will appear as an elevated or detached RPE is a drusenoid RPE detachment or extensive areas of large confluent drusen.[50] Drusenoid RPE detachments can be distinguished from serous detachments of the RPE in that drusenoid RPE detachments will fluoresce faintly during the transit and do not progress to *bright* hyperfluorescence in the late phase of the angiogram. In contrast, serous detachments of the RPE will fluoresce brightly in the early-transit phase and remain brightly hyperfluorescent in the late phase. In addition, serous detachments usually will have a smoother, sharper boundary compared with drusenoid RPE detachments. Drusenoid RPE detachments can be distinguished from fibrovascular PEDs in occult CNV by noting that fibrovascular PEDs will show areas of stippled hyperfluorescence with persistence of staining or leakage within a sensory retinal detachment overlying the area in the late phase of the angiogram. RPE detachments associated with large, soft, confluent drusen are usually smaller, more shallow, and more irregular in outline than are fibrovascular PEDs. In addition, the drusenoid RPE detachments will often have reticulated pigment clumping overlying the large, soft confluent drusen.

NATURAL COURSE AND INDICATIONS FOR TREATMENT

The interpretation of the fluorescein angiographic appearances of CNV secondary to AMD are used to determine whether or not laser treatment is indicated. The immediate goal of treatment in all clinical trials evaluating laser use for CNV[31, 32, 57–60] was to *photocoagulate the entire area of CNV*. In order to treat the entire area of CNV, the ophthalmologist has to be able to identify the boundaries of the choroidal neovascular lesion. Therefore, at the present time, treatment is indicated only when the boundaries of the CNV are well demarcated. The risks and benefits of treatment are further delineated depending on the location of the CNV with respect to the geometric center of the foveal avascular zone (FAZ).

Risks and Benefits of Treatment of Extrafoveal CNV (Posterior Boundary of CNV Between 200 and 2500 μ From Geometric Center of the FAZ)

In the MPS, laser treatment was beneficial at decreasing the risk of severe visual loss in eyes with extrafoveal CNV secondary to AMD when compared with no treatment.[59] The proportion of eyes with severe visual loss (6 lines or more of vision loss) 1 yr after presenting with extrafoveal CNV was 41 percent in the eyes assigned to no treatment and 24 percent in the eyes assigned to laser treatment. By 3 yr, 63 percent of the eyes assigned to no treatment and 45 percent of the eyes assigned to treatment had severe visual loss. This treatment benefit was maintained by 5 yr after treatment, at which time 64 percent of the eyes assigned to no treatment and 46 percent of the eyes assigned to treatment had severe visual loss (Fig. 65–11).[61] The relative risk of losing 6 lines or more of visual acuity from baseline among untreated eyes (n = 117) compared with laser-treated eyes (n = 119) was 1.5 from 6 mo through 5 yr after entry into the study (P = .001). Furthermore, after 5 yr, untreated eyes had lost a mean of 7.1 lines of visual acuity, whereas laser-treated eyes had lost 5.2 lines.

Recurrent CNV was observed in 54 percent of laser-treated eyes by the end of the 5-yr follow-up period (Fig. 65–12).[61] About 75 percent of all these recurrences occurred by the end of the first year after treatment. An additional 17 percent of all the recurrences occurred between 1 and 2 yr of follow-up. The remaining 7 percent of all recurrences occurred between the end of the second year and the fifth year of follow-up (Fig. 65–12). The effect of recurrence on visual acuity can be seen in Table 65–1; by 3 yr, only 10 percent of the treated eyes with no recurrence had severe visual loss compared with 80 percent of the treated eyes with recurrence. At the end of the third year of follow-up, the average visual acuity of the treated eyes with no recurrence was 20/50 and that of the treated eyes with

recurrence was 20/250.[61] This treatment benefit has been confirmed by two independent trials comparing treatment and the natural course.[57, 58]

Risks and Benefits of Treatment of Juxtafoveal CNV (Posterior Boundary of Neovascular Lesion 1 to 199 μ From Geometric Center of FAZ)

With the initial success of the MPS findings for CNV in which the posterior boundary was greater than 199 μ from the geometric center of the FAZ, the MPS investigators examined the role of photocoagulation in which treatment was permitted up to the geometric center of the FAZ. Specifically, lesions in this study included the following: (1) lesions in which the posterior edge of the CNV was between 1 and 199 μ from the center of the FAZ and (2) lesions in which the posterior edge of the CNV was between 200 and 2500 μ from the center with associated blood or blocked fluorescence, or both, in which the blood or blocked fluorescence extended to within 200 μ of the FAZ center. The treatment protocol differed from the MPS investigation of extrafoveal lesions. Specifically, for extrafoveal lesions treatment was required to extend 100 μ beyond all boundaries of the CNV. In the study of juxtafoveal lesions, the MPS investigators did not want to extend treatment *through* the foveal center. Therefore, the treatment protocol still called for treatment to extend 100 μ beyond the CNV on the *nonfoveal* side; however, on the *foveal* side of the lesion, treatment was to extend only up to the boundary of the CNV. When the posterior boundary of the CNV was greater than 100 μ from the foveal center *and* blood was present on the foveal side of the CNV, treatment was to extend 100 μ into the blood.[60]

In the MPS study of juxtafoveal CNV secondary to AMD, treatment was beneficial when compared with no treatment. Specifically, 45 percent of the eyes assigned to no treatment, compared with 31 percent of the eyes

Table 65–1. VISUAL ACUITY BY HISTORY OF RECURRENCE AFTER LASER TREATMENT OF EXTRAFOVEAL CHOROIDAL NEOVASCULARIZATION SECONDARY TO AGE-RELATED MACULAR DEGENERATION

Years Since Treatment	Recurrence	Number of Eyes	Average Visual Acuity	Eyes with 6-line Loss n (%)
1	No	62	20/40	4 (6)
	Yes	49	20/125	20 (41)
2	No	49	20/40	4 (8)
	Yes	54	20/160	31 (57)
3	No	48	20/50	5 (10)
	Yes	46	20/250	37 (80)
4	No	43	20/50	5 (12)
	Yes	47	20/250	37 (79)
5	No	42	20/50	7 (17)
	Yes	50	20/250	39 (78)

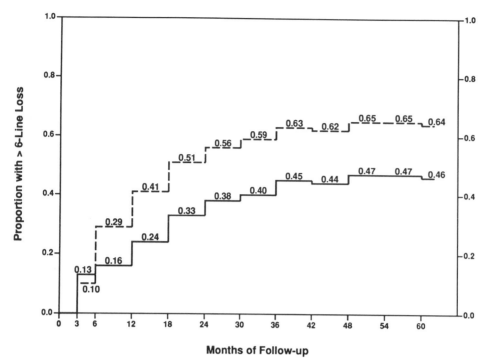

Figure 65–11. Proportion of eyes at each follow-up examination with decrease in visual acuity of six or more lines from baseline in the Senile Macular Degeneration Study of the MPS. *Dashed line* indicates eyes assigned randomly at entry to no treatment, and *solid line,* eyes assigned at entry to laser treatment. All eyes at baseline (time zero) had well-demarcated extrafoveal CNV. (From Macular Photocoagulation Study Group: Argon laser photocoagulation for neovascular maculopathy after five years. Results from randomized clinical trials. Arch Ophthalmol 109:1109–1114, 1991. Copyright 1991, American Medical Association.)

assigned to treatment, had severe visual loss by 1 yr after entry into the study. This treatment benefit was somewhat diminished by 3 yr after entry but persisted even after 5 yr from entry into the study (Fig. 65–13). As in the MPS trial of extrafoveal CNV, a high proportion of treated eyes had recurrence, often within the first year following treatment (Fig. 65–14).[62] Thirty-two percent of the treated eyes had evidence of leakage from CNV within 6 wk following treatment. An additional 22 percent of the treated eyes had recurrence within the first year.

The term *persistence* was used by the MPS group to indicate the presence of recurrent CNV, or more specifically the presence of fluorescein leakage on the *periphery* of the foveal side of the laser scar within 6 wk following treatment. The investigators felt that fluorescein leakage within this time might represent *persistence* of neovascularization. The MPS investigators chose to use the term *recurrence* when angiography confirmed no leakage for at least 6 wk following treatment, with leakage subsequently noted sometime after 6 wk following treatment.[62] These terms were strictly defined for

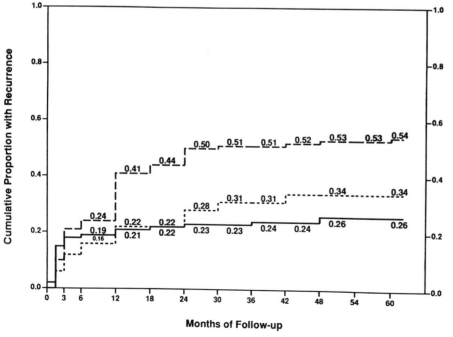

Figure 65–12. Cumulative proportion of laser-treated eyes ever having recurrent CNV documented after initial laser treatment. *Dashed line* indicates eyes assigned to laser treatment in the senile macular degeneration study in which patients had extrafoveal CNV secondary to age-related macular degeneration. For comparison to a cumulative proportion of recurrences following treatment of CNV secondary to other etiologies, *solid line* indicates eyes assigned to laser treatment in the ocular histoplasmosis study, and *dotted line,* eyes in the idiopathic neovascularization study. (From Macular Photocoagulation Study Group: Argon laser photocoagulation for neovascular maculopathy after five years. Results from randomized clinical trials. Arch Ophthalmol 109:1109–1114, 1991. Copyright 1991, American Medical Association.)

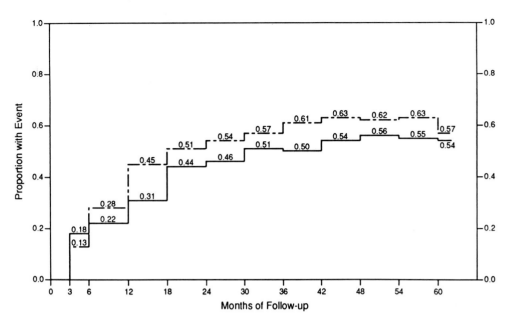

Figure 65–13. Mean change in lines of visual acuity from baseline at each specified time. *Broken line* indicates no-treatment group; *solid line,* treatment group. All eyes had juxtafoveal CNV secondary to age-related macular degeneration at time zero. (From Macular Photocoagulation Study Group: Krypton laser photocoagulation for neovascular lesions of age-related macular degeneration. Results of a randomized clinical trial. Arch Ophthalmol 108:816–824, 1990. Copyright 1990, American Medical Association.)

analysis of the data from these trials. However, one could consider using the term *recurrence* whenever the following conditions apply: (1) leakage is seen at the periphery of a laser scar and (2) one has previously documented unequivocal lack of peripheral leakage following treatment. A *persistence* could be defined as leakage at the periphery of the laser scar without any prior unequivocal documentation of lack of peripheral leakage on prior fluorescein angiograms. As with extrafoveal lesions, persistence or recurrence following treatment of juxtafoveal CNV had an adverse effect on visual acuity, as shown in Table 65–2. It is unknown whether a more extensive area of treatment, as was done for

extrafoveal lesions (in which treatment extended for 100 μ beyond the CNV boundaries, even on the foveal side), would have resulted in a better or worse treatment benefit.

Risks and Benefits of Treatment of Subfoveal CNV (CNV Lies Under the Geometric Center of the FAZ)

In 1986, the MPS group initiated two randomized clinical trials of laser treatment for subfoveal choroidal

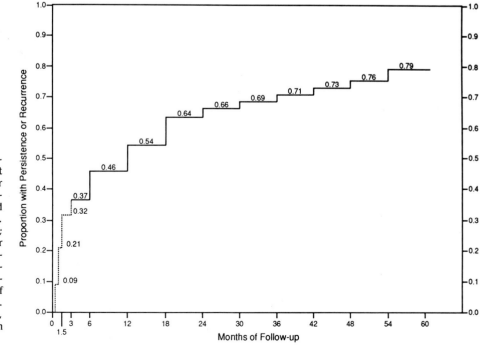

Figure 65–14. Cumulative proportion of treated eyes with persistent or recurrent CNV following laser treatment of well-demarcated juxtafoveal CNV secondary to age-related macular degeneration at time zero. *Dotted line* represents persistence; *solid line,* recurrence. (From Macular Photocoagulation Study Group: Persistent and recurrent neovascularization after krypton laser photocoagulation for neovascular lesions of age-related macular degeneration. Arch Ophthalmol 108:825–831, 1990. Copyright 1990, American Medical Association.)

Table 65–2. VISUAL ACUITY BY ANGIOGRAPHIC STATUS OF LEAKAGE AFTER LASER TREATMENT OF JUXTAFOVEAL CHOROIDAL NEOVASCULARIZATION SECONDARY TO AGE-RELATED MACULAR DEGENERATION

Time Since Treatment	Angiographic Status	Number of Eyes	Average Visual Acuity	Eyes With >5.5-line Loss n (%)
1	No previous leakage	58	20/80	6 (10)
	Persistence	74	20/160	28 (38)
	Recurrence	93	20/160	33 (36)
2	No previous leakage	52	20/100	7 (14)
	Persistence	64	20/200	35 (55)
	Recurrence	86	20/250	50 (58)
3	No previous leakage	44	20/100	9 (21)
	Persistence	53	20/200	29 (55)
	Recurrence	71	20/250	47 (66)
4	No previous leakage	25	20/80	4 (16)
	Persistence	36	20/200	21 (58)
	Recurrence	52	20/250	36 (69)

neovascular lesions secondary to AMD. One trial was initiated for subfoveal CNV in eyes with *no previous photocoagulation* in the macula, and a companion trial was initiated for subfoveal *recurrent* neovascularization that developed following laser treatment of extrafoveal or juxtafoveal neovascularization.

In the trial for subfoveal CNV in eyes with no previous laser treatment,[33] laser was beneficial with respect to visual acuity, reading speed, and contrast sensitivity compared with no treatment, although there was an immediate decrease in visual acuity following treatment. Three months after enrollment, 20 percent of laser-treated eyes, compared with 11 percent of untreated eyes, had lost 6 lines or more of visual acuity from the baseline level. However, 24 mo after enrollment, only 20 percent of laser-treated eyes, compared with 37 percent of untreated eyes, had lost 6 lines or more of visual acuity. Laser-treated eyes retained contrast threshold for large letters at or near baseline levels throughout 36 mo of follow-up examinations, whereas the contrast threshold of untreated eyes worsened. Furthermore, median reading speed was greater in laser-treated eyes when compared with untreated eyes at 24 mo after enrollment. Subsequent persistent or recurrent neovascularization was observed in 51 percent of the laser-treated eyes by 24 mo after initial treatment, but unlike the earlier MPS trials of extrafoveal or juxtafoveal lesions, persistence or recurrence in this subfoveal trial was not associated with a worse visual acuity outcome.

In the trial for subfoveal *recurrent* neovascularization,[34] laser treatment was beneficial with respect to visual acuity, reading speed, and contrast sensitivity when compared with no treatment, although there was an immediate decrease in visual acuity following treatment. Three months after enrollment, 14 percent of laser-treated eyes, compared with 9 percent of untreated eyes, had lost 6 or more lines of visual acuity from the baseline level. However, 24 mo after randomization, the findings were reversed: 9 percent of laser-treated eyes, compared with 28 percent of untreated eyes, had lost 6

lines or more of visual acuity ($P = .03$). On average, treated eyes maintained the initial level of contrast threshold for large letters, whereas the contrast threshold of untreated eyes worsened steadily throughout 24 mo of follow-up. Also, untreated eyes read fewer words per minute than did treated eyes by 24 mo after entry into the study. About half of the treated eyes had persistent or recurrent leakage at the periphery of the laser scar following treatment.

It should be emphasized that the results of these MPS clinical trials on subfoveal lesions may apply only to lesions that met the eligibility criteria of the study. Specifically, the subfoveal lesions in the MPS trials were to have evidence of classic CNV, well-demarcated lesion boundaries, and size less than or equal to 3.5 disc diameters (if no previous treatment of CNV had been performed in the macula). In the case of subfoveal recurrent CNV, the size had to be such that after treatment of the recurrence, the final treatment scar (prior treatment scar plus new treatment) would be no larger than 6 disc areas and would spare some retina within 1500 μ of the center of the FAZ. With these criteria in mind, a large number of lesions that present to ophthalmologists with subfoveal CNV still may not benefit from laser treatment. Specifically, eyes in which there is no evidence of classic CNV within the lesion (Fig. 65–15) or in which the boundaries of the neovascular lesion are not well demarcated (Fig. 65–16) or in which the lesion is larger than the size criteria used in the MPS trials may derive no benefit or may even be worse with laser treatment when compared with no treatment. Subgroup analysis of the subfoveal trials suggests that treatment benefit diminishes with larger lesions that were entered into the study, as well as with lesions that were deemed ineligible, mainly because the boundaries of the lesion were not well demarcated.[33] One would expect that had the MPS trials expanded eligibility to subfoveal lesions that were even larger than the maximal size criteria listed for the study, any treatment benefit might completely disappear. Similar lack of treatment benefit may have occurred had the trial been extended to include lesions with poorly demarcated boundaries. Therefore, when considering treatment of subfoveal lesions, the results of the MPS trials apply only to lesions that are similar to those that meet the eligibility criteria of the trial. When treatment is contemplated, the patient and ophthalmologist should realize that a large loss of visual acuity may occur immediately following treatment and that such a course is being recommended only because this large loss of visual acuity probably will be better than an even larger loss of visual acuity, contrast threshold, and ability to read large letters in eyes without treatment when followed for 2 yr or more.[33, 34]

LASER TREATMENT TECHNIQUE FOR CNV

The principle of photocoagulation is that laser light is absorbed by pigment in the RPE and choroid and is then converted into heat, which dissipates into the

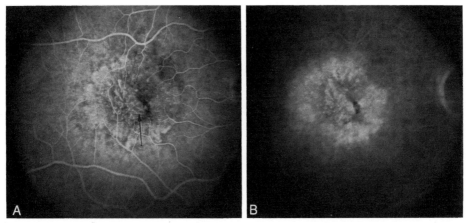

Figure 65–15. A, Lesion with occult CNV with well-demarcated boundaries, but no classic CNV. Early phase of angiogram shows hyperfluorescence from occult CNV with no evidence of classic CNV. Note retinal pigment epithelial folds *(arrow)*. Lesion does not meet eligibility criteria of the MPS because no part of the lesion has classic CNV, even though boundaries of the entire lesion are well demarcated. B, Late phase of angiogram confirms leakage of occult CNV and, again, no angiographic evidence of classic CNV. (A and B, From Macular Photocoagulation Study Group: Subfoveal neovascular lesions in age-related macular degeneration. Guidelines for evaluation and treatment in the Macular Photocoagulation Study. Arch Ophthalmol 109:1242–1257, 1991. Copyright 1991, American Medical Association.)

adjacent tissues. If CNV is adjacent to an area of photocoagulation, it may be ablated by coagulation necrosis. Clinicopathologic correlative studies[63] suggest that the CNV may not become ablated completely by the laser. Rather, the neovascular lesion may become enveloped by multiple layers of RPE fibrous tissue and that this laser-induced scar limits continued growth of the neovascular lesion and therefore limits the extent of retina that would otherwise be destroyed by the natural course of the neovascular lesion. Laboratory evidence suggests that proliferation of the RPE following laser

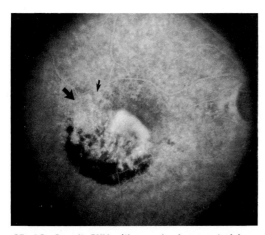

Figure 65–16. Occult CNV with poorly demarcated boundaries accompanied by classic CNV. Middle phase of angiogram demonstrates inability of determining boundaries of occult CNV. Borders of elevated RPE *(large arrow)* slope gradually downward to surrounding flat RPE *(small arrow)* so that sharp demarcation between elevated RPE and flat RPE cannot be determined with certainty. Lesion does not meet MPS criteria for consideration of treatment because the entire lesion is not well demarcated. (From Macular Photocoagulation Study Group: Subfoveal neovascular lesions in age-related macular degeneration. Guidelines for evaluation and treatment in the Macular Photocoagulation Study. Arch Ophthalmol 109:1242–1257, 1991. Copyright 1991, American Medical Association.)

treatment may play a role in treating CNV by enveloping the CNV and absorbing the fluid that separates the neovascularization from the overlying sensory retina.[64–66]

Preparation

An angiogram is projected onto a screen near the laser so that the ophthalmologist can make rapid and repeated extrapolations from the fluorescein's retinal vascular landmarks to the patient's fundus when identifying the location of the CNV with respect to these landmarks. Careful evaluation of vascular landmarks in the patient's fundus in comparison with landmarks concurrently viewed on a projection of a fluorescein angiogram during treatment should enable the ophthalmologist to identify the boundaries of the lesion with confidence and accuracy and avoid inadvertent treatment of retina that is not involved with the lesion.

Retrobulbar anesthesia may be used whenever necessary to ensure that neither ocular motility nor patient discomfort will compromise the success of treatment by preventing the ophthalmologist from delivering laser of sufficient intensity and duration of exposure to produce a uniform white treatment burn. This is especially true when treating near or within the FAZ, when there is a natural reluctance to treat on the foveal side of the lesion,[62, 67] and when small amounts of undertreatment may allow persistence of neovascularization[62, 67] or small amounts of overtreatment might obliterate foveal structures unnecessarily.

Treatment Parameters

Initial laser burns are placed along the boundary of the CNV using a 200-μ spot size and 0.2- to 0.5-sec duration. These parameters allow the ophthalmologist to get sufficient heat to the retina (with the long duration) without risking a sudden break in Bruch's membrane and minimize the frequency of bleeding (by spreading the intensity of the burn over a 200-μ spot rather than a 50- or 100-μ spot). The area to be covered, if one is following the protocol used in the MPS, differs depending on the location of the lesion and is outlined in Table 65–3. After the boundaries of the lesion have been treated, the area within the boundaries is treated subsequently with burns of the same spot size or larger, using a duration of 0.5 to 1 sec. The desired end-point for the intensity of the laser lesion is to create a uniformly white lesion. The ophthalmologist can achieve this end-point in either of the following ways: (1) by initially applying white laser burns that meet or exceed the intensity illustrated by a standard photograph from the MPS[60] or (2) by applying lighter gray-white laser spots that overlap again and again until the entire laser lesion is a uniform white treatment burn at least as white as the treatment intensity standard (Fig. 65–17).[30]

Wavelength Selection

When the MPS was begun in 1978, the argon blue-green laser was the one most commercially available to investigators. This laser is no longer recommended for treatment within the macular region because macular xanthophyll pigment directly absorbs the blue light of

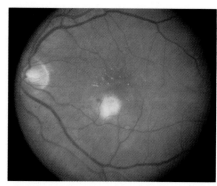

Figure 65–17. Treatment intensity standard. Treatment protocol of the MPS specified a uniform, white burn at least as intense as the treatment standard. (From Macular Photocoagulation Study Group: Persistent and recurrent neovascularization after krypton laser photocoagulation for neovascular lesions of ocular histoplasmosis. Arch Ophthalmol 107:344–352, 1989. Copyright 1989, American Medical Association.)

the argon blue-green laser, thereby inducing thermal damage to the inner retina.[68] In addition, the risk of inducing internal limiting membrane wrinkling, although rarely of clinical significance, is probably greatest with the argon blue-green laser.[69] Subsequent trials in the MPS for juxtafoveal lesions employed the krypton red laser because of its theoretical advantage of penetrating through xanthophyll and passing through thin layers of red hemorrhage, allowing the uptake of the laser to be concentrated within the RPE and melanocytes of the inner choroid. When the MPS trials for subfoveal lesions were designed, eyes randomized to the treatment group were further randomized to either the argon green or the krypton red wavelength for treatment. None of the findings from the subfoveal trials suggests a reason to favor either the argon green or the krypton red wavelength.[33, 34] If there was any theoretical advantage to using one wavelength over another for treatment of CNV, one might have expected to have detected a difference within the MPS subfoveal trials. Although these trials did not have sufficient power to demonstrate a small or moderate difference between the two wavelengths, a large difference has been ruled out by these studies.[33, 34] Recurrence and persistence rates also were similar between the two laser wavelengths. The recurrence and persistence rates were similar to those observed when the krypton red laser alone was used to treat neovascular lesions in the MPS trial of juxtafoveal neovascularization. Thus, no visible wavelength appears to have a *significant* advantage over other wavelengths. Small differences in convenience of achieving the end-point of a uniform white burn might be seen with red or yellow wavelengths when penetrating through the increased nuclear yellow in the older age group afflicted with CNV secondary to AMD, but any significant differences of clinical importance have not been shown.

Special Circumstances

When treating CNV that lies under a major retinal vessel, the laser burns should straddle the retinal vessel

Table 65–3. TREATMENT PROTOCOL FOR CHOROIDAL NEOVASCULARIZATION FROM THE MACULAR PHOTOCOAGULATION STUDY

All Lesions
Angiogram <96 hr old
Retrobulbar anesthesia as necessary
200–500-μ spot; 0.2–0.5-sec duration
Cover entire area of neovascular lesion
Intensity sufficient to produce uniform white burn

Extrafoveal Lesions
(>199 μ from Foveal Center)
Extend treatment additional 100 μ beyond any adjacent blood, pigment ring circumferentially surrounding the lesion, or other blocked fluorescence surrounding the lesion

Juxtafoveal Lesions
(1–199 μ from Foveal Center)
Extend treatment additional 100 μ beyond the neovascular lesion on border away from fovea
Extend treatment additional 100 μ into any blood present on the foveal side if the hyperfluorescence from the neovascular lesion itself is 100 μ or further from foveal center

Subfoveal Lesions
(CNV Underlies Foveal Center)
Extend treatment additional 100 μ beyond peripheral boundaries of all lesion components except blood
Cover, but not necessarily extend 100 μ beyond areas of blocked fluorescence into thick blood

Subfoveal Recurrent Lesions
(Prior Laser Treatment with Recurrent Lesion Underlying Foveal Center)
Extend treatment 300 μ into previous treatment scar–recurrent neovascular lesion interface
If feeder vessels present, extend treatment 100 μ beyond lateral borders of recurrent vessels and 300 μ radially beyond base (origin) of feeder vessel

to reduce the possibility of causing hemorrhage or damaging the vessel by thermal vasculitis. There is no evidence to suggest that this technique compromises the effectiveness of treatment.

When treating CNV that is contiguous with the optic nerve, one must consider that laser treatment directly over the optic nerve can cause thermal necrosis of disc tissue and nerve fiber bundle defects.[70] Therefore, one should consider refraining from treatment within 100 to 200 μ of the optic nerve. Similarly, when treating a parapapillary area of CNV, one may want to consider treatment only when at least 1½ clock hr of papillomacular bundle on the temporal side of the disc can be spared, as was done in several of the MPS trials.[59, 71]

Certain subgroups in the various trials had different treatment benefits, which should be considered when determining whether treatment would be beneficial for a particular patient. This subgroup analysis should probably not *completely* sway someone in recommending or denying treatment. Rather, the subgroup analysis data should serve as a *guideline* when trying to decide whether treatment should be recommended to a *particular individual*. For instance, in the krypton trial of juxtafoveal lesions,[60] patients who were normotensive had a marked treatment benefit. Patients who had evidence of hypertension, either by elevated systolic or diastolic blood pressures or by the use of antihypertensive medications, had no treatment benefit. Although similar trends were noted in the argon trial for patients with CNV secondary to the ocular histoplasmosis syndrome,[71] similar trends were *not* noted in the argon trial of CNV secondary to AMD[72] nor in the subfoveal trials in AMD.[33, 34] Therefore, although the data in the juxtafoveal trial were strikingly against a treatment benefit for hypertensive patients, lack of corroboration of this finding in two other prospective trials on CNV secondary to AMD cautions one from withholding treatment in patients who are hypertensive.

In the subfoveal trials, subgroup analysis showed that the greatest treatment benefit was noted in lesions that were less than 2 disc areas in size. The treatment benefit was smaller and took a longer time to become significantly different from no treatment when the lesions were larger than 2 disc areas.[33] Thus, one may want to consider treatment whenever the subfoveal lesion is small, even when the visual acuity is fairly good (20/40 to 20/100), since the likelihood of rapid, severe visual loss without treatment is so much greater than it is with treatment. However, one may want to consider withholding treatment from a patient with a large lesion centered on the foveal center in whom the visual acuity is relatively good (20/40 to 20/100), since treatment may cause a rapid, marked deterioration in vision and eyes with no treatment will take several years to become worse than treated eyes. Also, since the benefits of treatment in large lesions may not be realized until 18 mo following treatment, one may want to consider the general health of the patient and his or her likelihood of living long enough to benefit from the treatment.[73]

Treatment of RPE detachments may be indicated when one is treating a subfoveal lesion, and an RPE detachment is a component of that lesion. However, classic CNV should be the major component of the lesion, not the RPE detachment. Furthermore, the RPE detachment should have well-demarcated boundaries and include only serous detachments of RPE, fibrovascular RPE detachments, or elevated blocked fluorescence caused by a hemorrhagic RPE detachment or hyperplastic pigment or scarring. Drusenoid RPE detachments should not be included as a component to be treated in conjunction with subfoveal CNV.

Most RPE detachments are not eligible for treatment, even when they do not represent drusenoid RPE detachments, because the boundaries of the CNV usually are not well demarcated or classic CNV is not the major component of the lesion.

On rare occasion, a patient will present with extrafoveal classic CNV contiguous to a serous detachment of the RPE in which the serous detachment extends through the foveal center. There have been case reports in which only the extrafoveal CNV in these lesions is treated, resulting in prompt flattening of the RPE detachment with improvement of vision in selected cases.[74] Nevertheless, many of these eyes have acquired recurrent CNV with extensive scarring and visual loss, and more often the classic extrafoveal CNV is associated with fibrovascular PED through the foveal center in which treatment of the extrafoveal CNV alone has not been shown to be of any benefit.

POSTOPERATIVE MANAGEMENT

Evaluating Extent of Laser Treatment With Extent of CNV

Data from the MPS group have shown that eyes in which laser treatment did not cover the CNV completely on the foveal side or did not meet the required level of intensity (a uniform white burn, as shown in Fig. 65–17) had approximately three times the risk of having persistent CNV within 6 wk following treatment compared with eyes in which the CNV was covered completely by intense, confluent burns.[67] Because of this information, it is essential not only to obtain a uniform white laser burn during treatment but also to ensure that the extent of the intense confluent burns completely covers the extent of the CNV. This may be especially true for juxtafoveal lesions.

When CNV is not very close to the foveal center, it usually is not difficult for an ophthalmologist who is experienced in treating CNV to extend laser treatment over the entire extent of the CNV.[59, 71] There is probably little hesitancy in extending treatment slightly beyond the borders of the CNV in an effort to ensure adequate coverage when the CNV is far away from the foveal center. Slight extension of treatment should have little effect on the visual acuity, since the treatment in these situations will not affect central foveal photoreceptors.

Conversely, when one is treating a juxtafoveal lesion, even the most experienced ophthalmologist may be reluctant to treat the foveal perimeter of the CNV too extensively.[62, 67] Excessive treatment in this situation could easily contribute to visual loss. However, failure to cover the CNV in its entirety could lead to increased persistence within 6 wk following treatment, as was shown in the MPS trials.[62, 67]

In an attempt to minimize persistent CNV caused by inadequate coverage, one may evaluate the laser treatment by comparing the area of laser treatment from a posttreatment photograph (such as a 35-mm Polaroid transparency) to the area of the lesion to be covered from the pretreatment angiogram.[23, 75, 76] The MPS group has described their methods for this evaluation.[76] In step 1, the extent and location of the CNV with respect to the vascular landmarks (Fig. 65–18 A) is traced on a piece of plain white paper that is taped to the screen of a microfilm reader upon which the pretreatment angiogram is projected. Alternatively, a clear piece of acetate paper can be taped to a projection device such as a Topcon viewer. In step 2, immediately after treatment, a posttreatment 35-mm Polaroid transparency (Polaroid Polapan 35-mm film, CT–135–36) is taken. This Polaroid

transparency is then projected, and the area of heavy treatment and the same landmark vessels are outlined on a separate piece of plain white paper (with the microfilm reader) or acetate paper (with a projection viewer) (Fig. 65–18B). In step 3, the treatment drawing from step 2 is placed on a light box, and the pretreatment drawing from step 1 is placed over this, superimposing the landmark vessels. The area of heavy treatment can then be traced onto the pretreatment drawing to determine whether the treatment has covered the CNV in its entirety (Fig. 65–18C). Any areas not adequately treated can be "touched up" while the patient is still in the office. The MPS group proved the usefulness of this method *using 1-day posttreatment stereoscopic color photographs;* areas of inadequate treatment were identified, and these eyes did indeed have a higher rate of persistent CNV in the juxtafoveal trials.[62, 67] It is unknown whether *immediate* posttreatment Polaroid photographs or videotape image evaluations would be more, equally, or less accurate than the 1-day posttreatment stereoscopic color photographs used in the MPS trials.

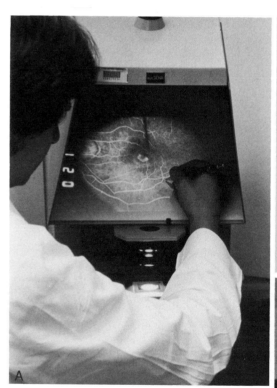

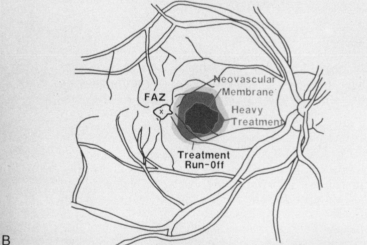

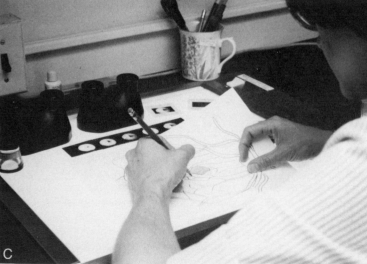

Figure 65–18. Evaluation of CNV treatment. Angiogram is projected onto an apparatus (such as a microfilm reader or slide viewer) such that the CNV and key landmarks around the CNV such as subretinal blood, retinal vessels, and foveal center can be drawn (A). FAZ indicates the foveal avascular zone and *x* indicates foveal center (B). A posttreatment photograph is then projected and the area of heavy treatment and the same landmark vessels can be outlined on a separate piece of paper (C). Evaluation of photocoagulation treatment can be determined by placing the treatment drawing (C) under the pretreatment drawing (A) on a lightbox. The area of heavy treatment can then be traced onto the pretreatment drawing to determine whether the treatment has covered the CNV entirely. (A–C, From Bressler NM, Bressler SB, Fine SL: Age-related macular degeneration. Surv Ophthalmol 32:375–413, 1988.)

Follow-up Evaluations

A follow-up evaluation that includes best-corrected vision, fluorescein angiography, and biomicroscopy of the fundus is obtained 2 or 3 wk following treatment. Follow-up earlier than 2 wk is often difficult to evaluate because swelling and leakage from the treatment itself may obscure persistent or recurrent CNV. At follow-up, an angiogram should be scrutinized for the presence of leakage at the periphery of the laser scar to identify the presence of persistent or recurrent CNV. Simultaneous projection of the fluorescein angiogram during biomicroscopy may help differentiate areas of atrophy, which stain from areas of recurrent leakage. If no residual or recurrent CNV is noted at this time, a similar evaluation is repeated 2 or 3 wk later because the risk of recurrent CNV is so high within the first 6 wk to 12 mo following treatment. By 6 wk following treatment, a patient should be encouraged to monitor the central vision of the treated eye daily for clarity of distance and near vision, as well as for any distortion, blurred vision, or increase in scotoma. These latter symptoms might indicate leakage from persistent or recurrent CNV and are an indication for prompt examination. The ophthalmologist's office staff also should be aware that these patients may need prompt reevaluation if such symptoms develop and not necessarily schedule such patients for the "next available opening" 2 or 3 wk later. Furthermore, although the risk of recurrent CNV following treatment in eyes with AMD is high, the recent results showing the benefits of treatment make follow-up warranted for identifying these recurrences before they become large.

Since many recurrences occur within 3 to 6 mo following treatment, an evaluation, including fluorescein angiography, is again repeated at 3 and 6 mo. Subsequent evaluations, probably with angiography, at 9 and 12 mo appear to be indicated for CNV secondary to AMD that has been treated because many recurrences develop between 6 and 12 mo following treatment. After 2 yr, recurrences are unusual; follow-up every 6 mo without angiography (unless signs or symptoms suggest a recurrence) is probably sufficient.

Predicting Recurrences

It may be possible to reduce the risk of persistent CNV after treatment by ensuring that a uniform white laser treatment covers the extent of the CNV in its entirety. However, in the MPS trials for extrafoveal and juxtafoveal lesions secondary to AMD, recurrences also were likely if the fellow eye already had CNV-scarring at the time of treatment of the study eye. If no CNV-scarring is present in the fellow eye at the time of treatment of the first eye, studies have suggested that the presence of large drusen in the macula of the fellow eye is associated with an increased risk of recurrence developing in the first eye. Other factors that might increase the rate of recurrence include cigarette smoking,[77] hypertension,[77] and CNV that is very lightly pig-

mented.[38] This last finding may be a reflection of the difficulty in obtaining a uniform white confluent treatment in CNV that is very lightly pigmented, and the inability to obtain a uniform white treatment burn is associated with an increased risk of persistent CNV following treatment.

Risk of Fellow Eye Involvement With Subsequent CNV-Scarring

It is important to have the patient monitor the vision in the fellow eye if its macula does not already have CNV-scarring. The MPS group has shown that if a patient presents with an extrafoveal CNV in one eye and no evidence of CNV or scarring in the fellow eye, about one third of these eyes will have CNV in the fellow eye within 5 yr.[78] The risk of CNV developing in these eyes may be further specified depending on the drusen and RPE abnormalities present in the fellow eye at baseline.[1] The risk of CNV developing in the fellow eye within 5 yr after presenting with extrafoveal CNV in the first eye was 10 percent for those eyes presenting with only small drusen, approximately 30 percent in eyes presenting with either large drusen or focal clumps of RPE hyperpigmentation, and approximately 60 percent for eyes presenting with both large drusen and focal clumps of RPE hyperpigmentation within 1500 μ of the foveal center.[1] As one might have suspected, for the fellow eyes that had no evidence of CNV or scarring at baseline and subsequently developed CNV within 5 yr, the average visual acuity loss was 8 lines of vision.[78] In contrast, for the two thirds of fellow eyes that had no evidence of CNV or scarring at baseline and did not have CNV within 5 yr, the average visual acuity loss was less than half a line of vision (specifically, 0.4 line).[78] Therefore, the risk of moderate or severe loss of visual acuity is highly correlated with the development of CNV during follow-up. Eyes that do not acquire CNV during follow-up have little or no visual acuity loss. This finding should be considered when evaluating the role of vitamins, minerals, or other treatment modalities in preventing visual acuity loss for eyes with drusen or RPE abnormalities without the presence of CNV or scarring.

If one couples this information of fellow eye involvement with success of treatment in the first eye from the extrafoveal argon MPS trial, one can determine the risk of legal blindness (visual acuity of 20/200 or worse in both eyes) when treating the first eye. The risk of legal blindness, again, is highly correlated with whether or not the fellow eye had CNV or scarring at baseline. If CNV or scarring was present in the fellow eye at baseline, it was likely that the fellow eye already had significant loss of visual acuity and that there was a high risk of recurrence developing in the treated eye. Forty-nine percent of patients in the argon AMD MPS trial were legally blind within 5 yr of follow-up when the fellow eye initially had CNV or scarring, whereas only 12 percent of patients were legally blind within 5 yr of follow-up when the fellow eye had no evidence of CNV or scarring initially.[78] Of course, if the visual acuity of the fellow eye is compromised at all, and the first eye has CNV, low-vision aids are probably indicated to assist with magnification for near visual tasks, as are telescopic aids for spotting at distance.

Low-vision Aids

Patients who have central visual impairment in both eyes should be advised about the availability of a variety of low-vision aids. A low-vision evaluation includes not only prescribing appropriate lenses, magnifying aids, and other items of assistance but also properly training and encouraging the patient to use them. Patients should also be told of community resources available to assist them with visual impairment such as might be obtained from the directory of agencies serving the visually handicapped in the United States provided by the American Foundation for the Blind. A realistic appraisal of the prognosis coupled with appropriate counseling and support is necessary to enable the visually impaired patient to continue functioning as normally as possible despite the central visual impairment. The American Foundation for the Blind can also inform patients as to which aids, such as talking books, large-print books, watches that "tell" time, closed circuit television readers, and other devices, are available through the directory of products for people with vision problems.

Visual aids for detailed near and distance tasks, such as reading, writing, typing, sedentary distance viewing, and distance spotting for street signs, can be prescribed with a thorough low-vision examination conducted in a room with glare-free high-intensity lighting and large trial lenses to allow for eccentric fixation. There is a wide range of magnification levels available in the present armamentarium of low-vision aids. Some incorporate their own illumination source. Each aid has certain advantages and limitations, so a patient must decide with a low-vision aid specialist what combination of aids is best for his or her visual objectives and visual needs.

There are four types of reading aids available: reading glasses, hand-held lenses, stand magnifiers, and electronic devices. Reading glasses (convex lenses) provide relatively large fields of vision, but the strongest lenses require short working distances. Telescopic reading glasses increase the working distance; however, they allow a relatively smaller field of view and shorter depth of focus than a simple high plus reader of comparable magnification. Hand-held magnifiers may suffice for quick, simple tasks that are conducted at arm's length, such as adjusting a stove dial. A stand magnifier consists of a mounted lens that will remain in focus if placed on the reading material and held so that its focal point corresponds to the focal point of the patient's near correction. This device offers an alternative to the high plus lens for the weak or tremulous patient; it is also useful when the patient wishes an increase in working distance or wants to have an illumination source incorporated into the magnifying system. Closed circuit television provides electronic magnification at greater levels than is possible with optical systems. It also provides

binocular viewing and can be used at a comfortable reading distance. Unfortunately, it is usually not portable and remains costly. Writing assistance may be provided with a weak hand lens or a +5.00 add-in spectacle. Additional invaluable and simple tools to aid in writing include signature guides, black felt-tip pens, and bold wide-ruled paper.

Distance vision may be enhanced with binocular field glasses and opera glasses. Lightweight telescopes can be hand-held or mounted onto spectacles. Unfortunately, these instruments distort distances and limit peripheral vision; therefore, their applicability is limited to tasks of sedentary distance viewing and distance spotting.

Finally, the success of each of these aids is highly variable, depending on the visual deficit and the motivation of the patient. They can only attempt to enhance lighting or magnification for the remaining vision. The patient should not look on them as a treatment for macular degeneration nor expect to regain central vision. Nevertheless, it is important to give these patients every opportunity to be evaluated for and trained in the use of optical and nonoptical systems that may serve to improve the quality of life.

CONCLUSIONS AND FUTURE RESEARCH

The decade of the 1980s provided enormous progress in the management of AMD. Specifically, laser treatment has been shown to be beneficial when compared with no treatment. However, the fact that laser treatment is more beneficial for preserving vision when compared with observation alone is only a start. Successful cases of laser treatment still result in central visual acuity loss for the patient, especially when treatment involves the foveal center as it so often does in AMD.

Therefore, future research will have to evaluate other modalities of treatment that do not cause destruction of the foveal center or therapies that prevent the development of CNV in the first place. Such investigations will require interdisciplinary approaches to this problem that will probably include epidemiologists, clinicians, psychophysicists, vitreoretinal surgeons, and cellular biologists. These investigations may include therapies to prevent the development of CNV or minimize the damage it causes. Medical interventions that affect angiogenesis may hold some promise. Surgical interventions that could remove the neovascular process before it destroys a large area of the central retina may also hold some promise.

REFERENCES

1. Bressler SB, Maguire MG, Bressler NM, Fine SL: Macular Photocoagulation Study Group: Relationship of drusen and abnormalities of the retinal pigment epithelium to the prognosis of neovascular macular degeneration. Arch Ophthalmol 108:1442–1447, 1990.
2. Gass JDM: Drusen and disciform macular detachment and degeneration. Arch Ophthalmol 90:206–217, 1973.

3. Smiddy WE, Fine SL: Prognosis of patients with bilateral macular drusen. Ophthalmology 91:271–277, 1984.
4. Strahlman E, Fine SL, Hillis A: The second eye of patients with senile macular degeneration. Arch Ophthalmol 101:1191–1193, 1983.
5. Green WR, McDonnell PH, Yeo JH: Pathologic features of senile macular degeneration. Ophthalmology 92:615–627, 1985.
6. Sarks SH: Ageing and degeneration in the macular region: A clinicopathologic study. Br J Ophthalmol 60:324–341, 1976.
7. Gass JDM: Pathogenesis of disciform detachment of the neuroepithelium. VI. Disciform detachment secondary to heredodegenerative, neoplastic and traumatic lesions of the choroid. Am J Ophthalmol 63:689, 1967.
8. Gass JDM, Clarkson JG: Angioid streaks and disciform macular detachment in Paget's disease (osteitis deformans). Am J Ophthalmol 75:576, 1973.
9. Heriot WJ, Henkind P, Bellhorn RW, Burns MS: Choroidal neovascularization can digest Bruch's membrane: A prior break is not essential. Ophthalmology 91:1603–1608, 1984.
10. Löffler KU, Lee WR: Basal linear deposit in the human macula. Graefes Arch Clin Exp Ophthalmol 224:493–501, 1986.
11. Penfold PL, Killingsworth MC, Sarks SH: Senile macular degeneration: The involvement of immunocompetent cells. Graefes Arch Clin Exp Ophthalmol 223:69–76, 1985.
12. Penfold PL, Provis JM, Billson FA: Age-related macular degeneration: Ultrastructural studies of the relationship of leucocytes to angiogenesis. Graefes Arch Clin Exp Ophthalmol 225:70–76, 1987.
13. Ryan SJ: Development of an experimental model of subretinal neovascularization in disciform macular degeneration. Trans Am Ophthalmol Soc 77:707–745, 1979.
14. Ryan SJ: Subretinal neovascularization: Natural history of an experimental model. Arch Ophthalmol 100:1804–1809, 1982.
15. Friedman E, Ivry M, Ebert E, et al: Increased scleral rigidity and age-related macular degeneration. Ophthalmology 96:104–108, 1989.
16. Broekhuyse RM: The lipid composition of the aging sclera and cornea. Ophthalmologica 171:82, 1975.
17. Bressler SB, Bressler NM, Alexander J, Green WR: Clinicopathologic correlation of occult choroidal neovascularization in age-related macular degeneration. Invest Ophthalmol Vis Sci 32:689, 1991.
18. Bressler SB, Bressler NM, Fine SL, et al: Natural course of choroidal neovascular membranes within the foveal avascular zone in senile macular degeneration. Am J Ophthalmol 93:157–163, 1982.
19. Bird AC: Macular disciform response and laser treatment. Trans Ophthalmol Soc UK 97:490–493, 1977.
20. Bressler NM, Frost LA, Bressler SB, et al: Natural course of poorly defined choroidal neovascularization associated with macular degeneration. Arch Ophthalmol 106:1537–1542, 1988.
21. Chandra SR, Gragoudas ES, Friedman E, et al: Natural history of disciform degeneration of the macula. Am J Ophthalmol 78:579–582, 1974.
22. Gragoudas ES, Chandra SR, Friedman E, et al: Disciform degeneration of the macula. II. Pathogenesis. Arch Ophthalmol 94:755–757, 1976.
23. Bressler NM, Bressler SB, Fine SL: Age-related macular degeneration. Surv Ophthalmol 32:375–413, 1988.
24. Boldt C, Bressler NM, Fine SL, Bressler SB: Age-related macular degeneration. Curr Opinion Ophthalmol 1:247–257, 1990.
25. Moisseiev J, Bressler NM: Asymptomatic neovascular membranes in the second eye of patients with visual loss from age-related macular degeneration (AMD). Invest Ophthalmol Vis Sci 31:462, 1990.
26. Fine AM, Elman MJ, Ebert JE, et al: Earliest symptoms caused by neovascular membranes in the macula. Arch Ophthalmol 104:513–514, 1986.
27. Nasrallah F, Jalkh AE, Trempe CL, et al: Subretinal hemorrhage in atrophic age-related macular degeneration. Am J Ophthalmol 107:38–41, 1989.
28. Small ML, Green WR, Alpar JJ, et al: Senile macular degeneration: Clinicopathologic correlation of two cases with neovascularization beneath the retinal pigment epithelium. Arch Ophthalmol 94:601–607, 1976.
29. Doyle WJ, Davidorf FH, Makley TA, Dieruf WJ: Histopathology of an active lesion of ocular histoplasmosis. Ophthalmic Forum 2:106–111, 1984.
30. Macular Photocoagulation Study Group: Subfoveal neovascular lesions in age-related macular degeneration: Guidelines for evaluation and treatment in the Macular Photocoagulation Study. Arch Ophthalmol 109:1242–1257, 1991.
31. Klein ML, Zorizzo PA, Watzke RC: Growth features of choroidal neovascular membranes in age-related macular degeneration. Ophthalmology 96:1416–1421, 1989.
32. Vander JF, Morgan CM, Schatz H: Growth rate of subretinal neovascularization in age-related macular degeneration. Ophthalmology 96:1422–1429, 1989.
33. Macular Photocoagulation Study Group: Laser photocoagulation of subfoveal neovascular lesions in age-related macular degeneration. Results of a randomized clinical trial. Arch Ophthalmol 109:1219–1231, 1991.
34. Macular Photocoagulation Study Group: Laser photocoagulation of subfoveal recurrent neovascular lesions in age-related macular degeneration. Results of a randomized clinical trial. Arch Ophthalmol 109:1232–1241, 1991.
35. Soubrane G, Coscas G, Francais C, Koenig F: Occult subretinal new vessels in age-related macular degeneration. Ophthalmology 97:649–657, 1990.
36. Jalkh AE, Nasrallah FP, Marinelli I, Van de Velde F: Inactive subretinal neovascularization in age-related macular degeneration. Ophthalmology 97:1614–1619, 1990.
37. Schatz H, McDonald HR, Johnson RN: Retinal pigment epithelial folds associated with retinal pigment epithelial detachments in macular degeneration. Ophthalmology 97:658–665, 1990.
38. Sorenson JA, Yannuzzi LA, Shakin JL: Recurrent subretinal neovascularization. Ophthalmology 92:1059–1075, 1985.
39. Bressler NM, Bressler SB, Alexander J, et al: Macular Photocoagulation Study Reading Center: Loculated fluid: A previously undescribed fluorescein angiographic finding in choroidal neovascularization associated with macular degeneration. Arch Ophthalmol 109:211–215, 1991.
40. Cantrill HL, Ramsay RC, Knobloch WH: Rips in the pigment epithelium. Arch Ophthalmol 101:1074–1079, 1983.
41. Decker WL, Sanborn GE, Ridley M, et al: Retinal pigment epithelial tears. Ophthalmology 90:507–512, 1983.
42. Gass JDM: Pathogenesis of tears of the retinal pigment epithelium. Br J Ophthalmol 68:514–519, 1984.
43. Green SN, Yarian D: Acute tear of the retinal pigment epithelium. Retina 3:16–20, 1983.
44. Hoskin A, Bird AC, Sehow K: Tears of detached retinal pigment epithelium. Br J Ophthalmol 65:417–422, 1981.
45. Yeo JH, Marcus S, Murphy RP: Retinal pigment epithelial tears: Patterns and prognosis. Ophthalmology 95:8–13, 1988.
46. Bressler NM, Finkelstein D, Sunness JS, et al: Retinal pigment epithelial tears through the fovea with preservation of good visual acuity. Arch Ophthalmol 108:1694–1697, 1990.
47. Marmor MF: Mechanisms of normal retinal adhesion. In Ryan SJ (ed): Retina. St Louis, CV Mosby, 1989, p 76.
48. Tani PM, Buettner H, Robertson DM: Massive vitreous hemorrhage and senile macular choroidal degeneration. Am J Ophthalmol 90:525–533, 1980.
49. Kreiger AE, Sterling JH: Vitreous hemorrhage in senile macular degeneration. Retina 3:318–321, 1983.
50. Caswell AG, Kohen D, Bird AC: Retinal pigment epithelial detachments in the elderly: Classification and outcome. Br J Ophthalmol 69:397–403, 1985.
51. Bird AC, Marshall J: Retinal pigment epithelial detachments in the elderly. Trans Ophthalmol Soc UK 105:674–682, 1986.
52. Elman MJ, Fine SL, Murphy RP, et al: The natural history of serous retinal pigment epithelium detachments in patients with age-related macular degeneration. Ophthalmology 93:224–230, 1986.
53. Gass JDM: Serous retinal pigment epithelial detachment with a notch. A sign of occult choroidal neovascularization. Retina 4:205–220, 1984.
54. Poliner LS, Olk RJ, Burgess D, Gordon ME: Natural history of retinal pigment epithelial detachments in age-related macular degeneration. Ophthalmology 93:543–550, 1986.
55. Teeters VW, Bird AC: The development of neovascularization in

senile disciform macular degeneration. Am J Ophthalmol 76:1–18, 1973.

56. Singerman L: Laser photocoagulation for choroidal new vessel membrane complicating age-related macular degeneration associated with pigment epithelial detachments. Retina 8:115–121, 1988.

57. Coscas G, Soubrane G: Photocoagulation des neovaisseaux sous-retiniens dans la degenerescence maculaire senile par laser a argon. Resultats de l'etude randomisee de 60 cas. Bull Mem Soc Fr Ophthalmol 94:149–154, 1982.

58. Moorfields Macular Study Group: Treatment of senile disciform macular degeneration: A single-blind randomized trial by argon laser photocoagulation. Br J Ophthalmol 66:745–753, 1982.

59. Macular Photocoagulation Study Group: Argon laser photocoagulation for senile macular degeneration: Results of a randomized clinical trial. Arch Ophthalmol 100:912–918, 1982.

60. Macular Photocoagulation Study Group: Krypton laser photocoagulation for neovascular lesions of age-related macular degeneration. Results of a randomized clinical trial. Arch Ophthalmol 108:816–824, 1990.

61. Macular Photocoagulation Study Group: Argon laser photocoagulation for neovascular maculopathy after five years. Results from randomized clinical trials. Arch Ophthalmol 109:1109–1114, 1991.

62. Macular Photocoagulation Study Group: Persistent and recurrent neovascularization after krypton laser photocoagulation for neovascular lesions of age-related macular degeneration. Arch Ophthalmol 108:825–831, 1990.

63. Green WR: Clinicopathologic studies of treated choroidal neovascular membranes: A review and report of two cases. Retina 11:328–356, 1991.

64. Miller H, Miller B, Ryan SJ: Correlation of choroidal subretinal neovascularization with fluorescein angiography. Am J Ophthalmol 99:263–271, 1985.

65. Miller H, Miller B, Ryan SJ: Newly-formed subretinal vessels: Fine structure and fluorescein leakage. Invest Ophthalmol Vis Sci 27:204–213, 1986.

66. Miller H, Miller B, Ryan SJ: The role of the retinal pigment epithelium in the involution of subretinal neovascularization. Invest Ophthalmol Vis Sci 27:1644–1652, 1986.

67. Macular Photocoagulation Study Group: Persistent and recurrent neovascularization after krypton laser photocoagulation for neovascular lesions of ocular histoplasmosis. Arch Ophthalmol 107:344–352, 1989.

68. Smiddy WE, Fine SL, Quigley HA, et al: Comparison of krypton and argon laser photocoagulation in simulated clinical treatment of primate retina. Arch Ophthalmol 102:1086–1092, 1984.

69. Han DP, Folk JC: Internal limiting membrane wrinkling after argon and krypton laser photocoagulation of choroidal neovascularization. Retina 6:215–219, 1986.

70. Goldberg MF, Herbst RW: Acute complications of argon laser photocoagulation. Arch Ophthalmol 89:311–318, 1973.

71. Macular Photocoagulation Study Group: Argon laser photocoagulation for ocular histoplasmosis. Results of a randomized clinical trial. Arch Ophthalmol 101:1347–1357, 1983.

72. Jampol LM: Hypertension and visual outcome in the Macular Photocoagulation Study. Arch Ophthalmol 109:789–790, 1991.

73. Schachat AP: Management of subfoveal choroidal neovascularization. Arch Ophthalmol 109:1217–1218, 1991.

74. Maguire JI, Benson WE, Brown GC: Treatment of foveal pigment epithelial detachments with contiguous extrafoveal choroidal neovascular membranes. Am J Ophthalmol 109:523–529, 1990.

75. Bressler NM, Bressler SB: Laser treatment in macular degeneration and histoplasmosis. Ophthalmol Clin North Am 4:565–581, 1989.

76. Chamberlin JA, Bressler NM, Bressler SB, et al: Macular Photocoagulation Study Group: The use of fundus photographs and fluorescein angiograms in the identification and treatment of choroidal neovascularization in the Macular Photocoagulation Study. Ophthalmology 96:1526–1534, 1989.

77. Macular Photocoagulation Study Group: Recurrent choroidal neovascularization after argon laser photocoagulation for neovascular maculopathy. Arch Ophthalmol 104:503–512, 1986.

78. Wilkinson CP, Bressler NM, Burgess D, et al: Five-year changes in visual acuity of fellow eyes of patients with extrafoveal choroidal neovascularization in age-related macular degeneration. Invest Ophthalmol Vis Sci 232:712, 1991.

Chapter 66

■

Angioid Streaks

DAVID R. GUYER, EVANGELOS S. GRAGOUDAS, and
DONALD J. D'AMICO

HISTORICAL PERSPECTIVE

Angioid streaks were first described by Doyne in 1889.[1] In 1892, Knapp[2] thought that they resembled vessels and coined the term *angioid streaks*. It was not until 1917 that Kofler[3] correctly stated that the main pathologic changes were at the level of Bruch's membrane. This finding was confirmed histopathologically in the late 1930s.[4, 5]

The recognition of angioid streaks is important because they can be associated with choroidal neovascularization (CNVM) and macular degeneration and can herald the presence of systemic disorders, such as pseudoxanthoma elasticum (PXE), Paget's disease, and the hemoglobinopathies (Table 66–1).

CLINICAL FINDINGS

Angioid streaks are irregular, spokelike, curvilinear streaks that radiate outward from the peripapillary area in all directions (Fig. 66–1). They lie beneath the retina and above the choroidal vasculature and thus can be distinguished from blood vessels. These lesions are almost always bilateral. Angioid streaks are within 2 disc diameters of the optic nerve in 27 percent of cases and are widespread in 73 percent of patients.[6] They usually do not go past the equator. The streaks can be wide or narrow and can vary in number from one to many. There is usually associated peripapillary chorioretinal changes.

The color of the streaks can range from red to dark

Table 66–1. COMMON ASSOCIATED SYSTEMIC
FINDINGS WITH ANGIOID STREAKS

Finding	Percentage
Pseudoxanthoma elasticum	34
Paget's disease	10
Hemoglobinopathy	6
Idiopathic	50

From Clarkson JG, Altman RD: Angioid streaks. Surv Ophthalmol 26:235–246, 1982.

brown; it is often dependent on the pigmentation of the fundus. They can appear gray if fibrovascular tissue is present. In one study,[6] 32 percent of streaks were gray, 23 percent were red, and 14 percent had pigment proliferation with a blackish coloration. In general, the color of the streaks was reddish-brown to reddish-gray. Hyperpigmentation or atrophy of the retinal pigment epithelium (RPE) may occur at the margin of the streak.

The streaks themselves are usually asymptomatic, but associated complications may cause vision loss. Subretinal hemorrhage may often occur after trauma.[7] However, the main cause of vision loss in these patients is CNVM, RPE detachment, and macular degeneration (Fig. 66–2). In one series,[6] macular degeneration was observed in 40 (72 percent) of 56 cases; 32 patients had exudative maculopathy and 8 patients had atrophic maculopathy. In another study of 110 cases, the occurrence of exudative macular degeneration was associated with the length of the streak, the distance of the streak from the fovea, and the diffuse or "cracked egg shell" type of streak.[8] A case of an RPE tear associated with angioid streaks has also been reported.[9]

Other associated findings include peau d'orange changes (Fig. 66–3), light margins along streaks, periph-

eral focal lesions (salmon spots), hemorrhage, paired red spots along the streaks, and disc drusen. In one series,[6] these lesions were observed in 61, 57, 44, 35, 19, and 10 percent of patients, respectively. Some of these lesions, such as disc drusen, salmon spots, and the peau d'orange changes, are exclusively or more commonly noted only in cases of angioid streaks associated with PXE.

FLUORESCEIN ANGIOGRAPHIC FINDINGS

Many authors[6, 10–17] have observed early hyperfluorescence of the streaks with late staining (see Fig. 66–1). Others,[6, 17–19] however, have reported hypofluorescence of the streaks themselves with hyperfluorescence of the margins of the streaks, which stain late. In these cases, the underlying choriocapillaris may separate and produce nonperfusion in the area of the streak itself, which may cause the hypofluorescence.[17] In some cases, the fluorescein angiography findings may reveal angioid streaks not observed clinically.[10, 20] The classic findings of associated CNVM, RPE detachments, and serous or hemorrhagic detachments may also be observed on fluorescein angiography.

The peau d'orange changes produce hypofluorescent areas on fluorescein angiography, which may represent focal defects of Bruch's membrane and the choriocapillaris.[17]

NATURAL HISTORY

Although patients with angioid streaks are usually asymptomatic early in the course of the condition, visual

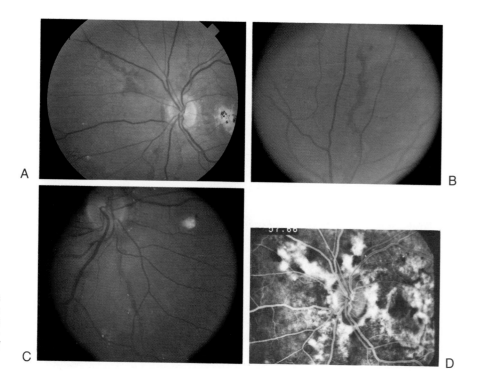

Figure 66–1. A–C, Angioid streaks are irregular, curvilinear, reddish-brown streaks that radiate outward from the peripapillary area. D, Fluorescein angiography reveals hyperfluorescence of the streaks.

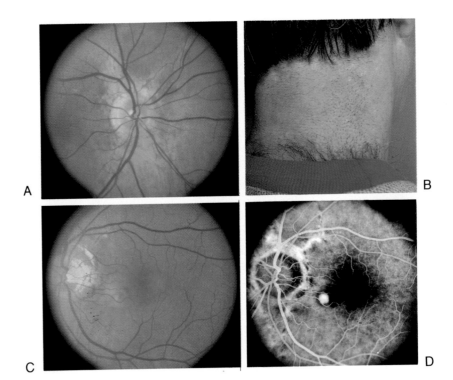

Figure 66–2. This patient with angioid streaks (A) has the characteristic "plucked-chicken" skin lesions (B) of pseudoxanthoma elasticum. The patient experienced choroidal neovascularization (C and D), which occurs in a high percentage of patients with angioid streaks.

loss usually occurs with time. In several studies,[21–23] vision of 20/200 or worse was noted in most eyes after 50 yr of age. In one series,[24] greater than 50 percent of patients had an initial visual acuity of 20/40 or better, but more than half of the patients were legally blind at an average follow-up of 3.6 yr. In another study of 29 cases, 66 percent of patients had a visual acuity of 20/200 or worse.

The cause of this vision loss is macular degeneration or CNVM, or both (see Fig. 66–2). Three separate studies have reported macular degeneration in approximately 70 percent of patients with angioid streaks.[6, 25, 26] The macular degeneration has even been observed in a patient 14 yr old.[25]

Unlike age-related macular degeneration, the exudative form is more common than the atrophic type of maculopathy in patients with angioid streaks.[24, 27] However, the exudative form is found less frequently in patients with angioid streaks and sickle cell disease than in patients with other associated systemic conditions.[28, 29] The macular degeneration is not always associated with

a foveal angioid streak, and it does not occur in all patients with a streak through the fovea.[30]

Piro and associates[24] studied 62 patients with angioid streaks and found that 86 percent had CNVM in at least one eye. Bilateral CNVM were noted in 49 percent of patients, and 37 percent of patients had unilateral CNVM. Five fellow eyes of 22 patients with unilateral CNVM developed CNVM during a mean follow-up period of 18 mo. Mansour and coworkers[8] reported that the CNVM was associated with streak length, streak distance from the fovea, and the diffuse type of streak in their series.

Minor trauma may cause subretinal hemorrhage, often with macular involvement.[5, 7, 28, 30, 31] Patients should be warned to avoid trauma and contact sports and to monitor their vision daily for the onset of CNVM.

SYSTEMIC ASSOCIATIONS

Clarkson and Altman[32] found an associated systemic disease in 50 percent of the 50 patients in their series.

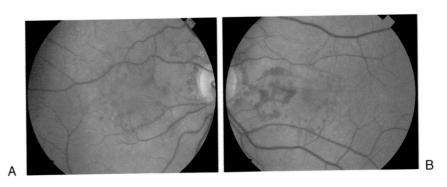

Figure 66–3. A and B, The peau d'orange lesion is a diffuse mottling of the retinal pigment epithelium in the temporal midperiphery. These changes appear as multiple, yellowish retinal pigment epithelial lesions that have the appearance of an orange skin (peau d'orange).

PXE, Paget's disease, and hemoglobinopathy were diagnosed in 34, 10, and 6 percent of the cases, respectively (see Table 66–1). Piro and associates[24] noted PXE in 61 percent of their patients and no systemic disease in 35 percent of the patients. Federman and colleagues[17] reported PXE in 30 (54 percent) of their 56 patients. In 1941, Scholz[26] reported that 59 percent of 131 patients with angioid streaks had PXE. Many other systemic disorders have been associated with angioid streaks, but some of these associations may be coincidental (Table 66–2). PXE, Paget's disease, and the hemoglobinopathies remain the most commonly found associated systemic diseases.

Pseudoxanthoma Elasticum (PXE)

PXE is a form of systemic elastorrhexis that affects mainly the skin, eyes, gastrointestinal (GI) system, and heart.[32] Females are affected twice as often as males. Patients usually are diagnosed in the third to fourth decades of life. The inheritance of this rare disorder is usually autosomal recessive but may be autosomal dominant.[33, 34] It has been thought that the condition is caused by elastic fiber abnormalities with secondary calcification. Recently, however, the earliest finding in PXE was determined by cytoimmunochemistry and x-ray analysis to be an accumulation of polyanions in the dermis.[35] These authors speculate that the polyanions attract calcium, which causes mineralization. Thus, the basic defect in PXE may not be one of calcium or elastin metabolism but rather of glycosaminoglycans and glycoproteins. These glycosylated molecules may attach to elastic fibers, mineralize, and cause abnormal collagen synthesis.

Table 66–2. OTHER SYSTEMIC DISORDERS ASSOCIATED WITH ANGIOID STREAKS

Acromegaly
Ehlers-Danlos syndrome
Facial angiomatosis
Heterotopic calcification with hyperphosphatemia
Idiopathic thrombocytic purpura
Multiple hamartoma syndrome with uterine cancer
Ocular melanocytosis
Lead poisoning
Familial polyposis
Hypo- and abetalipoproteinemia
Chronic familial hyperphosphatemia
Diabetes
Hemochromatosis
Acquired hemolytic anemia
Hypercalcinosis
Hyperphosphatemia
Myopia
Neurofibromatosis
Senile elastosis
Tuberous sclerosis
Diffuse lipomatosis
Dwarfism
Epilepsy
Trauma

The characteristic skin change in PXE is a redundant waxy, yellow, papule-like lesion, which commonly affects the neck, face, abdomen, axillary areas, inguinal regions, periumbilical area, and oral mucosa (see Fig. 66–2).[36] This skin lesion looks like a "plucked chicken." Skin biopsy results reveal elastic tissue staining of the deep dermis, often with calcification. Recently, Lebwohl and associates[37] performed biopsies on scar and normal flexural skin in patients suspected of having PXE without the typical clinical skin findings. Six of 10 scar biopsy results showed fragmentation of elastic tissue, and 3 normal flexural skin biopsy results showed signs of PXE. These authors concluded that scar biopsy is useful in suspected cases of PXE without the characteristic clinical skin lesions.

Other systemic findings in PXE include cerebral ischemia, cerebrovascular accidents, intracranial aneurysms, claudication, hypertension, myocardial infarction, and GI hemorrhage with or without ulceration. The GI hemorrhage may be life-threatening, can occur in up to 15 percent of patients, and may occur before the skin or eye findings.[38]

The first ocular findings in PXE were reported in 1903.[39] The first report of the association between PXE and angioid streaks was in 1929 by Groenblad[40] and Strandberg.[41] The ocular and cutaneous findings of PXE are referred to as the Groenblad-Strandberg syndrome in their honor. Angioid streaks are present in approximately 85 percent of patients with PXE.[25, 32] The streaks usually occur in early adulthood but can occur in patients as young as age 13 yr.[42–44]

The peau d'orange changes represent a diffuse mottling of the RPE in the temporal midperiphery and consist of multiple yellowish RPE lesions that have the appearance of the skin of an orange (peau d'orange) (see Fig. 66–3). These lesions may be observed prior to the occurrence of the angioid streaks.[45, 46] They are usually seen in association with PXE but occasionally can be present in cases of Paget's disease or sickle hemoglobinopathy.[32]

The salmon spot[43, 45] is a multiple focal, yellow, atrophic peripheral RPE lesion that appears "punched-out" like a histoplasmosis syndrome spot. Macular drusen and atypical drusen may be present in up to 75 percent of cases.[27, 48, 49] Gass[10] has reported five patients with a reticular pigment dystrophy of the macula with PXE and angioid streaks. Kadri and colleagues[20] have described intraretinal bands from the optic disc, peripheral retinal degeneration, and bilateral retinal detachments in one case. Multiple small crystalline bodies may be present in 75 percent of patients in the midperipheral or juxtapapillary regions.[10, 48] These crystalline bodies are associated with atrophic RPE changes and may resemble a comet when RPE atrophy occurs in a tail-like configuration next to it.[10]

Optic disc drusen are commonly associated with PXE and angioid streaks.[6, 43, 47, 50] Coleman and coworkers[50] state that the incidence of disc drusen is 20 to 50 times greater in patients with PXE than in normal individuals. Shields and associates[6] found disc drusen in 10 percent of the patients in their series, and Meislik and colleagues[48] observed them in 5.8 percent of their patients. Calcium-containing macromolecules may attach to the elastic fibers at the cribriform plate, disrupt axonal flow, and produce disc drusen.[50]

Coleman and coworkers[50] believe that disc drusen may be the first manifestation of ocular PXE. The peau d'orange and other pigmentary lesions may precede angioid streaks, which may not develop until the third to fourth decades of life. The angioid streaks then lead to CNVM, disciform scarring, and macular degeneration.

Paget's Disease

Paget's disease or osteitis deformans is a common chronic, progressive connective tissue disorder that involves the collagen matrix of bone.[32] Osteoelastic activity with an osteoblastic reaction occurs. The condition may be due to a slow virus related to measles or to the respiratory syncytial virus[51, 52] or may be transmitted in an autosomal dominant manner. Males and females are equally affected. Systemic findings include an enlarged bone mass affecting the pelvis, skull, spine, humeri, and femora, extraskeletal calcifications of the skin and arteries, pain, secondary osteoarthritis, neurologic damage, cardiac disease, decreased hearing, hyperparathyroidism, and claudication. The diagnosis is made by finding an elevated serum alkaline phosphatase level, increased urinary total peptide hydroxyproline levels, and characteristic radiographic findings.[32]

The first associations between Paget's disease and angioid streaks were made by Verhoeff in 1928[53] and Rowland in 1929.[54] Angioid streaks are found in 8 to 15 percent of patients with Paget's disease.[26, 32, 55, 56] However, others have recently suggested that the association may be less common.[57, 58] Dabbs and Skjodt[57] found only 1 (1.4 percent) of 70 patients with angioid streaks to also have Paget's disease.

Clarkson and Altman[32] studied 50 patients with active Paget's disease. Angioid streaks were found in 7 patients. Those with angioid streaks were found to have had a longer duration of Paget's disease, a high alkaline phosphatase level, more disease sites seen on x-ray film, and increased urinary hydroxyproline excretion. In addition, 6 of the 7 patients had skull involvement.

Occasionally patients with Paget's disease may have peau d'orange lesions and other RPE changes.[10, 32] Optic atrophy, sometimes secondary to bony compression, may also occur.

Hemoglobinopathies

The first association of angioid streaks with sickle cell disease was made in 1959 by Lieb and coworkers.[59] Paton also reported two cases in 1959.[29] In a selected population of patients with sickle cell disease, 5 (6 percent) of 69 patients were found to have streaks.[60] Condon and Serjeant[61] did not find any patients with angioid streaks in their study of 76 patients with hemo-

globin SS disease. In another study of 124 patients with hemoglobin SS disease, no patients with streaks were observed.[62] However, 5 (1.4 percent) of 356 patients in another series[63] had angioid streaks, and in Clarkson and Altman's report[32] six patients with hemoglobin SS disease and 1 patient with hemoglobin SC disease, had angioid streaks. The frequency of angioid streaks appears to be higher in elderly patients;[64] of 60 elderly patients with hemoglobin SS disease, 13 (22 percent) had streaks, whereas only 3 (2 percent) of 150 younger patients were observed to have angioid streaks.

Hamilton and associates[65] reported 21 of 242 patients with hemoglobin SS disease to have angioid streaks. Their patients had good prognoses, as only 2 individuals had macular disease.

Angioid streaks have also been reported in association with other hemoglobinopathies besides hemoglobin SS disease, such as hemoglobin SC disease;[66] hereditary spherocytosis;[67, 68] sickle trait (hemoglobin AS);[69] β-thalassemia major, minor, and intermedia;[70–75] hemoglobin H disease;[76] and sickle cell thalassemia.[77]

Thus, angioid streaks appear in 1 to 2 percent of patients with hemoglobinopathies, with the incidence increasing with age. Complications, such as CNVM or macular degeneration, are uncommon with angioid streaks associated with sickle cell disease.

Other Systemic Associations

PXE, Paget's disease, and the hemoglobinopathies are most commonly associated with angioid streaks. However, many other associated systemic conditions have been reported.

Green and colleagues[78] found angioid streaks in two individuals from the same family with the Ehlers-Danlos syndrome. This condition is a rare autosomal dominant connective tissue disorder with hyperextensible skin caused by a deficient collagen matrix. The other systemic conditions associated with angioid streaks probably represent coincidental findings. These disorders include acromegaly,[79–81] facial angiomatosis,[82] heterotopic calcification with hyperphosphatemia,[83] idiopathic thrombocytic purpura,[84] multiple hamartoma syndrome with uterine cancer,[85] ocular melanocytosis,[86] lead poisoning,[87] familial polyposis,[88] hypo- and abetalipoproteinemia,[89–91] chronic familial hyperphosphatemia,[92] diabetes,[32, 93] hemochromatosis,[32] acquired hemolytic anemia,[32] hypercalcinosis,[32] hyperphosphatemia,[83] myopia,[32] neurofibromatosis,[94] senile elastosis,[32] tuberous sclerosis,[32] diffuse lipomatosis,[95] dwarfism,[96] epilepsy,[97] and trauma[1] (see Table 66–2).

PATHOPHYSIOLOGY

The pathogenesis of angioid streaks is controversial, and there may be no common pathogenesis. In PXE and Paget's disease, Bruch's membrane may become calcified and brittle. Adelung[98] has studied the lines of force in the eye resulting from traction of the ocular muscles. Cracks may occur in a brittle Bruch's membrane because of the ocular muscles pulling the eye around a fixed origin. Calcification is observed in other parts of the body in both PXE and Paget's disease, and thus this mineralization may be a common mechanism.

The cause of angioid streaks in sickle cell disease is even more confusing. Calcification is not common in this disorder. One study[99] suggested that a diffuse elastic degeneration was present in patients with sickle cell disease; however, others report no evidence of elastic degeneration in this condition.[63] Another theory is that iron deposition in Bruch's membrane may occur from hemolysis.[5, 29, 43, 100] This iron deposition could cause mineralization of Bruch's membrane. However, only one study[5] has documented iron staining of Bruch's membrane. Other studies[65, 101, 102] could not confirm these findings. Jampol and associates[102] state that calcification may be more important than iron deposition. Another hypothesis for the occurrence of angioid streaks in patients with sickle cell disease states that the lesions occur from impaired nutrition caused by sickling and stasis.[103] Small vessel occlusion could also be important in the pathogenesis.[65]

PATHOLOGIC FEATURES

The first histopathologic studies of angioid streaks were reported in the late 1930s.[4, 5] Basophilia and calcification of a thickened Bruch's membrane were observed in both reports. Breaks in Bruch's membrane correlated with the clinical sites of the streaks. Elastic degeneration was noted, and some breaks were invaded by fibrovascular tissue from the choroid. Thus, angioid streaks appear to be linear cracks in a thickened, degenerated, and calcified Bruch's membrane.

It appears that the histopathologic appearance is similar regardless of the associated systemic condition.[32, 102] Iron deposition has not been found in cases of the associated sickle cell disease except for one report.[5, 65, 101, 102] Dreyer and Green[101] have studied the histopathologic features of 32 eyes from 21 cases. Two patients had PXE, 5 patients had Paget's disease, and 14 patients had no systemic disorder. These authors confirmed that angioid streaks are defects in the thickened, calcified elastic layer of Bruch's membrane. They found that the earliest change was a break in the elastic and collagenous layers of Bruch's membrane. Fibrovascular ingrowth occurred in some of the breaks. Secondary changes included thickening of the basement membrane of the RPE, RPE atrophy, choriocapillaris damage, photoreceptor loss, RPE hypertrophy or hyperplasia, serous retinal detachment, and disciform scar formation. CNVM and serous retinal detachment were observed in 2 cases, and disciform scars were present in 8 eyes. Salmon spots were found to be isolated breaks in Bruch's membrane with fibrovascular ingrowth.

Jensen[104] has studied Bruch's membrane in PXE using histochemical, ultrastructural, and x-ray microanalytic techniques. He found two types of calcification: hydroxyapatite and $CaHPO_4$. He also observed a "thready" material in the membrane and an increased amount of acid mucopolysaccharide. He stated that malformed collagen may be the underlying abnormality in PXE.

TREATMENT

Safety glasses should be considered for these patients with angioid streaks because trauma precipitates hemorrhage. In addition, these patients should not engage in contact sports. Low-vision aids may be useful, and in some cases genetic counseling should be considered. Prophylactic treatment of angioid streaks should not be performed, as it may induce CNVM.

The treatment of CNVM associated with angioid streaks has been reported in the literature as being disappointing.[32] However, recent studies have been somewhat more optimistic. Singerman and Hatem[74] treated eight eyes with extrafoveal CNVM with laser photocoagulation. Improved or stabilized vision was noted in seven of the eight cases. Recurrences occurred in four eyes. Successful results have also been reported by others.[105–107] Pece and colleagues[108] treated 17 eyes and noted improvement, although recurrences were frequent. Piro and associates[24] found a poor response to laser photocoagulation in their series because of recurrences.

Brancato and coworkers[109] treated 13 such eyes and stated that laser photocoagulation should be performed. Van Eijk and Oosterhuis[110] successfully treated 7 of 15 eyes. Eight eyes had subfoveal recurrences. Gelisken and associates[111] treated 30 such eyes. Sixteen of the eyes had stable or improved vision postoperatively. Twelve of the remaining 14 cases retained 20/200 vision or better during a mean follow-up period of 3.4 yr. Eleven untreated fellow eyes developed macular degeneration and the loss of central vision.

Although there have been no prospective randomized controlled trials of laser photocoagulation for CNVM associated with angioid streaks, it seems reasonable to consider treatment of well-defined CNVM outside the foveal avascular zone. However, the recurrence rate may be higher with CNVM associated with angioid streaks than with CNVM associated with other macular disorders.[32, 74, 106]

DIFFERENTIAL DIAGNOSIS

Only 39 percent of cases in one series[6] were correctly diagnosed as having angioid streaks prior to referral. Twenty-three percent of these cases were misdiagnosed as age-related macular degeneration. Other disorders that were confused with the angioid streaks included choroidal sclerosis, myopia and lacquer cracks, histoplasmosis, toxoplasmosis, retinal vasculitis and papilledema, and traumatic hemorrhage. Other entities to consider in the differential diagnosis include choroidal rupture and choroidal folds (Table 66–3).

Table 66–3. DIFFERENTIAL DIAGNOSIS OF ANGIOID STREAKS

Age-related macular degeneration
Choroidal sclerosis
Myopic lacquer cracks
Histoplasmosis
Toxoplasmosis
Retinal vasculitis and papilledema
Traumatic hemorrhage
Choroidal rupture
Choroidal folds

CONCLUSIONS

Angioid streaks are distinctive fundus lesions that are associated with systemic disorders in 50 percent of cases. The most commonly associated diseases include PXE, Paget's disease, and the hemoglobinopathies. Angioid streaks themselves are usually asymptomatic, but the occurrence of CNVM and macular degeneration can cause devastating visual loss. The streaks represent breaks in a calcified and thickened Bruch's membrane. Laser photocoagulation may be beneficial to treat CNVM associated with angioid streaks; however, the recurrence rate is high.

REFERENCES

1. Doyne RW: Choroidal and retinal changes. The result of blows on the eyes. Trans Ophthalmol Soc UK 9:128, 1889.
2. Knapp H: On the formation of dark angioid streaks as an unusual metamorphosis of retinal hemorrhage. Arch Ophthalmol 21:289–292, 1892.
3. Kofler A: Beitraege zur Kenntnis der angioid Streaks (Knapp). Arch Augenheilkd 82:134–149, 1917.
4. Bock J: Zur Klinik und Anatomic der gefaessehnlichen Streifen im Augenhintergrund. Z Augenheilkd 95:1–50, 1938.
5. Hagedoorn A: Angioid streaks. Arch Ophthalmol 21:746–774; 935–965, 1939.
6. Shields JA, Federman JL, Tomer TL, Annesley WH Jr: Angioid streaks. I. Ophthalmoscopic variations and diagnostic problems. Br J Ophthalmol 59:257–265, 1975.
7. Fine SL: Angioid streaks. Int Ophthalmol Clin 17:173–182, 1977.
8. Mansour AM, Shields JA, Annesley WH, et al: Macular degeneration in angioid streaks. Ophthalmologica 197:36–41, 1988.
9. Lim JI, Lam S: A retinal pigment epithelium tear in a patient with angioid streaks. Arch Ophthalmol 108:1672–1674, 1990.
10. Gass JDM: Stereoscopic Atlas of Macular Diseases, Diagnosis and Treatment, 2nd ed. St Louis, CV Mosby, 1977.
11. Gass JDM: Pathogenesis of disciform detachment of the neuroepithelium. VI. Disciform detachment secondary to heredodegenerative, neoplastic, and traumatic lesions of the choroid. Am J Ophthalmol 63:689, 1967.
12. Smith JL, Gass JDM, Justice J Jr: Fluorescein fundus photography of angioid streaks. Br J Ophthalmol 48:517–521, 1964.
13. Norton EWD, Gass JDM, Smith JL, et al: Fluorescein in the study of macular disease. Trans Am Acad Ophthalmol Otolaryngol 69:631–642, 1965.
14. Patniak B, Malik SRK: Fluorescein fundus photography of angioid streaks. Br J Ophthalmol 55:833–837, 1971.
15. Kolin J, Oosterhuis JA: Bruch's membrane lesions studied with fluorescein angiography. Opthalmologica 163:46–55, 1971.
16. Wessing A: Fluorescein Angiography of the Retina. St Louis, CV Mosby, 1969, pp 126–128.
17. Federman JL, Shields JA, Tomer TL: Angioid streaks. II. Fluorescein angiographic features. Arch Ophthalmol 93:951–962, 1975.
18. Gass JDM, Clarkson JG: Angioid streaks and disciform macular detachment in Paget's disease (osteitis deformans). Am J Ophthalmol 75:576–586, 1973.
19. Hull DS, Aaberg TM: Fluorescein study of a family with angioid streaks and pseudoxanthoma elasticum. Br J Ophthalmol 58:738–745, 1974.
20. Kadri W, Rosen E, Harcourt B: Intraretinal changes in the Groenblad-Strandberg syndrome. Br J Ophthalmol 57:588–592, 1973.
21. Streiff FH, Portmann UP: Une fratrie de stries angioides de la retine. Considerations sur l'heredite et l'evolution. Ophthalmologica 121:87–91, 1951.
22. Groenblad E: "Angioid streaks"—Pseudoxanthoma elasticum. De Zusammenhang zwischen diesen gleichzeitig auftretenden Augen- und Hautveran-derungen. Acta Ophthalmol 1(Suppl):1–114, 1932.
23. Groenblad E: Colour photographs of angioid streaks in the late stages. Acta Ophthalmol 36:472, 1958.
24. Piro PA, Scheraga D, Fine SL: Angioid streaks. Natural history and visual prognosis. In Fine SL, Owens S (eds): Management of Retinal Vascular and Macular Disorders. Baltimore, Williams & Wilkins, 1983, pp 136–139.
25. Connor PJ, Juergens JL, Perry HO, et al: Pseudoxanthoma elasticum and angioid streaks. A review of 106 cases. Am J Med 30:537, 1961.
26. Scholz RO: Angioid streaks. Arch Ophthalmol 26:677, 1941.
27. Verhoeff FH: Histological findings in a case of angioid streaks. Br J Ophthalmol 32:531, 1948.
28. Archer AB, Logan WC: Angioid streaks. In Krill AE (ed): Hereditary Retinal and Choroidal Diseases, vol. 2. Philadelphia, JB Lippincott, 1976, p 863.
29. Paton D: Angioid streaks and sickle cell anemia. A report of 2 cases. Arch Ophthalmol 62:852, 1959.
30. Gass JDM: Stereoscopic Atlas of Macular Diseases. Diagnosis and Treatment, 3rd ed. St Louis, CV Mosby, 1987.
31. Britten MJA: Unusual traumatic retinal haemorrhages associated with angioid streaks. Br J Ophthalmol 50:540–542, 1966.
32. Clarkson JG, Altman RD: Angioid streaks. Surv Ophthalmol 26:235–246, 1982.
33. McKusick VA: Heritable Disorders of Connective Tissue, 4th ed. St Louis, CV Mosby, 1972, pp 475–520.
34. Pope FM: Two types of autosomal recessive pseudoxanthoma elasticum. Arch Dermatol 110:209–212, 1974.
35. Walker ER, Frederickson RG, Mayes MD: The mineralization of elastic fibers and alterations of extracellular matrix in pseudoxanthoma elasticum. Arch Dermatol 125:70, 1989.
36. Pinnell SR, McKusick VA: Heritable changes of connective tissue with skin changes. In Fitzpatrick TB, Eisen AZ, Wolf K, et al (eds): Dermatology in General Medicine, 3rd ed. New York, McGraw-Hill, 1987, pp 1782–1785.
37. Lebwohl M, Phelps RG, Yannuzzi L: Diagnosis of pseudoxanthoma elasticum by scar biopsy in patients without characteristic skin lesions. N Engl J Med 317:347–350, 1987.
38. Goodman RM, Smith EW, Paton D, et al: Pseudoxanthoma elasticum. A clinical and histopathological study. Medicine 42:297, 1963.
39. Hallopeau L: Nouvelle note sur un cas de pseudoxanthome elastique. Ann Dermatol Syph (Paris) 4:595–596, 1903.
40. Groenblad E: Angioid streaks—Pseudoxanthoma elasticum; vorlaeufige Mitteilung. Acta Ophthalmol 7:329, 1929.
41. Strandberg J: Pseudoxanthoma elasticum. Z Haut Geschlechtski 31:689, 1929.
42. Grand MG, Issermann J, Miller CW: Angioid streaks associated with pseudoxanthoma elasticum in a 13-year-old patient. Ophthalmology 94:197–200, 1987.
43. Paton D: The relation of angioid streaks to systemic disease. Springfield, IL, Charles C Thomas, 1972, pp 3–37.
44. Whitmore PV: Skin and mucous membrane disorders. In Duane TD, Jaeger EA (eds): Clinical Ophthalmology, vol. 5. Philadelphia, JB Lippincott, 1986, pp 15–16.
45. Shimizu K: Mottled fundus in association with pseudoxanthoma elasticum. Jpn J Ophthalmol 5:111–113, 1961.
46. Gills JP Jr, Paton D: Mottled fundus oculi in pseudoxanthoma elasticum: A report on two siblings. Arch Ophthalmol 73:792–795, 1965.
47. Krill AE, Klein BA, Archer DB: Precursors of angioid streaks. Am J Ophthalmol 76:875, 1973.

48. Meislik J, Neldner K, Basil Reeve E, Ellis PP: Atypical drusen in pseudoxanthoma elasticum. Ann Ophthalmol 11:653, 1979.

49. McKusick VA: Heritable disorders of connective tissue. VI. Pseudoxanthoma elasticum. J Chronic Dis 3:263, 1956.

50. Coleman K, Ross MH, McCabe M, et al: Disk drusen and angioid streaks in pseudoxanthoma elasticum. Am J Ophthalmol 112:166–170, 1991.

51. Altman RD: Paget's Disease. In Talbot MD (ed): Clinical Rheumatology, 1st and 2nd eds. New York, Elsevier North-Holland, 1978, 1st ed, pp 184–190; and 1981, 2nd ed, pp 198–206.

52. Altman RD (ed): Proceedings of the Kroc Foundation Conference on Paget's disease of bone. Arthritis Rheum 23:1073–1240, 1980.

53. Verhoeff FH: The nature and pathogenesis of angioid streaks in the ocular fundus. Transactions of the Section on Ophthalmology of the American Medical Association, 1928, p 243.

54. Rowland WD: Bilateral caerulean cataract. Am J Ophthalmol 16:61, 1933.

55. Terry TL: Angioid streaks and osteitis deformans. Trans Am Ophthalmol Soc 32:555–573, 1934.

56. Berliner ML: Discussion of Newman DA: Angioid streaks of the retina with pseudoxanthoma elasticum. Arch Ophthalmol 10:709, 1933.

57. Dabbs TR, Skjodt K: Prevalence of angioid streaks and other ocular complications of Paget's disease of bone. Br J Ophthalmol 74:579–582, 1990.

58. Smith R: Paget's disease and angioid streaks: One complication less? [Editorial] Br J Ophthalmol 74:577–578, 1990.

59. Lieb WA, Geeraets WJ, Guerry D III: Sickle-cell retinopathy: Ocular and systemic manifestations of sickle-cell disease. Acta Ophthalmol (Copenh) Suppl 58:1–45, 1959.

60. Geeraets WJ, Guerry D III: Angioid streaks and sickle cell disease. Am J Ophthalmol 49:450–570, 1960.

61. Condon PI, Serjeant GR: Ocular findings in homozygous sickle cell anemia in Jamaica. Am J Ophthalmol 73:533–543, 1972.

62. Majekodunmi SA, Akinyanju OO: Ocular findings in homozygous sickle cell disease in Nigeria. Can J Ophthalmol 13:160–162, 1978.

63. Nagpal K, Asdourian G, Goldbaum M, et al: Angioid streaks and sickle haemoglobinopathies. Br J Ophthalmol 60:31–34, 1976.

64. Condon PI, Serjeant GR: Ocular findings in elderly cases of homozygous sickle cell disease in Jamaica. Br J Ophthalmol 60:361–364, 1976.

65. Hamilton AM, Pope FM, Condon PI, et al: Angioid streaks in Jamaican patients with homozygous sickle cell disease. Br J Ophthalmol 65:341–347, 1981.

66. Condon PI, Serjeant GR: Ocular findings in hemoglobin SC disease in Jamaica. Am J Ophthalmol 74:921–931, 1972.

67. McLane NJ, Grizzard WS, Kousseff BG, et al: Angioid streaks associated with hereditary spherocytosis. Am J Ophthalmol 97:444–449, 1984.

68. Singerman LJ: Angioid streaks associated with hereditary spherocytosis. Am J Ophthalmol 98:647–648, 1984.

69. Gerde LS: Angioid streaks in sickle cell trait hemoglobinopathy. Am J Ophthalmol 77:462–464, 1974.

70. Kinsella FP, Mooney DJ: Angioid streaks in beta thalassaemia minor. Br J Ophthalmol 72:303–304, 1988.

71. Theodossiadis G, Ladas I, Koutsandrea C, et al: Thalassaemia et neovaisseaux sous-retiniens maculaires. J Fr Ophtalmol 7:115–118, 1984.

72. Aessopos A, Stamatelos G, Savvides P, et al: Angioid streaks in homozygous β thalassemia. Am J Ophthalmol 108:356–359, 1989.

73. Gibson JM, Chaudhuri PR, Rosenthal AR: Angioid streaks in a case of beta thalassaemia major. Br J Ophthalmol 67:29–31, 1983.

74. Singerman LJ, Hatem GF: Laser treatment of choroidal neovascular membranes in angioid streaks. Retina 1:75–85, 1981.

75. Gartaganis S, Ismiridis K, Papageorgiou O, et al: Ocular abnormalities in patients with β thalassemia. Am J Ophthalmol 108:699–703, 1989.

76. Daneshmend TK: Ocular findings in a case of haemoglobin H disease. Br J Ophthalmol 63:842–844, 1979.

77. Goldberg MF, Charache S, Acadio I: Ophthalmologic manifestations of sickle cell thalassaemia. Arch Intern Med 128:33–39, 1971.

78. Green WR, Friedman-Kien A, Banfield WG: Angioid streaks in Ehlers-Danlos syndrome. Arch Ophthalmol 76:197–204, 1966.

79. Holloway TB: Angioid streaks: A report concerning two cases. Trans Am Ophthalmol Soc 25:173, 1927.

80. Howard GM: Angioid streaks and acromegaly. Am J Ophthalmol 56:137, 1963.

81. Paton D: Angioid streaks and acromegaly. Am J Ophthalmol 56:841, 1963.

82. Kalina RE: Facial angiomatosis with angioid streaks. Association of angioid streaks with a component of the Sturge-Weber syndrome. Arch Ophthalmol 84:528–531, 1970.

83. McPhaul JJ Jr, Engel F: Heterotopic calcification: Hyperphosphatemia and angioid streaks of the retina. Am J Med 31:488–492, 1961.

84. Yatzkan DN: Angioid streaks of the fundus in association with posthemorrhagic amaurosis. Am J Ophthalmol 43:219, 1957.

85. Allen BS, Fitch MH, Smith JG Jr: Multiple hamartoma syndrome. A report of a new case with associated carcinoma of the uterine cervix and angioid streaks of the eyes. J Am Acad Dermatol 2:303–308, 1980.

86. Awan KJ: Ocular melanocytosis and angioid streaks. J Pediatr Ophthalmol Strabismus 17:300–304, 1980.

87. DeSimone S, DeConciliis V: Strie angioidi della retina. Arch Ottalmologia 62:161, 1958.

88. Awan KJ: Familial polyposis and angioid streaks in the ocular fundus. Am J Ophthalmol 83:123–125, 1977.

89. Duker JS, Belmont J, Bosley TM: Angioid streaks associated with abetalipoproteinemia. Arch Ophthalmol 105:1173–1174, 1987.

90. Runge P, Muller DPR, McAllister J, et al: Oral vitamin E supplements can prevent the retinopathy of abetalipoproteinemia. Br J Ophthalmol 70:166–173, 1986.

91. Dieckert JP, White M, Christmann L, Lambert HM: Angioid streaks associated with abetalipoproteinemia. Ann Ophthalmol 21:173–175, 1989.

92. Iancu TC, Almagor G, Savir H: Ocular abnormalities in chronic familial hyperphosphatasemia. J Pediatr Ophthalmol Strabismus 17:220–223, 1980.

93. Johnson BW, Oshinskie L: Diagnosis and management of angioid streaks. J Am Optom Assoc 59:704–711, 1988.

94. McWilliam RJ: On the histology of angioid streaks. Trans Ophthalmol Soc UK 71:243–249, 1951.

95. Bonamour MG: Stries angioides de la retina et maladie de Launois-Bensaube (lipomatose diffuse). Bull Soc Ophtalmol 406:1959.

96. Yoneyama T, Yoneyama K: Angioid streaks and dwarfism. J Clin Ophthalmol 14:1013, 1960.

97. Blobner F: Angioid streaks and epilepsy. Klin Monatsbl Augenheilkd 95:12, 1935.

98. Adelung JC: Zur genese der angioid streaks (Knapp). Klin Monatsbl Augenheilkd 119:241–250, 1951.

99. Geeraets WJ, Guerry D: Elastic tissue degeneration in sickle cell disease. Am J Ophthalmol 50:213, 1960.

100. Klein BA: Angioid streaks: A clinical and histopathologic study. Am J Ophthalmol 30:955–968, 1947.

101. Dreyer R, Green WR: The pathology of angioid streaks: A study of twenty-one cases. Trans Pa Acad Ophthalmol Otolaryngol 31:158–167, 1978.

102. Jampol LM, Acheson R, Eagle RC, et al: Calcification of Bruch's membrane in angioid streaks with homozygous sickle cell disease. Arch Ophthalmol 105:93–98, 1987.

103. Hogan JF, Heaton CL: Angioid streaks and systemic disease. Br J Dermatol 89:411–416, 1973.

104. Jensen OA: Bruch's membrane in pseudoxanthoma elasticum. Histochemical, ultrastructural, and x-ray microanalytical study of the membrane and angioid streak areas. Graefes Arch Clin Exp Ophthalmol 203:311–320, 1977.

105. Meislik J, Neldner K, Reeve EB, Ellis PP: Laser treatment in

maculopathy of pseudoxanthoma elasticum. Can J Ophthalmol 13:210–212, 1978.
106. Deutman AF, Kovacs B: Argon laser treatment in complications of angioid streaks. Am J Ophthalmol 88:12–17, 1979.
107. Kayazawa F: A successful argon laser treatment in macular complications of angioid streaks. Ann Ophthalmol 13:581–584, 1981.
108. Pece A, Avanza P, Zorgno F, et al: Photocoagulation au laser des negvaisseaux sous-retiniens maculaires survenant au cours des stries angioides. J Fr Ophthalmol 12:687–689, 1989.
109. Brancato R, Menchini U, Pece A, et al: Laser treatment of macular subretinal neovascularizations in angioid streaks. Ophthalmologica 195:84–87, 1987.
110. Van Eijk AW, Oosterhuis JA: Kryptonlaserbehandlung von gefabneubildungen bei angioiden streifen. Klin Monatsbl Augenheilkd 191:443–448, 1987.
111. Gelisken O, Hendrikse F, Deutman AF: A long-term follow-up study of laser coagulation of neovascular membranes in angioid streaks. Am J Ophthalmol 105:299–303, 1988.

Chapter 67

■

Ocular Histoplasmosis Syndrome

LAWRENCE S. HALPERIN and R. JOSEPH OLK

The ocular histoplasmosis syndrome (OHS) causes permanent loss of central vision in 2000 young adults per year. The organism *Histoplasma capsulatum* has been suspected as a cause of granulomatous uveitis for many years. Krause and Hopkins[1] in 1951 reported a patient with atrophic chorioretinal lesions with pigment change and hemorrhage. A histoplasmin skin test result was positive and a chest x-ray film showed calcified lung nodules. Woods and Wahlen,[2] in 1960, published a report of a collection of patients who were residents of an area endemic for histoplasmosis and had clear vitreous, peripheral atrophic spots, disciform macular lesions, positive histoplasmin skin test results, and pulmonary calcifications.

The four signs of OHS are peripheral punched-out chorioretinal lesions, juxtapapillary atrophic pigmentary changes, disciform macular changes, and a clear vitreous.

This chapter reviews the epidemiology, clinical findings, evaluation, and treatment of OHS.

EPIDEMIOLOGY

Most individuals with OHS are between 30 and 40 yr of age. Fundus scars may occur with equal frequency among blacks and whites, although maculopathy is very rare in blacks. Baskin and associates[3] reported six blacks with OHS and macular lesions, five of whom had positive skin test results.

Epidemiologic Studies

The epidemiology of OHS has been studied by many investigators and yet the relationship between *H. capsulatum* infection and the manifestations of ocular disease remains an enigma. A review of several of these reports provides varying aspects of the debate.

Braunstein and coworkers[4] reported 15 individuals in the United Kingdom who had the clinical findings of OHS but in whom all skin test results were negative. They concluded that there could be a different causative factor in the United Kingdom.

Ellis and Schlaegel[5] found the Mississippi and Ohio river valleys to be highly infected; 80 percent of the adult population had positive skin test results. This area includes 80 million individuals, involving Missouri, Illinois, Indiana, Kentucky, Tennessee, and Mississippi (Fig. 67–1). Wheat and colleagues[6] collected worldwide patterns of skin sensitivity to histoplasmin. Feman and associates[7] noted that 60 percent of the Tennessee population had positive skin test results, but only 44 new cases of visual loss resulting from OHS occurred in a 6-mo period. Smith and Ganley and coworkers[8–10] studied 842 individuals in Walkersville, Maryland, where 60 percent had positive skin test results. One hundred percent of patients with highly suspicious lesions had positive skin test results, but only 4.4 percent of those who had positive results had typical fundus lesions. Only 1 individual had a disciform macular lesion. We conclude that OHS is relatively uncommon, even in endemic areas. Typically, 2 to 12 percent of the population in an endemic area has ocular findings consistent with OHS, and only 1 in 1000 experiences maculopathy.

Davidorf and Anderson[11] examined 353 school-aged children after an acute epidemic infection on Earth Day in 1970. Forty-one percent of the children became acutely ill from histoplasmosis infection, and 85 percent had elevated serum titers, compared with 10 percent of controls. Two years later, all children who had the infection had a positive skin test result, compared with 23.4 percent of controls. However, the incidence of fundus lesions was similar in infected children when

HISTOPLASMIN SENSITIVITY

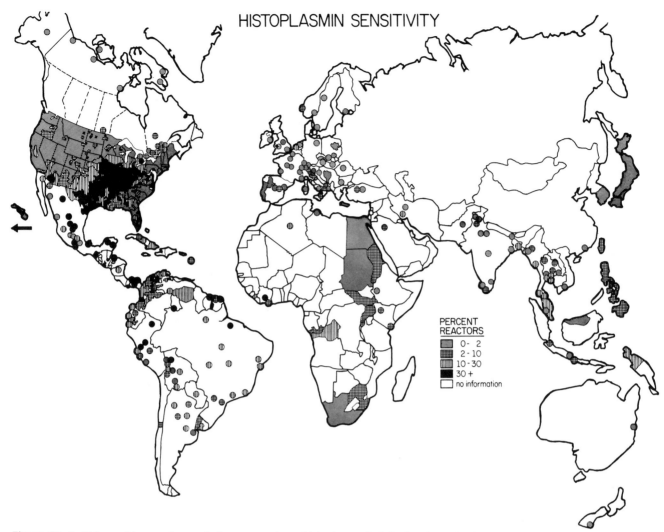

PERCENT
REACTORS
- 0 - 2
- 2 - 10
- 10 - 30
- 30 +
- no information

Figure 67–1. This world map demonstrates areas where histoplasmosis infection is endemic. (From Ellis FD, Schlaegel TF: The geographic localization of presumed histoplasmic choroiditis. Am J Ophthalmol 75:953–956, 1973. Published with permission from the American Journal of Ophthalmology. Copyright by The Ophthalmic Publishing Company.)

compared with controls, and this brought the association of histoplasmosis infection and OHS into question. A more likely explanation is that a 2-yr period after exposure to histoplasmosis is not sufficient time to assess the occurrence of OHS lesions.

Feman and Tilford[12] found that six of eight patients with positive systemic histoplasmosis cultures had chorioretinal scars consistent with OHS. This again lends support to the concept that *H. capsulatum* causes OHS.

Fellow Eye

Patients with a disciform process in one eye have posterior atrophic lesions in the fellow eye approximately 25 to 59 percent of the time.[13, 14] If one eye has a choroidal neovascular membrane, and a focal scar in the posterior pole is present in the second eye, that eye has between an 8 and a 27 percent chance of acquiring a subretinal neovascular membrane (SRNVM) in 3 yr.[13–17] More histoplasmosis spots in the posterior pole may lead to increased chances of activation. If no

macular scar is present in the posterior pole of the second eye, there is less than a 5 percent chance of an SRNVM developing in 5 yr; however, new spots may develop. Close follow-up is needed for the fellow eye, especially if posterior histoplasmosis spots are present. An individual with bilateral macular histoplasmosis spots has a 5 percent chance of an SRNVM developing in one eye within 5 yr.

HISTOPATHOLOGIC FEATURES

Organism and Systemic Infection

H. capsulatum is a fungus that is present in its yeast form. The fungus is carried and deposited by droppings from chickens, pigeons, blackbirds, and bats. The birds are not infected but carry the fungus on their feathers. Bats, however, are infected.

In humans, the fungus is first inhaled into the lungs and is then disseminated into the blood stream. Acute pneumonitis with fever may ensue and an acute, life-threatening disease may rarely occur. Pulmonary granulomas form and heal with calcification, and these may be seen on chest radiography. The systemic forms of disease rarely have ocular manifestations.

Ocular Histopathologic Features

There are several reports of *H. capsulatum* in eyes with OHS.[18, 19] However, Roth's[19] report was refuted by Gass and Zimmerman.[20]

Ocular histopathologic studies have shown *H. capsulatum* in disseminated histoplasmosis, often in immunocompromised hosts (Fig. 67–2).[21–25] Some of these patients exhibited clinical signs of OHS as well.[19, 26] These cases and others have been well summarized.[25]

Meredith and colleagues[27] reported cracks in Bruch's membrane related to the growth of choroidal blood vessels into the subretinal space. The overlying retina showed loss of outer layers and cystic degeneration. The retinal pigment epithelium (RPE) was lacking in the center of the lesion but was clumped at the edges. Subretinal pigment epithelium neovascularization ex-

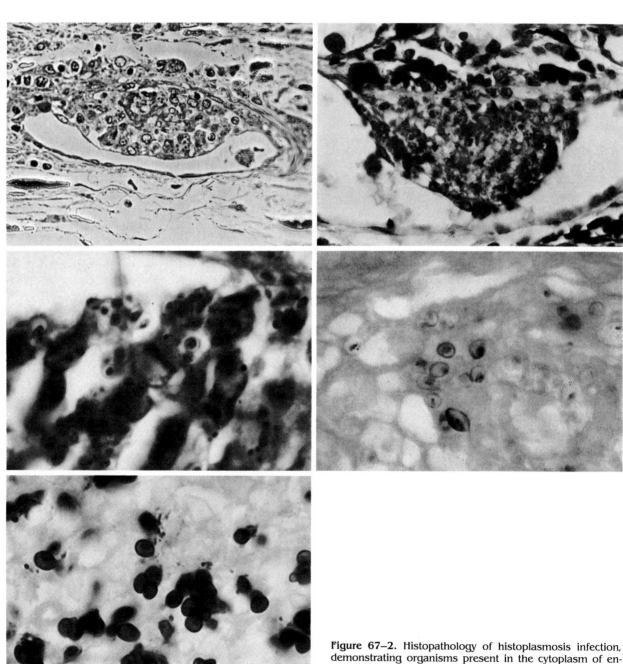

Figure 67–2. Histopathology of histoplasmosis infection, demonstrating organisms present in the cytoplasm of endothelial cells. (From Scholz R, Green WR, Kutys R, et al: *Histoplasma capsulatum* in the eye. Published courtesy of Ophthalmology [1984;91:1100–1104].)

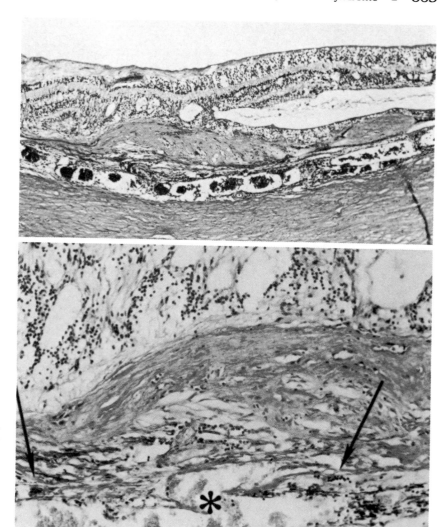

Figure 67–3. Histopathologic specimen from a case of ocular histoplasmosis. Discontinuities in Bruch's membrane *(between arrows in bottom figure)* allow choroidal vessels *(asterisk)* to grow in the subretinal or subretinal pigment epithelial space. (From Meredith TA, Green WR, Key SN, et al: Ocular histoplasmosis: Clinicopathologic correlation of 3 cases. Surv Ophthalmol 22:189, 1977.)

tended beyond the disciform process. The juxtapapillary changes resulted from loss of RPE, loss of photoreceptors, and discontinuities in Bruch's membrane. The peripheral lesions showed loss of the RPE, scarring, and occasional lymphocytic infiltration (Fig. 67–3).

Experimental Animal Model

Smith and associates developed an experimental animal model involving the injection of live fungus via the carotid artery.[28-30] Most animals had positive skin test results and early acute choroiditis resulting from mononuclear cell and macrophage infiltration with phagocytosis of yeast. Lymphocytes were found in the choroid, and damage to Bruch's membrane occurred. Six weeks later, yeast was rarely found. Atrophic lesions resulted from loss of RPE associated with altered Bruch's membrane and lymphocytes in the choroid. Subclinical lesions occurred in areas that were not detectable by clinical examination or fluorescein angiography, but lymphocytes were seen under the retina and RPE.

Disappearing lesions occurred where lesions were at one time visible but became invisible. There were lymphocytes in the choroid, but the RPE and retina were normal. Chronic choroiditis occurred, with organisms disappearing in 6 wk. This may be why amphotericin B has no effect on the disease. No macular disciform lesions developed. These laboratory data support clinical findings. Disseminated histoplasmosis causes acute lesions with yeast particles. Later, chronic OHS shows lesions without yeast, but inflammatory cells may still be present. Doubts concerning the cause and effect of *H. capsulatum* and OHS could be explained by these experimental data.

IMMUNOLOGY

Several theories exist that attempt to explain the pathogenesis of OHS, including the following:

1. Immunologic responses to previous infection causes OHS. The macular lesion may be a hypersensitivity reaction to dead organisms elsewhere in the eye.

2. Macular disease in OHS is the result of reinfection with histoplasmosis.

3. Some vascular decompensation in the choroid is responsible for the findings in OHS.

Lymphocyte Hyperreactivity

Schlaegel and coworkers[31] found altered skin test reactivity to certain antigens in patients with OHS. Lymphocytes are hyperreactive in patients with disciform lesions in OHS, and some investigators believe there is an increased rate of macular subretinal hemorrhage after histoplasmin skin testing. Others[32, 33] found that lymphocyte transformation may correlate with OHS activity. Patients with disciform lesions have stimulated lymphocytes in comparison with patients with only peripheral scars and controls. Brahmi and colleagues[34] found acute histoplasmin infection to be different from OHS in terms of T-cell studies.

Histocompatability Antigens

Meredith and associates,[35] in the Walkersville study, found no increase in HLA-B7 for peripheral lesions only but did find an association with HLA-DRw2. There was a definite association between HLA-B7 and macular lesions. Braley and coworkers[36] found that 78 percent of patients with OHS and macular disciform lesions were HLA-B7–positive compared with 20 percent of controls. Godfrey and colleagues[37] found that 54.8 percent of macular lesions were HLA-B7–positive.

All these studies support the concept that OHS is an immunologic disorder. However, refuting this theory is the fact that lymphocytes are found in scars and lesions in OHS, and they also are found in disciform lesions of age-related macular degeneration. Further, it is fairly uncommon to see simultaneous bilateral macular lesions in OHS, but if OHS is an immunologic disease, one would think these lesions would be more common. Unfortunately, there is no animal model for macular lesions in OHS to study these questions further.

CLINICAL CHARACTERISTICS
(Table 67–1)

Punched-out Chorioretinal Lesions

Smith and associates[38] found one to four punched-out chorioretinal lesions per eye, juxtapapillary changes in 28 percent of eyes, and bilateral changes in 62 percent of patients with OHS. Macular lesions are rarer but more visually devastating.

The atrophic spots are small, irregular, roundish lesions in the midperiphery and posterior pole. They may have pigment on the edge or in the center and range from 0.3 to 0.7 disc diameter. Choroidal vessels may be

Table 67–1. CLINICAL CHARACTERISTICS OF THE OCULAR HISTOPLASMOSIS SYNDROME

Punched-out chorioretinal lesions
Juxtapapillary chorioretinal atrophy
Subretinal neovascularization
No vitritis
No pigment epithelial detachment
Disseminated choroiditis—rare

seen throughout the atrophic lesions (Fig. 67–4). Watzke[42] found that atrophic lesions change shape, size, and pigmentation over time.

Linear streaks of chorioretinal lesions of variable length, width, and pigmentation may form (Fig. 67–5). They are usually equatorial, parallel to the ora, and average 3 clock hr in length. Bottoni and coworkers[39] found streaks in five patients who also had SRNVMs, and Fountain and Schlaegel[40] found streaks in 5 percent of their patients with OHS, but this was a skewed population.

New lesions may form in areas previously seen to be normal on clinical examination and fluorescein angiography. Schlaegel and colleagues[41] said 26 percent of spots were newly developed over 5 yr of follow-up, whereas other studies cited 9 and 16.6 percent.[14, 42, 43] Gass and Wilkinson[44] found only 1 out of 81 patients in whom a new peripheral lesion developed, but Lewis and Schiffman[14] reevaluated 99 of their patients with longer follow-up and found that 19 percent acquired new lesions, suggesting that longer follow-up leads to identification of more new lesions.

Juxtapapillary Chorioretinal Atrophy

The juxtapapillary changes in OHS are probably due to juxtapapillary choroiditis that goes unrecognized, and this leads to chorioretinal changes around the disc (Fig. 67–6). Various investigators have found that 85 to 94 percent of patients with OHS have juxtapapillary changes.[13, 31, 45] The atrophic juxtapapillary changes may lead to subretinal neovascularization that can decrease central vision (Fig. 67–7).[46] Lewis and associates[45] found 3.8 percent of patients with juxtapapillary changes experienced a juxtapapillary SRNVM, and Cantrill and Burgess[47] found that 15 percent of patients with symptoms from a juxtapapillary SRNVM in one eye had a juxtapapillary SRNVM in the fellow eye. Gass and Wilkinson[44] found that 10 percent of all SRNVMs in OHS were juxtapapillary, and despite the benign nature of many juxtapapillary SRNVMs, Gutman[13] reported that 58 percent of these patients had visual acuity of 20/200 or worse.

Macular Lesion

The classic macular lesion associated with OHS is a choroidal neovascular membrane with serous detach-

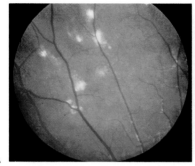
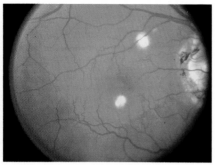

Figure 67–4. *A,* Fundus photograph of peripheral, punched-out lesions typical of the ocular histoplasmosis syndrome (OHS). *B,* Fundus photograph of atrophic macular lesions.

A

B

ment of the retina, subretinal hemorrhage, hard lipid exudate, and a pigment halo surrounding the active lesion (Fig. 67–8). The presence of subretinal blood may indicate a large SRNVM that is rapidly growing, thereby predicting a poorer prognosis.

Symptoms of a choroidal neovascular membrane include decreased vision, metamorphopsia, and blurring. Micropsia occasionally may be a subjective complaint.

Frequently, but not always, the SRNVM occurs at the edge of an old healed chorioretinal scar that is associated with a discontinuity in Bruch's membrane on histopathologic examination. Macular lesions can develop in previously normal retina. It is more common, however, that reactivation of old lesions accounts for new SRNVMs, with a 20 to 23 percent activation rate.[44, 45]

Emotional stress may induce serous detachment in eyes with an existing SRNVM.[44] Schlaegel and colleagues[31] found a relationship between skin test results and the activation of old macular lesions, but this is disputed by other investigators.

Choroidal neovascular membranes are classified by their location in relation to the center of the foveal avascular zone. The designations of *extrafoveal, juxtafoveal,* and *subfoveal* are described.

Extrafoveal SRNVMs have an edge of hyperfluorescence or blockage of fluorescence, as shown on fluorescein angiography, between 200 and 2500 μ from the center of the foveal avascular zone. Lewis and associates[45] found that 69 percent of patients with extrafoveal SRNVMs had visual acuity of 20/40 or better at presentation.

Juxtafoveal SRNVMs have either a hyperfluorescent edge 1 to 200 μ from the center of the foveal avascular zone, with or without blockage (blood, pigment) through the center of the foveal avascular zone, or an SRNVM 200 to 2500 μ from the center, with blood or blocked fluorescence within 200 μ of the center. Lewis and associates[45] found that 71 percent of patients with juxtafoveal SRNVMs from OHS had visual acuity measuring 20/200 or worse. Gutman[13] found that if the SRNVM was inside the foveal avascular zone, there was a 63 percent chance that visual acuity would be less than 20/200, but a 25 percent chance if the SRNVM was outside the foveal avascular zone. Olk and coworkers[17] found that 65 percent of patients with juxtafoveal membranes had a visual outcome of 20/200 or worse. Poor prognostic clinical signs include subretinal blood, poor initial vision, membrane close to the center of the foveal avascular zone, and large SRNVM size. Steroids have no effect on juxtafoveal lesions.

SRNVMs have active leakage under the center of the foveal avascular zone. Fourteen to 16 percent of these patients recover visual acuity of 20/40 spontaneously without laser treatment,[17, 45, 48] and laser treatment through the center of the foveal avascular zone would almost certainly decrease visual acuity to the 20/200 level immediately. Therefore, these patients should not be considered for laser treatment. Fifty percent or more of these eyes end up with very poor vision.[17, 44, 49] A good prognosis has been predicted by the following: age less than 30 yr, small SRNVM, and good fellow eye. Poor prognosis was found in eyes with initially excellent vision and an SRNVM that involved more than 50

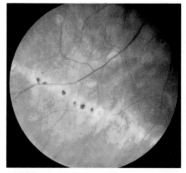

Figure 67–5. Fundus photograph shows peripheral linear streak of histoplasmosis spots.

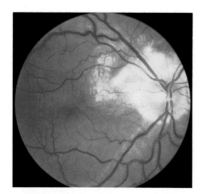

Figure 67–6. Juxtapapillary changes include retinal pigment epithelial hypertrophy and atrophy.

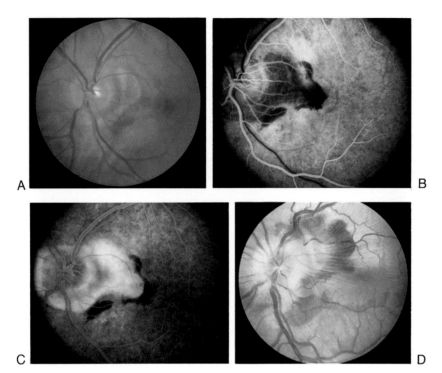

Figure 67–7. In this eye, juxtapapillary changes led to the development of subretinal neovascularization. *A,* The fundus photograph shows evidence of gray subretinal lesions along with subretinal blood, both of which are signs of subretinal neovascularization. *B,* An early frame of a fluorescein angiogram shows early hyperfluorescence. *C,* A later frame shows massive leakage from the new vessel membrane. *D,* In another patient, a juxtapapillary subretinal neovascular membrane causes extensive retinal striae.

percent of the foveal avascular zone. Thirty-six percent of patients less than 30 yr of age had visual acuity of 20/40 or better, establishing that the greater the area of foveal avascular zone covered by the SRNVM, or the further the SRNVM is beyond the center of the foveal avascular zone, the worse the prognosis.[17]

Vitritis and OHS

The presence of vitritis almost always rules out the diagnosis of OHS. Any time vitreous cells are present, entities other than OHS must be considered.

Pigment Epithelial Detachments

Gass[50] and others believe that pigment epithelial detachments are very rare in OHS. There may be sur-

rounding atrophy of the RPE. Patients with OHS who are older than 60 yr may prove exceptions to this "rule."

Disseminated Choroiditis

Disseminated choroiditis usually occurs in immunocompromised patients. The lesions present as yellow, circumscribed, elevated choroidal infiltrates with fuzzy edges and a surrounding ring of pigment (Fig. 67–9). The foci of choroiditis may develop into an SRNVM, with serous retinal detachment, hemorrhage, and retinal striae.

Optic Disc Edema

Optic disc edema occurs rarely in patients with OHS.[51, 52] The juxtapapillary findings in OHS may originate from undetected, transient papillitis.

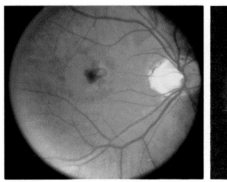
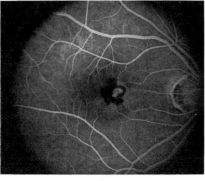

Fig. 67–8. Macular lesion of OHS. *A,* Fundus photograph of a subretinal neovascular membrane (SRNVM), with a gray membrane, subretinal hemorrhage, subretinal fluid, and pigment ring. *B,* An early frame of a fluorescein angiogram with early hyperfluorescence demonstrates a juxtafoveal SRNVM.

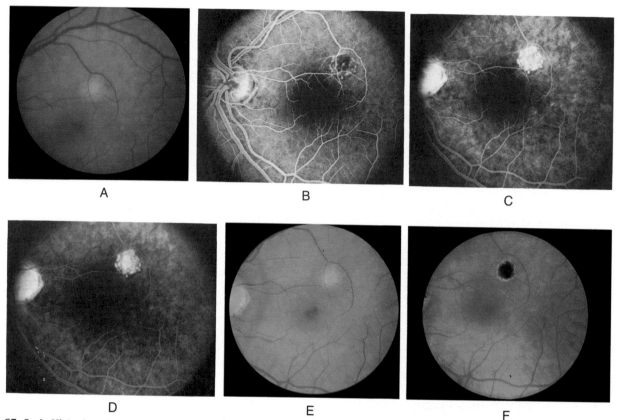

Fig. 67–9. A, Histoplasmic choroiditis causes yellow choroidal infiltrates with a surrounding pigment ring. Fluorescein angiography demonstrates early blocked fluorescence (B) and the intermediate (C) and late (D) staining of the lesion. These lesions can become atrophic with time (E) and ultimately may develop secondary reactive hyperplasia of the retinal pigment epithelium (F).

Exogenous Histoplasmic Endophthalmitis

One case of exogenous histoplasmic endophthalmitis following cataract extraction has been reported.[53]

Vitreous Hemorrhage

There has been one report of a patient with OHS in whom an SRNVM developed and resulted in breakthrough vitreous hemorrhage.[54] OHS can be considered in the differential diagnosis of vitreous hemorrhage.

FLUORESCEIN ANGIOGRAPHIC FINDINGS

Indications

Fluorescein angiography is crucial in the care of patients with OHS. Patients with no subjective complaints or findings of peripheral or macular chorioretinal scars do not require fluorescein angiography. The indications for fluorescein angiography include symptoms of an SRNVM, such as visual loss, metamorphopsia, or blurring; clinical signs of SRNVM; and the need to evaluate the fellow eye of a patient with OHS to check for the presence of macular chorioretinal scars that would indicate an increased risk to that eye (Table 67–2). It is vital to obtain a fluorescein angiogram in any patient with new symptoms.

Findings

The histoplasmosis "spots" show early hypofluorescence with faint late staining (Fig. 67–10). These areas can change to early staining with late leakage over time. Gass[50] believes the punched-out lesions fluoresce but that this is due to scleral reflection and not actual leakage of dye. The RPE and choriocapillaris between the histoplasmosis lesions are normal (in age-related macular degeneration, this is not the case).

Table 67–2. SYMPTOMS AND SIGNS OF SUBRETINAL NEOVASCULARIZATION

Metamorphopsia
Visual blurring
Serous detachment of retina
Subretinal hemorrhage
Hard lipid exudate
Pigment halo surrounding lesion

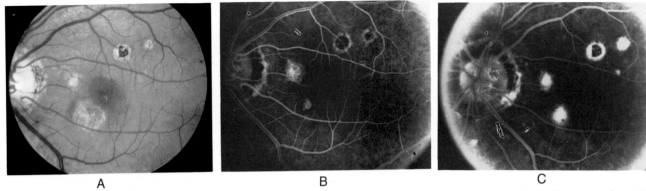

Fig. 67–10. *A,* Fundus photograph of an SRNVM (inferior to the fovea) and histoplasmosis spots (superior to the fovea). *B* and *C,* Fluorescein angiograms of histoplasmosis spots. *B* shows early hypofluorescence and *C* shows late staining. Note how the new vessel membrane leaks fluorescein dye and develops fuzzy margins late in the study. The histoplasmosis spots show staining of the sclera but stay sharply demarcated.

Acute, yellow choroidal lesions stain with fluorescein.[50]

An SRNVM stains early in a lacy pattern and leaks late, with the margins of the lesion becoming hazy. Subretinal fluid may collect dye late in the study and therefore show staining. Subretinal blood allows fluorescence of retinal vessels but blocks fluorescence of the choroidal vessels and SRNVM. The SRNVM may extend beyond the halo of hypofluorescence around the hyperfluorescent lesion.

DIFFERENTIAL DIAGNOSIS
(Table 67–3)

Multifocal Choroiditis and Panuveitis (Pseudo-Presumed OHS)

Dreyer and Gass[55] reported on 28 patients with multifocal choroiditis, old punched-out lesions, juxtapapillary atrophic changes, and SRNVMs. Most patients were from nonendemic areas and had vitritis and decreased electroretinogram signals. Of 16 patients who underwent skin testing, only 5 tested positive for histoplasmosis. This syndrome is especially difficult to differentiate from birdshot choroidopathy and diffuse unilateral subacute neuroretinopathy. Deutsch and Tessler[56] reported similar findings; 43 percent of their patients were black. The choroidal punched-out lesions in pseudo-presumed OHS are smaller than those in OHS, some of the spots represent an active choroiditis, and vitritis is present.

Table 67–3. DIFFERENTIAL DIAGNOSIS OF THE OCULAR HISTOPLASMOSIS SYNDROME

Multifocal choroiditis and panuveitis
Birdshot choroidopathy
Diffuse unilateral subacute neuroretinopathy
Acute posterior multifocal placoid pigment epitheliopathy
Vogt-Koyanagi syndrome
Behçet's disease

Systemic steroids may help the active lesions in pseudo-presumed OHS.

Birdshot (Vitiliginous) Choroidopathy

Birdshot choroidopathy presents in an older age group than does OHS. Choroidal lesions are creamy, active spots without atrophy or pigmentation, and there are no juxtapapillary changes. Optic disc pallor occurs, but choroidal neovascularization is rare. The electroretinogram is depressed and fluorescein angiography shows disc leakage and cystoid macular edema.

Diffuse Unilateral Subacute Neuroretinopathy

Diffuse unilateral subacute neuroretinopathy is a unilateral parasitic infestation. Early in the disease, there are clusters of white spots, vitritis, and retinal pigment epithelial changes between white lesions. The lesions are evanescent and change with the location of the parasite. Late in its course, optic atrophy and arterial narrowing develop.

Acute Posterior Multifocal Placoid Pigment Epitheliopathy

Usually occurring after upper respiratory infection, acute posterior multifocal placoid pigment epitheliopathy leads to clustered lesions in the posterior pole, often with severe loss of vision. The lesions disappear after a brief period, usually with return of good vision.

Vogt-Koyanagi Syndrome

The Vogt-Koyanagi syndrome is a granulomatous uveitis with infiltrative choroidal lesions. Exudative retinal detachment is frequently present. Systemic symptoms such as tinnitus, deafness, poliosis, vitiligo, and headache occur.

Behçet's Disease

Behçet's disease includes severe vasculitis with panuveitis. Aphthous oral ulcers and genital lesions usually accompany the attacks of uveitis.

TREATMENT

Steroids

Schlaegel and colleagues[41] considered systemic steroids to be appropriate for acute flare-ups and possibly for long-term use to prevent visual loss. Schlaegel[57, 58] believed that steroids, if used, should be given in high doses (prednisone 60 to 100 mg/day) and tapered very slowly over 1 to 2 yr. Makley and coworkers[59] found some benefit if steroids were used early in the course of macular lesions.

Steroid use is controversial, but there may be a role in subfoveal lesions, especially in acute choroidal neovascular membranes without a lot of subfoveal hemorrhage or in cases of acute choroiditis in the fovea. However, no controlled trial has proved the efficacy of steroids.

Before beginning steroid treatment, a tuberculin skin test should be performed. Blood pressure and serum blood glucose levels should be monitored during long-term use. There are many systemic side effects that must be monitored during use.

Desensitization

Schlaegel and colleagues[41] desensitized OHS patients by giving small doses of histoplasmin antigen subcutaneously. They found there was no difference between treated and control groups. Some investigators report that skin testing or desensitization may exacerbate macular lesions in OHS.

Laser Treatment of Inactive Macular Lesions

Gitter and Cohen[60] attempted to prevent SRNVM formation in fellow eyes by laser treatment of inactive macular lesions. Their study contained no controls, but no complications were reported. Later, one of the patients experienced an SRNVM in a treated scar. Others have reported similar cases.[61, 62] This procedure is not recommended, as it is not useful in preventing SRNVM formation.

Amphotericin B

Amphotericin B has been tried in the past in an attempt to obliterate a histoplasmosis infection. Makley and coworkers[59] found no treatment benefit. Most investigators believe that OHS lesions are probably sterile, inflammatory lesions containing no organisms and, therefore, antifungal agents play no role in the treatment of OHS.

Antihistamines

Antihistamines were at one time thought to play a regulatory role for choroidal capillaries and have been tried in OHS macular disciform lesions but without success.

6-Mercaptopurine

6-Mercaptopurine has been tried, but with no benefit.

MACULAR PHOTOCOAGULATION STUDY—OHS AND EXTRAFOVEAL SRNVM

The ocular histoplasmosis section of the Macular Photocoagulation Study was a multicenter, controlled clinical study designed to answer specific questions concerning whether laser treatment would prevent visual loss from SRNVMs. The subretinal neovascular complex includes hyperfluorescence, blood, pigment, and blocked fluorescence on fluorescein angiography. Extrafoveal SRNVMs are defined as having hyperfluorescence on fluorescein angiography 200 to 2500 μ from the center of the foveal avascular zone (Fig. 67–11). The diagnosis of OHS requires at least one atrophic chorioretinal scar. Entrance into the Macular Photocoagulation Study required visual acuity of 20/100 or better. Juxtapapillary SRNVMs were included in the study only if treatment would spare at least 1½ clock hr of nerve fiber layer in the maculopapular bundle.

Argon blue-green laser, which emits wavelengths of 488 (blue) and 514 (green) nm, was used in this study. Blue light is absorbed by xanthophyll (the yellow pigment around the fovea), the cataractous lens, hemoglobin, melanin, and the inner retina. Green laser light is absorbed by hemoglobin and melanin.[63] Although the Macular Photocoagulation Study used argon blue-green, argon green is currently used to avoid the complications of blue light. The advantages of green over blue-green include less xanthophyll absorption and less damage to the inner retina.

Before the Macular Photocoagulation Study, many investigators had tried laser photocoagulation in OHS. The studies varied in the patient populations, treatment protocol, and whether a fluorescein angiogram was obtained in every patient. Treating SRNVM with mild to moderate laser burns has no benefit.[41, 67] Gass[68] treated extrafoveal lesions and found that 50 percent of these patients had visual acuity of 20/30 or better with laser treatment. Sabates and associates[69] believed that the laser must be used to destroy the SRNVM completely. Forty-eight percent of their patients had visual acuity of

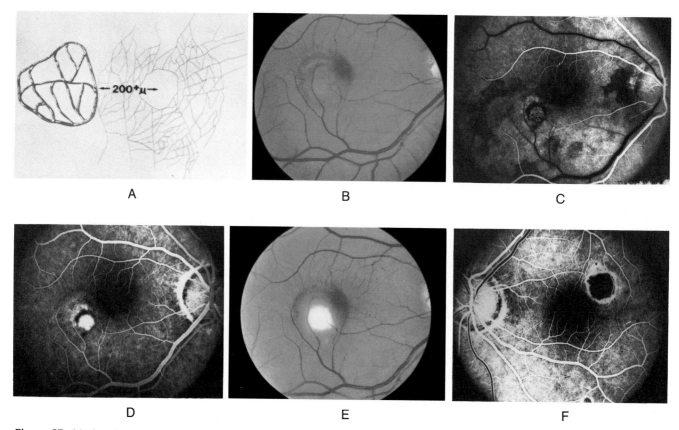

Figure 67–11. *A*, Schematic representation of an extrafoveal SRNVM, demonstrating the measurement from the center of the foveal avascular zone to the edge of the SRNVM, in this case 200 μ away. (From Poliner LS, Olk RJ: Ocular histoplasmosis syndrome. Semin Ophthalmol 2:238, 1987.) *B*, Fundus photograph of an SRNVM. *C*, Fluorescein angiogram demonstrating early, lacy hyperfluorescence. *D*, Middle frame of the angiogram showing leakage of dye. *E*, Posttreatment photograph. *F*, Fluorescein angiogram showing obliteration of the new vessel membrane. Note normal hyperfluorescence at edge of laser scar.

20/50 or better, and 30 percent had visual acuity of 20/200 or worse. Patz and Fine[70] treated SRNVMs that were more than 125 μ from the edge of the foveal avascular zone without blood into the foveal avascular zone. They extended laser treatment 125 μ past the edge of the SRNVM and felt that this resulted in better closure of the SRNVM. Inadequate treatment may stimulate bleeding and make visual results worse than if no treatment were performed. Maumenee and Ryan[71] treated SRNVMs with the xenon laser and found that 67 percent of patients had no change or improvement in vision. Klein and coworkers[72] found no statistical difference between treatment and observation. Okun[73] found that 76 percent of patients had the same or better vision with xenon laser treatment compared with 44 percent without treatment. Gitter and Cohen[60] reported that 63 percent of their patients had visual acuity of 20/40 or better when treated with argon laser. Olk and colleagues[74] treated SRNVM complex at least 125 μ from the edge of the foveal avascular zone with argon laser. Seventy-five percent of patients had visual acuity of 20/40 or better, and 19 percent had visual acuity of less than 20/200. Almost one third of their initial successes exhibited recurrence. Lewis and associates[45] had a 70 percent success with argon or xenon laser, treating SRNVM more than 375 μ from the center of the foveal avascular zone.

Results of the Macular Photocoagulation Study[64] showed that at 24 mo, a 6-line visual loss had occurred in 50 percent of the group receiving no treatment and in 22 percent of the treated group. At 36 mo, the results were 45 percent for the group receiving no treatment and 10 percent for the treated group.[65] The effectiveness of laser treatment when compared with controls was present in all subgroups at all stages of follow-up. Burgess[66] concluded that any SRNVM completely outside the foveal avascular zone should be treated with laser.

Our current recommendations for the evaluation and treatment of extrafoveal SRNVMs resulting from OHS are somewhat different from those of the Macular Photocoagulation Study trial. We recommend that juxtapapillary SRNVMs be considered for treatment if they are (1) more than halfway between the disc and the fovea, (2) causing serous detachment of the fovea, or (3) causing hemorrhage under the fovea. All others may be watched without laser treatment. Some extrafoveal SRNVMs may be followed with frequent examination and daily home use of the Amsler grid to assess visual acuity.

MACULAR PHOTOCOAGULATION STUDY—OHS AND JUXTAFOVEAL SRNVM

The Macular Photocoagulation Study[75] also looked at subretinal neovascular SRNVMs that are closer than 200 μ to the center of the foveal avascular zone. Fine and associates[76] reviewed the two branches of the Macular Photocoagulation Study studies. A juxtafoveal SRNVM was defined in this study as having a hyperfluorescent edge 1 to 200 μ from the center of the foveal avascular zone or an SRNVM 200 to 2500 μ from the center, with blood or blocked fluorescence within 200 μ of the center (Fig. 67–12).

Juxtafoveal SRNVMs have been studied by several investigators in addition to the Macular Photocoagulation Study. Gass and Wilkinson[44] found no clear benefit of laser using either the ruby or the xenon laser. They had variable techniques of intensity and found many patients did well without laser treatment. Yassur and coworkers[77] used krypton laser to treat SRNVMs in OHS. They found that krypton penetrates thin blood and is not absorbed by macular xanthophyll, and it creates less retinal whitening than does argon laser. Olk and coworkers[17] treated juxtafoveal SRNVMs and found that in 86 percent of patients, visual acuity ended up being 20/200 or worse. Sabates and associates[69] compared argon and krypton with observation in juxtafoveal SRNVMs in OHS. Twenty percent of eyes needed more than one treatment session. Patients with visual acuity of 20/40 or better were separated into the following treatment groups: 28.5 percent argon, 35.4 percent krypton, and 23 percent observation. Patients with 20/200 vision or worse were separated into the following treatment groups: 53.5 percent argon, 25.8 percent krypton, and 63 percent observation. These studies were not definitive, and this led to the organization of the Macular Photocoagulation Study.

The krypton section of the Macular Photocoagulation Study required vision to be at least 20/400. Patients with juxtapapillary membranes could be entered if treatment would allow 1½ clock hr of disc to be left untreated. The SRNVM was ineligible if it extended under the center of the foveal avascular zone. This branch of the Macular Photocoagulation Study used the krypton red laser (647 nm). There are several advantages of krypton red laser, including less lens scatter, less absorption by xanthophyll, and less inner retina damage.[63] Hemoglobin does not absorb red laser at all. There are several disadvantages to krypton red. This laser can crack Bruch's membrane more easily than can argon green, but the incidence of internal limiting membrane wrinkling is higher with argon. These advantages and disadvantages are created because the red laser is absorbed by melanin in the RPE and choroid.

The results of the juxtafoveal branch of the Macular Photocoagulation Study at 1 yr of follow-up showed that the risk of a 6-line visual loss was 24.8 percent in the group who received no treatment compared with 6.6 percent in the treated group.[75] The results were very similar at 3 yr follow-up.

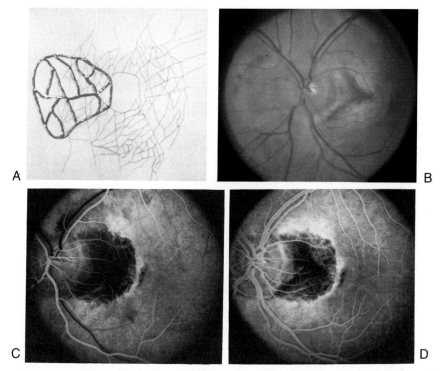

Figure 67–12. A, Schematic representation of juxtafoveal SRNVM inside 200 μ from the center of the foveal avascular zone. (From Poliner LS, Olk RJ: Ocular histoplasmosis syndrome. Semin Ophthalmol 2:238, 1987.) B–D, Photograph (B) and angiograms showing early (C) and middle frames (D) from the patient shown in Figure 67–7 after krypton red laser treatment. Note that choroidal vessels are visible through the laser scar.

Proximity to the fovea is crucial in juxtafoveal SRNVMs. Outside the foveal avascular zone, the chances of maintaining visual acuity of 20/40 or better is 60 percent compared with 15 percent if the SRNVM is inside the foveal avascular zone.

LASER TREATMENT TECHNIQUE

General Guidelines

There are some general rules that may guide laser photocoagulation of choroidal neovascular membranes.

The role of *anesthesia* in laser photocoagulation of SRNVMs is to provide comfort during the procedure and to increase the margin of safety when treating near the fovea. Topical anesthesia may be adequate for treatment in the cooperative patient with an extrafoveal SRNVM. For juxtafoveal SRNVMs, we recommend retrobulbar anesthesia in all but the most cooperative patients. If the patient squeezes the lids, Bell's phenomenon can move the eye superiorly, thereby risking photocoagulation of the fovea during treatment of an SRNVM superior to fixation. Further, juxtafoveal SRNVMs should be treated with krypton red, and this frequently causes some discomfort if local anesthesia is not given.

A recent *fluorescein angiogram* is essential for adequate treatment. It has been shown that SRNVMs may grow, especially those closer to the fovea, in the course of several days. The fluorescein angiogram being used to guide treatment should be less than 72 hr old, especially with juxtafoveal lesions. More latitude may be taken with extrafoveal SRNVMs that are greater than 500 μ from the center of the foveal avascular zone.

The fluorescein angiogram is essential for mapping the foveal avascular zone, as well as the SRNVM. The use of the aiming beam to map fixation is not a reliable way to define the foveal avascular zone. Because of eccentric fixation or distortion of the fovea, one may be fooled into treating the fovea.

The following procedural details may be helpful. Both the surgeon and the patient should be seated comfortably at the laser. An elbow rest should be used to stabilize the surgeon's arm. A fixation light for the fellow eye helps to stabilize the treatment eye. The patient should be introduced to the sound of the laser before treatment actually begins. We firmly believe that treatment should be guided by an early frame of a recent fluorescein angiogram. One should use a slide projector to project the fluorescein angiogram behind the patient, a tabletop viewer, or a stereo viewer taped to the top of the laser slit lamp.

Various fundus contact lenses are available for macular treatment. It must be remembered that some lenses reverse and invert the surgeon's view of the fundus (Mainster, Rodenstock). The fluorescein angiogram must be properly oriented so that the surgeon does not confuse the anatomy.

If *bleeding* occurs during the laser treatment, intraocular pressure should be increased with the contact lens and then laser treatment applied over the bleeding site, preferably with argon green.

Klein and coworkers[72] did not avoid *retinal vessels* in the treatment area. We recommend that heavy, long-duration burns not be placed directly over retinal vessels, especially if the vessel supplies the central fovea.

Sabates and colleagues[78] found that *hemorrhage* obscures the complete extent of the SRNVM and absorbs the laser energy, thus sparing the SRNVM. Intense treatment over areas of subretinal hemorrhage is not indicated, as energy absorption is quite superficial and will cause damage to the retina.

Argon Green Laser for Extrafoveal SRNVM

First, the SRNVM is outlined with burns of 100-μ size and 0.1-sec duration. Gass[68] recommends covering any pigment ring and subretinal neovascularization as shown by an early frame of the fluorescein angiogram. On the foveal side, 100- to 200-μ spots of 0.2-sec duration are delivered in a confluent fashion. These should be heavy white spots. The remainder of the lesion is covered confluently with heavy laser burns of 200- to 500-μ spots and 0.5-sec duration. The SRNVM should be covered 100 μ past the edge of the subretinal neovascular complex. On the foveal side, if the treatment will not enter the foveal avascular zone, the treatment should extend 100 μ. If the edge of the subretinal neovascular complex is close to the edge of the foveal avascular zone, coverage of the SRNVM by a full 100 μ beyond the edge is not required (Fig. 67–13).

Krypton Red Laser for Juxtafoveal SRNVM

The krypton red laser should be used with large spots (at least 200 μ) and long duration (at least 0.2 sec) to decrease the chance of rupturing Bruch's membrane. The retina will whiten less with krypton red than with argon green. It is not necessary to treat blood or blocked fluorescence (Fig. 67–14).

First, the foveal side of the lesion is treated with 200-μ spots of 0.2-sec duration. The remainder of the lesion is treated with 200- to 500-μ confluent burns of 0.5-sec duration.

1. If hyperfluorescence is more than 100 μ from the center of the foveal avascular zone, and if blood or blocked fluorescence is present, treatment extends 100 μ into the blocked fluorescence, but the center of the foveal avascular zone is not treated.

2. If hyperfluorescence is within 200 μ and if no blocked fluorescence is present, laser treatment should cover the hyperfluorescence, and treatment does not need to extend 100 μ past the edge.

Subfoveal Treatment of SRNVM

Subfoveal treatment of SRNVMs is contraindicated, as some patients with subfoveal subretinal neovascularization will undergo spontaneous regression with a good outcome.

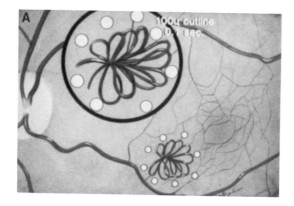
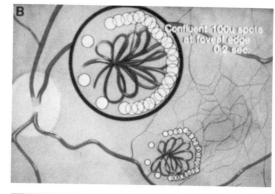
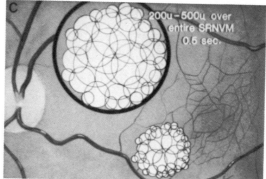

Figure 67–13. A–C, Schematic representation of treatment of extrafoveal SRNVM. (A–C, From Poliner LS, Olk RJ: Ocular histoplasmosis syndrome. Semin Ophthalmol 2:238, 1987.)

Surgical Removal of SRNVM

Several investigators are working with the removal of subfoveal SRNVMs in OHS. This is a research tool at this time and indications for this procedure have not yet been determined.

RECURRENT SRNVM IN OHS

Definition

After laser photocoagulation, interpretation of the posttreatment angiogram can be one of the most challenging facets in the treatment of macular disease. A *persistent* SRNVM shows hyperfluorescence (representing subretinal neovascularization) within 6 wk of treatment. A *recurrent* SRNVM is defined as leakage adjacent to or within the laser scar occurring more than 6 wk after treatment.

Incidence

The Macular Photocoagulation Study reviewed the incidence of recurrent SRNVMs.[77, 78] In the OHS–juxtafoveal segment of the study, 31 percent of the treated eyes had recurrent SRNVMs, and 65 percent of these recurrences were amenable to further treatment. The remainder were not retreatable because of subfoveal extension of the SRNVM. This compares with 59 percent of treated eyes with age-related macular degeneration and 33 percent of eyes with idiopathic SRNVM.

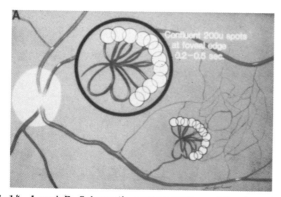
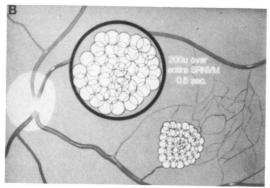

Figure 67–14. A and B, Schematic representation of treatment of juxtafoveal SRNVM. (A and B, From Poliner LS, Olk RJ: Ocular histoplasmosis syndrome. Semin Ophthalmol 2:238, 1987.)

Time Course

Most recurrences were noted within 12 mo after treatment, with the majority occurring within the first 6 mo.

Etiology

There are several factors that may contribute to the recurrence of SRNVMs after treatment: inadequate coverage or intensity of treatment, the presence of blood or pigment within 200 μ of the center of the foveal avascular zone, and location of the SRNVM less than 200 μ from the center. Further, the growth of an independent SRNVM may occur during the posttreatment follow-up period. This is believed to be unrelated to treatment. Several risk factors have been statistically associated with recurrences, including hypertension, cigarette smoking, proximity to fovea, young age, and female gender.

In relation to the original SRNVM, recurrences can occur on the margin of the treatment, in the center of the treatment scar, contiguous to the scar, from a feeder vessel originating from the original SRNVM, or as a completely new lesion greater than 250 μ from the margin of the laser scar (Fig. 67–15). Ninety percent of marginal recurrences are on the foveal side of the treatment, indicating that recurrences are largely responsible for visual loss from OHS after laser treatment.

MARGINAL RECURRENCE

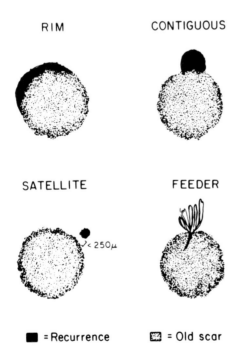

RIM   CONTIGUOUS

SATELLITE   FEEDER

< 250μ

■ = Recurrence   ▨ = Old scar

Figure 67–15. Schematic examples of locations of recurrent SRNVMs. (From Sorenson JA, Yannuzzi LA, Shakin JL: Recurrent subretinal neovascularization. Published courtesy of Ophthalmology [1985; 92:1059–1074].)

Table 67–4. COMPLICATIONS OF LASER TREATMENT

Recurrence of subretinal neovascular membrane
Retinal pigment epithelial rips
Acute choroidal hemorrhage
Nerve fiber layer field defects
Premacular fibroplasia

Presentation

The signs and symptoms of recurrent SRNVMs are similar to those of the original lesion. Visual loss and metamorphopsia are common subjective complaints. Clinical findings include sensory retinal detachment, subretinal hemorrhage, gray subretinal mass, cystoid macular edema, choroidal folds, and subretinal fibrosis (Fig. 67–16). The findings for recurrence can be more subtle than those for primary SRNVMs, making diagnosis more difficult. This creates the need for routine posttreatment fluorescein angiography.

Treatment

The laser treatment technique is the same for recurrences as for a primary SRNVM. In the Macular Photocoagulation Study, 62 percent of eyes had stabilized visual acuity after retreatment.[80] Olk and Burgess[81] reported 60 percent of their patients had stable or increased vision following treatment of recurrent SRNVMs, and 77 percent of the patients had visual acuity of 20/80 or better. Central recurrence does not need to be treated, as it rarely leads to subfoveal extension. Careful follow-up is indicated.

COMPLICATIONS OF TREATMENT AND RETREATMENT (Table 67–4)

The most important complication of the treatment of SRNVMs is recurrence of the membrane (see preceding discussion). This has a very high visual morbidity. Rips of the RPE may occur at the time of laser treatment or in the postoperative period. The rips are due to contraction of the RPE induced by laser energy. However, ripping of the RPE in the treatment of OHS is extremely rare.

Acute choroidal hemorrhage may create subretinal or sub–pigment epithelial hemorrhage, both of which are associated with a poor visual outcome. Laser treatment in the papillomacular bundle can result in nerve fiber layer visual field defects.

Premacular fibroplasia and internal limiting membrane contracture may occur (Fig. 67–17) and may lead to macular hole formation. Han and Folk[82] found more internal limiting membrane wrinkling in eyes treated with argon than with those treated with krypton. This was also dependent on intensity, area of SRNVM, and the presence of subretinal blood. Symptoms from premacular fibroplasia included metamorphopsia, macular dragging, and binocular diplopia.

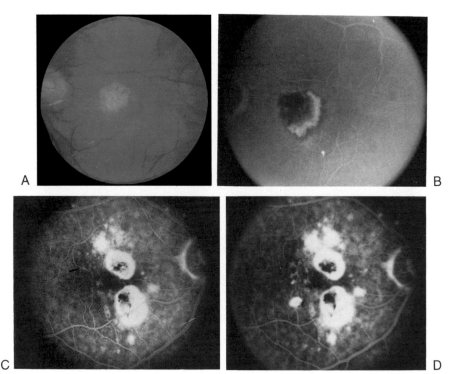

Figure 67–16. Examples of recurrent SRNVMs. *A,* Photograph of a laser scar with a pigmented halo temporally. *B,* Fluorescein angiography demonstrates a rim recurrence with hyperfluorescent leakage along the temporal edge of the laser scar. *C,* Frame of a fluorescein angiogram showing two treated new vessel membranes. *D,* Note the new small membrane temporal to the original areas. Thus, an area previously uninvolved can develop subretinal neovascularization.

FOLLOW-UP

Nonexudative OHS

Patients with histoplasmosis chorioretinal scars in the macula should be warned of the risk of the development of SRNVMs. Any symptoms of decreased vision or metamorphopsia should initiate immediate examination by a qualified ophthalmologist. These patients should follow an Amsler grid on a regular basis (Fig. 67–18). The onset of new symptoms warrants a careful ophthalmic examination and an immediate fluorescein angiogram.

Posttreatment Follow-up

Initially after laser treatment, very careful follow-up is essential. Our routine is to see patients at 2, 4, and 6 wk after treatment then at 3 and 6 mo. We obtain a fluorescein angiogram on all patients at the 2- and 6-wk visits, then on an "as needed" basis. These patients should follow an Amsler grid to check visual acuity on a regular basis.

Shah and associates[83] found that laser scars migrate an average of 150 μ toward the fovea yearly for the first 2 yr, then 22 μ/yr thereafter. They found eight patients who had scars expand under the foveal center, and six of them had vision better than or equal to their initial vision, indicating that this occurrence is not of poor prognostic value.

Fellow Eye

SRNVMs in OHS may appear in an area of previously normal retina.[13, 84, 85] There is no guarantee when the clinical examination and fluorescein angiogram of the fellow eye are clear that nothing can happen; the patient and ophthalmologist must follow both eyes carefully.

Interpretation of Posttreatment Fluorescein Angiogram

The posttreatment fluorescein angiogram can be very difficult to interpret. A stereo fluorescein angiogram

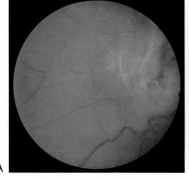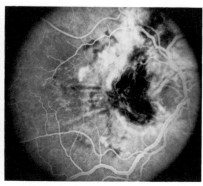

Figure 67–17. Example of a complication of laser treatment for SRNVMs in OHS. *A,* Fundus photograph. *B,* Fluorescein angiogram of a patient after treatment of a juxtapapillary SRNVM. This patient experienced premacular fibrosis.

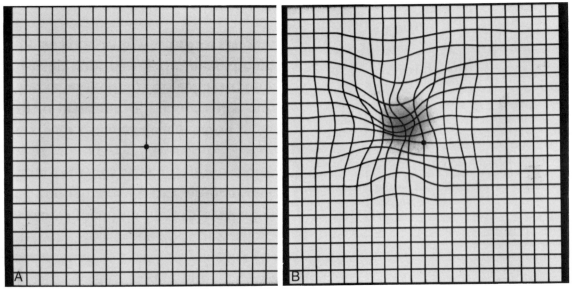

Figure 67–18. *A,* An Amsler grid is used for diagnosis of SRNVMs. This grid can be used at home by patients at risk for the development of new vessel membranes. *B,* An artist's demonstration of metamorphopsia and relative scotoma seen by a patient with a new SRNVM.

frequently will help to identify the source of hyperfluorescence. Of course, not everything that is hyperfluorescent on posttreatment fluorescein angiography is a recurrence of choroidal neovascularization. Heat damage to retinal vessel walls causes increased permeability, leading to leakage of fluorescein in the early posttreatment period. This occurs with argon green laser more frequently than with krypton red laser. Further, staining of fluorescein may occur at the edge of the laser scar because of heat damage to the RPE. Later, transmission defects and late scleral staining occur within the laser scar. Clinical examination is important in these cases. Lastly, persisting or recurring SRNVMs may be present and lead to leakage of fluorescein.

Visual Recovery

Jost and coworkers[86] reported visual recovery in eyes with OHS and subretinal SRNVMs. They found 10 of 22 patients who met their requirements. A decrease in vision in the fellow eye appeared to induce an improvement in vision in the first eye. Eccentric fixation was believed to be responsible for the recovery. Good prognosis for visual recovery included young age, short time interval between visual loss in the two eyes, smaller laser scars, and less fovea involved with the SRNVM.

CONCLUSION

OHS is a relatively common disease, especially in the endemic areas of the Ohio and Mississippi river valleys. Two symposia have been held to discuss OHS, and these reviews and discussions have been published previously.[87, 88] Patients with macular chorioretinal scars are at risk for the development of choroidal neovascularization that can threaten central vision.

The Macular Photocoagulation Study has provided valuable information on the evaluation and treatment of SRNVM due to OHS. Each patient needs to be evaluated on an individual basis, but guidelines for treatment are now available.

REFERENCES

1. Krause AC, Hopkins WG: Ocular manifestations of histoplasmosis. Am J Ophthalmol 34:564, 1951.
2. Woods AC, Wahlen HE: The probable role of benign histoplasmosis in the etiology of granulomatous uveitis. Am J Ophthalmol 49:205, 1960.
3. Baskin MA, Jampol LM, Huamonte FU, et al: Macular lesions in blacks with the presumed ocular histoplasmosis syndrome. Am J Ophthalmol 89:77, 1980.
4. Braunstein RA, Rosen DA, Bird AC: Ocular histoplasmosis syndrome in the United Kingdom. Br J Ophthalmol 58:893, 1974.
5. Ellis FD, Schlaegel TF: The geographic localization of presumed histoplasmic choroiditis. Am J Ophthalmol 75:953, 1973.
6. Wheat LJ, French MLV, Kohler RB, et al: The diagnostic laboratory test for histoplasmosis. Ann Intern Med 97:680, 1982.
7. Feman SS, Podgorski SF, Penn MK: Blindness from presumed ocular histoplasmosis in Tennessee. Ophthalmology 89:1295, 1982.
8. Smith RE, Ganley JP: An epidemiologic study of presumed ocular histoplasmosis. Trans Am Acad Ophthalmol Otolaryngol 75:994, 1971.
9. Smith RE, Ganley JP: Presumed ocular histoplasmosis. I. Histoplasmin skin test sensitivity in cases identified during a community survey. Arch Ophthalmol 87:245, 1972.
10. Ganley JP, Smith RE, Knox DL, Comstock GW: Presumed ocular histoplasmosis. III. Epidemiologic characteristic of people with peripheral atrophic scars. Arch Ophthalmol 89:116, 1973.
11. Davidorf FH, Anderson JD: Ocular lesions in the Earth Day histoplasmosis epidemic. Trans Am Acad Ophthalmol Otolaryngol 78:876, 1974.
12. Feman SS, Tilford RH: Ocular findings in patients with histoplasmosis. JAMA 253:2534, 1985.
13. Gutman FA: The natural course of active choroidal lesion in the presumed ocular histoplasmosis syndrome. Trans Am Acad Ophthalmol Soc 77:515, 1979.
14. Lewis ML, Schiffman JC: Long-term follow-up of the second eye in ocular histoplasmosis. Int Ophthalmol Clin 23:125, 1983.
15. Sawelson H, Goldberg RE, Annesley WH, Tomer TL: Presumed ocular histoplasmosis syndrome. Arch Ophthalmol 94:221, 1976.

16. Gass JDM: Pathogenesis of disciform detachment of the neuroepithelium. Am J Ophthalmol 63:661, 1967.
17. Olk RJ, Burgess DB, McCormick PA: Subfoveal and juxtafoveal subretinal neovascularization in the presumed ocular histoplasmosis syndrome—Natural history. Ophthalmology 91:1592, 1984.
18. Hoefnagels KLJ, Pijpers PM: *Histoplasma capsulatum* in a human eye. Am J Ophthalmol 63:715, 1967.
19. Roth AM: *Histoplasma capsulatum* in the presumed ocular histoplasmosis syndrome. Am J Ophthalmol 84:293, 1977.
20. Gass JDM, Zimmerman LE: Histopathologic demonstration of *Histoplasma capsulatum*. Am J Ophthalmol 85:725, 1978.
21. Macher A, Rodriques MM, Kaplan W, et al: Disseminated bilateral chorioretinitis due to *Histoplasma capsulatum* in a patient with the acquired immunodeficiency syndrome. Ophthalmology 92:1159, 1985.
22. Klintworth GK, Hollingsworth AS, Lusman PA, Bradford WD: Granulomatous choroiditis in a case of disseminated histoplasmosis: Histologic demonstration of *Histoplasma capsulatum* in choroidal lesions. Arch Ophthalmol 90:45, 1973.
23. Craig EL, Suie T: *Histoplasma capsulatum* in human ocular tissue. Arch Ophthalmol 91:285, 1974.
24. Schwarz J, Salfelder K, Viloria JE: *Histoplasma capsulatum* in vessels of the choroid. Ann Ophthalmol 9:633, 1977.
25. Scholz R, Green WR, Kutys R, et al: *Histoplasma capsulatum* in the eye. Ophthalmology 91:1100, 1984.
26. Khalil MK: Histopathology of presumed ocular histoplasmosis. Am J Ophthalmol 94:369, 1982.
27. Meredith TA, Green WR, Key SN, et al: Ocular histoplasmosis: Clinicopathological correlation of 3 cases. Surv Ophthalmol 22:189, 1977.
28. Smith RE: Natural history and reactivation studies of experimental ocular histoplasmosis in a primate pool. Trans Am Ophthalmol Soc 80:695, 1982.
29. Smith RE, Dunn S, Jester JV: Natural history of experimental histoplasmic choroiditis in the primate. I. Clinical features. Invest Ophthalmol Vis Sci 25:801, 1984.
30. Smith RE, Dunn S, Jester JV: Natural history of experimental histoplasmic choroiditis in the primate. II. Histopathologic features. Invest Ophthalmol Vis Sci 25:810, 1984.
31. Schlaegel TF, Weber JC, Helveston E, et al: Presumed histoplasmic choroiditis. Am J Ophthalmol 63:919, 1967.
32. Check IJ, Diddie KR, Jay WM, et al: Lymphocyte stimulation by yeast phase *Histoplasma capsulatum* in presumed ocular histoplasmosis. Am J Ophthalmol 87:311, 1979.
33. Ganley JP, Nemo GJ, Comstock GW, Brody JA: Lymphocyte transformation in presumed ocular histoplasmosis. Arch Ophthalmol 99:1424, 1981.
34. Brahmi Z, Wheat J, Rubin RH, et al: Humoral and cellular immune response in ocular histoplasmosis. Ann Ophthalmol 17:440, 1985.
35. Meredith TA, Smith RE, Braley RE, et al: The prevalence of HLA-B7 in presumed ocular histoplasmosis in patients with peripheral atrophic scars. Am J Ophthalmol 86:325, 1978.
36. Braley RE, Meredith TA, Aaberg TM, et al: The prevalence of HLA-B7 in presumed ocular histoplasmosis. Am J Ophthalmol 85:859, 1978.
37. Godfrey WA, Sabates R, Cross DE: Association of presumed ocular histoplasmosis with HLA-B7. Am J Ophthalmol 85:854, 1978.
38. Smith RE, Ganley JP, Knox DL: Presumed ocular histoplasmosis. II. Patterns of peripheral and peripapillary scarring in persons with nonmacular disease. Arch Ophthalmol 87:251, 1972.
39. Bottoni FG, Deutman AF, Aandekerk AL: Presumed ocular histoplasmosis syndrome and linear streak lesions. Br J Ophthalmol 73:528, 1989.
40. Fountain JA, Schlaegel TF: Linear streaks of the equator in the presumed ocular histoplasmosis syndrome. Arch Ophthalmol 99:246, 1981.
41. Schlaegel TF, Cofield DD, Clark G, Weber JC: Photocoagulation and other therapy for histoplasmic choroiditis. Trans Am Acad Ophthalmol Otolaryngol 72:355, 1968.
42. Watzke RC, Claussen RW: The long-term course of multifocal choroiditis (presumed ocular histoplasmosis). Am J Ophthalmol 91:750, 1981.
43. Miller SA, Stevens TS, de Venecia G: De novo lesions in presumed ocular histoplasmosis–like syndrome. Br J Ophthalmol 60:700, 1976.
44. Gass JDM, Wilkinson CP: Follow-up study of presumed ocular histoplasmosis. Trans Am Acad Ophthalmol Otolaryngol 76:672, 1972.
45. Lewis ML, Van Newkirk MR, Gass JDM: Follow-up study of presumed ocular histoplasmosis syndrome. Ophthalmology 87:390, 1980.
46. Meredith TA, Aaberg TM: Hemorrhagic peripapillary lesions in presumed ocular histoplasmosis. Am J Ophthalmol 84:160, 1977.
47. Cantrill HL, Burgess DB: Peripapillary neovascular membranes in presumed ocular histoplasmosis. Am J Ophthalmol 89:192, 1980.
48. Kleiner RC, Ratner CM, Enger C, et al: Subfoveal neovascularization in the ocular histoplasmosis syndrome. Retina 8:225, 1988.
49. Klein ML, Fine SL, Knox DL, Patz A: Follow-up study in eyes with choroidal neovascularization caused by presumed ocular histoplasmosis. Am J Ophthalmol 83:830, 1977.
50. Gass JDM: Stereoscopic Atlas of Macular Disease, 3rd ed. St Louis, CV Mosby, 1987.
51. Beck RW, Sergott RC, Barr CC, Annesley WH: Optic disc edema in the presumed ocular histoplasmosis syndrome. Ophthalmology 91:183, 1984.
52. Husted RC, Shock JP: Acute presumed histoplasmosis of the optic nerve head. Br J Ophthalmol 59:409, 1975.
53. Pulido JS, Folberg R, Carter KD, et al: *Histoplasma capsulatum* endophthalmitis after cataract extraction. Ophthalmology 97:217, 1990.
54. Kranias G: Vitreous hemorrhage secondary to presumed ocular histoplasmosis syndrome. Ann Ophthalmol 17:295, 1985.
55. Dreyer RF, Gass JDM: Multifocal choroiditis and panuveitis. Arch Ophthalmol 102:1776, 1984.
56. Deutsch TA, Tessler HH: Inflammatory pseudohistoplasmosis. Ann Ophthalmol 17:461, 1985.
57. Schlaegel TF: Ocular Histoplasmosis. New York, Grune & Stratton, 1977.
58. Schlaegel TF: Corticosteroids in the treatment of ocular histoplasmosis. Int Ophthalmol Clin 23:111, 1983.
59. Makley TA, Long JW, Suie T: Therapy of chorioretinitis presumed to be caused by histoplasmosis. Int Ophthalmol Clin 15:181, 1975.
60. Gitter KA, Cohen G: Photocoagulation of active and inactive lesions of presumed ocular histoplasmosis. Am J Ophthalmol 79:428, 1975.
61. Boucher MC, Dumas J, Labelle P, et al: Prophylactic argon laser photocoagulation of the second eye in presumed ocular histoplasmosis syndrome. Can J Ophthalmol 22:266, 1987.
62. Fine SL, Patz A, Orth DH, et al: Subretinal neovascularization developing after prophylactic argon laser photocoagulation of atrophic macular scars. Am J Ophthalmol 82:352, 1976.
63. Mainster MM: Wavelength selection in macular photocoagulation. Ophthalmology 93:952, 1986.
64. Macular Photocoagulation Study Group: Argon laser photocoagulation for ocular histoplasmosis. Arch Ophthalmol 101:1347, 1983.
65. Macular Photocoagulation Study Group: Argon laser photocoagulation for neovascular maculopathy—Three-year results. Arch Ophthalmol 104:594, 1986.
66. Burgess DB: Ocular histoplasmosis syndrome. Ophthalmology 83:967, 1986.
67. Watzke RC, Leaverton PE: Light coagulation in presumed histoplasmic choroiditis. Arch Ophthalmol 86:127, 1971.
68. Gass JDM: Photocoagulation of macular lesions. Trans Am Acad Ophthalmol Otolaryngol 75:580, 1970.
69. Sabates FN, Lee KY, Ziemianski MC: A comparative study of argon and krypton laser photocoagulation in the treatment of presumed ocular histoplasmosis syndrome. Ophthalmology 89:729, 1982.
70. Patz A, Fine SL: Argon laser photocoagulation in ocular histoplasmosis syndrome. Int Ophthalmol Clin 16:45, 1976.
71. Maumenee AE, Ryan SJ: Photocoagulation of disciform macular lesions in the ocular histoplasmosis syndrome. Am J Ophthalmol 75:13, 1973.

72. Klein ML, Fine SL, Patz A: Results of argon photocoagulation in presumed ocular histoplasmosis. Am J Ophthalmol 86:211, 1978.
73. Okun E: Photocoagulation treatment of presumed ocular histoplasmic choroidopathy. Trans Am Ophthalmol Soc 70:467, 1972.
74. Olk RJ, Fine SL, Scheraga D, et al: Long-term follow-up of presumed ocular histoplasmosis treated with argon laser photocoagulation. Retina 1:238, 1981.
75. Macular Photocoagulation Study Group: Krypton laser photocoagulation for neovascular lesions of ocular histoplasmosis. Arch Ophthalmol 105:1499, 1987.
76. Fine SL, Olk RJ, Murphy RP, Hillis A: Current status of clinical trials to evaluate argon (blue-green) laser and krypton (red) laser photocoagulation in the treatment of ocular histoplasmosis. Int Ophthalmol Clin 23:79, 1983.
77. Yassur Y, Gilad E, Ben-Sira I: Treatment of macular subretinal neovascularization with the red-light krypton laser in presumed ocular histoplasmosis syndrome. Am J Ophthalmol 91:172, 1981.
78. Sabates NF, Lee KY, Sabates R: Early argon laser photocoagulation of presumed histoplasma maculopathy. Am J Ophthalmol 84:172, 1977.
79. Macular Photocoagulation Study Group: Recurrent choroidal neovascularization after argon laser photocoagulation for neovascular maculopathy. Arch Ophthalmol 104:503, 1986.
80. Macular Photocoagulation Study Group: Persistent and recurrent neovascularization after krypton laser photocoagulation for neo-

vascular lesions of ocular histoplasmosis. Arch Ophthalmol 107:344, 1989.
81. Olk RJ, Burgess DB: Treatment of recurrent juxtafoveal subretinal choroidal neovascular membranes with krypton red laser photocoagulation. Ophthalmology 92:1035, 1985.
82. Han DP, Folk JC: Internal limiting membrane wrinkling after argon and krypton laser photocoagulation of choroidal neovascularization. Retina 6:215, 1986.
83. Shah SS, Schachat AP, Murphy RP, et al: The evolution of argon laser photocoagulation scars in patients with the ocular histoplasmosis syndrome. Arch Ophthalmol 106:1533, 1988.
84. Ryan SJ: De novo subretinal neovascularization in the histoplasmosis syndrome. Arch Ophthalmol 94:321, 1976.
85. Wilkinson CP: Presumed ocular histoplasmosis. Am J Ophthalmol 75:140, 1976.
86. Jost BF, Olk RJ, Burgess DB: Factors related to spontaneous visual recovery in the ocular histoplasmosis syndrome. Retina 7:1, 1987.
87. Schlaegel TF (ed): Ocular histoplasmosis. Int Ophthalmol Clin 15, 1975.
88. Schlaegel TF (ed): Update on ocular histoplasmosis. Int Ophthalmol Clin 23, 1983.
89. Poliner LS, Olk RJ: Update on ocular histoplasmosis syndrome. Semin Ophthalmol 2:238, 1987.
90. Sorenson JA, Yannuzzi LA, Shakin JL: Recurrent subretinal neovascularization. Ophthalmology 92:1059, 1985.

Chapter 68

■

Pathologic Myopia

RONALD C. PRUETT

The term *myopia* is derived from two Greek roots—*myein*, which means to close, and *ops*, which means eye. It describes the ancient observation that affected individuals habitually approximate their eyelids to form a stenopeic slit to improve image quality. In a myopic eye, rays of light from a distant source are focused anterior to the plane of the retina because of an optical mismatch between the anterior and the posterior segments of the globe. This may result from excessive convergent power caused by a steeply curved cornea, an abnormally spherical lens, or an increase in the lenticular index of refraction, as with nuclear sclerosis. Most frequently, myopia is due to axial elongation associated with expansion of the scleral shell.

In clinical practice, myopia often is classified as being physiologic or pathologic. Although not optically complementary, the dimensions and refractive powers of the ocular components in a physiologically myopic eye fall within normal limits. The refractive disparity in these eyes usually is less than -6.00 D. Pathologically myopic eyes have errors of -6.00 D or greater, sometimes in excess of -40.00 D. The classic works of Tron[1] and Stenstrom[2] demonstrated that axial length and refractive component measurements occurred in a bimodal gaussian distribution if eyes with pathologic dimensions were excluded from the population. Eyes with pathologic myopia are an eccentric group in which the myopia is more likely due to a disease than to a biologic variation. Such eyes show excessive axial length with equatorial scleral expansion, dehiscences, and posterior staphyloma formation. Global expansion can slowly progress during a person's lifetime and result in blinding complications. In addition to physiologic and pathologic myopia, Curtin[3] introduced the term *intermediate myopia* to indicate those eyes that represent neither extreme and share characteristics of both.

PREVALENCE

Myopia is the most common ocular abnormality. Its prevalence varies among different ethnic groups, being least in blacks and greatest in Asians. Among the mixed population of the United States, 25 percent of individuals were found to be myopic; among a subset of American blacks the percentage was 12.6 percent.[4] When 120,000 Chinese individuals were studied, 70 percent were found to be myopic.[5] Females are more likely than males to be myopic, as are those people in higher socioeconomic classes and those with greater academic training. Pathologic myopia also is influenced by ethnicity but is observed less frequently (i.e., in approximately 2 percent of Americans). A survey of international prevalence statistics[6] showed wide variation, from lows of 0.2 percent (Egypt) and 1.0 percent (Czechoslovakia) to highs of 9.6 percent (Spain) and 8.4 percent (Japan). Although they were less likely to survive in the hunter-gatherer period of early humankind, individuals with pathologic myopia have thrived and reproduced in more advanced civilizations.

PATHOGENESIS

Although in many cases myopia appears to be genetically determined, its precise pathophysiology and the influence of environmental factors in determining its development have yet to be elucidated. Etiologic theories are discussed in *Principles and Practice of Ophthalmology: Basic Sciences,* Chapter 56. Unfortunately, no animal model faithfully reproduces the human condition of pathologic myopia as we know it. Excessive myopia is one of the manifestations of a wide variety of established genetic disorders, such as the Marfan, Ehler-Danlos, and Stickler syndromes. In familial studies, both dominant and recessive modes of inheritance have been found. The fact that the sclera is grossly abnormal has suggested to many that it is biomechanically weak and subject to stretch (creep) in response to intraocular pressure, extraocular muscle tension, and other factors.[7–14] When compared with normal, the microscopic scleral architecture shows smaller diameter collagen bundles that are loosely woven, especially at the posterior pole, which is last to mature.[15–18] In addition, highly myopic globes have low ocular rigidity,[19] are prone to develop low-tension, pigmentary, and open-angle glaucoma,[20, 21] and often respond to topical steroid application with a rise in intraocular pressure.[22, 23]

Although unproved, the postulates of impaired scleral resistance and increased expansile force have served as the basis for treatment. Until we have a thorough understanding of genomic and biochemical mechanisms, efforts can be directed only toward mitigating the complications of pathologic myopia rather than toward its cause.

COMPLICATIONS

Visual disabilities due to myopia are protean; the greater the degree of myopia, the higher their incidence. Among these complications are image minification, anisometropic amblyopia, visual field defects, impaired dark adaptation, abnormal color discrimination, suboptimal binocularity, premature cataract formation, glaucoma, lattice degeneration, giant retinal tear, and retinal detachment. In this chapter, we focus on three manifestations of pathologic myopia that appear directly related to progressive axial elongation: posterior vitreous detachment, posterior retinal detachment, and posterior staphyloma.

Vitreous Detachment

Posterior detachment of the vitreous gel from the internal limiting membrane of the neurosensory retina can be seen following trauma, with occlusive retinal vascular disorders such as diabetic retinopathy and retinal vein obstruction, and in association with various types of chorioretinitis and other conditions. The most common cause of posterior vitreous detachment (PVD) is aging. Premature PVD also is characteristic of retinitis pigmentosa and pathologic myopia,[24] which prompts

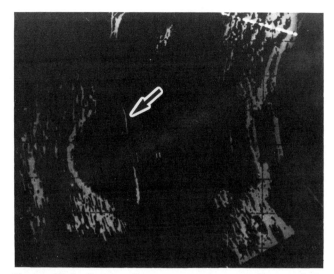

Figure 68–1. B-scan ultrasonogram demonstrating posterior staphyloma and posterior vitreous detachment *(arrow)* in an eye with an axial length of 31.1 mm.

speculation that disordered metabolism or demise of certain cellular elements of the sensory retina is responsible for failure of vitreous gel maintenance in the adult.

The incidence of PVD increases with the degree of myopia and with age. PVD usually is preceded by vitreous syneresis—formation of irregular fluid-filled cavities within the gel substance. If acute in onset, PVD may be accompanied by photopsia resulting from vitreoretinal traction and migratory small scotomata, or "floaters," which result from shadows cast on the retina by fibrillar condensations and discrete opacities in the gel, including its former ring attachment at the optic disc. Blood released from capillaries at the disc margin and along the vascular arcades or from vessels at the posterior vitreous baseline at the ora serrata can also cause this symptom. Although PVD can be demonstrated by B-scan ultrasonography (Fig. 68–1), vitreoretinal changes are best observed using indirect ophthalmoscopy with scleral depression and biomicroscopy with a mirrored contact lens. Occasionally, a retinal vessel will be avulsed by acute traction, or a full-thickness retinal tear will form, especially along the margin of vitreous adhesion to a peripheral strip of lattice degeneration.

These findings present an increased risk for recurrent vitreous hemorrhage and retinal detachment, particularly if located in the superior half of the fundus. Laser photocoagulation occlusion of an avulsed vessel and laser or cryocoagulation of retinal breaks and all other areas of retinal degeneration are recommended preventive measures. Actual retinal separation requires scleral buckling for definitive management in most eyes with pathologic myopia.

Posterior Retinal Detachment

The most frequent causes of macular hole formation are blunt trauma and extreme myopia. But retinal detachment caused by a foveal break is rare. Usually the eye has a history of poor visual acuity from prior foveal cyst formation and myopic posterior chorioretinal degeneration. Detachment is heralded by an enlarging central scotoma.

A posterior retinal detachment begins as a relatively shallow elevation confined within the temporal vascular arcades, but it can spread peripherally. Retinal breaks identified within a peripheral area of detachment can raise concerns about whether the detachment is caused by the foveal hole or the peripheral breaks, or both. Is the apparent foveal hole penetrating or only partially penetrating, a "pseudohole"? Thermal treatment of the macular defect to secure closure would increase the size and density of the postoperative central scotoma. Given these findings, most physicians treat the peripheral breaks only, using a conventional scleral buckling technique with drainage of subretinal fluid. If reaccumulation of fluid is noted at the posterior pole postoperatively, a second intervention is needed to treat the macula.

When no peripheral break exists in the area of detachment, or when the detachment is confined to the posterior fundus, the foveal hole is assumed to be the cause. Surgical repair can be either internal or external. Internal surgery consists of pars plana vitrectomy, endoevacuation of subretinal fluid through the foveal break, a vitreous fluid-gas exchange with filtered air, C_3F_8 or SF_6, and postoperative prone positioning of the head for internal tamponade. Some surgeons apply endolaser treatment to the gas-occluded break, whereas others omit thermal treatment.

If the internal approach fails, or if the surgeon is confronted by an extreme posterior staphyloma with advanced atrophy of the retina, pigment epithelium, and choroid, the external method[25] can be successful. Technically it is more difficult. Adequate exposure of the posterior region of a pathologically myopic eye usually requires a lateral canthotomy and temporary tenotomy of the lateral rectus muscle. Thermal treatment of the macular hole can be accomplished using a single application of cryocoagulation or transscleral diathermy with a fiberoptic-illuminated electrode[26] under indirect ophthalmoscopic control. A small, convex solid silicone rubber button explant is hand carved and fixed with polyester sutures to a No. 40 or 240 silicone band. The explant is positioned over the macular region while the two arms of the band are threaded episclerally into the lower nasal and upper temporal quadrants of the globe. Prefixed polyester slipknots, located anterior to the equator, are used to adjust tension in the partially encircling band while the position and height of the posterior buckling are observed by indirect ophthalmoscopy. If the break is closed, additional sutures or surgical glue is applied to secure the band and buckling device posteriorly. If the break remains elevated, a careful posterior sclerotomy is performed to release subretinal fluid from the staphylomatous region. Hypotony following release of fluid is reversed with a controlled pars plana injection of filtered air or synthetic gas and Schiøtz tonometer monitoring. In such a case, postoperative prone positioning is used for internal tamponade of the macular break against the posterior buckling indentation (Fig. 68–2).

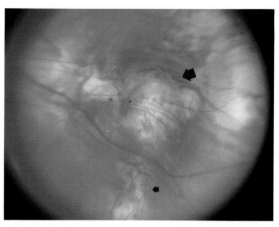

Figure 68–2. Posterior scleral buckling (sling operation) was used to repair a posterior retinal detachment caused by a macular hole in this highly myopic eye: buckling, *large arrow;* band, *small arrow.*

Posterior Staphyloma

With pathologic myopia, there is global expansion, scleral thinning with equatorial dehiscences, and its hallmark ectasia—a posterior staphyloma. First illustrated by Scarpa[27] in the early 19th century, posterior staphyloma contributes to macular hole formation and retinal detachment. In addition, it causes other cumulative damage that can be equally blinding. This is believed to result from slowly progressive chorioretinal stretching, mechanical tearing, and atrophy.

The earliest sign of tissue traction is seen at the lateral margin of the optic disc. Dragging of the pigment epithelium and choroid from the nerve produces a temporal crescent in which white sclera can be visualized through the transparent retinal nerve fiber layer. This change can surround the disc if the staphyloma incorporates, or extends nasal to, the optic nerve. Visual field testing will reveal an enlarged physiologic blind spot. Tilting and anatomic dispersal of receptor elements within the staphyloma can have other psychophysical consequences such as image minification, skewed visual direction, and impaired binocularity.[28]

Further tissue stress within the staphyloma can produce an acute break in Bruch's membrane. This may be accompanied by a subjective light flash followed by a positive scotoma caused by a small subretinal hemorrhage from the choriocapillaris. Bruch's membrane breaks and hemorrhages may be multiple and sequential and go unnoticed by the patient if they are not near the visual axis (Fig. 68–3). Such fractures, called *lacquer cracks*, are pathologically similar to ruptures seen following blunt ocular trauma and to angioid streaks. However, Myopic breaks form a distinctive reticular pattern within the base of the staphyloma with connections to the temporal crescent at the disc.[29] The subretinal hemorrhages reabsorb over a period of weeks to months, and vision returns to its former level unless a lacquer crack has involved the fovea. In that case there is permanent reduction in visual acuity.

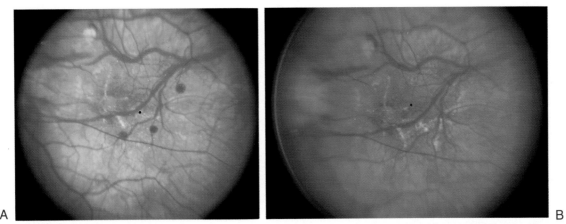

Figure 68–3. *A,* Pathologic myopia with multiple lacquer cracks and three asymptomatic macular hemorrhages. *B,* Extended lacquer cracks 15 mo later.

A secondary complication of lacquer crack formation, one that often occurs in young and middle-aged individuals, is submacular invasion by a choroidal neovascular membrane. Leakage of serum, blood, and subsequent pigmented cicatrix formation, a Förster-Fuchs spot, can cause a significant drop in visual acuity, even to the "counting fingers" level if the fovea is affected.

As time passes, lacquer cracks increase in number and width, subretinal hemorrhages affect the retinal sentient elements, and Förster-Fuchs scars become surrounded by a halo of retinal pigment epithelial and choroidal atrophy. Large choroidal vessels may show "sclerosis," whereas smaller choroidal circulatory lobules atrophy and disappear with their overlying pigment epithelium. As these areas grow and coalesce, wide atrophic patches cover the entire region of the staphyloma, and small remaining islands of vision become submerged in a "sea" of central darkness.

Clinical management of posterior staphyloma is hampered by ignorance of its pathophysiology and is sometimes controversial. A basic assumption is that the sclera is abnormally pliant and the victim of mechanical stress.[30] Advice to patients may be "commonsense" and unproved; therapies may be given to increase scleral resistance or decrease intraocular tension, or both—an extrapolation of the La Place equation:

$$S = \frac{r(p^i - p^e)}{2t}$$

This describes an ideal spherical container of uniform composition and thickness that is pressurized from within. The stress on its wall (S in grams/millimeter squared) is directly related to the radius of the sphere (r in millimeters) and the difference between its internal pressure (p^i in grams/millimeter square) and its external pressure (p^e in grams/millimeter square) and inversely related to the thickness of its wall (t in millimeters). Maximal stress would be expected in a large eye with elevated intraocular pressure and thin sclera.

Patients with pathologic myopia, particularly those with lacquer cracks, should avoid abrupt elevations in intraocular pressure from vigorous rubbing of the eyes and blunt trauma. Valsalva maneuvers and body inversion exercises also are inadvisable because of increased intraocular tension and choroidal congestion effects. Unless the risk of macular hemorrhage is outweighed by that of systemic complications, chronic use of aspirin and other anticoagulants is contraindicated. Medical treatment to maintain intraocular tension at a level as low as possible is important in individuals with open-angle glaucoma. Treatment is also advised for patients with low-tension glaucoma and for those who have suspected glaucoma and pathologic myopia. The use of pharmacologic ocular hypotension in nonglaucomatous individuals to retard the progression of myopia has received only preliminary evaluation.[31] The efficacy of this approach awaits testing of carefully selected subjects in a prospective double-blind study. Chronic cycloplegia can be effective to some degree,[32–37] but loss of accommodation, glare, photophobia, and concerns about light toxicity have prevented their general acceptance. Submacular choroidal neovascular networks are best left untreated unless there is significant leakage.[38, 39] In the latter case, laser photocoagulation is recommended, but long-term enlargement of the laser scar can be expected in many eyes.

Contact lens wear can produce essentially normal vision in many individuals with low degrees of myopia. For individuals with high myopia, successful fitting becomes more difficult because of increased thickness of the lens edge. Frustrated by image minification, prismatic effects, restricted peripheral visual field, and the unsightly appearance of spectacles, some seek relief through refractive surgical methods. In this case as well, the patient with pathologic myopia is a poor candidate. Extreme degrees of myopic error cannot be fully corrected by keratorefractive techniques such as radial keratotomy, keratomileusis, epikeratoprosthesis, and laser sculpting. Anterior chamber intraocular lens implantation and extraction of a clear lens for refractive purposes have as yet unmeasured potential risks of corneal decompensation and retinal detachment. Unfortunately, all these methods fail to address the basic problem of progressive scleral expansion in the individual with pathologic myopia and the likelihood that any refractive gain will be slowly eroded with time. Furthermore, the threats of posterior chorioretinal degeneration and retinal detachment remain.

To deal directly with posterior staphyloma formation, surgical approaches have been used to modify two factors in the La Place equation: the radius of curvature and the thickness of the globe. The radius and volume of the eye can be reduced by performing an equatorial scleral resection.[40, 41] The dangers of ocular rupture during surgery, massive choroidal hemorrhage, retinal detachment, and anterior segment ischemia limit the acceptance of this procedure.

Surgical reinforcement of the posterior pole was introduced in the 1950s to arrest staphyloma progression.[40] A number of materials have been employed, including donor sclera, fascia lata, dura mater, silicone rubber, Dacron mesh and polytetrafluoroethylene (Gore-Tex). Although thousands of operations have been performed in the former Soviet Union, Poland, and Japan with claims of success, studies have been poorly controlled and documented. The efficacy of the procedure is debated in the West, where there are believers[42–45] and skeptics.[46] If its value could be demonstrated by a long-term investigation of a standardized operation with biometric monitoring and internal controls, scleral reinforcement would be recommended early, before irreversible damage occurs. Of course, prevention of posterior staphyloma would be best. For this we are dependent on the genius of present and future molecular biologists to reveal its fundamental mechanisms of formation.

REFERENCES

1. Tron EJ: The optical elements of the refractive power of the eye. In Ridley F, Sorsby A (eds): Modern Trends of Ophthalmology. London, Butterworth, 1940, p 245.
2. Stenstrom S (Woolf D, translation): Untersuchungen uber die Variation und Kovariation der optischen Elemente des menschilichen Auges. Am J Optom 25:218, 1948.
3. Curtin BJ: The Myopias, Basic Science and Clinical Management. Philadelphia, Harper & Row, 1985, pp 169–234.
4. Sperduto RD, Seigel D, Roberts J, Rowland M: Prevalence of myopia in the United States. Arch Ophthalmol 101:405, 1983.
5. Rasmussen OD: Incidence of myopia in China. Br J Ophthalmol 20:359, 1936.
6. Fuchs AW: Frequency of myopia gravis. Am J Ophthalmol 49:1418, 1960.
7. Curtin BJ: Myopia: A review of its etiology, pathogenesis and treatment. Surv Ophthalmol 15:1, 1970.
8. Avetisov ES, Ferfilfain IL, Krush II: Rheologic properties of the sclera in high myopia. Vestn Oftalmol 90:43, 1974.
9. Greene PR, McMahon TA: Plastic deformation of the sclera. Invest Ophthalmol Vis Sci 17(ARVO Suppl):297, 1978.
10. Greene PR, McMahon TA: Scleral creep vs temperature and pressure in vitro. Exp Eye Res 29:527, 1979.
11. Greene PR: Mechanical considerations in myopia: Relative effects of accommodation, convergence, intraocular pressure and extraocular muscles. Am J Optom Physiol Opt 57:902, 1980.
12. Ku DN, Greene PR: Scleral creep in vitro resulting from cyclic pressure pulses: Application to myopia. Am J Optom Physiol Opt 58:528, 1981.
13. Battaglioli JL, Kamm RD: Measurements of the compressive properties of scleral tissue. Invest Ophthalmol Vis Sci 25:59, 1984.
14. Greene PR: Closed-form ametropic pressure-volume and ocular rigidity solutions. Am J Optom Physiol Opt 62:870, 1985.
15. Gorzino A: Modificazoni del collagene sclerale nella miopia maligna. Rass Ital Ottalmol 25:251, 1956.
16. Nikolaeva TE: Electron microscopic investigations of the sclera of eyes with emmetropia and myopia. Vestn Oftalmol 89:52, 1973.
17. Avetisov ES, Khoroshilova-Maslova IP, Andreeva LD: Ultrastructure changes of the medium in myopia. Vestn Oftalmol 97:36, 1980.
18. Curtin BJ, Iwamoto T, Renaldo DP: Normal and staphylomatous sclera of high myopia: An electron microscopic study. Arch Ophthalmol 97:912, 1979.
19. Draeger J: Untersuchungen Uber den Rigiditatskoeffizienten. Doc Ophthalmol 13:431, 1959.
20. David R, Zangwiel LM, Tessler Z, Yassur Y: The correlation between intraocular pressure and refractive status. Arch Ophthalmol 103:1812, 1985.
21. Ganley JB: Epidemiological aspects of ocular hypertension. Surv Ophthalmol 25:130, 1980.
22. Podos SM, Becker B, Morton WR: High myopia and primary open angle glaucoma. Am J Ophthalmol 62:1039, 1966.
23. Thomas JV, Pruett RC: Steroid provocation testing in high myopia. Proceedings of the Third International Conference on Myopia. Rome, Italy, May 1986.
24. Pruett RC, Albert DM: Vitreous degeneration in myopia and retinitis pigmentosa. In Schepens CL, Neetans A (eds): The Vitreous and Vitreoretinal Interface. New York, Springer-Verlag, 1987, pp 211–228.
25. Margherio RR, Schepens CL: Macular breaks, management. Am J Ophthalmol 74:233, 1972.
26. de Guillebon H, Schepens CL: A transilluminator scleral marker. Arch Ophthalmol 86:298, 1971.
27. Scarpa A, (Briggs J, translation): A Treatise on the Principal Diseases of the Eye, 2nd ed. London, Cadell Davies, 1818, p 392.
28. Pruett RC: Refractive surgery: Psychophysical considerations in progressive myopia. Ann Acad Med Singapore 19:131, 1989.
29. Pruett RC, Weiter JJ, Goldstein R: Myopic cracks, angioid streaks and traumatic tears in Bruch's membrane. Am J Ophthalmol 103:537, 1987.
30. Pruett RC: Progressive myopia and intraocular pressure: What is the linkage? A literature review. Acta Ophthalmol 185(Suppl) (66):117, 1988.
31. Jensen H: Timolol maleate in the control of myopia: A preliminary report. Acta Ophthalmol 185(Suppl)(66):128, 1988.
32. Bedrossian RH: Effect of atropine on myopia. Ann Ophthalmol 3:891, 1971.
33. Gimbel HV: The control of myopia with atropine. Can J Ophthalmol 8:527, 1973.
34. Kelly TSB, Chatfield C, Tustin G: Clinical assessment of the arrest of myopia. Br J Ophthalmol 59:529, 1975.
35. Dyer JA: Role of cycloplegics in progressive myopia. Ophthalmology 86:642, 1979.
36. Brodstein RS, Brodstein DE, Olson RJ, et al: The treatment of myopia with atropine and bifocals. Ophthalmology 91:1373, 1984.
37. Brenner RL: Further observations on use of atropine in the treatment of myopia. Ann Ophthalmol 17:137, 1985.
38. Avila MP, Weiter JJ, Jalkh AE, et al: Natural history of choroidal neovascularization in degenerative myopia. Ophthalmology 91:1573, 1984.
39. Jalkh AE, Weiter JJ, Trempe CL, et al: Choroidal neovascularization in degenerative myopia: Role of laser photocoagulation. Ophthalmic Surg 18:721, 1987.
40. Malbran J: Una nueva orientacion quirergica contra la miopia. Arch Soc Oftal Hisp Am 14:1167, 1954.
41. Borley WE, Miller WW: Surgical treatment of degenerative myopia. Trans Am Acad Ophthalmol Otolaryngol 62:791, 1958.
42. Miller WW, Borley WE: Surgical treatment of degenerative myopia. Am J Ophthalmol 57:796, 1964.
43. Miller WW: Surgical treatment of degenerative myopia: Scleral reinforcement. Trans Am Acad Ophthalmol Otolaryngol 78:896, 1974.
44. Snyder AA, Thompson FB: A simplified technique for surgical treatment of degenerative myopia. Am J Ophthalmol 74:273, 1972.
45. Thompson FB: Scleral reinforcement. In Thompson FB (ed): Myopia Surgery: Anterior and Posterior Segments. New York, MacMillan, 1990, pp 267–297.
46. Curtin BJ: The Myopias, Basic Science and Clinical Management. Philadelphia, Harper & Row, 1985, pp 415–421.

Chapter 69

∎

Idiopathic Macular Holes

DAVID R. GUYER and EVANGELOS S. GRAGOUDAS

Recent advances in the classification and pathogenesis of idiopathic macular holes and their precursor lesions have generated a renewed interest in this disorder (Table 69–1).[1–3] In addition, interest in the potential role of vitrectomy for either impending macular holes or full-thickness macular holes has created further controversy over the proper management of these patients.[4–7]

HISTORICAL PERSPECTIVE AND EARLY THEORIES ON PATHOGENESIS

The first case of a macular hole was reported in 1869 by Knapp;[8] however, the patient had a history of trauma and a macular hemorrhage.[9] Thus, the first true case of an idiopathic macular hole was described in 1871 by Noyes.[10] In 1900, the term *macular hole* was coined by Ogilvie.[11]

Initially, many investigators stated that trauma was the only, or most common, cause of macular holes.[8, 10–13] Several authors suggested that trauma could lead directly to a macular hole,[14] whereas others believed that the traumatic cystic changes progressed to form a macular hole.[15–20]

Table 69–1. CLASSIFICATION OF IDIOPATHIC MACULAR HOLES AND THEIR PRECURSOR LESIONS

Stage 1	Pre–macular hole lesions, macular cyst, impending macular hole
	Foveal detachment
	No or decreased foveal depression
	Stage 1A: Foveal yellow spot
	Stage 1B: Foveal yellow ring
	Retinal striae
	Lack of Watzke's sign
Stage 2	Eccentric early full-thickness macular hole
Stage 3	Full-thickness macular hole with vitreofoveal detachment
	Yellow deposits at the level of the retinal pigment epithelium
	Cuff of subretinal fluid
	Operculum
	Cystoid macular edema
	Positive Watzke's sign
Stage 4	Full-thickness macular hole with a posterior vitreous detachment

Data from Gass JDM: Idiopathic senile macular hole: Its early stages and pathogenesis. Arch Ophthalmol 106:629–639, 1988, Copyright 1988, American Medical Association; and Johnson RN, Gass JDM: Idiopathic macular holes. Observations, stages of formation, and implications for surgical intervention. Published courtesy of Ophthalmology (1988; 95:917–924).

Although traumatic macular holes can occur, we now know that these cases are rare. In several series, only 5 to 15 percent of macular holes were caused by trauma.[21–23] The idiopathic or senile macular hole, which usually occurs in elderly women, is by far the most common type. In one series,[23] 83 percent of cases were of this type.

Another early theory on the pathogenesis of macular holes suggested that macular cysts degenerated into macular holes.[24, 25] One author[24] in 1900 implicated a degenerated fovea as the culprit and termed this disorder *retinitis atrophicans sive rarificans centralis*.

A later theory stated that a macular hole was produced by rupture of a macular cyst caused by traction from a posterior vitreous detachment. As early as 1924, Lister[20] stated the importance of the vitreous in this condition. Several series showed signs of vitreoretinal traction in this disorder.[21, 22, 26, 27] For instance, Aaberg and associates[22] described opercula in 26 percent of the cases in their series. Many authors have also described a high incidence of posterior vitreous detachments in these patients.[23, 28]

An increased incidence of systemic estrogen use or a history of hysterectomy in patients with idiopathic macular holes has also been reported.[23, 28] McDonnell and coworkers[23] speculated that estrogen fluctuations could cause vitreous destabilization, traction, vitreous detachment, and finally a macular hole. However, this idea is highly speculative, and the preceding studies that showed a relationship with estrogen usage were not appropriately controlled.

McDonnell and coworkers[23] observed that a posterior vitreous detachment occurred whenever any of the pre-macular hole lesions (macular cysts) in their series progressed to a full-thickness macular hole. Morgan and Schatz[29, 30] reported that 10 of 12 (83 percent) eyes that had posterior vitreous detachments at follow-up examination also had a full-thickness macular hole. In their series, only 7 percent of eyes that initially had a posterior vitreous detachment progressed to develop a macular hole, whereas 44 percent of eyes without a posterior vitreous detachment initially developed a macular hole. These findings add support to the important role of the vitreous in this condition.

Other authors have used a special El Bayadi-Kajiura preset lens[31, 32] to study the vitreoretinal interface. In one of these reports,[32] 8 of 28 fellow eyes without posterior vitreous detachments developed macular holes, whereas none of the 21 fellow eyes with posterior vitreous detachments developed a macular hole. These authors concluded that a complete posterior vitreous detachment may protect the fellow eye from the formation of a macular hole. Recently, Fisher and Slakter[33] reported that the ultrasonic finding of attached vitreous faces in both eyes at the initial visit was a risk factor for the development of a macular hole in the second eye. Thus, attached vitreous may be ominous, whereas detached vitreous may be protective.

The role of a posterior vitreous detachment in the pathogenesis of an idiopathic macular hole, however, continues to be controversial. Recent surgical experience[4] has suggested that determining vitreoretinal interactions by slit-lamp biomicroscopy may be imprecise. In three patients,[4] a thin layer of cortical vitreous was present on the retina intraoperatively, despite the presence of a posterior vitreous detachment on slit-lamp biomicroscopic examination. Recent work has also suggested that posterior vitreous detachments are not as important as tangential vitreous traction in the pathogenesis of this condition.[1, 2]

Another theory on the pathogenesis of idiopathic macular holes has been advocated by Morgan and Schatz.[29, 30] These authors described a new pre–macular hole lesion termed *involutional macular thinning*. According to their theory, choroidal vascular changes lead to ischemia, which causes cystic changes in the macula. Atrophic changes follow, and vitreous traction on a thinned macula then produces a full-thickness macular hole. Inconsistent with this theory, however, is that choroidal changes have not been observed in histopathologic studies of this disorder.[34, 35]

CURRENT CONCEPTS OF PATHOGENESIS AND CLASSIFICATION

Although anterioposterior vitreous detachment, such as occurs with a posterior vitreous detachment, can create a macular hole, recent evidence suggests that this process is not the most common mechanism of macular hole formation.[1, 2, 36]

Gass[1] and Johnson and Gass[2] suggest that focal shrink-

age of the foveal cortical vitreous and subsequent tangential vitreous traction is crucial in the pathogenesis of macular holes. The vitreous nature of this contracting tissue has been confirmed by histopathologic study.[37]

These authors[1, 2] also described a new classification system for macular holes and their precursor lesions (see Table 69–1). In stage 1, a foveal detachment occurs with a lack of or decreased foveal depression. Vision is usually 20/25 to 20/70. Two types of stage 1 lesions have been described. A stage 1A lesion has a foveal yellow spot, whereas a stage 1B lesion consists of a yellow ring (Fig. 69–1). The yellow material is probably xanthophyll. Retinal striae may also be observed.

Fluorescein angiography of stage 1 lesions may be normal or may show mild early hyperfluorescence. Stage 1 lesions are probably identical to what other authors have described as macular cysts[23] or impending macular holes.[4] All of these entities are pre–macular hole lesions.

The stage 1B yellow ring enlarges over weeks to months in some cases and progresses to a macular hole. A stage 2 lesion is an early macular hole, which begins eccentrically at one edge of the lesion and enlarges with time (Fig. 69–2). A stage 3 lesion is a full-thickness macular hole with vitreofoveal detachment (Fig. 69–3). Yellow deposits at the level of the retinal pigment epithelium, cystoid macular edema, a cuff of subretinal fluid, and an operculum are often present. The lesion usually develops in 3 to 6 mos. Vision is usually between 20/70 and 20/400. Fluorescein angiography may show early hyperfluorescence in this stage and thus may be indistinguishable from a stage 1 or stage 2 lesion. A stage 4 lesion is a macular hole with a posterior vitreous detachment.

CLINICAL FINDINGS[1–3]

Pre–macular Hole Lesions

Pre–macular hole lesions have been described by different names in the literature, such as macular cyst, stage 1 lesion, impending macular hole, and involutional

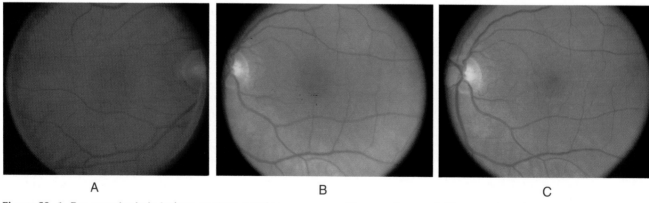

Figure 69–1. Pre–macular hole lesions or stage 1 lesions appear as either a yellow spot (A) or a yellow ring (B) lesion. This patient (B) with a stage 1B lesion initially presented with a visual acuity of 20/80. Sixteen months later, a flat, reddish lesion was present, and the yellow ring had disappeared (C). The visual acuity had improved to 20/30. (A–C, From Guyer DR, de Bustros S, Diener-West M, Fine SL: The natural history of idiopathic macular holes and cysts. Arch Ophthalmol 110:1264–1268, 1992. Copyright 1992, American Medical Association.)

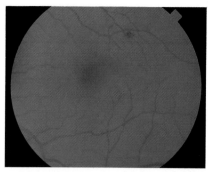

Figure 69–2. A stage 2 lesion is an early eccentric full-thickness macular hole, which often has a minimal accumulation of subretinal fluid. (Courtesy of Donald J D'Amico, M.D.)

macular thinning.[1–3, 9, 23, 29, 30] All of these lesions are probably identical. A 100- to 200-μ-diameter yellow spot (stage 1A) or a 200- to 350-μ-diameter yellow ring (stage 1B) is present, often with radiating retinal striae (see Fig. 69–1). The foveal depression is decreased or lacking. The center of the yellow ring may appear reddish. These patients have no Watzke's sign[3] (no interruption of the vertical slit beam on biomicroscopy). However, these patients may notice widening or narrowing of the slit beam.

Full-thickness Macular Holes

A stage 2 full-thickness macular hole is an early hole with an eccentric opening. Minimal subretinal fluid may be present (see Fig. 69–2).

A stage 3 full-thickness macular hole consists of an area devoid of retinal tissue that is approximately one third of a disc diameter in size (see Fig. 69–3). A 1200- to 1500-μ-diameter halo of detached retina with subretinal fluid usually surrounds the macular hole. Cystoid macular edema is also present. An operculum and yellow deposits at the level of the retinal pigment epithelium may also be observed. A positive Watzke sign is usually present[3] (interruption of a fine vertical slit beam focused on the hole). A stage 4 macular hole is identical to a stage 3 lesion but also has an associated posterior vitreous detachment.

Lamellar Macular Hole

This lesion is a partial-thickness macular hole with one or more "sharply circumscribed round, oval, or petal-shaped, red depressions in the inner retinal surface."[38]

Resolved Lesions

Spontaneous release of vitreous traction on a macular hole or stage 1 lesion may create partial resolution of the lesion. A flat, reddish lesion[3] or a lamellar macular hole[1, 2] may result (Fig. 69–4). A vitreofoveal opacity or pseudooperculum may be present.[1, 2]

DIFFERENTIAL DIAGNOSIS

Pre–macular hole lesions are often misdiagnosed. Gass and Joondeph[38] reported that only 1 of 18 patients referred to them with the diagnosis of a stage 1 lesion actually had such a lesion. The other cases had an aborted stage of macular hole formation (8 cases), stage 2 holes (4 cases), stage 3 holes (1 case), and unrelated lesions (4 cases). In determining the diagnosis of a lesion, it is important to search for very small eccentric holes, study the vitreoretinal interfaces, determine if a Watzke sign is present, and consider the visual acuity of the eye (Table 69–2).

Many other conditions should be considered in the differential diagnosis of macular holes and their precursor lesions. An epiretinal membrane with a pseudohole can be confused with a macular hole. The pseudohole usually allows better vision than does the macular hole. In addition, the pseudohole usually does not have a halo of fluid, an operculum, or yellow deposits at the level of the retinal pigment epithelium.

A foveal detachment due to central serous chorioretinopathy can be mistaken for a pre–macular hole lesion. Both appear as a yellow spot; however, fluorescein angiography can distinguish these two disorders. Central serous chorioretinopathy usually occurs in young to middle-aged men, whereas idiopathic macular holes usually affect elderly women.

The early yellow lesion of solar retinopathy can also

Figure 69–3. A stage 3 lesion is a full-thickness macular hole, which consists of a central area devoid of retinal tissue with a surrounding halo of subretinal fluid and cystoid macular edema (A). Yellow lesions at the level of the retinal pigment epithelium are often observed in patients with full-thickness macular holes (B).

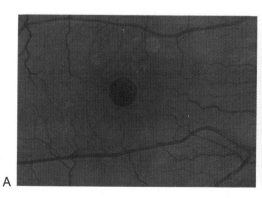

A

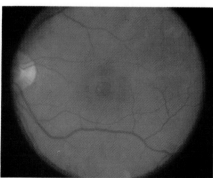

B

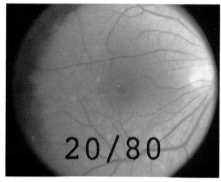 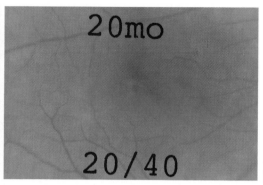

Figure 69–4. This patient presented with a full-thickness stage 3 macular hole. A cuff of subretinal fluid and yellow deposits at the level of the retinal pigment epithelium can be observed (A). Twenty months later, spontaneous release of vitreous traction occurred, and a flat reddish lesion without evidence of a macular hole was noted (B). Visual acuity had improved from 20/80 to 20/40. (A and B, From Guyer DR, de Bustros S, Dienet-West M, Fine SL: The natural history of idiopathic macular holes and cysts. Arch Ophthalmol 110:1264–1268, 1992. Copyright 1992, American Medical Association.)

appear similar to a stage 1 lesion. A history of sungazing should be searched for in these cases. Cystoid macular edema can also mimic the yellow spot of a stage 1 lesion.[38] Fluorescein angiography and a clinical history of cataract extraction can be useful in determining the correct diagnosis.

A central druse or retinal pigment epithelium depigmentation with a small amount of subretinal fluid and a central fibrocellular epiretinal membrane with a macular detachment have been described as mimicking an impending macular hole.[38] Failed attempts at macular hole formation should also be considered in the differential diagnosis of a pre–macular hole lesion.[38]

The vitreomacular traction syndrome[50, 51] can mimic an impending macular hole. Vitreous traction on the macula due to an incomplete vitreous detachment is responsible for this lesion. These disorders can be distinguished by examination of the vitreous. It is especially important to diagnose the vitreomacular traction syndrome because this condition can often be improved by vitrectomy.

NATURAL HISTORY

Pre–macular Hole Lesions

In one small retrospective series,[23] 50 percent of macular cysts progressed to a macular hole. However, the visual prognosis depended on the initial visual acuity; if vision was 20/40 or better, 23 percent of the cysts progressed to a macular hole 2 yr later, whereas if the vision was 20/50 or worse, 89 percent of the cysts progressed to a macular hole after 2 yr.

Morgan and Schatz[30] reported that 27 percent of their patients with a pre–macular hole lesion developed a macular hole. Retinal pigment epithelial changes on fluorescein angiography and the lack of a posterior vitreous detachment were risk factors in their study.

In Gass's series,[1] 10 of 18 (56 percent) stage 1 lesions progressed to a full-thickness macular hole, whereas 8 of 18 (44 percent) underwent spontaneous vitreofoveal separation without progression to a macular hole. In the

resolved cases, foveal reattachment was observed, the yellow spot or halo disappeared, and vision was usually 20/30 or better. Johnson and Gass[2] reported that 6 of 9 (67 percent) stage 1 lesions progressed to a macular hole. A prefoveal opacity or a lamellar hole, possibly consistent with unobserved resolved stage 1 lesions, was observed in 10 of 60 (16 percent) fellow eyes in their series.

Recently, however, other investigators[3] have reported that only 2 of 19 (10.5 percent) of the pre–macular hole lesions in their series had progressed to a macular hole at follow-up examination. A resolved flat, reddish lesion was observed in 15 of 19 (79 percent) of their patients (see Fig. 69–1).

All of the preceding series are small and retrospective in nature. A prospective natural history study is necessary to determine the actual frequency of progression of a pre–macular hole lesion to a macular hole. Our best current information suggests that the frequency of the development of a macular hole from a pre–macular hole lesion is between 10.5 and 67 percent.

Full-thickness Macular Holes

Patients with macular holes usually retain peripheral vision and have a visual acuity of approximately

Table 69–2. DIFFERENTIAL DIAGNOSIS

Epiretinal membrane with pseudohole
Foveal detachment secondary to central serous
    chorioretinopathy
Solar retinopathy
Cystoid macular edema
Central druse or retinal pigment epithelium depigmentation
    with subretinal fluid
Central fibrocellular epiretinal membrane with a macular
    detachment
Aborted attempts at macular hole formation
Vitreomacular traction syndrome

From Gass JDM, Joondeph BC: Observations concerning patients with suspected impending macular holes. Am J Ophthalmol 109:638–646, 1990. Published with permission from The American Journal of Ophthalmology. Copyright by The Ophthalmic Publishing Company.

20/200.[23] However, 5 to 12 percent of eyes with macular holes will show spontaneous improvement.[3, 22, 23, 29] Several investigators[3, 39, 40] have reported spontaneous partial resolution of macular holes. In one series,[3] 3 of 66 (5 percent) stage 3 macular holes appeared to have resolved at follow-up examination (see Fig. 69–4). A flat, reddish lesion was observed in these cases. These authors speculated that spontaneous release of vitreous traction could decrease the tension on the edges of the hole and thus decrease the actual size of the hole. In many cases, the hole might become so small that it could no longer be observed clinically. Resolution of subretinal fluid and cystoid macular edema could follow and allow improved vision in some cases. Recent surgical,[6, 7] histopathologic,[34] and scanning laser ophthalmoscopy[41] studies appear to support this hypothesis. However, it should be emphasized that the great majority of macular holes do not improve or worsen with time.

The occurrence of a retinal detachment in a patient with a macular hole is quite rare unless the patient is a high myope or has experienced ocular trauma.

Normal Fellow Eyes of Patients With Macular Holes or Pre–macular Hole Lesions

The risk of a macular hole developing in the normal fellow eye has been reported as being from 1 to 22 percent.[3, 9, 14, 22, 23, 28–31, 33, 36, 42–45] In one series,[3] only 1 (1.2 percent) and 2 (2.5 percent) of 80 normal fellow eyes developed a macular hole or pre–macular hole lesion, respectively, at follow-up examination. Therefore, the normal fellow eye of a patient with a macular hole or a pre–macular hole lesion has an excellent prognosis.

HISTOPATHOLOGY

On histopathologic examination a macular hole appears as a retinal defect in the foveal area surrounded by rounded edges, which are detached because of the accumulation of subretinal fluid (Fig. 69–5). Cystoid macular edema (79 percent) and epiretinal membranes (68 percent) were commonly observed in a recent histopathologic study of idiopathic macular holes.[34] Photoreceptor atrophy was variable.

Three cases of the probable histopathologic correlate of the resolved flat, reddish lesion were also noted. In these cases, the edges of the holes were reattached by glial cell or retinal pigment epithelium proliferation, or both.

In 50 percent of the lamellar (partial-thickness) macular holes, tangential traction by an epiretinal membrane on the internal limiting membrane was observed. Macular cysts were associated with cystoid macular edema in 67 percent of cases, and coalescence of edematous spaces may be important in the pathogenesis of this condition.

Study of the vitreous by histopathologic examination has been hampered by artifactious changes in the vitreous during gross examination and microscopic processing.

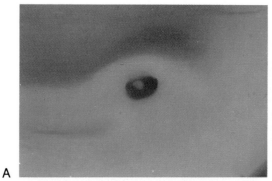

A

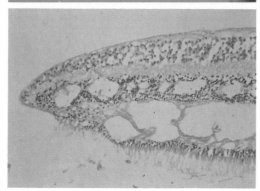

C

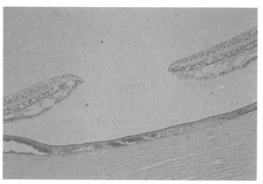

B

Figure 69–5. Gross examination of this autopsy eye reveals a full-thickness macular hole with an overlying operculum (A). Histopathologic examination of this macular hole demonstrates the rounded edges of retina at the edges of the hole (B). Underlying subretinal fluid and cystoid macular edema are present. Higher magnification of one edge of the macular hole shows marked cystoid macular edema and photoreceptor atrophy (C). (A–C, From Guyer DR, Green WR, de Bustros S, Fine SL: Histopathologic features of idiopathic macular holes and cysts. Ophthalmology 97:1045–1051, 1990.)

TREATMENT

The management of pre–macular hole lesions and full-thickness macular holes is highly controversial at present. Preliminary studies on the potential role of vitrectomy in this condition await confirmation by prospective randomized controlled clinical trials. Until these studies are completed, vitrectomy for pre–macular hole lesions and full-thickness macular holes must be considered experimental. The physician and patient must understand the preliminary nature of these studies and make an informed management decision on an individual basis.

Vitrectomy for Pre–macular Hole Lesions (Impending Macular Holes)

Several uncontrolled studies[4, 5, 46] have suggested that vitrectomy may be beneficial for the patient with an impending macular hole. In one study,[4] 15 patients with pre–macular hole lesions and decreased vision underwent pars plana vitrectomy. Progression to a macular hole was arrested in 12 of 15 (80 percent) eyes during a median follow-up time of 26 mo. Improved vision was noted in 5 of the 12 eyes. In another study,[5] 10 of 11 stage 1 lesions that underwent vitrectomy did not progress to macular holes. However, these small studies lacked control groups, and thus the role of surgery for this condition cannot be properly evaluated. In addition, vitrectomy is not without complications. In one of the series,[4] one peripheral retinal tear and progressive cataract formation in 5 of 14 (36 percent) phakic eyes were reported. Direct macular damage can also lead to an iatrogenic macular hole.

A prospective multicentered randomized controlled study of vitrectomy for patients with pre–macular hole lesions is currently under way.[47] This study should provide us with important information regarding this controversial topic in the near future.

Treatment of Full-thickness Macular Holes

Several investigators have attempted to cause reabsorption of the cuff of subretinal fluid or cystoid macular edema in patients with macular holes in order to improve visual function. Schocket and associates[48] applied laser photocoagulation to the rim of the hole in 18 patients. Visual improvement was observed in 10 (55.6 percent) eyes. However, this study had no control group and thus the results need to be confirmed. In addition, this type of treatment theoretically could damage potentially viable photoreceptors at the margins of the macular hole.

Kelly and Wendel[7] performed pars plana vitrectomies with removal of the prefoveal cortical vitreous and epiretinal membranes and a total gas-fluid exchange in 52 patients with full-thickness macular holes. These authors successfully reattached 30 (58 percent) of these eyes. Of these anatomically successful cases, improved vision was observed in 22 (73 percent) patients. Their overall success rate was 42 percent, whereas their complication rate was 15 percent. Glaser and associates[6] reported the use of vitrectomy with air-fluid gas exchange and application of transforming growth factor-β in the treatment of 12 macular holes. In 7 of 12 eyes, the edges of the hole flattened and visual improvement was noted in 5 cases.

Both of the preceding preliminary studies are small, uncontrolled series that need confirmation. Therefore, valid conclusions concerning the potential role of vitrectomy for full-thickness macular holes await the results of a prospective randomized controlled clinical trial. In addition to the well-known complications of vitreous surgery, retinal pigment epithelial changes have been reported to occur postoperatively in this disorder.[7, 49]

Normal Fellow Eyes of Patients With Macular Holes or Pre–macular Hole Lesions

Prophylactic treatment of normal fellow eyes of patients with macular holes and pre–macular hole lesions is not required because of the excellent visual prognosis for these eyes.

REFERENCES

1. Gass JDM: Idiopathic senile macular hole: Its early stages and pathogenesis. Arch Ophthalmol 106:629–639, 1988.
2. Johnson RN, Gass JDM: Idiopathic macular holes. Observations, stages of formation, and implications for surgical intervention. Ophthalmology 95:917–924, 1988.
3. Guyer DR, de Bustros S, Diener-West M, Fine SL: The natural history of idiopathic macular holes and cysts. Arch Ophthalmol 110:1264–1268, 1992.
4. Smiddy WE, Michels RG, Glaser BM, de Bustros S: Vitrectomy for impending macular holes. Am J Ophthalmol 105:371–376, 1988.
5. Jost BF, Hutton WL, Fullet DG, et al: Vitrectomy in eyes at risk for macular hole formation. Ophthalmology 97:843–847, 1990.
6. Glaser BM, Sjaarda RN, Kuppermann BD, et al: Transforming growth factor-beta in the treatment of full-thickness macular holes. Ophthalmology 98(Suppl):145, 1991.
7. Kelly NE, Wendel RT: Vitreous surgery for idiopathic macular holes: Results of a pilot study. Arch Ophthalmol 109:654–659, 1991.
8. Knapp H: Ueber isolirte Zerreissungen der Aderhaut in folge von Traumen auf dem Augapfel. Arch Augenheilk 1:6–29, 1869.
9. Aaberg TM: Macular holes. A review. Surv Ophthalmol 15:139–162, 1970.
10. Noyes HD: Detachment of the retina, with laceration at the macula lutea. Trans Am Ophthalmol Soc 1:128–129, 1871.
11. Ogilvie FM: On one of the results of concussion injuries of the eyes ("holes" at the macula). Trans Ophthalmol Soc UK 20:202–229, 1900.
12. Collins ET: Unusual changes in the macular region (the results of injury). Trans Ophthalmol Soc UK 20:196–197, 1900.
13. Haab O: Die traumatische Durchlocherung der macula lutea. Z Augenheilk 3:113–126, 1900.
14. Croll LF, Croll M: Hole in the macula. Am J Ophthalmol 33:248–253, 1950.

15. Alvarez-Luna RA: Edema de Belin y agupero de la macula. Arch Soc Oftal Hip Am 7:221–225, 1947.
16. Bonamour G: Letrou post-traumatique de la macula. Annee Ther Clin Ophtalmol 7:343, 1956.
17. Fuchs E: Zur Veranderung der Macula Lutea nach contusion. Z Augenheilk 6:181–186, 1901.
18. Zeeman WPC: Uber Loch-und Cystenbildung der fovea Centralis. Graefe Arch Clin Exp Ophthalmol 80:259–269, 1912.
19. Zentmayer W: Hole at the macula. Ophthalmic Rec 18:198–200, 1909.
20. Lister W: Holes in the retina and their clinical significance. Br J Ophthalmol 8:1–20, 1924.
21. Reese AB, Jones IS, Cooper WC: Macular changes secondary to vitreous traction. Am J Ophthalmol 64:544–549, 1967.
22. Aaberg TM, Blair CJ, Gass JDM: Macular holes. Am J Ophthalmol 69:555–562, 1970.
23. McDonnell PJ, Fine SL, Hillis AI: Clinical features of idiopathic macular cysts and holes. Am J Ophthalmol 93:777–786, 1982.
24. Kuhnt H: Ueber cine eigenthumliche veranderung der netzhaut ad maculam (retinitis atgrophicans sive rareficans centralis). Z Augenheilk 3:105–112, 1900.
25. Tower P: Observations on hole in the macula. Ophthalmologica 40(Suppl):1–60, 1954.
26. Yoshioka H: Clinical studies on macular hole. III. On the pathogenesis of the senile macular hole. Acta Soc Ophthalmol Jpn 72:575–584, 1968.
27. Jaffe NS: Vitreous traction at the posterior pole of the fundus due to alterations in the vitreous posterior. Trans Am Acad Ophthalmol Otolaryngol 71:642–652, 1967.
28. James M, Feman SS: Macular holes. Graefes Arch Clin Exp Ophthalmol 215:59–63, 1980.
29. Morgan CM, Schatz H: Idiopathic macular holes. Am J Ophthalmol 99:437–444, 1985.
30. Morgan CM, Schatz H: Involutional macular thinning. A premacular hole condition. Ophthalmology 93:153–161, 1986.
31. Avila MP, Jalkh AE, Murakami K, et al: Biomicroscopic study of the vitreous in macular breaks. Ophthalmology 90:1277–1283, 1983.
32. Trempe CL, Weiter JR, Furukawa H: Fellow eyes in cases of macular hole. Arch Ophthalmol 104:93–95, 1986.
33. Fisher YL, Slakter JS: Ultrasound evaluation of the vitreoretinal interface in macular hole formation. Ophthalmol 98(Suppl):146, 1991.
34. Guyer DR, Green WR, de Bustros S, Fine SL: Histopathologic features of idiopathic macular holes and cysts. Ophthalmology 97:1045–1051, 1990.
35. Frangieh GT, Green WR, Engel HM: A histopathologic study of macular cysts and holes. Retina 1:311–336, 1981.
36. Gass JDM: Macular dysfunction caused by vitreous and vitreoretinal interface abnormalities. In Gass JDM (ed): Stereoscopic Atlas of Macular Disease, vol. 2. St Louis, CV Mosby, 1987.
37. Smiddy WE, Michels RG, de Bustros S, et al: Histopathology of tissue removed during vitrectomy for impending idiopathic macular holes. Am J Ophthalmol 108:360–364, 1989.
38. Gass JDM, Joondeph BC: Observations concerning patients with suspected impending macular holes. Am J Ophthalmol 109:638–646, 1990.
39. Lewis H, Cowan GM, Straatsma BR: Apparent disappearance of a macular hole associated with development of an epiretinal membrane. Am J Ophthalmol 102:172–175, 1986.
40. Bidwell AE, Jampol LM, Goldberg MF: Macular holes and excellent visual acuity. Arch Ophthalmol 106:1350–1351, 1988.
41. Guyer DR, Sunness JS, Fine SL, et al: Idiopathic macular holes and cysts: A scanning laser ophthalmoscope analysis. Invest Ophthalmol 97(Suppl):152, 1990.
42. Margherio RR, Schepens CL: Macular breaks. 1. Diagnosis, etiology, and observations. Am J Ophthalmol 74:219–232, 1972.
43. Bronstein MA, Trempe CL, Freeman HM: Fellow eyes of eyes with macular holes. Am J Ophthalmol 92:757–761, 1981.
44. Yaoeda H: Clinical observations on macular hole. Acta Soc Ophthalmol Jpn 71:1723–1736, 1967.
45. Atmaca LS: Follow-up of macular holes. Ann Ophthalmol 16:1064–1065, 1986.
46. Margherio RR, Trese MT, Margherio AR, Cartright K: Surgical management of vitreomacular traction syndromes. Ophthalmology 96:1437–1445, 1989.
47. de Bustros S: Early stages of macular holes. To treat or not to treat? Arch Ophthalmol 108:1085–1086, 1990.
48. Schocket SS, Lakhanpal V, Xiaoping M, et al: Laser treatment of macular holes. Ophthalmology 95:574–582, 1988.
49. Poliner LS, Tornambe PE: Retinal pigment epitheliopathy following macular hole surgery. Ophthalmology 98(Suppl):146, 1991.
50. Smiddy WE, Michels RG, Green WR: Idiopathic macular disorders. Ophthalmology 96(Suppl):94, 1989.
51. Smiddy WE, Michels RG, Green WR: Morphology, pathology, and surgery of idiopathic vitreoretinal macular disorders. Retina 10:288–296, 1990.

Chapter 70

▪

Choroidal and Retinal Folds

THOMAS R. FRIBERG

Many disorders are associated with the formation of folds in the choroid and retina. For descriptive purposes, folds primarily involving the choroid, with the overlying retina only secondarily affected, are classified as *choroidal folds*, whereas folds occurring exclusively within the layers of the sensory retina are termed *retinal folds* (Fig. 70–1). Choroidal folds are often a sign of orbital or ocular disease, but they may develop after surgery or occur idiopathically.[1–5] Retinal folds found without the presence of choroidal folds develop in association with uveitis, in response to certain medications,[6] and as a result of proliferative vitreoretinopathy and macular pucker.

CHOROIDAL FOLDS

Description, Pathogenesis, and Symptoms

Choroidal folds are undulations of the choroid, Bruch's membrane, and pigment epithelium, with the overlying retina wrinkled to a lesser extent.[1] They develop secondary to mechanical stresses produced within these tissues. Because the choroid consists of a plexus of randomly oriented blood vessels, an interstitium of connective tissue, and multiple fluid-filled spaces, it has intrinsic elasticity and sponginess. In addition, Bruch's

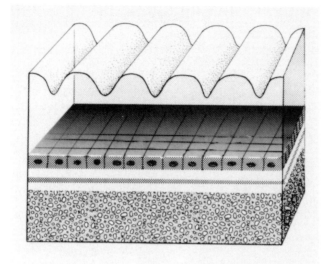

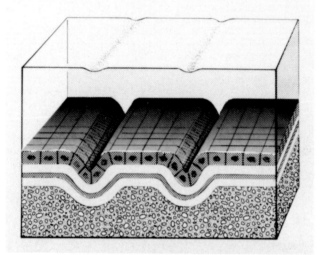

Figure 70–1. *Top,* Retinal folds involve the superficial layers of the retina and are usually secondary to tangential forces present on the retinal surface. The underlying retinal pigment epithelium (cuboidal cells) and choroid are not characteristically folded. *Bottom,* Choroidal folds are characterized by undulations of the choroid, Bruch's membrane, and overlying retinal pigment epithelial layers. The sensory retina is folded in the deeper layers, but these pleats do not extend completely to the superficial layers. Hence, retinal vessels are typically not included in the folding process.

membrane and the overlying retinal pigment epithelium (RPE) are firmly bonded to the inner surface of choroid at the choriocapillaris. This architecture is roughly analogous to that of a sponge onto which a thin elastic sheet has been fused. When such a sponge is compressed, folds form along its surface (Fig. 70–2). Analogously, if compressive forces of sufficient magnitude are induced in the choroid, it will be forced into pleats or folds, as will Bruch's membrane, the pigment epithelium, and the sensory retina. Hence, choroidal folds are a manifestation of biomechanical stresses present within the choroid, rather than being a sign of a particular disease.[2]

Symptoms of choroidal folds depend on the degree of folding of the overlying retina, particularly at the fovea,

and the amount of induced refractive error associated with the development of the choroidal folds. Retinal folds running through the fovea in association with choroidal folds may cause metamorphopsia and a reduction of visual acuity that cannot be eliminated by corrective lenses. Since choroidal folds are commonly found when the choroid is thickened or the globe has been flattened posteriorly, axial hyperopia is typical. If the globe is deformed more anteriorly from an intraorbital tumor, induced astigmatic errors along with the hyperopia are common.[7] Incidental equatorial folds created by encircling procedures to repair retinal detachments do not cause distortion or refractive errors themselves, but the scleral buckle in this situation produces relative myopia.

On funduscopic examination, choroidal folds appear as alternating dark and light streaks. Often, their appearance is subtle, especially if the fundus is lightly pigmented and the folds have not undergone any chronic changes. Choroidal folds are best viewed clinically by indirect ophthalmoscopy, as the field of view is usually large enough to allow observation of the entire fold pattern.

Histopathologic sections through choroidal folds demonstrate the reason for their striated appearance. Typically, Bruch's membrane and the RPE are tightly folded within the troughs of the folds (as viewed from the vitreous), whereas at the crests, the change in curvature is more gradual.[4] Hence, the melanocytes within the choroid and the RPE are compressed into a smaller than normal region in the troughs, whereas over the crest of the folds, these cells are stretched apart. This change in pigment density across the folds creates the alternating dark and light striae seen clinically.

Fluorescein Angiography and Choroidal Folds

Sodium fluorescein leaks quickly out of the fenestrations of the choroidal vessels and stains the choroid. Because the RPE effectively filters out most of this potential background choroidal fluorescence, however, the choroid appears gray rather than white on angiography. In the troughs of the choroidal folds, in which the RPE cells are compressed, the RPE becomes a more efficient filter. Conversely, when the choroid and RPE are stretched, the concentration of melanin granules per unit area is reduced. The net effect is that choroidal folds appear dramatically as alternating black and white striae on fluorescein angiography (Fig. 70–3).[8]

CHOROIDAL FOLDS AND SPECIFIC DISORDERS

Choroidal Tumors and Choroidal Detachments

When a choroidal tumor such as a melanoma, metastatic carcinoma, or choroidal hemangioma grows, it

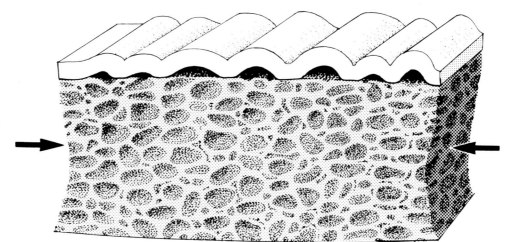

Figure 70–2. As an analog, the formation of choroidal folds may be compared with folds developing along the surface of a compressed sponge onto which an elastic membrane has been glued. The sponge represents the choroid, whereas the membrane represents Bruch's membrane and the retinal pigment epithelium.

compresses the adjacent choroid and may force it into folds. In this instance, folds develop parallel to the boundaries of the tumor (Fig. 70–4). Similarly, choroidal folds may develop at the edge of large choroidal detachments. The folds in these cases are not extensive because only local compressive stresses are produced. Folds typically do not form over the tumor surface at which point the choroid is stretched rather than compressed. Occasionally, however, folds develop over regions of localized choroidal hemorrhage.[9]

Orbital Tumors

INTRACONAL ORBITAL TUMORS

Tumors located within the muscle cone, such as cavernous hemangiomas, metastatic neoplasms, and optic nerve meningiomas, can press on the globe posteriorly, producing exophthalmos, flattening of the globe, and shifting of the refractive error toward hyperopia.[7] In addition, such a tumor often displaces the optic nerve to one side, inducing stresses within the globe at the disc (Fig. 70–5A). The choroid on one side of the optic nerve is compressed, whereas on the opposite side, the choroid is stretched, often resulting in a parabolic fold pattern with the nerve head located among the folds (Fig. 70–6).[7]

EXTRACONAL ORBITAL TUMORS

An extraconal tumor may press directly on the extraocular muscles and Tenon's capsule, as well as on the sclera. The forces generated tend to buckle the wall of the globe (Fig. 70–5B), creating choroidal folds. Because of anterior segment distortion, astigmatic refractive errors are commonly induced. With respect to the fold pattern, the convex side usually points toward the posterior pole and optic nerve, but the nerve head is usually located outside the region of folds (Fig. 70–7).[7] Typical extraconal tumors associated with choroidal folds include mucoceles, dermoids, tumors of the lacrimal gland, and orbital meningiomas.

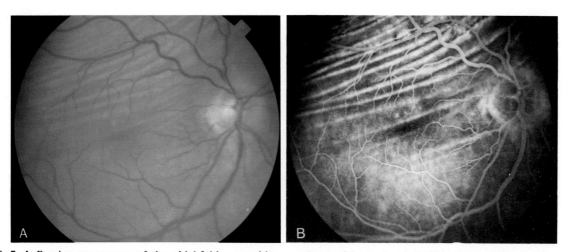

Figure 70–3. A, Fundus appearance of choroidal folds caused by an extraconal tumor located within the superior temporal quadrant of the orbit. B, On fluorescein angiography, the folds are much more dramatic, appearing as alternating light and dark streaks. Note that the retinal vessels are not distorted by the underlying choroidal folds.

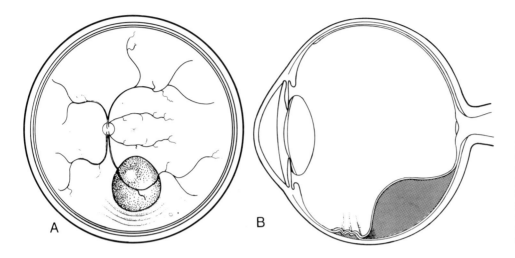

Figure 70–4. A, An expanding choroidal tumor compresses the choroid along its boundaries, forming folds parallel to its perimeter. B, Folds seldom form over the tumor surface, as the choroid is stretched uniformly over the mass, as seen in this vertical cross section.

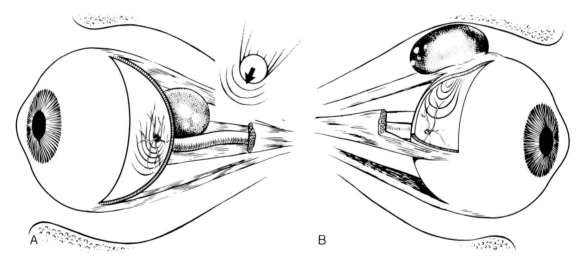

Figure 70–5. A, Intraconal orbital tumors typically displace the optic nerve, compressing the choroid in the direction of the nerve head displacement, and placing the choroid under tension on the opposite side. The result is a choroidal fold pattern, the convex side of which is directed away from the nerve head (arrow). B, Extraconal tumors buckle the wall of the globe equatorially, producing a curvilinear fold pattern with its convex side directed toward the optic nerve. (From Friberg TR: The etiology of choroidal folds. Graefes Arch Clin Exp Ophthalmol 227:459–464, 1989.)

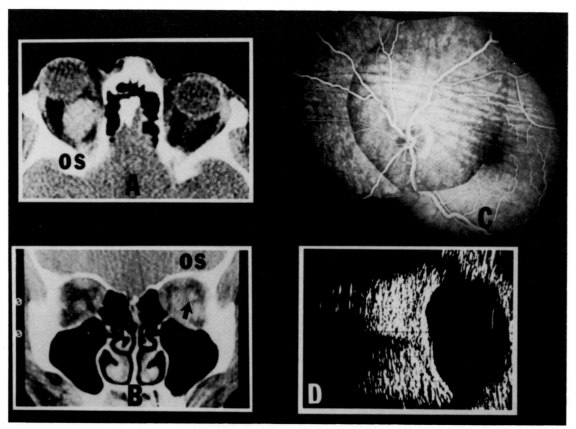

Figure 70–6. An intraconal tumor, in this case an orbital hemangioma, has displaced the left globe and optic nerve superiorly, as seen in computed tomograms (A and B). The associated choroidal folds (C) are primarily located superior to the optic nerve, whereas some folds radiate from the disc and extend into the macula. D, A B-scan ultrasonogram demonstrates characteristic flattening of the posterior sclera. (From Friberg TR, Grove AS: Choroidal folds and refractive errors associated with orbital tumors. An analysis. Arch Ophthalmol 101:598–603, 1983. Copyright 1983, American Medical Association.)

ORBITAL TUMORS AND THE PATTERN OF FOLDS

Although historically the choroidal fold pattern was said to have no relevance in localizing a tumor within the orbit,[1] in fact the pattern of folds often reflects the location of the orbital pathologic condition. The tumor is often located along the axis of symmetry drawn through the pattern of choroidal folds.[7] The location as indicated by the folds is only approximate, however, and must be corroborated by more sophisticated evaluations, such as computed tomography or B-scan ultrasonography.

Disorders of the Optic Nerve Head

As the optic nerve head swells, it expands centrifugally, compressing the peripapillary choroid and often creating choroidal folds concentric to the disc margins (Fig. 70–8). Thus, concentric folds are a sign of papilledema, disc edema, optic nerve head drusen, or a tumor within the nerve head. In these cases, the abnormality of the optic nerve is usually quite obvious, whereas the folds themselves are subtle.

Scleral Buckling Procedures

Encircling scleral buckling procedures are commonly associated with choroidal striae (Fig. 70–9A and B). In this case, the folds are confined to the vicinity of the buckle and are oriented perpendicular to the plane of the encircling element. The encirclement reduces the surface area available to the choroid, compressing the tissue together within the plane of the buckling element. In addition, radial buckling elements can also produce folds by compression (Fig. 70–9C and D). Folds associated with retinal surgery are typically prominent during the immediate postoperative period and fade over time. Furthermore, choroidal folds caused by buckling are smoothed out if the intraocular pressure rises.

Chorioretinal Scars

Dense, fibrotic, chorioretinal scars from trauma or intense choroidal inflammation contract as the scar tissue matures. Forces from this contraction pull on the surrounding choroid and may produce folds directed radially toward the center of the scar (Fig. 70–10). Scarring associated with subretinal neovascularization can also produce radially oriented folds.[10]

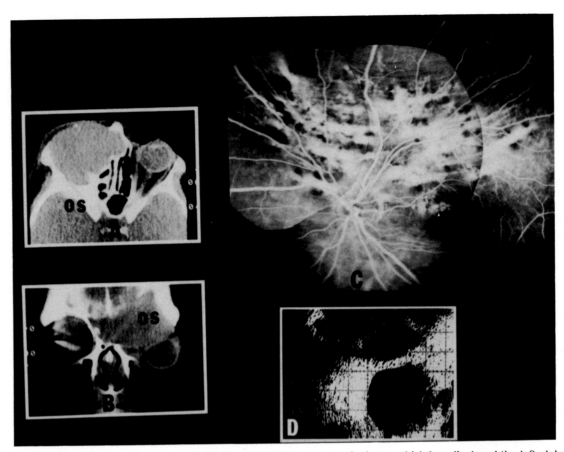

Figure 70–7. Choroidal folds caused by an extraconal tumor, in this case a meningioma, which has displaced the left globe inferiorly and temporally as seen on computed tomography *(A and B). C,* A curvilinear fold pattern typically associated with an extraconal tumor is seen on the fluorescein angiogram, with the convex side of the pattern directed toward the optic nerve head. A B-scan ultrasonogram shows equatorial flattening of the sclera by the meningioma *(D).* (From Friberg TR, Grove AS: Choroidal folds and refractive errors associated with orbital tumors. An analysis. Arch Ophthalmol 101:598–603, 1983. Copyright 1983, American Medical Association.)

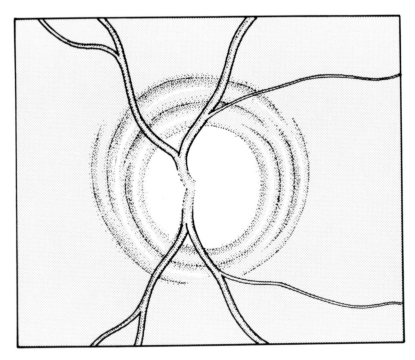

Figure 70–8. Swelling of the optic nerve from papilledema or tumor compresses the adjacent choroid, producing choroidal folds concentric to the disc.

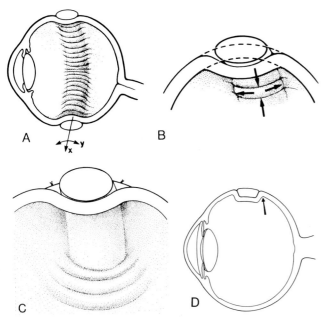

Figure 70–9. Choroidal folds secondary to an encircling scleral buckle (A). The choroid is compressed in the x direction along the plane of the buckle and stretched in the y direction (B), producing folds oriented perpendicular to the induced compressive stresses. (A and B, From Friberg TR: The etiology of choroidal folds. Graefes Arch Clin Exp Ophthalmol 227:459–464, 1989.) C and D, A radially placed scleral buckle element produces choroidal folds by compressing the adjacent choroid (C). The abrupt change in scleral contour (arrow) as seen on cross section (D) creates these compressive forces.

FOLDS ASSOCIATED WITH CHOROIDAL THICKENING

The choroid may thicken as a result of hypotony, inflammation, the uveal effusion syndrome, or venostasis such as that found after a central retinal vein occlusion. As its thickness increases, the surface area available to the choriocapillaris, Bruch's membrane, and the RPE is reduced because the choroid must expand inward toward the center of the eye, being confined by the sclera. Ultimately, the choroid may be forced into redundant folds (Fig. 70–11). Additionally, because the internal diameter of the globe has been decreased, the refractive error shifts toward hyperopia. It is important to remember that this hyperopia is secondary to the development of choroidal thickening and fold formation, rather than being the cause of the folds.

Hypotony

Hypotony or low intraocular pressure results in radial expansion of the choroid toward the vitreous cavity. Hypotony may result from an obvious cause such as uveitis, filtering procedures, or trauma. Choroidal folds developing shortly after anterior segment surgery suggest a wound leak or the presence of a cyclodialysis cleft.

Scleral Inflammations

Inflammatory diseases of the orbit and sclera such as Graves' exophthalmopathy, orbital pseudotumors, and orbital myositis can flatten the sclera and cause scleral and choroidal thickening. Choroidal compression and choroidal fold formation may be the result. Sometimes serous retinal detachments develop in association with the folds, presenting a confusing picture. Successful treatment of the inflammatory component will lead to resolution of the folds in most cases.

Uveal Effusion

Eyes with idiopathic choroidal folds and concomitant serous detachments may appear similar to eyes with the uveal effusion syndrome. Typically, this syndrome is characterized by poor vision, a thickened or detached choroid and ciliary body, and an extensive serous retinal detachment that dominates the clinical appearance.[11] In some cases, however, the choroid may be thickened uniformly without a significant serous detachment, and vision may be maintained. In these cases, choroidal folds may be the first sign of an abnormality. Decompression of the vortex veins and excision of scleral flaps has, in some severe cases, led to resolution of the choroidal detachments and folds with improvement of visual acuity.[11, 12]

IDIOPATHIC FOLDS

Choroidal folds may develop in one or both eyes of a patient with no apparent ocular or orbital disorder. These patients are usually male and often present with acquired hyperopia of 3D or less. Computed tomographic findings in these eyes may show thickening of the sclera, flattening of the posterior pole, enlargement

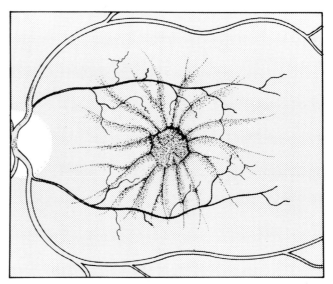

Figure 70–10. A dense chorioretinal scar draws the surrounding choroid inward toward its center as the scar tissue matures and contracts. Radially oriented folds are produced.

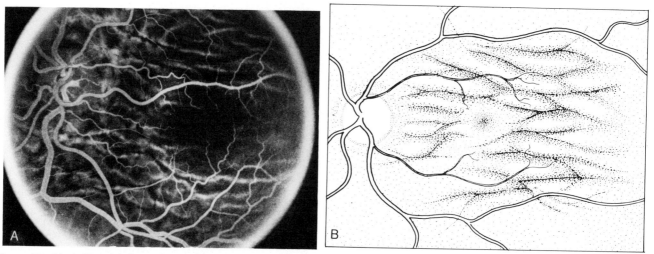

Figure 70–11. A, Fluorescein angiogram of choroidal folds associated with hypotony and secondary choroidal thickening. B, In these cases, the choroidal fold pattern is typically random, as the folds develop secondary to rather uniform swelling of the choroid.

of the optic nerve image, and the presence of a space seen between the optic nerve and its meninges. Occasionally, serous retinal detachments develop (Fig. 70–12). Patients usually retain good vision, and in some individuals the folds disappear spontaneously.[13] The cause of these alterations is unclear. Possibly, drainage through the choroidal venous plexus and into the vortex veins is compromised from structural alterations within the scleral wall. In other cases, posterior scleritis or other local inflammation may have initially produced the folds, which then persist long after the inflammation resolves.

IMPLICATIONS OF CHOROIDAL FOLDS

Choroidal folds are a sign of an ocular disorder or disease. Hence, the major consideration when presented with a patient with choroidal folds is to determine the cause of the folds. Of particular importance is an investigation to rule out the possibility of an orbital or choroidal tumor. B-scan ultrasonography and computed tomography are usually indicated, particularly in patients with unexplained unilateral folds.

If choroidal folds remain for months, the RPE in the troughs may undergo hypertrophy and hyperplasia from being mechanically compacted. Even if the folds resolve, this linear pigmentation may persist. RPE atrophy and apparent fractures of Bruch's membrane may also be seen along the folds, especially in older patients (Fig. 70–13). Such changes also occur along angioid streaks, which are sometimes confused with choroidal folds.[7] As with angioid streaks, subretinal neovascularization can develop along choroidal folds (Fig. 70–14).[14] Macular folds of the choroid should therefore be eliminated, if possible, to help avoid permanent visual loss.

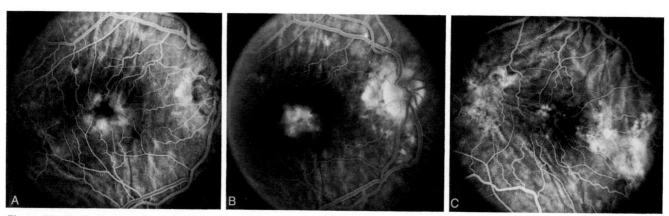

Figure 70–12. A, Fluorescein angiogram of the right eye in a woman with mild hyperopia and acquired chorioretinal folds. There is leakage of dye from the choriocapillaris, which pools within the fovea in the late-phase films (B). A serous retinal detachment is present overlying the area of leakage. C, Left eye of the same patient. Fluorescein angiography shows randomly oriented folds and retinal pigment epithelial window defects in the peripapillary region, at the fovea, and temporal to the macula.

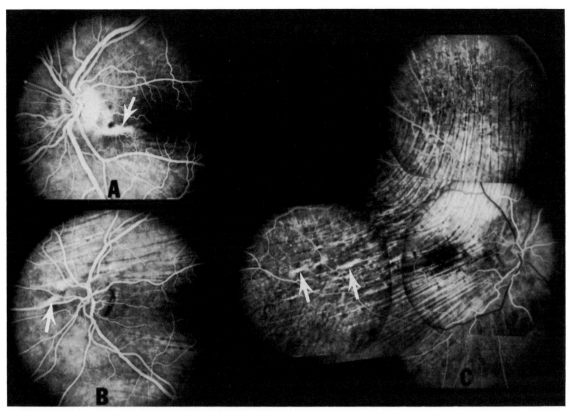

Figure 70–13. A–C, Retinal pigment epithelial clumping and atrophy *(arrows)* can occur along choroidal folds, making the folds appear similar to atrophic angioid streaks, both on clinical examination and particularly upon fluorescein angiography (From Friberg TR, Grove AS: Choroidal folds and refractive errors associated with orbital tumors. An analysis. Arch Ophthalmol 101:598–603, 1983. Copyright 1983, American Medical Association.)

RETINAL FOLDS

Retinal folds are commonly associated with epiretinal membrane formation. Such membranes exert stress on the underlying retina and promote wrinkle formation, leading to macular pucker and symptoms of metamor-

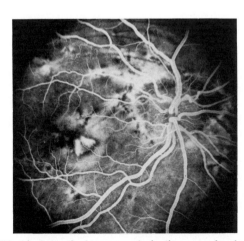

Figure 70–14. Subretinal neovascularization may develop along choroidal folds as demonstrated by this trapezoidal subretinal neovascular net found along a fold running through the macula. In this case, the choroidal folds developed secondary to an orbital tumor. (From Friberg TR, Grove AS: Subretinal neovascularization and choroidal folds. Ann Ophthalmol 12:245–250, 1980.)

phopsia. These cellophane-like membranes can best be seen on careful biomicroscopy of the fundus. Alternatively, in certain cases of rhegmatogenous retinal detachment, proliferative membranes grow along the retinal surface, creating star folds and retinal striae. In both instances, surgical removal of the membranes may be necessary.

Shallow superficial retinal folds may develop when choroidal folds are lacking whenever there is relative choroidal thickening, particularly in association with uveal inflammation. Reduction of the surface area available to the retina from the radial displacement of the choroidal surface is a likely cause. Retinal folds in conjunction with transient myopia may also be associated with the administration of sulfonamides. In this case, swelling of the ciliary body and vitreous traction may play a role.[6] Elimination of the uveal inflammation or discontinuation of the sulfonamides should promote resolution of the retinal folds in these cases.[6]

REFERENCES

1. Newell FW: Choroidal folds. Am J Ophthalmol 75:930–942, 1973.
2. Friberg TR: The etiology of choroidal folds. Graefes Arch Clin Exp Ophthalmol 227:459–464, 1989.
3. Cangemi FE, Trempe CL, Walsh JB: Choroidal folds. Am J Ophthalmol 86:380–387, 1978.
4. Wolter JR: Parallel horizontal choroidal folds secondary to an orbital tumor. Am J Ophthalmol 77:669–673, 1974.

5. Bullock JD, Egbert PR: The origin of choroidal folds: A clinical, histopathological and experimental study. Doc Ophthalmol 37:261–293, 1974.
6. Ryan EH, Jampol LM: Drug-induced acute transient myopia with retinal folds. Retina 6:220–223, 1986.
7. Friberg TR, Grove AS: Choroidal folds and refractive errors associated with orbital tumors. An analysis. Arch Ophthalmol 101:598–603, 1983.
8. Norton EWD: A characteristic fluorescein angiographic pattern in choroidal folds. Proc R Soc Med 62:119–128, 1969.
9. Morgan CM, Gragoudas ES: Limited choroidal hemorrhage mistaken for a choroidal melanoma. Ophthalmology 94:41–46, 1987.
10. Gass JDM: Radial chorioretinal folds: A sign of choroidal neovascularization. Arch Ophthalmol 99:1016–1018, 1982.
11. Schepens CL, Brockhurst RJ: Uveal effusion: Clinical picture. Arch Ophthalmol 70:189–201, 1963.
12. Ward RC, Gragoudas ES, Pon DM, Albert DM: Abnormal scleral findings in uveal effusion syndrome. Am J Ophthalmol 106:139–146, 1988.
13. Dailey RA, Mills RP, Stimac GK, et al: The natural history and CT appearance of acquired hyperopia with choroidal folds. Ophthalmology 93:1336–1342, 1986.
14. Friberg TR, Grove AS: Subretinal neovascularization and choroidal folds. Ann Ophthalmol 12:245–250, 1980.

Chapter 71

■

Cystoid Macular Edema After Ocular Surgery

NORMAN P. BLAIR and SANG H. KIM

HISTORY AND TERMINOLOGY

Although macular edema occurs in a variety of ocular conditions, this chapter focuses on macular edema following ocular surgery, especially cataract extraction. Macular edema unrelated to ocular surgery is discussed elsewhere in this book in association with the underlying disease. Macular edema occurs in a considerable percentage of eyes after surgery but usually is self-limited. Still, it is considered to be the most common cause of an unfavorable visual outcome after uncomplicated cataract extraction,[1, 2] and it may result in permanent visual loss. Jampol has estimated that this problem is responsible for disappointing visual results in 10,000 to 20,000 patients/year.[3] In 1953, Irvine described a syndrome occurring after cataract extraction that included vitreous and macular changes.[4] In 1966, Gass and Norton first described aphakic eyes with characteristic fluorescein angiographic features, which they called *cystoid macular edema*.[5] Thus, cystoid macular edema that occurs after cataract surgery has become known as the *Irvine-Gass syndrome*. The term *cystoid* is preferred over *cystic* because true cysts have an epithelial lining.[6]

We define *macular edema* as increased fluid within the sensory retina of the macula. Serous detachment of the sensory retina and retinal pigment epithelial detachment are not included because in these conditions the fluid accumulation is external to the sensory retina. Furthermore, these conditions differ from cystoid macular edema in pathogenesis, prognosis, and treatment. The excessive tissue fluid increases the retinal volume, and this is manifested as retinal thickening because the retina has minimal capacity to lengthen. Macular edema, particularly in the Irvine-Gass syndrome, is almost always associated with disruption of the blood-retinal barrier, as detected with high sensitivity by leakage on fluorescein angiography. In fact, in clinical practice, the diagnosis of cystoid macular edema is commonly made if fluorescein leakage is seen. However, the amount of leakage on fluorescein angiography and the degree of macular thickening do not correlate completely, and the latter appears more closely related to visual acuity.[7] If fluorescein leakage can occur without retinal thickening (as we have observed in diabetes [unpublished data]), in such cases, the term *cystoid macular edema* would be inaccurate. However, until the time that retinal thickness measurements are available in patients who have had surgery, we will use the term *cystoid macular edema* if angiographic leakage is present, as is the current convention.

Three categories of cystoid macular edema have been defined based on the severity of the clinical condition. Angiographic cystoid macular edema is present when there is leakage on fluorescein angiography but the patient has no symptoms. Clinically significant cystoid macular edema is present if the patient has reduced vision. If clinically significant cystoid macular edema persists for 6 mo, chronic cystoid macular edema is present.[8, 9]

CLINICAL CHARACTERISTICS

Symptoms

Eyes affected with cystoid macular edema often have undergone uncomplicated cataract surgery,[5] although the condition is more likely to occur when there have been complications. Angiographic cystoid macular edema is the most common type; therefore, many patients have no symptoms. The chief symptom is usually reduced central vision, with visual acuity occasionally as low as 20/200. Eyes with cystoid macular edema frequently have more ocular irritability and photophobia than usual after surgery.[10] Patients may complain of floaters.

Physical Findings

Circumcorneal injection and anterior chamber flare and cells may be seen, but the intraocular pressure is usually normal. Sometimes there is rupture of the anterior hyaloid face, particularly after intracapsular surgery (even without vitreous loss), and vitreous may adhere to the incision. Iris incarceration in the wound, a peaked pupil, vitreous adherence to the iris, or poor pupillary dilatation may be present. Vitreous cells, syneresis, liquefaction, fibrillation, and detachment are common. The frequency of vitreomacular adhesions with partial posterior vitreous detachment is controversial,[5, 8, 11, 12] and they may be difficult to identify with conventional techniques. In many patients, no abnormalities are found in the fundus. The foveal area may appear translucent with a granular surface. The inner foveal surface often bows forward with loss of the foveal reflex. A deep, soft, yellow-white spot in the fovea may be present. Intraretinal cystoid spaces demarcated by a stellate pattern of refractile lines may be seen (Fig. 71–1). These spaces are more easily visualized during slit-lamp biomicroscopy using a contact lens, particularly with red-free light (Fig. 71–2), or by retroillumination when the beam is focused adjacent to the fovea. Blurring of the disc margins may occur, and occasionally intraretinal or intracystoid space hemorrhages are visible.[13] Retinal periphlebitis, epiretinal membranes, serous retinal detachment, and subretinal precipitates can occur. Hard exudates are rarely seen. In chronic cases, atrophic or hyperpigmentary changes in the pigment epithelium may develop. In addition, cystoid degeneration of the fovea may progress to a lamellar or full-thickness mac-

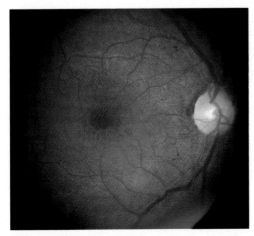

Figure 71–1. An eye with aphakic cystoid macular edema. Note the fine lines outlining the cystoid spaces in the foveal area, including a central cystoid space. A few small intraretinal hemorrhages are seen just inferior to the first branch of the major superotemporal vein near the bifurcation.

ular hole. These latter manifestations imply irreversible retinal damage and limited visual potential.

Ancillary Tests

A mild to moderate diffuse haze is common on color fundus photographs. Fluorescein angiography shows early, usually symmetric leakage from the perifoveal capillaries. The leakage eventually fills the intraretinal cystoid spaces, giving the classic pattern of hyperfluorescence resembling the petals of a flower (see Fig. 71–2).[5] Milder degrees of leakage give less-developed patterns (Fig. 71–3). The degree of leakage does not necessarily correlate with the visual acuity.[7] Leakage from the optic nerve head is common (see Fig. 71–2), and the iris may also leak abnormally.[14] There may be diffuse leakage into the ocular media, producing generalized hyperfluorescence on the photographs, particularly those taken a relatively long time after dye injection. This can reduce contrast and obscure fundus detail. Adequate fluorescein angiograms for the evaluation of cystoid macular edema can be obtained after the oral administration of fluorescein, which may be advantageous in selected patients.[15] The focal and pattern electroretinograms may be abnormal, but the visual evoked potentials tend to remain normal.[16]

COURSE AND PROGNOSIS

Cystoid macular edema usually occurs 4 to 12 wk after surgery, but in rare instances it has occurred many years later.[17] Accordingly, the clinician should consider cystoid macular edema in any patient who experiences a decline in vision in an eye that has had cataract surgery. The incidence of cystoid macular edema is low within the first postoperative week[18] and peaks around 4 to 6 wk after surgery. The visual symptoms may undergo recurrent exacerbations and remissions that do not necessarily correlate with fluorescein leakage.[19] Most cases of cystoid macular edema resolve spontaneously within a few weeks to months. However, chronic cystoid macular edema occurs in about 1 percent of cases.[3, 20] Optic disc leakage appears to be a risk factor for the development of chronic cystoid macular edema and a poorer visual outcome.[21] The best source of information on chronic cystoid macular edema is the Vitrectomy–Aphakic Cystoid Macular Edema Study.[8] This was a national, collaborative, prospective, randomized investigation on 115 eyes with chronic cystoid macular edema and vitreous adherent to the corneoscleral wound. Each eye had reduced vision for 6 mo to 4 yr, and each was followed for at least 6 mo. Of the 47 eyes observed without surgery, 27 percent attained a visual acuity of 20/50 or better if the vision had never fallen to 20/80 or worse. If the vision fell to this level, only 8 percent of the eyes spontaneously improved to at least 20/50. No systemic vascular factors were identified that correlated significantly with the prognosis. Furthermore, the investigators were not able to show that improvement after a short course of systemic antiprostaglandins, systemic

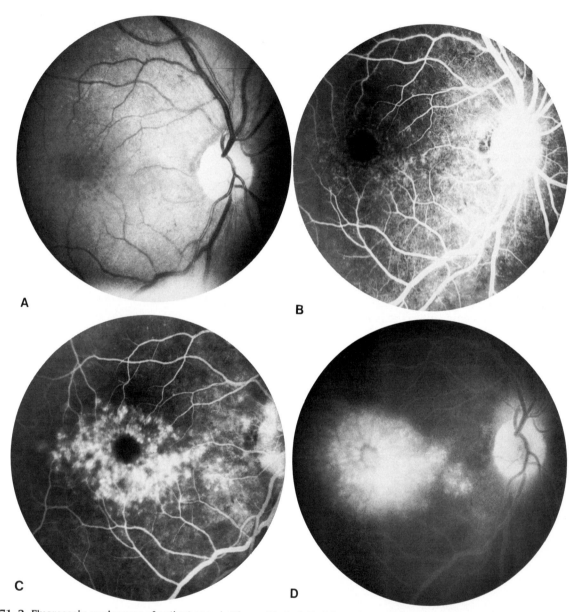

Figure 71–2. Fluorescein angiogram of patient seen in Figure 71–1. *A,* Red-free photograph. Note septae outlining the cystoid spaces. *B,* Early-phase photograph revealing some leakage from the perifoveal capillaries. *C,* Midphase photograph showing extensive, diffuse leakage from the perifoveal capillaries. Note also the leakage from the optic disc temporal to the disc. *D,* Late-phase photograph demonstrates well-developed petaloid pattern of cystoid macular edema. Note the central cystoid space and disc leakage.

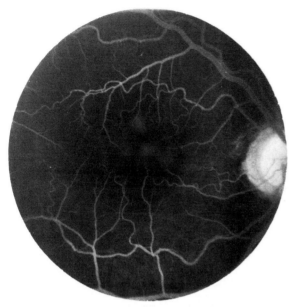

Figure 71–3. Late-phase fluorescein angiogram of an eye that had cataract surgery. Note mild perifoveal intraretinal fluorescein accumulation with a poorly developed petaloid pattern.

steroids, or topical steroids correlated with a more favorable outcome. Cystoid macular edema can improve spontaneously after periods of as long as 3 or 4 yr. However, resolution of the edema does not necessarily imply that the vision will improve.

DIFFERENTIAL DIAGNOSIS

Cystoid macular edema must be differentiated from other causes of reduced vision after surgery, including hypotony retinopathy, various types of optic neuropathy, preexisting age-related macular degeneration, and rhegmatogenous retinal detachment.[22] The fundus findings of cystoid macular edema in some cases may be confused with burns from the operating microscope,[23] a stage 1 macular hole,[24] cystoid macular degeneration without leakage in nicotinic acid toxicity, and the foveal abnormalities in congenital retinoschisis or the Goldmann-Favre syndrome. Cystoid macular edema may be present secondary to other conditions (Table 71–1).

Since diabetic patients frequently undergo cataract surgery, sometimes one must differentiate macular edema related to the surgery from that caused by the diabetes. Cystoid macular edema related to surgery tends to be located symmetrically around the fovea, whereas areas of diabetic macular edema tend to be located in patches scattered throughout the macula in association with leaking microaneurysms. If the diabetic process predominates, focal photocoagulation may be of benefit.

EPIDEMIOLOGY

Incidence

The reported incidence of cystoid macular edema after cataract surgery varies widely, particularly on the basis of the study design. Several early, large retrospective studies found an incidence of approximately 1 percent.[11, 25, 26] A prospective study done before fluorescein angiography was widely used found an incidence of 7.6 percent in patients who had intracapsular cataract surgery.[27] Prospective studies using angiography performed in the first few months after intracapsular surgery without intraocular lens implantation found incidences between 36 and 60 percent.[28–34] More recent prospective studies using angiography in patients undergoing extracapsular surgery have shown incidences of approximately 10 to 20 percent.[35–42] Since the majority of these patients were asymptomatic, the incidence of clinically significant cystoid macular edema must be less than 10 percent, and that of chronic cystoid macular edema is even lower, about 1 percent.[3, 20]

General Factors

Cystoid macular edema does not seem to have a predilection by eye or sex. It is generally believed that if one eye has developed cystoid macular edema, the other is at increased risk for its development after surgery.[34, 43] It is not clear whether race is a risk factor for cystoid macular edema.[42] Cystoid macular edema does occur more commonly among older patients[34, 35] and is uncommon in children having cataract surgery,[44–48] although Hoyt and Nickel found it in a substantial proportion of their patients.[49] Some evidence suggests an increased incidence of cystoid macular edema in eyes with glaucoma that undergo extracapsular cataract surgery.[50] Conversely, cystoid macular edema may be related to decreased intraocular pressure, although this remains to be established. Systemic vascular diseases such as hypertension and diabetes seem to predispose to cystoid macular edema after surgery.[34]

Type of Cataract Surgery

Most investigators have found a reduced incidence of cystoid macular edema after extracapsular surgery as opposed to intracapsular procedures.[1, 51–53] This advan-

Table 71–1. CLINICAL CONDITIONS ASSOCIATED WITH CYSTOID MACULAR EDEMA

Diabetic retinopathy
Retinal vein occlusion (branch or central)
Severe hypertensive retinopathy
Retinal telangiectasis (e.g., Coats' disease, juxtafoveolar)
Macroaneurysm
Angiomatosis retinae
Radiation retinopathy
Uveitis (e.g., pars planitis, birdshot retinochoroidopathy)
Hereditary retinal dystrophies (e.g., retinitis pigmentosa, autosomal dominant cystoid macular edema)
Epiretinal membranes
Intraocular tumors (e.g., malignant melanoma, choroidal hemangioma)
Choroidal neovascularization (e.g., age-related macular degeneration, angioid streaks)
Epinephrine use in aphakia
Previous ocular surgery

tage appears to be lost if the capsule is interrupted at surgery, either intentionally or unintentionally. The unfavorable effect of immediate capsulotomy on angiographic cystoid macular edema is supported by two large, randomized prospective studies.[37, 40] Placement of an intraocular lens does not alter the incidence of cystoid macular edema.[1, 52] However, iris-supported or iridocapsular-supported intraocular lenses are associated with more persistent cystoid macular edema.[54–56] Cystoid macular edema is more common in the presence of vitreous loss, interruption of the anterior hyaloid membrane, adherence of the vitreous to the inner surface of the operative wound, poor positioning of an intraocular lens, movement of an intraocular lens, or chronic inflammation.[52, 57] In intracapsular surgery, the anterior hyaloid face can rupture at some time after the operation even if the surgery was uncomplicated, and this predisposes to cystoid macular edema.[4]

Other Surgical Procedures Associated With Cystoid Macular Edema

Cystoid macular edema is the most common macular complication of scleral buckling surgery,[58–60] occurring in about 25 percent of phakic eyes and 50 percent of aphakic eyes. Ackerman and Topilow[61] presented evidence that it was more common when cryopexy rather than diathermy had been used, whereas no difference between procedures was found by Sabates and associates.[62] Cystoid macular edema can occur after penetrating keratoplasty in combination with cataract extraction or in eyes previously having had cataract surgery. It is rare after keratoplasty in eyes remaining phakic.[63] It occurs more frequently if cataract surgery had been performed previously, if the intracapsular technique is used, or if vitrectomy is performed.[63–65] When these risk

factors are present, the incidence can exceed 50 percent.[64] Cystoid macular edema can follow early or late posterior capsulotomy for opacification of the posterior capsule after extracapsular cataract surgery.[66] It appears to be less frequent after neodymium-yttrium-aluminum-garnet (Nd.YAG) laser capsulotomy than after discission with a knife.[67] Because of this fact and its noninvasiveness, laser capsulotomy has almost completely supplanted discission. The incidence of symptomatic cases appears to be about 1 percent.[68, 69] Delaying capsulotomy may reduce the risk of the development of cystoid macular edema.[68] This condition has also been seen after aphakic epikeratophakia,[70] corneal relaxing incisions,[71] glaucoma filtering operations,[20] laser iridotomy,[72] phakic scleral buckling with cryopexy for retinal breaks without detachment,[73] cryopexy alone,[74] and laser photocoagulation of the retina.[75]

PATHOLOGY

Histopathologic studies of eyes with cystoid macular edema have shown the accumulation of watery, proteinaceous material in spaces within the inner nuclear and outer plexiform layers (Fig. 71–4).[76–79] In more severe cases, these spaces may extend throughout most of the thickened retina between the internal and the external limiting membranes and also may extend considerable distances from the center of the fovea.[78] The cystoid spaces can distort the neural elements markedly; it is not surprising that cellular function may be compromised and vision may be impaired. Loss of photoreceptor cells is a consistent finding.[78] Several cases have shown adherence of the vitreous to the iris or surgical wound.[76, 80] Clear-cut traction on the perifoveal area by the vitreous has not been seen frequently. Chronic inflammatory cells have been observed in the ciliary body, the iris, and occasionally the retina.[76, 80] There appears to be some predilection for infiltration around

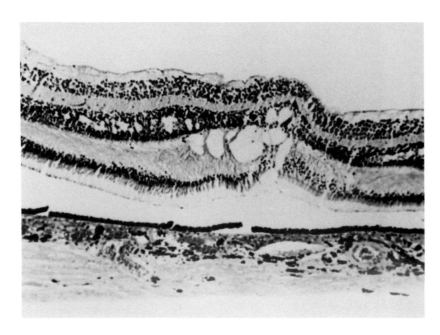

Figure 71–4. Photomicrograph of an eye with aphakic macular edema. There are large cystoid spaces in the outer plexiform layer. Smaller cystoid spaces are seen in the inner nuclear layer. Note the attenuation of the outer nuclear layer adjacent to the cystoid spaces. H&E, ×90. (From Tso MO: Pathology of cystoid macular edema. Ophthalmology 89:902–915, 1982.)

the retinal veins.[77] Mild vacuolization, atrophy, and reactive proliferation have been observed in the retinal pigment epithelium.[78]

Electron microscopic studies of cystoid macular edema after ocular surgery are not available, but two studies have been performed in eyes with cystoid macular edema due to choroidal melanoma or diabetes.[79, 81] Fine and Brucker, whose patients did not have well-developed cystoid spaces on angiography, found marked degeneration and swelling of the Müller cells with no enlargement of the extracellular space.[81] Gass and co-workers found polycystic expansion of the extracellular spaces that corresponded to the well-developed pattern of cystoid macular edema on angiography.[79] Additional studies are needed to settle the issue of the location of the excessive fluid in eyes after surgery.

The reason leakage in this condition so characteristically occurs in the foveal area is not clear. However, the unique anatomy of the perifoveal area probably contributes to its appearance. The foveal area has no inner nuclear, inner plexiform, ganglion cell, or nerve fiber layers. The Müller cells and bipolar and photoreceptor processes are not oriented perpendicular to the retinal surfaces, as they are elsewhere in the retina. This arrangement presumably reduces resistance to swelling. Furthermore, these cellular elements radiate centrifugally from the center of the fovea, so that fluid accumulating along them assumes the typical radiating petaloid pattern.

PATHOPHYSIOLOGY

Macular edema means excessive fluid in the retina. The amount of fluid normally in the retina presumably is maintained according to hydrostatic and osmotic pressures existing between the retina and the vasculature, which are compartmentalized by the blood-retinal barrier. This mainly consists of the cells of the retinal vascular endothelium and the retinal pigment epithelium—cells joined by tight junctions. This barrier is comparable to the blood-brain barrier and regulates the composition of the retinal extracellular space. This provides a stable, optimal milieu for the retinal cells, without which cellular dysfunction and visual impairment can supervene. Some molecules (e.g., oxygen) pass directly through the normal barrier with minimal interference, some are almost totally excluded (e.g., albumin), some are transported by specialized transport systems down a concentration gradient (e.g., glucose), and some are transported via specialized, energy-dependent transport systems (e.g., fluorescein) against an electrochemical gradient. The last type of transport often operates differently in the two directions (e.g., fluorescein is transported from retina to blood with far greater facility than from blood to retina).[82]

Very little is known of the precise derangements in these processes that underlie the occurrence of cystoid macular edema after ocular surgery. Fluorescein angiography shows convincingly that the perifoveal retinal capillaries are disturbed. It is unclear to what extent, if any, the pigment epithelium is involved. However, Tso

and Shih have observed disruption of the blood-retinal barrier at the level of the retinal pigment epithelium in monkeys undergoing cataract surgery.[83] Hypothesizing that there is a mild, generalized disturbance of the blood-retinal barrier, Blair and colleagues performed vitreous fluorophotometry in patients after cataract surgery.[84] Since fluorophotometry is quite sensitive to diffuse leakage, their finding of normal values in most patients suggests that the barrier is essentially intact except at the locations seen to be abnormal by angiography. The lack of hard exudates suggests that different types of molecules accumulate in the retina (possibly related to the molecular size, electrical charge, or other factors) in cystoid macular edema when compared with other conditions, such as diabetes. The accumulation of different types of molecules presumably would result from differences in the derangement of the blood-retinal barrier in these conditions.

Although disruption of the blood-retinal barrier incontestably plays a major role in cystoid macular edema, other processes may be involved. Pathologic evidence of cell loss and Müller cell abnormalities has suggested that microinfarction and defective removal of intraretinal plasma proteins by Müller cells may be contributing factors.[78, 85]

Several theories have been advanced to explain how ocular surgery leads to cystoid macular edema. First, inflammation in the anterior segment may liberate substances, particularly prostaglandins, that diffuse posteriorly and provoke cystoid macular edema. The rationale is based on the fact that affected eyes tend to have clinical signs and histopathologic evidence of inflammation, as well as leakage on iris angiography. Miyake[86] and several others[42, 87, 88] have shown that inhibitors of cyclooxygenase, such as indomethacin, can reduce the incidence of angiographic cystoid macular edema. Some of these studies were carefully conducted and convincingly indicate the role of prostaglandins in the pathogenesis of cystoid macular edema. Furthermore, Miyake has reported markedly elevated aqueous humor prostaglandin concentrations in patients with chronic cystoid macular edema and vitreous incarceration.[89] Pars plana vitrectomy usually reduced the prostaglandin levels, inflammatory signs, and macular dye leakage and improved the visual acuity. This theory does not clearly explain why the perifoveal retinal vessels are preferentially involved.

Another theory is that tractional forces on the foveal area exerted by the vitreous lead to cystoid macular edema. The vitreous is considered to be particularly adherent to the retina at the macular region and at the optic nerve head,[90, 91] both of which tend to show leakage after surgery. Since the vitreous inserts into the internal limiting membrane, which is attached to the Müller cells, these cells could be particularly affected by vitreous traction and edema may result.[91, 92] Partial posterior vitreous detachment with either a narrow or a broad attachment persisting at the fovea has been observed in patients with cystoid macular edema.[11, 12] Furthermore, Schepens and coworkers maintain that vitreous traction on the macula may be responsible for cystoid macular edema even if there is no posterior vitreous detachment.[12] However, not all investigators have been able to visualize these vitreomacular adhesions consistently. This theory does not readily explain why breakdown of the blood-retinal barrier should be so prominent. Furthermore, cystoid macular edema after surgery appears similar to that in various retinal vascular diseases such as diabetic retinopathy and branch retinal vein occlusion. In these conditions, the edema is clearly located in relation to vascular abnormalities in the retina and not to the normal sites of vitreous insertion.

It is well established that excessive light exposure can cause retinal damage, and several studies have been undertaken to determine if this could be responsible for cystoid macular edema. The normal crystalline lens filters near-ultraviolet radiation out of the light impinging on the retina. Since the filtering effect is lacking after cataract surgery, long-term exposure to this radiation after surgery may be injurious. Kraff and colleagues conducted a large, prospective, double-masked study in which each eye was randomized to receive an intraocular lens with or without a chromophore that markedly attenuated ultraviolet light.[38] They found that an approximately 50 percent reduction in angiographic cystoid macular edema was attributable to the filter. This led to the hypothesis that the cause of cystoid macular edema involves the ultraviolet light–induced formation of free radicals that stimulate the synthesis of prostaglandins beyond that induced by the surgical manipulation.[93] However, others have not been able to reproduce these results in smaller studies,[94, 95] and McIntyre found no reduction in clinically significant cystoid macular edema using ultraviolet light–absorbing intraocular lenses in 1731 cases.[96] The incidence of angiographic cystoid macular edema was not reduced by blocking near-ultraviolet light from the operating microscope or by using a pupillary light occluder during cataract surgery.[39, 41] Additional studies are needed to establish the role of photic injury in the pathogenesis of cystoid macular edema.

Roper and Nisbet provided evidence that hyaluronidase in the retrobulbar anesthetic could contribute to the development of cystoid macular edema.[97] This factor was evaluated systematically by Kraff and associates, who found no effect.[36]

A full understanding of the pathophysiology of cystoid macular edema will have to account for the peculiar time course seen in this disease. It is uncommon immediately after surgery,[18] but then develops with high frequency. There is a tendency of the disease to wax and wane,[19] and some cases do not occur until long after surgery.[17] Whether these phenomena are related to differences in pathophysiologic mechanisms remains a mystery.

TREATMENT

Pharmacologic Approaches

As noted earlier, many studies have been performed to assess the therapeutic efficacy of cyclooxygenase inhibitors. When these agents were given both preoperatively and for varying periods after surgery, they were found in most studies to be effective in reducing the incidence of angiographic cystoid macular edema,[87, 88, 98] even without topical steroids,[42] but were not effective in improving visual acuity or providing sustained benefit. The natural course of the disease is to improve spontaneously in most cases, so most untreated eyes eventually recover about the same visual level as do treated eyes. Most studies of patients in whom treatment was started after the development of cystoid macular edema have shown no benefit. An exception is the double-masked, randomized, placebo-controlled study of Flach and associates using topical ketorolac tromethamine.[9] They showed a highly significant visual improvement attributable to the drug. Because both clinically significant and chronic cystoid macular edema occur in such a small percentage of patients undergoing surgery (even though the total number of patients is substantial), large, collaborative trials may be necessary to enroll enough patients to demonstrate conclusively a meaningful therapeutic benefit of cyclooxygenase inhibitors.

Although the foregoing studies were of patients undergoing cataract surgery, Miyake and coworkers showed benefit from topical indomethacin in patients undergoing surgery for retinal detachment.[60] Corticosteroids have been used by many investigators to treat cystoid macular edema, but no benefit has been shown in rigorously conducted studies to date. Cox and associates used acetazolamide to treat cystoid macular edema associated with several conditions, and patients who had undergone cataract surgery tended to respond.[99] Additional studies are needed to confirm this finding. A preliminary report suggested that treatment with hyperbaric oxygen might ameliorate macular edema.[100] In summary, no pharmacologic therapy has been established to prevent or treat clinically significant cystoid macular edema at this time.

Surgical Approaches

Vitreous adhesions to the cataract incision are associated with cystoid macular edema, regardless of whether they act by irritation of the iris, by traction on the macula, or by some other mechanism. This raises the question of whether sectioning the vitreous strands would be of benefit in cystoid macular edema. This issue was formally addressed by the Vitrectomy—Aphakic Cystoid Macular Edema Study.[8] The investigators found a statistically significant improvement in visual acuity in the eyes undergoing surgery. They recommended (1) delaying intervention until the visual acuity was stable for 2 or 3 mo, (2) considering vitrectomy if the visual acuity was 20/80 or less, (3) performing vitrectomy before the visual acuity was 20/80 or less for 2 yr, and (4) performing vitrectomy via the pars plana approach or via a combination of pars plana and limbal approaches.

The Nd.YAG laser has been used to section vitreous strands to the wound in patients with cystoid macular edema, with encouraging visual results.[101, 102] Complete section may be technically difficult and require repeated treatment, especially when the adherent vitreous is broad and thick. Laser photocoagulation has not been effective in the management of cystoid macular edema.[19]

Current Treatment Recommendations

Since the therapeutic options are limited, we recommend reducing the risk of cystoid macular edema after cataract extraction by performing extracapsular surgery and avoiding interruption of the posterior capsule and vitreous loss. If an eye with cystoid macular edema shows significant inflammatory signs and symptoms, it seems reasonable to treat with antiinflammatory agents such as topical steroids,[103] although quieting the eye may not reduce the edema. We do not recommend using any of the available antiprostaglandin agents because evidence of their efficacy in clinically significant or chronic cystoid macular edema is insufficient, and there is no clinical benefit in preventing or treating angiographic cystoid macular edema. There is even less evidence to support the use of other pharmacologic agents at this time. When there is chronic cystoid macular edema with vitreous adherent to the cataract incision, we advocate vitrectomy according to the recommendations of the Vitrectomy—Aphakic Cystoid Macular Edema Study,[8] as indicated earlier. In our hands, this has been more effective than the Nd.YAG laser.

References

1. The Miami Study Group: Cystoid macular edema in aphakic and pseudophakic eyes. Am J Ophthalmol 88:45, 1979.
2. Stark WJ, Worthen DM, Holladay JT, et al: The FDA report on intraocular lenses. Ophthalmology 90:311, 1983.
3. Jampol LM: Cystoid macular edema following cataract surgery. Arch Ophthalmol 106:894, 1988.
4. Irvine SR: A newly defined vitreous syndrome following cataract surgery. Am J Ophthalmol 36:599, 1953.
5. Gass JDM, Norton EWD: Cystoid macular edema and papilledema following cataract extraction: A fluorescein funduscopic and angiographic study. Arch Ophthalmol 76:646, 1966.
6. Yanoff M, Fine BS: Ocular Pathology: A Text and Atlas, 2nd ed. Philadelphia, Harper & Row, 1982, p 477.
7. Nussenblatt RB, Kaufman SC, Palestine AG, et al: Macular thickening and visual acuity. Measurement in patients with cystoid macular edema. Ophthalmology 94:1134, 1987.
8. Fung WE: Vitrectomy for chronic aphakic cystoid macular edema. Results of a national, collaborative, prospective, randomized investigation. Ophthalmology 92:1102, 1985.
9. Flach AJ, Dolan BJ, Irvine AR: Effectiveness of ketorolac tromethamine 0.5% ophthalmic solution for chronic aphakic and pseudophakic cystoid macular edema. Am J Ophthalmol 103:479, 1987.
10. Gass JDM, Norton EWD: Fluorescein studies of patients with macular edema and papilledema following cataract extraction. Trans Am Ophthalmol Soc 64:232, 1966.
11. Tolentino FI, Schepens CL: Edema of the posterior pole after cataract extraction: A biomicroscopic study. Arch Ophthalmol 74:781, 1965.
12. Schepens CL, Avila MP, Jalkh AE, et al: Role of the vitreous in cystoid macular edema. Surv Ophthalmol 28(Suppl):499, 1984.
13. Bovino JA, Kelly TJ Jr, Marcus DF: Intraretinal hemorrhages in cystoid macular edema. Arch Ophthalmol 102:1151, 1984.
14. Kottow M, Hendrickson P: Iris angiography in cystoid macular edema after cataract extraction. Arch Ophthalmol 93:487, 1975.
15. Kelley JS, Kincaid M: Retinal fluorography using oral fluorescein. Arch Ophthalmol 97:2331, 1979.
16. Salzman J, Seiple W, Carr R, et al: Electrophysiological assess-
ment of aphakic cystoid macular oedema. Br J Ophthalmol 70:819, 1986.
17. Mao LK, Holland PM: "Very late onset" cystoid macular edema. Ophthalmic Surg 19:633, 1988.
18. Klein RM, Yannuzzi L: Cystoid macular edema in the first week after cataract extraction. Am J Ophthalmol 81:614, 1976.
19. Yannuzzi LA: A perspective on the treatment of aphakic cystoid macular edema. Surv Ophthalmol 28:540, 1984.
20. Gass JDM: Stereoscopic Atlas of Macular Diseases, 3rd ed. St Louis, CV Mosby, 1987, p 368.
21. Barbera LG, Kung JS, Kimmel AS, et al: Optic disc leakage as a prognostic indicator in aphakic cystoid macular edema. CLAO J 14:51, 1988.
22. Lakhanpal V, Schocket SS: Pseudophakic and aphakic retinal detachment mimicking cystoid macular edema. Ophthalmology 94:785, 1987.
23. McDonald HR, Irvine AR: Light-induced maculopathy from the operating microscope in extracapsular cataract extraction and intraocular lens implantation. Ophthalmology 90:945, 1983.
24. Gass JD: Idiopathic senile macular hole. Arch Ophthalmol 106:629, 1988.
25. Welch RB, Cooper JC: Macular edema, papilledema and optic atrophy after cataract extraction. Arch Ophthalmol 59:665, 1958.
26. Keerl G: Maculaodem nach Kataraktoperation. Klin Monatsbl Augenheilkd 156:850, 1970.
27. Gehring JR: Macular edema following cataract extraction. Arch Ophthalmol 80:626, 1968.
28. Irvine AR, Bresky R, Crowder BM, et al: Macular edema after cataract surgery. Ann Ophthalmol 3:1234, 1971.
29. Satake Y: Studies on macular circulation after cataract operation with fluorescein angiography. Folia Ophthalmol Jpn 22:993, 1971.
30. Yoshioka H, Kawashima K: Macular edema following cataract extraction. Acta Soc Ophthalmol Jpn 75:2269, 1971.
31. Yoshioka H, Kawashima K, Sugita T: Macular edema following cataract extraction. Acta Soc Ophthalmol Jpn 76:1118, 1972.
32. Hitchings RA, Chisholm IH: Incidence of aphakic macular edema: A prospective study. Br J Ophthalmol 59:444, 1975.
33. Hitchings RA, Chisholm IH, Bird AC: Aphakic macular edema, incidence and pathogenesis. Invest Ophthalmol 14:68, 1975.
34. Meredith TA, Kenyon KR, Singerman LJ, et al: Perifoveal vascular leakage and macular oedema after intracapsular cataract extraction. Arch Ophthalmol 60:765, 1976.
35. Kraff MC, Sanders DR, Jampol LM, et al: Prophylaxis of pseudophakic cystoid macular edema with topical indomethacin. Ophthalmology 89:885, 1982.
36. Kraff MC, Sanders DR, Jampol LM, et al: Effect of retrobulbar hyaluronidase on pseudophakic cystoid macular edema. Am Intraocular Implant Soc J 9:184, 1983.
37. Kraff MC, Sanders DR, Jampol LM, et al: Effect of primary capsulotomy with extracapsular surgery on the incidence of pseudophakic cystoid macular edema. Am J Ophthalmol 98:166, 1984.
38. Kraff MC, Sanders DR, Jampol LM, et al: Effect of an ultraviolet-filtering intraocular lens on cystoid macular edema. Ophthalmology 92:366, 1985.
39. Jampol LM, Kraff MC, Sanders DR, et al: Near-UV radiation from the operating microscope and pseudophakic cystoid macular edema. Arch Ophthalmol 103:28, 1985.
40. Wright PL, Wilkinson CP, Balyeat HD, et al: Angiographic cystoid macular edema after posterior chamber lens implantation. Arch Ophthalmol 106:740, 1988.
41. Kraff MC, Lieberman HL, Jampol LM, et al: Effect of a pupillary light occluder on cystoid macular edema. J Cataract Refract Surg 15:658, 1989.
42. Flach AJ, Stegman RC, Graham J, et al: Prophylaxis of aphakic cystoid macular edema without corticosteroids. Ophthalmology 97:1253, 1990.
43. Gass JDM, Norton EWD: Follow-up study of cystoid macular edema following cataract extraction. Trans Am Acad Ophthalmol Otolaryngol 73:665, 1969.
44. Poer DV, Helveston EM, Ellis FD: Aphakic cystoid macular edema in children. Arch Ophthalmol 99:249, 1981.
45. Gilbard SM, Peyman GA, Goldberg MF: Evaluation for cystoid maculopathy after pars plicata lensectomy-vitrectomy for congenital cataracts. Ophthalmology 90:1201, 1983.

46. Schulman J, Peyman GA, Raichand M, et al: Aphakic cystoid macular edema in children after vitrectomy for anterior segment injuries. Ophthalmic Surg 14:848, 1983.

47. Morgan KS, Franklin RM: Oral fluorescein angioscopy in aphakic children. J Pediatr Ophthalmol Strabismus 21:33, 1984.

48. Pinchoff BS, Ellis FD, Helveston EM, et al: Cystoid macular edema in pediatric aphakia. J Pediatr Ophthalmol Strabismus 25:240, 1988.

49. Hoyt CS, Nickel B: Aphakic cystoid macular edema: Occurrence in infants and children after transpupillary lensectomy and anterior vitrectomy. Arch Ophthalmol 100:746, 1982.

50. Handa J, Henry JC, Krupin T, et al: Extracapsular cataract extraction with posterior chamber lens implantation in patients with glaucoma. Arch Ophthalmol 105:765, 1987.

51. Jaffe NS, Luscombe SM, Clayman HM, et al: A fluorescein angiographic study of cystoid macular edema. Am J Ophthalmol 92:775, 1981.

52. Jaffe NS, Clayman HM, Jaffe MS: Cystoid macular edema after intracapsular and extracapsular cataract extraction with and without an intraocular lens. Ophthalmology 89:25, 1982.

53. Severin TD, Severin SL: Pseudophakic cystoid macular edema: A revised comparison of the incidence with intracapsular and extracapsular cataract extraction. Ophthalmic Surg 19:116, 1988.

54. Winslow RL, Taylor BC, Harris WS: A one-year follow-up of cystoid macular edema following intraocular lens implantation. Ophthalmology 85:190, 1978.

55. Wilkinson CP: A long-term follow-up study of cystoid macular edema in aphakic and pseudophakic eyes. Trans Am Ophthalmol Soc 79:810, 1981.

56. Taylor DM, Sachs SW, Stern AL: Aphakic cystoid macular edema. Long-term clinical observations. Surv Ophthalmol 28(Suppl):437, 1984.

57. Stark WJ Jr, Maumenee AE, Fagadau W, et al: Cystoid macular edema in pseudophakia. Surv Ophthalmol 28(Suppl):442, 1984.

58. Lobes LA Jr, Grand MG: Incidence of cystoid macular edema following scleral buckling procedure. Arch Ophthalmol 98:1230, 1980.

59. Meredith TA, Reeser FH, Topping TM, et al: Cystoid macular edema after retinal detachment surgery. Ophthalmology 87:1090, 1980.

60. Miyake K, Miyake Y, Maekubo K, et al: Incidence of cystoid macular edema after retinal detachment surgery and the use of topical indomethacin. Am J Ophthalmol 95:451, 1983.

61. Ackerman AL, Topilow HW: A reduced incidence of cystoid macular edema following retinal detachment surgery using diathermy. Ophthalmology 92:1092, 1985.

62. Sabates NR, Sabates FN, Sabates R, et al: Macular changes after retinal detachment surgery. Am J Ophthalmol 108:22, 1989.

63. Nirankari VS, Karesh JW: Cystoid macular edema following penetrating keratoplasty: Incidence and prognosis. Ophthalmic Surg 17:404, 1986.

64. West CE, Fitzgerald CR, Sewell JH: Cystoid macular edema following aphakic keratoplasty. Am J Ophthalmol 75:77, 1973.

65. Kramer SG: Penetrating keratoplasty combined with extracapsular cataract extraction. Am J Ophthalmol 100:129, 1985.

66. Liesegang TJ, Bourne WJ, Ilstrup DM: Secondary surgical and neodymium-YAG laser discissions. Am J Ophthalmol 100:510, 1985.

67. Keates RH, Steinert RF, Puliafito CA, et al: Long-term follow-up of Nd:YAG laser posterior capsulotomy. J Am Intraocular Implant Soc 10:164, 1984.

68. Stark WJ, Worthen D, Holladay JT, et al: Neodymium:YAG lasers. An FDA report. Ophthalmology 92:209, 1985.

69. Shah GR, Gills JP, Durham DG, et al: Three thousand YAG lasers in posterior capsulotomies: An analysis of complications and comparison to polishing and surgical discission. Ophthalmic Surg 17:473, 1986.

70. Rosenfeld SI: Cystoid macular edema following epikeratophakia. Am J Ophthalmol 106:746, 1988.

71. Carter J, Barron BA, McDonald MB: Cystoid macular edema following corneal-relaxing incisions. Arch Ophthalmol 105:70, 1987.

72. Choplin NT, Bene CH: Cystoid macular edema following laser iridotomy. Ann Ophthalmol 15:172, 1983.

73. Ryan SJ: Cystoid macular edema in phakic retinal detachment procedures. Am J Ophthalmol 76:519, 1973.

74. Kimball RW, Morse PH, Benson WE: Cystoid macular edema after cryotherapy. Am J Ophthalmol 86:572, 1978.

75. McDonald HR, Schatz H: Macular edema following panretinal photocoagulation. Retina 5:5, 1985.

76. Norton AL, Brown WJ, Carlson M, et al: Pathogenesis of aphakic macular edema. Am J Ophthalmol 80:96, 1975.

77. Martin NF, Green WR, Martin LW: Retinal phlebitis in the Irvine-Gass syndrome. Am J Ophthalmol 83:377, 1977.

78. Tso MO: Pathology of cystoid macular edema. Ophthalmology 89:902, 1982.

79. Gass JD, Anderson DR, Davis EB: A clinical, fluorescein angiographic, and electron microscopic correlation of cystoid macular edema. Am J Ophthalmol 100:82, 1985.

80. Michels RG, Green WR, Maumenee AE: Cystoid macular edema following cataract extraction (the Irvine-Gass syndrome): A case studied clinically and histopathologically. Ophthalmic Surg 2:217, 1971.

81. Fine BS, Brucker AJ: Macular edema and cystoid macular edema. Am J Ophthalmol 92:466, 1981.

82. Blair NP, Zeimer RC, Rusin MM, et al: Outward transport of fluorescein from the vitreous in normal human subjects. Arch Ophthalmol 101:1117, 1983.

83. Tso MO, Shih CY: National Eye Institute Symposium on Experimental Pathology—Part II: Experimental macular edema after lens extraction. Invest Ophthalmol Vis Sci 16:381, 1977.

84. Blair NP, Elman MJ, Rusin MM: Vitreous fluorophotometry in patients with cataract surgery. Graefes Arch Clin Exp Ophthalmol 225:441, 1987.

85. Bellhorn RW: Analysis of animal models of macular edema. Surv Ophthalmol 28(Suppl):520, 1984.

86. Miyake K: Prevention of cystoid macular edema after lens extraction by topical indomethacin (I). A preliminary report. Graefes Arch Clin Exp Ophthalmol 203:81, 1977.

87. Jampol LM: Pharmacologic therapy of aphakic cystoid macular edema. Ophthalmology 89:891, 1982.

88. Mishima H, Masuda K, Miyake K: The putative role of prostaglandins in cystoid macular edema. Prog Clin Biol Res 312:251, 1989.

89. Miyake K: Indomethacin in the treatment of postoperative cystoid macular edema. Surv Ophthalmol 28(Suppl):554, 1984.

90. Grignolo A: Fibrous components of the vitreous body. Arch Ophthalmol 47:760, 1952.

91. Sebag J, Balazs EA: Pathogenesis of cystoid macular edema: An anatomic consideration of vitreoretinal adhesions. Surv Ophthalmol 28(Suppl):493, 1984.

92. Schubert HD: Cystoid macular edema: The apparent role of mechanical factors. Prog Clin Biol Res 312:277, 1989.

93. Jampol LM: Aphakic cystoid macular edema. A hypothesis. Arch Ophthalmol 103:1134, 1985.

94. Clarke MP, Yap M, Weatherill JR: Do intraocular lenses with ultraviolet-absorbing chromophores protect against macular oedema? Acta Ophthalmol 67:593, 1989.

95. Komatsu M, Kanagami S, Shimizu K: Ultraviolet-absorbing intraocular lens versus non–UV-absorbing intraocular lens: Comparison of angiographic cystoid macular edema. J Cataract Refract Surg 15:654, 1989.

96. McIntyre DJ: Phototoxicity—The ultraviolet question. Trans New Orleans Acad Ophthalmol 323, 1988.

97. Roper DL, Nisbet RM: Effect of hyaluronidase on the incidence of cystoid macular edema. Ann Ophthalmol 10:1673, 1978.

98. Jampol LM: Pharmacologic therapy of aphakic and pseudophakic cystoid macular edema. 1985 update. Ophthalmology 92:807, 1985.

99. Cox SN, Hay E, Bird AC: Treatment of chronic macular edema with acetazolamide. Arch Ophthalmol 106:1190, 1988.

100. Pfoff DS, Thom SR: Preliminary report on the effect of hyperbaric oxygen on cystoid macular edema. J Cataract Refract Surg 13:136, 1987.

101. Katzen LE, Fleischman JA, Trokel S: YAG laser treatment of cystoid macular edema. Am J Ophthalmol 95:589, 1983.

102. Steinert RF, Wasson PJ: Neodymium:YAG laser anterior vitrolysis for Irvine-Gass cystoid macular edema. J Cataract Refract Surg 15:304, 1989.

103. Jampol LM: In reply: Cystoid macular edema following cataract surgery. [Letter] Arch Ophthalmol 107:166, 1089.

Chapter 72

∎

Acute Posterior Multifocal Placoid Pigment Epitheliopathy

STEVEN J. ROSE and PETER L. LOU

Acute posterior mutifocal placoid pigment epitheliopathy (APMPPE) is a term first used by Gass[1] in 1968 to describe a specific fundus picture seen in three young women. Although the clinical findings of this disease may have been reported earlier,[2] Gass was the first to link the clinical findings with a proposed pathogenesis.

APMPPE is a disease that typically affects young, otherwise healthy adults. There is a fairly rapid loss of central vision in one or both eyes, with the concomitant development of multiple gray-white, flat lesions that are located primarily in the posterior pole at the level of the retinal pigment epithelium (RPE) or choriocapillaris. Spontaneous resolution, with recovery of vision, usually follows within 2 to 3 wk, leaving behind well-demarcated pigment epithelial scars.

Unilateral cases have been observed,[3, 5, 12] although the fellow eyes were thought to have evidence of abnormal choroidal perfusion.

APMPPE is generally considered to be nonrecurrent, although recurrences have been reported.[3, 4, 6, 15]

CLINICAL PRESENTATION

As already mentioned, APMPPE is usually seen in young, healthy adults between the ages of 20 and 50 yr (average age approximately 25 yr).[3, 4] Patients experience a rapid visual loss that may be central or paracentral in one or both eyes. The visual acuity may reach the level of "counting fingers." The characteristic acute-phase fundus changes include the presence of multifocal, creamy, yellow-white lesions at the level of the pigment epithelium of the posterior pole. The retina itself appears normal (Fig. 72–1A). The lesions are usually well circumscribed and discrete. They may be few in number (Fig. 72–2) or multiple, with large confluent patches

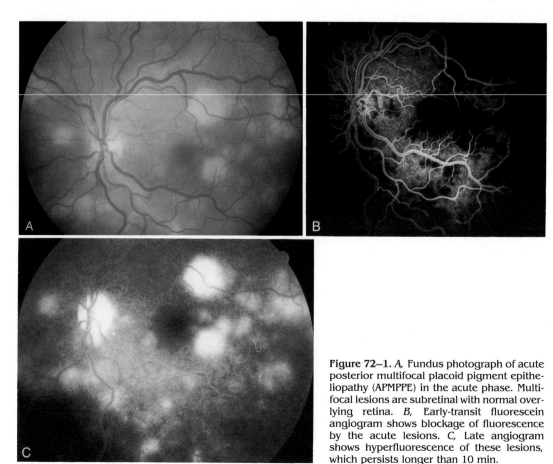

Figure 72–1. *A,* Fundus photograph of acute posterior multifocal placoid pigment epitheliopathy (APMPPE) in the acute phase. Multifocal lesions are subretinal with normal overlying retina. *B,* Early-transit fluorescein angiogram shows blockage of fluorescence by the acute lesions. *C,* Late angiogram shows hyperfluorescence of these lesions, which persists longer than 10 min.

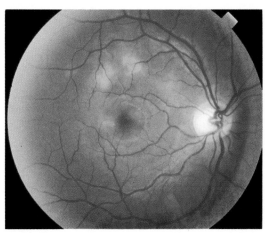

Figure 72–2. Fundus photograph of a patient with a few isolated APMPPE lesions.

(Fig. 72–3A). Within 1 wk, the acute lesions begin to fade and after 2 to 3 wk, these areas are replaced by scattered areas of depigmentation and fine to coarse clumping of the pigment epithelium (Fig. 72–4). A typical patient is seen in Figures 72–5 and 72–6.

Spontaneous recovery is the rule, and in one study 80 percent of patients had recovery of visual acuity to 20/40 or better.[4] In a long-term follow-up study by Gass,[3] less

than 4 percent of eyes achieved a visual acuity worse than 20/30 after 5 yr.

FLUORESCEIN ANGIOGRAPHY

The fluorescein angiogram appearance of APMPPE is fairly characteristic. In 1973, Annesley and coworkers[5] performed fluorescein angiography on patients both upon initial presentation and during follow-up visits.

During the acute, active stage, the lesions block fluorescence in the early frames of the angiogram (see Figs. 72–1B and 72–3B). In the later frames, the lesions show a diffuse hyperfluorescence that reaches a peak a few seconds later (see Figs. 72–1C and 72–3C), with fluorescence persisting up to 30 min.

Occasionally, large choroidal vessels can be seen in the background of the lesion (Fig. 72–7, *arrow*), but they are not always apparent.

In the inactive, resolved stage of APMPPE, fluorescein angiography demonstrates early transmission of the background fluorescence through the areas of RPE atrophy and depigmentation (see Fig. 72–7). The late angiograms are remarkable for the lack of persistent fluorescence.

In those patients in whom acute lesions begin to resolve, the transition from the active to the inactive lesion can be useful in determining the presence and

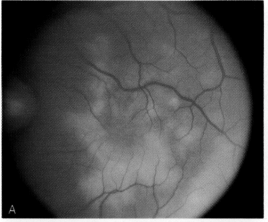

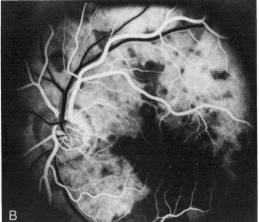

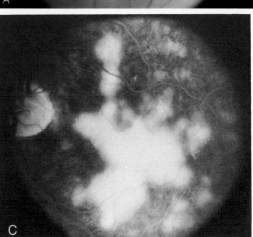

Figure 72–3. *A,* Fundus photograph of a patient with multiple, confluent patches of APMPPE. Visual acuity is 20/400. *B,* Early angiogram shows blockage corresponding to the exact pattern of the acute lesions. *C,* Late staining is evident in this angiogram. (*A–C,* Courtesy of Robert J. Brockhurst, M.D.)

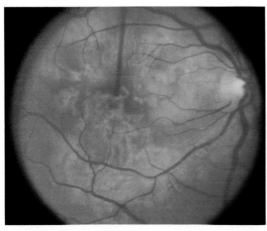

Figure 72—4. Fundus photograph of a patient with APMPPE 1 mo after the acute onset. Scattered areas of retinal pigment epithelial atrophy and pigment changes are evident. Visual acuity is 20/30. (Courtesy of Robert J. Brockhurst, M.D.)

amount of residual activity. According to Annesley and coworkers,[5] the central portion of the placoid lesion shows angiographic features similar to the active lesion with early blockage and late fluorescence. The peripheral portion of the lesion was similar to the inactive stage, showing irregular transmission without late staining.

ELECTROPHYSIOLOGIC TESTING

Fishman and associates[6] and others[7] described a case of APMPPE with electroretinography, electrooculography, dark adaptation, and color vision abnormalities. They found a marked and persistently abnormal electrooculogram (EOG) with only a moderately and transiently abnormal electroretinogram (ERG) in the acute phase of APMPPE. Blue-green color vision deficiency was apparent on pseudoisochromatic plates. Dark adaptation was normal.

According to Gass,[8] most patients tested at the Bascom Palmer Eye Institute have had normal ERGs and EOGs.

Retinal densitometry measurements, a function of RPE photopigment kinetics, have been reported in patients with APMPPE. During the active stage, the amount of pigment in the RPE was reduced and subsequently improved in eight of ten eyes following resolution of the fundus lesions. Another study[10] described normal photopigment kinetics 6 mo following the acute onset of APMPPE.

ASSOCIATED OCULAR AND SYSTEMIC MANIFESTATIONS

Despite the fact that the majority of patients with APMPPE show only ocular findings, many patients have presented with APMPPE in conjunction with various ocular and systemic manifestations.

Other ocular manifestations of APMPPE besides the characteristic fundus lesions include papillitis[11-16] and uveitis,[5, 12, 14, 17-19] including sarcoidosis.[20] Peripheral corneal thinning,[16] episcleritis,[8] retinal vasculitis,[15, 21, 22] hemorrhagic retinal detachment,[21] and serous retinal detachment[23] have also been described.

Systemic manifestations are limited mainly to the central nervous system and include severe headache,[1, 12, 24-26] optic neuritis,[15, 16, 27] episodes of transient cerebral ischemia producing strokelike symptoms,[17] permanent homonymous hemianopia,[24, 28] and cerebrospinal fluid pleocytosis.[12, 17, 24-26, 28, 29]

Other rare systemic manifestations include erythema nodosum,[14, 18] thyroiditis,[16] subclinical renal disease,[13] and transient hearing loss.[30]

The cause of APMPPE is not known, but many patients have presented with a prodromal viral-like upper respiratory syndrome.[1, 3, 5, 19, 29, 31] Azar and colleagues[31] were able to document concurrent adenovirus, type 5 infection in one patient with APMPPE, although extensive serologic testing for viral and other infectious agents has not been helpful.[17]

Other viral-like associations include a mild hypersensitivity reaction to swine flu vaccine,[22] lymphadenopathy,[3] hepatomegaly,[8] and regional enteritis.[3]

A study by Wolf and coworkers[32] of 30 patients with APMPPE found an association with HLA-B7 and HLA-DR2, which may suggest an immunogenetic predisposition to the acquisition of this disease.

PATHOGENESIS

Although there is widespread acceptance of the clinical and angiographic manifestations of this disease, the exact anatomic location of the precipitating events remains controversial.

Since his initial report, Gass[1] has favored the RPE cell as the primary cell involved. Gass feels that the disease causes multifocal areas of color change in the RPE and possibly in the retinal and receptor cells. The RPE cell cytoplasm apparently becomes sufficiently cloudy that it blocks out all background choroidal fluorescence. This damaged pigment epithelium later absorbs fluorescein, implying a breakdown in the integrity of the metabolic barrier at Bruch's membrane. Even with marked changes in the pigment content, most of the retinal receptors recover, and visual acuity returns to near normal.

Most authors now favor the choroid or, more specifically, the choriocapillaris, as the initial site of involvement in APMPPE.

Van Buskirk and associates[14] were the first to present evidence implicating APMPPE as a primary choroidal vasculopathy. They interpreted the fluorescein changes to represent delayed choriocapillary filling rather than blockage by swollen RPE cells.

In 1972, Deutman and coworkers[18] agreed that the overlying swollen RPE cells were the most likely explanation for the obscuring of choroidal fluorescence, but they felt that APMPPE represented an acute inflam-

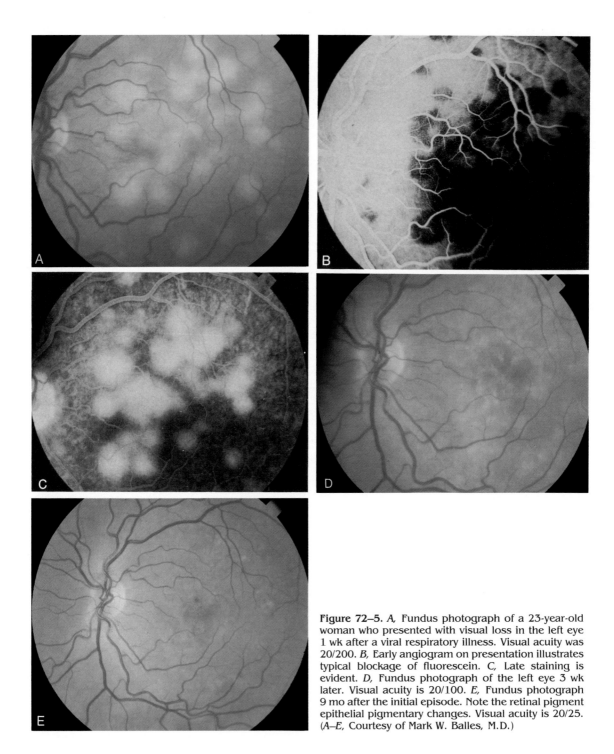

Figure 72–5. *A,* Fundus photograph of a 23-year-old woman who presented with visual loss in the left eye 1 wk after a viral respiratory illness. Visual acuity was 20/200. *B,* Early angiogram on presentation illustrates typical blockage of fluorescein. *C,* Late staining is evident. *D,* Fundus photograph of the left eye 3 wk later. Visual acuity is 20/100. *E,* Fundus photograph 9 mo after the initial episode. Note the retinal pigment epithelial pigmentary changes. Visual acuity is 20/25. (*A–E,* Courtesy of Mark W. Balles, M.D.)

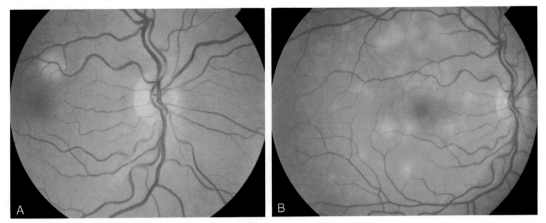

Figure 72–6. *A,* Fundus photograph of the right eye in the same patient in Figure 72–5. One week after symptoms began in the left eye, the patient noted metamorphopsia and mildly decreased visual acuity. *B,* Two weeks later, the patient's visual acuity decreased with a concomitant increase in the number of lesions.

matory process of the choriocapillaris, which quickly affected the pigment epithelium without affecting the intermediate or large choroidal vessels.

Ryan and Maumenee[29] lent support to the RPE theory in that the lesions in their patients did not involve the retina or the choroid beyond the area of affected pigment epithelium and were flat without associated serous detachment of the overlying retina. In contrast to this, Bird and Hamilton[23] described cases of APMPPE presenting with bilateral serous retinal detachments that resolved rapidly. They felt that in the acute stage of the disease reduced blood flow in the choriocapillaris caused focal RPE swelling from ischemia. They felt that the dye subsequently leaked into the RPE and subretinal fluid.

Hayreh's studies of the anatomy of the choroidal vasculature provided more support for investigators who favored the vascular theory.[33] He felt APMPPE represented an occlusive disorder of a terminal choroidal arteriole because the lesions in the disease resembled a unit or lobule of choriocapillaris in size and shape. In widespread confluent APMPPE lesions, a single sub-

macular arteriole may be the site of involvement. Similar lesions were seen in Hayreh's experimental posterior ciliary artery occlusions in rhesus monkeys.[34]

In 1977, Deutman and Lion[35] provided some solid evidence implicating the choriocapillaris as the structure primarily affected in APMPPE. They demonstrated nonperfusion of some of the lobules of the choriocapillaris but showed perfusion of the larger choroidal vessels. They interpreted this to mean that the hypofluorescence could not be due to swollen RPE cells because this would not allow transmission of larger choroidal vessels. They felt the RPE changes were secondary to the choriocapillaris filling defects.

Fishman and associates[6] addressed the controversy with electrophysiologic testing of APMPPE patients. They concluded that APMPPE was most consistent with a primary pigment epithelial disease because their subjects had normal ERGs but persistently abnormal EOGs. They argued that if the choriocapillaris was involved primarily, the ERG findings should parallel the EOG findings.

Gass[3, 8] also feels that the vascular theory is difficult to prove. He believes the variability in APMPPE lesions bears little or no resemblance to the anatomy of the choriocapillaris. In addition, he would expect that the acute lesions stain from the periphery inward, as the normally perfused choriocapillaris affects the nonperfused areas. Gass argues that recovery of visual function is more compatible with disease of the pigment epithelium, but other conditions that appear related to choriocapillaris damage, such as toxemia of pregnancy caused by accelerated hypertension,[36] are compatible with recovery of visual function after the acute phase.

MANAGEMENT

As APMPPE is generally self-limiting, there is no rationale for treatment. If the cause of the disease can be linked to an immunogenetic predisposition, as has been reported,[32] steroids may offer a theoretical advan-

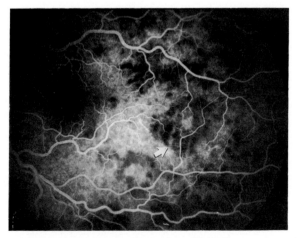

Figure 72–7. Early blockage of choriocapillaris fluorescence with larger choroidal vessels is evident *(arrow).*

tage toward shortening the disease course or modifying its effects on central vision.

DIFFERENTIAL DIAGNOSIS

Although most cases of APMPPE are readily diagnosed, some similarities among disease entities can present a problem in diagnosis.

Serpiginous or geographic choroiditis, multiple evanescent white dot syndrome, diffuse unilateral subacute neuroretinitis, neoplasms of the choroidal space, birdshot chorioretinopathy, and other syndromes that may cause focal inflammatory infiltrates of the choroid need to be considered.

CONCLUSION

APMPPE is a disease of otherwise healthy young adults, becoming manifested as multiple creamy lesions at the level of the RPE with characteristic fluorescein angiographic findings. In most cases, the disease process affects central vision early but resolves within 1 mo, with good recovery of visual function. The cause and location of the disease process remain controversial, and there is currently no treatment that has been proved effective.

REFERENCES

1. Gass JDM: Acute posterior multifocal placoid pigment epitheliopathy. Arch Ophthalmol 80:177, 1968.
2. Bonnin P, Lavat P: In connection with a case of Gass placoid epitheliopathy in 1860. Bull Soc Ophthalmol Francais 83:49, 1983.
3. Gass JDM: Acute posterior multifocal placoid pigment epitheliopathy: A long-term follow-up study. In Fine SL, Owens SL (eds): Management of Retinal Vascular and Macular Disorders. Baltimore, Williams & Wilkins, 1983.
4. Lewis RA, Martonyi CL: Acute posterior multifocal placoid epitheliopathy: A recurrence. Arch Ophthalmol 93:235, 1975.
5. Annesley WH, Tomer TL, Shields JA: Multifocal placoid pigment epitheliopathy. Am J Ophthalmol 76:511, 1973.
6. Fishman GA, Rabb MF, Kaplan J: Acute posterior multifocal placoid pigment epitheliopathy. Arch Ophthalmol 92:173, 1974.
7. Smith VC, Dokorny J, Ernest JT, et al: Visual function in acute posterior placoid pigment epitheliopathy. Am J Ophthalmol 85:192, 1978.
8. Gass JDM: Inflammatory diseases of the retina and choroid. In Stereoscopic Atlas of Macular Diseases: Diagnosis and Treatment, 3rd ed. St Louis, CV Mosby, 1987.
9. Keunen JEE, van Meel GJ, van Norren D, et al: Retinal densitometry in acute posterior multifocal placoid pigment epitheliopathy. Invest Ophthalmol Vis Sci 30:1515, 1989.
10. Hansen RM, Fulton AB: Cone pigments in acute posterior multifocal placoid pigment epitheliopathy. Am J Ophthalmol 91:465, 1981.
11. Deutman AF: Choriocapillaris filling patterns in health and disease. Trans Ophthalmol Soc UK 100:553, 1968.
12. Savino PJ, Weinberg RJ, Yassin JG, et al: Diverse manifestations of acute posterior multifocal placoid pigment epitheliopathy. Am J Ophthalmol 77:659, 1974.
13. Priluck IA, Robertson DM, Buettner H: Acute posterior multifocal placoid pigment epitheliopathy: Urinary findings. Arch Ophthalmol 99:1560, 1980.
14. Van Buskirk EB, Lessell S, Friedman E: Pigment epitheliopathy and erythema nodosum. Arch Ophthalmol 85:369, 1972.
15. Kirkham TH, Ffytche TJ, Sanders MD: Placoid pigment epitheliopathy with retinal vasculitis and papillitis. Br J Ophthalmol 56:875, 1972.
16. Jacklin HN: Acute posterior multifocal placoid pigment epitheliopathy and thyroiditis. Arch Ophthalmol 95:995, 1977.
17. Holt WS, Regan CDJ, Trempe C: Acute posterior multifocal placoid pigment epitheliopathy. Am J Ophthalmol 81:403, 1976.
18. Deutman AF, Oosterhuis JA, Boen-Tan TN, et al: Acute posterior multifocal placoid pigment epitheliopathy: Pigment epitheliopathy or choriocapillaritis. Br J Ophthalmol 56:863, 1972.
19. Fitzpatrick PJ, Robertson DM: Acute posterior multifocal placoid pigment epitheliopathy. Arch Ophthalmol 89:373, 1973.
20. Dick DJ, Newman PK, Richardson J, et al: Acute posterior multifocal placoid pigment epitheliopathy and sarcoidosis. Br J Ophthalmol 72:74, 1988.
21. Isashiki M, Koide H, Yamashita T, et al: Acute posterior multifocal placoid pigment epitheliopathy associated with diffuse retinal vasculitis and late hemorrhagic macular detachment. Br J Ophthalmol 70:255, 1986.
22. Hector RE: Acute posterior multifocal placoid pigment epitheliopathy. Am J Ophthalmol 86:424, 1978.
23. Bird AC, Hamilton AM: Placoid pigment epitheliopathy presenting with bilateral serous retinal detachments. Br J Ophthalmol 56:881, 1972.
24. Sigelman J, Behrens M, Hilal S: Acute posterior multifocal placoid pigment epitheliopathy associated with cerebral vasculitis and homonymous hemianopia. Am J Ophthalmol 88:919, 1979.
25. Bullock JD, Thomas ER, Fletcher RL: Cerebrospinal fluid abnormalities in acute posterior multifocal placoid pigment epitheliopathy. Am J Ophthalmol 84:45, 1977.
26. Fishman GA, Baskin M, Jednick N: Spinal fluid pleocytosis in acute posterior placoid pigment epitheliopathy. Ann Ophthalmol 9:33, 1977.
27. Jenkins RB, Savino PJ, Pilkerton AR: Placoid pigment epitheliopathy with swelling of the optic discs. Arch Neurol 29:204, 1973.
28. Smith CH, Savino PJ, Beck RW, et al: Acute posterior multifocal placoid pigment epitheliopathy and cerebral vasculitis. Arch Neurol 40:48, 1983.
29. Ryan SJ, Maumenee AE: Acute posterior multifocal placoid pigment epitheliopathy. Am J Ophthalmol 74:1066, 1972.
30. Clearkin LG, Hung SO: Acute posterior multifocal placoid pigment epitheliopathy associated with transient hearing loss. Trans Ophthalmol Soc UK 103:562, 1983.
31. Azar P, Gold RS, Waltman D, et al: Acute posterior multifocal placoid pigment epitheliopathy associated with an adenovirus type 5 infection. Am J Ophthalmol 80:1003, 1975.
32. Wolf MD, Folk JC, Panknen CA, et al: HLA-B7 and HLA-DR2 antigens and acute posterior multifocal placoid pigment epitheliopathy. Arch Ophthalmol 108:698, 1990.
33. Hayreh SS: Segmental nature of the choroidal vasculature. Br J Ophthalmol 59:631, 1975.
34. Hayreh SS: Occlusion of the posterior ciliary arteries. Trans Am Acad Ophthalmol Otolaryngol 77:300, 1973.
35. Deutman AF, Lion F: Choriocapillaris nonperfusion in acute multifocal placoid pigment epitheliopathy. Am J Ophthalmol 84:652, 1977.
36. Gaudric A, Coscas G, Bird AC: Choroidal ischemia. Am J Ophthalmol 94:489, 1982.

Chapter 73

Multiple Evanescent White Dot Syndrome

JOHN A. SORENSON and LAWRENCE A. YANNUZZI

The multiple evanescent white dot syndrome (MEWDS) was first described in 1984 by Jampol and associates.[1] In the Japanese literature, Takeda and co-workers also reported on four patients who had manifestations that were indistinguishable from MEWDS.[2] They termed the condition *acute disseminated retinal pigment epitheliopathy.* Since these initial reports, at least 50 patients with MEWDS have been described in the ophthalmic literature.[1-16] The subjective, demographic, clinical, fluorescein angiographic, and electrophysiologic findings of MEWDS represent a distinct clinical entity.

SUBJECTIVE COMPLAINTS

The usual presenting symptom is the acute onset of decreased or blurred vision often accompanied by dark or black spots in the periphery. Virtually all patients also note photopsia, described as flickering or shimmering lights. The photopsia sometimes seems to emanate from temporal scotomas. Two patients reported headaches accompanying the visual symptoms,[1, 10] and another complained of ocular discomfort.[7] Eleven of 50 patients have had a preceding "flulike" illness.[1, 6, 7, 13, 16]

DEMOGRAPHICS

Most patients are female (39 of 50 reported cases) with an average age of 25.8 yr (range 14 to 47 yr). The condition does not seem to have a racial predilection.

CLINICAL FINDINGS

Visual acuity on presentation ranges from 20/20− to 20/400. Some of these patients have an afferent pupillary defect. The anterior segment examination is normal except for the occasional presence of mild iritis. The most striking findings on posterior slit-lamp biomicroscopic examinations are the white spots, approximately 100 to 200 μ in size and located at the level of the retinal pigment epithelium (RPE) or deep retina. They are most prominently seen encircling the posterior pole and in the perifoveal region, but the fovea is spared (Figs. 73–1*A* and *B*, 73–2, and 73–3*A* and *B*). The spots are discrete and are not associated with overlying exudative changes. They are sometimes migratory, clearing in one area while appearing in another over a period of several days. A characteristic foveal RPE granularity is evident in most cases (Fig. 73–4). Other findings sometimes include a few cells in the posterior vitreous, mild blurring of the disc margin, and isolated areas of perivascular sheathing. When seen, the cellular reaction in the posterior vitreous is mild and transient in the early stages of the disease. Cotton-wool spots have been seen in one patient.[9]

VISUAL FIELDS

The visual field findings are variable, ranging from normal to a generalized depression (Fig. 73–5). Large blind spots are a frequent finding. Arcuate scotomas, cecocentral scotomas, and central depression have also been reported.[1, 7, 9, 13, 14] The field loss is sometimes exaggerated when compared with the clinical findings in the retina and at the disc.

FLUORESCEIN ANGIOGRAPHY

The fluorescein angiographic findings are characteristic. Early punctate hyperfluorescence at the level of the RPE is present, corresponding to the white dots. A cluster of hyperfluorescent dots often corresponds to the clinically evident white spots. The early punctate hyperfluorescence is often in a wreathlike configuration. The late-phase fluorescein angiogram reveals staining in the area of the spots and the optic nerve head (see Figs. 73–1*C* and *D* and 73–3*C* and *D*).[1, 5, 8] Late capillary leakage in the perifoveal area and focal areas of vasculitis are occasionally noted.

ELECTROPHYSIOLOGY

The electrophysiologic findings were described for three of the original patients reported to have MEWDS.[17] During the acute phase of the illness, the electroretinogram (ERG) a-wave and early receptor potential amplitudes were profoundly decreased. Both returned to normal with resolution of the disease. Subsequent reports have also noted abnormal ERGs.[2, 4, 8, 13, 14] Electrooculography results have also been reported to be abnormal.[2, 4, 12] Abnormal foveal densitometry has been reported for a patient with MEWDS who had normal ERG findings.[15]

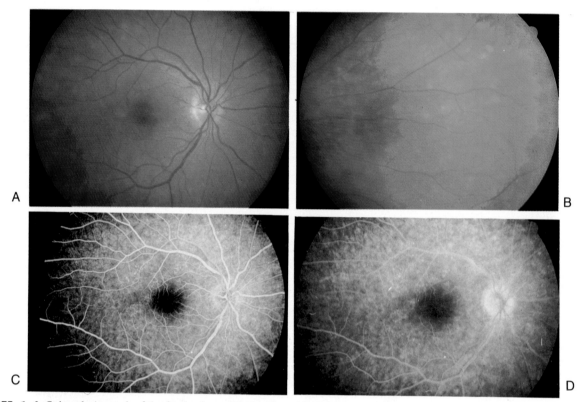

Figure 73–1. *A,* Color photograph of the fundus in a patient with multiple evanescent white dot syndrome (MEWDS). Note the scattered deep retinal spots in the posterior pole. *B,* Color photograph of the nasal posterior retina of the same patient. Additional spots are evident extending toward the midperipheral retina. *C,* Early fluorescein angiogram reveals multiple pinpoint dots, most of which correspond to the white lesions. *D,* The late-stage angiogram reveals no significant leakage associated with the punctate hyperfluorescent dots. Disc edema is evident. The left eye was completely normal clinically and angiographically in this patient.

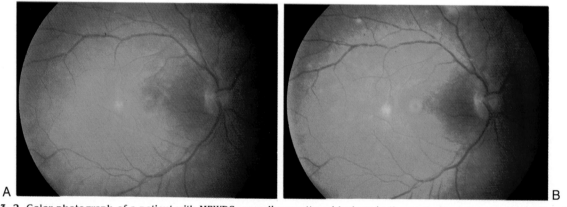

Figure 73–2. Color photograph of a patient with MEWDS, revealing scattered lesions in the posterior pole, most prominently evident in the inferior and superior nasal juxtapapillary regions. There were a few cells in the posterior vitreous. *B,* Color photograph of the same patient 4 days later. Note the disappearance of the white spots in the nasal juxtapapillary regions and the appearance of new spots in the temporal macula. There were no vitreous cells noted at this time.

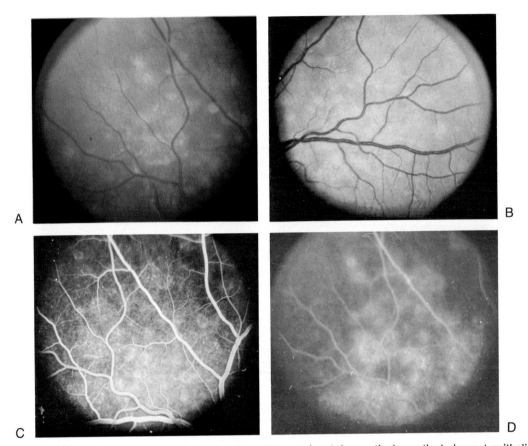

Figure 73–3. *A*, Color photograph of a patient with MEWDS. Note the prominent deep retinal or retinal pigment epithelial lesions, or both. These are more conspicuously evident than in the patient in Figure 73–1. *B*, A monochromatic photograph of the same patient highlights the white spots in the fundus. *C*, Early fluorescein angiogram in this patient reveals the characteristic hyperfluorescent dots in the region of the pigment epithelium. *D*, Late-stage fluorescein angiogram reveals staining of the retinal pigment epithelium and outer retina. In this patient, there has been alteration of the posterior blood-retinal barrier from extensive neuroretinitis involving the pigment epithelium.

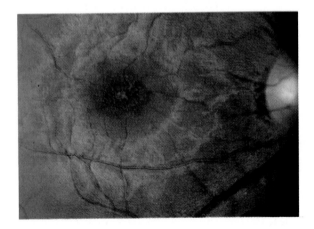

Figure 73–4. Color photograph of a patient with MEWDS. Note the granular appearance of the macula, which is characteristic of this disease and is exceedingly prominent in this patient. This is presumably due to a perifoveal neuroretinitis.

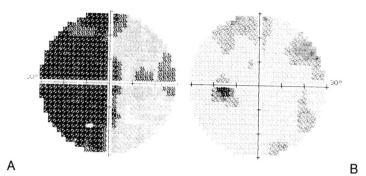

A

B

Figure 73–5. A, Humphrey's visual field of a 24-year-old woman with MEWDS involving the left eye 1 wk after the onset of symptoms. The field demonstrates marked visual loss in the entire visual field, most profound temporally (giant blind spot). The visual acuity was 20/40 – . B, Visual field of the same patient 4 mo later. The field is now nearly normal, although the patient still complained of dim vision. The visual acuity had returned to 20/20 and the white spots were completely gone. Eight months after the initial onset of symptoms, this patient still complained of dim vision in the left eye.

COURSE

Most patients with MEWDS have a relatively short course with recovery of vision within 3 to 10 wk. The vision returns to 20/30 or better, with the majority of patients regaining 20/20 vision. The white spots also disappear during this time; however, the foveal granularity usually persists. Some patients will have visual symptoms for much longer periods following resolution of the white spots. Even though visual acuity returns, some patients are aware of visual field defects, photopsia, or dim vision for extended periods. One patient experienced a subfoveal choroidal neovascular membrane approximately 4 mo after complete recovery from an episode of MEWDS.[16]

Only 6 of 50 patients reported in the literature have had bilateral involvement.[3, 4, 9, 10, 12] When both eyes are involved, one eye is usually involved minimally and is asymptomatic. In five of the six bilateral cases, the asymptomatic eye had 20/20 vision or better and only a few white spots peripheral to the arcades. Only one reported case was symptomatic in both eyes simultaneously.[4] This patient experienced visual loss in the right eye after 7 wk of visual loss in the left eye. Vision in the left eye was 20/300, and vision in the right eye was 20/50. The right eye had 1+ vitreous cells, foveal granularity, and an occasional white spot. Only two patients have been reported to have a recurrence of MEWDS.[3] One patient had a recurrence in the same eye nearly 3 yr after the original episode, and the other patient had a recurrence in the fellow eye nearly 4 yr after the initial episode.

PATHOPHYSIOLOGY

MEWDS is a distinct clinical syndrome that has only recently been recognized. Since it has an acute onset and is sometimes preceded by a "flulike" illness, a viral cause seems likely. One case has been reported with increased serum levels of total IgG and IgM during the acute phase.[11] Clinically and angiographically, the disease process involves the RPE and outer retina. The electrophysiologic results also confirm the abnormality at the level of the pigment epithelium–photoreceptor complex.

DIFFERENTIAL DIAGNOSIS

MEWDS must be differentiated from other inflammatory disorders of the RPE, choroid, or retina. In most instances, the diagnosis of MEWDS can be made confidently on clinical examination, and other disorders can be excluded.

Acute posterior multifocal placoid pigment epitheliopathy can also present with rapid loss of vision in a young patient.[18] However, this condition is usually bilateral, and the fundus lesions are characteristic. Multiple, flat gray-white lesions are present at the level of the RPE. These lesions are much larger than the spots of MEWDS. The lesions are hypofluorescent in the early-stage fluorescein angiogram and stain late. Extensive RPE alterations develop as lesions resolve.

Acute retinal pigment epitheliitis was described by Krill and Deutman in 1972.[19] Chittum and Kalina more recently reported the findings of eight patients with acute retinal pigment epitheliitis.[20] This condition is also characterized by acute loss of vision in a young patient. The ages of the first nine reported patients ranged from 18 to 45 yr.[19, 21] Three of the nine patients had bilateral involvement. The acute findings have been described as discrete clusters of dark spots surrounded by hypopigmented halos. These spots are localized to the perifoveal region. Fluorescein angiography can reveal blockage of choroidal fluorescence from the pigmented center with a surrounding zone of hyperfluorescence corresponding to the hypopigmented halo. Gradual resolution of the fundus findings with complete recovery of vision within 7 to 10 wk is typical. Subtle RPE alterations may remain. If acute retinal pigment epitheliitis still exists as a distinct clinical entity, it must be very rare. We have not seen a case in the New York area.

Birdshot retinochoroidopathy or vitiliginous chorioretinitis is characterized by white or depigmented spots at the level of the RPE scattered throughout the fundus.[22, 23] The older age at presentation, chronic course, bilateral involvement, and significant vitreous involvement all help to easily distinguish this syndrome from MEWDS.

Several papers have described a group of patients that can probably best be lumped together as cases of multifocal chorioretinitis. They include the following: punctate inner choroidopathy,[24] multifocal choroiditis and pan uveitis,[25] multifocal choroiditis associated with progressive subretinal fibrosis,[26] and recurrent multifocal choroiditis.[27] The patients described in these papers are similar. As in MEWDS, they are usually young females who present with acute visual loss in one eye and spots in the fundus. Punctate inner choroidopathy was described by Watzke and associates in 1984.[24] Ten moderately myopic women (aged 21 to 37 yr) presented with blurred vision, paracentral scotomas, or light flashes. The characteristic fundus lesions are small gray-yellow spots approximately 100 to 200 μ in diameter at the level of the RPE and inner choroid scattered throughout the posterior pole. Many lesions had an overlying serous detachment. Neither vitreous nor anterior chamber inflammation is present. The fluorescein angiogram reveals early hyperfluorescence and late staining or leakage into an overlying sensory retinal detachment. Eight of 10 patients had bilateral involvement, although symptoms were usually unilateral. The lesions developed into atrophic scars. Some scars became pigmented over time. Four of 10 patients eventually experienced subretinal neovascularization in association with perifoveal scars. Dreyer and Gass described 28 patients with multifocal choroiditis and pan uveitis.[25] Besides the characteristic RPE lesions resembling those seen in the presumed ocular histoplasmosis syndrome, these patients also had vitreous cells and anterior segment inflammation. Many of these patients experienced peripapillary or subfoveal subretinal neovascularization. Cantrill and Folk reported five female patients in whom progressive subretinal fibrosis developed in association with multifocal choroiditis.[26] Doran and Hamilton[28] and Palestine and coworkers[29] had previously reported similar cases. Morgan and Schatz described a similar group of female patients with multifocal choroiditis who had multiple recurrences.[27]

All these papers describe a multifocal chorioretinitis that is generally seen in young myopic females. The disorder can be chronic and recurrent. Although often presenting with unilateral symptoms, findings are usually bilateral. The RPE and inner choroidal spots vary in size but are generally larger than those seen in MEWDS. Papillitis, retinal phlebitis, vitritis, anterior uveitis, cystoid macular edema, and subretinal neovascularization can all be part of the disease process. One or more of these manifestations may predominate in a given patient. Following resolution of the spots in the acute stage, there is some degree of permanent RPE and choroidal damage, which can be atrophic, pigmentary, or cicatricial in nature. Since many disorders may mimic this idiopathic condition, a full medical work-up is needed, especially to rule out treatable infectious or inflammatory conditions such as syphilis or sarcoidosis. One paper has associated the Epstein-Barr virus with patients having multifocal chorioretinitis;[30] however, another report did not.[31] It is our feeling that this ubiquitous organism is not likely to be the causative agent in the majority of these cases. Hopefully, more specific serologic testing and ocular tissue analysis will serve to differentiate these disorders into more specific entities in the future. Although these patients may resemble those with MEWDS on presentation, the constellation of physical findings and subsequent course should make it easy to differentiate patients with multifocal chorioretinitis from those with MEWDS.

Another cause of retinochoroiditis that must be differentiated from MEWDS is toxoplasmosis. Ocular toxoplasmosis can present with multifocal gray-white lesions at the level of the deep retina and RPE, with little or no overlying vitreous reaction.[32, 33] These lesions typically resolve slowly and can recur. The diagnosis of punctate outer retinal toxoplasmosis is difficult to confirm. The presence of satellite lesions and positive serologic findings for toxoplasmosis can help to make the diagnosis in the appropriate clinical setting.

The early stage of diffuse unilateral subacute neuroretinitis (DUSN) can be characterized by recurrent crops of evanescent gray-white lesions at the level of the outer retina and RPE.[34] The chronic course of DUSN with eventual development of visual loss, optic atrophy, diffuse RPE degeneration, and retinal vessel narrowing easily differentiates this disorder from MEWDS. DUSN is caused by a nematode that can sometimes be visualized in the subretinal space.[35, 36]

Acute macular neuroretinopathy is another cause of loss of vision and paracentral scotomas in young patients.[37–39] This disorder can be bilateral and is characterized by cloverleaf, wedge-shaped, grayish lesions in the macular area, probably in the outer retinal layers. Interestingly, two patients have been reported with acute macular neuroretinopathy and MEWDS in the same eye, suggesting some similarity in their origins.[8]

The preceding chorioretinal disorders can, for the most part, be easily differentiated from cases of MEWDS. Perhaps the biggest difficulty in diagnosis is identifying a case of MEWDS after the retinal spots have faded. At this point in the disease process, the signs and symptoms can be indistinguishable from those of primary optic nerve disease, which include the presence of an afferent pupillary defect, defective color vision, disc edema, and visual field defects, particularly large blind spots and paracentral scotomas. The visual field defects in MEWDS may last for many months following the resolution of the retinal spots. Patients with MEWDS have initially been diagnosed as having optic neuritis or retrobulbar neuritis.[9] Identification of the typical foveal granularity seen in MEWDS or the subtle fluorescein angiographic findings consistent with MEWDS can help in identifying these cases. Testing visual evoked potentials and color vision may also be useful in distinguishing between retinal and optic nerve disease. Fletcher and colleagues described a syndrome occurring primarily in young females consisting of blind spot enlargement without optic disc edema.[40] The acute idiopathic blind spot enlargement (AIBSE) syndrome has features suggesting retinal dysfunction as its cause, including the presence of positive visual symptoms in the region of the scotoma, steep borders of the scotoma, and prolonged recovery time with photostress testing. Hamed and colleagues suggested that patients with AIBSE represent a subset of those with MEWDS, presenting for examination after the retinal spots have faded.[6, 41] More recently, Singh and associates suggested that MEWDS is one of several conditions that may be characterized by blind spot enlargement.[42] Some cases of AIBSE, but not all, may be due to MEWDS.

CONCLUSIONS

In summary, MEWDS is a unilateral, idiopathic, inflammatory disease with a constellation of well-described subjective, clinical, fluorescein angiographic, and electrophysiologic features. It occurs as a unilateral phenomenon, predominantly in young females. The most characteristic manifestation is that of outer retinal or superficial pigment epithelial white spots, which vary in their dimension but are usually confined to the posterior pole or midretinal areas. These fleeting disturbances are migratory in nature and relatively silent on fluorescein angiography except in some patients who presumably have involvement of the pigment epithelium with a permeability breakdown in the outer retinal-blood barrier. A consistent foveal granularity and mild papillitis are hallmarks of the disorder. Similarly, there are characteristic electroretinographic findings and visual field loss. The field changes exceed what might be expected on the basis of the clinical findings in the retina and at the optic nerve. The natural course is generally benign with spontaneous disappearance of the lesions and improvement of the visual function. MEWDS is easily differentiated from other categorized intraocular inflammatory diseases, although the presenting features are uniformly a reduction in acuity and photopsia. Although there is considerable information available on the subjective, demographic, clinical, and fluorescein angiographic and electrophysiologic features of this disease, a causative agent is still unknown. Further clinical research is needed to identify the precise pathogenesis.

REFERENCES

1. Jampol LM, Sieving PA, Pugh D, et al: Multiple evanescent white dot syndrome. I. Clinical findings. Arch Ophthalmol 102:671, 1984.
2. Takeda M, Kimura S, Tamiya M: Acute disseminated retinal pigment epitheliopathy. Folia Ophthalmol Jpn 35:2613, 1984.
3. Aaberg TM, Campo RV, Joffe L: Recurrences and bilaterality in the multiple evanescent white-dot syndrome. Am J Ophthalmol 100:29, 1985.
4. Jost BF, Olk RJ, McGaughey A: Bilateral symptomatic multiple evanescent white-dot syndrome. [Letter] Am J Ophthalmol 101:489, 1986.
5. Mamalis N, Daily MJ: Multiple evanescent white dot syndrome. A report of eight cases. Ophthalmology 94:1209, 1987.
6. Hamed LM, Glaser JS, Gass JDM, et al: Protracted enlargement of the blind spot in multiple evanescent white dot syndrome. Arch Ophthalmol 107:194, 1989.
7. Kimmel AS, Folk JC, Thompson HS, et al: The multiple evanescent white-dot syndrome with acute blind spot enlargement. [Letter] Am J Ophthalmol 107:425, 1989.
8. Gass JDM, Hamed LM: Acute macular neuroretinopathy and multiple evanescent white dot syndrome occurring in the same patients. Arch Ophthalmol 107:189, 1989.
9. Dodwell DG, Jampol LM, Rosenberg M, et al: Optic nerve involvement associated with the multiple evanescent white-dot syndrome. Ophthalmology 97:862, 1990.
10. Meyer RJ, Jampol LM: Recurrences and bilaterality in the multiple evanescent white-dot syndrome. [Letter] Am J Ophthalmol 101:338, 1986.
11. Chung Y, Yeh T, Liu J: Increased serum IgM and IgG in the multiple evanescent white-dot syndrome. [Letter] Am J Ophthalmol 104:187, 1987.
12. Laatikainen L, Immomen I: Multiple evanescent white dot syndrome. Graefes Arch Clin Exp Ophthalmol 226:37, 1988.
13. Slusher MM, Weaver RG: Multiple evanescent white dot syndrome. Retina 8:132, 1988.
14. Nakao K, Isashiki M: Multiple evanescent white dot syndrome. Jpn J Ophthalmol 30:376, 1986.
15. Keunen JEE, van Norren D: Foveal densitometry in the multiple evanescent white-dot syndrome. [Letter] Am J Ophthalmol 105:561, 1988.
16. Wyhinny GJ, Jackson JL, Jampol LM, et al: Subretinal neovascularization following multiple evanescent white-dot syndrome. [Case report] Arch Ophthalmol 108:1384, 1990.
17. Sieving PA, Fishman GA, Jampol LM, et al: Multiple evanescent white dot syndrome. II. Electrophysiology of the photoreceptors during retinal pigment epithelial disease. Arch Ophthalmol 102:675, 1984.
18. Gass JDM: Acute posterior multifocal placoid pigment epitheliopathy. Arch Ophthalmol 80:177, 1968.
19. Krill AE, Deutman AF: Acute retinal pigment epitheliitis. Am J Ophthalmol 74:193, 1972.
20. Chittum ME, Kalina RE: Acute retinal pigment epitheliitus. Ophthalmology 94:1114, 1987.
21. Deutman AF: Acute retinal pigment epitheliitis. Am J Ophthalmol 78:571, 1974.
22. Ryan SJ, Maumenee AE: Birdshot retinochoroidopathy. Am J Ophthalmol 89:31, 1980.
23. Gass JDM: Vitiliginous chorioretinitis. Arch Ophthalmol 99:1778, 1981.
24. Watzke RC, Packer AJ, Folk JC, et al: Punctate inner choroidopathy. Am J Ophthalmol 98:572, 1984.
25. Dreyer RF, Gass JDM: Multifocal choroiditis and panuveitis. A syndrome that mimics ocular histoplasmosis. Arch Ophthalmol 102:1776, 1984.
26. Cantrill HL, Folk JC: Multifocal choroiditis associated with progressive subretinal fibrosis. Am J Ophthalmol 101:170, 1986.
27. Morgan CM, Schatz H: Recurrent multifocal choroiditis. Ophthalmology 93:1138, 1986.
28. Doran RML, Hamilton AM: Disciform macular degeneration in young adults. Trans Ophthalmol Soc UK 102:471, 1982.
29. Palestine AG, Nussenblatt RB, Parven LM, et al: Progressive subretinal fibrosis and uveitis. Br J Ophthalmol 68:667, 1984.
30. Tiedeman JS: Epstein-Barr viral antibodies in multifocal choroiditis and panuveitis. Am J Ophthalmol 103:659, 1987.
31. Sugin S, Spaide R, Yannuzzi L, DeRosa J: Multifocal choroiditis and panuveitis and the Epstein-Barr virus. [Poster] Presented at The Association for Research in Vision and Ophthalmology (Annual Meeting), Sarasota, Florida, April 1991.
32. Doft BH, Gass JDM: Punctate outer retinal toxoplasmosis. Arch Ophthalmol 103:1332, 1985.
33. Matthews JD, Weiter JJ: Outer retinal toxoplasmosis. Ophthalmology 95:941, 1988.
34. Gass JDM, Scelfo R: Diffuse unilateral subacute neuroretinitis. J R Soc Med 71:95, 1978.
35. Gass JDM, Braunstein RA: Further observations concerning the diffuse unilateral neuroretinitis syndrome. Arch Ophthalmol 101:1689, 1983.
36. Kazacos KR, Raymond LA, Kazaces EA, et al: The raccoon ascarid. A probable cause of human ocular larva migrans. Ophthalmology 92:1735, 1985.
37. Bos PJ, Deutman AF: Acute macular neuroretinopathy. Am J Ophthalmol 80:573, 1975.
38. Rush JA: Acute macular neuroretinopathy. Am J Ophthalmol 83:490, 1977.
39. Priluck IA, Buettner H, Robertson DM: Acute macular neuroretinopathy. Am J Ophthalmol 86:775, 1978.
40. Fletcher WA, Imes RK, Goodman D, et al: Acute idiopathic blind spot enlargement. A big blind spot syndrome without optic disc edema. Arch Ophthalmol 106:44, 1988.
41. Hamed LM, Schutz NJ, Glaser JS, et al: Acute idiopathic blind spot enlargement without optic disc edema. [Letter] Arch Ophthalmol 106:1030, 1988.
42. Singh K, de Frank MP, Shults WT, et al: Acute idiopathic blind spot enlargement. A spectrum of disease. Ophthalmology 98:497, 1991.

Chapter 74

■

Epiretinal Macular Membranes

RAYMOND R. MARGHERIO

The proliferation of epiretinal membranes on the inner retinal surface along the internal limiting membrane was first described by Iwanoff in 1865.[1] These membranes have been shown to be relatively common. In 1971, Roth and Foos reported that in a series of autopsied eyes, epiretinal membranes were present in 2 percent of patients aged 50 yr and in more than 20 percent of patients by age 75 yr.[2] Clarkson and coworkers, in reviewing some 1612 postmortem eyes, noted epiretinal membranes in 1.7 percent of eyes that had not undergone previous ocular surgery.[3] Pearlstone reported an incidence of 6.4 percent in 1000 consecutive routine eye examinations in patients older than 50 yr, with 20 percent being bilateral.[4] Other authors report bilateral involvement in 10 to 20 percent of cases.[5-7]

The wrinkling of the retinal surface caused by epiretinal membranes in the macular region has been termed *surface wrinkling retinopathy,*[2] *macular pucker,*[8-10] *cellophane maculopathy,*[11, 12] *wrinkling of the internal limiting membrane,*[13] *preretinal macular fibrosis,*[13, 14] *epiretinal macular membrane, primary retinal folds,*[15] *internoretinal fibrosis,*[16] *idiopathic preretinal macular gliosis,*[6, 17, 18] *undetected central retinal vein occlusion,*[19] and *silkscreen retinopathy.* The term *macular pucker* has most frequently been applied to the condition when retinal surface wrinkling occurs following reattachment of a rhegmatogenous retinal detachment. This condition complicates 4 to 8 percent of otherwise successful primary retinal reattachments.[20, 21]

The presence of epiretinal membranes in the macular region has been associated with numerous clinical conditions including (1) postretinal detachment repair, (2) nonproliferative retinovascular disorders, (3) ocular inflammatory disorders, (4) certain proliferative retinopathies, (5) vitreous hemorrhage, (6) congenital conditions,[22] (7) idiopathic or spontaneous conditions, as well as (8) following trauma, and (9) after cryopexy or photocoagulation. The membranes develop because of proliferation of cells and collagen on the surface of the retina. The clinical appearance depends to some degree on cell type, membrane thickness, and the presence or lack of vessels. Vinores and colleagues found a correlation between the disease process and the amount of extracellular matrix, with proliferative vitreoretinopathy having a thicker membrane than postdetachment macular pucker, which, in turn, was thicker than an idiopathic macular pucker.[23] These ultrastructural findings correlate well with the clinical appearance of the various entities.

CLINICAL FEATURES

Patients with epiretinal membranes peripheral to the macula are generally asymptomatic. When the membranes involve the macula or are perimacular, however, the type and degree of symptoms experienced will depend on the membrane thickness, the degree of retinal distortion caused by the overlying membrane, the presence or lack of significant traction that can cause a microdetachment of the posterior pole, and the presence or lack of edema in the macular and perimacular regions.

Thin epiretinal membranes usually cause few symptoms. The condition appears to be relatively stable or slowly progressive with only a small number of patients, approximately 5 percent, having a vision of 20/200 or worse.[5, 24, 25] In more advanced cases, there is a reduction in vision, micropsia, metamorphopsia, Amsler grid distortion, and occasionally monocular diplopia. Spontaneous separation of an epiretinal macular membrane, although uncommon, can occur; when this happens, there is a general decrease in symptoms and a concomitant improvement in visual acuity.[12, 15, 26-29]

The clinical appearance is variable and may present as only a mild sheen or glint in the macular region, which can best be seen with red-free or monochromatic green or blue light (Fig. 74–1). In more severe cases, there is increased vascular tortuosity, and the perimacular vessels are seen to be pulled toward an epicenter, with striae and heterotopia of the macula. The superior and inferior arcuate vessels are also closer together and straighter than in an uninvolved eye (Fig. 74–2). Other findings that may be present include small intraretinal hemorrhages, cystic changes in the macula, and macular edema. Pseudoholes or macular cysts have been noted in up to 8 percent of idiopathic cases (Fig. 74–3).[6, 30] Thin membranes may be completely translucent, whereas thicker membranes are frequently opaque or pigmented and generally obscure details of the underlying fundus (Fig. 74–4).[31-33] The thicker and occasionally pigmented membranes are often seen following retinal detachment surgery, severe inflammatory conditions, and trauma.

An apparent posterior vitreous separation has been reported by most authors to exceed 75 percent in cases of idiopathic epiretinal membranes.[2-6, 11, 23, 24, 34-37] We have found that even experienced observers frequently cannot accurately determine the vitreoretinal relationships preoperatively. These relationships are evaluated more accurately during vitreous surgery using oblique

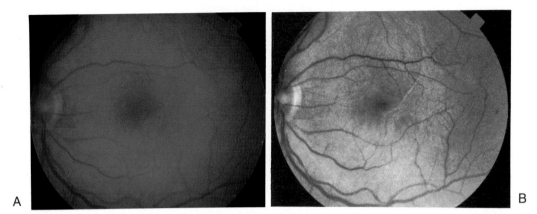

Figure 74–1. *A*, An idiopathic epiretinal membrane in a 65-year-old man. Visual acuity was 20/25. *B*, Black-and-white fundus photograph taken with a green 540-nm filter. Note increased definition of the epiretinal membrane.

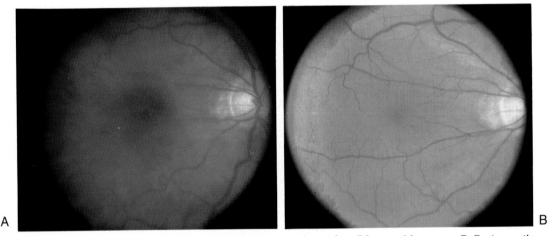

Figure 74–2. *A*, Preoperative appearance of an idiopathic epiretinal membrane in a 56-year-old woman. *B*, Postoperative appearance after removal of an intact thin membrane. Visual acuity improved from 20/200 to 20/30.

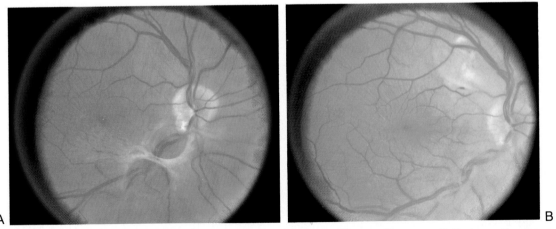

Figure 74–3. *A*, Idiopathic epiretinal membrane with a macular pseudohole in a 35-year-old woman. *B*, Postoperative appearance with disappearance of macular pseudohole and improvement in vision from 20/100 to 20/40.

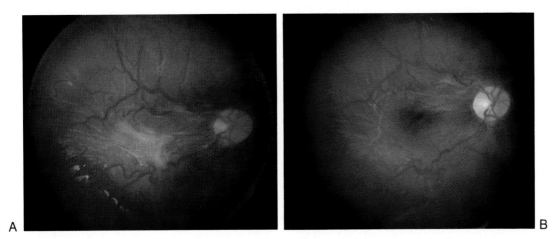

Figure 74–4. *A*, Preoperative appearance of a thick epiretinal membrane in a 10-year-old boy following trauma. *B*, Postoperative appearance after removal of epiretinal tissue. Vision improved from counting fingers to 20/100.

intraocular illumination and noting the effects of surgical manipulation on the underlying retina.[38] In some cases, a large, optically empty space was thought to be a posterior vitreous detachment preoperatively. Intraoperatively, however, epiretinal membrane peeled from the macular region because of an impending macular hole was clinically consistent with posterior hyaloid (Fig. 74–5).[38] This observation was supported by ultrastructural study of the tissue.[39] Kishi and Shimizu noted the presence of this ocular empty space in 84 autopsied eyes.[40] They termed this area the *posterior precortical vitreous pocket* (PPVP). They found this pocket in 48 of 84 eyes with either an incomplete or no posterior vitreous detachment and in 19 of 36 eyes with a posterior vitreous detachment. They noted that in eyes with advanced liquefaction of the vitreous, a large PPVP appeared to be a complete posterior vitreous detachment. In all their cases, the posterior layer of the PPVP was composed of a thin layer of cortical vitreous. The presence of this PPVP strengthens the hypothesis that its contraction causes tangential traction on the macula, giving the clinical appearance of an idiopathic epiretinal membrane or in some cases an idiopathic macular cyst or hole. The presence of epiretinal membranes has been thought to play a role in the formation of idiopathic macular holes.[30, 38, 41–43] These impending holes or "cysts" have been noted to resolve with spontaneous or surgical stripping of the membranes.[30, 38, 42]

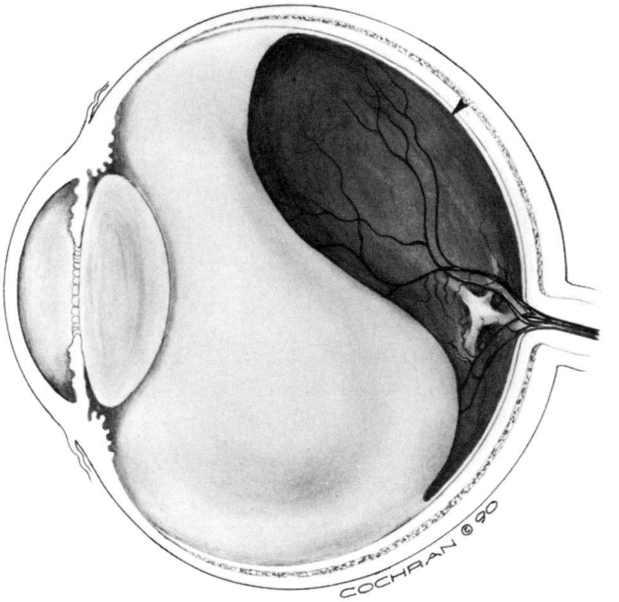

PATHOLOGY

The cellular origin of epiretinal membranes has long been debated, and almost every possibility has been considered. Iwanoff, in 1865, implicated the endothelial cell in the formation of the membranes.[1] Manschot, in 1958, thought that the membrane was an extension of the Müller cell processes,[44] whereas Wolter considered the cells to originate from fibroblasts in the vascular connective tissue.[45] Smith suggested that the cells in the membrane originated from the pigmented or nonpigmented cells of the pars ciliaris, retinal pigment epithelial cells, mesodermal elements of the vascular system, normal vitreous cells, inflammatory cells within the vitreous, or retinal glial cells.[46] In 1962, Kurz and Zimmerman felt that the cells originated from migration of retinal pigment epithelial cells.[47] Ashton later suggested that they originated from a transformation of vascular mesenchymal cells into fibroblasts,[48] and in 1969, Von Gloor proposed that hyalocytes were the cells of origin.[49]

The development of vitreous surgery has provided an opportunity to advance our understanding of the clinicopathologic relationships of epiretinal membranes. Constable reported on the histopathologic characteristics of membranes obtained by open-sky vitrectomy. He found proliferating fibroblasts interspersed with extra-

Figure 74–5. Large syneretic cavity simulating a complete posterior vitreous separation but with a thin layer of posterior hyaloid still attached to posterior pole (*arrowhead*).

cellular material and clumps of pigment.[50] Since then, numerous authors have attempted to characterize the cells of origin based on the suspected cause of the membrane obtained by pars plana vitrectomy. The general consensus has been that membranes in eyes that have retinal breaks or previous detachments were composed of cells of retinal pigment epithelial origin and that cells of glial origin predominated in the thin idiopathic epiretinal membranes.[23, 39, 51–61] However, other studies have demonstrated a high incidence of the retinal pigment epithelial type of cell, even in the idiopathic epiretinal membranes.[59] This finding is supported by Vinores and colleagues, who studied the ultrastructural and electron immunocytochemical characterization of cells in epiretinal membranes. Their work suggests that both retinal pigment epithelial cells and retinal glial cells are most likely to be the major participants in the pathogenesis of epiretinal membranes.[23] Foos suggested that the glial cells found in the thin idiopathic membranes were derived from the glial cells of the superficial retina and had migrated through breaks in the internal limiting lamina to proliferate on the retinal surface.[62] This hypothesis was subsequently supported by Bellhorn and associates.[63] The dispersion of retinal pigment epithelial cells on the retinal surface has been demonstrated clinically and experimentally in cases of retinal breaks and detachment.[64–68] However, the finding of retinal pigment epithelial cells in idiopathic membranes is more difficult to explain. Smiddy and associates suggest that the retinal pigment epithelial cells gain access to the retinal surface by various methods, including migration through occult breaks, inactivation of developmental rests of retinal pigment epithelial cells already on the surface of the retina, transformation from other cell types, or via transretinal migration.[59] The exact mechanism or combination of mechanisms is yet to be elucidated. Stern and coworkers[69] suggested that the contractile forces of the membranes were related to their constituent cell types and were not dependent on intercellular collagen as suggested by previous investigators.[70]

TREATMENT

The majority of patients with epiretinal macular membranes have symptoms that are mild and either nonprogressive or slowly progressive; therefore, treatment is rarely indicated. In a few cases, the membrane may spontaneously release with a marked decrease in symptoms and improvement in acuity. For patients with significant symptoms and substantially reduced visual acuity, bimanual vitrectomy with epiretinal membrane peeling can diminish the severity of the symptoms and improve acuity in 75 percent or more of cases.

There is no effective treatment available for mild forms of epiretinal macular membranes. In the past, photocoagulation of the leaking capillaries has been suggested.[24] This technique has not been proved effective, however, and is probably contraindicated.[71] Treatment of peripheral lesions with photocoagulation has been reported to increase the visual status of eyes with epiretinal macular membranes in rare cases.[31]

In 1978, Machemer[72] first reported on the surgical management of advanced cases of epiretinal macular membranes using the technique of pars plana vitrectomy. Subsequent authors reported on larger series and attempted to identify preoperative factors that appeared to influence the postoperative visual prognosis.[30, 33, 34, 56, 57, 73–93] Modern vitreous surgeons use conventional pars plana vitreous surgical techniques with either a three-port system or a two-port system utilizing a fiberoptic light pipe fitted with an infusion sleeve. We prefer a two-port system utilizing an irrigating light pipe, which may reduce complications by eliminating the need for an infusion port.

The technique of pars plana vitrectomy is now used extensively to remove epiretinal macular membranes. Although technique and instrumentation have improved over the years, almost eliminating complications such as iatrogenic retinal tears and detachments, the problems of membrane recurrence[94] and accelerated nuclear sclerosis remain unsolved. Also, although improvement in acuity is achieved in most cases, it may be less than expected, and it is rare to completely eliminate metamorphopsia. This appears to be especially true in eyes with relatively good preoperative vision;[89, 95] therefore, when vision is better than 20/70, surgery should be approached with caution.

A contact lens placed over the cornea and sutured in place has proved very useful in the surgical management of epiretinal macular membranes. It provides excellent, motionless visualization of the posterior pole, and the lack of manipulation of the lens by the assistant during the procedure reduces the incidence of epithelial edema, which may necessitate denuding of the surface epithelium.

The surgical technique for removing epiretinal macular membranes includes first performing a limited posterior core vitrectomy (Fig. 74–6). There is no need to remove the anterior vitreous, which may cause inadvertent lens damage in phakic patients and may increase the incidence of peripheral retinal tears or detachments, or both, in aphakic or pseudophakic patients.

Following the core vitrectomy, a 23-gauge 1.5-in needle is prepared by bending the tip toward its lumen approximately 80 degrees. The needle is then attached to a tuberculin syringe that is partially filled with a balanced salt solution. The salt solution is used to fill the hub and shaft of the needle to avoid the introduction of air bubbles into the vitreous, which could interfere with visualization. If there is an obvious edge to the membrane, the tip of the bent needle can slide under it and the membrane can be removed (Fig. 74–7). This should be accomplished with tangential rather than anteroposterior force. As the membrane is lifted off the surface of the neurosensory retina, great care must be used to avoid creating retinal tears. This is especially true when peeling the membrane off the fovea. When the membrane has been lifted off the posterior pole, it can be removed from the eye using vitreous forceps or a vitrector.

In eyes in which there is no obvious edge to the epiretinal membrane, one may use the oblique illumination of the light pipe to cast a "shadow" of the retinal

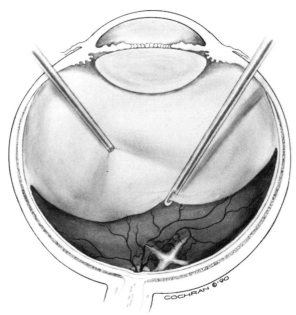

Figure 74–6. A limited-core vitrectomy removing the posterior one third to one half of vitreous gel.

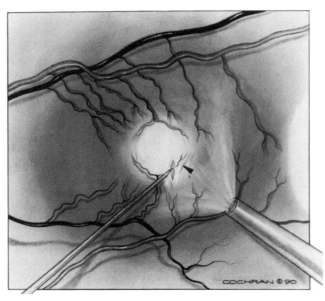

Figure 74–8. Opening created in epiretinal membrane with tip of bent 23-gauge needle. Dissection performed over small retinal vessel to guard against creating retinal hole. *Arrowhead* shows area of maximal vascular shadowing that identifies area of greatest elevation of the neurosensory retina from the retinal pigment epithelium.

vessels on the retinal pigment epithelium. This will readily enable one to identify the area of maximal elevation of the neurosensory retina. The bent needle is then used over a small retinal vessel in that area to open a small hole in the membrane. It can then be removed as previously described (Fig. 74–8).

When removing thick, opaque membranes, especially in cases secondary to previous retinal detachment surgery, one may encounter a fibrous "plug" in the epicenter. A vitreous pick with a moderately blunt tip or a blunt-tipped right-angle spatula may be useful in these cases.[96]

Dissection should always be carried out with the tip of the needle facing the light source to avoid working

in a shadow (Fig. 74–9). After initial removal of the membrane, an attempt should be made to determine whether or not a multilayered membrane is present. If so, the layers must be sequentially peeled, or the expected visual and anatomic results will be compromised. Incomplete removal of a multilayered membrane can sometimes be confused with a recurrence. Following complete removal of the membrane, the peripheral retina is inspected for tears and detachments, which, if present, can be subsequently repaired.

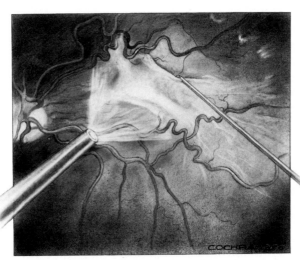

Figure 74–7. In cases with an obvious edge, the tip of the bent needle engages the membrane and gently peels it from the retinal surface.

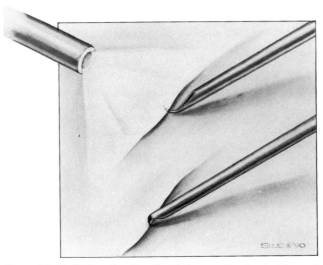

Figure 74–9. By keeping the tip of the needle directed toward the source of endoillumination, one avoids working in shadow and improves visualization during dissection of epiretinal membrane.

RESULTS

Following surgical removal of epiretinal macular membranes, there is a tendency toward normalization of the appearance of the retina in most cases, although there is almost never a complete resolution of the vascular tortuosity and retinal striae. Similarly, vision is improved in most eyes, but a return to normal acuity is rare even in eyes without a previous underlying pathologic condition. In our experience of treating 328 eyes, there was an overall improvement in visual acuity of at least two lines in 74 percent of cases, with 24 percent being unchanged and 2 percent becoming worse. Better visual results were generally found in the 184 idiopathic cases.[30] This was expected because of the lack of a preexisting macular pathologic condition from a previous retinal detachment, retinal vascular disease, and so on. Other series, however, report greater improvement in nonidiopathic cases than in idiopathic cases.[95]

Numerous authors have attempted to define prognostic indicators of postoperative vision in vitrectomy for treatment of epiretinal membranes of the macula. Indicators that have been mentioned include (1) the preoperative visual acuity, (2) the duration of diminished acuity prior to surgery, (3) the presence of preoperative cystoid macular edema, (4) the age of the patient, (5) the thickness of the epiretinal membrane, (6) idiopathic versus nonidiopathic epiretinal membranes, and (7) the presence of retinal pigment epithelial window defects on fluorescein angiography. Trese and coworkers reported that transparent membranes had a better visual prognosis than opaque ones.[93] They also felt that the presence of cystoid macular edema was a poor prognostic sign. Rice and associates, however, found that eyes with thin, transparent membranes had a poorer prognosis than eyes with thicker membranes.[95] McDonald and colleagues found no association between the transparency of the membrane and the final postoperative vision.[82] Ferencz and coworkers, in a study of 167 cases of idiopathic epiretinal membranes, found no association between the transparency of the membrane and the final visual outcome. Likewise, they found no association between the presence or lack of cystoid macular edema or a retinal pigment epithelial defect and the final visual outcome. Only preoperative vision had a predictive value with regard to the ultimate visual prognosis.[75] Other studies have also suggested that the presence of cystoid macular edema is a poor prognostic sign.[34, 57, 82, 85, 93, 95, 97] However, larger series have shown no relationship between the presence of preoperative cystoid macular edema and the ultimate visual prognosis.[30, 75, 80, 89]

COMPLICATIONS

The most frequently occurring intraoperative complications with pars plana vitrectomy for epiretinal membrane surgery include vitreous hemorrhage and peripheral and posterior iatrogenic retinal breaks. The vitreous hemorrhage is generally small and is easily removed with the vitrectomy instrument. Posterior breaks are rare and occur in less than 1 percent of cases in most series.[30, 34, 74, 78, 86] In some series, however, the occurrence of posterior breaks has been as high as 9 percent.[90] The retinal tears are treated with transscleral cryosurgery or photocoagulation.

Postoperative complications can include the development of accelerated nuclear sclerosis, retinal tears or detachment, rubeosis iridis, and endophthalmitis. Retinal detachments can generally be repaired without further loss of vision. Rubeosis and endophthalmitis have occurred in less than 0.5 percent of cases.[30, 57] The most troublesome postoperative complication has been the development of accelerated nuclear sclerosis, which has ranged from 12 to more than 60 percent.[30, 57, 82, 85, 89, 90] The reasons for this are unclear, but possible factors are the influence of the operating microscope light, the chemical composition of infusion fluid, infusion via an anterior infusion port, or change in intraocular temperature, or a combination of these factors.[30, 98]

The membrane recurs in less than 5 percent of idiopathic cases. In eyes with membranes from known causes, recurrence is much higher and can approach 100 percent in eyes of young patients in whom epimacular membranes develop following trauma or inflammatory disease.[30, 94]

SUMMARY

Epiretinal membranes are relatively common. They occur in 2 to 6 percent of patients. The incidence of idiopathic membranes increases with age and may approach 20 percent by age 70 yr.

Many cell types have been implicated in the origin of epiretinal macular membranes. Retinal pigment epithelial cells and retinal glial cells are most likely the major participants in the pathogenesis of epiretinal membranes. The epidemiology of the membranes includes proliferative diseases, trauma, inflammation, retinal surgery, and idiopathic causes. The clinical appearance is variable and depends on cell type, membrane thickness, presence of vessels, and cause. In most cases, the condition is relatively stable or slowly progressive with only 5 percent of eyes progressing to a visual acuity of 20/200 or worse. Membranes involving the macular or perimacular regions can cause a reduction in vision, metamorphopsia, micropsia, or occasionally, monocular diplopia. The contractile forces of the membranes appear to be more closely related to their cellular constituents than to the extracellular collagen matrix. The contraction of epiretinal membranes may be implicated in the development of macular cysts or holes, or both. Occasionally, the membrane may spontaneously separate with relief of symptoms.

Bimanual pars plana vitrectomy surgery can successfully remove epiretinal macular membranes in virtually all advanced cases. Following surgical removal, vision improves in approximately 75 percent of cases. However, a return to normal vision is unlikely. Postoperatively, retinal complications such as tears and detachment are rare in idiopathic cases but are somewhat more common in cases associated with other causes. The most frequent postoperative complication is the development of accelerated nuclear sclerosis in 12 to 68 percent of cases. The reasons for this have yet to be defined. Epiretinal membranes recur in about 5 percent of cases.

REFERENCES

1. Iwanoff A: Beiträge zur normalen und pathologischen Anatomie des Auges. Graefes Arch Clin Exp Ophthalmol 11:135–170, 1865.
2. Roth AM, Foos RY: Surface wrinkling retinopathy in eyes enucleated at autopsy, Trans Am Acad Ophthalmol Otolaryngol 75:1047–1059, 1971.
3. Clarkson JG, Green WR, Massof D: A histopathologic review of 168 cases of preretinal membrane. Am J Ophthalmol 84:1–17, 1977.
4. Pearlstone AD: The incidence of idiopathic preretinal macular gliosis. Ann Ophthalmol 17:378–380, 1985.
5. Scudder MJ, Eifrig DE: Spontaneous surface wrinkling retinopathy. Ann Ophthalmol 7:333–336, 339–341, 1975.
6. Sidd RJ, Fine SL, Owens SL, and Patz A: Idiopathic preretinal gliosis. Am J Ophthalmol 94:44–48, 1982.
7. Spitznas M, Leuenbeer R: Die primare epiretinale gliose. Klin Monatsbl Augenheilkd 171:410–420, 1977.
8. François J, Verbraeken H: Relationship between the drainage of the subretinal fluid in retinal detachment surgery and the appearance of macular pucker. Ophthalmologica 179:111–114, 1979.
9. Tanenbaum HL, Schepens CL, Elzeneiny I, Freeman HM: Macular pucker following retinal detachment surgery. Arch Ophthalmol 83:286–293, 1970.
10. Tanenbaum HL, Schepens CL, Elzeneiny I, Freeman HM: Macular pucker following retinal surgery: A biomicroscopic study. Can J Ophthalmol 4:20–23, 1969.
11. Jaffe NS: Macular retinopathy after separation of vitreoretinal adherence. Arch Ophthalmol 78:585–591, 1967.
12. Maumenee AE: Further advances in the study of the macula. Arch Ophthalmol 68:151–165, 1967.
13. Wise GN: Preretinal macular fibrosis (an analysis of 90 cases). Trans Ophthalmol Soc UK 92:131–140, 1972.
14. Mills PV: Preretinal macular fibrosis. Trans Ophthalmol Soc UK 99:50–53, 1979.
15. Kleinert H: Primäre Netzhaufältelung im Maculabereich. Graefes Arch Clin Exp Ophthalmol 155:350–358, 1954.
16. Von Gloor B, Werner H: Postkoagulative und spontan aufretende internoretinale Fibroplasie mit Maculadegeneration. Klin Monatsbl Augenheilkd 151:822–845, 1967.
17. Noble KG, Carr RE: Idiopathic preretinal gliosis. Ophthalmology 89:521–523, 1982.
18. Yagoda AD, Walsh JB, Henkind P: Idiopathic Preretinal Macular Gliosis. Boston, Little, Brown, 1981.
19. Wise GN: Macular changes after venous obstruction. Arch Ophthalmol 58:544–557, 1957.
20. Hagler WS, Aturaliya U: Macular puckers after retinal detachment surgery, Br J Ophthalmol 55:451–457, 1971.
21. Lobes LA Jr, Burton TC: The incidence of macular pucker after retinal detachment surgery. Am J Ophthalmol 85:72–77, 1978.
22. Wise GN: Congenital preretinal macular fibrosis. Am J Ophthalmol 79:363–365, 1975.
23. Vinores SA, Campochiaro PA, Conway BP: Ultrastructural and electron-immunocytochemical characterization of cells in epiretinal membranes. Invest Ophthal Vis Sci 31:14–28, 1990.
24. Wise GN: Clinical features of idiopathic preretinal macular fibrosis. Am J Ophthalmol 79:349–357, 1975.
25. Wiznia RA: Natural history of idiopathic preretinal macular fibrosis. Ann Ophthalmol 14:876–878, 1982.
26. Allen AW Jr, Gass JDM: Contraction of a perifoveal epiretinal membrane simulating a macular hole. Am J Ophthalmol 82:684–691, 1976.
27. Barr CC, Michels RG: Idiopathic nonvascularized epiretinal membranes in young patients: Report of six cases. Ann Ophthalmol 14:335–341, 1982.
28. Messner KH: Spontaneous separation of preretinal macular fibrosis. Am J Ophthalmol 83:9–11, 1977.
29. Sumers KD, Jampol LM, Goldberg MF, Huamonte FU: Spontaneous separation of epiretinal membranes. Arch Ophthalmol 98:318–320, 1980.
30. Margherio RR, Cox MS Jr, Trese MT, et al: Removal of epimacular membranes. Ophthalmology 92:1075–1083, 1985.
31. Dellaporta A: Macular pucker and peripheral retinal lesions. Trans Am Ophthalmol Soc 71:329–340, 1973.
32. Laqua H: Pigmented macular pucker. Am J Ophthalmol 86:56–58, 1978.
33. Robertson DM, Buettner H: Pigmented preretinal membranes. Am J Ophthalmol 83:824–829, 1977.
34. deBustros S, Thompson JT, Michels RG, et al: Vitrectomy for idiopathic epiretinal membranes causing macular pucker. Br J Ophthalmol 72:692–695, 1988.
35. Foos RY: Surface wrinkling retinopathy. In Freeman HM, Hirose T, Schepens CL (eds): Vitreous Surgery and Advances in Fundus Diagnosis and Treatment. New York, Appleton-Century-Crofts, 1977, pp 23–38.
36. Hirokawa H, Jalkh AE, Takahashi M, et al: Role of the vitreous in idiopathic preretinal macular fibrosis. Am J Ophthalmol 101:166–169, 1986.
37. Wise GN: Relationship of idiopathic preretinal macular fibrosis to posterior vitreous detachment. Am J Ophthalmol 79:358–362, 1975.
38. Margherio RR, Trese MT, Margherio A, Cartright K: Surgical management of vitreomacular traction syndromes. Ophthalmology 96:1437–1444, 1989.
39. Trese MT, Margherio RR, Hartzer M, et al: Macular cysts associated with subtle epimacular membranes. Vitreoretinal Surg Technol 2:2–3, 1990.
40. Kishi S, Shimizu K: Posterior precortical vitreous pocket. Arch Ophthalmol 108:979–982, 1990.
41. Gass JDM: Stereoscopic Atlas of Macular Diseases. St Louis, CV Mosby, 1987, pp 694–712.
42. Gass JDM: Idiopathic senile macular hole. Its early stages and pathogenesis. Arch Ophthalmol 106:629–639, 1988.
43. Johnson RN, Gass JDM: Idiopathic macular holes. Observations, stages of formation and implications for surgical intervention. Ophthalmology 95:917–924, 1988.
44. Manschot WA: Persistent hyperplastic primary vitreous; special reference to preretinal glial tissue as a pathological characteristic and to the development of the primary vitreous. Arch Ophthalmol 59:188, 1958.
45. Wolter JR: Glia of human retina. Am J Ophthalmol 48:370, 1959.
46. Smith TR: Pathologic findings after retina surgery. In Schepens CL (ed): Importance of the Vitreous Body in Retina Surgery with Special Emphasis on Reoperations. St Louis, CV Mosby, 1960, pp 61–75.
47. Kurz GH, Zimmerman LE: Vagaries of the retinal pigment epithelium. Int Ophthalmol Clin 2:441, 1962.
48. Ashton N: Oxygen and the growth and development of retinal vessels; in vivo and in vitro studies. The XX Francis I Proctor Lecture. Am J Ophthalmol 62:412, 1966.
49. Von Gloor BP: Mitotic activity in the cortical vitreous cells (hyalocytes) after photocoagulation. Invest Ophthalmol 8:633, 1969.
50. Constable IJ: Pathology of vitreous membranes and the effect of haemorrhage and new vessels on the vitreous. Trans Ophthalmol Soc UK 95:382–386, 1975.
51. Green WR, Kenyon KR, Michels RG, et al: Ultrastructure of epiretinal membranes causing macular pucker after retinal reattachment surgery. Trans Ophthalmol Soc UK 99:63–77, 1979.
52. Kampik A, Green WR, Michels RG, Nase PK: Ultrastructural features of progressive idiopathic epiretinal membrane removed by vitreous surgery. Am J Ophthalmol 90:797–809, 1980.
53. Kampik A, Kenyon KR, Michels RG, et al: Epiretinal and vitreous membranes: Comparative study of 56 cases. Arch Ophthalmol 99:1445–1454, 1981.
54. Kenyon KR, Michels RG: Ultrastructure of epiretinal membrane removed by pars plana vitreoretinal surgery. Am J Ophthalmol 83:815–823, 1977.
55. Letson AD, Davidorf FH, McDonald C: Scanning electron microscopy of an epiretinal membrane. Ophthalmic Forum 1:44–47, 1983.
56. McDonald HR, Abrams GW, Burke JM, Neuwirth J: Clinicopathologic results of vitreous surgery for epiretinal membranes in

patients with combined retinal and retinal pigment epithelial hamartomas. Am J Ophthalmol 100:806–813, 1985.

57. Michels RG: A clinical and histopathologic study of epiretinal membranes affecting the macula and removed by vitreous surgery. Trans Am Ophthalmol Soc 80:580–656, 1982.

58. Rentsch FJ: The ultrastructure of preretinal macular fibrosis. Graefes Arch Clin Exp Ophthalmol 203:321–337, 1977.

59. Smiddy WE, Maguire AM, Green R, et al: Idiopathic epiretinal membranes. Ophthalmology 96:811–821, 1989.

60. Trese MT, Chandler DB, and Machemer R: Macular pucker. II. Ultrastructure. Graefes Arch Clin Exp Ophthalmol 221:16–26, 1983.

61. Van Horn DL, Aaberg TM, Machemer R, Fenzl R: Glial cell proliferation in human retinal detachment with massive periretinal proliferation. Am J Ophthalmol 84:383–393, 1977.

62. Foos RY: Vitreoretinal juncture—Simple epiretinal membranes. Graefes Arch Clin Exp Ophthalmol 189:231–250, 1974.

63. Bellhorn MB, Friedman AH, Wise GN, Henkind P: Ultrastructure and clinicopathologic correlation of idiopathic preretinal macular fibrosis. Am J Ophthalmol 79:366–373, 1975.

64. Campochiaro PA, Kaden IH, Vidaurri-Leal J, Glaser BM: Cryotherapy enhances intravitreal dispersion of viable retinal pigment epithelial cells. Arch Ophthalmol 103:434–436, 1985.

65. Machemer R, Laqua H: Pigment epithelium proliferation in retinal detachment (massive periretinal proliferation). Am J Ophthalmol 80:1–23, 1975.

66. Machemer R, van Horn D, Aaberg TM: Pigment epithelial proliferation in human retinal detachment with massive periretinal proliferation. Am J Ophthalmol 85:181–191, 1978.

67. Newsome DA, Rodrigues MM, Machemer R: Human massive periretinal proliferation. In vitro characteristics of cellular components. Arch Ophthalmol 99:873–880, 1981.

68. Wallow IHL, Miller SA: Preretinal membrane by retinal pigment epithelium. Arch Ophthalmol 96:1643–1646, 1978.

69. Stern WH, Fisher SK, Anderson DH, et al: Epiretinal membrane formation after vitrectomy, Am J Ophthalmol 93:757–772, 1982.

70. Daicker B, Guggenheim R: Rasterelektronenmikroskopische untersuchungen an fibrösen und fibro-gliösen epiretinalen fibroplasien. Graefes Arch Clin Exp Ophthal 207:229–242, 1978.

71. Gass JDM: Stereoscopic Atlas of Macular Diseases: Diagnosis and Treatment. St Louis, CV Mosby, 1977, pp 344–366.

72. Machemer R: Die chirurgische entfernung von epiretina en makulamembranen (macular puckers). Klin Monatsbl Augenheilkd 173:36–42, 1978.

73. Cairns JD: Surgical treatment of epiretinal macular membranes. Aust J Ophthalmol 10:129–134, 1982.

74. deBustros S, Rice TA, Michels RG, et al: Vitrectomy for macular pucker after treatment of retinal tears or retinal detachment. Arch Ophthalmol 106:758–760, 1988.

75. Ferencz JR, Nussbaum JJ, Richards SC, et al: Predictive variables in vitrectomy for idiopathic epimacular membranes. Submitted for publication.

76. Fisher YL, Shafer DM, Yannuzzi LA: Microsurgical management of macular epiretinal membranes (macular pucker). Dev Ophthalmol 5:122–130, 1981.

77. Haut J, Larricart P, Sfeir T, van Effenterre G: Treatment of epiretinal membranes: Report of 40 operated cases. Ophthalmologica 183:190–196, 1981.

78. Mandelcorn MS, Liao R: Preretinal membranectomy in idiopathic preretinal macular fibrosis. Can J Ophthalmol 18:321–324, 1983.

79. Margherio AR, Nachazel DP, Murphy PL, et al: The surgical management of epiretinal membranes. [Scientific exhibit] American Academy of Ophthalmology Annual Meeting, 1981. Ophthalmology 88(Suppl):82, 1981.

80. Margherio RR: Discussion. Ophthalmology 91:1387–1388, 1984.

81. McDonald HR, Aaberg TM: Idiopathic epiretinal membranes. Semin Ophthalmol 1:189–195, 1986.

82. McDonald HR, Verre WP, Aaberg TM: Surgical management of idiopathic epiretinal membranes. Ophthalmology 93:978–983, 1986.

83. Michels RG: Surgical management of epiretinal membranes. Trans Ophthalmol Soc UK 99:54–62, 1979.

84. Michels RG: Surgery of epiretinal membranes. Dev Ophthalmol 2:175–184, 1981.

85. Michels RG: Vitreous surgery for macular pucker. Am J Ophthalmol 92:628–639, 1981.

86. Michels RG: Vitrectomy for macular pucker. Ophthalmology 91:1384–1388, 1984.

87. Michels RG, Gilbert HD: Surgical management of macular pucker after retinal reattachment surgery. Am J Ophthalmol 88:925–929, 1979.

88. Nolthenius PAT, Deutman AF: Surgical removal of epiretinal membranes. Int Ophthalmol 3:155–159, 1981.

89. Pessin SR, Olk RJ, Grand MG, et al: Vitrectomy for premacular fibroplasia: Prognostic factors, long-term follow-up and time course of visual improvement. Ophthalmology 98:1109–1114, 1991.

90. Poliner LS, Olk RJ, Grand MG, et al: The surgical management of premacular fibroplasia. Arch Ophthalmol 106:761–764, 1988.

91. Shea M: The surgical management of macular pucker. Can J Ophthalmol 14:110–113, 1979.

92. Shea RJ: The surgical management of macular pucker in rhegmatogenous retinal detachment. Ophthalmology 87:70–74, 1980.

93. Trese MT, Chandler DB, Machemer R: Macular pucker. I. Prognostic criteria. Graefes Arch Clin Exp Ophthalmol 221:16–26, 1983.

94. Wilkinson CP: Recurrent macular pucker. Am J Ophthalmol 88:1029–1031, 1979.

95. Rice TA, deBustros S, Michels RG, et al: Prognostic factors in vitrectomy for epiretinal membranes of the macula. Ophthalmology 93:602–610, 1986.

96. Michels RG, Rice TA, Ober RR: Vitreoretinal dissection instruments. Am J Ophthalmol 87:836–837, 1979.

97. Charles S: Epimacular proliferation. In Schachet WS (ed): Vitreous Microsurgery. Baltimore, Williams & Wilkins, 1981, pp 131–133.

98. deBustros S, Thompson JT, Michels RG, et al: Nuclear sclerosis after vitrectomy for idiopathic epiretinal membranes. Am J Ophthalmol 105:160–164, 1988.

Chapter 75

■

Acute Macular Neuroretinopathy

LUCY H. Y. YOUNG and DONALD J. D'AMICO

Acute macular neuroretinopathy was first described in 1975 by Bos and Deutman.[1] In their six patients, this entity was characterized by a sudden onset of paracentral scotomas and the presence of cloverleaf, wedge-shaped, darkish red lesions centered around the fovea. Only a small number of cases have been added subsequently.

Characteristically, visual acuity remains normal or is slightly reduced.[1-15] The chief complaint is usually related to the sudden appearance of paracentral scotomas. This rare macular disease can occur unilaterally or bilaterally, and the majority of patients are young adults, mostly women. Many of these patients are taking birth control pills.[1, 3–5, 11–15] The visual disturbance is often preceded by a bout of a flulike syndrome, such as influenza, pharyngitis, or enteritis.[1, 4, 5, 9, 11, 12, 14] The clinical features of the 28 patients reported to date are summarized in Table 75–1.

When patients are tested with the Amsler grid, they can usually outline parafoveal negative scotomas, frequently in the shape of teardrops, corresponding exactly with the fundus lesions (Fig. 75–1).[9, 11–13] In patients whose fundus lesions are less prominent, examination with red-free light may be useful in highlighting the lesions. As mentioned by Guzak and colleagues,[4] this enhancement is probably related to the color of the lesion rather than to the surface changes in the retina. Although Bos and Deutman[1] suggested that the fundus lesions seen in their six patients were located in the superficial retina, subsequent reports relying on biomicroscopic examination, stereophotographs, fluorescein angiography, and electrodiagnostic testing indicate that the acute macular neuroretinopathy lesions are located in the outer retinal layers.[9, 11, 13] In addition to the deep, reddish brown lesions, a few small, superficial retinal hemorrhages may be present in the macula.[2, 9] The retinal vasculature, nerve fiber layer, retinal pigment epithelium, and optic disc are normal, and there are no vitreous cells.

Fluorescein angiography studies are essentially normal. Questionably dilated perimacular capillaries with-

Table 75–1. CLINICAL FEATURES OF ACUTE MACULAR NEURORETINOPATHY: SUMMARY OF 28 CASES

Mean age	28
Number of females	25 (89%)
History of a flulike syndrome	19 (68%)
Bilateral involvement	19 (68%)
Number of patients on contraceptives or other estrogen preparations	18 (64%)

out leakage and subtle hypofluorescence corresponding to the fundus lesions have been reported.[1, 2, 9]

Electrical testing such as electroretinogram and electrooculogram studies of patients afflicted with acute macular neuroretinopathy are normal.[1, 7, 9, 12] This is not unexpected because both tests measure mass physiologic responses and are not sensitive to pathologic processes confined to the macula alone. To address this issue, Sieving and associates[13] recorded the early retinal potential responses from the posterior fundi in one patient with unilateral acute macular neuroretinopathy. The early retinal potential is generated in the photoreceptor outer segments, and by restricting the recording to the posterior fundus, the investigators made the recording more sensitive to localized lesions in the macula. They found a reduced amplitude in the affected eye when compared with the normal fellow eye. This recording was done 13 mo following the initial onset of visual disturbances. A follow-up early retinal potential measurement 7 mo later, or 20 mo after the onset of symptoms, showed similar amplitude reduction. Their find-

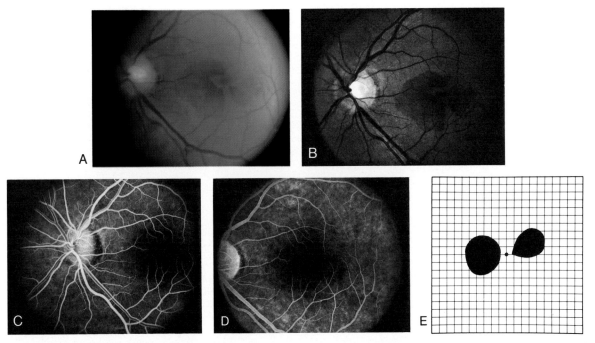

Figure 75–1. This 42-year-old woman presented with a 3-wk history of a flulike syndrome before the onset of paracentral scotomas in the left eye. Her past medical history was significant for she had undergone hysterectomy and oophorectomy 2 yr previously and had since been using estradiol transdermal (Estroderm) patch. Her visual acuity was 20/20 in the left eye. Note the darkish red lesions centered around the fovea (A). These lesions are better appreciated with red-free light (B). Angiography results were normal (C and D). Amsler grid testing showed two paracentral scotomas (E). (A–E, Courtesy of Jack F. Bowers, M.D.)

ings would suggest that the abnormality is located in the outer segments, but to date only one patient has been analyzed with this test.

Although acute macular neuroretinopathy is associated with minimal, if any, decline in visual acuity, patients with this disorder rarely report improvement of symptoms. The paracentral scotomas may become less dense but usually persist despite resolution of the fundus lesions. Most of the follow-up examinations reported to date range from months to a few years only.[1, 2, 4–6, 9, 11–15] However, one patient[5] with bilateral involvement was followed for up to 9 yr. This patient had resolution of paracentral scotomas in the right eye but persistence of a large scotoma in the left eye 2 yr later. During the following 7 yr, the large paracentral scotoma remained but slowly became smaller.

Both the histopathologic features and the pathogenesis of these rare macular lesions are unknown. Although a large number of patients reported had experienced a flulike syndrome prior to the onset of their visual symptoms, a relationship to viral infection has not yet been established. It has also been suggested that there is an association with oral contraceptives because the condition affects predominantly healthy young women, many of whom are taking this medication. However, since the majority of women with this condition are of child-bearing age, it is highly likely that the use of birth control pills is only coincidental; in addition, cases have been reported without birth control pill use. Furthermore, acute macular neuroretinopathy has been reported in three male patients, although it is interesting to note that one of them was being treated with fosfestrol (an estrogen preparation), for a prostatic carcinoma at the time of the onset of visual symptoms.[6]

O'Brien and coworkers[8] reported three patients in whom acute macular neuroretinopathy developed following acute hypertension caused by intravenous sympathomimetics. Guzak and associates[4] reported two cases, and both of their patients experienced macular neuroretinopathy following intravenous injections of epinephrine for adverse reactions to contrast agents. However, blood pressure readings were not reported in these two cases. The temporal relationship between the development of acute macular neuroretinopathy and the acute elevation of blood pressure in the three patients described by O'Brien and coworkers suggests an association with either the hypertensive episodes or the sympathomimetics themselves. However, this would not explain the cause of the other 23 cases reported to date.

Gass and Hamed[3] have reported acute macular neuroretinopathy and multiple evanescent white dot syndrome occurring in the same patients. They compared the clinical features of acute macular neuroretinopathy and multiple evanescent white dot syndrome and suggested that these two rare syndromes may be related pathogenetically and etiologically.

The milder forms of acute macular neuroretinopathy, i.e., when the characteristic macular lesions are not prominent, may be mistaken for acute retinal pigment epitheliitis because both entities cause loss of central vision in young adults. A list of the differential diagnos-

tic features of these two entities is shown in Table 75–2. The peculiar macular lesions may also be mistaken for subretinal hemorrhage; this is probably what happened in the case reported by Weinberg and Nerney.[15] No recurrence of this entity has been reported.

Table 75–2. DIFFERENTIAL DIAGNOSTIC FEATURES OF PIGMENT EPITHELIITIS AND ACUTE MACULAR NEURORETINOPATHY

Feature	Pigment Epitheliitis[16–18]	Acute Macular Neuroretinopathy
Ophthalmoscopy	Clusters of round, dark lesions surrounded by hypopigmented halos	Red-brown wedges
Lesion distribution	Macular	Macular
Location	Retinal pigment epithelium	Sensory retina
Laterality	Usually unilateral	Either
Associated vitritis	None	None
Diminished visual acuity	Moderate	Mild
Sex predilection	None	Female
Age of onset	Young adults	Young adults
Associated systemic infection	None	Often preceded by a flulike syndrome
Visual recovery	Complete in 7–10 wk	Minimal
Etiology	Unknown	Unknown
Fluorescein angiography	Normal or halos of hyperfluorescence	Normal

REFERENCES

1. Bos PJM, Deutman AF: Acute macular neuroretinopathy. Am J Ophthalmol 80:573, 1975.
2. Gass JDM: Stereoscopic Atlas of Macular Diseases: Diagnosis and Treatment, 3rd ed. St Louis, CV Mosby, 1987, p 512.
3. Gass JDM, Hamed LM: Acute macular neuroretinopathy and multiple evanescent white dot syndrome occurring in the same patients. Arch Ophthalmol 107:189, 1989.
4. Guzak SV, Kalina RE, Chenoweth RE: Acute macular neuroretinopathy following adverse reaction to intravenous contrast media. Retina 3:312, 1983.
5. Miller MH, Spalton DJ, Fitzke FW, Bird AC: Acute macular neuroretinopathy. Ophthalmology 96:265, 1989.
6. Nagasawa N, Hommura S: A case of acute macular neuroretinopathy—An optical consideration on the peculiar features of fundus oculi. Acta Soc Ophthalmol Jpn 86:2044, 1982.
7. Neetens A, Burvenich H: Presumed inflammatory maculopathies. Trans Ophthalmol Soc UK 98:160, 1978.
8. O'Brien DM, Farmer SG, Kalina RE, Leon JA: Acute macular neuroretinopathy following intravenous sympathomimetics. Retina 9:281, 1989.
9. Priluck JA, Buettner H, Robertson DM: Acute macular neuroretinopathy. Am J Ophthalmol 86:775, 1978.
10. Putteman A, Toussaint D, Deutman AF: Neuroretinopathie maculaire aigue. Bull Soc Belge Ophtalmol 199–200:35, 1982.
11. Rait JL, O'Day J: Acute macular neuroretinopathy. Aust NZ J Ophthalmol 15:337, 1987.
12. Rush JA: Acute macular neuroretinopathy. Am J Ophthalmol 83:490, 1977.

13. Sieving PA, Fishman GA, Salzano T, Rabb MF: Acute macular neuroretinopathy: Early receptor potential change suggests photoreceptor pathology. Br J Ophthalmol 68:229, 1984.
14. van Herck M, Leys A, Missotten L: Acute macular neuroretinopathy. Bull Soc Belge Ophtalmol 210:119, 1984.
15. Weinberg RJ, Nerney JJ: Bilateral submacular hemorrhages associated with an influenza syndrome. Ann Ophthalmol 15:710, 1983.
16. Deutman AF: Acute retinal pigment epitheliitis. Am J Ophthalmol 78:571, 1974.
17. Eifrig DE, Knobloch WH, Moran JA: Retinal pigment epitheliitis. Ann Ophthalmol 9:639, 1977.
18. Friedman MW: Bilateral recurrent acute retinal pigment epitheliitis. Am J Ophthalmol 79:567, 1975.
19. Krill AE, Deutman AF: Acute retinal pigment epitheliitis. Am J Ophthalmol 74:193, 1972.

Chapter 76

■

Toxoplasmosis

RICHARD R. TAMESIS and C. STEPHEN FOSTER

Toxoplasmosis is one of the leading causes of infectious necrotizing retinitis.[1] It is produced by the coccidian parasite *Toxoplasma gondii,* and the cat is the definitive host. Humans and other animals act as intermediate hosts. Congenital toxoplasmosis, as well as toxoplasmosis in immunocompromised patients, is serious and potentially fatal.

T. gondii is ubiquitous in nature. The parasite has three forms: tachyzoite, bradyzoite, and sporozoite.[2] The tachyzoite is the infectious form of the parasite; it multiplies intracellularly and causes host cell death and the release of more tachyzoites. The host's immune response causes it to transform into the slowly dividing bradyzoite, which is the encysted, intracellular form of the parasite found in tissue cysts. These cysts may remain in any organ, such as the retina, for years without provoking an immune response in the host. When tissue cysts rupture, parasites are released into the surrounding tissues, resulting in a recurrence of clinical disease. The sporozoite or oocyst is produced only in the young cat. Millions of oocysts are released into the environment for 2 to 3 wk after primary infection until the cat becomes immune.[3] The oocysts undergo sporulation within a few days and may remain infectious for up to 2 yr.

Human infection may occur by either the congenital or the acquired route. The acquired disease occurs by the ingestion of either oocysts or tissue cysts in improperly cooked infected meat and is usually asymptomatic in immunocompetent persons. Infected livestock are a prominent source of infection for humans. Congenital infection occurs through transplacental transmission from a mother, infected just prior to or during pregnancy, to the developing fetus.[4] The severity of congenital infection is highest when acquired during the first trimester of pregnancy, although the frequency of transmission to the fetus is greatest during the third trimester, when contact of the maternal and the fetal circulations is more likely to occur. Once maternal immunity has developed, it is believed that all future fetuses are protected from the development of congenital toxoplasmosis.

CLINICAL FEATURES OF OCULAR TOXOPLASMOSIS

The majority of cases of ocular toxoplasmosis are congenital.[1] Cases of acquired ocular toxoplasmosis, however, have been reported, suggesting that this route may be more important than previously thought.[5–7] In one study of 300 cases of congenital toxoplasmosis in newborns, ocular lesions were present in 76 percent, neurologic involvement was present in 51 percent, intracranial calcifications were present in 32 percent, and microcephaly or hydrocephalus was present in 26 percent.[8] Among the clinical manifestations of congenital ocular toxoplasmosis reported in infants are microphthalmia, enophthalmos, ptosis, nystagmus, choroidal colobomas, and strabismus.[9]

Ocular toxoplasmosis frequently presents as a focal necrotizing retinitis, usually adjacent to a large, atrophic chorioretinal scar (Fig. 76–1), which is often located in the macula in congenital cases. The scar is typically yellow-white and unevenly pigmented. The areas of retinitis are the result of tissue cysts bursting and releasing bradyzoites that transform into tachyzoites, which, in turn, invade neighboring cells. These destructive lesions are usually larger than 1 disc diameter and are surrounded by retinal edema.[10] When the tachyzoites come under increasing attack by the immune response, they gradually transform back into bradyzoites. Inflammatory cells will be found in the vitreous overlying the active lesion (Fig. 76–2). Perivascular inflammatory exudates may be present around retinal vessels peripheral to an area of active inflammation. Patients will frequently complain of pain, blurred vision, floaters, and photophobia. More than a third of patients with active ocular toxoplasmosis will have macular involvement, resulting in severe visual loss.[11] Ocular toxoplasmosis may also present as gray-white punctate lesions in the outer retina and retinal pigment epithelium (Fig. 76–3).[11, 12] Occasionally, patients will present initially with severe unilateral papillitis and vitreal inflammation (Fig. 76–4).[13]

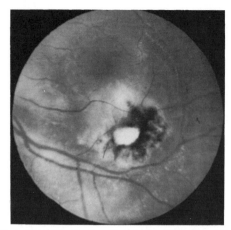

Figure 76–1. Atrophic chorioretinal scar with surrounding retinal pigment epithelial proliferation, a chorioretinal scar quite typical of *Toxoplasma* chorioretinitis. Note also, however, the fresh satellite lesion at the edge of the pigmented chorioretinal scar (at the 11 o'clock position) threatening the fovea.

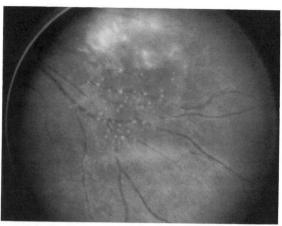

Figure 76–3. *Toxoplasma* retinitis without typical choroidal involvement. Note the multifocal nature of the lesions, with an area of active retinitis at the 11 o'clock position in the photograph. Note also the associated vasculitis.

COMPLICATIONS OF OCULAR TOXOPLASMOSIS

Secondary complications arising from ocular toxoplasmosis include choroidal neovascularization,[14, 15] chorioretinal vascular anastomoses,[16] branch artery occlusion,[17] secondary glaucoma, cystoid macular edema, cataracts, traction retinal detachment, and optic atrophy.[11] The most frequent complication seen is secondary glaucoma. There is a well-known association between Fuchs' heterochromic iridocyclitis and ocular toxoplasmosis, but the reasons for this remain unclear.[18]

HISTOPATHOLOGIC AND IMMUNOLOGIC FEATURES OF OCULAR TOXOPLASMOSIS

Histopathologically, there is necrosis of the involved retina with destruction of the retinal architecture and the underlying choroid.[10] Since the parasite has a propensity for neural tissue, tissue cysts and trophozoites

are usually found in the superficial layers of the retina within the area of necrosis (Figs. 76–5 and 76–6). The infiltrate consists predominantly of lymphocytes, macrophages, and epithelioid cells, with plasma cells in the periphery of the lesion.

Cell-mediated immunity is felt to be the major defense mechanism against *Toxoplasma* infection.[19] Several purified antigens from tachyzoites have been identified, including the major surface protein antigen p 30,[20] which can participate in antibody-dependent complement-mediated lysis of the tachyzoite.[20, 21] In patients with ocular toxoplasmosis, the cellular immune response appears to be directed predominantly against the cell surface protein p 22.[22] However, some evidence also indicates that part of the disease may be mediated by an autoimmune mechanism directed against certain retinal antigens.

The role of the humoral response to toxoplasmosis is unclear. Although an intact cellular component of the immune system is necessary for the resolution of active

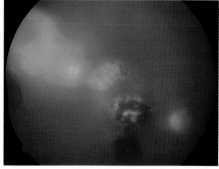

Figure 76–2. Multiple atrophic and hyperpigmented chorioretinal scars from previous toxoplasmosis. Note the fresh area of chorioretinitis with overlying vitreal inflammatory cells and vitreal "haze."

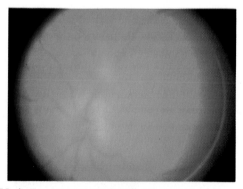

Figure 76–4. *Toxoplasma* papillitis with vitreal inflammatory cells anterior to the optic nerve, making visualization of the optic nerve slightly difficult. The enzyme-linked immunosorbent assay (ELISA) test for *Toxoplasma* antibodies gave the following results: the IgG titer was 1:496; the IgM titer at the time this photograph was taken was 1:64; 2 wk later the anti-*Toxoplasma* IgM antibody titer was 1:256.

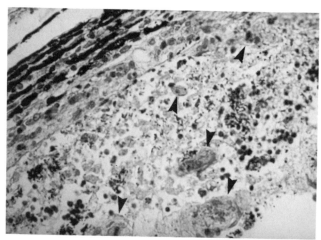

Figure 76–5. *Toxoplasma* feline retinochoroiditis. Histopathologic appearance of the retina and choroid. Note the *Toxoplasma gondii* cysts *(arrows)*.

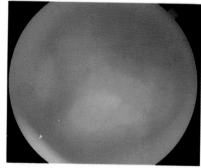

Figure 76–7. Diffuse retinitis with probable underlying choroiditis in an immunocompromised patient with toxoplasmosis. Note the overlying vitreal inflammatory cellular response with vitreal "haze."

disease, antibody may be important in establishing a state of immunity in the host.[23] Antibodies directed against a cytoplasmic protein designated F3G3[24] can protect passively immunized mice from a lethal challenge of *T. gondii*.[25]

OCULAR TOXOPLASMOSIS IN THE IMMUNOCOMPROMISED HOST

Although *T. gondii* is a common opportunistic pathogen with a penchant for attacking the central nervous system in immunocompromised patients, including those with AIDS,[26–31] ocular toxoplasmosis appears to be uncommon.[32] Ocular toxoplasmosis occurs in approximately 1 percent of patients with AIDS.[32, 33] Systemically, these patients are prone to the development of encephalitis, myocarditis, or pneumonitis.

AIDS-related *Toxoplasma* retinochoroiditis may have

several atypical clinical manifestations, including single or multifocal discrete lesions[33–35] or diffuse areas of retinal necrosis (Fig. 76–7).[36] Vascular sheathing may be present, and prominent inflammatory reactions in the vitreous and anterior chambers are common (Fig. 76–8).[37] Lesions may occur adjacent to retinal blood vessels and are rarely associated with preexisting retinochoroidal scars. These findings suggest that the ocular lesions in AIDS patients are the result of newly acquired disease or organisms that have disseminated to the eye from extraocular sites. There is no evidence to date that immunologic alterations initiate recurrent ocular toxoplasmosis. The retina can be infected by both *T. gondii* and cytomegalovirus in AIDS patients.[37] Anti-*Toxoplasma* IgG antibodies are present in these patients, although IgM antibodies against *Toxoplasma* are uncommon.

Infection usually produces a full-thickness retinal necrosis, but early lesions may be confined to either the inner or the outer layers. Large numbers of trophozoites and cysts with scanty inflammatory reaction are seen within the necrotic retina and optic nerve head.[33, 37] Although involvement of anterior segment structures

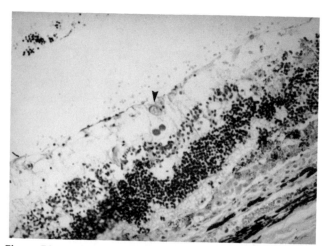

Figure 76–6. Same specimen as in Figure 76–5. Note the *Toxoplasma* cyst *(arrow)*.

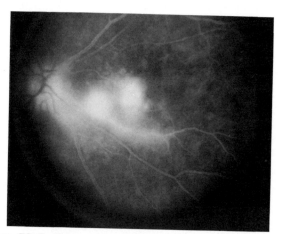

Figure 76–8. Fluorescein angiogram in a patient with active toxoplasmosis. Note not only the dye accumulation in the two foci representing the areas of active *Toxoplasma* chorioretinitis but also the papillitis with dye staining of the nerve head and the associated retinal vasculitis with late vascular staining.

and uveal tissue with *Toxoplasma* is rarely seen in otherwise healthy patients,[38] parasites may be present in these structures in patients with AIDS and ocular toxoplasmosis.[37]

DIAGNOSIS OF OCULAR TOXOPLASMOSIS

The definitive diagnosis of ocular toxoplasmosis requires the demonstration of the proliferative form of *T. gondii* in ocular tissues.[39] The presence of cysts in tissue samples only suggests but does not prove acute infection. *Toxoplasma* retinochoroiditis is, therefore, usually a presumptive diagnosis based on a compatible lesion in the fundus and positive serologic results for *Toxoplasma* antibodies. Additionally, other causes of focal exudative retinitis, including syphilis, tuberculosis, sarcoidosis, cytomegalovirus, and fungal infections, must be excluded.

Because of their ease of performance and their relatively high sensitivity and specificity, serologic methods are often preferred for the diagnosis of toxoplasmosis. Serologic diagnosis is complicated by the high prevalence of *T. gondii*–specific antibodies in the human population persisting for years and therefore frequently reflecting past infection. Classic serodiagnosis of acute infection requires the demonstration of a seroconversion, a significant antibody titer rise in paired sera taken 4 to 6 wk apart, or the presence of anti-*Toxoplasma* IgM antibody in a single serum sample. Because sera are often submitted late after infection, it is difficult to detect an antibody titer rise. Establishing the presence of *Toxoplasma* antibodies in a patient's serum is considered essential in the diagnosis of *Toxoplasma* retinochoroiditis. In this case, any titer of antibody is significant because no correlation exists between the level of *Toxoplasma* titers and activity of the ocular disease in recurrent ocular toxoplasmosis.[40]

The most widely used serologic methods for detecting anti-*Toxoplasma* antibodies are the Sabin-Feldman test, the complement fixation test, agglutination tests, the indirect immunofluorescence assay (IFA), and more recently, the enzyme-linked immunosorbent assay (ELISA). Although the Sabin-Feldman dye test represents the standard against which all other tests are measured, it is no longer performed routinely. This test is now rarely used because it requires the constant maintenance of virulent organisms in the laboratory with the associated risk to laboratory personnel.

The IFA test, which has largely replaced the Sabin-Feldman dye test, has become the most widely used test for the detection of anti-*Toxoplasma* IgG or IgM antibodies.[41] Although it is easy to perform, the interpretation of results can be misleading. False-negative IgM titers may occur because of competitive inhibition by anti-*Toxoplasma* IgG, which is present simultaneously.[42] False-positive IgM titers can occur because of the presence of rheumatoid factor.[43] Rheumatoid factor (which is an IgM anti-IgG) can bind to specific anti-*Toxoplasma* IgG. Finally, the presence of antinuclear antibodies may produce false-positive IgM and IgG titers.[44] This may

occur because *Toxoplasma* organisms contain antigens that are indistinguishable, by immunologic techniques, from those found in human leukocyte nuclei. Because IgM titers in ocular toxoplasmosis become significant only in cases of acquired retinochoroiditis,[45, 46] the specificity limitations of the IFA tests are restricted, for practical purposes, to false-positive IgG titers produced by the presence of antinuclear antibodies.

Commercially available IFA tests for *Toxoplasma* begin with a 1:16 serum dilution because specificity decreases when more concentrated dilutions are used. Since any titer of antibody is considered significant in establishing the diagnosis of *Toxoplasma* retinochoroiditis, it is logical to expect a significant percentage of false-negative titers using this serologic method. One report cited three documented cases of *Toxoplasma* retinochoroiditis with positive Sabin-Feldman dye titers and negative immunofluorescent titers (titer <1:16).[47]

The double-sandwich ELISA for anti-*Toxoplasma* antibodies eliminates IgM specificity problems associated with the IFA test.[48, 49] False-positive reactions resulting from rheumatoid factor and false-negative reactions because of competing IgG are avoided because only IgM of the test serum adheres to plates precoated with anti-IgM antiserum. The ELISA for *Toxoplasma* antibodies is believed to be as specific and sensitive as the Sabin-Feldman dye test.[40] Therefore, in cases in which ocular toxoplasmosis is strongly suspected despite negative immunofluorescent titers, a Sabin-Feldman titer or an ELISA titer, or both, should be obtained before excluding the diagnosis of toxoplasmosis.[47]

THERAPY FOR OCULAR TOXOPLASMOSIS

Since available agents against *T. gondii* are ineffective against the tissue cysts, the major aim of therapy is to stop the multiplication of tachyzoites during active retinochoroiditis. It is important for the clinician to realize this and to inform patients that drug therapy does not totally eradicate the parasite. *Toxoplasma* organisms lack the transmembrane transport systems for physiologic folates and thus synthesize this substance instead. Folic acid antagonists inhibit this biochemical pathway and thus prevent the organism from replicating by impairing DNA synthesis.[50] A combination of sulfadiazine (2 g loading dose, then 1 g p.o. four times/day) with pyrimethamine (25 mg three times/day for the first day, then 25 mg daily) and folinic acid (3 to 5 mg twice weekly) is considered the most effective treatment for toxoplasmosis;[51] however, many toxic side effects have been reported, most notably bone marrow depression with subsequent hematologic complications. Weekly white blood cell counts and platelet counts are mandatory in these patients.

A less toxic means of treatment consists of clindamycin (300 mg p.o. four times/day) in combination with sulfadiazine. We generally treat patients for 4 to 6 wk on this drug regimen. This combination was repeatedly shown to be effective in patients with ocular toxoplasmosis.[52–54] Some studies, however, have reported disappointing results.[55, 56] Diarrhea, colitis, and pseudomembranous colitis remain potential problems with clindamycin use.

Scattered case reports showed that co-trimoxazole (trimethoprim with sulfamethoxazole) was effective for the treatment of toxoplasmosis in humans,[57, 58] but others report no difference with untreated controls using this approach.[56] There are no randomized, controlled studies to demonstrate the superiority of one regimen over the other. Thus, it remains to be seen which therapeutic combination is more effective in treating the acute disease and preventing recurrences.

The addition of corticosteroids to the therapeutic regimen may diminish the degree of damage from the inflammatory response, but this has not been definitively established. Some experts advocate adding prednisone 12 to 24 hr after initiating the antiparasitic therapy if the Toxoplasma lesion is in the posterior pole or is threatening the optic nerve head or if the vitreal inflammation is extreme, starting with 80 mg of prednisone with breakfast daily for 1 wk, then rapidly tapering the prednisone before discontinuing the anti-Toxoplasma therapy. Corticosteroids should never be used without concurrent antimicrobial therapy. Several cases of fulminant ocular toxoplasmosis have been described after the use of corticosteroids alone.[59, 60] Other recommendations for ocular toxoplasmosis therapy in various situations are given in Table 76–1.

Standard antitoxoplasmosis drug regimens can control AIDS-related ocular lesions. A combination of pyrimethamine and clindamycin is reported to be more effective than either pyrimethamine alone or in combination with sulfadiazine for patients with AIDS.[61] Toxoplasmosis in patients with AIDS frequently recurs when medical treatment is discontinued.[62–64] It may be necessary to continue treatment indefinitely to maintain control of the disease, but adequate maintenance treatment regimens have not been established. Zidovudine (azidothymidine or AZT), however, antagonizes the anti-Toxoplasma activity of pyrimethamine both in vivo and in vitro.[65] Co-trimoxazole has been employed in patients sensitive to pyrimethamine, but this has been associated with failure of treatment.[66]

The role of laser photocoagulation in the treatment of ocular toxoplasmosis appears to be limited.[67] Although photocoagulation can destroy Toxoplasma cysts and tachyzoites, Toxoplasma cysts can reside in ophthalmoscopically normal-appearing retina. Furthermore, photocoagulation of active lesions can be complicated by retinal or vitreous hemorrhage, or even by retinal detachment. Vitrectomy and lensectomy can be performed to remove vitreous and lens opacities in these patients.[68] Patients undergoing surgery should probably be treated with anti-Toxoplasma agents preoperatively and the medication should be continued postoperatively.

REFERENCES

1. Perkins ES: Ocular toxoplasmosis. Br J Ophthalmol 57:1, 1973.
2. Krick JA, Remington JS: Toxoplasmosis in the adult—An overview. N Engl J Med 298:550, 1978.
3. van Knapen F: Toxoplasmosis, old stories and new facts. Int Ophthalmol 13:371, 1989.
4. Swartzenberg JE, Remington JS: Transmission of Toxoplasma. Am J Dis Child 129:777, 1975.
5. Teutsch SM, Juranek DD, Sulzer A, et al: Epidemic toxoplasmosis associated with infected cats. N Engl J Med 300:695, 1979.
6. Akstein RB, Wilson LA, Teutsch SM: Acquired toxoplasmosis. Ophthalmology 89:1299, 1982.
7. Silveira C, Belfort R Jr, Burnier M Jr, Nussenblatt R: Acquired toxoplasmosis infection as the cause of toxoplasmic retinochoroiditis in families. Am J Ophthalmol 106:363, 1988.
8. Couvreur J, Desmonts G: Congenital and maternal toxoplasmosis. A review of 300 congenital cases. Dev Med Child Neurol 4:519, 1962.
9. de Jong PTVM: Ocular toxoplasmosis: Common and rare symptoms and signs. Int Ophthalmol 13:391, 1989.
10. Jabs DA: Ocular toxoplasmosis. Int Ophthalmol Clin 30:264, 1990.
11. Friedman CT, Knox DL: Variations in recurrent active toxoplasmic retinochoroiditis. Arch Ophthalmol 81:481, 1969.
12. Doft BH, Gass JD: Outer retinal layer toxoplasmosis. Graefes Arch Clin Exp Ophthalmol 224:78, 1986.
13. Folk JC, Lobes LA: Presumed toxoplasmic papillitis. Ophthalmology 91:64, 1984.
14. Fine SL, Owens SL, Haller JA, et al: Choroidal neovascularization as a late complication of ocular toxoplasmosis. Am J Ophthalmol 91:318, 1981.
15. Skorska I, Soubrane G, Coscas G: Toxoplasmic choroiditis and subretinal neovessels. J Fr Ophtalmol 7:211, 1984.
16. Kennedy JE, Wise GN: Retinochoroidal vascular anastomoses in uveitis. Am J Ophthalmol 71:1221, 1971.
17. Braunstein RA, Gass JDM: Branch artery occlusion caused by acute toxoplasmosis. Arch Ophthalmol 98:512, 1980.
18. Toledo de Abreu M, Belfort R Jr, Hirata PS: Fuchs' heterochromic cyclitis and ocular toxoplasmosis. Am J Ophthalmol 93:739, 1982.
19. Williams DM, Grumet FC, Remington JS: Genetic control of murine resistance to Toxoplasma gondii. Infect Immunol 19:416, 1978.
20. Kasper LH, Crabb JH, Pfefferkorn ER: Purification of a major membrane protein of Toxoplasma gondii by immunoabsorption with a monoclonal antibody. J Immunol 130:2407, 1983.
21. Kasper LH, Crabb JH, Pfefferkorn ER: Isolation and characterization of a monoclonal antibody–resistant antigenic mutant of Toxoplasma gondii. J Immunol 129:1694, 1982.

Table 76–1. RECOMMENDED THERAPY FOR OCULAR TOXOPLASMOSIS

Clinical Features	Recommended Treatment
Peripheral lesion; mild to moderate vitreal cells	Clindamycin, 300 mg p.o. q.i.d. and Sulfadiazine, 2 g p.o. loading, then 1 g p.o. q.i.d.
Peripheral lesion; moderate to severe vitreal cells	As above plus Prednisone, 1 mg/kg p.o./day with taper based on clinical response
Juxtamacular lesion	Clindamycin and sulfadiazine as above plus Pyrimethamine, 75 mg p.o. loading, then 25 mg p.o./day and Folinic acid, 5 mg p.o. twice a week Prednisone use based on vitreal cells, as in the case of peripheral lesions

22. Nussenblatt RB, Mittal KK, Fuhrman S, et al: Lymphocyte proliferative responses of patients with ocular toxoplasmosis to parasite and retinal antigens. Am J Ophthalmol 107:632, 1989.

23. Hafizi A, Modabber FZ: Effect of cyclophosphamide on *Toxoplasma gondii* infection: Reversal of the effect by passive immunization. Clin Exp Immunol 33:389, 1978.

24. Naot Y, Remington JS: Use of enzyme-linked immunosorbent assays (ELISA) for detection of monoclonal antibodies. Experience with antigens of *Toxoplasma gondii*. J Immunol Methods 43:333, 1981.

25. Sharma SD, Araujo FG, Remington JS: *Toxoplasma* antigen isolated by affinity chromatography with monclonal antibody protects mice against lethal infection with *Toxoplasma gondii*. J Immunol 133:2818, 1984.

26. Cohen SN: Toxoplasmosis in patients receiving immunosuppressive therapy. JAMA 211:657, 1970.

27. Rushkin J, Remington JS: Toxoplasmosis in the compromised host. Ann Intern Med 84:193, 1976.

28. Ryning FW, Mills J: *Pneumocystis carinii, Toxoplasma gondii,* cytomegalovirus and the compromised host. West J Med 130:18, 1979.

29. Wong B, Gold JWM, Brown AE, et al: Central nervous system toxoplasmosis in homosexual men and parenteral drug abusers. Ann Intern Med 100:36, 1984.

30. Luft BJ, Brooks RG, Conley FK, et al: Toxoplasmic encephalitis in patients with acquired immune deficiency syndrome. JAMA 252:913, 1984.

31. Araujo FG, Remington JS: Toxoplasmosis in immunocompromised patients. Eur J Clin Microbiol 6:1, 1987.

32. Jabs DA, Green WR, Fox R, et al: Ocular manifestations of acquired immune deficiency syndrome. Ophthalmology 96:1092, 1989.

33. Friedman AH: The retinal lesions of the acquired immune deficiency syndrome. Trans Am Ophthalmol Soc 82:447, 1984.

34. Schuman JS, Friedman AH: Retinal manifestations of the acquired immune deficiency syndrome (AIDS). Cytomegalovirus, *Candida albicans, Cryptococcus,* toxoplasmosis and *Pneumocystis carinii*. Trans Ophthalmol Soc UK 103:177, 1983.

35. Heinemann MH, Gold JMW, Maisel J: Bilateral *Toxoplasma* retinochoroiditis in a patient with acquired immune deficiency syndrome. Retina 6:224, 1986.

36. Parke DW, Font RL: Diffuse toxoplasmic retinochoroiditis in a patient with AIDS. Arch Ophthalmol 104:571, 1986.

37. Holland GN, Engstrom RE, Glasgow BJ, et al: Ocular toxoplasmosis in patients with the acquired immunodeficiency syndrome. Am J Ophthalmol 106:653, 1988.

38. Zimmerman LE: Ocular pathology of toxoplasmosis. Surv Ophthalmol 6:832, 1961.

39. Remington JS, Miller MJ, Brownlee I: IgM antibodies in acute toxoplasmosis. II. Prevalence and significance in acquired cases. J Lab Clin Med 71:855, 1968.

40. Schlaegel TF Jr: Ocular Toxoplasmosis and Pars Planitis. New York, Grune & Stratton, 1978, pp 138–172.

41. Kelan AE, Ayllon-Leindl L, Labzoffsky NA: Indirect fluorescent antibody method in serodiagnosis of toxoplasmosis. Can J Microbiol 8:545, 1962.

42. Pyndiah N, Krech U, Price P, Wilhelm J: Simplified chromatographic separation of immunoglobulin M from G and its application to *Toxoplasma* indirect immunofluorescence. J Clin Microbiol 9:170, 1979.

43. Fucillo DA, Madden DL, Tzan N, Sever JL: Difficulties associated with serological diagnosis of *Toxoplasma gondii* infections. Diagn Clin Immunol 5:8, 1987.

44. Araujo FG, Barnett EV, Gentry LO, Remington JS: False-positive anti-*Toxoplasma* fluorescent-antibody tests in patients with antinuclear antibodies. Appl Microbiol 22:270, 1971.

45. Akstein RB, Wilson LA, Teutsch SM: Acquired toxoplasmosis. Ophthalmology 89:1299, 1982.

46. Asbell PA, Vermund SH, Hofeldt AJ: Presumed toxoplasmic retinochoroiditis in four siblings. Am J Ophthalmol 94:656, 1982.

47. Weiss MJ, Velazquez N, Hofeldt AJ: Serologic tests in the diagnosis of presumed toxoplasmic retinochoroiditis. Am J Ophthalmol 109:407, 1990.

48. Naot Y, Desmonts G, Remington JS: IgM enzyme-linked immunosorbent assay test for the diagnosis of congenital *Toxoplasma* infection. J Pediatr 98:32, 1981.

49. Tomas JP, Schlit AF, Staatbaeder S: Rapid double sandwich enzyme-linked immunosorbent assay for detection of human immunoglobulin anti–*Toxoplasma gondii* antibodies. J Clin Microbiol 24:849, 1986.

50. Giles CL: Pyrimethamine (Daraprim) and the treatment of toxoplasmic uveitis. Surv Ophthalmol 16:88, 1971.

51. Smith RE, Nozik RA (eds): Toxoplasmic retinochoroiditis. *In* Uveitis, A Clinical Approach to Diagnosis and Management. Baltimore, Williams & Wilkins, 1989, pp 128–134.

52. Tate GW, Martin RG: Clindamycin in the treatment of human ocular toxoplasmosis. Can J Ophthalmol 12:188, 1977.

53. Chandra J, Donaldson EJ: Clindamycin in human ocular toxoplasmosis: A preliminary report. Aust J Ophthalmol 6:135, 1978.

54. Goldstein H: Clindamycin and sulphonamides in the treatment of ocular toxoplasmosis. Acta Ophthalmol 61:51, 1983.

55. Acers TE: Toxoplasmic retinochoroiditis: A double-blind therapeutic study. Arch Ophthalmol 71:58, 1964.

56. Rothova A, Buitenhuis HJ, Meenken C, et al: Therapy of ocular toxoplasmosis. Int Ophthalmol 13:415, 1989.

57. Norby R, Eilard T, Svedhem A. Lycke E: Treatment of toxoplasmosis with trimethoprim-sulphamethoxazole. Scand J Infect Dis 7:72, 1975.

58. Williams M, Savage DCL: Acquired toxoplasmosis in children. Arch Dis Child 53:829, 1978.

59. Nicholson DH, Wolchok EB: Ocular toxoplasmosis in an adult receiving long-term corticosteroid therapy. Arch Ophthalmol 94:248, 1976.

60. Sabates R, Pruett RC, Brockhurst RJ: Fulminary ocular toxoplasmosis. Am J Ophthalmol 92:497, 1981.

61. Rolston KVI, Hoy J: Role of clindamycin in the treatment of central nervous system toxoplasmosis. Am J Med 83:551, 1987.

62. Heinemann MH, Gold JMW, Maisel J: Bilateral *Toxoplasma* retinochoroiditis in a patient with acquired immune deficiency syndrome. Retina 6:224, 1986.

63. Luft BJ, Conley F, Remington JS, et al: Outbreak of central nervous system toxoplasmosis in Western Europe and North America. Lancet 1:781, 1983.

64. Levy RM, Bredesen DE, Rosenblum ML: Neurological manifestations of the acquired immunodeficiency syndrome (AIDS). Experience at UCSF and review of the literature. J Neurosurg 62:475, 1985.

65. Israelski DM, Tom C, Remington JS: Zidovudine antagonizes the action of pyrimethamine in experimental infection with *Toxoplasma gondii*. Antimicrob Agents Chemother 33:30, 1989.

66. Holliman RE: Toxoplasmosis and the acquired immune deficiency syndrome. J Infect 16:121, 1988.

67. Ghartey KN, Brockhurst RJ: Photocoagulation of active toxoplasmic retinochoroiditis. Am J Ophthalmol 89:858, 1980.

68. Fitzgerald CR: Pars plana vitrectomy for vitreous opacity secondary to presumed toxoplasmosis. Arch Ophthalmol 98:321, 1980.

Chapter 77

Retinal Manifestations of AIDS: Diagnosis and Treatment

MICHAEL K. PINNOLIS, W. WYNN McMULLEN, and
DONALD J. D'AMICO

During the decade of the 1980s, AIDS evolved into a major epidemic. Through August 1991, there were 191,601 reported cases of AIDS and 122,905 reported deaths from AIDS in the United States.[1] There are numerous ocular lesions associated with AIDS, but retinal manifestations account for some of the most commonly seen abnormalities in this disease and certainly are the most threatening to vision. Many different types of pathogens will give rise to similar-appearing fundus lesions. Because of the difficulty involved with retinal biopsy and vitreous culture and the inaccuracy of serologic testing for ocular pathogens, clinical diagnosis remains the major method of differentiating the cause of an AIDS-related retinopathy.

HIV-ASSOCIATED RETINOPATHY

The most common retinal manifestation of AIDS is a microangiopathy clinically manifested by the appearance of single or multiple cotton-wool spots (cytoid bodies) (Fig. 77–1). This microangiopathy has been reported in approximately 50 percent of all patients with AIDS (range 25 to 92 percent).[2–12] The lesions are usually found in the posterior pole and are distributed either along the major arcades or near the optic nerve. There may also be scattered hemorrhages, Roth spots, microaneurysms, or other microvascular changes seen throughout the retina, but these findings are less frequent. The cotton-wool spots are transient and nonprogressive in nature, usually resolving within 6 to 8 wk, which distinguishes them from the infectious retinopathies. HIV microvasculopathy is rarely symptomatic or clinically significant, even with the presence of cotton-wool spots in the macula; one should consider other causes in patients with symptoms of scotomata or visual loss (Table 77–1). Conversely, the appearance of cotton-wool spots in an otherwise healthy individual should suggest consideration of HIV infection.

Although the microangiopathy may be seen in patients who are HIV-positive or who have either AIDS or AIDS-related complex, it is probably a marker for a more advanced stage of the illness. HIV retinopathy has been shown to be related to a decreasing CD4:CD8 (T helper:T suppressor) ratio; this ratio decreases as AIDS progresses and further damages the immune system. Therefore, the presence of HIV microangiopathy may herald a worsening prognosis.[2, 11, 13]

Cotton-wool spots are due to swollen axons in the nerve fiber layer of the retina, probably associated with areas of focal ischemic injury. Cotton-wool spots occur in a variety of systemic diseases that affect small vessels, including diabetes mellitus, hypertension, collagen vascular diseases, anemia, and leukemia. Although the exact cause of the cotton-wool spots in AIDS has not been elucidated, possible causes for the focal ischemia include direct infection of the vascular endothelium with HIV,[14–17] circulating immune complex deposition on the vascular endothelium,[6] or rheologic difficulties resulting from increased red blood cell aggregation with resultant sludging of blood flow.[18]

No specific treatment other than observation is indicated for this clinical finding. Cotton-wool spots are significant mainly for the fact that they must be differentiated from other forms of infectious retinopathy, such as cytomegalovirus (CMV) infection of the retina.

CMV RETINITIS

Epidemiology and Pathogenesis

CMV retinitis is the most common retinal infection seen in AIDS. Although the reported prevalence of CMV retinitis varies from 5.7 to 40 percent, it is prob-

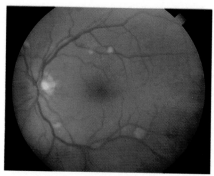

Figure 77–1. HIV microangiopathy: cotton-wool spots.

Table 77–1. HIV MICROANGIOPATHY

Prevalence: more than 50% of patients with AIDS
Multiple cotton-wool spots in posterior pole
Nonprogressive: usually resolve in 6 to 8 wk
Visual symptoms rare; occasional paracentral scotoma

935

ably accurate to state that about one third of AIDS patients will present with CMV retinitis during the course of their illness.[2, 3, 12, 19–21]

It is generally thought that CMV retinitis is hematogenously seeded into the retina by infected monocytes. HIV-infected endothelial cells in the retinal capillaries may facilitate access of the virus to the retina; the monocytes are more easily able to migrate through the damaged wall of the retinal vessels. This hypothesis is supported by the finding that CMV retinitis is 10 times more common in AIDS patients than in immunosuppressed transplant patients. Microangiopathy is a common feature in AIDS, possibly because of endothelial cell damage, but it is uncommon in transplant patients.[14, 17, 22, 23] Rarely, the infection may spread to the retina directly from primary involvement of the optic nerve.[23–25]

Clinical Presentation and Diagnosis

CMV retinitis may be bilateral or unilateral and may demonstrate multifocal sites of infection in an individual eye. Presenting symptoms of CMV retinitis vary depending on the location of the lesions (Table 77–2). Posterior lesions may give rise to paracentral scotomata or decreased visual acuity, especially for lesions located in the macula or involving the optic nerve. Metamorphopsia may be associated with an advancing edge of retinal edema for lesions near the macula. Symptoms of vitreous floaters may be present.[23, 26, 27] In our experience, vitreous floaters are the most common symptom associated with CMV retinitis and are more common than suggested by the literature. On careful questioning, most patients with CMV retinitis will report the presence of floaters. The symptoms may be subtle however, and therefore unrecognized by the patient for many weeks. Patients and their attending physicians should be alerted to watch for symptoms of floaters. CMV retinitis may occasionally be the initial manifestation of AIDS, but this is rare.[28–30]

Clinically, there are two presentations of CMV retinitis described. The first is the classically described form. It is usually seen in or near the posterior pole. This presentation may be referred to as the hemorrhagic type and has a "crumbled cheese and ketchup" appearance. Large areas of retinal hemorrhage associated with areas of thick, whitish retinal necrosis are seen alongside blood vessels (Fig. 77–2). The second form, which is most

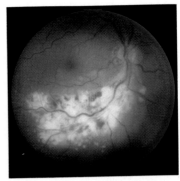

Figure 77–2. Posterior hemorrhagic cytomegalovirus (CMV) retinitis.

often seen peripherally, is the granular type. In this granular form, the lesions typically spread out from a central focus. The advancing border has a yellow, granular appearance, often with little or no hemorrhage. Behind the advancing border is an area of atrophic and thinned retina, which gives this lesion the so-called brush-fire appearance (Fig. 77–3). Both forms of retinitis are associated with infection of the inner retina. There is no ocular pain or conjunctival injection seen in either form of CMV retinitis. Anterior segment inflammation is rare but may present as a mild iritis with small, fine keratic precipitates. Usually, one will see a few anterior vitreous cells, although rarely, dense vitreous debris and inflammation can be present. Perivascular sheathing is often seen in the immediate vicinity of the retinitis but can on occasion be seen in other areas of the retina as well.[6, 8, 23, 26, 27, 31–34] The differential diagnosis for CMV retinitis includes cotton-wool spots, toxoplasmosis, syphilitic retinitis, herpes simplex virus, varicella-zoster virus, and *Pneumocystis carinii* infection (Table 77–3). It may be especially difficult to differentiate early CMV from cotton-wool spots. Serial examinations on patients with suspected cotton-wool spots should allow one to differentiate these entities, since CMV will progress and the cotton-wool spots will resolve in a few weeks.

The diagnosis of CMV retinitis is a clinical one. Serum titers are not helpful. Many patients with AIDS will demonstrate elevated titers to CMV, but that may be reflective of a previous infection or a current infection elsewhere. Likewise, vitreous aspirates for culture and

Table 77–2. CYTOMEGALOVIRUS RETINITIS

Posterior Type
Found in posterior pole along retinal vessels
Thick, whitish infiltrate with associated retinal hemorrhages
"Crumbled cheese and ketchup" appearance

Peripheral Type
Granular edge surrounding area of retinal necrosis
Little or no retinal hemorrhage
Satellite lesions
"Brush-fire" appearance

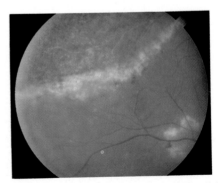

Figure 77–3. Peripheral "brush-fire" CMV retinitis.

Table 77–3. AIDS-ASSOCIATED RETINOPATHIES: DIFFERENTIAL DIAGNOSIS

Microangiopathy (noninfectious)
Cytomegalovirus
Pneumocystis carinii
Syphilis
Acute retinal necrosis (herpes zoster or herpes simplex)
Toxoplasmosis
Mycobacterium avium–intracellulare complex
Cryptococcus

titers have not yet proved helpful because the amount of infected material is small. Retinal biopsy remains too complex to use routinely.[27]

Natural History

CMV retinitis is an indolent infection spreading slowly over the course of many weeks or months to eventually involve the entire retina. Without treatment, vision is usually lost because of optic nerve involvement, spread of the lesions into the macula with macular necrosis, or retinal detachment. Rarely, visual acuity may be impaired because of media opacification from dense vitreous inflammatory debris. Spontaneous remission of CMV retinitis is reported but rare and may result from an improvement in the immune status of the patient, possibly related to the use of zidovudine (azidothymidine, AZT).[35–37] The presence of CMV retinitis generally implies that the patient is severely immunocompromised. In an early report, CMV retinitis was regarded as a preterminal infection with a rather dismal life expectancy of 6 wk from the time of initial diagnosis.[12] Recent studies have reported an increased survival time of 5.5 to 8 mo from the time of diagnosis.[20, 38, 39] We have seen several patients who have survived more than 2 yr from the time of diagnosis. This is probably due to a combination of factors. Diagnosis, prophylaxis, and treatment of AIDS-related illnesses, such as *Pneumocystis carinii* pneumonia, have improved overall survival considerably. There may be a bias toward earlier diagnosis, since both patients and clinicians have become more aware of the subtle presenting symptoms of CMV retinitis. Finally, ganciclovir (Cytovene, DHPG), which is used to treat CMV infections, may also play a role by improving the prognosis of life-threatening CMV infections, such as CMV colitis.[20, 38] It is unlikely that AZT has played any role in the increased survival. Most patients must stop AZT while on ganciclovir because the combination of both drugs can lead to severe bone marrow suppression.

Treatment (Table 77–4)

CMV is a DNA virus in the Herpesviridae family. However, systemic acyclovir has been ineffective in treating CMV infections. An acyclic nucleoside such as acyclovir is normally converted by viral thymidine kinase

to its triphosphate form, which then competitively inhibits viral DNA synthesis. However, because CMV lacks viral thymidine kinase, acyclovir does not provide an effective substrate for enzymatic conversion. Ganciclovir is an antiviral acyclic nucleoside analog of acyclovir that has been shown to have an effect against CMV. Ganciclovir is also a prodrug and has proved to be virustatic for CMV. The exact mechanism of how CMV converts ganciclovir to the triphosphate form is unknown.[31] (Ganciclovir has received United States Food and Drug Administration [FDA] approval as effective treatment for CMV retinitis.)

In 1985, Felsenstein and associates were the first to report success in treating CMV retinitis in AIDS patients by using ganciclovir.[40] Since then there have been a number of reports that have confirmed the efficacy of ganciclovir for treatment of CMV retinitis. Ganciclovir stabilizes the retinitis, halting or delaying progression and visual loss, and decreases viral shedding.[38, 41–53] In order to obtain adequate blood concentrations, the drug must be administered intravenously, and because ganciclovir is virustatic, patients must be put on continuous intravenous (IV) maintenance therapy for the rest of their lives. In early studies, in which the drug was discontinued, almost all patients had a recurrence of the retinitis.[44, 48, 50]

Patients begin therapy with a 2- or 3-wk induction of ganciclovir: 5 mg/kg given IV b.i.d. After induction, patients continue on maintenance therapy of 5 to 6 mg/kg/day IV given 5 to 7 days during the week. Since ganciclovir is excreted by the kidneys, the dose may need to be adjusted in patients with compromised renal function. Therapy is continued indefinitely unless the patient experiences a resistant CMV infection or is unable to take the drug because of side effects. Neutropenia is the most common side effect of ganciclovir and is reported to occur in 20 to 40 percent of all patients taking the drug.[19, 45, 49, 52, 53] The neutropenia is usually reversible upon cessation of drug therapy. Other side effects include thrombocytopenia and anemia. Recently, a new drug, GCSF (granulocyte colony–stimulating factor, Neupogen), was approved by the FDA. GCSF stimulates the production of granulocytes and may counteract the neutropenic effects of ganciclovir. GCSF has

Table 77–4. TREATMENT OF CMV RETINITIS

Ganciclovir (Cytovene, DHPG)
  Induction: 5 mg/kg IV b.i.d.
  Maintenance: 5 mg/kg IV q.d.
  Side effects:
    Neutropenia
    Thrombocytopenia
    Anemia

Foscarnet (Foscavir, phosphoformic acid)
  Induction: 60 mg/kg IV t.i.d.
  Maintenance: 60 mg/kg IV b.i.d. or 90 mg/kg IV q.d.
  Side effects:
    Nephropathy
    Seizures
    Hypocalcemia or other electrolyte imbalances
    Nausea

proved quite useful as an adjunct to ganciclovir therapy; many patients are now able to tolerate higher doses of ganciclovir and are able to stay on the drug for longer periods.

Initially, 78 to 100 percent of patients with CMV retinitis will respond to ganciclovir.[19, 52, 53] Relapses usually occur when the patient must stop ganciclovir because of neutropenia. However, recurrent CMV during maintenance therapy occurs in approximately 30 to 50 percent of patients.[19, 20, 38, 47, 49, 52, 53] If the patient experiences a reactivation of the retinitis while taking ganciclovir, a reinduction is performed. Attempts at reinduction may occur several times during the course of treatment with ganciclovir unless the patient becomes intolerant to the medication.

Patients should be followed every 2 to 3 wk to assess the efficacy of the treatment. Gross and colleagues describe a "smoldering" retinitis in which the infection progressively damages retina without significant clinical signs of activity.[38] Serial photography is extremely important in these patients to enable the clinician to determine whether there has been progression of the retinitis; subtle changes are often otherwise impossible to ascertain. Final visual outcome depends on the initial location of the CMV lesions and the ability to maintain the patients on therapy. Fourteen to 26 percent of patients will lose vision while on treatment.[38, 47] However, ganciclovir has been shown to halt progression of the retinitis and improve visual outcome.[20, 31] We currently begin treatment in patients with any evidence of CMV retinitis, even those who have only peripheral lesions, shortly after diagnosis is made. Since the retinitis always progresses, it seems prudent to treat the infection early rather than wait until it is close to the macula and threatening vision.

Bilateral disease may develop in about 50 percent of patients. Because of this, Jabs and coworkers have advocated prophylactic therapy with ganciclovir for the uninvolved eye in patients who have lost vision in one eye from CMV retinitis.[20] Additionally, many of these patients have a concomitant systemic infection, such as CMV colitis. We have preferred not to treat if one eye is lost to CMV, the other eye is uninvolved, and there are no systemic manifestations of CMV. Ganciclovir is a highly toxic medication, the benefits of prophylaxis remain uncertain, and patients may experience CMV retinitis despite ganciclovir therapy.[54] Instead, the patients are followed closely with serial examinations and are treated at the first signs of retinitis. Treatment failure with ganciclovir may be due to intractable neutropenia, inadequate drug dosage,[44, 47] or possibly, resistant CMV retinitis.[55] One should be cautious in discontinuing treatment. CMV retinitis is often associated with other systemic CMV infections, such as colitis and pneumonitis. It is prudent to remember that one is not treating the eye alone, and maintenance therapy may be beneficial. Foscarnet, another antiviral drug, has been shown to prolong the life expectancy of AIDS patients with CMV.[56] This information, although preliminary, may suggest another reason in favor of prophylactic therapy.

The primary alternative treatment to ganciclovir is foscarnet (phosphonoformic acid, Foscavir). Foscarnet is a potent inhibitor of herpes simplex virus DNA polymerases, as well as retrovirus reverse transcriptase. Although the mechanism of action is different from that of ganciclovir, foscarnet is also virustatic for CMV and requires continuous intravenous maintenance therapy. Several studies have demonstrated its effectiveness against CMV infections.[42, 57–61] (Foscarnet was recently approved by the FDA for use in CMV retinitis.) We have been treating patients with a 2-wk induction period of 60 mg/kg given IV three times a day followed by maintenance treatment of 90 mg/kg IV q.d. or 60 mg/kg IV b.i.d. The most troubling side effect of foscarnet is nephrotoxicity. Hypocalcemia, nausea, tremors, seizures, and anemia have also been reported. Treatment and follow-up on patients treated with foscarnet is basically similar to those for ganciclovir. Frequent examinations are performed and serial photographs are used to assess for recurrences.

The potential for anti-HIV activity with foscarnet may be an additional benefit. The multicenter Study of Ocular Complications in AIDS (SOCA) sponsored by the National Institutes of Health has demonstrated a prolonged survival in AIDS patients treated with foscarnet when compared with those treated with ganciclovir.[56] Physicians should consider using foscarnet as the primary treatment for CMV retinitis and switch to ganciclovir as a secondary drug. The disadvantages of foscarnet include a more difficult induction with infusions three times a day, a longer length of infusion (about 2 hr), and some nausea. These issues should be discussed with the patient and his or her physician so that the patient may make an informed decision as to the most appropriate course of treatment. We are currently looking at inducing with ganciclovir, which is much easier for the patient, and then using maintainence therapy of foscarnet as long as possible.

Another alternative for treatment of CMV retinitis is direct intraocular injection of ganciclovir. Several authors have reported good success with intravitreal ganciclovir therapy. The patients are given intravitreal injections of 200 to 400 μg of ganciclovir through the pars plana. There is usually a 2- to 3-wk induction period of intravitreal injections twice weekly and maintenance therapy with weekly injections thereafter. Reported complications include endophthalmitis and retinal detachment. Although not yet reported, there is also the theoretical possibility of cataract formation and direct retinal toxicity from the drug.[62–69]

Other possible treatments are currently under investigation. One is the combined use of ganciclovir with GM-CSF (granulocyte-macrophage colony-stimulating factor), which is similar to GCSF and is used in an attempt to circumvent the neutropenic effects of the ganciclovir.[70] Oral ganciclovir is also currently in phase 2 trials, but its efficacy is still unknown.

Several treatment modalities have proved unsuccessful. Stevens and associates failed to halt progression of CMV retinitis by treating around peripheral lesions with laser photocoagulation. They had hoped to prevent cell-to-cell spread of the virus by creating a "fire-break" in the retina.[71] Other treatment failures include the use of interferon α[72] and intravenous CMV immunoglobulin as an adjunct to ganciclovir.[54]

PNEUMOCYSTIS CARINII CHOROIDITIS

Pathogenesis

Pneumocystis carinii pneumonia (PCP) is one of the most common opportunistic infections seen in patients with AIDS. It is also the most common cause of death in these patients. Macher and coworkers reported the first reliable evidence of *Pneumocystis* infection of the choroid.[73] There have been several subsequent reports in the literature describing a choroiditis secondary to disseminated *Pneumocystis* infection.[74–79] In recent years, treatment for PCP has improved. Currently, standard treatment includes the prophylactic use of pentamidine inhalation on a monthly basis to control the *Pneumocystis* infection when the patient is not experiencing an active pneumonia. Although this may suppress pulmonary *Pneumocystis* infection and prolong life expectancy, it apparently does not provide systemic protection. In fact, several authors have reported disseminated *Pneumocystis* infections in other organ systems, including the eye, while pentamidine inhalation therapy was being used.[74, 76, 80]

Clinical Diagnosis and Treatment

In general, patients with *Pneumocystis* choroiditis tend to have advanced AIDS. Signs and symptoms of *Pneumocystis* choroiditis are often minimal. Sometimes they may be attributable to other intraocular infections related to AIDS. Several of the reported patients had concurrent CMV retinitis.[75, 77, 78] Patients may be asymptomatic at the time of diagnosis or may, occasionally, present with symptoms of decreased visual acuity. Floaters are rarely noted. Examination usually shows no conjunctival injection or anterior segment inflammation, and vitritis is minimal. The characteristic appearance of *Pneumocystis* choroiditis is that of yellowish or cream-colored choroidal lesions in the posterior pole. They are typically large, plaquelike lesions ranging from 500 to 2000 μ in size. They may be slightly elevated. Early lesions are round or ovoid. However, they may coalesce or grow as time progresses, forming large, geographic infiltrates (Fig. 77–4). Satellite lesions are not a feature of this condition. The retinal pigment epithelium overlying larger lesions may take on a mottled appearance. Typically, growth is slow but the infection does tend to progress over time. Vision may be affected if the choroiditis spreads into the macula. Diagnosis of choroidal involvement is extremely important, since the presence of *Pneumocystis* choroiditis is evidence of life-threatening systemic infection. Treatment should be instituted and may include oral trimethoprim-sulfamethoxazole or

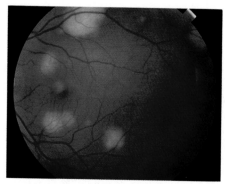

Figure 77–4. Pneumocystis choroiditis with deep choroidal lesions.

IV pentamidine. The choroidal lesions will usually respond to therapy.

Several studies have demonstrated the presence of trophozoites and cysts of *P. carinii* in the choroid on pathologic examination.[77, 78] However, the diagnosis is based on the clinical appearance: No useful diagnostic tests have yet been developed, and retinal biopsy is problematic. Differential diagnosis includes reticulum cell sarcoma, cryptococcal choroiditis,[33, 79, 81, 82] atypical *Mycobacterium* infections,[79, 83] metastatic carcinoma, secondary syphilis, sarcoid granulomas, and Dalen-Fuchs nodules of the Vogt-Koyanagi-Harada syndrome or sympathetic ophthalmia.[78]

SYPHILITIC RETINITIS

Secondary syphilis is well known to cause a fulminant vitritis and retinitis. Many of the patients infected with HIV also have a high incidence of sexually transmitted diseases such as syphilis. Although not common, there have been several reports of syphilitic retinitis in patients with AIDS.[82, 84–87]

The clinical presentation of syphilitic retinitis may take on various features depending on the immune status of the patient. Usually there is evidence of anterior segment inflammation with fine keratic precipitates and anterior chamber cells. There may be a mild vitritis, but often the vitreous inflammation is quite marked. The retina will usually have some vascular sheathing, and the vasculitis may be extensive. There can be geographic areas of whitish retinal infiltrates consistent with acute retinal necrosis (ARN). These areas may be single, multiple, or confluent. This retinitis usually affects the inner retinal layers; hemorrhage may also be seen. Serous macular detachment has been reported. Optic perineuritis is a common finding, and syphilis may also present as an isolated papillitis or in combination with retinitis.[82, 84, 85, 88, 89] Rhegmatogenous retinal detachment is a late finding in some patients. Differential diagnosis includes CMV, toxoplasmosis, herpes zoster retinitis (ARN), and tuberculous retinitis. The suspicion of syphilitic retinitis should be increased with a history of syphilis, prominent vitreous inflammation, a prominent retinal vasculitis associated with retinal necrosis, or a combination of these conditions. Laboratory work-up to rule out syphilis is mandatory if the diagnosis is suspected or the cause of retinitis is uncertain.

All patients with syphilitic retinitis should be presumed to have associated neurosyphilis. One series reported that 66 percent of AIDS patients with ocular manifestations of syphilis had accompanying neurosyphilis.[85] Therefore, lumbar puncture should be performed in patients in whom one suspects syphilitic retinitis or vitritis. Testing must include the fluorescent treponemal antibody absorption (FTA-ABS) or micro-hemagglutination–*Treponema pallidum* (MHA-TP) test in order to rule out the diagnosis of syphilis; The Venereal Disease Research Laboratory (VDRL) or rapid plasma reagin (RPR) test may not be positive in AIDS patients infected with *T. pallidum*.

Patients with AIDS and diagnosed ocular syphilis should be treated with a regimen recommended for concurrent neurosyphilis and HIV, type I infection. Benzathine penicillin has proved ineffective in some of these cases.[85] The treatment consists of high-dose intravenous penicillin G for 10 to 14 days. In patients with AIDS, the syphilitic infection tends to recur, and some form of maintenance therapy with penicillin may be indicated. It is still uncertain whether any kind of maintenance therapy is necessary. The following guidelines for treatment of neurosyphilis have been recommended by the Centers for Disease Control: (1) appropriate clinical response, (2) serial monthly reagin titers for 3 mo and every 6 mo thereafter, and (3) a two-dilution decrease in titers after 6 mo. In patients allergic to penicillin, alternative antibiotics include IV doxycycline, chloramphenicol, and ceftriaxone.[90]

ARN—PRESUMED HERPES ZOSTER RETINITIS

ARN, consisting of severe vitritis and a necrotizing retinitis, has been well documented in nonimmunocompromised patients. It is presumed to have a viral cause probably secondary to herpes zoster (varicella-zoster) or herpes simplex viruses.[91–94] There have now been several reports of ARN presumed to be herpetic in origin in patients with AIDS.[95–98] The clinical presentation of ARN in AIDS patients may vary and may not demonstrate the severe, extensive inflammation classi-

cally seen in ARN patients. The lesions may be unilateral or bilateral. The retinitis may affect the outer retinal layers, sparing the inner layers until very late in the disease process. The initial lesions, if seen early, can be small, yellowish lesions in the outer retina, typically between 100 and 300 μ in size (Fig. 77–5A). The spread of the lesions is often quite dramatic and rapid: The lesions coalesce to form large, geographic areas of outer retinal necrosis within 2 to 6 wk (Fig. 77–5B). Often, one can see smaller satellite lesions at the edge of the involved areas. There may be hemorrhage associated with these lesions, but this appearance is variable. Early in the course, the retinal vasculature is commonly spared. These lesions, unlike CMV lesions, do not spread out in a "brush-fire" pattern. They more typically demonstrate large, geographic areas of infiltrate. Several patients have been reported to have had a simultaneous or prior episode of dermal herpes zoster.

The natural course is for rapid progression and destruction of the outer retina. Some patients have extensive areas of retinal necrosis, retinal detachment, and proliferative vitreoretinopathy.

Differential diagnosis includes CMV, syphilis, *Pneumocystis* infection, toxoplasmosis, and fungal choroiditis. CMV is usually associated with more hemorrhage and tends to spread slowly from one nidus of infection. Its course is typically indolent, taking several months to spread centrally to the macula. Syphilis tends to involve the inner retina, and negative results on laboratory work-up should rule out this diagnosis. Retinal biopsy may need to be considered for diagnosis if uncertainty exists in sight-threatening cases.

At least one group has reported success in the treatment of early retinal necrosis with IV acyclovir.[95] However, the experience in treating more advanced lesions with acyclovir has been disappointing.[96–98] Herpes-like virus particles in the retina of these patients have been found on retinal biopsy, but further specific typing was not possible. It is conceivable that the infectious agent may either be herpes zoster or herpes simplex, or even CMV, which has a similar appearance. One study demonstrated the presence of varicella-zoster virus through culture and immunochemistry of biopsy specimens.[98] Although ganciclovir and foscarnet are more toxic than acyclovir, they are effective against herpesviruses as well as CMV. If the retinitis has failed to respond to acyclovir in one eye, one may wish to consider the use of ganciclovir or foscarnet.

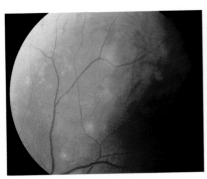
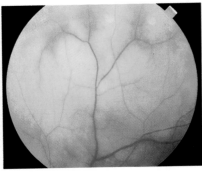

Figure 77–5. *A,* Acute retinal necrosis: early, small outer retinal lesions. *B,* Acute retinal necrosis: diffuse necrosis seen within 3 wk.

TOXOPLASMIC RETINITIS

Toxoplasmic retinitis has long been described in the ophthalmic literature. In general, it is felt that most cases of toxoplasmic retinitis are congenitally acquired. *Toxoplasma gondii* is another of the many opportunistic pathogens that can infect patients with AIDS. Toxoplasmosis is a frequent cause of nonviral, intracranial infections seen in AIDS patients. Surprisingly, despite the quite common reports of toxoplasmic meningitis in AIDS patients, the number of reports of toxoplasmic retinitis is small.[33, 99-105]

Clinical Findings and Diagnosis

The clinical features may be variable. There is often vitritis in patients with toxoplasmosis, but this is not always the case. The retinal lesions may be similar to the classic lesions seen in nonimmunocompromised hosts. They are large, yellowish lesions in the inner retina, between 500 and 2000 μ in size with surrounding vitreous inflammation. These patients may have single or multiple inner retinal lesions with overlying vitreous inflammation. However, there may also be very little inflammation in more severely immunocompromised patients. A form of outer retinal toxoplasmosis has also been reported. Again, these lesions tend to be somewhat larger and whiter and in general are not multifocal (Fig. 77-6). Differential diagnosis includes CMV, ARN, syphilitic retinitis, and *Pneumocystis* choroiditis. Toxoplasmosis serum titers may or may not be helpful in the diagnosis of these patients. Severely immunocompromised patients may not be able to mount an antibody response to the infection. Computed tomography scanning of the head with contrast medium may be helpful in differentiating this from other forms of retinitis: The finding of an enhancing ring lesion should confirm the diagnosis. Sometimes vitreous biopsy may be needed to make the diagnosis.[103]

Standard treatment consists of pyrimethamine, sulfa drugs, or clindamycin, or a combination. Systemic steroids may be considered for macular lesions, but their role is uncertain. Spiramycin is a macrolide antibiotic widely used in Europe for toxoplasmosis. It may be obtained from the FDA for compassionate use. Unlike

Table 77–5. RETINAL DETACHMENT IN CMV RETINITIS

Problems with conventional surgical approach
  Multiple, small holes in one or more quadrants
  Recurrent detachments common:
    Progression of retinitis after surgery
    Temporary tamponade with gas
  Prolonged recovery of vision with gas tamponade

Advantages of primary silicone oil
  Permanent tamponade
  Rapid visual recovery
  One-time surgery

toxoplasmosis in the non–AIDS patient, toxoplasmosis in AIDS patients should be treated regardless of location in the retina.[102]

MYCOBACTERIUM

Mycobacterium avium–intracellulare (MAI complex) is a frequently reported pathogen in patients with AIDS. One pathologic study demonstrated the presence of MAI forms in the choroid of patients with AIDS.[6] There has been some suggestion in the literature that MAI could be involved in a choroidal granuloma formation, but as yet this is unproved.[79]

Tuberculous choroiditis has also been described in a patient with AIDS.[83] Clinical findings included a granulomatous uveitis and a low-grade vitritis. There were numerous small, yellow-white choroidal infiltrates present. Some had coalesced into larger elevated nodules. This diagnosis should be considered in any disseminated choroiditis in AIDS patients. If the diagnosis of disseminated tuberculosis is made, appropriate therapy should be instituted.

CRYPTOCOCCAL CHOROIDITIS

Cryptococcus is a common fungal agent, most often responsible for causing meningitis in AIDS patients. *C. neoformans* can infect the uveal tract, and cryptococcal choroiditis has been reported in several patients with AIDS.[6, 33, 79, 81, 82, 106] The most common ocular manifestation of cryptococcus is severe papilledema, usually secondary to meningeal involvement. Choroiditis may present as yellowish "fluff balls" in the choroid or as elevated, depigmented lesions in patients with cryptococcal meningitis. The diagnosis of cryptococcal choroiditis implies meningeal involvement, and appropriate systemic treatment should be started with that in mind.

VITREORETINAL SURGERY IN AIDS PATIENTS

Vitreoretinal surgery may be necessary in patients with AIDS, because of either retinal detachment or the need for diagnostic retinal biopsy (Table 77-5). Both CMV retinitis and ARN have been shown to cause

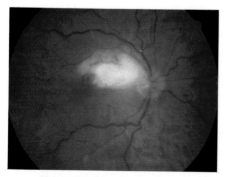

Figure 77–6. Toxoplasmosis.

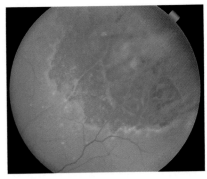

Figure 77–7. Retinal detachment with multiple breaks.

retinal detachments in patients with AIDS. Retinal detachment is a common complication of CMV retinitis and may occur in 5 to 29 percent of patients with CMV retinitis.[20, 53, 107] The decision whether to operate depends on several factors, including the status of the patient's other eye, the degree of retinitis, the prognosis for good visual outcome in the involved eye, and the patient's general health and prognosis for life expectancy. In general, surgery may be indicated in a patient in whom the retinitis is not threatening to involve the optic nerve or macula and in whom the prognosis for somewhat extended life expectancy is good.

Retinal detachments caused by ARN or CMV retinitis, or both, are problematic: There tend to be multiple small retinal holes in widely scattered areas of the retina (Fig. 77–7). Additionally, the retinitis may progress and cause further retinal breaks after the patient has been successfully treated with a scleral buckle procedure or vitrectomy.[26, 107]

Several authors have recommended a vitrectomy with silicone oil tamponade as the primary procedure in AIDS patients with retinitis and retinal detachment.[26, 107–109] Silicone oil provides a permanent tamponade that will keep the retina in place despite further hole formation. It allows a more rapid visual rehabilitation than does intraocular gas, which can be important in patients with somewhat limited life expectancy. The most common complications seen with silicone oil, cataract and corneal decompensation, do not seem to occur frequently in AIDS patients. This is partly because of the fact that patients often do not live long enough to experience these complications. Additionally, patients will become hyperopic ($+5.00$ to $+7.00$ D) if silicone oil is used in a phakic eye. Nevertheless, we have had some reasonable success in rehabilitating and maintaining vision in patients whose only hope for sight was such a procedure.

Our general approach is to perform a standard pars plana vitrectomy leaving the crystalline lens in place. A small cushion of anterior vitreous is left during the vitrectomy to provide some protection from the silicone oil. Care is taken to remove the posterior vitreous gel from the retina in the area of intended internal drainage. Often, these young patients will not have a posterior vitreous detachment. An air-fluid exchange is performed using internal drainage. The retinotomy is treated with endolaser. The other retinal breaks are not treated. A complete air–silicone oil exchange is then performed; care is taken to drain all of the subretinal fluid in order to avoid a visible postoperative meniscus.

Retinal biopsy may be indicated for cases of atypical retinitis in which the diagnosis is important for treatment purposes. The technique of retinal biopsy in AIDS patients with retinitis has been described and has been shown to be useful in certain circumstances.[107, 110, 111]

During surgery, care must be taken to protect both the surgeon and the operating room personnel. Although the risk may seem highest for surgery on patients with AIDS, in actuality, the risk is probably greatest for those patients in whom the HIV status is unknown. Therefore, it is advisable to use universal precautions in all cases, including in patients with AIDS. We employ a system for protecting both surgeon and scrub nurse during our surgery on HIV-infected patients. The number of sharp instruments on the instrument stand is kept to an absolute minimum. Needles and sharp instruments are not passed from hand to hand during the procedure but are placed on a table and then retrieved by the surgeon or scrub nurse. This table becomes a "neutral zone" in which only one hand can be placed at any given time. Whenever practical, needles are not reused, and they are always mounted using instruments, never fingers. The practice of removing shoes and wearing only socks in the operating room is discouraged and probably should be discontinued for safety reasons.

REFERENCES

1. Centers for Disease Control: HIV/AIDS Surveillance Report 1991. September pp 1–18. Atlanta, Centers for Disease Control.
2. Jabs DA, Green WR, Fox R, et al: Ocular manifestations of acquired immune deficiency syndrome. Ophthalmology 96:1092–1099, 1989.
3. Turu AC, Civera AA, Latorre X: Ophthalmic manifestations of acquired immunodeficiency syndrome. A study of thirty-four patients. Ophthalmologica 197:113–119, 1988.
4. Humphry RC, Parkin JM, Marsh RJ: The ophthalmological features of AIDS and AIDS-related disorders. Trans Ophthalmol Soc UK 105:505–509, 1986.
5. Kestelyn P, Van de Perre P, Rouvroy D, et al: A prospective study of the ophthalmologic findings in the acquired immune deficiency syndrome in Africa. Am J Ophthalmol 100:230–238, 1985.
6. Pepose JS, Holland GN, Nestor MS, et al: Acquired immune deficiency syndrome. Pathogenic mechanisms of ocular disease. Ophthalmology 92:472–484, 1985.
7. Newsome DA, Green WR, Miller ED, et al: Microvascular aspects of acquired immune deficiency syndrome retinopathy. Am J Ophthalmol 98:590–601, 1984.
8. Palestine AG, Rodrigues MM, Macher AM, et al: Ophthalmic involvement in acquired immunodeficiency syndrome. Ophthalmology 91:1092–1099, 1984.
9. Khadem M, Kalish SB, Goldsmith J, et al: Ophthalmologic findings in acquired immune deficiency syndrome (AIDS). Arch Ophthalmol 102:201–206, 1984.
10. Rosenberg PR, Uliss AE, Friedland GH, et al: Acquired immunodeficiency syndrome. Ophthalmic manifestations in ambulatory patients. Ophthalmology 90:874–878, 1983.
11. Freeman WR, Chen A, Henderly DE, et al: Prevalence and significance of acquired immunodeficiency syndrome–related retinal microvasculopathy. Am J Ophthalmol 107:229–235, 1989.
12. Holland GN, Pepose JS, Pettit TH, et al: Acquired immune deficiency syndrome. Ocular manifestations. Ophthalmology 90:859–873, 1983.

13. Pezzi PP, Tamburi S, Doffizi GP, et al: Retinal cotton-wool–like spots: A marker for AIDS? Ann Ophthalmol 21:31–33, 1989.
14. Schmitt Graff A, Neuen Jacob E, Rettig B, Sundmacher R: Evidence for cytomegalovirus and human immunodeficiency virus infection of the retina in AIDS. Virchows Arch 416:249–253, 1990.
15. Cantrill HL, Henry K, Jackson B, et al: Recovery of human immunodeficiency virus from ocular tissues in patients with acquired immune deficiency syndrome. Ophthalmology 95:1458–1462, 1988.
16. Cantrill HL, Henry K, Sannerud K, Balfour HH: HIV infection of the retina. N Engl J Med 318:1539, 1988.
17. Pomerantz RJ, Kuritzkes DR, de la Monte SM, et al: Infection of the retina by human immunodeficiency virus type I. N Engl J Med 317:1643–1647, 1987.
18. Engstrom RE Jr, Holland GN, Hardy D, Meiselman HJ: Hemmorheologic abnormalities in patients with human immunodeficiency virus infection and ophthalmic microvasculopathy. Am J Ophthalmol 109:153–161, 1990.
19. Jacobson MA, O'Donnell JJ, Porteous D, et al: Retinal and gastrointestinal disease due to cytomegalovirus in patients with the acquired immune deficiency syndrome: Prevalence, natural history, and response to ganciclovir therapy. Q J Med 67:473–486, 1988.
20. Jabs DA, Enger C, Bartlett JG: Cytomegalovirus retinitis and acquired immunodeficiency syndrome. Arch Ophthalmol 107:75–80, 1989.
21. Nussenblatt R: Ocular complications of the acquired immunodeficiency syndrome. Nat Immun Cell Growth Regul 7:131–134, 1988.
22. Skolnik PR, Pomerantz RJ, de la Monte SM, et al: Dual infection of retina with human immunodeficiency virus type 1 and cytomegalovirus. Am J Ophthalmol 107:361–372, 1989.
23. Culbertson WW: Infections of the retina in AIDS. Int Ophthalmol Clin 29:108–118, 1989.
24. Grossniklaus HE, Frank KE, Tomsak RL: Cytomegalovirus retinitis and optic neuritis in acquired immune deficiency syndrome. Report of a case. Ophthalmology 94:1601–1604, 1987.
25. Gross JG, Sadun AA, Wiley CA, Freeman WR: Severe visual loss related to isolated peripapillary retinal and optic nerve head cytomegalovirus infection. Am J Ophthalmol 108:691–698, 1989.
26. Kreiger AE, Holland GN: Ocular involvement in AIDS. Eye 2:496–505, 1988.
27. Bloom JN, Palestine AG: The diagnosis of cytomegalovirus retinitis. Ann Intern Med 109:963–969, 1988.
28. Freeman WR, Henderly DE, Lipson BK, et al: Retinopathy before the diagnosis of AIDS. Ann Ophthalmol 21:468–474, 1989.
29. Henderly DE, Freeman WR, Smith RE, et al: Cytomegalovirus retinitis as the initial manifestation of the acquired immune deficiency syndrome. Am J Ophthalmol 103:316–320, 1987.
30. Sison RF, Holland GN, MacArthur LJ, et al: Cytomegalovirus retinopathy as the initial manifestation of the acquired immunodeficiency syndrome. Am J Ophthalmol 112:243–249, 1991.
31. Jacobson MA, Mills J: Serious cytomegalovirus disease in the acquired immunodeficiency syndrome (AIDS). Clinical findings, diagnosis, and treatment. Ann Intern Med 108:585–594, 1988.
32. Schuman JS, Orellana J, Friedman AH, Teich SA: Acquired immunodeficiency syndrome (AIDS). Surv Ophthalmol 31:384–410, 1987.
33. Schuman JS, Friedman AH: Retinal manifestations of the acquired immune deficiency syndrome (AIDS): cytomegalovirus, *Candida albicans,* cryptococcus, toxoplasmosis and *Pneumocystis carinii.* Trans Ophthalmol Soc UK 103:177–190, 1983.
34. Palestine AG: Clinical aspects of cytomegalovirus retinitis. Rev Infect Dis 10(Suppl 3):S515–S521, 1988.
35. Fay MT, Freeman WR, Wiley CA, et al: Atypical retinitis in patients with the acquired immunodeficiency syndrome. Am J Ophthalmol 105:483–490, 1988.
36. Guyer DR, Jabs DA, Brant AM, et al: Regression of cytomegalovirus retinitis with zidovudine. A clinicopathologic correlation. Arch Ophthalmol 107:868–874, 1989.
37. D'Amico DJ, Skolnik PR, Kosloff BR, et al: Resolution of cytomegalovirus retinitis with zidovudine therapy. Arch Ophthalmol 106:1168–1169, 1988.
38. Gross JG, Bozzette SA, Mathews WC, et al: Longitudinal study of cytomegalovirus retinitis in acquired immune deficiency syndrome. Ophthalmology 97:681–686, 1990.
39. Holland GN, Sison RF, Jatulis DE, et al: Survival of patients with the acquired immune deficiency syndrome after development of cytomegalovirus retinopathy. UCLA CMV Retinopathy Study Group. Ophthalmology 97:204–211, 1990.
40. Felsenstein D, D'Amico DJ, Hirsch MS, et al: Treatment of cytomegalovirus retinitis with 9-[2-hydroxy-1-(hydroxymethyl)-ethoxymethyl]guanine. Ann Intern Med 103:377–380, 1985.
41. Weisenthal RW, Sinclair SH, Frank I, Rubin DH: Long-term outpatient treatment of CMV retinitis with ganciclovir in AIDS patients. Br J Ophthalmol 73:996–1001, 1989.
42. Mills J, Jacobson MA, O'Donnell JJ, et al: Treatment of cytomegalovirus retinitis in patients with AIDS. Rev Infect Dis 10(Suppl):S522–S531, 1988.
43. Jacobson MA, O'Donnell JJ, Brodie HR, et al: Randomized prospective trial of ganciclovir maintenance therapy for cytomegalovirus retinitis. J Med Virol 25:339–349, 1988.
44. Rosecan LR, Stahl Bayliss CM, Kalman CM, Laskin OL: Antiviral therapy for cytomegalovirus retinitis in AIDS with dihydroxy propoxymethyl guanine. Am J Ophthalmol 101:405–418, 1986.
45. Collaborative DHPG Treatment Study Group: Treatment of serious cytomegalovirus infections with 9-(1,3-dihydroxy-2-propoxymethyl)guanine in patients with AIDS and other immunodeficiencies. N Engl J Med 314:801–805, 1986.
46. Bach MC, Bagwell SP, Knapp NP, et al: 9-(1,3-Dihydroxy-2-propoxymethyl)guanine for cytomegalovirus infections in patients with the acquired immunodeficiency syndrome. Ann Intern Med 103:381–382, 1985.
47. Holland GN, Buhles WC, Mastre B, Kaplan HJ: A controlled retrospective study of ganciclovir treatment for cytomegalovirus retinopathy. Use of a standardized system for the assessment of disease outcome. UCLA CMV Retinopathy Study Group. Arch Ophthalmol 107:1759–1766, 1989.
48. Holland GN, Sakamoto MJ, Hardy D, et al: Treatment of cytomegalovirus retinopathy in patients with acquired immunodeficiency syndrome. Use of the experimental drug 9-[2-hydroxy-1-(hydroxymethyl)ethoxymethyl]guanine. Arch Ophthalmol 104:1794–1800, 1986.
49. Henderly DE, Freeman WR, Causey DM, Rao NA: Cytomegalovirus retinitis and response to therapy with ganciclovir. Ophthalmology 94:425–434, 1987.
50. Palestine AG, Stevens G, Lane HC, et al: Treatment of cytomegalovirus retinitis with dihydroxy propoxymethyl guanine. Am J Ophthalmol 101:95–101, 1986.
51. Masur H, Lane HC, Palestine A, et al: Effect of 9-(1,3-dihydroxy-2-propoxymethyl) guanine on serious cytomegalovirus disease in eight immunosuppressed homosexual men. Ann Intern Med 104:41–44, 1986.
52. Jabs DA, Newman C, De Bustros S, Polk BF: Treatment of cytomegalovirus retinitis with ganciclovir. Ophthalmology 94:824–830, 1987.
53. Holland GN, Sidikaro Y, Kreiger AE, et al: Treatment of cytomegalovirus retinopathy with ganciclovir. Ophthalmology 94:815–823, 1987.
54. Jacobson MA, O'Donnell JJ, Rousell R, et al: Failure of adjunctive cytomegalovirus intravenous immune globulin to improve efficacy of ganciclovir in patients with acquired immunodeficiency syndrome and cytomegalovirus retinitis: A phase 1 study. Antimicrob Agents Chemother 34:176–178, 1990.
55. Erice A, Chou S, Biron KK, et al: Progressive disease due to ganciclovir-resistant cytomegalovirus in immunocompromised patients. N Engl J Med 320:289–293, 1989.
56. National Institutes of Health: Clinical Alert: October 17, 1991. Washington, DC, National Institutes of Health, 1991.
57. Jacobson MA, Crowe S, Levy J, et al: Effect of foscarnet therapy on infection with human immunodeficiency virus in patients with AIDS. J Infect Dis 158:862–865, 1988.
58. Lehoang P, Girard B, Robinet M, et al: Foscarnet in the treatment of cytomegalovirus retinitis in acquired immune deficiency syndrome. Ophthalmology 96:865–873, 1989.
59. Singer DR, Fallon TJ, Schulenburg WE, et al: Foscarnet for cytomegalovirus retinitis. [Letter] Ann Intern Med 103:962, 1985.

60. Walmsley SL, Chew E, Read SE, et al: Treatment of cytomegalovirus retinitis with trisodium phosphonoformate hexahydrate (foscarnet). J Infect Dis 157:569–572, 1988.

61. Fanning MM, Read SE, Benson M, et al: Foscarnet therapy of cytomegalovirus retinitis in AIDS. J Acquir Immune Defic Syndr 3:472–479, 1990.

62. Orellana J, Lieberman RM, Peairs R, Restreppo S: Intravitreal therapy with ganciclovir for posterior pole cytomegalovirus retinitis in AIDS patients. [Letter] Br J Ophthalmol 74:511, 1990.

63. Heinemann MH: Long-term intravitreal ganciclovir therapy for cytomegalovirus retinopathy. Arch Ophthalmol 107:1767–1772, 1989.

64. Cantrill HL, Henry K, Melroe NH, et al: Treatment of cytomegalovirus retinitis with intravitreal ganciclovir. Long-term results. Ophthalmology 96:367–374, 1989.

65. Buchi ER, Fitting PL, Michel AE: Long-term intravitreal ganciclovir for cytomegalovirus retinitis in a patient with AIDS. Case report. Arch Ophthalmol 106:1349–1350, 1988.

66. Ussery F III, Gibson SR, Conklin RH, et al: Intravitreal ganciclovir in the treatment of AIDS-associated cytomegalovirus retinitis. Ophthalmology 95:640–648, 1988.

67. Daikos GL, Pulido J, Kathpalia SB, Jackson GG: Intravenous and intraocular ganciclovir for CMV retinitis in patients with AIDS or chemotherapeutic immunosuppression. Br J Ophthalmol 72:521–524, 1988.

68. Henry K, Cantrill H, Fletcher C, et al: Use of intravitreal ganciclovir (dihydroxy propoxymethyl guanine) for cytomegalovirus retinitis in a patient with AIDS. Am J Ophthalmol 103:17–23, 1987.

69. Cochereau-Massin I, Lehoang P, Lautier-Frau M, et al: Efficacy and tolerance of intravitreal ganciclovir in cytomegalovirus retinitis in acquired immune deficiency syndrome. Ophthalmology 98:1348–1355, 1991.

70. Grossberg HS, Bonnem EM, Buhles WC: GM-CSF with ganciclovir for the treatment of CMV retinitis in AIDS. N Engl J Med 320:1560, 1989.

71. Stevens G, Palestine AG, Rodrigues MM, et al: Failure of argon laser to halt cytomegalovirus retinitis. Retina 6:119–122, 1986.

72. Chou SW, Dylewski JS, Gaynon MW, et al: Alpha-interferon administration in cytomegalovirus retinitis. Antimicrob Agents Chemother 25:25–28, 1984.

73. Macher AM, Bardenstein DS, Zimmerman LE, et al: *Pneumocystis carinii* choroiditis in a male homosexual with AIDS and disseminated pulmonary and extrapulmonary *P. carinii* infection. [Letter] N Engl J Med 316:1092, 1987.

74. Hagopian WA, Huseby JS: *Pneumocystis* hepatitis and choroiditis despite successful aerosolized pentamidine pulmonary prophylaxis. Chest 96:949–951, 1989.

75. Koser MW, Jampol LM, MacDonell K: Treatment of *Pneumocystis carinii* choroidopathy. Arch Ophthalmol 108:1214–1215, 1990.

76. Dugel PU, Rao NA, Forster DJ, et al: *Pneumocystis carinii* choroiditis after long-term aerosolized pentamidine therapy. Am J Ophthalmol 110:113–117, 1990.

77. Freeman WR, Gross JG, Labelle J, et al: *Pneumocystis carinii* choroidopathy. A new clinical entity. Arch Ophthalmol 107:863–867, 1989.

78. Rao NA, Zimmerman PL, Boyer D, et al: A clinical, histopathologic, and electron microscopic study of *Pneumocystis carinii* choroiditis. Am J Ophthalmol 107:218–228, 1989.

79. Rosenblatt MA, Cunningham C, Teich SA, Friedman AH: Choroidal lesions in patients with AIDS. Br J Ophthalmol 74:610–614, 1990.

80. Hardy WD, Northfelt DW, Drake TA: Fatal, disseminated *Pneumocystis* in a patient with acquired immunodeficiency syndrome receiving prophylactic aerosolized pentamidine. N Engl J Med 322:936–937, 1989.

81. Carney MD, Combs JL, Waschler W: Cryptococcal choroiditis. Retina 10:27–32, 1990.

82. Winward KE, Hamed LM, Glaser JS: The spectrum of optic nerve disease in human immunodeficiency virus infection. Am J Ophthalmol 107:373–380, 1989.

83. Blodi BA, Johnson MW, McLeish WM, Gass JD: Presumed choroidal tuberculosis in a human immunodeficiency virus infected host. Am J Ophthalmol 108:605–607, 1989.

84. Passo MS, Rosenbaum JT: Ocular syphilis in patients with human immunodeficiency virus infection. Am J Ophthalmol 106:1–6, 1988.

85. McLeish WM, Pulido JS, Holland S, et al: The ocular manifestations of syphilis in the human immunodeficiency virus type 1–infected host. Ophthalmology 97:196–203, 1990.

86. Levy JH, Liss RA, Maguire AM: Neurosyphilis and ocular syphilis in patients with concurrent human immunodeficiency virus infection. Retina 9:175–180, 1989.

87. Stoumbos VD, Klein ML: Syphilitic retinitis in a patient with acquired immunodeficiency syndrome–related complex. Am J Ophthalmol 103:103–104, 1987.

88. Carter JB, Hamill RJ, Matoba AY: Bilateral syphilitic optic neuritis in a patient with a positive test for HIV. Arch Ophthalmol 105:1485–1486, 1987.

89. Kleiner RC, Najarian L, Levenson J, Kaplan HJ: AIDS complicated by syphilis can mimic uveitis and Crohn's disease. Arch Ophthalmol 105:1486–1487, 1987.

90. Centers for Disease Control: Recommendations for diagnosing and treating syphilis in HIV-infected patients. MMWR 37:600–608, 1988.

91. Willerson D Jr, Aaberg TM, Reeser FH: Necrotizing vaso-occlusive retinitis. Am J Ophthalmol 84:209–219, 1977.

92. Young NJA, Bird AC: Bilateral acute retinal necrosis. Br J Ophthalmol 62:581–590, 1978.

93. Fisher JP, Lewis ML, Blumenkranz M, et al: The acute retinal necrosis syndrome. Part 1. Clinical manifestations. Ophthalmology 89:1309–1316, 1982.

94. Sternberg P Jr, Knox DL, Finkelstein D, et al: Acute retinal necrosis syndrome. Retina 2:145–151, 1982.

95. Fabricius EM, Lipp T, Kaboth W: Acute retinal necrosis and herpes encephalitis. The key role of the ophthalmologist in diagnosing opportunistic infections in AIDS, successful therapy with acyclovir (Zovirax). [German, English abstract] Klin Monatsbl Augenheilkd 196:160–165, 1990.

96. Chess J, Marcus DM: Zoster-related bilateral acute retinal necrosis syndrome as presenting sign in AIDS. Ann Ophthalmol 20:431–435, 438, 1988.

97. Forster DJ, Dugel PU, Frangieh GT, et al: Rapidly progressive outer retinal necrosis in the acquired immunodeficiency syndrome. Am J Ophthalmol 110:341–348, 1990.

98. Margolis TP, Lowder CY, Holland GN, et al: Varicella-zoster virus retinitis in patients with the acquired immunodeficiency syndrome. Am J Ophthalmol 112:119–131, 1991.

99. Bottoni F, Gonnella P, Autelitano A, Orzalesi N: Diffuse necrotizing retinochoroiditis in a child with AIDS and toxoplasmic encephalitis. Graefes Arch Clin Exp Ophthalmol 228:36–39, 1990.

100. Dennehy PJ, Warman R, Flynn JT, et al: Ocular manifestations in pediatric patients with acquired immunodeficiency syndrome. Arch Ophthalmol 107:978–982, 1989.

101. Hansen LL, Nieuwenhuis I, Hoffken G, Heise W: Retinitis in AIDS patients: Diagnosis, follow-up and treatment. [German, English abstract] Fortschr Ophthalmol 86:232–238, 1989.

102. Holland GN, Engstrom RE Jr, Glasgow BJ, et al: Ocular toxoplasmosis in patients with the acquired immunodeficiency syndrome. Am J Ophthalmol 106:653–667, 1988.

103. Heinemann MH, Gold JM, Maisel J: Bilateral toxoplasma retinochoroiditis in a patient with acquired immune deficiency syndrome. Retina 6:224–227, 1986.

104. Parke D, Font RL: Diffuse toxoplasmic retinochoroiditis in a patient with AIDS. Arch Ophthalmol 104:571–575, 1986.

105. Friedman AH: The retinal lesions of the acquired immune deficiency syndrome. Trans Am Ophthalmol Soc 82:447–491, 1984.

106. Lipson BK, Freeman WR, Beniz J, et al: Optic neuropathy associated with cryptococcal arachnoiditis in AIDS patients. Am J Ophthalmol 107:523–527, 1989.

107. Freeman WR, Henderly DE, Wan WL, et al: Prevalence, pathophysiology, and treatment of rhegmatogenous retinal detachment in treated cytomegalovirus retinitis. Am J Ophthalmol 103:527–536, 1987.

108. Jabs DA, Enger C, Haller J, deBustros S: Retinal detachments in patients with cytomegalovirus retinitis. Arch Ophthalmol 109:794–799, 1991.

109. Dugel PU, Liggett PE, Lee MB, et al: Repair of retinal detachment caused by cytomegalovirus retinitis in patients with the acquired immunodeficiency syndrome. Am J Ophthalmol 112:235–242, 1991.
110. Freeman WR, Wiley CA, Gross JG, et al: Endoretinal biopsy in immunosuppressed and healthy patients with retinitis. Indi-cations, utility, and techniques. Ophthalmology 96:1559–1565, 1989.
111. Schneiderman TE, Faber DW, Gross JG, et al: The agar-albumin sandwich technique for processing retinal biopsy specimens. Am J Ophthalmol 108:567–571, 1989.

Chapter 78

▪

Acute Retinal Necrosis

MARK S. BLUMENKRANZ, JAY S. DUKER, and
DONALD J. D'AMICO

Acute retinal necrosis (ARN) is a clinical syndrome consisting of the presence of vitreous inflammation, retinal periarteritis, optic neuropathy, and confluent peripheral necrotizing retinal infiltrates.[1–7] Initially described in Japan in 1971 by Uryama and colleagues and termed *Kirisawa's uveitis,* the disease has only recently been documented to represent the consequences of acute infection of the retina and associated ocular tissues by certain types of Herpesvirus hominis.[8, 9] The demonstration of a viral cause for this disease led to the development of specific pharmacologic therapies, although late retinal detachment continues to be a serious complication. Modern vitreoretinal surgical techniques have improved the prognosis for retinal reattachment and visual improvement.[13] Prompt treatment with antiviral agents and prophylactic retinal photocoagulation may lessen the risk of disease in the fellow eye and the incidence of late retinal detachment in the initially involved eye.[14, 15] Experimental animal studies have shed further light on the mode of viral transmission between the eye and the central nervous system and the contribution of immunoregulatory events to the pathophysiology of this disease.[16, 17] In selected instances in which optic neuropathy is a conspicuous feature, optic nerve sheath decompression may be of value.[18]

EPIDEMIOLOGY

Initially described in Asia,[1] ARN has now been documented in Europe[3, 19–21] and North America.[4–9] Prevalence data are not available for this disease, but the incidence does appear to be rising. There were no reported cases prior to 1971, although it now seems likely that previously cases either were not recognized or were misclassified as other forms of posterior uveitis. By 1982, there were 41 cases reported in the world literature,[6] and by 1991 more than 80 articles were devoted to the subject.[22]

The disease affects both men and women and adults and children, although it is more common in the former of each group. In one report, 63 percent of patients were male and 37 percent were female; none was younger than 13 yr of age.[6] The disease may affect one or both eyes, with the initial presentation being unilateral in approximately two thirds of cases.[6, 19] When involvement is bilateral, there is generally a delay between involvement of the first and second eyes, ranging on average from 1 to 6 wk.[6, 19] This is consistent with theories on the propagation and transfer of virus from one eye to the other via the optic nerve and central nervous system.[16, 17] Delays as long as 12 yr between involvement of the first and the second eyes have been reported in patients not treated with acyclovir.[10, 19, 23] The risk of development of disease in the fellow eye in patients not treated with intravenous acyclovir has been estimated to be as high as 65 percent 2 yr after the onset of the disease.[14]

The disease was initially described in healthy patients,[1–10] and immunocompetence was judged to be one criterion for establishing this diagnosis.[10] This characteristic distinguished ARN from other forms of opportunistic retinitis in patients with competent immune systems or in those with concurrent herpetic disease of the central nervous system.[24, 25] Subsequent reports have documented that immunosuppressed patients may experience ocular disease that is identical to that seen in classic ARN and is readily distinguished from other forms of opportunistic retinitis, including cytomegalovirus (CMV) inclusion disease.[26, 28]

HOST FACTORS

Most cases of ARN probably represent primary infection of the retina with virus reactivated from dormant sites, including ganglionic tissue. Serum neutralizing antibodies to the herpes zoster varicella virus group are present in up to 95 percent of adults,[8, 29] and it is likely that host factors predispose certain individuals to the development of clinical disease. For example, although in excess of 3 million persons each year experience chickenpox, to date there have been fewer than 10 patients reported with ARN as a short-term complication of varicella.[30–32] Similarly, although ARN has been reported to occur as an early complication of herpes zoster in a small number of patients, this is also thought to be an extremely infrequent problem.[33, 34] In one prospective randomized series of patients with herpes zoster ophthalmicus, none of the 71 patients treated with either acyclovir or placebo experienced ARN, although in other large series, 10 to 33 percent of patients with herpes zoster ophthalmicus demonstrated other forms of viral dissemination.[35] It is possible that patients who experience ARN may have an underlying immunogenetic predisposition to the disease. Holland and associates demonstrated a statistically significant increase in the frequency of HLA-DQw7 (55 percent) in patients with ARN versus control patients without ARN (19 percent) ($P < .0004$; relative risk, 5.2). In this study, the HLA phenotype Bw62,DR4 was also more frequent than in normal control populations (16 percent versus 2.6 percent; relative risk, 7.49).[36]

In addition to differences in underlying genetic predisposition, there is evidence that other host factors and viral factors may play a role in the development of ARN and an unfavorable clinical outcome. Patients with diffuse retinal arteritis, reduced electroretinographic a- and b-waves, elevated levels of circulating immune complex, and larger zones of necrosis and exudation are reported to have an especially unfavorable prognosis.[37]

CLINICAL FEATURES

Although the most dramatic and visually devastating aspect of this disease is the confluent necrotizing retinitis from which it draws its name, most ocular tissues are concurrently affected. The disease can be divided into two different phases: (1) the *acute herpetic phase,* which lasts approximately 4 to 8 wk, and (2) the *late cicatricial phase,* occurring 4 to 8 wk after the onset of the disease and characterized by organization of the vitreous and the development of large retinal tears, retinal detachment, and proliferative vitreoretinopathy.

Disease Types

Increased awareness and recognition of ARN have enabled clinicians to make increasingly subtle distinctions between the "classic" form of the disease initially described by Uryama and colleagues in healthy adults, presumably caused by the herpes zoster varicella virus group,[1] and other disease variants. These variants include a "mild form which is more indolent in character and not associated with retinal detachment"[38] and a severe, rapidly progressive form seen in immunosuppressed patients, which is distinct from CMV retinitis.[39, 40] Moreover, there is some evidence to suggest that the disease course and clinical profile of patients with this syndrome may differ, depending on whether the causative agent is herpes simplex virus or the herpes zoster varicella virus group.[9, 40]

Acute Herpetic Phase

PRESENTING SYMPTOMS

The onset of ARN is frequently heralded by the development of ocular pain, diminished vision, floaters, and external ocular injection. The patient may give a history of recent or remote herpes zoster or varicella infection in the majority of cases or may occasionally volunteer no history of prior herpetic infection.

ANTERIOR SEGMENT EXAMINATION

The conjunctiva is invariably injected with limbal flush, episcleritis, or scleritis. Anterior chamber cell and flare are frequent in conjunction with granulomatous, keratinous precipitates (Fig. 78–1). Although a plasmoid aqueous or mild fibrin strands may be seen, iris nodules or hypopyon is rare. One clinical feature that may assist in the differentiation of the early phases of ARN from other causes of acute granulomatous anterior uveitis is the frequent occurrence of ocular hypertension, which is also seen in herpes zoster keratouveitis. Herpetic corneal epithelial dendrites or disciform corneal lesions are not encountered, although some patients with concurrent herpes zoster ophthalmicus may demonstrate typical vesicular lesions in the distribution of the affected fifth dermatome. The lens is typically unaffected aside from the presence of inflammatory precipitates on its surfaces, which are responsive to steroid therapy. If untreated, posterior synechiae and pupillary seclusion may occur in addition to complicated cataract.

VITREOUS EXAMINATION

Vitreous cellular infiltration and protein exudation are characteristic features of the acute phases of the disease. In the earliest stages, the inflammatory infiltrate in the vitreous may be relatively mild, increasing as cellular

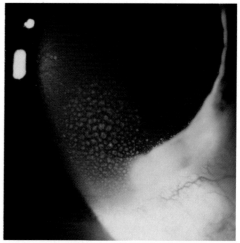

Figure 78–1. Granulomatous keratic precipitates seen in a slit-lamp photomicrograph of a middle-aged man with the early phases of acute retinal necrosis (ARN).

immunity to the virus develops. The vitreous cellular infiltrate is composed predominantly of mononuclear cells, including lymphocytes and plasma cells, paralleling the infiltrates seen in other ocular tissues.[8] A viral cytopathic effect has been obtained from culture of vitreous specimens obtained at the time of enucleation in the acute phase of the disease.[8, 12, 40] Polyclonal anti–herpes simplex virus antibodies have been identified from vitrectomy specimens in patients with the active phase of the disease.[11] Aqueous specimens from patients with the disease similarly demonstrate antibodies to both herpes simplex virus, type 1 and the herpes zoster varicella virus group in ratios suggesting local intraocular antibody production.[8, 11, 12, 40]

RETINA EXAMINATION

Retinal involvement consists of two characteristic features: (1) confluent zones of opaque necrotizing retinitis predominantly involving the periphery and (2) generalized retinal arteritis associated with capillary vasoocclusion.

Necrotizing Retinitis

The earliest retinal lesions are subtle, isolated outer retinal opacities that may assume a patchy, granular or nummular configuration, depending on their stage of evolution. Although usually seen in the midperiphery and preequatorial regions, small nummular lesions may also be seen in the posterior retina, generally sparing the macula (Fig. 78–2). In distinction from the granular white dots frequently associated with cytomegalic inclusion disease of the retina, the early retinal lesions of ARN are not prominently associated with venules or perivenous hemorrhage (Fig. 78–2). With progression of the disease, the granular and nummular lesions increase in size and coalesce to form confluent zones of full-thickness retinal necrosis. These lesions, which are typically situated in the retinal periphery, may occupy

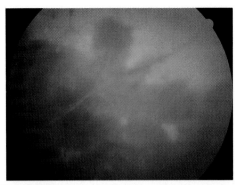

Figure 78–3. Typical lesion of ARN involving the periphery. Note the confluent white-yellow appearance with irregular scalloped posterior margin and sharp transition between involved and noninvolved portions.

as little as 1 to 2 clock hours or may extend to completely encircle the retina over 360 degrees (Fig. 78–3). The mature lesions have a yellow to white homogeneous color with a somewhat jagged or dentate posterior border in portions extending more posteriorly (Fig. 78–4). They obstruct visualization of the underlying retinal pigment epithelium and choroid. The lesions end abruptly at the ora serrata anteriorly and do not appear to parallel or otherwise respect the retinal vasculature, as is frequently seen in cytomegalic inclusion disease. The retinal lesions, which are seen early in the disease, arise abruptly and may progress in size and number over approximately a 2-wk period in untreated patients. The lesions then begin a period of regression characterized by loss of retinal opacification, thinning, and pigmentary scarring (Fig. 78–5). The loss of opacification, which correlates with the resolution of the inflammatory and viral infiltration of the retina, may initially be seen as perivascular curvilinear lucencies within zones of confluent necrosis. This has been termed a *Swiss cheese* appearance (Fig. 78–6).[10] Over the course of several ensuing weeks, these zones of retinal lucency enlarge in conjunction with the development of pigmentary changes in the RPE and the neural retina.

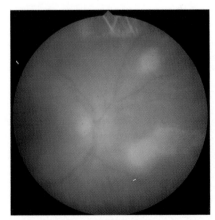

Figure 78–2. Nummular lesion of ARN superonasal and inferonasal to the optic nerve in a middle-aged man with associated herpes zoster involving the upper extremity.

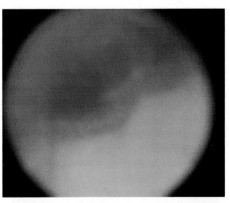

Figure 78–4. Area of confluent necrotizing retinitis with early depigmentation at the posterior margin signifying the beginning of resolution phase.

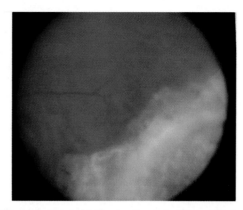

Figure 78–5. The same region as shown in Figure 78–4, approximately 4 mo later demonstrating clearing of ocular media opacity and better visualization of retinal vascular detail. Note the atrophic pigmented zone corresponding to the area of prior necrosis with some fibroglial proliferative change overlying the center of scar.

The pigmentary changes that characterize the convalescent phase of ARN are most prominent initially at the posterior margins of the lesions and progress outward in a centrifugal fashion coincident with the development of lucencies. The character of the pigmentary response associated with the resolution of ARN is similar to that associated with other forms of viral retinitis, including rubella and CMV, and is distinct from either the heavily pigmented hyperplastic response typical of toxoplasmosis or the atrophic scalloped appearance associated with presumed ocular histoplasmosis. In zones in which there has been particularly severe retinal inflammation and underlying choroidal inflammation, the degree of postnecrotic thinning and pigment epithelial atrophy may be prominent. In other zones in which the necrotizing retinitis was more mild, it may be difficult to identify the original margins of involvement in the later phases of the disease. In some instances, the acute phase of the disease may be accompanied by the development of a peripheral exudative retinal detachment. This may be distinguished from a rhegmatogenous or complex detachment by the lack of retinal holes, its

presence beneath areas of opaque retina, and the presence of shifting subretinal fluid or xanthochromia.

Retinal Vasculitis

The second major feature of retinal involvement in this disorder is the development of severe vasoocclusive changes predominantly involving the arterial system. The presence of arteritis, rather than phlebitis, and the associated peripheral vasoocclusion seen in this disease help to distinguish it from CMV infection of the retina on ophthalmoscopic grounds. Although occasionally seen in ocular toxoplasmosis and syphilis, retinal arteritis is particularly striking and severe in ARN and was recognized to be a characteristic feature of herpes zoster infection of the retina even prior to the widespread recognition of this syndrome in the English literature (Fig. 78–7; see also Fig. 78–4).[43] Fluorescein angiographic and histopathologic studies on eyes with ARN confirm that the arteritis is not confined to the retinal vessels and may be seen in virtually all tissues studied, including the iris, ciliary body, choroid, and optic nerve. The ophthalmoscopic features of retinal periarteritis include opacification and refractile changes in the walls of the larger retinal arterioles, ophthalmoscopically visible nonperfusion and obliteration of the smaller more distal ramifications, and retinal capillary nonperfusion as best demonstrated by fluorescein angiography. The retinal opacification seen in this syndrome is distinct from the cloudy swelling commonly associated with retinal arteriole obstruction, although the latter may contribute to this phenomenon in addition to the cellular infiltration seen histopathologically.[2] Despite the presence of peripheral retinal capillary nonperfusion, retinal, optic nerve, and iris neovascularization are distinctly uncommon in this disease, as contrasted with other forms of vasoocclusive retinopathy.[44, 45] The reasons for this are unknown but may reflect the concurrent development of retinal and pigment epithelial necrosis in conjunction with nonperfusion, resulting in a lessened angiogenic stimulus. Although large zones of intraretinal hemorrhage are not a characteristic feature of ARN,

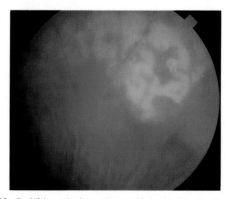

Figure 78–6. Midresolution phase of ARN with development of curvilinear perivascular lucencies within zones of necrosis prior to the development of late pigmentary changes (Swiss cheese appearance).

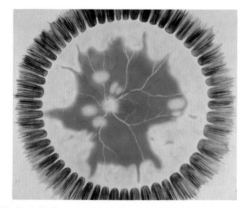

Figure 78–7. Artist's representation of a patient with the classic features of ARN, including confluent necrotizing retinitis, posterior nummular infiltrates, and retinal arteritis (with involved vessels seen in yellow).

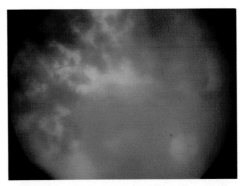

Figure 78–8. A patient with confirmed herpes zoster infection of the retina producing ARN. Note the prominent hemorrhagic component suggestive of concomitant retinal venous obstruction.

they may occur in patients in association with zones of phlebitis or venous occlusion. Rarely, the fundus appearance may be that of a combined central retinal artery and vein occlusion when there has been severe involvement of the optic nerve and associated vasculature (Fig. 78–8).

CHOROIDAL INVOLVEMENT

The choroidal vasculature is actively involved in this disease. Prior to the development of opaque confluent retinal lesions, it is possible to identify more subtle opacifications in the outer retina and underlying choroid and pigment epithelium. Early-frame angiograms document the presence of focal areas of choroidal hypoperfusion with intense late staining suggestive of infiltration and ischemia (Fig. 78–9). These frequently presage overlying zones of necrotizing retinitis. In histopathologic specimens, the choroidal thickness may be increased three- to fourfold in conjunction with diffuse plasma, cell, macrophagic, and lymphocytic stromal infiltrates and perivascular cuffing (Fig. 78–10). To date, despite the marked inflammatory changes seen in the choroid, herpesvirus particles have not been identified by either electron microscopy or culture, suggesting that the choroidal changes are immunocytopathologic.

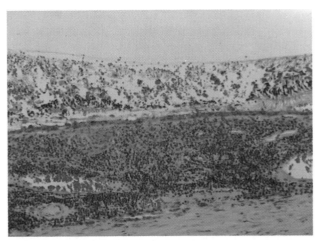

Figure 78–10. Histopathologic specimen demonstrating marked choroidal stromal thickening and lymphocytic infiltration including larger choroidal vessels. H&E, ×100.

OPTIC NERVE

Optic neuropathy is a frequent and serious complication of ARN. Some degree of optic disc swelling is seen in most cases (Fig. 78–11) and may be associated with engorgement of the disc capillaries, swelling of the neural tissue, and distention of the optic nerve sheath.[18, 46] In some instances, this may result in profound vision loss. The mechanism of vision loss associated with optic neuropathy remains somewhat uncertain. It may reflect one of multiple causes, including direct viral infection of the optic nerve,[9, 16, 17] optic nerve ischemia secondary to vasoocclusion,[6, 8] or the result of compression by distention of the nerve sheath.[18, 46] Optic nerve sheath fenestration has been proposed as a method of therapy for patients who demonstrate optic nerve sheath distention by neuroradiologic imaging studies. This has been associated with dramatic visual improvement in some instances. In one clinical series, 47 percent of eyes in patients with ARN demonstrated neuropathy severe enough to warrant consideration of

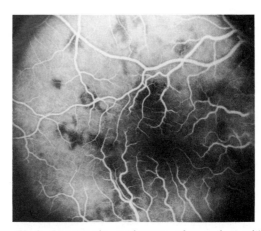

Figure 78–9. Fluorescein angiogram of a patient with ARN. (Courtesy of Jay Duker.)

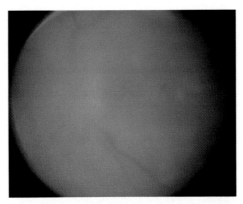

Figure 78–11. Photograph of severe optic nerve involvement in a patient with ARN. Visual acuity is reduced to light perception despite the lack of obvious macular involvement. Media opacity secondary to vitritis is not consistent with the level of vision dysfunction.

surgical intervention.[46] Similar to patients with other forms of ischemic and inflammatory optic neuropathy, some patients with optic neuropathy associated with ARN may demonstrate considerable improvement in macular function in response to medical or surgical therapy. Optic neuropathy in ARN that is sufficiently severe to warrant consideration of surgical optic nerve sheath decompression has been defined as (1) the presence of an afferent pupillary defect not consistent with retinal findings, (2) poor correlation between retinal findings and visual acuity and visual field, and (3) sudden deterioration of visual acuity not corresponding to retinal changes.[46]

Cicatricial Phase

With or without therapy, ARN appears to be a self-limited disease, with resolution of the acute inflammatory changes occurring over the course of 1 to 3 mo, depending on the severity of the initial infection and other factors. Following resolution of the active phase of the disease, secondary cicatricial changes occur, which frequently lead to development of late retinal tears, retinal detachment, and loss of useful visual function. The phase of active viral replication is thought to be controlled by normal host humoral and cellular immune mechanisms. In patients not treated with oral acyclovir, corticosteroids, or other pharmacologic agents, the time course for resolution of the acute phase may be 6 to 12 wk. In patients treated with oral acyclovir, this phase may be shortened to 4 to 6 wk, although to date no prospective randomized studies confirming this have been performed.[10] It is thought that the breakdown in the blood-ocular barrier and secondary cellular and humoral infiltration of the vitreous contribute to the development of late organizational changes in the vitreous body. Collagenous and cellular membranes composed of pigment epithelial cells and fibroblastic ele-

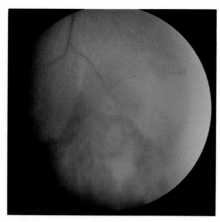

Figure 78–13. Large tear in the inferior posterior retina of a patient with ARN.

ments develop.[19, 47] Additionally, secondary growth of pigment epithelial, glial, and fibroblastic membranes on the surface of the retina and continuous with the organized vitreal membranes occurs in the periphery. The concurrence of peripheral retinal thinning, membrane formation, and vitreous contraction contributes to the development of severe proliferative vitreoretinopathy frequently seen in patients in the cicatricial stages of ARN (Figs. 78–12 to 78–14). Irrespective of acyclovir therapy, late retinal detachment occurs in 75 to 86 percent of eyes with ARN.[6, 10] Prophylactic photocoagulation during the acute phase of the disease may reduce this risk in some patients.[12, 15] Although retinal detachment in this condition has previously been associated with a generally unfavorable prognosis,[3–7] more recent advances in vitreoretinal surgical therapy have improved the outlook (see Management of Retinal Detachment). Other late cicatricial complications of this disease include iris atrophy, cataract, ciliary body fibrosis and hyposecretion, visually significant vitreous opacities, and macular pucker.

Disease Variants

In addition to the "classic" form of this disease, patients may exhibit both more benign and more ful-

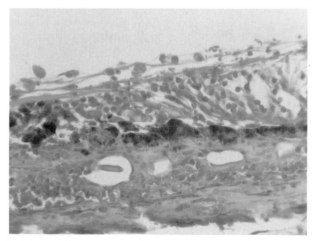

Figure 78–12. Zone of retinal pigment epithelial proliferation and migration underlying thinned necrotic peripheral retina. Note the presence of nonpigmented epiretinal membrane on the surface of the necrotic retina. H&E, × 250.

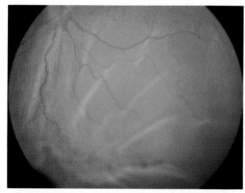

Figure 78–14. Retinal folds in stage C2 proliferative vitreoretinopathy associated with ARN. Note the pigmented epiretinal membranes in the lower left corner of this photograph.

minant variants. Matsuo and coworkers described six patients with isolated midperipheral nonconfluent retinal infiltrates and serologic evidence of herpes zoster varicella infection in whom disease did not progress to retinal detachment. The role of early acyclovir treatment of these patients in the prevention of more severe phases of the disease is unclear.[37] More indolent forms of the disease have also been reported in patients with varicella.[30–32] Varicella-associated ARN appears to be limited predominantly to adults rather than to children who contract the disease, with five of six reported patients being 26 yr of age or greater. In contrast, more than 90 percent of all cases of varicella affect persons between the ages of 1 and 14 yr.[48] Varicella-associated retinal necrosis is thought to occur within 1 mo of the onset of primary infection (ranging from 5 to 28 days), to be limited primarily to adults, to involve fewer quadrants, to have less vitritis, and infrequently to lead to retinal detachment.[30]

ARN has also been associated with cutaneous herpes zoster, reflecting reactivation of latent virus rather than primary disease as in varicella. In contrast to varicella-associated ARN, patients with herpes zoster–associated ARN demonstrate typical features, including confluent peripheral necrosis, severe vitritis, optic nerve involvement, and late retinal detachment.[33, 34] The time interval between cutaneous eruption and ARN ranges from 5 days to 3 mo and has been unilateral in eight of nine cases reported to date. Slightly less than half of cases reported to date have involved cranial nerves V or VII, with the remainder of sites being remote from the eye.

Although typical ARN has been reported in immunocompromised patients, including those with AIDS,[26–28] a subgroup of patients experience a more fulminant, rapidly progressive form of the disease, distinct from either CMV retinitis or typical ARN and consistent with herpes zoster infection of the retina. This syndrome, termed *rapidly progressive outer retinal necrosis,* has been seen exclusively in patients with AIDS and is associated with an unfavorable outcome. This syndrome is characterized by primary involvement of the outer retina, with sparing of the inner retina and retinal vasculature until later in the disease. Patients exhibit a fulminant downhill course, with optic atrophy, lesser degrees of vitreal and choroidal inflammation, and a poor response to acyclovir therapy.[38, 39] Not all patients with AIDS and ARN demonstrate this variant, and further clinical experience will help to define underlying factors that predispose to the development of this condition.

PATHOPHYSIOLOGY

Viral Etiology

Although initial reports noted the similarities between the clinical findings of ARN and those of both Behçet's disease and certain viral infections, the viral etiology of the disorder was not definitively established until 1982.[8] Several lines of evidence implicate the Herpesvirus hominis class of viral retinal infection as the cause of this syndrome. These data include direct viral culture,[8, 9, 49] detection of viral antigens in intraocular fluid specimens by direct or indirect immunofluorescence,[27, 50] elevated or serially increasing intraocular or serum antibody titers to herpesviruses,[41, 51, 52] immunocytochemical staining of viral antigens in fixed tissue from biopsy or enucleation specimens,[8, 39, 53, 54] Herpesvirus hominis particles in glutaraldehyde-fixed retinal tissue,[8, 10, 38, 39, 53] herpesvirus antigens amplified by polymerase chain reaction,[38] and clinical disease coincident with or immediately following herpes infection in other sites.[30–34] Several members of the Herpesvirus hominis family have been implicated in the pathogenesis of this disease, including the herpes zoster varicella virus group,[8, 39, 49, 53] herpes simplex, types 1 and 2,[9, 40–42, 51] and in one instance, CMV.[54] The herpes zoster varicella virus group is thought to account for the majority of cases and the typical syndrome.

Herpesvirus hominis viruses, although exhibiting different immunocytochemical staining characteristics, appear morphologically similar by electron microscopy. The herpes zoster varicella viruses are relatively large, measuring approximately 150 to 200 nm when fully enveloped by an outer lipid coat with a central core of double-stranded DNA measuring approximately 100 nm. The central core is covered by an icosahedral capsid composed of 162 tubular capsomers, which in turn, are covered by the lipid bilayered envelope. The DNA contains approximately 125,000 base pairs and weighs 80 megadaltons. At least five families of varicella-zoster virus glycoproteins have been identified by immunochemical studies that represent the primary markers for both humoral and cell-mediated immunity (Figs. 78–15 and 78–16). The varicella-zoster virus group is highly cell-associated and spreads from cell to cell by direct contact. These viruses are fastidious and are difficult to culture, having been successfully transferred from ocular specimens to human embryonal lung fibroblasts and human embryonal kidney cells in vitro.[8, 29, 55]

Herpes simplex virus, types 1 and 2 are responsible for oral and genital ulcerations in humans. The virus, which appears structurally similar to the herpes zoster varicella virus group by transmission electron microscopy, is transmitted by direct contact between skin surfaces and mucous membranes. The virus consists of four major components: a centrally located core surrounded by three concentric structures—capsid, tegumen, and envelope. The core contains DNA coiled around proteins. The capsid (162 capsomers) is a tubular structure measuring approximately 100 nm, and the tegumen is composed of fibrillar material lying between the capsid and the envelope. The fully enveloped particle has an approximate diameter of 150 to 200 nm, with the envelope composed of lipid and protein components conveying the antigenicity of the virus and thereby dictating the host immunologic responses.

Both the herpes zoster varicella virus group and the herpes simplex virus code for two unique herpes-specific enzymes, an isofunctional deoxynucleoside kinase (herpes-specific thymidine kinase) and a herpes-specific DNA polymerase. These enzymes are coded by the herpesvirus genome and are not normally encountered

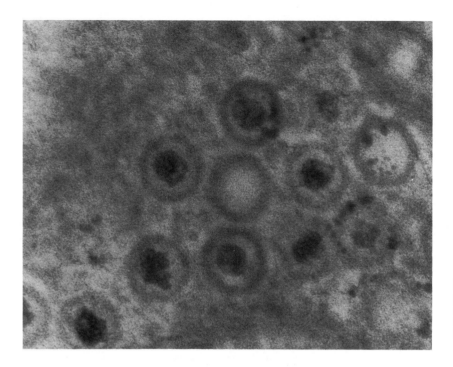

Figure 78–15. Transmission electron micrograph of viral particles in necrotic retina of a middle-aged man with ARN. Note complete and incomplete viral particles, including central nucleocapside and outer lipid envelope. ×87,000.

in mammalian cells.[57] Acyclovir (9[(2-hydroxy-ethoxy) methyl]guanine) is selectively phosphorylated by the herpes-coded thymidine kinase to its monophosphate form. Mammalian cellular enzymes are then capable of converting acyclovir monophosphate to acyclovir triphosphate. This represents the active antiviral form of the drug, which becomes a selective substrate and inhibitor of herpesvirus DNA polymerase. As a result, acyclovir inhibits viral application in two ways: first, by prevention of the incorporation of deoxynucleotide triphosphates into herpesvirus DNA and, second, by the incorporation of altered nucleotide analogs. Since mammalian cells do not contain the virus-specific enzyme that converts acyclovir to its monophosphate form, this sequence of inhibitory events is not initiated in non–virally infected cells, and the drug is therefore relatively nontoxic contrasted with other antiviral agents such as adenine arabinoside (Fig. 78–17).[24, 57]

Histopathology

Histopathologic studies in the acute phases of ARN have been performed on a relatively small number of

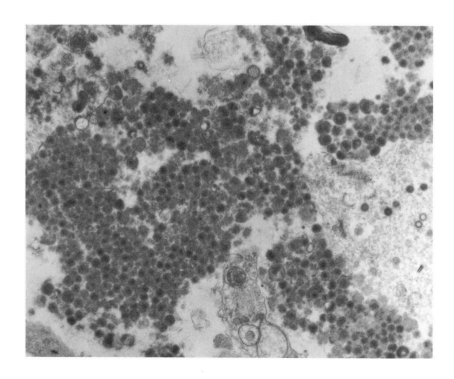

Figure 78–16. Another portion of the retina seen in Figure 78–15 demonstrates a large number of tightly packed viral particles in varying stages of assembly. ×30,000.

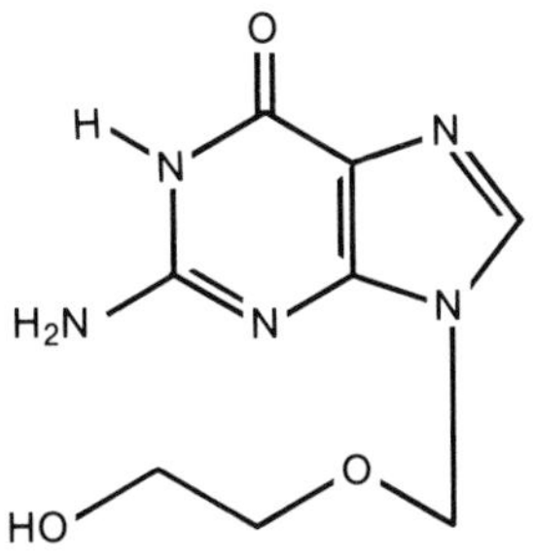

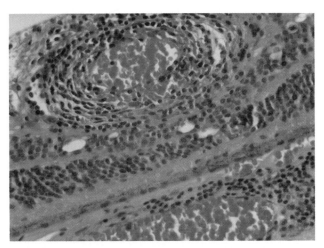

Acyclovir

Figure 78–17. Structural formula of acyclovir, a substituted purine nucleoside that is active against various members of the Herpesvirus hominis family.

Figure 78–18. Histopathologic specimen of thrombotic vascular occlusion in ARN. Note engorgement of the underlying choroidal vessel as well as severe perivascular cuffing and occlusion of the lumen in the vessel by erythrocytes. H&E, ×25.

eyes, either following enucleation or on retinal biopsy specimens taken during vitrectomy.[8, 27, 39, 53, 54] Initial reports based on eyes undergoing either vitrectomy for late retinal detachment or enucleation for intractable pain with chronic retinal detachment demonstrated extensive atrophy and degeneration of the outer retinal layers and pigment epithelium, occlusion of the retinal blood vessels, and massive choroidal lymphocytic infiltration and engorgement. Membranes associated with proliferative vitreoretinopathy demonstrated a prominent pigment epithelial component with intraretinal and subretinal cysts seen and ossification in the subretinal space. No viral particles were identified.[19, 47]

Eyes in the acute phases of the disease show widespread profound changes in virtually all ocular structures. Granulomatous, keratic precipitates line the corneal endothelium, and chronic and acute inflammatory cells infiltrate the iris and ciliary body in which perivascular lymphocytic cuffing is evident in conjunction with focal edema of the iris root and adjacent ciliary muscle. Chronic inflammatory cells are seen infiltrating the sclera, accounting for the pain and scleral injection commonly seen clinically. The histopathologic hallmarks are (1) retinal vasoocclusion, (2) sharply demarcated zones of necrotizing retinitis, (3) choroidal lymphocytic infiltration and thickening, and (4) optic neuropathy.

RETINAL VASOOCCLUSION

Both large- and small-caliber arterioles demonstrate perivascular cuffing, endothelial cell swelling, and fibrinoid or thrombotic occlusion to variable degrees.[17, 18] In some instances, the lumina may be nearly or totally occluded through a combination of endothelial swelling, red blood cell and platelet thrombi, and fibrin (Figs. 78–18 and 78–19). Despite the fact that the retinal and choroidal vascular changes are a conspicuous feature of the disease, to date no viral particles or antigen has been detected within vessel walls, suggesting that the changes seen are immunologically mediated.

CONFLUENT NECROTIZING RETINITIS

Another characteristic feature of ARN is the abrupt demarcation of necrotic and normal retina. Areas of relatively well-preserved retina containing inflammatory infiltrates and hemorrhages in the inner and outer layers may be immediately adjacent to other zones of full-thickness necrosis with partial or complete obliteration of the normal retinal architecture (see Fig. 78–10). High-power views disclose the presence of eosinophilic intranuclear inclusion bodies in infected retinal cells characteristic of herpes. These changes, termed *Cowdry A inclusions*, contain complete and incomplete viral particles and marginally displace the host nuclear chromatin, which is basophilic in H&E-stained sections (see Fig. 78–19). The pigment epithelial proliferation and migration from the normal monolayer through necrotic retina and onto the surface are frequently associated with reactive gliosis and epiretinal membrane formation

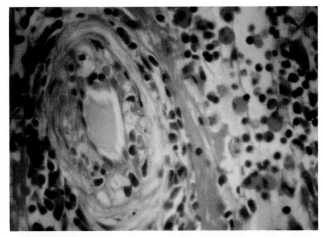

Figure 78–19. Cowdry A intranuclear eosinophilic nuclear inclusions in the retina in a zone of severe necrosis. Note the marked swelling of endothelial cells and the encroachment on lumen by fibrinoid change seen adjacent to a zone of inclusion bodies. H&E, ×400.

(see Fig. 78–12). These represent the sites of future retinal tears in response to contracting preretinal and transvitreal membranes. Pigmented macrophages are commonly encountered, and cytomegaly is not a conspicuous feature.

CHOROIDAL THICKENING AND LYMPHOCYTIC INFILTRATION

Another feature that differentiates ARN from CMV retinitis histologically is the relatively severe thickening and lymphocytic infiltration of the choroid seen in the former condition. The infiltrate is mononuclear, consisting predominantly of lymphocytes and plasma cells with associated occlusion of the choriocapillaris and, to a lesser extent, the larger choroidal vessels. Areas of granulomatous inflammation may be seen, although to date viral particles have not been identified in the choroid.

OPTIC NEUROPATHY

Involvement of the optic nerve is variable, ranging from patchy areas of chronic inflammation along the pia to broad zones of neuronal necrosis, plasma cell infiltration, and vascular occlusion (Fig. 78–20). To date, viral particles have not been identified in the optic nerves available for study, although there is experimental evidence to suggest that transmission from one eye to another in bilateral cases may occur via the optic nerve.[16, 17]

ELECTRON MICROSCOPIC AND IMMUNOCYTOLOGIC FEATURES

Viral particles found within individual retinal cells demonstrate nucleocapsids of 80 to 100 nm, which can be seen undergoing assembly within retinal cell nuclei to form poorly enveloped virus. These measure 150 to 200 nm in diameter and are adherent to retinal cell

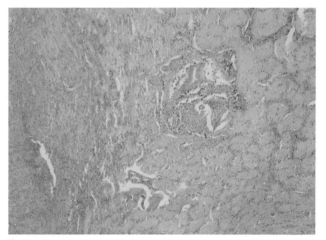

Figure 78–20. Cross section of the optic nerve from a patient with ARN. Note central zone of necrosis. H&E, × 100.

membranes. The virus appears most abundant in the inner retinal layers and in the transition zone between necrotic and preserved retina. In areas of greatest cytopathic effect, there is marked disruption of retinal tissue, with bare nuclei and fragmented cell membranes present. Viral antigens have been identified by immunocytochemical techniques employing a variety of murine monoclonal antibodies and avidin-biotin-peroxidase methods specific for the major GP98/GP62 varicella-zoster glycoprotein complex. Viral antigens have been detected in transitional zones between normal and necrotic retina, pigment epithelial cells, and inner and outer retinal cells, but not in vascular endothelium, choroid, ciliary body, or optic nerve. However, immunoglobulins G and M, fibrinogen, and complement component C3c have been detected in retinal arteriolar walls and in surrounding retinal tissue adjacent to zones of zoster antigens.[53]

Experimental ARN in an Animal Model

Although it is well established that the primary pathogenetic event of ARN is Herpesvirus hominis infection of the retina, a number of issues remain unresolved, including the route of transmission to the eye, the mechanism of bilateral disease in some patients, and the underlying mechanisms responsible for the variability and severity of the disease. The development of a murine model of herpes simplex retinitis has provided some insights into these questions.[16, 17, 58, 59]

It has been shown that intracameral injection of herpes simplex virus, type 1 (KOS strain) in Balb/c mice produces the picture of acute hemorrhagic necrotizing retinitis. Interestingly, the retinitis does not occur in the injected eye but rather in the contralateral (noninjected) eye 9 to 10 days following injection and is completed over the course of 12 to 48 hr.[58, 59] ARN develops only in immunocompetent animals and only when viral titers in the contralateral eye exceed a threshold level (4 $\log_{10}$, PFU [plaque-forming units]). This confirms that viral infection is essential for the development of this syndrome. Following injection into the anterior chamber of one eye, herpes simplex virus reaches the contralateral eye in two waves. The first, which fails to replicate, arrives within 24 hr. The second arrives within 5 to 7 days and reaches the eye after retrograde spread down the optic nerve from the brain. Within 24 to 48 hr of the arrival of the second wave of replicating virus, the characteristic picture of hemorrhagic and necrotizing retinitis develops.[59]

In this murine model, immunologic factors play an important role in the development of ARN. It is known that, paradoxically, immunocompetence is a prerequisite for the development of ARN in several different regards. First, immunoincompetent (athymic) mice do not develop the characteristic fundus picture of ARN, although viral replication takes place in the contralateral eye at a comparable time point and in similar quantity to immunocompetent animals. Second, ARN does not develop unless there is suppression of virus-specific delayed hypersensitivity. This phenomenon is termed *anterior chamber–associated immune deviation* and is genetically determined in certain strains of mice in which humoral antiviral antibody production remains unaffected. These findings are consistent with a report on humans that documented *magnetic resonance imaging* (MRI) evidence of bilateral high-intensity optic tract lesions involving the lateral geniculate ganglia, temporal lobes, and midbrain in a patient with ARN caused by herpes simplex virus. This, along with concurrent generalized malaise and fever, suggests a neural route of spread.[9] Similarly, studies of intraocular and serum antibody responses to herpes simplex and the herpes zoster varicella virus group have been positive and within expected ranges.[20, 41, 42, 50–53]

The requirement for immunocompetence appears to be based on the participation of precursor cytotoxic T cells in the development of retinal necrosis. T cells harvested from lymph nodes ipsilateral to the injected eye and from the contralateral eye proliferate in vitro when exposed to viral antigens and are thought to mediate the destruction of retinal cells infected by herpes simplex virus.[17] It has also been shown that herpes simplex virus–specific effector T cells, when promptly injected into the contralateral eye of animals undergoing intracameral injection of herpes simplex virus, will prevent the development of ARN, although injection of effector cells delayed by more than 1 day after virus injection will not. Moreover, herpes simplex virus, type 1–specific immune effector cells restimulated with virus in vitro are more effective in producing cytotoxicity to herpes simplex virus, type 1–infected target cells than are herpes simplex virus, type 1–specific immune effector cells that are not restimulated.[62]

Host Factors

Although these data provide a theoretical basis for the apparent differences in susceptibility to the development of ARN seen in large populations, as evidenced by HLA markers,[36] as well as the propensity for untreated patients to experience disease in the fellow eye, possibly through optic nerve spread,[6, 8, 9, 18, 39, 46] the initial route of infection of the first eye remains uncertain. Both hematogenous and neural spread have been proposed. A hematogenous mechanism would be most plausible if the disease occurred frequently in association with primary infection, such as during varicella when viremia is prevalent.[29] This is not typically the case, although rare instances have been reported.[30–32] In some patients, however, hematogenous dissemination of virus may occur even during reactivation of latent zoster varicella virus infection. Reactivation of latent viral disease in neural ganglionic tissue and direct cell-to-cell propagation along neural pathways appears more likely based on the well-documented association between herpes zoster and ARN and the available data regarding the natural history and method of propagation of the virus. It is known that in the United States as many as

90 percent of adults show serologic evidence of antibody response to the herpes zoster varicella virus group by adulthood.[29] Moreover, it has been shown that among subjects who tested seropositive for antibody to the herpes zoster varicella virus group on postmortem examination, both viral origin replication and gene 29 sequences could be detected in 87 percent of trigeminal ganglia examined and in 53 percent of thoracic ganglia examined.[63] Farrel and colleagues (personal communication) presented MRI evidence of bilateral trigeminal ganglionitis in a patient with ipsilateral herpes zoster ophthalmicus and concurrent contralateral ARN. It is possible that Herpesvirus hominis, which resides dormantly in various orbital and cranial ganglionic tissue, may become reactivated, propagate, and migrate to the eye, inducing the onset of ARN in response to systemic factors modified by underlying immunogenetic parameters.

DIFFERENTIAL DIAGNOSIS

Ophthalmoscopy

Because of its characteristic fundus appearance, the diagnosis of ARN can be established in the healthy immunocompetent patient on ophthalmoscopic grounds, which include (1) the presence of granulomatous anterior uveitis, (2) vitreous cellular reaction, (3) retinal arteritis, (4) multiple patchy or confluent areas of necrotizing retinitis with or without associated hemorrhage predominantly located in the retinal periphery, and (5) optic disc swelling of variable degree.

The conditions to be considered in the differential diagnosis of ARN are listed in Table 78–1. The clinical syndromes most commonly misdiagnosed as ARN in healthy patients are syphilitic neuroretinitis and acute multifocal hemorrhagic retinal vasculitis.[22, 44] The former can be distinguished on the basis of appropriate serologic testing, and the latter by the presence of a greater degree of retinal hemorrhage, initial venous involvement, and a subsequent clinical course that includes a failure to respond to acyclovir, a failure to experience retinal detachment, and the likelihood of ocular neovascularization. In some instances, the differentiation between ARN and CMV retinitis or toxoplasmic retinochoroiditis may be problematic in immunocompromised patients. Sarcoidosis, *Candida albicans* endophthalmitis, and Behçet's disease can generally be distinguished from

Table 78–1. DIFFERENTIAL DIAGNOSIS OF ACUTE RETINAL NECROSIS

Syphilitic neuroretinitis
Cytomegalovirus retinitis
Toxoplasmic retinochoroiditis
Candida albicans endophthalmitis
Acute multifocal hemorrhagic retinal vasculitis
Behçet's disease
Sarcoidosis
Ocular lymphoblastic lymphoma

ARN by the clinical history. It has been recognized recently that some patients with intraocular lymphoblastic lymphoma may present with retinal hemorrhages, pseudoretinal vasculitis, and infiltrates mimicking ARN.[65]

Laboratory Evaluation

It is recommended that patients with suspected ARN undergo baseline laboratory evaluation to help establish the diagnosis and facilitate treatment. These studies are outlined in Table 78–2. Patients should have a complete blood count, sedimentation rate determination, and basic serologic studies, including rheumatoid factor and antinuclear antibody determinations to exclude systemic vasculitis or coagulopathy. Abnormal platelet hyperaggregation in response to adenosine diphosphate administration has been detected in patients with ARN.[66] In addition to acute and convalescent serum (IgG and IgM) drawn for the herpes zoster varicella virus group, herpes simplex, types 1 and 2, and CMV, consideration should be given to exclusion of HIV positivity, toxoplasmosis, and Lyme disease. Serum creatinine and blood urea nitrogen determinations, as well as urinalysis, should be performed to evaluate the patient's suitability for acyclovir administration, and a chest x-ray study and a purified protein derivative (PPD) test should be performed to exclude the possibility of tuberculous disease, contraindicating the use of oral corticosteroids (see Table 78–2).

Optional studies should be performed in specialized circumstances, including a computed tomography (CT) scan or MRI study in patients who have clinical evidence

Table 78–2. SUGGESTED LABORATORY EVALUATION FOR PATIENTS WITH ARN

Recommended Tests
Complete blood count, sedimentation rate, antinuclear antibody, rheumatoid factor, prothrombin time, partial thromboplastin time,* platelet count, platelet aggregation,† Venereal Disease Research Laboratory test, fluorescent treponemal antibody absorption test, Lyme titer, HIV antibody, antitoxoplasmosis IgG and IgM titers, acute and convalescent immunoglobulins (IgG and IgM) against herpes simplex virus, types 1 and 2, herpes zoster varicella virus group, cytomegalovirus, and Epstein-Barr virus, blood urea nitrogen, creatinine, urine analysis, chest x-ray study, and purified protein derivative

Optional (Special Circumstances)
Computed tomography (CT) scan or magnetic resonance imaging to exclude optic nerve sheath distention in cases with severe vision loss (according to criteria of Sergott and coworkers),[46] lumbar puncture (in cases with systemic symptoms or abnormal CT scan), aqueous tap (for antibody titers to previously noted viruses; polymerase chain reaction technique when available)

Vitrectomy with culture and biopsy in immunocompromised patients, those with therapeutic failure, or atypical disease

Modified from Duker JS, Blumenkranz MS: Diagnosis and management of the acute retinal necrosis syndrome (ARN). Surv Ophthalmol 35:327–343, 1991.
*When available.
†If abnormal obtain screen for lupus anticoagulant factor.

of severe optic nerve dysfunction or central nervous system symptoms such as headache, meningismus, or altered mental status. Patients who demonstrate distention of the optic nerve sheaths may benefit from early surgical decompression.[18, 46] Additionally, MRI evidence (which may be enhanced by gadolinium) of optic nerve tract, ganglionic, or cerebral disease may have an impact on the dosage and duration of acyclovir therapy. Consideration should be given to lumbar puncture in patients with either neurologic symptoms or an abnormal neuroradiologic imaging study (after exclusion of hydrocephalus). Appropriate cerebrospinal cultures, antibodies, and cytologic studies should be performed only in rare instances to exclude other causes of central nervous system disease and retinal infiltration such as syphilis or lymphoblastic lymphoma. When available, assay for detection of aqueous viral antibody or antigen, particularly employing newer polymerase chain reaction techniques,[39, 67] and appropriate recalculations to correct for serum antibody levels by the Goldmann-Wittmer coefficient may be valuable in difficult cases. Rarely, in complex cases such as patients with underlying immunocompromise, atypical findings, or those who are refractory to initial antiviral therapy, diagnostic vitrectomy or retinal biopsy, or both, may be indicated. In addition to conclusively establishing the diagnosis, it may permit testing for antiviral sensitivities.[9, 39, 40, 49, 50] Diagnostic vitrectomy may be combined with therapeutic infusion of intravitreal acyclovir in concentrations of 10 to 40 µg/ml.[11]

CURRENT THERAPY

Current management of ARN consists of five primary components in the acute phase of the disease, in addition to treatment of retinal detachment if it occurs in the cicatricial phases of the disease. These five components include (1) antiviral therapy, (2) antiinflammatory therapy, (3) antithrombotic therapy, (4) retinal detachment prophylaxis, and (5) optic nerve therapy.

Antiviral Therapy

The demonstration of herpesvirus particles in eyes with ARN facilitated the development of more specific treatment regimens. Prior to this finding, treatment consisted primarily of supportive measures, including the use of antiinflammatory agents, oral and intravenous corticosteroid preparations, transfer factor, and rarely, immunosuppressive agents.[1-7] Subsequent to the demonstration of the viral cause of the disease, both intravitreal acyclovir[11] and intravenous acyclovir[10, 14] have been reported to be of benefit in the treatment of this disorder (see Fig. 78–17).

ACYCLOVIR

Acyclovir remains the drug of choice for the initial treatment of ARN and has selective advantages over other purine and pyrimidine nucleoside antimetabolites with antiviral activity in vitro, including phosphonoformate, bromovinyldeoxyuridine, and fluoroiodoaracytosine.[68] Because of the relative sensitivity of the herpes simplex virus (ED_{50} of 0.1 to 1.6 μM), and to a lesser extent the herpes zoster varicella virus group (ED_{50} of 3 to 4 μM) to acyclovir, the drug theoretically is effective in ARN associated with either agent.[57, 68] Because ARN is generally not thought to be caused by strains of CMV, which is typically more resistant to acyclovir (ED_{50} to 200 μM), more toxic agents, including vidarabine[24, 68] and the newer agents ganciclovir[69] and foscarnet,[70] are not generally required.

Following intravenous administration of 5 mg/kg of acyclovir in humans, peak plasma levels of 30 to 40 μM are reached with a half-life of 2 to 4 hr. These levels contrast with a peak concentration of 8.7 μM in the serum, and 3.3 μM in the aqueous humor following five oral 400-mg doses in volunteers undergoing cataract extraction.[71] Because there is a significant correlation between plasma and aqueous concentrations of the drug described by the following formula

$$\text{acyclovir [in aqueous humor (μM)]} = 1.2 + 0.24 \times \text{acyclovir in plasma (μM)}$$

it can be inferred that intraocular concentrations of acyclovir are considerably higher following intravenous administration than after oral administration. At present, initial therapy with intravenous acyclovir for a minimum of 1 wk is recommended. This dosage predicts aqueous concentrations in the noninflamed eye in the range of 9 to 10 μM based on projected serum concentrations of 30 to 40 μM (6.8 to 9.1 μg/ml).[57, 71] Because active viral particles have been identified in eyes with ARN subsequent to intravenous acyclovir therapy,[10] and the greatest period of risk for involvement of the fellow eye is within the first 6 wk after presentation of the first eye, oral acyclovir should be administered at a dosage of 2 to 4 g daily for 4 to 6 wk following completion of intravenous acyclovir as a precautionary measure. The role of oral acyclovir in higher dosage ranges (4 g daily) as an alternate treatment to intravenous acyclovir at present remains unsettled and awaits further study.

Intravenous acyclovir is generally administered at a total dosage of 1500 mg/sq m/day based on calculation of the body index in square meters from the height and weight; 500 mg/sq m/day is administered intravenously every 8 hr. Oral acyclovir is available in capsules of either 200-mg or 800-mg strength, which are administered five times daily in dosages ranging from 1000 mg to 4 g daily, depending on the severity of the disease process and the age and weight of the patient. We have encountered intravitreal acyclovir concentrations of approximately 3 μM 6 hr following oral administration in patients undergoing fluid-gas exchange subsequent to vitrectomy for ARN (Blumenkranz and Verstraeten, personal observation, 1991). Studies of antiviral sensitivities of the herpes zoster varicella virus group isolated from the vitreous of a patient with ARN indicated in vitro susceptibility of the isolate to both acyclovir (ED_{50} of 5.3 μM) and dehyroxyphenylglycol (ED_{50} of 4.7 μM).

Acyclovir has a large therapeutic index, and complications reported to date have been relatively minor. They include local irritation at the intravenous entry site and, rarely, reversible elevation of the serum creatinine concentration, presumably through crystallization. Central nervous system toxic reactions, including delirium, tremors, abnormal electroencephalograms, as well as elevation of liver transaminase levels, have been reported, although also rarely and in complex cases in which a causal relationship has not been clearly established. To date, acyclovir has not been found to be carcinogenic, mutagenic, or teratogenic.[57]

In one clinical series, treatment of patients with ARN with 1500 mg/sq m/day of acyclovir in conjunction with aspirin and corticosteroids resulted in regression of active retinal lesions of presumed viral origin beginning on average 3.9 days after initiation of therapy. Lesions completely regressed on an average of 32.5 days after initiation of therapy, and no eye developed new retinal lesions or progressive optic nerve involvement 48 hr or more after initiation of therapy. Acyclovir treatment does not appear to ameliorate vitritis or retard the rate of retinal detachment in advanced cases, although it may do so in cases treated at an earlier time point, prior to the development of severe confluent lesions.[10, 37] Retrospective analysis of patients treated both prior to the era of acyclovir therapy and subsequent to the introduction of acyclovir suggests a benefit of treatment with regard to prevention of new lesions in the fellow eye. Of 31 patients treated with acyclovir, 87.1 percent were disease-free in the fellow eye at the time of last examination, in contrast to only 30.4 percent of fellow eyes in patients not treated with acyclovir. Two years following treatment using multivariate methods, the cumulative proportion of patients who remained disease-free in the fellow eye was 75.3 percent for the group treated with acyclovir and 35.1 percent for the group not treated with acyclovir.[14] Since the patients involved in this study were evaluated retrospectively and treated in a nonrandomized fashion at different time points and at multiple different institutions, these data should be interpreted with appropriate caution (Figs. 78–21 and 78–22).

In patients who are unable to tolerate acyclovir or who demonstrate clinical disease progression suggestive of acyclovir drug resistance, consideration may be given to administration of intravenous ganciclovir as an alternate form of therapy. Recommended guidelines for treatment with ganciclovir at present are 5 mg/kg every 12 hr for 7 to 14 days by intravenous infusion. Patients undergoing ganciclovir administration should have a twice-weekly complete blood count with differential and platelet count to identify early signs of hematopoietic suppression. The dosage of ganciclovir should be reduced in patients with evidence of impaired creatinine clearance, and the drug should be discontinued upon signs of severe leukopenia (less than 1000 cells/μl) or thrombocytopenia (Foscarnet/Ganciclovir/Cytomegalovirus Retinitis Trial/SOCA. NEI, 1991).[49, 69, 71]

In addition to oral and intravenous routes, acyclovir may also be administered as an intravitreal infusate

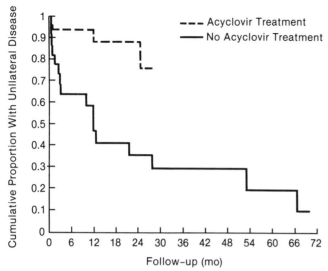

Figure 78–21. Life table analysis of lesions treated with and without acyclovir and the resultant cumulative risk of disease development in the fellow eye. The *broken line* represents treated patients with unilateral disease, whereas the *solid line* represents untreated patients with unilateral disease over time. The group of patients treated with acyclovir is less likely than the group not treated to develop ARN in the fellow eye (P = 0013). (From Palay DA, Sternberg P, Davis J, et al: Decrease in the risk of bilateral ARN by acyclovir therapy. Am J Ophthalmol 112:250–255, 1991. Published with permission from The American Journal of Ophthalmology. Copyright by The Ophthalmic Publishing Company.)

during the course of vitrectomy. Concentrations of 10 to 40 μg/ml have been reported to be safe.[11, 72] This form of therapy may be effective as an adjunct to oral and intravenous therapy in patients requiring vitrectomy during the acute phase of viral replication within the eye. The benefit of this therapy at a later stage for patients undergoing retinal reattachment procedures in the cicatricial phase of the disease remains uncertain.

Antiinflammatory Therapy

Inflammatory cells, including cytotoxic lymphocytes, are thought to play an important role both in the primary

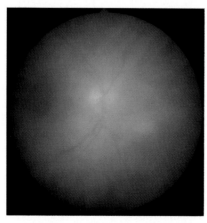

Figure 78–22. The same region as shown in Figure 78–2 following 10 days of intravenous administration of acyclovir. Note the nearly complete resolution of nummular lesions nasal to the optic nerve.

phases of the disease, when they may contribute to both retinal necrosis and vasculitis,[16, 17, 58–62] and secondarily, when vitreous cellular infiltrates contribute to organization of the vitreous that predisposes to late retinal detachment.[1–9] As a result, antiinflammatory therapy is an important component of treatment for this disease. Administration of oral prednisone or equivalent agents in dosages of 0.5 to 1.5 μg/kg/day is recommended in the early phases of the disease during the period of greatest intraocular inflammation. Because steroids are known to enhance viral replication under selected conditions, the initiation of steroid therapy should be delayed 24 to 48 hr following administration of acyclovir to avoid potential enhancement of viral replication. However, in cases in which the severity of intraocular inflammation is great, particularly when the optic nerve is involved, consideration may be given to earlier administration of oral steroids and at higher dosages, ranging up to 2 mg/kg daily. The exact duration of the antiinflammatory therapy is dictated by the severity of the intraocular inflammation and any associated conditions or limitations to therapy. In patients in whom there is no contraindication to prednisone, consideration should be given to treatment for up to 6 to 8 wk, with gradually tapering doses to reduce anterior and posterior segment inflammation and speed clearing of the vitreous cellular infiltrates. At present, no other form of antiinflammatory therapy, including cyclosporine or various antimetabolites, has been shown to be of benefit in this condition. In addition to treatment with oral prednisone, topical prednisolone every 2 to 6 hr should be administered in conjunction with a cycloplegic agent in the early phases of the disease. There has been no established benefit demonstrated for topical acyclovir.

Antithrombotic Therapy

Periarteritis and intraluminal narrowing are conspicuous features of ARN on both clinical examination and histologic study. Viral particles have not been demonstrated in the vascular endothelial cells, although the cells themselves may be markedly swollen, nearly obliterating the vascular lumina in some patients.[8, 53] These events are thought to be secondary to humoral and cell-mediated mechanisms and contribute to stasis and vascular thrombosis in patients with ARN. This may result in vision loss from both optic nerve dysfunction and retinal infarction. In addition to treatment with antiinflammatory agents, both antiplatelet agents and anticoagulation have been previously recommended.[10, 66] Platelet hyperaggregation has been detected in patients with ARN and may be treated with aspirin, 500 to 650 mg daily. The benefits of more aggressive forms of anticoagulation, including both heparin and coumadin, do not appear warranted at present.

Retinal Detachment Prophylaxis

Retinal detachment continues to be the most serious late complication of ARN, even with the prompt administration of acyclovir and steroid therapy.[1-10] Peripheral argon laser photocoagulation to demarcate zones of retinitis during the active phase of the disease (media permitting) has been recommended as a potentially effective prophylactic measure.[12] In one retrospective clinical series, 12 eyes in 10 patients undergoing prophylactic laser photocoagulation suffered a total of 2 retinal detachments (17 percent). During that same time period, 4 of 6 patients not receiving photocoagulation (66.6 percent) experienced retinal detachment as a complication of ARN.[15] Because it is likely that eyes with less severe forms of ARN have the clearest media and are therefore more likely to be able to undergo photocoagulation when compared with more severely affected eyes, it cannot be definitively concluded that the difference in these two rates is solely the result of photocoagulation. Nonetheless, it seems likely that photocoagulation does have some prophylactic value against the development of retinal detachment and should be administered in all patients at the earliest stage possible. Recommended treatment guidelines at present include the placement of at least three rows of argon, krypton, or dye laser at the junctional zones demarcating peripheral confluent necrosis from normal retina. When possible, photocoagulation should be extended into zones of necrosis in which retinal tears usually occur. The benefit of photocoagulation in isolated thumbprint lesions in the posterior segment is less certain. In some instances, longer wavelengths and retrobulbar anesthesia may be helpful in permitting successful applications in eyes with media opacities (Fig. 78–23). Despite photocoagulation, it can be estimated that up to 50 percent of eyes with ARN will develop retinal detachment.

One alternative strategy for retinal detachment prophylaxis has been the use of vitrectomy combined with endophotocoagulation and scleral buckling.[11, 12, 73] One difficulty encountered in the performance of a vitrectomy in such eyes is the tight adherence between the nondetached vitreous gel and the atrophic peripheral retina. Additionally, eyes with ARN associated with severe intraocular inflammation may develop severe ocular hypertension, fibrin response, and choroidal detachment following scleral buckling in certain instances.[74] The prophylactic benefit of combined vitrectomy and scleral buckling with endolaser for this has been debated and remains uncertain.[10, 11, 73, 74] In one series, three of four eyes undergoing prophylactic vitrectomy and photocoagulation experienced detached retinas despite this therapy and appeared to have a more unfavorable course than did eyes not undergoing prophylactic vitrectomy and photocoagulation.[10, 74]

Treatment of Acute Optic Neuropathy

In addition to the zones of frank neural necrosis seen histopathologically,[18, 46] it has been suggested that in some instances optic nerve sheath distention and compression of the optic nerve may contribute to the visual dysfunction associated with ARN. In one series, eight eyes in six patients with optic neuropathy thought to be secondary to ARN underwent optic nerve sheath decompression in addition to intravenous acyclovir therapy. These patients had a more favorable long-term visual prognosis than did patients with lesser degrees of neuropathy not undergoing decompression.[46] Clinical experience with this form of therapy remains limited, but it appears to be a potentially useful way to reduce visual disability in this condition in conjunction with appropriate antiviral, antiinflammatory, and antithrombotic therapy. This diagnosis may be established on the basis of CT or MRI scanning in patients with clinical or visual evidence of optic neuropathy in association with ARN.

MANAGEMENT OF RETINAL DETACHMENT

Retinal detachment continues to be a difficult problem in patients with late-stage ARN. In initial series of patients undergoing the combination of intravenous acyclovir therapy, corticosteroid administration, and antithrombotic therapy, 11 of 13 eyes experienced retinal detachment (84.6 percent).[10] This is comparable to a 75 percent rate of retinal detachment seen prior to the introduction of acyclovir.[17]

Retinal detachment complicating ARN is particularly severe. The majority of retinal detachments occur within 3 mo of the onset of symptoms. In one review, 41 of 55 eyes (75 percent) affected by the virus experienced retinal detachment. The time interval ranged from 1 to 10 mo, with only 4 of 41 eyes experiencing a retinal detachment more than 3 mos after the onset of the disease.[6] In a series of 12 patients (13 eyes) treated with intravenous acyclovir, 83.6 percent of eyes experienced retinal detachment an average of 59 days after initiation of therapy, with a range of 30 to 145 days.[10] Eyes with retinal detachment complicating ARN have a more unfavorable visual and anatomic prognosis for several

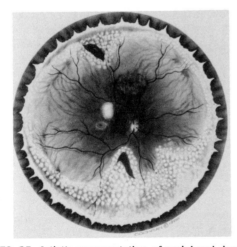

Figure 78–23. Artist's representation of peripheral demarcating photocoagulation, following vitrectomy and fluid-gas exchange in a patient with retinal holes and detachment secondary to ARN, seen in Figure 78–24.

reasons. The retinal breaks contributing to the rheg-matogenous components of these detachments are often-times multiple, large, and posteriorly located, either in necrotic retina or at the junction between normal and necrotic retina. Proliferative vitreoretinopathy is fre-quent, and eyes that demonstrate severe preexisting intraocular inflammation and vascular compromise are predisposed to fibrin response, choroidal detachment, and ocular hypertension (Fig. 78–24).[3, 13, 74, 75]

Proliferative vitreoretinopathy is a frequent occur-rence in eyes with ARN that experience retinal detach-ment. In one series, 72.7 percent of eyes with retinal detachment demonstrated grade C-1 or greater prolif-erative vitreoretinopathy.[10] The high frequency with which proliferative vitreoretinopathy occurs in this group of patients can be understood in view of the pathophysiology of the disease, including marked thin-ning of the peripheral retina and migration of pigment epithelial cells through necrotic retina onto the surface of the retina associated with metaplasia and epiretinal membrane formation (see Fig. 78–12). These changes occur in conjunction with cellular infiltration and secon-dary fibrotic changes in the vitreous, including adher-ence in the peripheral zones. It is known that the breakdown of the blood-ocular barrier encountered in patients with uveitis contributes to the development of proliferative vitreoretinopathy, possibly through libera-tion of serum-derived growth factors within the eye.[76] It is also known that fibrin, which is known to be more common in eyes undergoing retinal reattachment sur-gery for ARN,[74] is capable of producing mesenchymal transformation of pigment epithelial cells,[7] which may further contribute to the development of proliferative vitreoretinopathy.[77] As a result of these factors, retinal detachment repair in patients with ARN has been more difficult than other forms of retinal reattachment, al-though success rates appear to be improving as a result of evolving techniques.

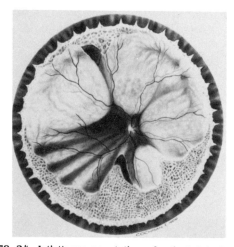

Figure 78–24. Artist's representation of retinal detachment in a patient with ARN, including a large superior retinal tear at the junction of involved and noninvolved retina as well as multiple smaller pinpoint defects in areas of postnecrotic zones. Note the presence of fixed folds radiating through the posterior pole from the periphery superotemporally.

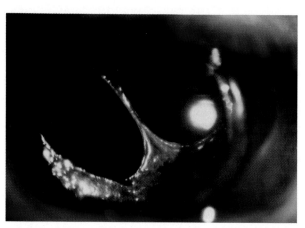

Figure 78–25. Slit-lamp photograph of pupillary fibrin response in a patient who underwent lensectomy, vitrectomy, scleral buck-ling, and endolaser treatment for an ARN-related retinal detach-ment.

Prior to 1982, retinal reattachment was attempted in only 18 of 41 eyes, with only 4 of 18 procedures being successful (22 percent).[6] Employing a combination of scleral buckling and vitrectomy in selected instances, Clarkson and associates reported an improved success rate, with 13 of 16 eyes that experienced retinal detach-ment from ARN requiring operation and 7 retinas remaining reattached (53.8 percent).[75] Similar results have been reported by other authors employing a com-bination of vitreoretinal surgery and scleral buckling.[78]

Other reports suggest that a combination of vitrec-tomy, lensectomy, internal fluid-gas exchange, and en-dolaser treatment without scleral buckling may provide a more favorable anatomic and visual outcome in eyes with retinal detachment complicating ARN.[13] In one series, eyes undergoing this procedure were compared with eyes undergoing conventional scleral buckling in association with vitrectomy. Overall, a combined final success rate of 93.8 percent (15 of 16 eyes) was reported. Complete retinal reattachment with one operation was achieved for all eyes not previously subjected to a prophylactic procedure.[13, 74] In this series of patients, perioperative complications, including ocular hyperten-sion (75 percent), fibrin response (87.5 percent), and choroidal detachment (62.5 percent) were common in patients undergoing scleral buckling. Without scleral buckling and cryotherapy, only one of eight eyes (12.5 percent) experienced fibrin response and none had cho-roidal detachment or ocular hypertension (intraocular pressure greater than 35 mmHg) (Fig. 78–25). The rate of reoperation and the final visual acuity rate also appeared to be more favorable in those patients undergoing vitrectomy without scleral buckling, with 87.5 percent of patients achieving a visual acuity of 20/200 or better and 62.5 percent achieving visual acuity of 20/70 or better. This was contrasted with only 25 percent of patients with visual acuity of 20/200 or better of those undergoing scleral buckling in conjunction with vitrectomy for this condition. This may be related to the higher rate of retinal reoperation and silicone oil in this group.[74] Silicone oil, other tamponade, and retinotomy may be required in some eyes with severe forms of retinal detachment.

Acknowledgments

The authors thank Ms. Sue Toto for editorial assistance and Dr. Victor Curtin for his assistance in the preparation and interpretation of histopathologic material.

REFERENCES

1. Uryama A, Yamada N, Sasaki Y, et al: Unilateral acute uveitis with retinal periarteritis and detachment. Jpn J Clin Ophthalmol 25:607–619, 1971.
2. Wilkerson D, Aaberg TM, Reeser FH: Necrotizing vaso-occlusive retinitis. Am J Ophthalmol 84:209–219, 1977.
3. Young NJA, Bird AC: Bilateral ARN. Br J Ophthalmol 62:581–590, 1978.
4. Price FW, Schlaegel TF: Bilateral ARN. Am J Ophthalmol 89:419–424, 1980.
5. Sternberg P, Knox DL, Finkelstein D, et al: Acute retinal necrosis syndrome. Retina 2:145–151, 1982.
6. Fisher JP, Lewis ML, Blumenkranz MS, et al: The ARN syndrome. Part 1: Clinical manifestations. Ophthalmology 89:1309–1316, 1982.
7. Gorman BD, Nadel AJ, Coles RS: Acute retinal necrosis. Ophthalmology 89:809–814, 1982.
8. Culbertson WW, Blumenkranz MS, Haines H, et al: The ARN syndrome. Part 2: Histopathology and etiology. Ophthalmology 89:1317–1325, 1982.
9. Lewis ML, Culbertson WW, Post JD, et al: Herpes simplex virus type I. A cause of the ARN syndrome. Ophthalmology 96:875–878, 1989.
10. Blumenkranz MS, Culbertson WW, Clarkson JG, et al: Treatment of the ARN syndrome with intravenous acyclovir. Ophthalmology 93:296–300, 1986.
11. Peyman GA, Morton FG, Uninsky E, et al: Vitrectomy and intravitreal antiviral drug therapy in ARN syndrome. Arch Ophthalmol 102:1618–1621, 1984.
12. Culbertson WW, Clarkson JG, Blumenkranz MS, Lewis ML: Acute retinal necrosis. Am J Ophthalmol 96:683–685, 1983.
13. Blumenkranz MS, Clarkson J, Culbertson WW, et al: Vitrectomy for retinal detachment associated with ARN. Am J Ophthalmol 106:426–429, 1988.
14. Palay DA, Sternberg P, Davis J, et al: Decrease in the risk of bilateral ARN by acyclovir therapy. Am J Ophthalmol 112:250–255, 1991.
15. Sternberg P, Han DP, Yeo JH, et al: Photocoagulation to prevent retinal detachment in ARN. Ophthalmology 95:1389–1393, 1988.
16. Atherton SS, Kanter MY, Streilein JW: ACAID requires early replication of HSV-1 in the injected eye. Curr Eye Res 10:75–80, 1990.
17. Streilein JW, Igietseme JU, Atherton SS: Evidence that precursor cytotoxic T cells mediate acute necrosis in HSV-1 infected retinas. Curr Eye Res 10:81–86, 1990.
18. Sergott RC, Belmont JB, Savino PJ, et al: Optic nerve involvement in the ARN syndrome. Arch Ophthalmol 103:1160–1162, 1985.
19. Saari KM, Boke W, Manthey KF, et al: Bilateral ARN. Am J Ophthalmol 93:403–411, 1982.
20. Gartry DS, Spalton DJ, Tilzey A, Hykin PG: Acute retinal necrosis syndrome. Br J Ophthalmol 75:292–297, 1991.
21. Kelly SP, Rosenthal AR: Chickenpox chorioretinitis. Br J Ophthalmol 74:698–699, 1990.
22. Duker JS, Blumenkranz MS: Diagnosis and management of the ARN syndrome. Surv Ophthalmol 35:327–343, 1991.
23. Martenet AC: Frequence et aspects cliniques des complications retiniennes de l'veite intermediare. Mem Soc Ophthalmol 92:410–412, 1980.
24. Egbert P, Pollard RB, Gallagher JG, Merigan T: Cytomegalovirus retinitis in immunosuppressed hosts. Natural history and effects of treatment with adenine arabinoside. Ann Intern Med 93:655–664, 1980.
25. Bloom JN, Katz JI, Kaufman HE: Herpes simplex retinitis and encephalitis in an adult. Arch Ophthalmol 95:1798–1799, 1977.
26. Friberg TR, Jost BF: Acute retinal necrosis in an immunosuppressed patient. Am J Ophthalmol 98:515–517, 1984.
27. Chambers RB, Derick RJ, Davidorf FH, et al: Varicella-zoster retinitis in human immunodeficiency virus infection. Arch Ophthalmol 107:960–961, 1989.
28. Jabs DA, Schachat AP, Liss R, et al: Presumed varicella-zoster retinitis in immunocompromised patients. Retina 7:9–13, 1987.
29. Englund JA, Balfour HH: Varicella and herpes zoster. In Hoeprich PD, Jordan MC (eds): Infectious Diseases, 4th ed. Philadelphia, JB Lippincott, 1989.
30. Culbertson WW, Brod RD, Flynn HW, et al: Chickenpox-associated ARN syndrome. Ophthalmology 98:1641–1646, 1991.
31. Matsuo T, Kuyama M, Matsuo N: Acute retinal necrosis as a novel complication of chickenpox in adults. Br J Ophthalmol 74:443–444, 1990.
32. Matsuo T, Morimoto K, Matsuo N: Factors associated with poor visual outcome in ARN. Br J Ophthalmol 75:450–454, 1991.
33. Yeo JH, Pepose JS, Stewart JA, et al: Acute retinal necrosis syndrome following herpes zoster dermatitis. Ophthalmology 93:1418–1422, 1986.
34. Browning DJ, Blumenkranz MS, Culbertson WW, et al: Association of varicella-zoster dermatitis with ARN syndrome. Ophthalmology 94:602–606, 1987.
35. Cobo LM, Foulks GN, Liesegant T, et al: Oral acyclovir in the treatment of acute herpes zoster ophthalmicus. Ophthalmology 93:763–770, 1986.
36. Holland GN, Cornell PJ, Park MS, et al: An association between retinal necrosis syndrome and HLA-DQw7 and phenotype Bw62,DR4. Am J Ophthalmol 108:370–374, 1989.
37. Matsuo T, Nakayama T, Koyama T, et al: A proposed mild type of ARN syndrome. Am J Ophthalmol 105:579–583, 1988.
38. Forster DJ, Dugel PU, Frangieh GT, et al: Rapidly progressive outer retinal necrosis in the acquired immunodeficiency syndrome. Am J Ophthalmol 110:341–348, 1990.
39. Margolis TP, Lowder CY, Holland GN, et al: Varicella-zoster virus retinitis in patients with the acquired immunodeficiency syndrome. Am J Ophthalmol 112:119–131, 1991.
40. Duker JS, Nielsen JC, Eagle RC, et al: Rapidly progressive ARN secondary to herpes simplex virus, type I. Ophthalmology 97:1638–1643, 1990.
41. Sarkies N, Gregor Z, Forsey T, Darougar S: Antibodies to herpes simplex virus type I in intraocular fluids of patients with ARN. Br J Ophthalmol 70:81–84, 1986.
42. Matsuo T, Nakayama T, Koyama T, Matsuo N: Cytological and immunological study of the aqueous humor in ARN syndrome. Ophthalmologica 195:38–44, 1987.
43. Brown RM, Mendis U: Retinal arteritis complicating herpes zoster ophthalmicus. Br J Ophthalmol 57:344–346, 1973.
44. Blumenkranz MS, Kaplan HJ, Clarkson JG, et al: Acute multifocal hemorrhagic retinal vasculitis. Ophthalmology 95:1663–1672, 1988.
45. Han DP, Abrams GW, Williams GA: Regression of disc neovascularization by photocoagulation in the ARN syndrome. Retina 8:244–246, 1988.
46. Sergott RC, Anand R, Belmont JB, et al: Acute retinal necrosis neuropathy. Clinical profile and surgical therapy. Arch Ophthalmol 107:692–696, 1989.
47. Topilow H, Nussbaum JJ, Freeman HM, et al: Bilateral ARN. Clinical and ultrastructural study. Ophthalmology 100:1901–1908, 1982.
48. Blumenkranz MS: Discussion of chickenpox-associated ARN syndrome. Ophthalmology 98:1645–1646, 1991.
49. Pepose JS, Biron K: Antiviral sensitivities of the ARN syndrome virus. Curr Eye Res 6:201–205, 1987.
50. Soushi S, Ozawa H, Matsuhashi M, et al: Demonstration of varicella-zoster virus antigens in the vitreous aspirates of patients with ARN syndrome. Ophthalmology 95:1394–1398, 1988.
51. Margolis T, Irvine AR, Hoyt WF, Hyman R: Acute retinal necrosis syndrome presenting with papillitis and arcuate neuroretinitis. Ophthalmology 95:937–940, 1988.
52. Suttorp-Schulten MS, Zaal MJ, Luyendijk BS, et al: Aqueous

chamber tap and serology in ARN. Am J Ophthalmol 108:327–328, 1989.

53. Culbertson WW, Blumenkranz MS, Pepose JS, et al: Varicella-zoster virus is a cause of the ARN syndrome. Ophthalmology 93:559–569, 1986.

54. Rugger-Brandle E, Roux L, Leuenberger PM: Bilateral ARN: Identification of the presumed infectious agent. Ophthalmology 91:1648–1658, 1984.

55. Whitley RJ: Varicella-zoster virus. Infectious diseases and their etiologic agents. Part III. *In* Mandell GL, Goudlas RG, Bennet JE (eds): Principles and Practice of Infectious Diseases, 3rd ed. New York, Churchill Livingstone, 1991, pp 1153–1159.

56. Easty DL: Virology of the Herpes Viruses in Virus Diseases of the Eye. Chicago, Year Book Medical, 1985, pp 76–78.

57. Laskin OL: Acyclovir. Pharmacology and clinical experience. Arch Intern Med 144:1241–1246, 1984.

58. Whittum JW, McCulley JP, Niederkorn JT, Streilein JW: Ocular disease induced in mice by anterior chamber inoculation of herpes simplex virus. Invest Ophthalmol Vis Sci 25:1065–1073, 1984.

59. Cousins SW, Gonzalez A, Atherton S: Herpes simplex retinitis in the mouse: Clinicopathologic correlations. Invest Ophthalmol Vis Sci 30:1485, 1989.

60. Whittum JA, Niederkorn JT, McCulley JP, Streilein JW: Intracameral inoculation of herpes simplex virus type I induces anterior chamber–associated immune deviation. Curr Eye Res 2:691–697, 1983.

61. Igietseme JU, Calzada PJ, Gonzalez AR, et al: Protection of mice from herpes simplex virus–induced retinitis by in vitro-activated immune cells. J Virol 63:4808–4813, 1989.

62. Igietseme JU, Streilein JW, Miranda F, et al: Mechanisms of protection against herpes simplex virus type I–retinal necrosis by in vitro–activated T lymphocytes. J Virol 65:763–768, 1991.

63. Mahalingham R, Wellish M, Wolf W, et al: Latent varicella-zoster viral DNA in human trigeminal and thoracic ganglia. N Engl J Med 323:627–631, 1990.

64. Duker JS, Blumenkranz MS: Diagnosis and management of the acute retinal necrosis syndrome (ARN). Surv Ophthalmol 35:327–343, 1991.

65. Ridley ME, McDonald HR, Sternberg P, et al: Retinal manifestations of ocular lymphoma (reticulum cell sarcoma). Ophthalmology 99:1153–1160, 1992.

66. Ando F, Kato M, Goto S, et al: Platelet function in bilateral ARN. Am J Ophthalmol 96:27–32, 1983.

67. Fox GM, Crouse GA, Chuang EL, et al: Detection of herpes viruses DNA in vitreous and aqueous specimens by the polymerase chain reaction. Arch Ophthalmol 109:266, 1991.

68. Hirsch MS, Schooley RT: Treatment of herpes virus infections. (Second of two parts.) N Engl J Med 309:1034–1039, 1983.

69. Holland GN, Sakamoto MJ, Hardy D, et al: CMV retinopathy study group: Treatment of cytomegalovirus retinopathy in patients with acquired immunodeficiency syndrome. Arch Ophthalmol 104:794, 1984.

70. Jacobson MA, Drew WL, Feinberg J, et al: Foscarnet therapy for ganciclovir-resistant cytomegalovirus in patients with AIDS. J Infect Dis 163:1348–1351, 1991.

71. Hung SO, Patterson A, Rees PJ: Pharmacokinetics of oral acyclovir (Zovirax) in the eye. Br J Ophthalmol 68:192–195, 1984.

72. Pulido JS, Palacio MN, Peyman GA, et al: Toxicity of antiviral drugs. Ophthalmic Surg 15:666–669, 1984.

73. Carney MD, Peyman GA, Goldberg MF, et al: Acute retinal necrosis. Retina 6:85, 1984.

74. Blumenkranz MS, Clarkson J, Culbertson WW, et al: Visual results and complications after retinal reattachment in the ARN syndrome: The influence of operative technique. Retina 9:170–174, 1989.

75. Clarkson JG, Blumenkranz MS, Culbertson WW, et al: Retinal detachment following the ARN syndrome. Ophthalmology 91:1665–1668, 1984.

76. Campochiaro P, Jerdan JA, Glaser BM: Serum contains chemoattractants for human retinal pigment epithelial cells. Arch Ophthalmol 102:1376–1379, 1984.

77. Vidaurri JS, Glaser BM: Effect of fibrin on retinal pigment epithelial cells. Arch Ophthalmol 102:1376–1379, 1984.

78. McDonald HR, Lewis H, Kreiger AE, et al: Surgical management of retinal detachment associated with the ARN syndrome. Br J Ophthalmol 75:455–458, 1991.

Chapter 79

■

Viral Infections of the Retina in the Pediatric Patient

SHALOM J. KIEVAL

RUBELLA

Rubella is a contagious disease caused by an RNA virus of the togavirus group. Postnatal infection generally causes a mild, self-limited illness characterized by fever, lymphadenopathy, and a distinctive rash. Transmission occurs through close contact and by aerosol droplet. Except in rare instances, lifelong immunity develops following primary infection. Maternal infection during the first trimester of pregnancy may produce severe damage to the fetus and result in spontaneous abortion, stillbirth, or multiple congenital deformities.[1–3]

Australian ophthalmologist Norman Gregg was the first to make the association between characteristic congenital defects and first-trimester maternal rubella infec-tion.[4–5] In 1941, he described 78 children with congenital cataracts, deafness, and cardiac anomalies, most of whom had evidence of maternal rubella infection early in gestation. Others soon confirmed this relationship and expanded the spectrum of findings, which collectively came to be known as the *congenital rubella syndrome*.

Isolation of the rubella virus in 1962 and a severe pandemic between 1962 and 1964 brought further understanding of the biologic features of the rubella virus and of the congenital syndrome and paved the way for the development of a vaccine in 1969. The widespread availability of a safe vaccine dramatically reduced the incidence of rubella in the United States (US). A total of 26 cases was reported in the US for the 5-yr period

1983 to 1987 compared with an estimated 20,000 affected infants during the 1962 to 1964 epidemic.[1]

An important feature of congenital rubella infection is the persistence of virus and chronicity of infection. Rubella virus may be retrieved from children years after birth. This may help explain the progression of established defects with time and the development of late manifestations of the disease. Infection that may be silent or mild at birth may later give rise to clinical disease. Of a group of neonates with subclinical infection, 71 percent subsequently manifested clinical signs of infection during a 5-yr follow-up.[1, 6]

Nonocular Manifestations

Hearing loss is the single most common feature of congenital rubella, and unlike other defects, it may occur in isolation. Deafness is usually bilateral, but unilateral cases occur. The hearing loss is most commonly of the sensorineural type. Cardiac defects occur frequently. Patent ductus arteriosus, pulmonary artery stenosis, and pulmonary valvular stenosis are most commonly reported. Other features of the congenital rubella syndrome include mental retardation, microcephaly, growth retardation, thrombocytopenia with purpura, hepatitis and hepatomegaly, splenomegaly, interstitial pneumonitis, and bony and dental abnormalities. Diabetes mellitus and other endocrine deficiencies may develop as late manifestations of the disease.[1-3]

Ocular Manifestations

Ocular involvement is common in congenital rubella.[7-12] Two prospective series found eye disease in 42.5 percent and 49 percent, of children with documented intrauterine infection.[8, 9]

Rubella retinopathy consists of a generalized pigmentary disturbance with a somewhat variable appearance.[10, 11] Pigmentary mottling of the "salt-and-pepper" type is commonly described and may affect both the macula and the periphery (Fig. 79–1). The pigment deposits may be more prominent in the posterior retina.

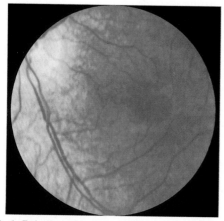

Figure 79–1. Rubella retinopathy with "salt-and-pepper" pigmentary disturbance. (Courtesy of Robert Petersen, M.D.)

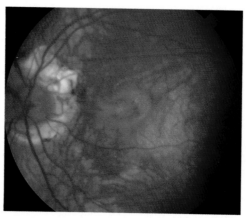

Figure 79–2. Rubella retinopathy with subretinal neovascular membrane in the macula.

The foveal reflex is frequently lost. The retinal vessels are of normal appearance. The optic nerve may be healthy or atrophic. Unilateral cases occur, although both eyes are generally involved. The incidence has been reported at 24 to 62 percent.

When no significant coexisting pathologic condition is present, visual acuity is generally good. Wolff reported a median vision of 20/25 (range 20/20 to 20/60).[8] The small group of children in his series with visual acuity in the 20/40 to 20/60 range appeared to have a more severe pigmentary disturbance. Most patients have normal electroretinograms and electrooculograms.[13] Histopathologic changes principally involve the retinal pigment epithelium. Foci of increased and decreased pigmentation and cellular loss are seen.[14]

Although once thought to be stationary, there is evidence that the retinopathy may be progressive, with pigmentary changes developing in eyes previously observed to be free of retinopathy.[8, 15] Several authors have also reported the late development of macular choroidal neovascular membranes in patients with rubella retinopathy (Fig. 79–2).[16-18]

The rubella cataract may show the typical pearly-white nucleus with surrounding clear zone, or it may be totally opaque. It may be unilateral or bilateral.[7] Other common ocular abnormalities include microphthalmia, glaucoma,[19, 20] corneal clouding, and iris hypoplasia.[8, 21] Strabismus and nystagmus also occur.[22]

When suspected on clinical grounds, the diagnosis may be confirmed by serologic testing and viral culture. The differential diagnosis includes the hereditary retinal degenerations, syphilitic chorioretinitis, choroideremia, the carrier state of X-linked albinism, and toxic retinopathies.

CYTOMEGALOVIRUS

Cytomegalovirus (CMV), a DNA virus of the herpes group, is a common pathogen capable of producing severe disease in the developing fetus and newborn and in the immunocompromised host. Conversely, infection in healthy children and adults may be asymptomatic or manifested by a mononucleosis-like syndrome, with fever, lymphadenopathy, and hepatitis. The virus is ubiquitous. In the US and Europe, estimates of seropositivity among young women for antibodies to CMV range from 50 to 80 percent, with prevalence rates being higher in lower socioeconomic groups.[24] Live virus is present in body fluids of actively infected individuals and may be shed for years following perinatally acquired infection. Transmission occurs through close person-to-person contact, transplacental spread, sexual contact, blood transfusion, and organ transplantation. Primary infection does not confer immunity, and maternal antibodies do not protect the fetus from intrauterine infection. Recurrent infection may result from exposure to exogenous virus or reactivation of latent endogenous virus.

Although congenital infection is common, most cases are not clinically apparent. It is estimated that congenital infection occurs in 1 percent of live births in the US.[24] Of these, approximately 10 percent will show clinical evidence of infection early in life. With primary maternal infection during pregnancy, the risk of fetal infection is estimated to be 30 to 40 percent.[24]

Nonocular Manifestations

Spontaneous abortion, stillbirth, intrauterine growth retardation, and premature birth may occur. The microcephaly that is present in approximately 50 percent of symptomatic infants reflects diffuse central nervous system involvement.[25] Periventricular calcifications may be seen on skull radiographs. Psychomotor retardation is seen in 70 percent of symptomatic children according to one study.[25] Neuromuscular problems, seizures, and hydrocephalus also occur.

Hepatomegaly and jaundice are characteristic findings in infants with prenatal CMV infection. Splenomegaly and thrombocytopenia with purpura and a petechial rash are commonly seen. Hearing loss of varying degree may be stable or progressive. Dental abnormalities have also been described.[26]

Ocular Manifestations

Ocular involvement is common in congenitally acquired CMV infection.[27-39] The most frequently described lesion is chorioretinitis, occurring in some 15 percent of children with clinically apparent prenatally acquired infection.[28, 29, 37] A typical description is that given by Lonn[34] in reporting a 3-month-old infant with bilateral posterior fundus involvement "characterized by discrete, circular areas of scarring and inflammation of the retina, with damage to the pigment epithelium and marginal pigmentation." There was contiguous, localized vitreous involvement as well. In some cases, involvement is limited to the fundus periphery.[27, 32] The ophthalmoscopic appearance of these lesions is similar to the chorioretinal scars of congenital toxoplasmosis. In contrast to congenital toxoplasmosis and rubella, typical lesions have not been noted to develop in previously uninvolved fundi.[37, 39] Optic atrophy, optic neuritis, optic nerve hypoplasia, and colobomas with microphthalmia have been reported.[36] Strabismus and nystagmus are additional frequent findings.[39] Two patients with anophthalmia and one with Peters' anomaly have been described.[38]

The diagnosis may be suspected in infants with the distinctive clinical features of congenital CMV disease. Virus isolation and persistence of antibody may confirm the diagnosis. Differential diagnosis includes congenital infection from toxoplasmosis, syphilis, rubella and varicella, and perinatal herpes simplex.

HERPES SIMPLEX

Herpes simplex virus (HSV; herpesvirus hominis) is a widespread DNA virus responsible for a variety of clinical disease presentations. Most common are the cutaneous orolabial lesions generally caused by HSV, type 1, and the genital lesions caused, in the majority of cases, by HSV, type 2. One of the characteristic features of herpesviruses is their ability to lie dormant and periodically become reactivated. As a result, both primary and secondary recurrent infections occur.

In both the adult and the child eye, HSV may cause severe keratitis, conjunctivitis, and uveitis as a result of primary and reactivation infection.

In the newborn infant, HSV can cause serious, life-threatening infection, with central nervous system, visceral, and ocular involvement. Intrauterine transplacental transmission of the virus has been demonstrated to occur and is characterized by microcephaly or hydranencephaly, chorioretinitis, and vesicular or cicatricial skin disease.

Most neonatal infections, however, are acquired at the time of delivery by exposure to virus shed by the mother as the baby passes through the birth canal. In some cases, intrauterine infection may occur through the ruptured amniotic membrane and the ascent of virus into the uterus. Maternal gestational HSV infection has been estimated to occur in 1 percent of pregnancies, and the incidence of live viral excretion at time of birth is estimated to occur up to 0.39 percent of the time.[40] In the presence of active maternal genital herpes infection at the time of delivery, there is at least a 40 percent risk of neonatal disease, unless cesarean section is performed prior to or within 4 hr of membrane rupture.[41] It is noteworthy, though, that in the majority of cases of neonatal HSV infection, there is no history of either primary or recurrent infection in the mother or her sexual partner. Up to 1000 cases of neonatal HSV infection occur annually in the US.[40]

Infants with natally acquired infection generally present at about 10 days of age, although signs of disease may be present as early as 4 days postpartum. Three forms of disease are recognized. In the first type, apparent involvement is limited to the skin, eye, or oral cavity. Vesicular lesions occur in 90 percent of these cases. Conjunctivitis and keratitis occur and may be the sole clinical manifestations. Encephalitis is the principal feature of the second type, although skin, eye, and mouth lesions may also be present. The third form is characterized by disseminated visceral involvement, generally with neurologic disease, and frequently with ocular, cutaneous, and oral disease as well. One half to two thirds of neonatal cases are of this type. Hepatic and adrenal involvement is common, but any organ may be affected. Signs include irritability, jaundice, respiratory distress, seizures, clotting abnormalities, and vesicular eruption. Without treatment, mortality approaches 80 percent, and most of the survivors suffer neurologic deficits.[40]

Ocular Manifestations

Ocular involvement with neonatal HSV infection occurs in 17 to 40 percent of cases.[42, 43] Eye findings may occur alone or in association with other localized or disseminated forms of the disease.[44] The spectrum of involvement ranges from a mild conjunctivitis to severe necrotizing retinitis. Conjunctivitis typically develops between 3 and 14 days postpartum.[45] It may be unilateral or bilateral, and unless accompanied by typical cutaneous lesions, it may not be readily differentiated from other causes of conjunctivitis in the neonate. Keratitis similar to that seen in the adult, with diffuse punctate staining, dendritic figures, or larger geographic ulcerations, may develop. Disciform stromal keratitis may also occur. Cataract is a less common, and generally late, finding.

Posterior segment involvement takes the form of a bilateral, often necrotizing chorioretinitis.[46–50] Acutely, small, punctate, yellow-white retinal lesions; large areas of exudation; hemorrhage; retinal edema; and perivasculitis may be seen. Both the periphery and the posterior retina may show extensive involvement. Vitreous reaction is present and may be severe. It seems likely that the fulminant necrotizing retinitis with uveitis represents the severe end of the spectrum and that some cases of milder disease may go unrecognized. Although most cases are caused by HSV, type 2, both the fulminant and the milder forms of chorioretinitis have been documented with the type 1 virus.[43, 50]

In most reported cases of perinatal infection, chorioretinitis has first been detected at 1 to 3 mo of age. It may develop when earlier ocular surface infection is either present or lacking. Of ten cases of chorioretinitis reviewed by Nahmias and Hagler,[45] only two patients had a history of prior keratitis or conjunctivitis. Retinitis may also be a feature of infantile HSV encephalitis acquired after the perinatal period,[51] and of localized herpetic uveitis.[52]

Healed inactive lesions are characterized by geographic, well-demarcated areas of chorioretinal atrophy with hyperpigmented borders. They are most commonly found in the fundus periphery but may affect the macula. Optic atrophy may develop in severe cases (Fig. 79–3).[53] Visual prognosis is related to the severity of the disease and to the integrity of critical ocular and neurologic structures.

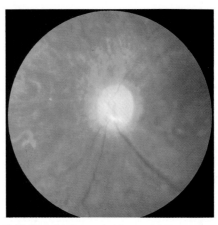

Figure 79–3. Perinatal herpes simplex retinitis with optic atrophy. (Courtesy of Robert Petersen, M.D.)

The incidence of chorioretinitis in neonatal HSV infection was found to be 4 percent in a large series of 297 patients.[42] A more recent study found signs of old chorioretinitis in 9 of 32 patients (28 percent) with perinatal HSV infection examined later in childhood.[43] These findings were notable in that they were concentrated in the subgroup of children who had had encephalitis and who had no antecedent history of uveitis or posterior segment involvement. Many of these children also had optic atrophy and cortical blindness. Bilateral active retinitis has developed 5 yr after neonatal HSV infection.[53] Other late manifestations of neonatal infection include corneal scarring, cataract, ocular motility disturbances, and retinal neovascularization.

The differential diagnosis of herpetic chorioretinitis includes CMV infection, toxoplasmosis, rubella infection, and syphilis. Since the chorioretinitis develops some time after the infection is established, the diagnosis must be suspected on the basis of the characteristic clinical presentation. The ophthalmologist may be of help to the pediatrician in identifying the typical keratitis, when present. Diagnosis is confirmed by virus isolation when possible or by cytologic study of scrapings from active cutaneous or ocular surface lesions.

Treatment consists of systemic antiviral therapy with vidarabine or acyclovir and administration of topical antiviral agents such as trifluorothymidine, vidarabine, or idoxuridine for ocular surface disease.[54]

SUBACUTE SCLEROSING PANENCEPHALITIS

Subacute sclerosing panencephalitis (SSPE) is a neurodegenerative disease typically affecting school-age children and caused by the measles (rubeola) virus. It was first described by Dawson in the early 1930s, who suspected a viral cause on the basis of the pathologic finding of inclusion bodies in neurons and glial cells from the brain of a 16-year-old individual with subacute progressive encephalitis. Much evidence now supports the identification of the measles virus as the causative agent.[55]

Most affected children have a history of measles infection during the first 2 yr of life. Immunization against measles lowers the risk of later developing SSPE. Among immunized children, the risk is estimated at 1 in 1 million as compared with a 10- to 20-fold greater risk in children with natural measles infection.[55] The disease itself generally develops between 5 and 13 yr of age, with an average of 7 yr. There is a striking male preponderance with a ratio of 3:1. Clinically, there is an insidious onset of intellectual deterioration and personality change. Tremors and involuntary muscular movements may develop early as well. Seizures and rhythmic myoclonic jerks are seen as the disease advances. The latter symptoms are quite characteristic of SSPE and are accompanied by distinctive electroencephalographic changes. Progressive neurologic deterioration ultimately leads to decerebration and in most cases death within 1 to 2 yr of onset of symptoms. Elevated levels of gamma globulin may be found in the cerebrospinal fluid. High titers of antibody to measles virus are present in the cerebrospinal fluid and serum.[55, 56]

Ocular Manifestations

Ophthalmic findings occur in some 50 percent of cases.[56–64] Chorioretinitis, nystagmus and other ocular motility disturbances, papilledema, optic atrophy, and cortical blindness have been described. Ocular manifestations may develop early or late in the course of the disease and may in fact be the first sign of the general neurologic deterioration yet to come. When such is the case, visual system abnormalities generally predate the neurologic signs by a few weeks to several months, although this time interval may be considerably longer.[63]

The characteristic ocular lesion is a focal retinitis or chorioretinitis. Both the macula and the periphery may be involved. Discrete areas of pigmentary disturbance, hemorrhage, retinal edema, and serous retinal detachment may be found. Cotton-wool spots, optic nerve edema, and optic atrophy are additional findings. There is little associated inflammatory reaction, and the vitreous is clear. Inactive lesions manifest thin, atrophic retina and associated pigmentary abnormalities. Macular holes may form. It may be clinically difficult, however, to differentiate low-grade active chorioretinitis from inactive quiescent scars except through serial observations.[57] A case of necrotizing retinitis like that seen in SSPE has also been reported in a teenaged boy with acute measles encephalopathy.[65] This patient was in an immunosuppressed state as a result of chemotherapy for testicular cancer.

Histopathologic findings include retinal atrophy, disorganization, and gliosis with minimal inflammatory reaction. Eosinophilic intranuclear inclusion bodies are seen in retinal glia and in all three neuronal layers, and intraretinal measles virus antigens have been demonstrated by immunologic techniques.[60] Filamentous, tubular structures of characteristic paramyxovirus morphology have been revealed by electron microscopy.[60]

VARICELLA

The varicella-zoster virus is a member of the herpes group of DNA viruses. Primary infection with this highly contagious agent commonly occurs in childhood and results in the generally benign and self-limited disease chickenpox. Herpes zoster eruptions arise from reactivation of latent virus in older individuals.

Primary maternal varicella infection or herpes zoster eruption during the first or early second trimester of pregnancy may result in a distinctive set of developmental malformations. This congenital varicella syndrome, first described by Laforet and Lynch in 1947,[66] consists variably of cicatricial skin lesions, limb deformities, psychomotor retardation, cortical atrophy, intrauterine growth retardation, failure to thrive, and early death.[67] Seizures, bulbar palsy, hemiparesis, and neurotrophic bladder may be associated findings.[68–70]

Ocular abnormalities occurred in 62 percent of 37 cases of congenital varicella syndrome reported prior to 1986.[67, 71–73] The eye findings included chorioretinitis (27 percent), microphthalmos (27 percent), cataract (24 percent), Horner's syndrome (19 percent), and nystagmus (19 percent). Optic nerve hypoplasia may also occur. The chorioretinal scars may be large and confluent, involving both the peripheral and the posterior retina. The most distinctive feature of these lesions is an intense, heavy pigmentation, particularly along the outer perimeter with central or adjacent areas of hypopigmentation (Fig. 79–4).[73] The vitreous is clear. The differential diagnosis includes congenital toxoplasmosis, syphilis, CMV infection, and HSV infection. Diagnosis is made by maternal history of gestational varicella-zoster infection, by the characteristic constellation of findings, and by the persistence of IgG antibodies to the virus.

Acquired chickenpox in childhood may rarely be complicated by encephalitis. A unilateral whitish-yellow, flat macular lesion has been described in a 3-year-old boy with chickenpox encephalitis and optic neuritis.[74] The macular spot appeared 3 wk after the rash, enlarged

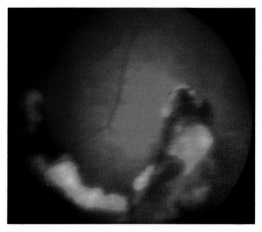

Figure 79–4. Congenital varicella syndrome with pigmented chorioretinal scars.

to two thirds of a disc diameter in size, and disappeared within 3 wk, evidently with good visual recovery.

AIDS

The first cases of AIDS in children were reported in 1982. By April of 1990, some 2000 cases had been reported to the Centers for Disease Control, representing approximately 2 percent of identified patients in the US. The incidence of pediatric AIDS is increasing rapidly, and 10,000 to 20,000 cases are expected in the US by the early 1990s.[75] Worldwide, the problem is worse. It is estimated that children constitute 15 to 20 percent of all AIDS cases in developing countries, and that by 1992, there would be more than 250,000 infants with HIV infection in Africa alone.[75]

In the US, 80 percent of affected children have acquired the disease perinatally from HIV-infected mothers.[76] Most of the rest were recipients of contaminated blood products. In children, the time from infection to the manifestation of disease is shorter than in the adult, with many patients presenting during the first year of life. Progression of the disease also tends to occur at a more rapid rate than in adults.

There is little information currently available concerning ocular involvement in pediatric AIDS. In a study of 40 children with AIDS,[77] 20 percent had ocular findings. Only two patients had CMV retinitis, and one had isolated cotton-wool spots. This contrasts with an incidence of up to 28 percent and 64 percent for these findings, respectively, in the adult population.[78] Two cases of molluscum contagiosum were included in this group, as were one case of bilateral macular toxoplasmosis and one of preseptal cellulitis. Of 16 children with AIDS examined by this author, 1 showed signs of localized perivasculitis, and the rest had normal examinations. Toxoplasmosis and necrotizing retinitis of the CMV type have been reported by others.[79, 80] In older children with AIDS, Palestine and deSmet have noted the findings of cotton-wool spots, CMV retinitis, toxoplasmosis, and herpes zoster retinitis.[81]

It appears that the frequency of ophthalmic disease in pediatric AIDS is lower than in the adult population. It seems likely that as the epidemic spreads in the pediatric age group and clinical experience grows, an expanded spectrum of ocular complications will be recognized.

REFERENCES

1. Preblud SR, Alford CA Jr: Rubella. *In* Remington JS, Kelin JO (eds): Infectious Diseases of the Fetus and Newborn Infant, 3rd ed. Philadelphia, WB Saunders, 1990.
2. Hanshaw JB, Dudgeon JA, Marshall WC: Viral Diseases of the Fetus and Newborn, 2nd ed. Philadelphia, WB Saunders, 1978.
3. Cherry JD: Rubella. *In* Feigin RD, Cherry JD (eds): Textbook of Pediatric Infectious Diseases, 2nd ed. Philadelphia, WB Saunders, 1987.
4. Gregg NM: Congenital cataract following German measles in the mother. Trans Ophthalmol Soc Aust 3:34, 1941.
5. Gregg NM: Rubella during pregnancy of the mother with its sequelae of congenital defects in the child. Med J Aust 1:313, 1945.
6. Schiff GM, Sutherland J, Light I: Congenital rubella. *In* Thalhammer O (ed): Prenatal Infection. International Symposium of Vienna. September 2–3, 1970. Stuttgart, Georg Thieme, 1971.
7. Alfano JE: Ocular aspects of the maternal rubella syndrome. Trans Am Acad Ophthalmol Otolaryngol 70:235, 1966.
8. Wolff SM: The ocular malformations of congenital rubella. Trans Am Ophthalmol Soc 70:577, 1972.
9. Geltzer AI, Guber D, Sears ML: Ocular manifestations of the 1964–65 rubella epidemic. Am J Ophthalmol 63:221, 1967.
10. Krill AE: The retinal disease of rubella. Arch Ophthalmol 77:445, 1967.
11. Krill AE: Retinopathy secondary to rubella. Int Ophthalmol Clin 12:89, 1972.
12. Hertzberg R: Twenty-five year follow-up of ocular defects in congenital rubella. Am J Ophthalmol 66:269, 1968.
13. Obenour LC: The electroretinogram in rubella retinopathy. Int Ophthalmol Clin 12:105, 1972.
14. Boniuk M, Zimmerman LZ: Ocular pathology in the rubella syndrome. Arch Ophthalmol 77:455, 1967.
15. Collis WJ, Cohen DN: Rubella retinopathy: A progressive disorder. Arch Ophthalmol 84:33, 1970.
16. Frank KE, Purnell EW: Subretinal neovascularization following rubella retinopathy. Am J Ophthalmol 86:462, 1978.
17. Deutman AF, Grizzard WS: Rubella retinopathy and subretinal neovascularization. Am J Ophthalmol 85:82, 1978.
18. Orth DH, Fishman GA, Segall M, et al: Rubella maculopathy. Br J Ophthalmol 64:201, 1980.
19. Sears ML: Congenital glaucoma in neonatal rubella. Br J Ophthalmol 51:744, 1967.
20. Boniuk M: Glaucoma in the congenital rubella syndrome. Int Ophthalmol Clin 12:121, 1972.
21. Boniuk V: Systemic and ocular manifestations of the rubella syndrome. Int Ophthalmol Clin 12:67, 1972.
22. O'Neill JF: Strabismus in the rubella syndrome. Int Ophthalmol Clin 12:111, 1972.
23. Gass JD: Stereoscopic Atlas of Macular Diseases, 3rd ed. St Louis, CV Mosby, 1987.
24. Stagno S: Cytomegalovirus. *In* Remington JS, Kelin JO (eds): Infectious Diseases of the Fetus and Newborn Infant, 3rd ed. Philadelphia, WB Saunders, 1990.
25. Pass RF, Stagno S, Myers GJ, et al: Outcome of symptomatic congenital cytomegalovirus infection: Results of a long-term longitudinal follow-up. Pediatrics 66:758, 1980.
26. Stagno S, Pass RF, Thomas JD, et al: Defects of tooth structure in congenital cytomegalovirus infections. Pediatrics 69:646, 1982.
27. Christensen L, Beeman HW, Allen A: Cytomegalic inclusion disease. Arch Ophthalmol 57:90, 1957.
28. Weller TH, Hanshaw JB: Virologic and clinical observations in cytomegalic inclusion disease. N Engl J Med 266:1233, 1962.
29. Eichenwald HF, Shinefield HR: Viral infections of the fetus and of the premature and newborn infant. Adv Pediatr 12:249, 1962.
30. Manschot WA, Daamen CBF: A case of cytomegalic inclusion disease with ocular involvement. Ophthalmologica 143:137, 1962.
31. Miklos G, Orban T: Ophthalmic lesions due to cytomegalic inclusion disease. Ophthalmologica 148:98, 1964.
32. Smith ME, Zimmerman LE, Harley RD: Ocular involvement in congenital cytomegalic inclusion disease. Arch Ophthalmol 76:696, 1966.
33. Boniuk I: The cytomegaloviruses and the eye. Int Ophthalmol Clin 12:169, 1972.
34. Lonn LI: Neonatal cytomegalic inclusion disease chorioretinitis. Arch Ophthalmol 88:434, 1972.
35. Nicholson DH: Cytomegalovirus infection of the retina. Int Ophthalmol Clin 15:151, 1975.
36. Hittner HM, Desmond MM, Montgomery JR: Optic nerve manifestations of human congenital cytomegalovirus infection. Am J Ophthalmol 81:661, 1976.
37. Stagno S, Reynolds DW, Amos CS, et al: Auditory and visual defects resulting from symptomatic and subclinical congenital cytomegalovirus and *Toxoplasma* infections. Pediatrics 59:669, 1977.
38. Frenkel LD: Unusual eye abnormalities associated with congenital CMV infections. Pediatrics 66:763, 1980.

39. Berenberg W, Nankervis G: Long-term follow-up of cytomegalic inclusion disease of infancy. Pediatrics 46:403, 1970.
40. Whitley RJ: Herpes simplex virus infections. *In* Remington JS, Klein JO (eds): Infectious Diseases of the Fetus and Newborn Infant, 3rd ed. Philadelphia, WB Saunders, 1990.
41. Nahmias AJ, Josey WC, Naib ZM, et al: Perinatal risk associated with maternal genital herpes simplex virus infections. Am J Obstet Gynecol 110:825, 1971.
42. Nahmias AJ, Visintine AM, Caldwell DR, Wilson LA: Eye infections with herpes simplex viruses in the neonates. Surv Ophthalmol 21:100, 1976.
43. el-Azzai M, Malm G, Forsgren M: Late ophthalmologic manifestations of neonatal herpes simplex virus infection. Am J Ophthalmol 109:1, 1990.
44. Whitley RJ, Hutto C: Neonatal herpes simplex virus infection. Pediatr Rev 7:119, 1985.
45. Nahmias AJ, Hagler WS: Ocular manifestations of herpes simplex in the newborn (neonatal ocular herpes). Int Ophthalmol Clin 12:191, 1972.
46. Cogan DF, Kuwabara T, Young GF, Knox DL: Herpes simplex retinopathy in an infant. Arch Ophthalmol 72:641, 1964.
47. Yanoff M, Allman MI, Fine BS: Congenital herpes simplex virus, type 2, bilateral endophthalmitis. Trans Am Ophthalmol Soc 75:325, 1977.
48. Cibis GW: Neonatal herpes simplex retinitis. Graefes Arch Clin Ophthalmol 39:196, 1978.
49. Hagler WS, Walters PV, Nahmias AJ: Ocular involvement in neonatal herpes simplex virus infection. Arch Ophthalmol 82:169, 1969.
50. Reersted P, Hansen B: Chorioretinitis of the newborn with herpes simplex virus type 1. Report of a case. Acta Ophthalmol (Stockh) 57:1096, 1979.
51. Cibis GW, Flynn JT, Davis EB: Herpes simplex retinitis. Arch Ophthalmol 96:299, 1978.
52. Pavan-Langston D, Brockhurst RJ: Herpes simplex panuveitis. Arch Ophthalmol 81:783, 1969.
53. Tarkkanen A, Laatikainen L: Late ocular manifestations in neonatal herpes simplex infection. Br J Ophthalmol 61:608, 1977.
54. Fischer DH: Viral disease and the retina. *In* Tabbara KF, Hyndiuk RA (eds): Infections of the Eye. Boston, Little, Brown, 1986.
55. Cherry JD: Measles. *In* Feigin RD, Cherry JD (eds): Textbook of Pediatric Infectious Diseases, 2nd ed. Philadelphia, WB Saunders, 1987.
56. Garner A, Klintworth GK: Pathobiology of Ocular Disease. New York, Marcel Dekker, 1982.
57. Robb RM, Watters GV: Ophthalmic manifestations of subacute sclerosing panencephalitis. Arch Ophthalmol 83:426, 1970.
58. Raymond LA, Kerstine RS, Shelburne SA: Preretinal vitreous membranes in subacute sclerosing panencephalitis. Arch Ophthalmol 94:1412, 1976.
59. Landers MB, Klintworth GK: Subacute sclerosing panencephalitis: A clinicopathologic study of the retina lesions. Arch Ophthalmol 86:156, 1971.
60. Font RL, Jenis EH, Tuck KD: Measles maculopathy associated with subacute sclerosing panencephalitis (SSPE). Arch Pathol 96:168, 1973.
61. La Piana FG, Tso MOM, Jenis EH: The retinal lesions of subacute sclerosing panencephalitis. Ann Ophthalmol 6:603, 1974.
62. Nelson DA, Weiner A, Yanoff M, dePeralta J: Retinal lesions in subacute sclerosing panencephalitis. Arch Ophthalmol 84:613, 1970.
63. Gravina RF, Nakanishi AS, Faden A: Subacute sclerosing panencephalitis. Am J Ophthalmol 86:106, 1978.
64. Green SH, Wirtschafter JO: Ophthalmoscopic findings in subacute sclerosing panencephalitis. Br J Ophthalmol 62:356, 1978.
65. Haltia M, Tarkkanen A, Vaheri A, et al: Measles retinopathy during immunosuppression. Br J Ophthalmol 62:356, 1978.
66. Laforet EG, Lynch CL: Multiple congenital defects following maternal varicella. Report of a case. N Engl J Med 236:534, 1947.
67. Gershon AA: Chickenpox, measles and mumps. *In* Remington JS, Klein JO (eds): Infectious Diseases of the Fetus and Newborn Infant, 3rd ed. Philadelphia, WB Saunders, 1990.
68. Savage MO, Moosa A, Gordon RR: Maternal varicella infection as a cause of fetal malformations. Lancet 1:352, 1973.
69. McKendry JBS, Bailey JD: Congenital varicella associated with multiple defects. Can Med Assoc J 108:66, 1973.
70. Alkalay AL, Pomerance JS, Rimoin DL: Fetal varicella syndrome. J Pediatr 111:320, 1987.
71. Charles NC, Bennet TW, Margolis S: Ocular pathology of the congenital varicella syndrome. Arch Ophthalmol 95:2034, 1977.
72. Cotlier E: Congenital varicella cataract. Am J Ophthalmol 86:627, 1978.
73. Lambert SR, Taylor D, Kriss A, et al: Ocular manifestations of the congenital varicella syndrome. Arch Ophthalmol 107:52, 1989.
74. Copenhaver RM: Chickenpox with retinopathy. Arch Ophthalmol 75:199, 1966.
75. Pizzo PA, Wilfert CM (eds): Pediatric AIDS. Baltimore, Williams & Wilkins, 1991.
76. Oxtoby MJ: Perinatally acquired HIV infection. *In* Pizzo PA, Wilfert CM (eds): Pediatric AIDS. Baltimore, Williams & Wilkins, 1991.
77. Dennehy PJ, Warman R, Flynn JT, et al: Ocular manifestations in pediatric patients with acquired immunodeficiency syndrome. Arch Ophthalmol 107:978, 1989.
78. Jabs DA, Green WR, Fox R, et al: Ocular manifestations of acquired immune deficiency syndrome. Ophthalmology 96:1092, 1989.
79. Levin AV, Zeichner S, Duke JS, et al: Cytomegalovirus retinitis in an infant with acquired immunodeficiency syndrome. Pediatrics 84:683, 1989.
80. Bottoni F, Gonnella P, Autelitano A, et al: Diffuse necrotizing retinochoroiditis in a child with AIDS and toxoplasmic encephalitis. Graefes Arch Clin Exp Ophthalmol 228:36, 1990.
81. Palestine AG, deSmet M: Retinitis and ophthalmic problems. *In* Pizzo PA, Wilfert CM (eds): Pediatric AIDS. Baltimore, Williams & Wilkins, 1991.

Chapter 80

■

Ocular Syphilis

C. STEPHEN FOSTER and RICHARD R. TAMESIS

Syphilis is a sexually transmitted, chronic, systemic infection caused by the spirochete *Treponema pallidum.* Primary infection is followed by an incubation period of about 3 wk, usually followed by the appearance of a primary skin or mucous membrane lesion, the chancre. This lesion, which may appear from 8 days to 6 wk after infection with *T. pallidum,* is usually painless and associated with regional lymph node enlargement. The chancre typically heals within a few weeks. The secondary stage of syphilis ensues. Symptoms of this stage (fever, malaise, headache, generalized lymph node enlargement, and rash) generally appear within a few weeks or, at most, a few months after the primary chancre has disappeared. This spirochetemic stage of the disease then subsides, even without antibiotic therapy, and the infection becomes "latent." Individuals with historical or serologic evidence of syphilis but with no clinical manifestations by definition have latent syphilis. Secondary syphilitic relapses may develop during this state of latency. Approximately one third of untreated cases will progress to tertiary syphilis, with syphilitic inflammatory lesions of the heart, aorta, brain, kidney, bone, eye, or skin.

ETIOLOGY

The organism responsible for syphilis, *T. pallidum*, was discovered by Schaudinn and Hoffman of Hamburg in 1905 in inflammatory lesions from a patient with syphilis. This organism is a thin, spiral-shaped parasite for whom the only known natural host is *Homo sapiens*. Other mammals can be infected with the organism. The origins are unknown, and several hypotheses exist regarding the development of syphilis in humans. Two main theories, one tracing the development from the tropics and the other tracing the development from Native Americans, are most commonly espoused. The first clear descriptions of clinical evidence of syphilis were recorded at the end of the 15th century, when a pandemic known as the Great Pox, as distinguished from smallpox, swept over Europe and Asia.[1] Warfare in the 15th century, including the seige of Naples by Charles VIII of France, was associated with the spread of what today is known as syphilis among soldiers, prostitutes, and other women who followed the warriors. The disease became known as the *French disease* among Italians and the *Italian disease* among the French. It supposedly received its present name from a poem written in 1530 by Fracastoro about an infected shepherd named Sifilis.[2]

EPIDEMIOLOGY

Transmission

With the notable exception of transplacental transmission from an infected mother to her fetus, the transmission of *T. pallidum* is almost exclusively sexual. Transmission requires a break in the skin, but *T. pallidum* can penetrate intact mucous membranes. The primary mode of transmission is through sexual intercourse, but transmission during oral sexual practices may also occur. Transmission following blood transfusions is, in essence, unheard of in civilized societies today because of the screening of blood and blood products for transfusion. The likelihood of transmission of an infectious dose of *T. pallidum* from an infected to a noninfected individual during sexual intercourse is undoubtably multifactorial. One study based on a pla-

cebo-controlled trial of antibiotic efficacy in aborting syphilis in known contacts, however, suggested a 30 percent incidence of transmission with a single sexual encounter.[3] Few organisms are needed to survive, proliferate, and produce disease. It is estimated that the ID_{50} inoculum is 57 spirochetes.[4]

With the exception of two periods of a rising incidence of syphilis, the incidence of this disease has been steadily decreasing since 1940. Infant deaths resulting from syphilis and new admissions of patients with syphilitic psychoses have fallen 99 percent since 1940 in the United States, and the total number of cases of late and latent syphilis has fallen 98 percent since 1943. A decrease of 98 percent in the number of congenital syphilitic cases has occurred since 1941.[1] An increase in the incidence of syphilis in World War II was noted in all Western countries; this incidence rapidly fell in the 1950s. A smaller rise occurred between 1971 and 1980, which can be accounted for primarily by the increasing incidence of syphilis in the promiscuous homosexual community. The incidence in this population began to decline as partner-changing decreased with the increased understanding of AIDS and its causes and modes of transmission.[4]

Age-related data show early syphilis to be concentrated in young adults, with many more male than female cases reported;[2] the reported incidence is higher among nonwhites than among whites, higher in urban areas than in rural areas, higher in the southern and southwestern United States, and higher in those states with large urban populations. Recent studies have suggested clustering within towns; a study from Seville, Spain, suggests that enhanced opportunity for spread accounts for this clustering of syphilis.[5] Special political and sociologic factors can also affect the epidemiology of this disease. For instance, Singapore experienced an increase of early infectious syphilis from 1980 to 1984; the factors blamed for this increase included prostitution, the reduced prescribing of penicillin for gonorrhea because of the emergence of penicillin-resistant strains of *Neisseria gonorrhoeae,* the loss of "herd" immunity following elimination of nonvenereal treponemal disease, and mobility of the population at risk.[6] By 1988, there were 40,275 new cases of primary and secondary syphilis reported in the United States, and syphilis, including congenital and tertiary cases, now accounts for about 100,000 new sexually transmitted disease cases annually.[4]

OCULAR MANIFESTATIONS

Uvea

Syphilis was believed to be a common cause of iritis prior to the antibiotic era. In the decade from 1970 to 1980 in a large referral uveitis practice, Schalegel and Kao estimated that only 1.1 percent of their uveitis cases were secondary to syphilis.[7] They emphasized, however, one of the most important points for ophthalmologists to remember: They did not initially suspect syphilis in most of their 28 patients who were ultimately shown to have this disease, and many of their patients had a nonreactive Venereal Disease Research Laboratory (VDRL) test. The authors emphasized, once again, the "great imitator" capabilities of syphilis and also emphasized the importance of the fluorescent treponemal antibody absorption test (FTA-ABS) in the routine testing of all patients with intraocular inflammation; if this test had not been used in their investigations, three fourths of their syphilitic iritis cases would have gone undiagnosed. We reemphasized this point as a result of our experience with 25 of 1020 new uveitis referral cases seen between January 1, 1983, and January 30, 1989.[8] This 2.45 percent portion of our new uveitis referral population had previously undiagnosed syphilis as the cause of their chronic or recurrent intraocular inflammation. More than one third of these patients had a nonreactive serum VDRL; all had a positive FTA-ABS and, on further testing, a positive micro-hemagglutination–*T. pallidum* (MHA-TP) test; all had total resolution of their uveitis with systemic intravenous penicillin therapy at doses adequate for neurosyphilis.

The iritis of syphilis has no remarkably distinguishing features. Although some authors have stated that ocular manifestations of syphilis are more likely to arise in the secondary stage of acquired syphilis, we would emphasize that in almost every instance in our referral practice, the patients have had latent syphilis with no clinical manifestations prompting a suspicion of this disease. In addition, although the older literature divided syphilitic iritis into three types according to iris features, we are impressed that in only one of our cases did we find an iris pathologic condition that prompted a specific suspicion for syphilis. We suspect that iritis roseati, with small dilated collections of capillaries in the iris; or iritis papulosa, with the iris roseati increasing in size to resemble a papule; or iritis nodosa, with increasing size of iris papulosa forming a yellow-red nodule, may be relatively restricted to cases of syphilitic uveitis that are associated with classic secondary syphilis with extraocular manifestations. Although we typically think of syphilis as being a "granulomatous" disease, and hence imagine that the iritis of syphilis should be a "granulomatous" one with mutton fat keratic precipitates (KP) on the corneal endothelium, in fact approximately one half of our patients exhibited no KP or fine KP on the endothelium. The one case with iritis nodosa has been previously reported,[8] and the iris lesion in the right eye of this patient, shown in Figure 80–1, is a good example of syphilitic uveitis nodosa.

Inflammatory cells may accumulate in the vitreous body to varying degrees (including nearly to the point of vitreal opacification) in syphilitic panuveitis or posterior uveitis. It may be difficult to evaluate the choroid and retina in such instances, but if and when the retina can be seen, sectors or foci of active choroiditis will usually be found. A diffuse retinitis or neuroretinitis without choroiditis can also occur, as can papillitis. Indeed, a healthy dictum for all ophthalmologists to follow would be that any patient with iritis and papillitis should be considered to have syphilis unless proved

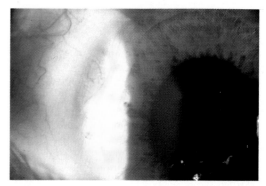

Figure 80–1. Iris nodule, syphilitic uveitis. Note the true mass in the substance of the iris periphery at the 8 to 9 o'clock positions.

otherwise. An example of sectoral neuroretinitis secondary to undiagnosed syphilis is shown in Figure 80–2, and an example of undiagnosed syphilitic multifocal chorioretinitis is shown in Figure 80–3. Figure 80–4 depicts syphilitic uveitis and associated papillitis.

Neuroophthalmic Manifestations

In addition to the possibility of papillitis previously described, optic neuritis,[9–11] optic perineuritis,[12–13] and papilledema[14] have been described as ocular manifestations in patients with ocular syphilis. Zambrano and associates reported the occurrence of bilateral syphilitic optic neuritis in a bisexual man with AIDS; this patient's visual acuity deteriorated over a period of approximately 12 hr from 20/20 bilaterally to total bilateral blindness.[15] Toshniwal reported optic perineuritis, characterized by swollen optic discs without raised intracranial pressure and visual dysfunction in a patient with secondary syphilis and a complaint of recurrent headache.[13]

Cornea and Sclera

Syphilis can cause corneal inflammation, and unlike the multifaceted uveitis presentations possible with syph-

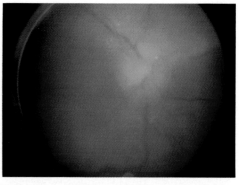

Figure 80–2. Sector retinitis, syphilitic uveitis, retinal vasculitis, and retinitis. Note sector of retina, beginning at the disc and extending superiorly, with infiltrate retinitis and associated retinal vasculitis.

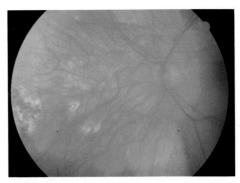

Figure 80–3. Syphilitic multifocal choroiditis. Multifocal chorioretinal lesions, now healed, with scarring in a patient with previous active syphilis with multifocal choroiditis.

Table 80–1. CAUSES OF INTERSTITIAL KERATITIS

Bacterial	Viral
Syphilis	Herpes simplex
Leprosy	Herpes zoster
Tuberculosis	Epstein-Barr virus
Chlamydia	Rubella
Lyme agent	Rubeola
	Vaccinia
Protozoal	Variola
Acanthamoeba	Mumps
Malaria	
Trypanosomiasis	**Helminthic**
Leishmaniasis	Cysticercosis
	Onchocerciasis
Other	
Cogan's syndrome	
Sarcoidosis	
Lymphoma	

ilis, syphilitic keratitis is typically an interstitial keratitis (i.e., a nonulcerative and nonsuppurative inflammation of the corneal stroma). Untreated, this stromal keratitis frequently is accompanied by stromal neovascularization. A variety of agents may cause interstitial keratitis (Table 80–1), but syphilis may be the second most common cause after herpes simplex virus. Approximately 10 percent of cases of interstitial keratitis secondary to syphilis are associated with acquired syphilis; 90 percent are seen in association with congenital syphilis. Syphilitic interstitial keratitis may be diffuse and generalized, or it may be localized. When localized, the area affected is commonly a sector of cornea (Fig. 80–5). The keratitis may be subtle, and in the photophobic patient with minimal circumlimbal injection, patience and practice are required to discover the subtle, diffuse patina of tiny, tan-colored inflammatory cells in the affected area of the corneal stroma. As the inflammatory process increases, the density of the inflammatory cell population rises, and the "infiltrate" is easier to see, as is the associated corneal edema. An associated iritis with or without KP may develop, and peripheral corneal neovascularization may ensue. Untreated, the keratitis may progress to involve the entire cornea, with progressive neovascularization of the stroma, enormous photophobia, and discomfort and decreased visual acuity for the patient. The inflammatory process may slowly regress over the ensuing 2 yr, leaving a scarred cornea

with emptied or "ghost" stromal vessels (Fig. 80–6). One or both eyes may be affected. In congenital syphilitic keratitis both eyes are affected, either simultaneously or sequentially, in more than 75 percent of patients.[16]

Syphilitic scleritis may be nodular or diffuse; we have never seen a case of necrotizing scleritis secondary to syphilis. Syphilitic scleritis has no distinguishing features and hence is diagnosed only because the ophthalmologist has cleverly included, as routine, an FTA-ABS test as part of the diagnostic survey in all patients with scleritis, interstitial keratitis, or uveitis.

DIAGNOSIS

Syphilis may be definitively diagnosed by direct or indirect techniques. Direct techniques include the darkfield examination, in which exudate from a suspected syphilitic lesion is examined by microscopy with a darkfield technique; the cork screw–shaped *T. pallidum* motile organisms are seen directly. Fluorescein-labeled anti–*T. pallidum* antibodies may be used in an immunofluorescence analysis of exudate or material taken from a suspected syphilitic lesion; the antibody will stick to syphilitic organisms in the exudate or specimen and

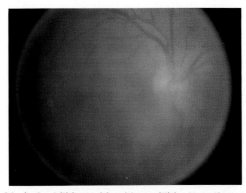

Figure 80–4. Syphilitic uveitis with papillitis. Note the swelling of the optic nerve and the hazy view of the nerve secondary to the associated inflammatory cells in the vitreous anterior to the disc.

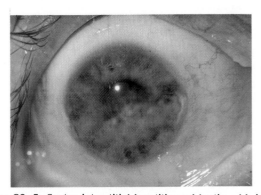

Figure 80–5. Sector interstitial keratitis and luetic, old, inactive sector interstitial keratitis with stromal scarring in the inferonasal quadrant in a patient with previously treated syphilis.

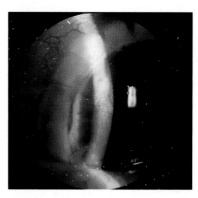

Figure 80–6. Luetic sector interstitial keratitis with ghost vessels in the deep corneal stroma (extremely difficult to capture on film and reproduce).

will be seen by the characteristic apple-green fluorescence when the specimen is examined under the fluorescence microscope. Detection of spirochetes in tissue specimens can be accomplished, through special staining techniques, including the Warthin-Starry method. The spirochetes are seen directly in the tissue specimens as shown in Figure 80–7.

Indirect techniques depend on serologic studies, some of which are *Treponema*-specific and others of which are nontreponemal tests; these nontreponemal tests detect antibodies directed against lipoidal antigens. The primary nontreponemal test used in the United States is the VDRL. This test is typically positive in patients with active syphilis and negative in patients with successfully treated syphilis. In patients with latent syphilis, however, the serum VDRL is only about 70 percent sensitive. As discussed before, 35 percent of Schalegel and Kao's patients with ocular syphilis would have been misdiagnosed if the authors had relied solely on the VDRL as the diagnostic test for syphilis.[7] More than a third of our patients had nonreactive serum VDRL tests.[8] These findings dramatically emphasize the importance of never relying on the VDRL as the sole screening test for the possibility of ocular syphilis. The standard

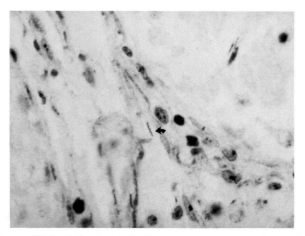

Figure 80–7. Spirochetes in the cornea, as demonstrated by silver stain, following penetrating keratoplasty in a patient with secondary syphilis and active interstitial keratitis.

treponemal tests for syphilis in the United States are the FTA-ABS and the MHA-TP. The FTA-ABS test is 98 percent sensitive, even in latent syphilis. This test will remain positive for life, regardless of whether the patient has been treated. The VDRL titer, in contrast, reflects the systemic activity of the disease and hence its major value, in our opinion, lies in monitoring the response to treatment. A persistent fall in VDRL titers following treatment provides essential evidence of an adequate response to therapy.

Evaluation for Asymptomatic Neurosyphilis

Patients with positive serologic tests for syphilis should have their cerebrospinal fluid (CSF) examined for VDRL titers, total protein, and cell counts including a differential count. Without a positive CSF VDRL test, an elevated white blood cell count with a predominance of lymphocytes in the CSF or an elevated total protein level is indicative of neurologic involvement, and the patient should be treated accordingly as for neurosyphilis.

Evaluation for HIV

There have been reports in the literature of HIV-positive young adult patients with concurrent ocular syphilis.[17] This is not surprising given the similar mode of transmission in both disease entities. There is evidence that syphilis may pursue a more aggressive course in patients who are concurrently infected with HIV, rendering standard therapy for primary and secondary syphilis inadequate.[18] In view of these reports, we believe that all patients with ocular syphilis should now be evaluated for HIV and vice versa.

TREATMENT

Patients Without Penicillin Allergy

We believe that patients with ocular syphilis should be treated in the same way that patients with neurosyphilis are treated, even without CSF evidence of neurosyphilis. We have adopted this philosophy for two reasons: (1) The blood-ocular barrier is as much a hindrance to adequate spirochetocidal doses of penicillin as is the blood-brain barrier and (2) some evidence exists suggesting that patients with syphilitic ocular inflammation may have CNS syphilis without VDRL-positive CSF. Therefore we suggest that all patients with ocular syphilis be hospitalized and given high-dose intravenous penicillin therapy. We suggest 24 million units of aqueous crystalline penicillin G intravenously every day for 10 days, followed by 2.4 million units of benzathine penicillin G intramuscularly each week for 3 wk. Close follow-up in collaboration with an infectious disease specialist and repeat serum and CSF VDRL titers to monitor the adequacy of treatment remain essential in these patients.

Patients With Penicillin Allergy

Some authors have recommended doxycycline,[19] tetracycline, or erythromycin in the treatment of penicillin-allergic patients with syphilis. It is as yet unclear whether this therapeutic approach is sufficient therapy in most patients with neurosyphilis, and little to no experience exists with these treatment regimens in patients with ocular syphilis. Some investigators believe that "penicillin-allergic" patients should be carefully evaluated and possibly desensitized and then treated with penicillin. Many patients with penicillin "allergy," in fact, do not have a true allergy at all. We would advocate careful allergy testing in patients with syphilis who claim to have a penicillin allergy. Such patients who have negative skin test results can safely undergo the aforementioned penicillin treatment program with close in-hospital monitoring. In addition, although penicillin allergy desensitization can be lengthy, costly, and complex, this alternative for treating the individual with ocular syphilis or neurosyphilis that has been proved to be allergic to penicillin is not without merit.

REFERENCES

1. Poitevin M, Collart P, Bolgert M: Syphilis in 1986. J Clin Neuro Ophthalmol 7:11, 1987.
2. Fracastoro: Le mal français ou syphilis. Extrait du livre de "contagionibus et contagiosis morbis" (1546) avec commentaires de A. Fournier. 1869.
3. Martin JP: Conquest of general paresis. Br Med J 2:159, 1972.
4. Centers for Disease Control: Summary—Cases of specified notifiable disease—United States. MMWR 37:802, 1989.
5. Alvarez-Dardet C, Marquez S, Perea EJ, et al: Urban clusters of sexually transmitted diseases in the city of Seville, Spain. Sex Transm Dis 12:166, 1985.
6. Thirumoorthy T, Lee CT, Lim KB: Epidemiology of infectious syphilis in Singapore. Genitourin Med 62:75, 1986.
7. Schalegel TF Jr, Kao SF: A review (1970–1980) of 28 presumptive cases of syphilitic uveitis. Am J Ophthalmol 93:412, 1982.
8. Tamesis RR, Foster CS: Ocular syphilis. Ophthalmology 97:1281, 1990.
9. Graveson GS: Syphilitic optic neuritis. J Neurol Neurosurg Psychiatry 13:216, 1950.
10. Walsh FB: Syphilis of the optic nerve. Ophthalmology 60:39, 1956.
11. Weinstein JM, Lexow SS, Ho P, Spickards A: Acute syphilitic optic neuritis. Arch Ophthalmol 99:1392, 1981.
12. Rush JA, Ryan EJ: Syphilitic optic perineuritis. Am J Ophthalmol 91:404, 1981.
13. Toshniwal P: Optic perineuritis with secondary syphilis. J Clin Neuro Ophthalmol 7:6, 1987.
14. Schatz NJ, Smith JL: Non-tumor causes of the Foster-Kennedy syndrome. J Neurosurg 27:37, 1967.
15. Zambrano W, Perez GM, Smith JL: Acute syphilitic blindness in AIDS. J Clin Neuro Ophthalmol 7:1, 1987.
16. Duke-Elder SS, Leigh AG: Diseases of the Outer Eye. System of Ophthalmology Series, vol. 8. St Louis, CV Mosby, 1965, p 790.
17. Passo MS, Rosenbaum JT: Ocular syphilis in patients with human immunodeficiency virus infection. Am J Ophthalmol 106:1, 1988.
18. Johns DR, Tierney M, Felsenstein D: Alteration in the natural history of neurosyphilis by concurrent infection with the human immunodeficiency virus. N Engl J Med 316:1569, 1987.
19. Tramont EC: Syphilis in the AIDS era. N Engl J Med 316:1600, 1987.

Chapter 81

■

Subretinal Fibrosis and Uveitis Syndrome

DAVID R. GUYER and EVANGELOS S. GRAGOUDAS

HISTORICAL PERSPECTIVE

The subretinal fibrosis and uveitis syndrome is a rare distinctive posterior uveitis, which was first described by Palestine and associates.[1] In 1984, these authors described three patients with the unusual findings of progressive subretinal fibrosis and uveitis. The condition most commonly occurs in healthy, young myopic females, usually with only minimal signs of ocular inflammation. Early in the disorder, multiple small, whitish-yellow retinal pigment epithelial or choroidal lesions are observed in the posterior pole and midperiphery. In the later stages of the disease, progressive subretinal fibrosis occurs. The histopathologic and immunohistopathologic features of this condition were subsequently described by the same group.[2, 3]

Alternatively, the subretinal fibrosis and uveitis syndrome may simply be a rarely observed late stage in the spectrum of the disorder termed *multifocal choroiditis,* rather than being a unique entity itself.[4] Thus, the spectrum of this disease may include reports describing the early stage of this condition with a recurrent multiple choroiditis and uveitis. These early findings have been described as *multifocal choroiditis and panuveitis* by Dreyer and Gass,[5] *punctate inner chorioretinopathy* by Watzke and coworkers,[6] and *recurrent multifocal inner choroiditis* by Morgan and Schatz.[7] In at least one case from each of these series,[5–7] there was evidence of later findings of lesion enlargement or subretinal fibrosis. The late findings of this disease have been described as *progressive subretinal fibrosis and uveitis* by Palestine and associates,[1, 2] *chorioretinopathy with anterior uveitis*

Table 81–1. THE SPECTRUM OF ACUTE MULTIFOCAL CHOROIDITIS AND PROGRESSIVE SUBRETINAL FIBROSIS

Acute Findings	Late Findings
Multifocal choroiditis and panuveitis[5]	Progressive subretinal fibrosis and uveitis [1-3]
Punctate inner chorioretinopathy[6]	Chorioretinopathy with anterior uveitis[8]
Recurrent multifocal inner choroiditis[7]	Multifocal choroiditis with disciform macular degeneration[9]
	Progressive subretinal fibrosis[10]

by Nozik and Dorsch,[8] *multifocal choroiditis with disciform macular degeneration* by Doran and Hamilton,[9] and *multifocal choroiditis associated with progressive subretinal fibrosis* by Cantrill and Folk[10] (Table 81–1).

PATIENT CHARACTERISTICS

The subretinal fibrosis and uveitis syndrome occurs predominantly in young, healthy myopic females. The patients are usually less than 35 yr of age.[1-10] In one series of 11 patients, the age range was 24 to 43 yr, with a mean age of 30.2 yr.[7] The disease has been described in patients as young as 6 yr and as old as 69 yr.[5, 8] In several series, all of the patients were females.[1, 2, 6, 7, 10] The patients usually have a myopic refractive error.[6, 7, 9] In Morgan and Schatz's series,[7] 10 of 11 patients were myopic, with a range of −2.75 to −8.50 D. Systemic evaluation of these patients is almost always unremarkable.[1-10] Cases have been associated with Reiter's syndrome; migraine; atopy; schizoid syndrome; gastric bypass surgery; positive skin, serologic, and biopsy findings of histoplasmosis; and a positive purified protein derivative test for tuberculosis. However, these associations are probably unrelated to the ocular condition.[1-10] Six of 11 patients in one series were taking oral contraceptives.[7] Patients with this condition do not respond to the retinal S antigen.[1]

SYMPTOMS

Patients usually complain of acute vision loss, often with metamorphopsia. Scotomas and photopsias also may be reported.

OBJECTIVE FINDINGS (Table 81–2)

The vision loss may be very mild or severe, depending on which stage of the disease the patient presents with. Patients with mild disease can have 20/20 vision, and severe disease may reduce visual acuity to the counting fingers to light perception level. In one series,[10] the initial visual acuity ranged from 20/20 to 20/400. These patients already had signs of subretinal fibrosis. In another series, patients with the early findings of this condition without subretinal fibrosis[7] also had initial visual acuity that ranged from 20/40 to 20/400. The condition is usually bilateral (45 to 100 percent of cases);[1-10] however, the fellow eye may be asymptomatic. In one series of five patients,[10] one case remained unilateral, one case presented with bilateral involvement, and in three cases the second eye became involved in 3 to 6 mo.

Slit-lamp examination may reveal an anterior or posterior uveitis (Fig. 81–1).[1-10] Usually, however, the inflammation is mild. A mild chronic vitritis is often associated with transient, multiple, small (100 to 500 μ), round, discrete, yellowish-white lesions of the retinal pigment epithelium or choriocapillaris in the posterior pole and midperiphery (see Fig. 81–1).[1-10] These lesions may fade or enlarge and coalesce to create multiple areas of whitish subretinal fibrosis (Fig. 81–2; see also Fig. 81–1).[1-10] The progression of subretinal fibrosis may occur over months to years.

Other findings may include optic disc edema, serous and hemorrhagic macular detachment, macular hole, cystoid macular edema, and choroidal neovascularization (CNV).[1-10] Although CNV was not reported in the series of Palestine and associates,[1] it has been reported in 36 to 100 percent of other series.[4-7, 9] In addition, Cantrill and Folk[10] reported an atypical type of CNV in their series.

FLUOROANGIOGRAPHIC AND ELECTROPHYSIOLOGIC FINDINGS

Retinal pigment epithelium window defects or mottled hyperfluorescence of the acute lesions are observed by fluorescein angiography in the early stages of this disorder.[1-10] The subretinal fibrosis shows late staining.[1, 2, 10] Optic disc leakage and macular edema may be present. CNV is commonly observed.

Electroretinographic signals may be depressed.[1, 2] The electrooculogram may be markedly decreased[1, 2] or normal.[7, 10] Three patients in one series[7] had normal color vision testing results.

NATURAL HISTORY

In all but one series,[7] the visual prognosis of these patients was poor. In Cantrill and Folk's series,[10] severe vision loss occurred in at least one eye. Many of these

Table 81–2. FINDINGS IN THE SUBRETINAL FIBROSIS AND UVEITIS SYNDROME

Anterior uveitis
Vitritis
Multifocal choroiditis
Subretinal fibrosis
Optic disc edema
Serous and hemorrhagic macular detachment
Cystoid macular edema
Choroidal neovascularization

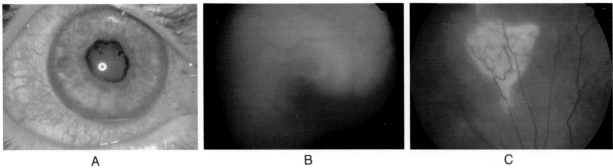

Figure 81–1. This 26-year-old woman presented with decreased vision, redness, and pain in both eyes. Slit-lamp examination revealed conjunctival injection, anterior chamber reaction, posterior synechiae, and a cataract *(A)*. Examination of the fundus showed subretinal fibrosis *(B and C)*.

patients had final visual acuities of 20/200 to the counting fingers level. This poor visual prognosis was confirmed in all of the other reports except for the series of Morgan and Schatz.[7] These authors noted a final vision of 20/20 to 20/70 in patients treated with steroids and vision of 20/400 in patients who were not treated. However, as is discussed further on, this beneficial effect of steroids upon the visual prognosis of this condition was not always noted in other reports.

Recurrences are common in this disorder and may range from two to seven recurrences per patient.

HISTOPATHOLOGIC AND IMMUNOHISTOPATHOLOGIC FINDINGS

Two histopathologic reports of this condition have been published (Fig. 81–3).[2, 3] In one chorioretinal biopsy specimen,[2] inflammation of the choroid was noted with B-cell lymphocytes and plasma cells. Complement C3, immunoglobulin G, and fibrin were present in the subretinal area. The retina and retinal pigment epithelium were replaced by amorphous connective tissue. The

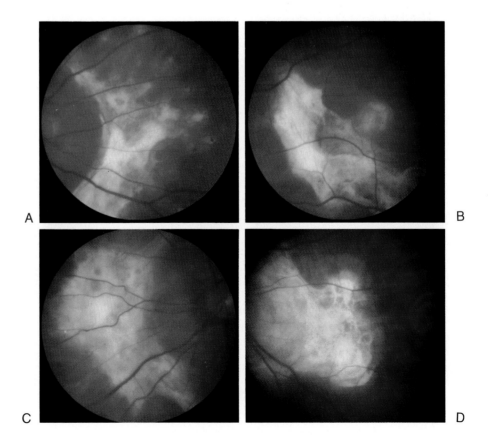

Figure 81–2. *A–D,* The extensive subretinal fibrosis that occurs in this syndrome is illustrated in this patient. *(A–D,* Courtesy of Robert Nussenblatt, M.D.)

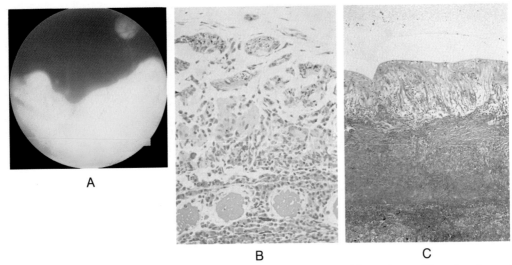

Figure 81–3. This 18-year-old woman presented with the subretinal fibrosis and uveitis syndrome (A) and underwent a chorioretinal biopsy. Histopathologic examination (B) revealed a thickened choroid that contained numerous lymphocytes and plasma cells. Connective tissue replaced the normal retina. C, Histopathologic study in another patient with the subretinal fibrosis and uveitis syndrome revealed thick, fibrous tissue interposed between the markedly gliotic retina and the choroid. (A–C, Courtesy of Chi-Chao Chan, M.D., and Robert Nussenblatt, M.D.)

subretinal fibrosis showed characteristics of both retinal pigment epithelium and Müller cells. No virus or circulating antiretinal antibody was found. A second specimen of an enucleated eye[3] revealed an extremely gliotic retina with subretinal tissue and a granulomatous inflammation of the choroid. Electron microscopy suggested that the subretinal tissue was derived from the retinal pigment epithelium.

PATHOPHYSIOLOGY

This condition is probably due to a localized autoimmune antibody-mediated inflammation with destruction of the retinal pigment epithelium.[1–3, 10] These patients do not typically show systemic abnormalities or respond to the retinal S antigen. The antibodies may be produced by plasma cells, which then destroy the retinal pigment epithelium and produce subretinal fibrosis.

TREATMENT

Once the subretinal fibrosis occurs, there appears to be no beneficial treatment.[1, 4] However, there is controversy over whether steroids may be useful in the acute phase of this condition. Responses to steroids during the acute phase have been reported; however, many patients will show no improvement.[1–10] In one series,[7] there was a dramatic response to systemic and periocular steroids. All nine treated patients showed visual improvement after treatment (final visual acuity 20/20 to 20/70), whereas the two untreated patients had a poor visual prognosis (visual acuity of 20/400). In this same series, a case of CNV appeared to respond to steroid treatment. However, this may represent a spontaneous

improvement. Thus, it seems reasonable to consider steroid treatment for acute cases but not for cases in which subretinal fibrosis has already occurred.

In some cases, the macular edema was improved by steroid administration, but again the number of cases was too small to make definitive conclusions. One patient was treated with cyclophosphamide without improvement.[3] Laser photocoagulation has also been attempted without apparent success in this condition.[5, 6, 9] Since B-cell lymphocytes have been found in the choroid, appropriate chemotherapy could be considered in severe cases.

DIFFERENTIAL DIAGNOSIS

The acute phase of this condition can be confused with many entities, although the disease is easy to

Table 81–3. DIFFERENTIAL DIAGNOSIS IN THE SUBRETINAL FIBROSIS AND UVEITIS SYNDROME

Sarcoidosis
Presumed ocular histoplasmosis syndrome
Tuberculosis
Syphilis
Birdshot chorioretinopathy
Toxoplasmosis
Fungal infections
Acute posterior placoid pigment epitheliopathy
Serpiginous choroidopathy
Multiple evanescent white dot syndrome
Diffuse unilateral subacute neuroretinitis
Punctate outer retinal toxoplasmosis
Sympathetic ophthalmia
Acute retinal pigment epitheliitis
Acute macular neuroretinopathy
Inflammatory pseudohistoplasmosis

identify once the progressive subretinal fibrosis occurs (Table 81–3). Acutely, the differential diagnosis includes sarcoidosis, presumed ocular histoplasmosis syndrome, tuberculosis, syphilis, birdshot chorioretinopathy, toxoplasmosis, fungal infections, acute posterior placoid pigment epitheliopathy, serpiginous choroidopathy, multiple evanescent white dot syndrome, diffuse unilateral subacute neuroretinitis, punctate outer retinal toxoplasmosis, sympathetic ophthalmia, acute retinal pigment epitheliitis, acute macular neuroretinopathy, and inflammatory pseudohistoplasmosis. The clinical history, inflammatory reaction, and progression to subretinal fibrosis can distinguish the subretinal fibrosis and uveitis syndrome from these conditions. In the later stages of this disease, choroidopathies with CNV and disciform scarring, such as seen in serpiginous choroidopathy, may be confused with this entity.

CONCLUSIONS

The subretinal fibrosis and uveitis syndrome is a condition in which progressive subretinal fibrosis occurs following an acute episode of recurrent multifocal choroiditis, usually in young, healthy myopic females. CNV and macular edema may also occur. The visual prognosis is generally poor. Steroid treatment may be beneficial during the acute stages of the disorder, and chemotherapy may be considered in severe cases.

The disease is probably caused by a localized autoimmune reaction in which antibodies destroy the retinal pigment epithelium and produce subretinal fibrosis. The condition probably represents the rarely observed late stages of disorders described as multifocal choroiditis and panuveitis, punctate inner chorioretinopathy, and recurrent multifocal inner choroiditis. Although the acute stages of this condition may be confused with other types of choroiditis, the progressive subretinal fibrosis observed at late stages distinguishes this disorder from most other diseases.

REFERENCES

1. Palestine AG, Nussenblatt RB, Parver LM, Knox DL: Progressive subretinal fibrosis and uveitis. Br J Ophthalmol 68:667–673, 1984.
2. Palestine AG, Nussenblatt RB, Chan CC, et al: Histopathology of the subretinal fibrosis and uveitis syndrome. Ophthalmology 92:838–844, 1985.
3. Kim MK, Chan CC, Belfort R, et al: Histopathologic and immunohistopathologic features of subretinal fibrosis and uveitis syndrome. Am J Ophthalmol 104:15–23, 1987.
4. Singerman LJ: Discussion of Morgan CM, Schatz H: Recurrent multifocal choroiditis. Ophthalmology 93:1143–1147, 1986.
5. Dreyer RF, Gass JDM: Multifocal choroiditis and panuveitis: A syndrome that mimics ocular histoplasmosis. Arch Ophthalmol 102:1776–1784, 1984.
6. Watzke RC, Packer AJ, Folk JC, et al: Punctate inner choroidopathy. Am J Ophthalmol 98:572–584, 1984.
7. Morgan C, Schatz H: Recurrent multifocal choroiditis. Ophthalmology 93:1138–1143, 1986.
8. Nozik RA, Dorsch W: A new chorioretinopathy associated with anterior uveitis. Am J Ophthalmol 76:758–762, 1973.
9. Doran RML, Hamilton AM: Disciform macular degeneration in young adults. Trans Ophthalmol Soc UK 102:471–480, 1982.
10. Cantrill HL, Folk JC: Multifocal choroiditis associated with progressive subretinal fibrosis. Am J Ophthalmol 101:170–180, 1986.

Chapter 82

▪

Diffuse Unilateral Subacute Neuroretinopathy

THOMAS R. HEDGES III

The term *diffuse unilateral subacute neuroretinopathy (DUSN)* was initially used by Gass and Scelfo to describe a syndrome characterized by widespread, unilateral, insidious, and inflammatory destruction of the neuroretina. It was originally categorized at the Bascom Palmer Eye Institute as the "unilateral wipe-out syndrome."[1] The cases described by Gass and coworkers,[1, 2] as well as previously reported similar cases,[3–6] indicate that the causative agent is one or more nematodes, which have been observed in many cases, but as yet have eluded definite serologic or pathologic identification.

CLINICAL FEATURES (Table 82–1)

In more than 50 percent of cases, the usual onset is striking loss of vision following apparently subacute loss of enough retinal function to cause an afferent pupillary defect and electroretinographic abnormalities. This is accompanied by diffuse and focal pigment epithelial derangement with relative sparing of the macula, optic atrophy, and narrowing of the retinal blood vessels. The age of patients so far reported has ranged from 7 to 65 yr. There does not appear to be a sexual or racial predilection. Most patients have been in generally good

Table 82–1. CLINICAL FEATURES OF DIFFUSE UNILATERAL SUBACUTE NEURORETINOPATHY (DUSN)

Occasional Early Features
Loss of visual acuity
Mild optic disc swelling
Relative afferent pupillary defect
Vitreous cells (few)
Anterior chamber cells (very unusual)
Subretinal or intraretinal tracks
Worm visible

Chronic Features
Insidious loss of vision in one eye
Loss of visual acuity and patchy loss of visual field
Relative afferent pupillary defect
Multifocal and diffuse retinal pigment epithelial derangement
(relative macular sparing)
Optic atrophy
Narrowing of retinal blood vessels
Abnormal electroretinogram

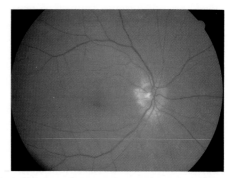

Figure 82–1. Fundus photograph showing mild optic disc swelling and peripapillary pigment thinning in the active phase of diffuse unilateral subacute neuroretinopathy (DUSN).

health without exposure to a specific animal vector. The syndrome has been seen primarily in the United States in Miami but also in the Midwest and New England (Table 82–2).

Early Stage

The early stage of the disease is recognized when the macular damage causes loss of visual acuity before more peripheral retina is affected. The resulting loss of visual acuity is either apparent to the patient or is identified in school, driving license, or ocular examinations. In this stage, the visual loss is out of proportion to visible changes in the retina or optic nerve. However, an afferent pupillary defect and mild optic disc swelling (Fig. 82–1) or pallor are present in most individuals, suggesting optic neuritis as an early part of the syndrome. Vitreous cells are seen in the early stages, indicating active inflammation, which is usually mild. Only rarely is the anterior segment of the eye involved, with mild to moderate ciliary flush, anterior chamber cells and flare, and keratitic precipitates (4 of 19 patients in one of Gass and associates' series).[7] Fundus fluorescein angiography tends to be normal in the early stages, except for mild optic disc staining and a few areas of hypofluorescence throughout the retina.

During observation, patients in the active phase will show multiple gray or yellow-white lesions involving deep or external layers of the retina one-quarter to one disc diameter in size, which may fade from view within days, leaving scattered areas of depigmentation (Fig. 82–2). It is in the early stages when a motile subretinal worm may be seen in an area of active inflammation.

Table 82–2. PATIENT CHARACTERISTICS IN DUSN

Age 7–65 yr
No sex or racial predilection
Most affected individuals healthy
Most reports from southeastern and midwestern
United States, Puerto Rico

However, the worm disappears within days to weeks and may be very difficult to find again. Two types of worm have been observed and differentiated by size. One is 400 to 1000 μm (Fig. 82–3) and the other is 1500 to 2000 μm in length.[2] Both have been measured to be 25 μm in diameter. Usually the worm is seen moving beneath the retina, occasionally within the retina, and rarely, in the vitreous. Even more rarely "tracks" are seen where the worm has traveled within the retina. Therefore, seeing the worm is difficult and requires multiple observations over weeks to months. There is some evidence that the worm can live within the eye up to 3 yr or more.[2] The examining light of the slit-lamp biomicroscope seems to stimulate the worm to move in a series of "slow coiling and uncoiling, and less often, slithering, snake-like movements."[2] Occasionally, the worm is seen only in photographs or by the photographer.

One of the most important diagnostic findings is an abnormal electroretinogram (ERG). Although the ERG may be normal in the early stages in some patients, it soon becomes characterized by loss of the b-wave with relative preservation of the a-wave. Even in the latter stages of the syndrome, the ERG rarely becomes extinguished. Electrooculographic abnormalities are also present in about half of affected individuals, but these are nonspecific.

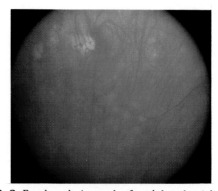

Figure 82–2. Fundus photograph of peripheral patches of retinal pigment epithelial atrophy in later stages of DUSN.

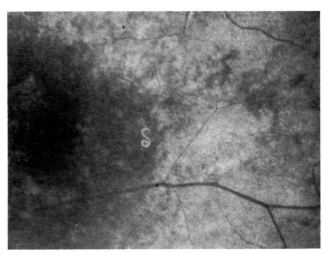

Figure 82–3. Photograph of presumed worm in the retina from a patient with DUSN. (Courtesy of J. Donald M. Gass, M.D.)

Late and Inactive Stage

As the disease progresses, more areas of retinal pigment epithelial atrophy develop. Vision declines to 20/200 or less, and dense central and patchy peripheral visual field loss becomes apparent. The optic disc becomes pale, and the retinal blood vessels become narrow. At this stage, there are many similarities to what has been described as unilateral retinitis pigmentosa or the final outcome of retinal and choroidal ischemia following compression of the eye during systemic hypotension. Choroidal neovascularization occurs extremely rarely, and retinal hemorrhages are hardly ever seen. Fundus fluorescein angiography in the late stages shows widespread hypofluorescence in areas in which retinal pigment epithelial loss has occurred. Also, retinal circulation time is prolonged on the angiogram.

DIFFERENTIAL DIAGNOSIS
(Table 82–3)

A variety of diagnoses may be considered by referring physicians, including retrobulbar optic neuritis, papillitis, and papilledema. Electroretinographic abnormalities readily distinguish these disorders from the retinopathy of DUSN. Occasionally, the patchy retinal pigment epithelial abnormalities are reminiscent of acute posterior multifocal plaquoid pigment epitheliopathy or active choroiditis caused by histoplasmosis or toxoplasmosis. However, the retinal pigment epithelial abnormalities of DUSN are milder than those seen in these conditions, and the lack of any retinal findings such as retinal necrosis or hemorrhage helps rule out cytomegalic inclusion retinitis, the retinopathy of subacute sclerosing panencephalitis, and choroiditis or retinopathy due to fungus or bacteria. An initial diagnosis of pars planitis may be made, but the eventual involvement of the retina helps identify the condition as a neuroretinitis.

DUSN may be confused with posttraumatic retinop-

athy, but the degree of trauma required to produce the widespread involvement typical of DUSN should be severe enough to be identified by history. The diffuse degeneration of the retina, with the electroretinographic characteristics of loss of the b-wave with relative preservation of the a-wave may suggest the possibility of retinal toxicity from intraocular iron. Again, the history may be useful in this situation, and careful examination of the retina and vitreous, together with computed tomography if necessary, should rule out the presence of an intraocular foreign body. In many ways, DUSN is reminiscent of combined central retinal artery and choroidal ischemia following compression of the eye, especially during periods of hypotension, such as during back surgery. Again, the history should be helpful. In elderly individuals, the remote possibility of ophthalmic artery occlusion might be considered. Another differential diagnostic consideration is unilateral retinitis pigmentosa. In fact, Gass and Scelfo have speculated that some previously reported cases of unilateral retinitis pigmentosa may actually have been cases of DUSN.[1] True unilateral retinitis pigmentosa is usually seen in patients who have a positive family history, and it is also characterized by more severe pigment epithelial abnormalities, with bone spicule formation, an extinguished ERG, and cataract. Furthermore, visual acuity is relatively preserved in retinitis pigmentosa but is lost in DUSN.

PATHOGENESIS

The pathogenesis of DUSN seems to involve local toxic effects on the outer retina caused by the worm, manifested by gray-white outer retinal lesions. More diffuse toxic damage to both inner and outer retina seems to cause loss of both visual function and the b-wave of the ERG. Eventual inner retinal destruction leads to optic atrophy, along with narrowing of the retinal blood vessels.

At least two nematodes are felt to be responsible for DUSN based on two distinct sizes of the worms seen thus far. Furthermore, the smaller, 400- to 1000-μm worm has been found predominantly in patients from the southeastern United States and Puerto Rico, whereas the larger 1500- to 2000-μm worm has been seen in patients predominantly from the midwestern United States.[2] The larger worm also seems to have a tendency to cause coarser clumping and "tracks" in the

Table 82–3. DIFFERENTIAL DIAGNOSIS OF DUSN

Optic neuritis
Acute posterior multifocal placoid pigment epitheliopathy
Histoplasmosis
Toxoplasmosis
Subacute sclerosing panencephalitis
Pars planitis
Posttraumatic retinal and choroidal ischemia
Central retinal artery occlusion (giant cell arteritis)
Iron toxicity
Unilateral retinitis pigmentosa

subretinal pigment, whereas the smaller worm tends to cause more chorioretinal atrophic scarring.

Both worms are larger than *Toxocara canis,* which is usually no more than 400 μm in length and most often causes a granulomatous mass. However, several reports have suggested that *Toxocara* is the most likely causative organism. A case reported by Rubin and colleagues showed indirect serologic evidence of *T. canis.*[5] Oppenheim and associates reported a patient with DUSN and eosinophilia in whom the enzyme-linked immunoabsorbent assay (ELISA) was strongly positive for *T. canis.*[8] Although Gass and Scelfo initially speculated that *Toxocara* was responsible,[1] they subsequently showed the ELISA for *Toxocara* to be negative in 14 cases and concluded that another, yet to be identified, nematode is responsible for DUSN.[2]

In an early report of this syndrome, Parsons suggested that the causative agent was *Ascaris lumbricoides.*[3] Price and Wadsworth made no definite conclusions regarding the type of worm in their case but did mention a number of worms that might have been responsible, including *Wuchereria bancrofti* filaria, *Onchocerca,* loa loa, *Dirofilaria* (*immitis* and *terminis*), and *Ascaris.*[4] Raymond and associates added *Dipetalonema arbuta* and *Brugia malayi* (from Korea).[6] Kazacos and associates, from Raymond's group, later speculated that the worm most likely to cause DUSN is *Baylisascaris,* especially *B. procyonis.*[9, 10] This nematode is a common intestinal round worm of lower carnivores, including raccoons and skunks. Most often *B. procyonis* causes central nervous system infection along with visceral larva migrans and ocular larva migrans. In affected primates, ocular lesions, which may occur without central nervous system infection,[10] resemble the early stages of DUSN. Kazacos and coworkers also suggested that the two different sizes of organisms observed in humans with DUSN may represent two ranges on a growth continuum for a single species, reflecting different ages of larvi.[10] *Baylisascaris* is 300 μm long after hatching and grows to 1500 to 2000 μm in its later stages. However, Kazacos believes that several nematodes, including *Toxocara,* hookworms, and *Strongyloides,* as well as *Bayosascaris,* may be responsible for DUSN (Kazacos, personal communication). An ELISA that is sensitive to this organism is being developed (Kazacos, personal communication) (Table 82–4).

Table 82–4. POSSIBLE ORGANISMS RESPONSIBLE FOR DUSN*

More likely organisms	Least likely
Ancylostoma canium[7-11]	*Ascaris lumbricoides*[3]
Baylisascaris procyonis[9, 10]	*Wuchereria bancrofti* filaria[4]
Less likely	*Onchocerca*[4]
Toxocara[1, 2, 8]	*Loa loa*[4]
Strongyloides	*Dirofilaria*[4]
	Dipetalonema arbuta[6]
	Brugia malayi[6]

*The nematodes responsible are of two sizes. Those found in the southeastern United States and Puerto Rico are 400 to 1000 μm in length and 25 μm in diameter. The nematodes found in the midwestern United States are 1500 to 2000 μm in length and 25 μm in diameter.

At least two attempts to obtain the worm by transscleral biopsy have been made[2] (Gass, personal communication). Pathologic sectioning of one eye removed from a patient with DUSN failed to reveal the exact nature of the organism on either histopathologic or electron microscopic studies.[7] However, Gass has indicated that the features found in the biopsy resembled a hookworm found in dogs, *Ancylostoma canium.* This parasite is a common cause of visceral larva migrans in the southeastern United States. The infective third stage of *A. canium* is about 650 μm in length, which is the size of the worm seen in patients with DUSN.[11]

INVESTIGATIONS

Considering the differential diagnosis and the type of worms potentially responsible in a patient with suspected DUSN, the following investigations might be considered. The patient should be asked specifically about travel history and exposure to animals, especially raccoons and skunks. History of ocular trauma, including the possibility of intraocular iron, should be specifically addressed. Risk factors for carotid and ophthalmic artery disease should be raised in elderly patients. In individuals older than 60 yr, an erythrocyte sedimentation rate determination to rule out the remote possibility of giant cell arteritis, as well as noninvasive studies of the carotid and ophthalmic artery blood flow, should also be considered. Magnetic resonance imaging might be worthwhile for identifying the possibility of retrobulbar optic neuropathy, but electroretinography usually indicates that the retina is the primary site of the disorder. When evaluating the results of the ERG, one should look for loss of the b-wave with relative preservation of the a-wave. Although electrooculographic abnormalities have been noted, they are nonspecific.

If the initial examination fails to reveal the presence of the worm, repeated slit-lamp biomicroscopic evaluation over a period of days to weeks is required. If the worm can be identified, all other differential diagnostic considerations, aside from an intraocular worm, can be disregarded. Once the worm has been visualized or other diagnostic considerations have been ruled out, or both, attempts to identify the nature of the worm should be pursued. Stool should be obtained for examination for ova and parasites. Liver function studies to rule out liver involvement, which may occur in a variety of nematode infections, should be performed. A complete blood count along with an eosinophil count should be obtained to help identify more systemic infection. An ELISA test for *T. canis* and other parasites is also appropriate. However, this has been shown to be positive only in a few cases and assay for other nematodes, when available, may allow for specific diagnoses to be made in the future.

TREATMENT

Prednisone has been tried to control the inflammation but is no longer felt to be useful in the treatment of

DUSN.[2] Thiabendazol, a drug used to control nematode infections, has shown no effect on the worm, either in terms of its mobility or in the progression of the syndrome.[2] Diethylcarbamazine citrate has likewise been ineffective in the few patients so treated.[2]

Laser has been the only effective way to eliminate the worm, and fortunately no severe toxic reaction appears to occur from the death of the worm.[2, 6, 7] However, in most cases, the worm has spontaneously disappeared, although the vast majority of patients who are untreated experience later stages of the disease with severe loss of vision.[2-5, 7, 8]

REFERENCES

1. Gass JDM, Scelfo R: Diffuse unilateral subacute neuroretinitis. J R Soc Med 71:95, 1978.
2. Gass JDM, Braunstein RA: Further observations concerning the diffuse unilateral subacute neuroretinitis syndrome. Arch Ophthalmol 101:1689, 1983.
3. Parsons HE: Registry of interesting cases. Nematode chorioretinitis. Report of a case, with photographs of a viable worm. Arch Ophthalmol 47:799, 1952.
4. Price JA, Wadsworth JAC: Registry of interesting cases. An intraretinal worm. Report of a case of macular retinopathy caused by invasion of the retina by a worm. Arch Ophthalmol 83:768, 1970.
5. Rubin ML, Kaufman HE, Tierney JP, et al: An intraretinal nematode. A case report. Trans Am Acad Ophthalmol Otol 72:855, 1968.
6. Raymond LA, Gutierrez Y, Strong LE, et al: Living retinal nematode (filarial-like) destroyed with photocoagulation. Ophthalmology 85:944, 1978.
7. Gass JDM, Gilbert WR, Guerry RK, et al: Diffuse unilateral subacute neuroretinitis. Ophthalmology 85:521, 1978.
8. Oppenheim S, Rogell G, Peyser R: Diffuse unilateral subacute neuroretinitis. Ann Ophthalmol 17:336, 1985.
9. Kazacos KR, Vestre WA, Kazacos EA, et al: Diffuse unilateral subacute neuroretinitis syndrome: Probable cause. Arch Ophthalmol 102:967, 1984.
10. Kazacos KR, Raymond LA, Kazacos EA, et al: The raccoon ascarid. A probable cause of human ocular larva migrans. Ophthalmology 92:1735, 1985.
11. Gass JDM: Stereoscopic Atlas of Macular Diseases, 3rd ed, St Louis, CV Mosby, 1987, p 472.

Chapter 83

■

Frosted Branch Angiitis

CAROL M. LEE and HENRY J. KAPLAN

Frosted branch angiitis was first described in 1976 by Ito in a 6-year-old boy with severe sheathing of all the retinal vessels, resembling the frosted branches of a tree.[1] Since then, eight other bilateral cases have been reported in the literature.[2-6] The initial clinical presentation of this rare entity may be similar to those of other more common retinal vasculitides. Because the differential diagnosis of retinal vasculitis encompasses many conditions, it is important to recognize the unique characteristics of this newly described disease. The term frosted branch angiitis has been used synonymously with diffuse acute retinal periphlebitis.[6]

CLINICAL CHARACTERISTICS

Acute frosted branch angiitis is a bilateral retinal vasculitis seen in young, otherwise healthy patients who range in age from 6 to 29 yr and present with a chief complaint of decreased visual acuity. Vision is usually profoundly affected, with the majority of reported cases presenting with 20/200 vision or worse (range 20/20 to light perception). On examination, both anterior chamber and vitreous inflammation is seen in almost all cases without pars plana deposits. Bilateral retinal phlebitis and arteritis are present, extending from the posterior pole to the periphery with uninterrupted severe sheathing of all the vessels, resembling the frosted branches of a tree (Fig. 83–1). The inflammation may predominantly affect the veins only, as 5 of the reported cases

had only venous involvement; 3 of the reported cases had extensive involvement of the arteries.

Fluorescein angiography shows normal blood flow without evidence of occlusion or stasis but with late staining and leakage of dye from affected vessels (Fig. 83–2). Additional fundus findings may include intraretinal hemorrhages, punctuate hard exudates, and serous exudative detachments of the macula or periphery. The retina can appear diffusely thickened and edematous.

DIAGNOSTIC TESTS

Electrophysiologic testing shows a reduction in the amplitude of the electroretinogram, which remains reduced even after convalescence. In contrast, the visual evoked response is initially reduced but may return to normal.[5] Visual field testing reveals concentric constriction or relative central defects that improve after clinical resolution of the vasculitis.

Laboratory investigations have not revealed an etiologic agent in this disease. Included among the normal laboratory studies were the following: complete blood cell count and differential; erythrocyte sedimentation rate; skin test for tuberculin delayed-type hypersensitivity; determination of serum antibodies for syphilis, HIV, herpes simplex, herpes zoster, and cytomegalovirus; urine and blood cultures for both bacteria and virus; antinuclear antibody determination; serum protein electrophoresis; immunoelectrophoresis; and determination

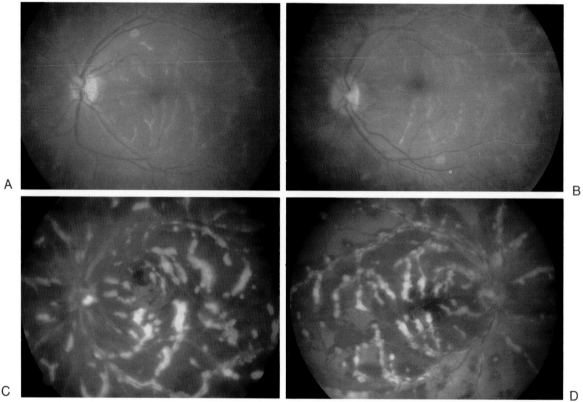

Figure 83–1. *A,* Bilateral retinal phlebitis extends from the posterior pole to the periphery with uninterrupted severe sheathing of all the vessels, resembling the frosted branches of a tree. Extensive perivenous exudates associated with intraretinal hemorrhage are noted in this patient. *B,* The most frequent presentation, however, is bilateral extensive venous sheathing. There is mild pallor of the left optic disc. *(Left figures,* right eye; *right figures,* left eye.)

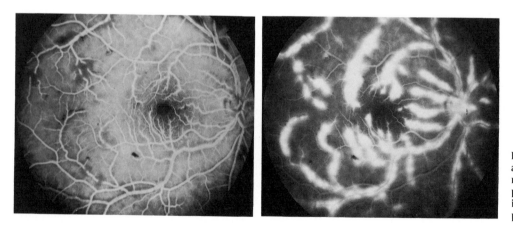

Figure 83–2. The fluorescein angiogram demonstrates normal venous flow in the early phase *(left),* with diffuse staining of the vein walls in the late phase *(right).*

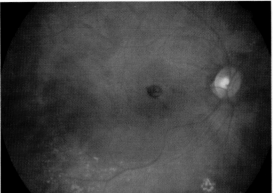 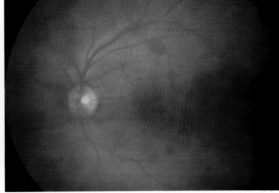

Figure 83–3. Systemic steroids are associated with the rapid resolution of the vascular sheathing, intraretinal hemorrhages, and associated exudative neurosensory retinal detachments. A residual scar in the right macula *(left figure)* of this patient resulted in a permanent decrease in vision to 20/300.

of serum angiotensin converting enzyme levels. Chest x-ray films, lumbosacral x-ray films, cerebrospinal fluid examination, and computed tomographic scan or magnetic resonance imaging scan of the head and orbits have all been normal. One patient demonstrated an increased serum anti-streptolysin O titer.[6]

CLINICAL CHARACTERISTICS

Frosted branch angiitis responds to systemic steroids with a rapid resolution of the vascular sheathing, retinal hemorrhages, and exudative neurosensory retinal detachment (Fig. 83–3). Systemic steroids (initial dose 80 to 100 mg oral prednisone for 10 days) should be initiated once treatable causes in the differential diagnosis are excluded. Funduscopic sequelae include attenuation of both the arteries and the veins, the development of sharply demarcated atrophic lesions in the periphery, and the deposition of yellow subretinal deposits in areas of previously detached retina. No recurrences have been noted.

Recovery to normal vision usually occurs, with a range of 20/15 to 20/40, the majority of cases being 20/20 or better. An exception was reported in one eye in which a fibrotic macular scar developed with a resultant final visual acuity of 20/300.[6] Remote sequelae have included a horseshoe tear in one patient and multiple bilateral branch vein occlusions in another. It is not known whether these complications are adverse sequelae of frosted branch angiitis or are fortuitous in their occurrence.[6]

DIFFERENTIAL DIAGNOSIS

Although no specific etiologic agent has been identified in frosted branch angiitis, treatable causes of retinal vasculitis should be excluded before the initiation of corticosteroid treatment (Table 83–1). Conditions associated with a predominant periphlebitis include tuberculosis, Eales' disease, sarcoidosis, multiple sclerosis,

and HIV infection, whereas systemic lupus erythematosus (SLE) and syphilis have been associated with a predominant inflammation of the arterial tree.

The ocular manifestations of sarcoidosis occur in 15 to 25 percent of cases.[7-9] Posterior segment involvement is seen frequently (14 to 28 percent), usually in association with anterior segment disease. The perivascular sheathing of ocular sarcoid is seen in the midperiphery, usually without vascular occlusion, and affects mainly the veins. Severe perivascular sheathing appears as "candle wax drippings." Occasionally branch or central retinal vein occlusion may occur, with subsequent peripheral retinal or disc neovascularization.

The vitritis of sarcoidosis consists of clumps of vitreal inflammatory cells—"snowballs" or "strings of pearls." Sarcoid granuloma can be seen in the deep retina or choroid or on the optic nerve head. Although the diagnosis of sarcoid should be excluded by a chest x-ray

Table 83–1. DIFFERENTIAL DIAGNOSIS OF
FROSTED BRANCH ANGIITIS

Disease	Laboratory Tests
Sarcoidosis	Chest x-ray film, serum calcium and phosphorus levels, serum angiotensin converting enzyme determination
Multiple sclerosis	Magnetic resonance imaging, cerebrospinal fluid examination
Pars plantis	
Eales' disease	
Tuberculosis	Chest x-ray film, tuberculin skin test
Syphilis	Venereal Disease Research Laboratory test, fluorescent treponemal antibody test
Systemic lupus erythematosus	Antinuclear antibody, anti-DNA determinations
AIDS	HIV antibody determination
Bone marrow tumefaction	Complete blood count with differential, vitreous biopsy, cerebrospinal fluid examination, magnetic resonance imaging

film and determinations of serum angiotensin converting enzyme, serum calcium, and phosphorus levels, the associated ophthalmic findings should help differentiate ocular sarcoidosis from frosted branch angiitis.

Retinal venous sheathing is observed in 10 to 20 percent of patients with multiple sclerosis[10-12] and is seen either as active periphlebitis, with white patchy cuffs surrounding the blood vessel, or as venous sclerosis. Periphlebitis in multiple sclerosis is occasionally accompanied by pars planitis and frequently resolves spontaneously without visual symptoms or hemorrhages. The diagnosis of multiple sclerosis can be made readily by magnetic resonance imaging or cerebrospinal fluid examination with oligoclonal banding. Additionally, the fluffy perivenous cuffs in multiple sclerosis are quite small and interrupted, in contrast to the widespread sheathing of the vessels in frosted branch angiitis.

Retinal periphlebitis can be found in association with peripheral uveitis or pars planitis.[13, 14] Snowbanks consisting of fibroglial proliferation and vascular exudation are seen over a broad area of the inferior peripheral retina; retinal edema and cystoid macular edema are also observed. The *peripheral* terminal branches of the retinal veins are cuffed with white inflammatory material, differentiating this entity from the diffuse periphlebitis of frosted branch angiitis.

Tuberculosis commonly produces focal perivenous sheathing in the peripheral venules, which only occasionally involves the central retinal vein.[20] Eales' disease, which has been associated with tuberculosis,[21] characteristically produces early capillary closure in the periphery of multiple quadrants of the retina, with sheathing of the peripheral retinal veins and intraretinal hemorrhages. Neovascularization of the retinal periphery results from the ensuing ischemia, usually at the clearly defined border between perfused and nonperfused retina. The characteristic picture of extensive peripheral capillary nonperfusion in Eales' disease and the focal perivenular sheathing in tuberculosis should help differentiate these entities from frosted branch angiitis.

The vasculitis of ocular syphilis is generally a periarteritis with arteriolar sheathing, exudates, and intraretinal and preretinal hemorrhages,[15-17] although isolated venous periphlebitis has also been described.[18] The arteriolitis may become occlusive, with eventual sclerosis of the involved arterioles and the development of peripheral retinal neovascularization. Other more common manifestations of posterior syphilis include neuroretinitis, chorioretinitis, and papillitis. The course of ocular syphilis has been noted to be more aggressive in patients with associated HIV disease, and as such it is recommended that patients being evaluated or treated for ocular syphilis be tested for HIV infection.[16, 19] Because ocular syphilis can mimic many diseases, patients with a vasculitis resembling frosted branch angiitis should have antibody tests for syphilis (the Venereal Disease Research Laboratory test and the fluorescent treponemal antibody test).

Retinal vasculitis is a common ophthalmic manifestation of SLE. Although the most common findings are cotton-wool spots with or without intraretinal hemorrhages, almost 30 percent of patients with SLE will have retinal vasculitis with microangiopathic small vessel occlusion most often affecting the arterioles. Occasionally, severe retinal occlusive disease can occur, affecting both the arteries and the veins in association with anticardiolipin antibodies,[23] with subsequent peripheral retinal neovascularization. Retinal arterial inflammation is also seen in segmental periarteritis of the retina, in which whitish plaques are scattered along the main arterial branches. Surprisingly, fluorescein leakage is seen from the venous but not from the arterial wall.[24] It can be distinguished from frosted branch angiitis by the generally more limited involvement of the retinal vascular tree.

The perivasculitis in AIDS retinopathy should also be included in the differential diagnosis of frosted branch angiitis.[25-29] Diffuse perivasculitis of the far peripheral veins and focal periarteritis can be seen in patients with AIDS or AIDS-related complex[27, 28] without concomitant infectious retinopathy. These conditions are more commonly seen, however, with an associated infectious component such as cytomegalovirus retinopathy.[26, 29] Frosted branch angiitis has been described in AIDS patients accompanying small areas of cytomegalovirus retinopathy.[29] In these cases treatment for cytomegalovirus infection provided resolution of the vasculitis component of their retinopathy.

Finally, bone marrow tumefactions such as leukemia and non-Hodgkin's lymphoma (i.e., reticulum cell sarcoma) should be considered in the presence of diffuse retinal vascular sheathing. Intraretinal hemorrhages and cotton-wool spots are more frequently seen in leukemia, whereas retinal cell sarcoma can present as a diffuse vitritis. Underlying the vitreal inflammation may be a diffuse retinal vasculitis resembling frosted branch angiitis. The diagnosis can be established by a vitreous biopsy if there is no obvious systemic evidence of disease.

CONCLUSIONS

In summary, frosted branch angiitis is a bilateral inflammation of the retinal arteries and veins, with the veins being more severely affected. No cause has been identified. Vision is profoundly diminished in the acute phase, with dramatic improvement following oral corticosteroid administration. The differential diagnosis is extensive, but frosted branch angiitis can frequently be distinguished by its unique clinical presentation and course.

REFERENCES

1. Ito Y, Nakano M, Kyu N, et al: Frosted branch angiitis in a child. Jpn J Clin Ophthalmol 30:797, 1976.
2. Sakanishi Y, Kanagami S, Ohara K: Frosted retinal angiitis in children. Jpn J Clin Ophthalmol 38:803, 1984.
3. Yamane S, Nishiuchi T, Nakagawa Y, et al: A case of frosted branch angiitis of the retina. Folia Ophthalmol Jpn 36:1822, 1985.
4. Higuchi K, Maeda K, Uji T, et al: A case of infantile uveitis with frosted branch angiitis. Jpn Rev Clin Ophthalmol 79:2660, 1985.

5. Watanabe Y, Takeda N, Adachi-Usami E: A case of frosted branch angiitis. Br J Ophthalmol 71:553, 1987.
6. Kleiner RC, Kaplan HJ, Shakin JL, et al: Acute frosted retinal periphlebitis. Am J Ophthalmol 106:27, 1988.
7. Obenauf CD, Shaw HE, Sydnor CF, et al: Sarcoidosis and its ophthalmic manifestations. Am J Ophthalmol 86:648, 1978.
8. Jabs DA, Johns CJ: Ocular involvement in chronic sarcoidosis. Am J Ophthalmol 102:297, 1986.
9. Spalton DJ, Sanders MD: Fundus changes in histologically confirmed sarcoidosis. Br J Ophthalmol 65:348, 1981.
10. Arnold AC, Pepose JS, Hepler RS, et al: Retinal periphlebitis and retinitis in multiple sclerosis. Ophthalmology 91:255, 1984.
11. Barnford CR, Ganley JP, Sibley WA, et al: Uveitis, perivenous sheathing and multiple sclerosis. Neurology 28:119, 1978.
12. Rucker CW: Sheathing of the retinal veins in multiple sclerosis: Review of the pertinent literature. Mayo Clin Proc 47:335, 1972.
13. Brockhurst RJ, Schepens CL, Okamura ID, et al: Uveitis II. Peripheral uveitis: Clinical description, complications, and differential diagnosis. Am J Ophthalmol 49:1257, 1966.
14. Wetzig RP, Chan CC, Nussenblatt RB, et al: Clinical and immunopathological studies of pars planitis in a family. Br J Ophthalmol 72:5, 1988.
15. Crouch ER, Goldberg MF: Retinal periarteritis secondary to syphilis. Arch Ophthalmol 93:384, 1975.
16. Tamesis RR, Foster CS: Ocular syphilis. Ophthalmology 97:1281, 1990.
17. Schlaegel RF, Kao SF: A review (1970–1980) of 28 presumptive cases of syphilitic uveitis. Am J Ophthalmol 93:412, 1982.
18. Lobes LA, Folk JC: Syphilitic phlebitis simulating branch vein occlusion. Ann Ophthalmol 13:825, 1981.
19. McLeish WM, Pulido JS, Holland S, et al: The ocular manifestations of syphilis in the human immunodeficiency virus type I–infected host. Ophthalmology 97:196, 1990.
20. Fountain JA, Werner RB: Tuberculous retinal vasculitis. Retina 4:48, 1984.
21. Renie WA, Murphy RP, Anderson KC, et al: The evaluation of patients with Eales' disease. Retina 3:243, 1983.
22. Lanham JG, Barrie T, Kohner EM, et al: SLE retinopathy: Evaluation by fluorescein angiography. Ann Rheum Dis 41:473, 1982.
23. Jabs DA, Fine SL, Hochberg MC, et al: Severe retinal vaso-occlusive disease in systemic lupus erythematosus. Arch Ophthalmol 104:558, 1986.
24. Orzalesi N, Ricciardi L: Segmental retinal periarteritis. Am J Ophthalmol 72:55, 1971.
25. Holland GN, Pepose JS, Pettit TH, et al: Acquired immune deficiency syndrome—Ocular manifestations. Ophthalmology 90:859, 1983.
26. Jabs DA, Green WR, Fox R, et al: Ocular manifestations of acquired immune deficiency syndrome. Ophthalmology 96:1092, 1989.
27. Kestelyn P, Van de Perre P, Rouvroy D, et al: A prospective study of the ophthalmologic findings in the acquired immune deficiency syndrome in Africa. Am J Ophthalmol 100:230, 1985.
28. Kestelyn P, Lepage P, Van de Perre P: Perivasculitis of the retinal vessels as an important sign in children with AIDS-related complex. Am J Ophthalmol 100:614, 1985.
29. Spaide RF, Vitale AT, Toth IR, et al: Frosted branch angiitis associated with cytomegalovirus retinitis. Am J Ophthalmol 113:522, 1992.

Chapter 84

■

Collagen Disorders: Retinal Manifestations of Collagen Vascular Diseases

E. MITCHEL OPREMCAK

Rheumatologic disorders are a collection of inflammatory diseases involving the connective tissues. These disorders are typically multisystemic with protean manifestations. Rheumatologic diseases are also called *collagen vascular* or *connective tissue diseases* because of the involvement of these supportive structures. Despite many clinical and pathologic presentations, these diseases primarily affect the joints, muscles, bursae, and tendons. It is not uncommon, however, for the eyes to be inflamed in many of these rheumatologic syndromes. Ocular inflammation is often considered a major diagnostic criterion for establishing a clinical diagnosis in several of these disorders (Table 84–1).

An accurate understanding of the connective tissue proper is required to appreciate ocular involvement in rheumatic diseases. Connective tissues and structures are the matrix that support individual cells, tissues, and organs. This ground substance is produced by specialized connective tissue cells that secrete various fibers (colla-

gens, reticulin, and elastin), as well as a group of mucopolysaccharides called *proteoglycans*.[1] Hyaluronic acid, chondroitin sulfate, dermatan sulfate, keratan sulfate, and heparin sulfate are the common polysaccharides found in the connective tissue proteoglycans.[2] Collagen fibers can also be further subdivided by their polypeptide structure into six types (collagen types I to VI).[3] Each tissue and organ maintains a distinct connective tissue environment by varying these individual components, thereby effecting optimal structure and function. In rheumatologic diseases, inflammation of these supportive structures and milieu results in tissue and organ dysfunction.

The eye, perhaps more than any other organ, maintains a unique connective tissue environment. In the cornea, keratocytes secrete both type II and type IV collagen, as well as chondroitin and keratan sulfate.[1, 4] This connective tissue combination results in strong tissue that becomes transparent as a result of unique

**Table 84–1. RHEUMATIC DISEASES WITH OCULAR
INVOLVEMENT**

Diffuse connective tissue diseases
  Rheumatoid arthritis
  Juvenile rheumatoid arthritis
  Systemic lupus erythematosus
  Progressive systemic sclerosis
  Polymyositis-dermatomyositis
  Necrotizing vasculitis and other vasculopathies
    Polyarteritis nodosa group
      Classic polyarteritis nodosa
      Churg-Strauss syndrome
    Wegener's granulomatosis
    Temporal arteritis
    Behçet's disease
  Sjögren's syndrome
  Relapsing polychondritis
Arthritis associated with spondylitis (HLA-B27–associated)
  Ankylosing spondylitis
  Reiter's syndrome
  Psoriatic arthritis
  Arthritis associated with chronic inflammatory bowel disease
    (Crohn's disease, ulcerative colitis)

lamellar fiber orientation and active endothelial cell dehydration. Hyalocytes in the vitreous produce hyaluronic acid and type II collagen, which forms a clear gel allowing transmission of light and provides support for the globe and retina.[1, 5] The retina and choroid possess connective tissue and a complex vascular system that is composed of type III and type IV collagen.[1] These circulations are critical for retinal function and general nutrition of the eye. Each of these ocular tissues performs critical functions in the visual system and is exquisitely sensitive to inflammation.

Separate connective tissues and structures within the eye can become inflamed in the various rheumatic diseases. Wegener's granulomatosis, rheumatoid arthritis (RA), and polyarteritis nodosa (PAN) can affect the cornea and produce peripheral ulcerative keratopathy. Reiter's syndrome is defined by the triad of urethritis, arthritis, and inflammation of the conjunctiva and iris. Juvenile rheumatoid arthritis (JRA) commonly produces a chronic iridocyclitis. Ankylosing spondylitis, Reiter's syndrome, psoriatic arthritis, and the chronic inflammatory bowel diseases produce an acute inflammation of the iris and ciliary body. It is important, therefore, to evaluate all patients who present with ocular inflammation or uveitis for symptoms and signs of an underlying connective tissue disease.

Often, rheumatic diseases present in the eye before the onset of significant systemic involvement. The eye may even be the primary target of several diseases such as Behçet's syndrome, Reiter's disease, and ankylosing spondylitis. The importance of performing a careful review of systems and physical examination cannot be underestimated. Particular attention should be paid to the skin, joints, central nervous system, lungs, gastrointestinal tract, and kidneys. Often, involvement of these systems can lead the ophthalmologist to establish the existence of an underlying collagen vascular disease as the cause for the ocular inflammation. For example, iritis in a patient complaining of large joint arthritis could represent JRA, systemic lupus erythematosus (SLE), Wegener's granulomatosis, or Behçet's disease. Oral ulcers, malaise, skin rash, and uveitis may be found in SLE, Behçet's disease, and sarcoidosis. Genital-urethral pain and uveitis may represent Behçet's disease, polyarteritis nodosa, or Reiter's syndrome. Laboratory evaluation and consultation with an internist-rheumatologist can help confirm the presence of a collagen vascular disease and result in diagnosis and the initiation of proper systemic therapy. Local ocular therapy in rheumatic disorders without attention to the underlying systemic process universally results in suboptimal control of the ocular inflammation and risks potentially life-threatening complications of uncontrolled systemic disease.

In summary, rheumatic diseases provide an opportunity for the ophthalmologist to interface with both the patient and the internist. The expertise of the ophthalmologist in determining the specific ocular tissue involved and the rheumatologist's knowledge of the systemic manifestations not only can facilitate the proper diagnosis but also can provide optimal care for these diseases of vision, often which are life-threatening.

RHEUMATOID ARTHRITIS

RA is a chronic systemic inflammatory disease of unknown cause, producing a distinct form of polyarticular and symmetric arthritis. It is more common in women (3:1) and typically begins between the ages of 30 and 40 yr.[6] RA is thought to have a strong autoimmune pathogenesis. Patients with RA have IgM, IgG, and IgA antibodies that are directed against the Fc portion of IgG.[7] The resulting immune complexes are postulated to mediate both the articular and the extraarticular manifestations of the disease through activation of complement.

Patients with RA complain of malaise, fatigue, weight loss, and arthralgia. The joint disease is symmetric and often involves the small joints of the wrist and hand, excluding the distal interphalangeal joints.[1] Morning stiffness is characteristic. Extraarticular involvement in RA, including pleurisy, neuropathy, and ocular inflammation, is thought to be secondary to systemic vasculitis and may represent a change from a local joint disease to a more serious systemic form of RA.

Keratoconjunctivitis sicca, marginal keratitis, peripheral ulcerative keratopathy, and anterior scleritis are the most common anterior segment findings in RA.[8] Uveitis and direct involvement of the retina are rare. The retina can be involved secondarily following the development of posterior scleritis. Forty-six percent of patients with scleritis will have an associated underlying connective tissue disease.[9] Although the differential diagnosis includes conditions such as Wegener's granulomatosis, relapsing polychondritis, and PAN, 30 percent of such patients will have RA.

Posterior scleritis is not as common as anterior forms of scleral inflammation. This condition is defined as scleritis, posterior to the equator of the eye, and in one series accounted for only 2 percent of all cases.[10, 11] It is important to recognize, however, that posterior scleritis is much more difficult to detect. In one report on 30 eyes enucleated for ocular inflammation, 40 percent had previously undetected posterior scleritis.[12] Unlike anterior scleritis, posterior scleritis can be unilateral and is often associated with a profound decrease in visual acuity. There is pain and tenderness with motion or palpation. On biomicroscopic examination, the anterior segment is often normal or may show only a narrow angle resulting from displacement by the posterior structures.

Fundus examination reveals choroidal thickening or choroidal nodules overlying the area of scleritis. Secondary choroidal folds and effusions may develop. The retina may demonstrate secondary striae and exudative retinal separations (Fig. 84–1).[11] A high index of suspicion is often required to make a clinical diagnosis of posterior scleritis. Ultrasonography or computed tomography can support this diagnosis by showing thickening of the sclera and choroid. There may be fluid in the contiguous Tenon's space. Fluorescein angiography illustrates the choroidal and retinal striae. A characteristic linear pattern of alternating hypo- and hyperfluorescent streaks can be seen as a result of folds in the retinal pigment epithelial layer (see Fig. 84–1B). Multifocal, punctate, hyperfluorescent choroidal lesions can also be noted and may evolve into areas of exudative retinal detachment. The retinal circulation is typically unaffected.

Once a clinical diagnosis of posterior scleritis is established, a search for an underlying cause is in order. A general physical examination and review of systems can help establish extraocular involvement. Patients with the characteristic deforming arthritis associated with RA seldom present a diagnostic challenge. Mild anemia, elevation of the erythrocyte sedimentation rate (ESR), and a positive result for rheumatoid factor in serum may support the clinical diagnosis. Without obvious systemic findings, scleritis may be the initial manifestation of occult rheumatic disease.

Therapy for rheumatoid scleritis should be directed at controlling the underlying systemic disease.[10] Local ocular therapy and regional steroids should be used with caution and only as adjuncts to systemic treatment. Regional steroids have been reported to cause scleral melting and ocular perforation and should be used only in extenuating circumstances. Mild cases can often be effectively managed by nonsteroidal antiinflammatory agents. Indomethacin (50 to 150 mg/day) has been reported to be particularly effective for scleritis.[9] In more severe cases, oral corticosteroids, gold salts, and second-generation immunosuppressive drugs such as methotrexate, azathioprine, and so on should be considered.

The ocular and systemic prognoses depend in part on establishing the proper diagnosis and detecting the underlying rheumatic disease. In a report by Foster and associates, the development of necrotizing scleritis forbode a more severe form of RA.[13] They noted an 8-yr mortality rate of 20 percent in patients with this extraarticular involvement.

JUVENILE RHEUMATOID ARTHRITIS

JRA is a multisystemic childhood disease associated with chronic arthritis. The cause of JRA is unknown but is thought to be a primary autoimmune disease. Children with the pauciarticular form of JRA have the highest risk for the development of ocular inflammation.[14] JRA is much more common in girls and occurs typically between the ages of 4 and 6 yr.

Chronic iridocyclitis develops in 5 to 17 percent of children with JRA.[15] Eye disease may precede the development of arthritis by several years. Ocular involvement may be insidious because of the lack of symptoms and ocular signs early in the disease. JRA-associated iridocyclitis is typically chronic and bilateral (70 percent). The inflammation is nongranulomatous and involves primarily the iris and ciliary body. Chronic inflammation commonly results in band keratopathy (41 percent), posterior synechiae, glaucoma (19 percent), and cataract formation (42 to 92 percent).[16]

Figure 84–1. Posterior scleritis in a patient with rheumatoid arthritis with secondary thickening of the choroid in the posterior pole and peripapillary area. A, Chorioretinal striae in the macula. B, Alternating hypofluorescent and hyperfluorescent linear streaks corresponding to folding of the retinal pigment epithelium.

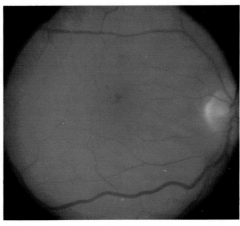

A

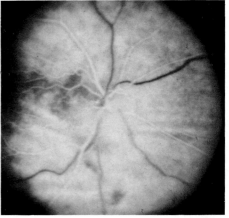

B

The anterior segment is involved to a much greater extent in JRA than are the retina and choroid. Cystoid macular edema may develop in patients with JRA. As a result of chronic cyclitis, organization and fibrosis of the anterior vitreous may occur, resulting in further media opacification. Cyclitic membrane formation and ocular hypotony can develop spontaneously following standard cataract surgery. True retinitis, retinal vasculitis, or choroiditis are uncommon in JRA.

JRA can be diagnosed in children with a characteristic arthritic and ocular picture. The diagnosis can be further supported by documenting a positive antinuclear antibody (ANA) level (79 percent) and a negative result for rheumatoid factor in serum.[17] Topical corticosteroids and cycloplegics are the mainstay of therapy for children with JRA. Oral nonsteroidal antiinflammatory agents have been shown to help control both the systemic and the ocular symptoms and signs.[18] Regional corticosteroids can be useful but are difficult to deliver in this age group and often require general anesthesia. Oral corticosteroids (1 mg/kg/day) can be used in severe cases and tapered according to the clinical response. Second-generation immunosuppressive agents should be considered in patients with otherwise unresponsive disease. The consequences of systemic immunosuppression in this age group are considerable, and these agents should therefore be used with caution and under the direction of physicians experienced with their use.

The overall visual prognosis in JRA is poor. Seventy-five percent of children with JRA have moderate or severe inflammation with loss of vision due to glaucoma, cataract, or phthisis.[1, 19] Lens and vitreous opacification should be addressed via pars plana lensectomy-vitrectomy to afford better control of the inflammation and prevent cyclitic membrane formation and hypotony.[15, 20]

SYSTEMIC LUPUS ERYTHEMATOSUS

SLE is a collagen vascular disease with truly protean manifestations. Ninety percent of patients with SLE are women at or around child-rearing age.[21] The pathogenesis of SLE appears to be an autoimmune systemic necrotizing vasculitis. Patients with SLE have ANAs and elevated levels of circulating immune complexes that appear to play a role in the disease.[21] Immune complexes composed of these autoantibodies and DNA have been found in the walls of inflamed blood vessels and in the areas of fibrinoid necrosis.

Clinically, patients with SLE present with malaise, fatigue, anorexia, and low-grade fever. On examination they may have arthritis, facial rash, alopecia, and pleurisy.[22] Raynaud's phenomenon, oral ulcers, and central nervous system complaints are also common. Laboratory evaluation may reveal anemia, an elevated ESR, the presence of ANAs, proteinuria, and a falsely positive Venereal Disease Research Laboratory (VDRL) result. Lupus nephritis and central nervous involvement represent serious and potentially fatal developments in SLE.

SLE may involve the eye in up to 50 percent of all cases, depending on the series and the nature of the clinic reporting the findings.[23] Anterior segment findings include keratoconjunctivitis sicca, scleritis, and keratitis. The retina and choroid may be primarily involved; however, it is important to separate lupus-associated retinal vasculitis from the secondary retinal and choroidal changes of SLE-mediated hypertension and anemia. Severe hypertension can occur in lupus as a result of nephritis. Arteriolar narrowing, intraretinal hemorrhages, exudate, and disc edema are characteristic of hypertensive retinopathy.

The mechanism of primary lupus retinopathy is unknown but is thought to be secondary to circulating immune complexes found in the disease. Ten percent of patients with SLE also have lupus anticoagulant antibodies that are known to increase the incidence of thrombosis. The relationship between this factor and lupus retinopathy is unclear but provocative.[24] Retinal manifestations of SLE are a result of focal ischemia and necrotizing retinal vasculitis. Three fundus presentations have been described.[25–27] The most common form is focal ischemia resulting in multiple cotton-wool spots. Intraretinal hemorrhages and mild disc edema can also be associated with this form of lupus retinopathy. A second form of retinopathy noted in SLE is a severe retinal vasoocclusive disease without evidence of retinal vasculitis.[26] Retinal infarction and hemorrhage can result in severe and sudden loss of vision. The third form of retinopathy in SLE is proliferative lupus retinopathy (Fig. 84–2A and B). Retinal vasculitis and secondary ischemia produce neovascularization of the optic nerve and elsewhere in the retina.[27] This neovascularization can result in vitreous hemorrhage and even retinal detachment. The choroidal circulation may be involved in this process as well (Fig. 84–2C and D).[28] Choroidal infarction, exudative changes, and subretinal neovascular membranes have been reported in this form of SLE.

SLE is a clinical diagnosis. The American Rheumatologic Association defines the disease by the presence of 4 of the 14 major symptoms and signs. Laboratory testing may support the clinical diagnosis by revealing the presence of ANAs, elevated circulating immune complexes, proteinuria, anemia, and a falsely positive VDRL test result. Fluorescein angiography may help define the extent of retinal involvement and may assist in differentiating secondary hypertensive retinopathy from the true retinal vasculitis noted in lupus retinopathy.

Therapy for SLE varies according to the severity of the systemic symptoms. It is important to note that lupus may present in the eye 1 to 5 yr prior to the onset of other systemic findings.[29] Lupus retinopathy may respond to systemic therapy, including nonsteroidal antiinflammatory agents, oral corticosteroids, hydroxychloroquil sulfate, gold, and cyclophosphamide. Proliferative lupus retinopathy can be treated with panretinal laser ablation to help control the consequences of ocular neovascularization.

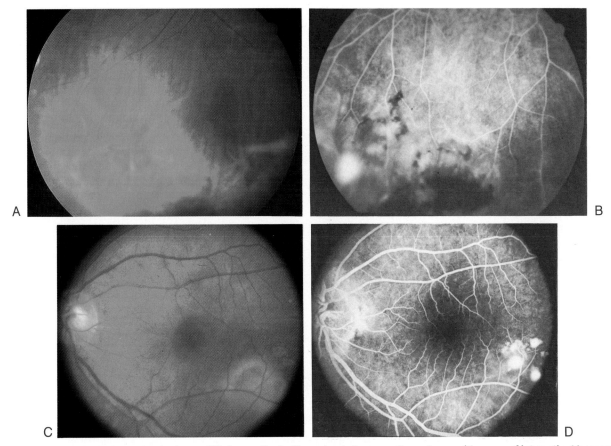

Figure 84–2. *A* and *B*, Peripheral retinal vasculitis in a patient with systemic lupus erythematosus with areas of intraretinal hemorrhage, retinal nonperfusion, and neovascularization on fluorescein angiography. *C* and *D*, Another patient with systemic lupus erythematosus with focal areas of serous elevation of the retinal pigment epithelium and sensory retina as a result of lupus-associated choroidopathy.

PROGRESSIVE SYSTEMIC SCLEROSIS

Progressive systemic sclerosis (PSS) or scleroderma is a chronic autoimmune disorder resulting in inflammation and fibrosis of the skin and other organs. Women in the fourth decade of life are affected more often than are men (4:1).[30] The immune defect in PSS is not completely understood, but circulating immune complex deposition, vasculitis, and secondary fibrosis of the vessels are thought to produce the typical clinical picture. Clinically, patients may present with scleroderma or may manifest other symptoms of the CREST syndrome, including calcinosis, Raynaud's phenomenon, esophageal symptoms, scleroderma, and telangiectasia.

The eye is commonly involved in scleroderma. Keratoconjunctivitis sicca occurs in up to 70 percent of patients with PSS as a result of lacrimal gland fibrosis.[31] Filamentary keratitis, eyelid edema, and conjunctival shrinkage can also be noted. Patients with PSS have also been seen to have fundus findings similar to those in SLE. Intraretinal hemorrhages, cotton-wool spots, and retinal vasculitis, as well as choroidal infarctions have been reported.[32]

The diagnosis can be established by the characteristic clinical picture of the scleroderma, with or without the other CREST findings. These systemic findings in association with retinal microvascular infarctions and retinal vasculitis support the clinical diagnosis. Laboratory testing may reveal the presence of ANAs with a speckled pattern. Fluorescein angiography can be used to document the cotton-wool spots and define the extent of choroidal nonperfusion. Long-term systemic therapy has not been useful in controlling PSS, and therapy is chiefly supportive.[33] Localized scleroderma has a relatively good prognosis. Systemic involvement has a worse prognosis, with an 80 percent 10-yr mortality rate.

DERMATOMYOSITIS AND POLYMYOSITIS

Dermatomyositis and polymyositis are autoimmune forms of inflammatory diffuse myopathy. The pathogenesis of these diseases appears to be mediated via microvascular damage from immune complex formation. Patients with dermatomyositis show ischemic necrosis and loss of capillary beds in the perifascicular region of the involved muscles.[34] Both children and adults are affected by this disease.

Ocular involvement in dermatomyositis includes a lilac discoloration and edema of the eyelids, conjunctivitis, iritis, blepharoptosis, scleritis, uveitis, and extraocular muscle paralysis.[35] Cotton-wool spots, intraretinal hemorrhages, venous engorgement and disc edema, and optic atrophy have been observed primarily in childhood dermatomyositis.[36]

Corticosteroids and immunosuppressive agents have proved helpful in managing these diseases. The prognosis is better for childhood forms of the disease, with a 90 percent 5-yr survival rate.[1] Adult-onset disease fares worse, with a 53 percent survival at 5 yr.

POLYARTERITIS NODOSA

PAN is a multisystemic disease associated with a necrotizing vasculitis. Medium- to small-sized vessels are characteristically affected with all stages of necrosis noted in the involved tissues.[37] The cause of PAN is unknown. Thirty to 70 percent of patients with PAN have anti–hepatitis B antibodies.[38] The significance of this virus in the pathogenesis has not been established. This is a rare disease that affects 20- to 50-year-old adults. Men are affected more frequently than are women (3:1).

Systemically, patients with PAN may note fatigue, myalgia, weight loss, fever, arthralgia, and testicular pain. The kidneys, liver, and gastrointestinal and central nervous systems are commonly involved. Renal involvement is one of the more serious and potentially fatal complications of PAN. Abdominal pain from intestinal infarction and headaches from central nervous system vasculitis are also serious and potentially life-threatening complications of this disease.

Ten to 20 percent of patients with PAN will have ocular involvement.[39] Peripheral ulcerative keratitis and mild iritis can be found in this disease. A mild vitritis may also be noted. The most common ocular findings in PAN are choroidal and retinal vasculitis.[40] Fundus examination will show retinal vasculitis with associated intraretinal hemorrhages, cotton-wool spots, and retinal edema (Fig. 84–3). Central retinal artery occlusion and optic atrophy have also been reported in PAN. Patients with PAN may also experience anterior or posterior scleritis. Posterior scleritis will manifest with pain and chorioretinal folds similar to those in RA.

Any patient with occlusive retinal vasculitis should be examined for evidence of systemic findings that may help establish the presence of a collagen vascular disease. Often, a biopsy of an involved artery or lesion will demonstrate a hemorrhagic vasculitis and fibrinoid necrosis and establish the diagnosis. Laboratory tests may show elevated white blood cell and eosinophil counts, decreased complement, elevated circulating immune complexes, and negative rheumatoid factor and ANA determinations. Hepatitis B surface antigen has been found in up to 70 percent of patients with PAN. Angiography in patients with abdominal pain may reveal aneurysmal dilatation of the hepatic and renal arteries.

PAN is a potentially fatal disease. Without therapy, it carries an 80 to 90 percent 5-yr mortality rate. Corticosteroids reduce this mortality rate to 50 percent.[41] The combination of corticosteroids with cyclophosphamide (1 to 2 mg/kg/day) results in an 80 percent 5-yr survival rate. Patients may require high doses of intravenous steroids and cyclophosphamide early in the course to gain control of severe disease.

WEGENER'S GRANULOMATOSIS

Wegener's granulomatosis is a multisystem disease associated with a necrotizing granulomatous vasculitis.[42] The cause is unknown. It is uncommon and occurs between the ages of 40 and 50 yr. Men are affected more often than are females (3:2). Immune complex formation and deposition are thought to result in vasculitis of small- to middle-sized vessels. Acute and chronic lesions can be found simultaneously in the involved tissues and organs.

Characteristically, Wegener's granulomatosis involves

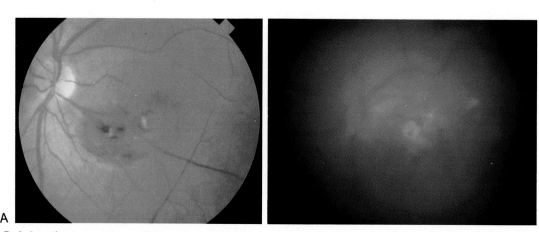

Figure 84–3. *A,* Localized area of necrotizing retinal vasculitis associated with polyarteritis nodosa. The patient refused immunosuppressive therapy and lost central acuity in the left eye over a 5-mo period because of progressive ischemic retinal vasculitis (*B*). Note the development of vitritis as well as further retinal involvement.

the upper and lower respiratory tracts.[43] Epistaxis, rhinorrhea, sinusitis, otitis, chronic cough, and saddle nose deformity are frequently observed. Chronic pulmonary infiltrates, nodules, and cavitary lesions are found in the lungs. Wegener's granulomatosis also commonly affects the kidneys and the central nervous system. A granulomatous glomerulitis can be found in 80 percent of patients with this collagen vascular disorder.

Wegener's granulomatosis may involve the eye in 40 to 50 percent of cases.[44] Eye involvement may precede other organ involvement. Proptosis and orbital pain from a pseudotumor is the most common finding. Scleritis, peripheral ulcerative keratitis, conjunctivitis, and dacryocystitis are also frequently noted ocular manifestations of Wegener's vasculitis. Posterior scleritis in Wegener's granulomatosis behaves similarly to scleritis in other rheumatologic disorders and presents with decreased vision and pain. Secondary chorioretinal thickening and striae can be seen both clinically and on fluorescein angiography. Although uveitis, retinitis, and retinal vasculitis have been reported, intraocular disease is rare. Retinitis and retinal vasculitis in Wegener's granulomatosis may present as a geographic area of retinal edema and intraretinal hemorrhage (Fig. 84–4), which may increase in size and can be difficult to distinguish from a secondary opportunistic or viral retinitis.

Wegener's granulomatosis should be suspected in patients with these ocular findings and respiratory, renal, or central nervous system involvement. The diagnosis can be supported by finding pneumonitis or cavitary lesions on chest x-ray film. Laboratory testing will demonstrate an elevated white blood cell count, ESR, and serum IgA. Antineutrophilic cytoplasmic antibodies have been found in this disease and have proved useful in advancing a diagnosis of Wegener's granulomatosis.[45] Biopsy of the involved tissue often establishes the diagnosis by revealing a granulomatous vasculitis.

Wegener's granulomatosis is a serious and potentially fatal disease. Therapy should be designed to address both the ocular and the systemic inflammation. Without therapy, the average survival is 5 mo, with an 80 percent mortality rate by 1 yr.[46] Corticosteroids prolong survival to 12½ mo. Cyclophosphamide (1 to 2 mg/kg/day) in combination with corticosteroids is the treatment of choice, with a 90 percent remission rate. Maintenance therapy may be required for 1 to 2 yr.

TEMPORAL ARTERITIS

Temporal arteritis (TA) or giant cell arteritis is a systemic vasculitis that involves medium- to large-sized muscular arteries.[47] The cause is unknown. TA affects an older population with an average age of 70 yr. The pathophysiology of this collagen vascular disease appears to be a panarteritis. Affected blood vessels demonstrate a mononuclear cell infiltration and giant cell formation within the vessel wall, with subsequent destruction and fragmentation of the internal elastic membrane.

Patients with TA commonly complain of fever, weight loss, malaise, and headaches. The most common ocular complication of TA is ischemic optic neuropathy.[48] The larger vessels supplying the optic nerve become inflamed and effect an infarction of the optic nerve. Rarely, the retinal vessels may be involved, producing a branch or central retinal artery occlusion.[49] Attenuation of the retinal arterioles, disc pallor, and optic atrophy may develop late. Primary uveitis or retinitis is uncommon.

The diagnosis can be made in the clinical setting of an older patient with malaise, fever, weight loss, headache, and sudden loss of vision in one or both (65 percent) eyes as a result of ischemic optic neuropathy. The diagnosis can be supported by finding a markedly elevated ESR and C-reactive protein level. Temporal artery biopsy will demonstrate a granulomatous vasculitis with infiltration of the vessel wall with mononuclear cells, histiocytes, and giant cells and loss of the internal elastic membrane.

Untreated, this disease has a poor prognosis with irreversible loss of vision secondary to ischemic optic neuropathy and death from coronary or cerebral vasculitis.[50] Therapy should be initiated when TA is suspected in order to prevent bilateral optic nerve involvement. Prednisone (1 to 2 mg/kg/day) is the treatment of

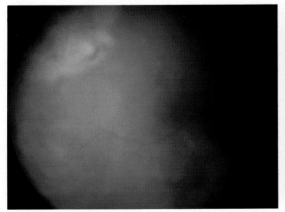 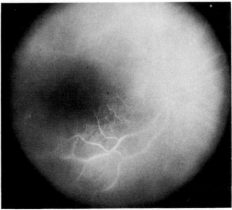

Figure 84–4. *A,* An area of retinitis and retinal vasculitis associated with biopsy-proven Wegener's granulomatosis. *B,* The fluorescein angiogram illustrates an area of segmental vascular staining and leakage of dye into the vitreous.

choice in TA, and maintenance doses may be required for 1 to 2 yr.

BEHÇET'S DISEASE

Behçet's disease is a systemic necrotizing vasculitis with diverse manifestations. The cause is unknown but is thought to have a strong autoimmune component. HLA associations have been established in other countries for Behçet's disease but have not proved useful in the United States.[51] HLA-B51, HLA-B12, and HLA-B27 have all been associated with certain forms of Behçet's disease. The disease is much more common in Asia and the Middle East.[52] In the United States, there is an equal gender distribution, and the disease is found in 20- to 40-year-old adults.

Behçet's vasculitis involves small- to medium-sized vessels. A perivascular infiltrate with polymorphonuclear neutrophils and mononuclear cells can be found around the veins and arteries. This is often associated with vessel thrombosis and tissue hemorrhage.

Clinically, there may be a 6- to 10-yr prodrome with recurrent or chronic malaise, fever, and sore throat.[53] The classic triad of recurrent aphthous oral ulcers (100 percent), genital ulcers (84 percent), and uveitis (66 percent) establishes the clinical diagnosis of Behçet's disease. Erythema nodosum (66 percent), arthritis (66 percent), and meningoencephalitis (22 percent) are also common. The gastrointestinal, renal, pulmonary, and cardiovascular systems may also be involved and are considered "minor" findings in this syndrome.

The eye may be the first or predominant organ involved in Behçet's disease. More characteristically, uveitis follows the other systemic findings by 1 to 3 yr. Systemic and ocular symptoms typically wax and wane. Patients will often present with an acute loss of vision associated with a bilateral (80 percent) uveitis.[54] The ocular inflammation may be severe and relapsing. A nongranulomatous iridocyclitis with hypopyon, posterior synechiae, and hyphema is common. On fundus examination, there may be a severe vitritis, disc edema, and attenuation of the arterioles.[55] An essential finding in Behçet's disease is the presence of an occlusive retinal vasculitis with surrounding intraretinal hemorrhage and retinal edema (Fig. 84–5). Cystoid macular edema, cataract, glaucoma, and retinal detachment can occur as secondary complications of the uveitis and retinal vasculitis.[56]

The complete form of Behçet's disease consists of oral ulcers, genital ulcers, uveitis, and nonulcerative skin lesions. Several systems have been proposed for diagnosing partial or incomplete forms of Behçet's disease.[57] Because of the prevalence of Behçet's disease in Japan, the Japanese classify this disease into four forms: (1) complete—all four major findings, (2) incomplete—three major findings or uveitis with one other major finding, (3) suspect—two major findings, and (4) possible—one major finding.

The presence of other minor findings associated with the multisystemic involvement can assist in the diagnosis. Laboratory testing may help by demonstrating an elevated ESR, elevated levels of C-reactive protein, immune complexes, and a positive ANA determination. HLA typing can also be helpful in incomplete forms of Behçet's disease. Properdin factor B, serum lysozyme, and α_1-acid glycoprotein are also elevated in Behçet's disease.[58] Pathergy and dermatographia, although much extolled, have not proved to be helpful measures for Behçet's disease in the United States. Fluorescein angiography can be employed to help document the ischemic retinal vasculitis and follow response to therapy. Cystoid macular edema and disc edema often result from the chronic inflammation. Choroidal vessels may be involved and show delayed filling or localized choroidal infarction.

Treatment of Behçet's disease is characteristically challenging. The disease is relapsing and may persist for many years. Behçet's disease can have explosive exacerbations following periods of relative inactivity or remission. Central nervous system involvement may be fatal in up to 40 percent of treated cases. Mild forms may be controlled initially with prednisone and colchicine (0.6 mg P.O. b.i.d.).[59] Usually, Behçet's disease

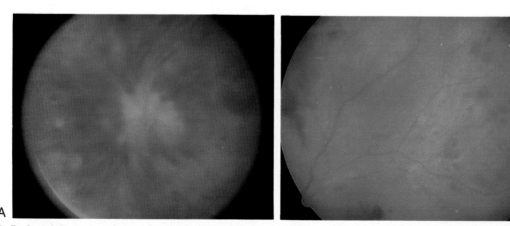

Figure 84–5. *A* and *B*, Two patients with Behçet's disease illustrating the profound involvement of the retinal vessels. A bilateral occlusive retinal vasculitis results in intraretinal edema, hemorrhage, and retinal nonperfusion. Progressive damage to the sensory retina results in marked attenuation of the arterioles.

requires more aggressive therapy. Periocular steroids can assist in controlling severe bouts of ocular inflammation. Chlorambucil (0.1 to 0.15 mg/kg/day) or cyclophosphamide (1 to 2 mg/kg/day) has been the mainstay of therapy.[60] Cyclophosphamide has fewer systemic side effects and therefore has been in favor for the treatment of ocular Behçet's disease in the United States.[61] Cyclosporine (4 mg/kg/day) also proved effective in controlling this disease and has become the treatment of choice at some centers.[62] Therapy may be required for several years. Careful monitoring for side effects and complications of immunosuppressive therapy is required. Even with treatment, up to 74 percent of patients lose useful visual acuity.

SJÖGREN'S SYNDROME

Sjögren's syndrome is a constellation of clinical disorders that have in common keratoconjunctivitis sicca and xerostomia.[62] Twenty-five to 50 percent of patients with RA have Sjögren's syndrome. This syndrome is more common in postmenopausal women. Exocrine glands, including the lacrimal gland, demonstrate infiltration with lymphocytes and secondary fibrosis. These patients have antinucleoprotein antibodies—anti-SSA (anti-Ro) and anti-SSB (anti-La).

Patients with Sjögren's syndrome complain of dryness of the mouth and eyes. Other manifestations of primary Sjögren's syndrome include pneumonitis, renal tubular acidosis, polymyositis, and gastritis.

Keratoconjunctivitis sicca is the most common ocular finding.[63] Secondary filamentary keratitis can also be problematic. In one series, eight patients with a clinical picture compatible with Sjögren's syndrome had anterior or intermediate uveitis but did not have chorioretinal involvement.[64] In another report, two patients with progressive retinal vasculitis were found to have anti-SSA antibodies, suggesting a Sjögren-like syndrome.[65] Their disease was unresponsive to corticosteroid, immunosuppressive, and panretinal photocoagulation therapy.

RELAPSING POLYCHONDRITIS

Relapsing polychondritis is a collagen vascular disease affecting primarily the cartilaginous tissues. The cause is unknown but appears to be an autoimmune disease directed against type II collagen.[66] Patients with polychondritis have circulating anti–type II collagen antibodies. These autoantibodies are thought to play a mediating role in the recurrent, granulomatous inflammation noted in this disease. Relapsing polychondritis occurs in adults aged 20 to 60 yr and affects both men and women.

Systemically, patients will have bilateral ear pinna inflammation and nasal cartilage destruction (72 percent).[67] Nasal septal damage typically results in a saddle nose deformity. Secondary otitis, vertigo, tinnitus, and deafness may be noted. A nonerosive polyarthralgia may also bring the patient to medical attention. Laryngeal and tracheal ring cartilage may be involved and can cause acute respiratory distress as a result of upper airway collapse.

Ocular involvement in relapsing polychondritis may occur in as many as 20 to 50 percent of cases.[68] This involvement is typically in the form of episcleritis, scleritis, or conjunctivitis. Anterior uveitis can be found in 20 percent of patients. Primary retinal or choroidal involvement is unusual. Retinal pigment epithelial and sensory retinal detachments as well as choroidal thickening can be noted as a result of localized posterior scleritis.[69]

The diagnosis can be established by the pathognomonic bilateral ear pinna inflammation. Biopsy of involved cartilage demonstrates the characteristic granulomatous chondritis. Relapsing polychondritis is a potentially fatal disease with a 30 percent mortality rate.[71] Prednisone, in combination with dapsone or cyclophosphamide, has proved to be the most effective agent in controlling this disease. Dapsone does not appear to be as effective in patients with severe necrotizing forms of scleritis.[71] Destructive changes in the cartilage are not reversible, and the goal of therapy should be to limit further disease progression.

ARTHRITIS ASSOCIATED WITH SPONDYLITIS (HLA-B27–ASSOCIATED)

The group of collagen vascular diseases have in common spondylitis and a strong association with HLA-B27. Ankylosing spondylitis, Reiter's syndrome, psoriatic arthritis, and arthritis associated with chronic inflammatory bowel disease (Crohn's and ulcerative colitis) compose this group. Patients with these disorders experience an acute, alternating, recurrent, nongranulomatous iridocyclitis. This anterior segment inflammation can be severe, with hypopyon and posterior synechiae formation. Secondary glaucoma and cataract are not uncommon. These collagen vascular diseases do not have marked posterior segment involvement in the form of primary choroiditis, retinitis, or retinal vasculitis. Cystoid macular edema can occur with prolonged or severe cases of anterior uveitis, which typically responds to therapies designed to address the iridocyclitis. Crohn's disease has been reported with uveitis and severe bilateral obliterative retinal vasculitis.[71–73] In these reports, the retinal vasculitis was responsive to corticosteroids or cyclophosphamide therapy, or a combination.

SUMMARY

The rheumatic diseases are a collection of inflammatory and autoimmune disorders that have multisystemic involvement and protean manifestations. Ocular inflammation may occur in many of these syndromes. The retina and choroid may be affected primarily as a result of retinal or choroidal vasculitis. Retinal ischemia, cotton-wool spots, intraretinal hemorrhages, retinal edema, and retinal vasculitis are the typical findings in these collagen vascular diseases. Posterior scleritis may result in secondary chorioretinal involvement.

The ophthalmologist should be aware of the association between ocular inflammation and the various connective tissue disorders. Many of these diseases either involve the eye primarily or present initially in the eye, preceding other organ system involvement by several years. A careful review of systems and general physical examination should be performed to ascertain systemic involvement. The prognosis for many of these vision- and life-threatening disorders depends on accurate diagnosis and institution of appropriate therapy. Until the pathophysiology and exact causes of the collagen vascular diseases are defined, antiinflammatory and immunosuppressive agents remain the mainstays of therapy. As such, the rheumatic diseases are best managed by a multidisciplinary approach, not infrequently negotiated by the ophthalmologist and the temper of the eye.

REFERENCES

1. Rodnan GP, Schumacher RH: The connective tissues: Structure, function and metabolism. *In* Rodnan GP, and Schumacher RH (eds): Primer on the Rheumatic Diseases, 8th ed. Atlanta, Arthritis Foundation, 1983.
2. Hascall VC, Hascall GK: Proteoglycans. *In* Hay ED (ed): Cell Biology of Extracellular Matrix. New York, Plenum, 1981.
3. Sanberg LB, Gray WR, Franzblau C (eds): Elastin and Elastic Tissue. New York, Plenum, 1977.
4. Friend J: Physiology of the cornea. *In* Smolin G, Thoft RA (eds): Cornea, 2nd ed. Boston, Little, Brown, 1987.
5. Fine BS, Yanoff M: The vitreous body. *In* Fine BS, Yanoff M (eds): Ocular Histology, 2nd ed. New York, Harper & Row, 1979.
6. Kelgren HJ: Epidemiology of rheumatoid arthritis. *In* Dutker JJR, Alexander WRM (eds): Rheumatic Diseases. Baltimore, Williams & Wilkins, 1968.
7. Torrigiana G, Roitt IM: Antiglobulin factors in sera from patients with rheumatoid arthritis and normal subjects. Ann Rheum Dis 3:315, 1977.
8. Barr CC, Davis H, Culbertson WW: Rheumatoid scleritis. Ophthalmology 88:1269, 1981.
9. Waston PG, Hayreh SS: Scleritis and episcleritis. Br J Ophthalmol 60:163, 1976.
10. Benson WE, Sheilds JA, Tasman W, et al: Posterior scleritis: A cause of diagnostic confusion. Arch Ophthalmol 97:1482, 1979.
11. Singh G, Guthoff R, Foster CS: Observation on long-term follow-up of posterior scleritis. Am J Ophthalmol 101:570, 1986.
12. Fraunfelder FT, Watson PG: Evaluation of eyes enucleated for scleritis. Br J Ophthalmol 60:227, 1976.
13. Foster CS, Forstot SL, Wilson LA: Mortality rate in rheumatoid arthritis patients developing necrotizing scleritis or peripheral ulcerative keratitis. Ophthalmology 91:1253, 1984.
14. Kanski JJ: Juvenile arthritis and uveitis. Surv Ophthalmol 34:253, 1990.
15. Kanski JJ, Shun-Shin GA: Systemic uveitis syndromes in childhood: An analysis of 340 cases. Ophthalmology 91:1247, 1984.
16. Giles CL: Uveitis in childhood: Part I. Anterior. Ann Ophthalmol 21:13, 1989.
17. Kanski JJ: Anterior uveitis in juvenile rheumatoid arthritis. Arch Ophthalmol 95:1794, 1977.
18. Olson NY, Lindsley CB, Godfrey WA: Nonsteroidal anti-inflammatory drug therapy in chronic childhood iridocyclitis. Am J Dis Child 142:1289, 1988.
19. Kanski JJ: Uveitis in juvenile rheumatoid arthritis: Incidence, clinical features and prognosis. Eye 2:641, 1988.
20. Diamond JG, Kaplan HL: Lensectomy and vitrectomy for complicated cataract secondary to uveitis. Arch Ophthalmol 96:1798, 1978.
21. Mintz G, Fraga A: Arteritis in systemic lupus erythematosus. Arch Intern Med 116:55, 1965.
22. Estes D, Christian CL: The natural history of systemic lupus erythematosus by prospective analysis. Medicine 50:85, 1971.
23. Baehr G, Klemperer R, Schifrin A: A diffuse disease of the peripheral circulation (usually associated with lupus erythematosus and endocarditis). Trans Assoc Am Phys 50:139, 1935.
24. Levine SR, Crofts JW, Lesse GR, et al: Visual symptoms associated with the presence of a lupus anticoagulant. Ophthalmology 95:686, 1988.
25. Gold DH, Morris DA, Henkind P: Ocular findings in systemic lupus erythematosus. Br J Ophthalmol 56:800, 1972.
26. Gold D, Feiner L, Henkind P: Retinal arterial occlusive disease in systemic lupus erythematosus. Arch Ophthalmol 95:1580, 1977.
27. Vine AK, Barr CC: Proliferative lupus retinopathy. Arch Ophthalmol 102:852, 1984.
28. Jabs DA, Hanneken AM, Schachat AP, et al: Choroidopathy in systemic lupus erythematosus. Arch Opthalmol 106:230, 1988.
29. Wong K, Everett A, Jones JV, et al: Visual loss as the initial symptom of systemic lupus erythematosus. Am J Ophthalmol 92:238, 1981.
30. Maricq HR, LeRoy EC: Progressive systemic sclerosis: Disorders of the microcirculation. Clin Rheum Dis 5:81, 1979.
31. Horan EC: Ophthalmic manifestations of progressive systemic sclerosis. Br J Ophthalmol 53:388, 1969.
32. Pollack IP, Becker B: Cytoid bodies of the retina in a patient with scleroderma. Am J Ophthalmol 54:655, 1962.
33. Medsger TA, Masi AT, Rodnan GP, et al: Survival with systemic sclerosis (scleroderma): A life-table analysis of 309 patients. Ann Intern Med 75:369, 1971.
34. Kissel JT, Mendell JR, Rammohan KW: Microvascular deposition of complement membrane attack complex in dermatomyositis. N Engl J Med 314:329, 1986.
35. Harrison SM, Frenkel M, Grossman BJ, et al: Retinopathy in childhood dermatomyositis. Am J Ophthalmol 76:786, 1973.
36. Bruce GM: Retinitis in dermatomyositis. Trans Am Ophthalmol Soc 36:282, 1938.
37. Christain CL, Sargent JS: Vasculitis syndromes, clinical and experimental models. Am J Med 61:385, 1976.
38. Gocke DJ, HSU K, Morgan C, et al: Association between polyarteritis and Australia antigen. Lancet 2:1149, 1970.
39. Stillerman ML: Ocular manifestations of diffuse collagen disease. Arch Ophthalmol 45:239, 1951.
40. Goar EL, Smith LS: Polyarteritis nodosa of the eye. Am J Ophthalmol 35:1619, 1952.
41. Fauci AS, Doppman JL, Wolff SM: Cyclophosphamide-induced remissions in advanced polyarteritis nodosa. Am J Med 64:890, 1978.
42. Goodman GC, Churg J: Wegener's granulomatosis: Pathology and review of the literature. Arch Pathol 58:533, 1954.
43. Robin JB, Schanzlin DJ, Meisler DM, et al: Ocular involvement in the respiratory vasculitides. Surv Ophthalmol 30:127, 1985.
44. Bullen CL, Liesegang TJ, McDonald TJ, et al: Ocular complications of Wegener's granulomatosis. Ophthalmology 90:279, 1083.
45. Pulido JS, Goeken JA, Nerad JA, et al: Ocular manifestations of patients with circulating antineutrophilic cytoplasmic antibodies. Arch Ophthalmol 108:845, 1990.
46. Fauci AS, Haynes BF, Katz P: The spectrum of vasculitis: Clinical, pathologic, immunologic and therapeutic considerations. Ann Intern Med 89:660, 1978.
47. Huston KA, Hunder GC, Lie JT, et al: Temporal arteritis. A 25-year epidemiological, clinical and pathological study. Ann Intern Med 88:162, 1978.
48. Keltner JL: Giant-cell arteritis. Ophthalmology 89:1101, 1982.
49. Whitfield JH, Bateman M, Cooke WT: Temporal arteritis. Br J Ophthalmol 47:555, 1963.
50. Cullen JF, Colier JA: Ophthalmic complications of giant cell arteritis. Surv Ophthalmol 20:247, 1976.
51. Numaga J, Kazumasas M, Mochizuki M, et al: An HLA-D region restriction fragment associated with refractory Behçet's disease. Am J Ophthalmol 105:528, 1988.
52. Aoki K, Fujioka K, Katsumata H, et al: Epidemiologic studies on Behçet's disease in Hokkaido district. [Japanese] J Clin Ophthalmol 25:2239, 1971.
53. Chajek T, Fainaru M: Behçet's disease: Report of 41 cases and a review of the literature. Medicine 54:179, 1975.

54. Michelson JB, Chisari VF: Behçet's disease. Surv Ophthalmol 26:190, 1982.
55. James DG, Spiteri MA: Behçet's disease. Ophthalmology 89:1279, 1982.
56. Colvard DM, Robertson DM, O'Duffy JD: The ocular manifestations of Behçet's disease. Arch Ophthalmol 95:1813, 1977.
57. Behçet's Disease Research Committee of Japan: Behçet's disease: Guide to diagnosis of Behçet's disease. Jpn J Ophthalmol 18:291, 1974.
58. Lehner T, Adinolfi M: Acute phase proteins, C9, factor B and lysozyme in recurrent oral ulceration and Behçet's syndrome. J Clin Pathol 33:269, 1980.
59. Hijakata K, Masuda K: Visual prognosis in Behçet's: Effects of cyclophosphamide and colchicine. Jpn J Ophthalmol 22:506, 1978.
60. O'Duffy JD, Robertson DM, Goldstein NP: Chlorambucil in the treatment of uveitis and meningoencephalitis of Behçet's disease. Am J Med 76:75, 1984.
61. Nussenblatt RB, Palastine AG, and Chan CC: Effectiveness of cyclosporin therapy in Behçet's disease. Arthritis Rheum 28:671, 1985.
62. Manthorpe R, Frost-Larson K, Isager H, et al: Sjögren's syndrome. Allergy 36:139, 1981.
63. Brown SI, Grayson M: Marginal furrows: A characteristic corneal lesion of rheumatoid arthritis. Arch Ophthalmol 79:563, 1968.
64. Rosenbaum JY, Bennett RM: Chronic anterior and posterior uveitis and primary Sjögren's syndrome. Am J Ophthalmol 104:346, 1987.
65. Farmer SG, Kinyoun MD, Nelson JL, et al: Retinal vasculitis associated with autoantibodies to Sjögren's syndrome A antigen. Am J Ophthalmol 100:814, 1985.
66. Foidart J-M, Abe S, Marin GR, et al: Antibodies to type II collagen in relapsing polychondritis. N Engl J Med 299:1203, 1978.
67. McAdam LP, O'Hanllan MA, Bluestone R, et al: Relapsing polychondritis: Prospective study of 23 patients and a review of the literature. Medicine 55:193, 1976.
68. Isaak BL, Liesang TJ, Michet CJ: Ocular and systemic findings in relapsing polychondritis. Ophthalmology 93:681, 1986.
69. Magargal LE, Donoso LA, Goldberg RE, et al: Ocular manifestations of relapsing polychondritis. Retina 1:96, 1981.
70. Hoang-Xuan T, Foster CS, Rice BA: Scleritis in relapsing polychondritis: Response to therapy. Ophthalmology 97:892, 1990.
71. Salmon JF, Wright JP, Bowen RM, et al: Granulomatous uveitis in Crohn's disease. Arch Ophthalmol 107:718, 1989.
72. Duker JS, Brown GC, Brooks, L: Retinal vasculitis in Crohn's disease. Am J Ophthalmol 103:664, 1987.
73. Ruby AJ, Jampol LM: Crohn's disease and vascular disease. Am J Ophthalmol 110:349, 1990.

Chapter 85

▪

Retinopathy Associated With Blood Anomalies

JOHN I. LOEWENSTEIN

ANEMIA

Fundus findings in anemia may include hemorrhages, cotton-wool spots, and retinal edema. The hemorrhages are typically superficial and flame-shaped, but they may also have a white center (Figs. 85–1 and 85–2). Rarely, preretinal or vitreous hemorrhage or a macular star may occur. The retinal vessels are usually normal, although pale arterioles and dilated veins may be seen.[1] Fluorescein angiography may reveal an increased retinal transit time.

The picture as a whole is suggestive, but not diagnostic, of anemia. It usually is not possible to determine the type of anemia from the fundus findings. Some authors feel that white-centered hemorrhages are more common in pernicious anemia than in other types of anemia;[2] others state that a picture of numerous preretinal hemorrhages, together with white-centered hemorrhages, is characteristic of aplastic anemia,[3] but systematic quantitative studies have not been undertaken. Vision is not affected unless there are changes at the macula, and such changes are unusual. Retinopathy resolves with treatment of the underlying anemia.

There is controversy in the literature regarding the most important factors related to the prevalence of retinopathy in anemia. Age, sex, type of anemia, he-

matocrit values, and platelet counts have all been invoked, but only a few quantitative studies have been performed. Foulds[3] studied 30 cases of pernicious anemia. He found retinopathy in all patients with a hemoglobin concentration of less than 5 g/dl, one third of patients with a hemoglobin concentration of 5 to 6 g/dl, and in no patients with a hemoglobin concentration of more than 6 g/dl. On this basis, he states that retinopathy is most likely associated with a hemoglobin concentration of less than 6 g/dl. Wise and associates[1] state that

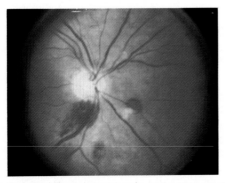

Figure 85–1. Intraretinal hemorrhages and cotton-wool spots in a case of severe anemia.

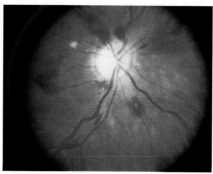

Figure 85–2. Intraretinal hemorrhages, white-centered hemorrhage, and cotton-wool spots in a case of aplastic anemia.

a hemoglobin concentration of 2.5 g/dl or less is usually associated with retinopathy. Merin and Freund[4] studied 89 patients with anemia in Africa. The majority of their patients had anemia secondary to nutritional deficiency and hookworm infestation. None of their patients with a hemoglobin level more than 8 g/dl had retinopathy, whereas 46 percent of those with a hemoglobin concentration of less than 8 g/dl showed hemorrhages or "exudates," or both. Aisen and colleagues[5] examined 35 anemic patients and 35 age- and sex-matched controls. Twenty percent of the anemic patients had hemorrhages or cotton-wool spots, but there was no correlation with the hematocrit value. Rubinstein and coworkers[6] studied two groups of patients with anemia. Group 1 consisted of 67 patients, each having a hemoglobin concentration of less than 12 g/dl or a platelet count of less than 100,000, or both. A variety of diseases was present in this group, including many cases of leukemia. Some of the leukemic patients were receiving chemotherapy. It was demonstrated that in these patients for a given platelet level, a lower hematocrit value was more likely to be associated with retinal hemorrhages. Similarly, for a given hemoglobin concentration, more severe thrombocytopenia was more likely to be associated with retinal hemorrhage. The data for group 1 are summarized in Table 85–1.

Group 2 consisted of 123 hemophiliacs and 42 patients with Cooley's anemia. All patients in this group had a hemoglobin concentration of less than 8 g/dl at some point in the course of disease, but none had thrombocytopenia. No patient in this group had retinal hemorrhages. Not all members of group 2 had a dilated fundus examination by an ophthalmologist, whereas all members of group 1 did have such an evaluation. It is therefore possible that the number of retinal hemorrhages in the patients in group 2 was underestimated. Since many leukemic patients were included in group 1, it is not possible to determine from their data whether the relationship among anemia, thrombocytopenia, and retinopathy holds true for nonleukemic cases. Holt and Gordon-Smith[7] examined a large number of patients with a variety of blood diseases. They studied 33 patients with leukemia and found that 18 of them had retinopathy, which was more likely with increasing anemia and thrombocytopenia. These authors did not report platelet levels in their other cases of anemia, but they did give the impression that the combination of anemia and thrombocytopenia was more likely to yield retinopathy. They found that more profound anemia was required to produce cotton-wool spots than was required to produce hemorrhages.

Merin and Freund,[4] in their study of anemia in Africa, could find no cases of retinopathy in children despite very low hemoglobin levels. This has led to speculation that age is a factor in the prevalence of retinal abnormalities in anemia. Aisen and colleagues,[5] however, could not confirm a correlation between age and retinopathy in their population. These two studies also suggested that hemorrhages and cotton-wool spots in anemia were more common in males than in females. Aisen and colleagues subjected this hypothesis to statistical analysis and failed to find significance despite the trend.

In summary, a precise level of anemia at which retinal abnormalities will occur cannot be given. Retinal abnormalities in anemia without accompanying thrombocytopenia are rare, however, unless the anemia is profound. The combination of thrombocytopenia and anemia makes retinopathy more likely. Young children may be less likely to show retinal changes with anemia, unless it is caused by leukemia. Different types of anemia may show varying thresholds of hemoglobin that must be reached to produce retinopathy; it is unclear how much of this variation can be accounted for by platelet levels.

Aisen and colleagues[5] measured venous tortuosity (as a function of venous length over distance traveled) in their anemic patients and controls. They found that the anemic patients had greater venous tortuosity than did the controls. Fletcher and associates[8] reanalyzed their data and found that no correlation was present between the degree of venous tortuosity and hematocrit value within each study group. They hypothesized that factors other than the hematocrit value contributed to tortuosity.

The pathophysiology of retinopathy in anemia is poorly understood. It is possible that dilatation of retinal vessels occurs as a response to retinal hypoxia in profound anemia. The resulting increase in transmural pressure, or perhaps the hypoxia itself, may damage

Table 85–1. DATA FOR GROUP 1 IN RUBENSTEIN AND COWORKERS' STUDY

Platelets/sq mm	Hemoglobin g/dl	Number of Patients	Patients With Retinal Hemorrhage
<50,000	<8	10	7
	8–12	14	5
	>12	1	0
50,000–100,000	<8	7	3
	8–12	8	2
	>12	5	0
>100,000	<8	19	2
	8–12	3	0

Data from Rubenstein RA, Yanoff M, Albert DM: Thrombocytopenia, anemia, and retinal hemorrhage. Am J Ophthalmol 65:435, 1968.

vascular walls. Thrombocytopenia might contribute by retarding healing. Aging changes in retinal blood vessels may play a role. This scheme might explain vascular leakage that produces hemorrhage and edema. Cotton-wool spots are infarcts of the nerve fiber layer of the retina. It is possible that they are produced by relative hypoxia in anemia; vascular spasm might explain their focal nature.

LEUKEMIA

The fundus in leukemia may show venous dilatation, tortuosity, and irregularity, and vessels may show abnormal color and sheathing. Flame, white-centered, preretinal and vitreous hemorrhages; cotton-wool spots; and leukemic infiltrates may occur (Figs. 85–3 to 85–5). The latter appear as white clumps or masses in the retina. Microaneurysms, venous occlusions, and neovascularization are sometimes seen, typically in chronic leukemia. Serous detachment of the retina may occur as a result of choroidal infiltration.[9]

Curiously, the presence of retinal abnormalities in leukemia does not correlate well with the white cell count. Autopsy studies show a high agonal white cell count in patients with leukemic infiltration,[10] but the relationship between the white cell count and infiltration is difficult to demonstrate in clinical studies.

The anemia, thrombocytopenia, and hyperviscosity that may accompany leukemia probably account for most of the retinal findings. Retinal hemorrhages are likely the result of anemia and thrombocytopenia. As discussed in the section on anemia, for a given platelet level, a lower hematocrit value is more likely to be associated with retinal hemorrhages.[6, 7] Similarly, for a given hemoglobin level, more severe thrombocytopenia is more likely to be associated with retinal hemorrhage. A prospective study of retinopathy in leukemia by Guyer and colleagues[11] demonstrated significantly lower platelet counts in patients with retinal hemorrhages in comparison with those without such lesions, regardless of the type of leukemia. In this study, patients with acute lymphocytic leukemia and retinal hemorrhages showed lower hematocrit levels than did those without retinal

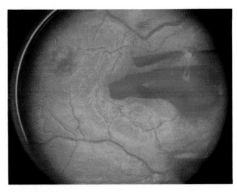

Figure 85–4. Intraretinal and preretinal hemorrhages in a case of acute lymphatic leukemia. Right eye.

hemorrhages. This relationship was not demonstrated in patients with myeloid leukemia. In patients with acute nonlymphocytic leukemia, however, the presence of anemia was related to the presence of white-centered hemorrhages. Hemorrhages (with or without white centers) and cotton-wool spots were more common in adults than in children. There was no correlation between fundus findings and mean leukocyte counts. Karesh and coworkers[12] in a prospective evaluation of the fundi of patients with myeloid leukemia, demonstrated significantly lower platelet counts in patients with retinopathy than in those without fundus lesions. They found no difference in hematocrit levels and white cell counts in groups with and without retinopathy. They did not do a separate analysis for different types of retinal lesions. Most of their patients with retinopathy had retinal hemorrhages.

Venous dilatation, tortuosity, and irregularity seen in leukemia may be caused by a combination of anemia and hyperviscosity. Venous occlusions are likely to result from hyperviscosity. Cotton-wool spots are caused by occlusion of precapillary arterioles, but the reason for these occlusions in leukemia has not been established. Ischemia secondary to anemia, direct occlusion by leukemic cells, occlusion by platelet-fibrin aggregates, or sludging resulting from hyperviscosity may all be factors. In their prospective study, Guyer and colleagues[11] did not find an association between hematologic variables and cotton-wool spots.

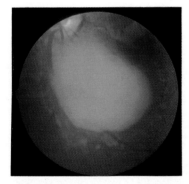

Figure 85–3. Large leukemic infiltrate. (From Schachat AP, Markowitz JA, Guyer DR, et al: Ophthalmic manifestations of leukemia. Arch Ophthalmol 107:698, 1989. Copyright 1989, American Medical Association.)

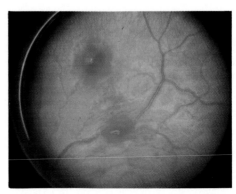

Figure 85–5. Left eye of patient in Figure 85–4.

Table 85–2. PREVALENCE OF RETINAL FINDINGS IN SCHACHAT AND ASSOCIATES' STUDY

Retinal Finding	Myeloid Patients (%)	Lymphoid Patients (%)	Total Affected (%)
Intraretinal hemorrhage	33	13	24
Cotton-wool spot	24	6	16
White-centered hemorrhage	13	8	11
Central vein occlusion	7	0	4
Vitreous hemorrhage	4	0	2
Leukemic infiltrate			3

From Schachat AP, Markowitz JA, Guyer DR, et al: Ophthalmic manifestations of leukemia. Arch Ophthalmol 107:697, 1989. Copyright 1989, American Medical Association.

Microaneurysms are seen in cases of chronic leukemia and may be related to hyperviscosity.[13, 14] In Jampol and associates'[14] study of 25 patients with chronic leukemia, 8 individuals had microaneurysms. Neovascularization may also be seen in cases of chronic leukemia[15] but is quite rare. It is usually accompanied by capillary closure.[16] The white centers of some hemorrhages seen in leukemia may consist of leukemic cells and debris, platelet-fibrin aggregates, or septic emboli.[17]

The prevalence of retinal involvement in leukemia varies widely in the literature. Almost all studies suffer from their retrospective nature and a variety of selection biases. Schachat and colleagues[18] performed a prospective ophthalmic study of patients with newly diagnosed leukemia. A summary of the prevalence of retinal findings in their patients is given in Table 85–2. They found a 5 percent prevalence of visual loss caused by vitreoretinal disease in those patients in whom a reliable acuity determination was possible. Karesh and coworkers[12] prospectively evaluated the fundi of patients with myeloid leukemia and found that 53 percent of their subjects had retinopathy. Five of 53 patients in their study had visual loss in one or both eyes related to macular hemorrhage.

Alterations in the retinal pigment epithelium caused by leukemia have been reported by several authors.[19–22] The appearance is one of pigment clumping or a reticular pattern of pigment change. Pathologic examination demonstrates leukemic infiltration of the choroid and retina, with destruction and hyperplasia of the pigment epithelium.

Burns and associates reported a single case of bilateral central serous retinopathy in acute lymphocytic leukemia.[23] It is difficult to know whether this represented a chance occurrence of two conditions or a manifestation of leukemia, perhaps secondary to infiltration of the choroid. Kuwabara and Aiello described the pathologic findings in a case of leukemic miliary nodules of the retina.[24]

POLYCYTHEMIA

Foulds[2] points out that whole blood viscosity is considerably influenced by the number of red cells present.

He finds clinical signs of hyperviscosity begin with a hematocrit value greater than 50 percent. Wise and associates[1] note that there is a linear relationship between viscosity and hematocrit value up to a hematocrit of 50 percent. When the level is greater than this, viscosity increases exponentially with the rising hematocrit value. Blood flow in retinal vessels is typically laminar, and Foulds notes that this may be responsible for the proportionality of whole blood viscosity to the shear rate; thus, whole blood viscosity is greater when blood flow is slower and hyperviscosity therefore results in greater changes in the venous system.

In polycythemia, the fundus typically shows dark, dilated, tortuous veins (Figs. 85–6 and 85–7). The disc is usually hyperemic and swollen, intraretinal hemorrhages are frequently seen, and there may be retinal edema. Central or branch vein retinal occlusions may occur. Patients may lose vision because of retinal edema or vein occlusion. Abnormalities are almost always present in both eyes; the patient with a central vein occlusion in one eye and a normal fellow eye rarely has underlying polycythemia.

Primary polycythemia is more likely to produce retinopathy than is secondary polycythemia, probably because of higher red cell counts and hyperviscosity in the former.[1] Treatment will reverse most of the findings unless venous occlusion has occurred.

DYSPROTEINEMIAS

Dysproteinemia that results in hyperviscosity of the serum from a variety of causes can produce a dramatic retinopathy.[25] Carr and Henkind[25] reported similar retinal findings in cases of hyperviscosity caused by cryomacroglobulinemia, hypergammaglobulinemia, Waldenström's macroglobulinemia, chronic lymphocytic leukemia with macroglobulinemia, and multiple myeloma with hyperglobulinemia. Waldenström's macroglobulinemia may be the most likely dysproteinemia to produce retinopathy, possibly because the large size of the protein molecules in this condition lead to very high viscosity levels.[1] Holt and Gordon-Smith,[7] however, found no correlation between total serum protein and retinopathy in their series. Rather, they felt that presence of retinopathy correlated with the degree of anemia present

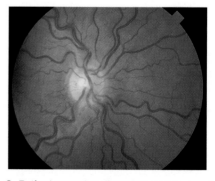

Figure 85–6. Retinal vascular dilatation and tortuosity in a case of secondary polycythemia. Right eye.

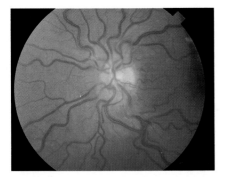

Figure 85–7. Left eye of patient in Figure 85–6.

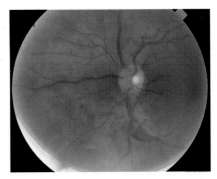

Figure 85–9. Left eye of patient in Figure 85–8. There is disc hyperemia in addition to vascular dilatation, tortuosity, and intra-retinal hemorrhage.

in their patients. They noted that their patients, as well as others reported in the literature with Waldenström's macroglobulinemia and retinopathy, exhibited severe anemia.

In retinopathy of dysproteinemia, the retinal veins are dark, dilated, and tortuous; intraretinal hemorrhages and cotton-wool spots are seen, and the disc is hyperemic (Figs. 85–8 and 85–9). The retinal hemorrhages may be of the superficial flame or deep punctate type and extend to the periphery. Retinal edema may occur. Central or branch vein retinal occlusion may be found, as in polycythemia. Visual loss may be due to vascular occlusion or retinal edema. Abnormalities are usually found bilaterally.

Retinal microaneurysms (Figs. 85–10 and 85–11) may be seen in more chronic cases.[26] Exudative retinal detachment has been described in multiple myeloma.[27, 28] Neovascularization of the retina or iris with vitreous hemorrhage or neovascular glaucoma can occur. Fibrous proliferation has been described.

Retinopathy may be reversible with treatment of the underlying disease if frank vein occlusion has not occurred.[29]

HEMORRHAGIC DISORDERS

The retina is not typically involved in hemorrhagic disorders unless there is ocular trauma. Thrombocytopenia is an exception, particularly if there is accompanying anemia (as described earlier). Idiopathic thrombocytopenic purpura rarely results in retinopathy.[7]

Thrombotic thrombocytopenic purpura may cause retinal hemorrhages and serous retinal detachment; the relative roles of thrombosis, hypertension, and renal disease in producing the retinal findings are uncertain.[30, 31]

APPROACH TO THE PATIENT WITH RETINAL HEMORRHAGES OF UNKNOWN CAUSE

The patient who presents with retinal hemorrhages can be a diagnostic dilemma, as the list of conditions involved in the differential diagnosis is very long. The first task is to decide whether the hemorrhages are intraretinal, subretinal, or preretinal. Intraretinal hemorrhages are of two types: dot and blot and flame. Dot and blot hemorrhages are located deep in the retina and are confined by the anteroposterior orientation of the rods and cones, bipolar cells, and Müller's cells. When viewed end-on through the ophthalmoscope, they appear as round, red dots or somewhat larger round "blots." Flame hemorrhages are located in the superficial retina and are confined by the mediolateral, arcing orientation of the nerve fiber layer. When viewed with the ophthalmoscope, they are flame-shaped, with feathery borders. Flame hemorrhages tend to occur mainly in the posterior portion of the retina. In the periphery, hemorrhages appear as dots and blots regardless of their level in the retina.[32] Intraretinal hemorrhages occur in a

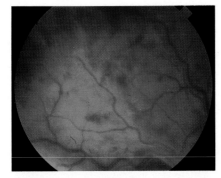

Figure 85–8. Retinal vascular dilatation and tortuosity, with intra-retinal hemorrhage, in a case of hyperviscosity due to dysproteinemia. Right eye.

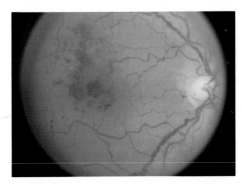

Figure 85–10. Waldenström's macroglobulinemia with venous dilatation and beading, as well as intraretinal hemorrhage. Right eye.

1000 ■ Retina and Vitreous

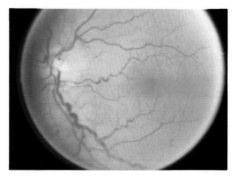

Figure 85–11. Left eye of patient in Figure 85–10.

wide variety of disorders, including many systemic diseases and retinal venous occlusions. Subretinal hemorrhages are amorphous in shape and are deep to the retinal vessels. These hemorrhages occur in trauma or with subretinal neovascularization (e.g., from age-related maculopathy). Preretinal hemorrhages may also be amorphous, or they may be boat-shaped, with a horizontal upper border and a curved lower border (caused by settling of red cells). These hemorrhages cover retinal vessels. Preretinal hemorrhages occur with retinal neovascularization (e.g., in diabetic retinopathy or sickle cell disease), vitreous detachment or retinal breaks, and trauma. Occasionally they are seen in other disorders (e.g., vein occlusion without neovascularization, leukemia, subarachnoid hemorrhage).

Bilateral intraretinal hemorrhages pose the greatest challenge to the differential diagnosis. Unilateral intraretinal hemorrhages are most frequently due to venous occlusive disease. Bilateral findings suggest systemic disease as the cause. The distribution of the hemorrhages may be helpful. If they occur mainly in the posterior fundus, systemic disease is likely. Extension to the far periphery suggests venous occlusive disease. Confinement to the peripapillary retina suggests optic nerve disease (including papilledema). Accompanying findings may be helpful in the differential diagnosis. Venous dilatation suggests obstructed flow, which may be due to venous occlusion or hyperviscosity. Microaneurysms are the hallmark of diabetic retinopathy, but they occur with hypertension, venous occlusion, leukemia, and other disorders. They are, however, a sign of chronicity. Arteriolar narrowing and sclerotic changes suggest systemic hypertension. Flame hemorrhages are more frequent in hypertension, with dot and blot lesions more common in diabetes, but both lesions occur in either disorder, as well as in vein occlusion and retinopathy associated with blood disorders. Cotton-wool spots or white-centered hemorrhages often accompany retinal hemorrhages, and they may be seen in so many disorders that they are of little help in the differential diagnosis. A thorough medical history, general physical examination, complete blood count, and blood glucose determination will reveal the cause of bilateral, posterior intraretinal hemorrhages in the majority of cases. Study of serum protein levels may be useful when hyperviscosity is suspected. Fluorescein angiography may be useful in demonstrating subtle abnormalities of the retinal and choroidal vasculature.

REFERENCES

1. Wise GN, Dollery CT, Henkind P: The Retinal Circulation. New York, Harper & Row, 1971.
2. Foulds WS: "Blood is thicker than water." Some haemorheological aspects of ocular disease. 50th Bowman lecture. Eye 1:343, 1987.
3. Foulds WS: The ocular manifestations of blood diseases. Trans Ophthalmol Soc UK 83:345, 1963.
4. Merin S, Freund M: Retinopathy in severe anemia. Am J Ophthalmol 66:1102, 1968.
5. Aisen ML, Bacon BR, Goodman AM, et al: Retinal abnormalities associated with anemia. Arch Ophthalmol 101:1049, 1983.
6. Rubenstein RA, Yanoff M, Albert DM: Thrombocytopenia, anemia, and retinal hemorrhage. Am J Ophthalmol 65:435, 1968.
7. Holt JM, Gordon-Smith EC: Retinal abnormalities in diseases of the blood. Br J Ophthalmol 53:145, 1969.
8. Fletcher ME, Farber MD, Cohen SB, et al: Retinal abnormalities associated with anemia. [Letter] Arch Ophthalmol 102:358, 1984.
9. Kincaid MC, Green WR, Kelley JS: Acute ocular leukemia. Am J Ophthalmol 87:698, 1979.
10. Robb RM, Ervin LD, Sallan SE: A pathologic study of eye involvement in acute leukemia of childhood. Trans Am Ophthalmol Soc 76:90, 1978.
11. Guyer DR, Schachat AP, Vitale S, et al: Leukemic retinopathy. Ophthalmology 96:860, 1989.
12. Karesh JW, Goldman EJ, Reck K, et al: A prospective ophthalmic evaluation of patients with acute myeloid leukemia: Correlaion of ocular and hematologic findings. J Clin Oncol 7:1528, 1989.
13. Duke JR, Wilkinson CP, Sigelman S: Retinal microaneurysms in leukemia. Br J Ophthalmol 52:368, 1968.
14. Jampol LM, Goldberg MF, Busse B: Peripheral retinal microaneurysms in chronic leukemia. Am J Ophthalmol 80:242, 1975.
15. Morse PH, McReady JL: Peripheral retinal neovascularization in CML. Am J Ophthalmol 72:975, 1971.
16. Schachat AP: The leukemias and lymphomas. In Ryan SJ, Ogden TE, Schachat AP (eds): Retina, vol. 1. St Louis, CV Mosby, 1989.
17. Kincaid MC, Green WR: Ocular and orbital involvement in leukemia. Surv Ophthalmol 27:211, 1983.
18. Schachat AP, Markowitz JA, Guyer DR, et al: Ophthalmic manifestations of leukemia. Arch Ophthalmol 107:697, 1989.
19. Clayman HM, Flynn JJ, Koch K, et al: Retinal pigment epithelial abnormalities in leukemic disease. Am J Ophthalmol 74:416, 1972.
20. Jakobiec F, Behrens M: Leukemic retinal pigment epitheliopathy, with report of a unilateral case. J Pediatr Ophthalmol 12:10, 1975.
21. Inkeles DM, Friedman AH: Retinal pigment epithelial degeneration, partial retinal atrophy and macular hole in acute lymphocytic leukemia. Graefes Arch Clin Exp Ophthalmol 194:253, 1975.
22. Verbraak FD, van den Berg W, Bos PJM: Retinal pigment epitheliopathy in acute leukemia. Arch Ophthalmol 111:111, 1991.
23. Burns CA, Blodi FC, Williamson BK: Acute lymphocytic leukemia and central serous retinopathy. Trans Am Acad Ophthalmol Otolaryngol 69:307, 1965.
24. Kuwabara T, Aiello L: Leukemic miliary nodules in the retina. Arch Ophthalmol 72:494, 1964.
25. Carr RE, Henkind P: Retinal findings with serum hyperviscosity. Am J Ophthalmol 56:23, 1963.
26. Gates RF, Richards RD: Macroglobulinemia with unusual vascular changes. Arch Ophthalmol 77:64, 1960.
27. Ashton N: Ocular changes in multiple myelomatosis. Arch Ophthalmol 73:487, 1965.
28. Franklin RM, Kenyon KR, Green WR, et al: Epibulbar IGA plasmacytoma occurring in multiple myeloma. Arch Ophthalmol 100:451, 1982.
29. Schwab PJ, Okun E, Fahey JL: Reversal of retinopathy in Waldenström's macroglobulinemia by plasmapheresis. Arch Ophthalmol 64:515, 1960.
30. Lambert SR, High KA, Cotlier E, et al: Serous retinal detachments in thrombotic thrombocytopenic purpura. Arch Ophthalmol 103:1172, 1985.
31. Percival SPB: Ocular findings in thrombotic thrombocytopenic purpura (Moschcowitz's disease). Br J Ophthalmol 54:73, 1970.
32. Ballantyne AJ, Michaelson IC: Textbook of the Fundus of the Eye, 2nd ed. Baltimore, Williams & Wilkins, 1970.

Chapter 86

■

Retinal Lesions in Sarcoidosis

CHARLES D. J. REGAN

This chapter discusses retinal lesions found in patients with confirmed or presumed sarcoidosis (Table 86–1). The systemic disease is described in Chapter 254, and the role of sarcoidosis in the production of uveitis is considered in Chapter 27.

When fundus lesions are the only ocular signs of sarcoidosis, there may be no symptoms to lead to their early detection. Consequently, patients with proven or suspected systemic sarcoidosis should have careful fundus examinations to permit the early recognition and management of existing lesions. The identification of posterior ocular lesions is also important because they are associated relatively frequently (37 percent) with central nervous system lesions of sarcoidosis.[1]

In many cases, it is difficult to establish a definite diagnosis of sarcoidosis, and repeated periodic testing may be necessary because ocular signs and symptoms may appear before laboratory and systemic manifestations of the disease.[2, 3] Nevertheless, a firm diagnosis is important for the selection of appropriate treatment, as well as for forming a reliable prognosis.

Diagnostic difficulties and variously accepted criteria may account for the considerable differences in the reported incidences of ocular and retinal involvement in sarcoidosis. Ocular involvement is reported in up to 30 percent of patients with systemic sarcoidosis, and retinal lesions occur in about 25 percent of those patients.[2, 4–6] Retinal lesions occur most often in association with anterior uveitis and vitritis, but in some cases they may be the only manifestation of sarcoidosis.[1, 3, 7, 8] When there is severe associated vitritis, it is sometimes impossible to identify retinal lesions, and their incidence may be higher than suspected, particularly if the retinal abnormalities are eliminated by the same treatment that clears the vitreous and makes the retina visible.[9] In the presence of vitreous haze, retinal lesions may be visualized in fluorescein angiograms when they cannot be appreciated by ophthalmoscopy or biomicroscopy, so angiography should be a regular component of serial examinations in these patients.

Retinal vasculitis is the most common retinal abnormality associated with sarcoidosis, and the complications of retinal vasculitis account for many of the other retinal lesions seen, such as perivascular exudation, vascular sheathing, macular edema, and retinal neovascularization. In addition, chorioretinitis, choroidal nodules or granulomas with overlying sensory retinal detachments, disc neovascularization, subretinal neovascularization with subretinal leakage, epiretinal membrane proliferation, and traction retinal detachments occur as complications in ocular sarcoidosis.[1–10]

RETINAL VASCULITIS

Vascular inflammation may be caused by vasoactive products such as prostaglandins, leukotrienes, and kinins released into the vitreous from other sites of ocular inflammation.[10–12] In those cases, the inflammation is not specific for sarcoid and occurs in the vessels of the posterior pole, as well as at the equator, and frequently is associated with cystoid macular edema (Fig. 86–1). The inflammation is patchy or extensive in the walls of affected venules and often is not detectable by ophthalmoscopy or biomicroscopy, although it may be inferred through recognition of concurrent macular edema. It is demonstrable by fluorescein angiography, however, and serial angiograms may be the most accurate means of assessing the efficacy of treatment. This form of "secondary vasculitis" does not progress to vascular occlusion, although it may produce permanent sheathing of the involved venules.

The form of vasculitis considered characteristic of sarcoidosis affects venules and capillaries, usually outside the posterior pole, and is sometimes associated with focal perivascular exudates that produce the appearance of "candle-wax drippings" when they extend along a segment of the vein wall (Figs. 86–2 and 86–3). Often they are associated with superficial retinal hemorrhages, focal retinal exudates in the area of the involved veins, and large vitreous nodules ("snowballs"; Fig. 86–4).[7, 13] On resolution, the perivascular exudates leave spotty defects in retinal pigment epithelium along the course of the sheathed vessel, but in a few cases, persistent vasculitis leads to branch retinal vein occlusion and focal retinal infarction, which occurs in most cases at the level of the equator.

Table 86–1. RETINAL LESIONS IN SARCOIDOSIS

Retinal vasculitis
  Macular edema
  Perivascular exudation
  Vascular sheathing
    Branch occlusion
    Ischemia
    Retinal neovascularization
Retinal granulomas
  Appearance of chorioretinitis or choroidal granulomas
Disc neovascularization
Juxtapapillary neovascularization
Epiretinal membranes
  Traction retinal detachment
  Retinal tears

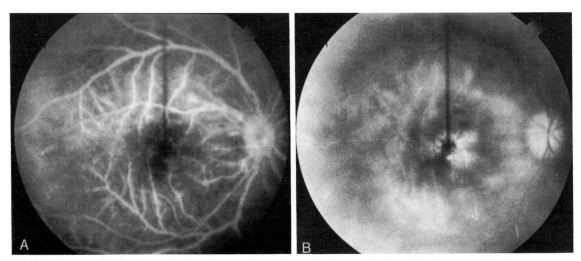

Figure 86–1. *A,* Diffuse vasculitis of macular branch vessels seen in early fluorescein transit. *B,* Late transit in the same eye, showing prominent cystoid macular edema.

RETINAL NEOVASCULARIZATION

Hypoxia in the area of infarcted retina can be the stimulus for neovascular proliferation (Fig. 86–5),[15] although retinal neovascularization related to peripheral retinal vasculitis without capillary obstruction in sarcoid patients has been reported.[10] In those cases, it is postulated that T lymphocytes, macrophages, or other inflammatory cells may be angiogenic.[16] Whatever its cause, neovascular proliferation may result in intravitreal bleeding with severe impairment of the patient's visual acuity and interference with the examiner's visualization of the fundus.

Neovascularization is reported in 1 to 5 percent of sarcoid patients with posterior segment involvement and is indistinguishable from the neovascular "sea fans" in sickle cell anemia.[5, 6, 9] In one report, both sarcoidosis and sickle cell anemia were diagnosed in a single patient with peripheral retinal neovascularization.[17] Given the prevalence of black Americans in the sarcoid population of the United States, it is essential to include hemoglobin electrophoresis in the initial studies of black patients with retinal neovascularization, even if sarcoidosis is proved. It has been reported on the basis of a small number of patients[9, 17] that the presence of a patent retinal vessel traversing the ischemic zone adjacent to the neovascularization may be characteristic of sarcoidosis, but the reliability of that sign requires more extensive corroboration.

GRANULOMATOUS LESIONS

A fortuitous histologic study of an eye with active lesions of sarcoidosis suggests that cellular exudates occur at all retinal levels but do not invade the choroid.[7] Traditionally, the literature cites chorioretinitis, chorioretinal nodules, and large choroidal granulomas as in-

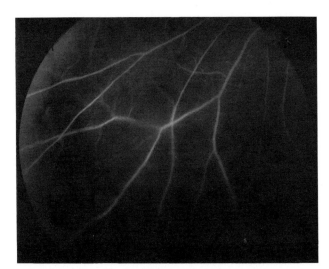

Figure 86–2. Vasculitis. Irregular areas of hyperfluorescence (staining) in walls of vessels near the equator seen in the late phase of a fluorescein angiogram.

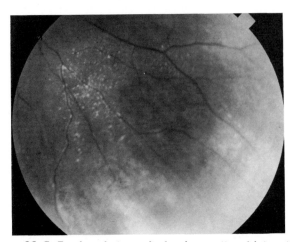

Figure 86–3. Fundus photograph showing scattered intraretinal exudates in a patient with presumed sarcoidosis. Many exudates are distributed along the branches of a venule in the form of a "string of pearls."

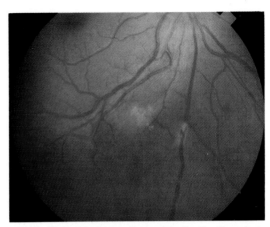

Figure 86–4. Retinal lesions of sarcoidosis. Fundus photograph showing a plaque of granulomatous material wrapped around a venule. A small intraretinal hemorrhage is seen to the right of the plaque, and an irregular granulomatous infiltrate is present in the retina to the left.

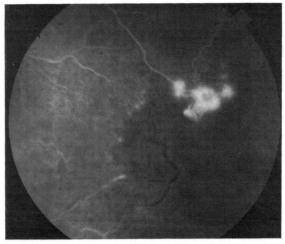

Figure 86–5. Retinal neovascularization seen in the late transit of a fluorescein angiogram. The new vessels show prominent hyperfluorescence and are located at the edge of an area of retinal capillary obstruction. An occluded branch vessel is present in the ischemic retinal area.

frequent findings in patients with sarcoidosis.[2, 3, 5, 6] The chorioretinitis is described as nonspecific and indistinguishable from that caused by other diseases, and the presumed chorioretinal nodules may be associated with overlying secondary detachments of the sensory retina.[5, 14] In one study, a granulomatous mass large enough to be mistaken for an amelanotic melanoma was noted but disappeared, leaving only a moderate retinal pigment epithelial disturbance after systemic steroid therapy.[3]

Extensive chorioretinal scarring usually is not found after the resolution of granulomatous lesions of any size, and the visual prognosis is good even after the occurrence of macular detachments overlying chorioretinal nodules, as long as epiretinal membranes do not form.[6, 8, 14] Usually a mottled disruption of retinal pigment epithelium remains, sometimes with small, focal, punched-out spots that appear to extend into the choroid; however, dense or deep chorioretinal scars are not

sequelae of sarcoid lesions. This is consistent with the histopathologic description of the nodules as clusters of epithelioid and giant cells surrounded by lymphocytes and neutrophils present in the retina and retinal pigment epithelial layer but not in the choroid.[7]

NEOVASCULARIZATION

Proliferation of new vessels on the optic nerve head has been noted in association with intraocular inflammation of several causes, including sarcoidosis.[8, 10, 15] The new vessels are usually sparse, and the proliferative tufts are delicate without the prominent glial components seen in diabetic disc neovascular proliferation (Fig. 86–6). As a consequence, the inflammatory neovascular tufts may be difficult to see and are often noted initially in fluorescein angiograms or are found by careful search-

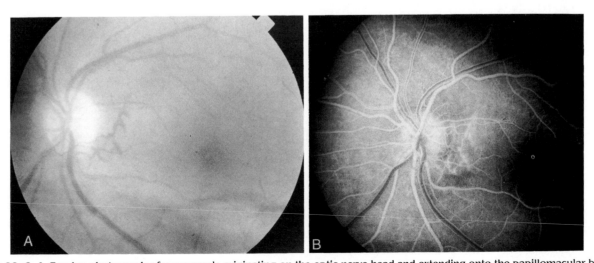

Figure 86–6. A, Fundus photograph of new vessels originating on the optic nerve head and extending onto the papillomacular bundle. B, Fluorescein angiogram in the early venous phase showing fluorescence of the neovascular net.

ing after a vitreous hemorrhage has cleared. They may remain static for long periods, depending on the degree of associated inflammatory activity elsewhere in the eyes, and many regress with remission of the inflammation.

Granulomas of the optic nerve head are observed clinically and histologically in sarcoidosis,[1, 5, 7, 8] but neovascularization is seen arising from the optic disc without any suggestion of granulomatous infiltration of the nerve. The same is true of the rarer complication of juxtapapillary subretinal neovascularization noted in sarcoidosis.[18] Ophthalmoscopically, this resembles papilledema, which occurs when the anterior portion of the optic nerve is involved with active inflammation, and fluorescein angiography is required to identify the neovascular net present under the juxtapapillary serous retinal elevation (Fig. 86–7). Early identification is important because limited experience suggests that subretinal nets are more likely than disc vessels to proliferate and threaten involvement of the macular area.

MEMBRANE PROLIFERATION

Chronic macular edema or serous elevation of the macula over an inflammatory nodule can stimulate the formation of an epiretinal membrane that may distort and blur central vision even after active inflammation has subsided.[7, 10, 19] Epiretinal membranes, or more extensive vitreoretinal membranes that result in proliferative vitreoretinopathy, can occur in many severe inflammatory diseases, especially when there is also hemorrhaging into the vitreous cavity. These lesions are not characteristic of the particular inflammatory disease that produces them but occur as complications of several diseases, including sarcoidosis. Although rare, traction retinal detachments may result from contraction of intravitreal membranes, which can also produce retinal breaks, causing complicated rhegmatogenous detachments.

TREATMENT

Sarcoidosis usually responds favorably to steroid therapy, which is basically the only effective treatment for the disease.[4, 10, 14, 21] The nature of sarcoidosis requires long-term treatment, which introduces the risk of serious complications associated with prolonged steroid use. Chief among these complications are cataract production, weight gain, behavioral changes, gastric ulcers, aseptic necrosis of the hip, hyperglycemia, osteoporosis, hypertension, and opportunistic infections. Consequently, exhaustive efforts to establish a definite diagnosis are justifiable before the patient is committed to an extended course of steroids.

The retinal manifestations of sarcoidosis are usually only one element in a spectrum of ocular involvement, and treatment is determined by the extent and severity of the total picture in an individual patient. The details of steroid therapy are specified elsewhere (Chap. 27) and pertain to the treatment of retinal vasculitis and granulomatous lesions of the fundus as well.

Retroseptal injections of triamcinolone acetonide (Kenalog) or methylprednisolone acetate (Depo-Medrol) into the orbit below the inferior rectus muscle are useful adjuncts to systemic therapy, particularly when macular edema is a prominent feature of retinal vasculitis or when the presentation of uveitis is acute. Injections may be repeated every few weeks if the vehicle is soluble (triamcinolone acetate), and they do not cause the systemic complications seen with oral steroids. Their use will usually permit effective treatment with smaller doses of oral steroids and will often shorten the course of oral therapy.

A similar modifying effect may be achieved with the use of nonsteroidal antiinflammatory agents. By themselves, they are not effective in controlling sarcoid uveitis, but their use in conjunction with oral and retroseptal steroid therapy may minimize the amount of oral steroid required to treat patients with active disease or to maintain patients in remission for long periods. In

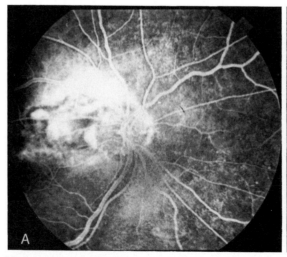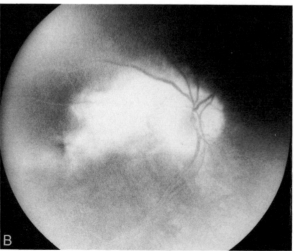

Figure 86–7. A, Fluorescein angiogram in early venous phase in a patient with presumed sarcoidosis. Hyperfluorescent subretinal vessels are seen adjacent to the temporal rim of the optic disc. B, Late fluorescein angiogram of the neovascular net showing leakage of subretinal fluid and extension of edema into the adjacent macular area.

our experience, diflunisal (Dolobid) and indomethacin (Indocin SR) have been the most effective nonsteroidal antiinflammatory agents in patients with sarcoidosis, particularly when retinal vasculitis and macular edema are present.

Successful management of retinal sarcoidosis depends on finding the combination of agents and the minimal dosage, of steroids in particular, that will eliminate the inflammation and maintain it in remission. Initially, intensive therapy with high-dose systemic and retroseptal steroids and nonsteroidal agents is often required to establish control. Once this is achieved, slow tapering of steroids will lead to the minimal dosage required, in conjunction with the supplementary medications, to prevent recurrence of the disease.

Both neovascularization of the retina and disc neovascularization have been observed to regress with systemic medical therapy alone in up to 50 percent of patients treated.[10, 15] In some eyes, persistent or progressive neovascularization has led to intravitreal hemorrhage. When bleeding occurs, however, photocoagulation is appropriate. Local grid treatment to cover the area of retinal capillary nonperfusion adjacent to retinal neovascular tufts is usually sufficient to cause regression of the abnormal vessels in the retina. When disc neovascularization causes recurrent hemorrhage, panretinal photocoagulation, as recommended for the treatment of proliferative diabetic retinopathy, may be required to eliminate the disc vessels.

The rare complication of juxtapapillary neovascularization does not appear to be influenced by systemic steroid therapy and is likely to advance toward the macula. Consequently, it is advisable to treat it directly with strong photocoagulation in an effort to obliterate the subretinal vessels completely.[18]

Vitrectomy also has a place in the treatment of sarcoid retinitis.[12, 20, 22] First, it is useful to clear the vitreous cavity after large hemorrhages that fail to absorb. Active neovascularization may be found in the course of vitrectomy in such eyes and may be treated at that time with endophotocoagulation or peripheral cryopexy, depending on the location and extent of the neovascularization. Vitrectomy is also useful in selected cases to remove epiretinal membranes, although the visual prognosis must be more guarded when there is evidence of extensive fibrosis from the inflammation. Vitrectomy is an essential part of the surgical procedure indicated when a traction or rhegmatogenous retinal detachment is caused by proliferation of vitreoretinal membranes, and in those complicated cases, vitrectomy is combined with scleral buckling procedures and intravitreal injections of gas or oil, depending on the nature and extent of the detachment.

Finally, vitrectomy may be considered to lessen the burden of inflammatory stimuli within the eye. This is still a controversial and unproven therapy, but there is increasing evidence that removal of vitreous from eyes with intractable uveitis can decrease the level of intraocular inflammation and make control easier with lower levels of medication.[10, 12, 16, 18, 20, 22–24] In addition, vitreous body and retinochoroidal biopsy have been recommended to diagnose posterior uveitis and determine appropriate therapy.[25]

REFERENCES

1. Chumley LC, Kearns TP: Retinopathy of sarcoidosis. Am J Ophthalmol 73:123, 1972.
2. Jabs DA, John CJ: Ocular involvement in chronic sarcoidosis. Am J Ophthalmol 102:297, 1986.
3. Letocha CE, Shields JA, Goldberg RE: Retinal changes in sarcoidosis. Can J Ophthalmol 10:184, 1975.
4. Karma A, Huhti E, Poukkula A: Course and outcome of ocular sarcoidosis. Am J Ophthalmol 106:467, 1988.
5. Jabs DA: Sarcoidosis. In Ryan SJ (ed): Retina, vol. 2. St Louis, CV Mosby, 1989.
6. Obenauf CD, Shaw HE, Sydnor CF, Klintworth GK: Sarcoidosis and its ophthalmic manifestations. Am J Ophthalmol 86:648, 1978.
7. Gass JDM, Olson CL: Sarcoidosis with optic nerve and retinal involvement. Arch Ophthalmol 94:945, 1976.
8. Spolton DJ, Sanders MD: Fundus changes in histologically confirmed sarcoidosis. Br J Ophthalmol 65:348, 1981.
9. Asdourian GK, Goldberg MF, Busse BJ: Peripheral retinal neovascularization in sarcoidosis. Arch Ophthalmol 93:787, 1975.
10. Graham EM, Stanford MR, Shilling JS, Sanders MD: Neovascularisation associated with posterior uveitis. Br J Ophthalmol 71:826, 1987.
11. Regan CDJ, Foster CS: Retinal vascular diseases: Clinical presentation and diagnosis. Int Ophthalmol Clin 26:25, 1986.
12. Foster CS: Vitrectomy in the management of uveitis. Ophthalmology 95:1011, 1988.
13. Kohner EM: Retinal ischemia. In Ryan SJ (ed): Retina, vol. 2. St Louis, CV Mosby, 1989, p 92.
14. Marcus BF, Bovino JA, Burton TC: Sarcoid granuloma of the choroid. Ophthalmology 89:1326, 1982.
15. Duker JS, Brown GC, McNamara JA: Proliferative sarcoid retinopathy. Ophthalmology 95:1680, 1988.
16. Lutty GA, Lin SH, Prendergast RA: Angiogenic lymphokines of activated T-cell origin. Invest Ophthalmol Vis Sci 24:1595, 1983.
17. Madigan JC Jr, Gragoudas ES, Schwartz PL, et al: Peripheral retinal neovascularization in sarcoidosis and sickle cell anemia. Am J Ophthalmol 83:387, 1977.
18. Gragoudas ES, Regan CDJ: Peripapillary subretinal neovascularization in presumed sarcoidosis. Arch Ophthalmol 99:1194, 1981.
19. Appiah AP, Hirose T: Secondary causes of perimacular fibrosis. Ophthalmology 96:389, 1989.
20. Mieler WF, Will BR, Lewis H, Aaberg TM: Vitrectomy in the management of proliferative uveitis. Ophthalmology 95:859, 1988.
21. Foster CS, Regan CDJ: Retinal vascular diseases: Management. Int Ophthalmol Clin 26:55, 1986.
22. Algvere P, Alanko H, Dickhoff K, et al: Pars plana vitrectomy in the management of intraocular inflammation. Acta Ophthalmol 59:727, 1981.
23. Nolthenius PAT, Deitman AF: Surgical treatment of the complications of chronic uveitis. Ophthalmologica 186:11, 1983.
24. Kaplan HJ, Diamond JG, Brown SA: Vitrectomy in experimental uveitis. Arch Ophthalmol 96:1798, 1978.
25. Fujikawa LS, Haugen JP: Immunopathology of vitreous and retinochoroidal biopsy in posterior uveitis. Ophthalmology 97:1644, 1990.

Chapter 87

■

Sickle Cell Retinopathy

GEORGE K. ASDOURIAN

Sickling hemoglobinopathies are caused by the presence of one or a combination of abnormal hemoglobins in the red blood cells. The normal hemoglobin, which is referred to as hemoglobin A, is composed of two α- and two β-peptide chains. A genetic mutation can lead to a single amino acid substitution in the sixth position of the β-chain (valine for glutamic acid), producing hemoglobin S, whereas a different substitution at the same position (lysine for glutamic acid) will produce hemoglobin C. The abnormal hemoglobins can occur as such or in combination with each other and with normal hemoglobin, resulting in different hemoglobins such as hemoglobin AS (sickle cell trait), hemoglobin SS (sickle cell disease or anemia), hemoglobin SC (sickle cell hemoglobin C disease), and others. A genetic mutation can also induce failure or defective production of one of the two peptide chains (α or β) which, in combination with sickle hemoglobin, leads to sickle cell thalassemia (S-thal) disease.

Normal red blood cells are round or oval, are rather pliable and flexible, and can squeeze through capillaries. Under conditions of hypoxia and other metabolic conditions, the red blood cells become rigid and adopt an elongated sickle-shaped configuration. As the sickle cells increase in number in the circulation, they increase the viscosity of the blood and lead to sluggish blood flow, erythrocytic aggregation, and eventual vasoocclusion of the vessel. Using fluorescein angiographic techniques, sluggish, prolonged transition times of blood have been well documented in the peripheral retina of sickle cell patients.[1, 2]

The systemic and ocular manifestations of the different hemoglobinopathies do not go hand in hand. Although patients with hemoglobin SS disease manifest the worse systemic symptoms, patients with hemoglobin SC and hemoglobin S-thal hemoglobinopathies exhibit the most severe ocular complications.

The sickling process can produce vasoocclusion and secondary tissue changes in all the vascular structures of the eye, including the conjunctiva[3–9] (conjunctival sickling sign), the iris[10, 11] (iris atrophy), the choroid[12, 13] (occlusion of the posterior ciliary vessels), the optic disc,[14–17] and the retina. The constellation of retinal abnormalities observed in these patients constitutes the retinopathy of sickle cell disease.[14–32]

The posterior segment abnormalities can be divided into the following categories:

Optic disc changes
Macular changes
Nonproliferative retinal changes
Proliferative retinal changes

OPTIC DISC CHANGES

Similar to vascular occlusions elsewhere, the small vessels on the surface of the optic disc can exhibit intravascular occlusions.[14–17] These occlusions are seen ophthalmoscopically as dark red intravascular spots (Fig. 87–1), similar to the changes seen in the conjunctival vessels of these patients (the conjunctival sickling sign). These changes are referred to as the *disc sign of sickling* and probably represent plugs of deoxygenated erythrocytes occurring in the small surface vessels of the disc. Fluorescein angiography (Fig. 87–2) shows linear or Y-shaped segments of hypofluorescence corresponding to these red spots. Angiography, however, does not reveal any substantial impairment of blood flow in these vessels.

These occlusions are found to be transient and do not produce any clinically detectable visual impairment. Although disc changes have been found to occur in patients with hemoglobin SS, hemoglobin SC, and hemoglobin S-thal diseases, they are most common in patients with hemoglobin SS disease.

MACULAR CHANGES (SICKLING MACULOPATHY)

Acute and chronic vascular changes of the posterior pole have been reported in patients with hemoglobin SS, hemoglobin SC, hemoglobin S-thal, and hemoglobin AS diseases.[33–44]

Acute major retinal vascular occlusions—i.e., central and branch retinal artery occlusions and peripapillary

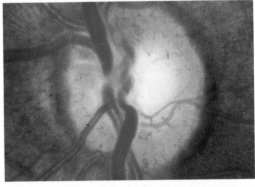

Figure 87–1. The disc sign of sickling. Blocked small vessels are seen as dark spots or lines. (From Goldbaum MH, Jampol LM, Goldberg MF: The disc sign in sickling hemoglobinopathies. Arch Ophthalmol 96:1597, 1978. Copyright 1978, American Medical Association.)

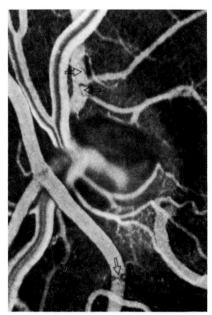

Figure 87–2. Fluorescein angiography of the optic disc showing several plugged vessels *(arrows)*. (From Goldbaum MH, Jampol LM, Goldberg MF: The disc sign in sickling hemoglobinopathies. Arch Ophthalmol 96:1599, 1978. Copyright 1978, American Medical Association.)

and macular arteriolar occlusions—although infrequent, have been reported (Fig. 87–3).[33-38] These occlusions cause acute retinal infarction, resulting in either complete loss of vision or debilitating central and paracentral scotomas.

Chronic macular vascular occlusions are more common and are reported to occur in approximately 30 percent of patients with sickle cell disease.[40, 41] These occlusions are clinically more difficult to detect and consist of alterations in the normal architecture of the fine vasculature of the macula, perimacular region, and region of the horizontal raphe lying temporal to the macula. These macular changes have an insidious, progressive course. Careful direct ophthalmoscopy, contact lens examination, and especially fluorescein angiography are necessary to detect these posterior pole changes. These microvascular changes include microaneurysm resembling dots, dark and enlarged segments of terminal

arterioles, hairpin-shaped vascular loops, an abnormal foveal avascular zone (FAZ), pathologic avascular zones, and areas of retinal depression (Fig. 87–4). Fluorescein angiography reveals the dark enlarged segments to be occluded precapillary arterioles, whereas the hairpin loops are associated with adjacent areas of capillary nonperfusion. Angiography also reveals enlargement of the FAZ, with several areas of adjacent beds of capillary nonperfusion (pathologic avascular zones) (Fig. 87–5). The areas of retinal depression are best seen by direct ophthalmoscopy and are thought to be the result of atrophy and thinning of the inner retina (secondary to capillary closures) (Fig. 87–6). These depressed areas produce a concavity that appears as a dark retinal area with a bright central reflex.

Even when the innermost arcades of the FAZ are occluded, these chronic macular vascular changes seldom seem to produce any clinically detectable visual defects. The visual acuity, color vision, and central visual fields may be normal in these patients; however, with more sophisticated clinical tests and static perimetry, absolute and relative scotomas can be detected that correspond to these areas of vascular abnormalities. These macular vascular changes may be the cause of unexplained visual loss or amblyopia in young patients with sickle cell disease.

NONPROLIFERATIVE RETINAL CHANGES

Changes in the retina referred to as nonproliferative or background sickle retinopathy include the following.

Venous Tortuosity

Although venous tortuosity (Fig. 87–7) was one of the first ophthalmoscopic signs of sickling to be described, it is neither pathognomonic nor of any diagnostic value, since it occurs in a great number of other ocular diseases. The tortuosity may be due to arteriovenous shunting that occurs in the retinal periphery of these patients.

Figure 87–3. *A,* Several cotton-wool spots in a patient with sickle cell disease. *B,* Macular infarction in a patient with sickle cell thalassemia. (*B,* From Asdourian GK, Goldberg MF, Rabb MF: Macular infarction in sickle cell B+ thalassemia. Retina 2:155, 1982.)

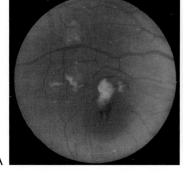

A

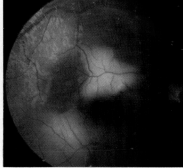

B

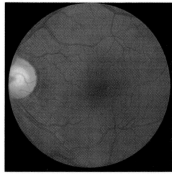

Figure 87–4. The left macula of a patient with sickle cell hemoglobin C (SC) disease with enlarged foveal avascular zone (FAZ).

Salmon-patch Hemorrhage, Schisis Cavity, and Iridescent Spots

Salmon-patch hemorrhages are preretinal or superficial intraretinal hemorrhages that occur mainly in the midperipheral retina, adjacent to a retinal arteriole.[45] Because of their peripheral location, they do not pro-

duce any visual symptoms. These hemorrhages are thought to occur following sudden arteriolar occlusions, with subsequent "blowout" of the vessel wall presumably from ischemic necrosis. These hemorrhages are round or oval and are initially bright red (Fig. 87–8). Over several days, however, they acquire an orange-red coloration and have been referred to as salmon patches or salmon hemorrhages (Fig. 87–9). Histologic studies have shown these hemorrhages to be limited by the internal limiting membrane, although some may dissect internally into the vitreous cavity or into the retina and the subretinal space (Fig. 87–10).[46] With the resorption of the hemorrhages, the retina may resume a normal appearance at the site of the hemorrhage, may be marked by a subtle retinal facet or dimple (usually highlighted by the light reflection from the internal limiting membrane), or more frequently may show a schisis cavity with multiple glistening yellow spots (Fig. 87–11). The schisis cavity represents the space created by the resorption of the intraretinal portion of the hemorrhage, whereas the glistening refractive bodies in the schisis cavity, referred to as *iridescent spots*, represent macrophages that are filled with iron and blood breakdown products (Fig. 87–12).

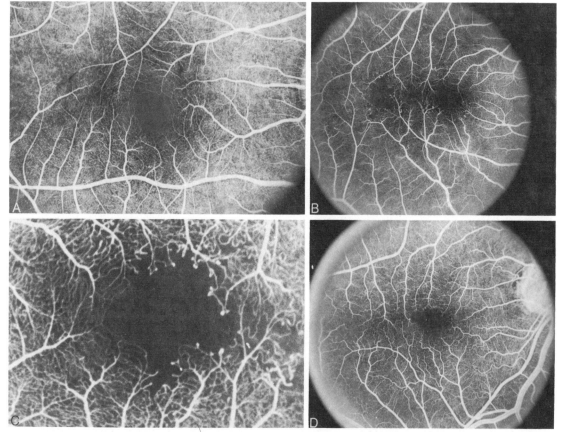

Figure 87–5. *A,* Fluorescein angiography of the macular area showing an occluded vessel. *B,* Fluorescein angiography showing pathologic avascular zone (PAZ), as well as microaneurysmal formation of the perifoveal capillaries. *C,* Fluorescein angiography showing an enlarged FAZ. (*A–C,* From Asdourian GK, Nagpal KC, Busse B, et al: Macular and perimacular vascular remodeling in sickling hemoglobinopathies. Br J Ophthalmol 60:431, 1976.) *D,* Fluorescein angiography of the macular area showing enlarged FAZ, microaneurysmal formation, and hairpin loops.

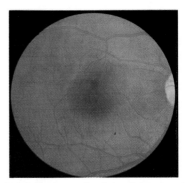

Figure 87–6. Color photograph of the right macula showing the retinal depression sign.

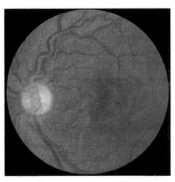

Figure 87–7. The left fundus of patient with sickle cell (SS) disease showing vascular tortuosity.

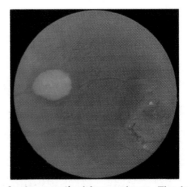

Figure 87–8. Acute preretinal hemorrhage. The hemorrhage is bright red. Anterior to the hemorrhage, a black sunburst lesion is seen.

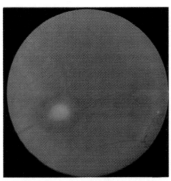

Figure 87–9. Same lesion as in Figure 87–8, 4 wk later. The hemorrhage has a pinkish color (salmon patch) with surrounding schisis cavity.

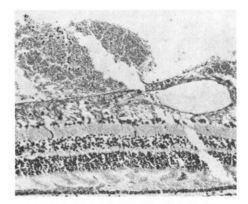

Figure 87–10. Histopathologic appearance of acute superficial retinal hemorrhage (salmon patch). (From Romayananda N, Goldberg MF, Green RW: Histopathology of sickle cell retinopathy. Trans Am Acad Ophthalmol Otolaryngol 77:OP652–76, 1973.)

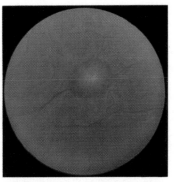

Figure 87–11. Same lesion as in Figure 87–8, 6 wk later. A schisis cavity is seen with multiple iridescent spots.

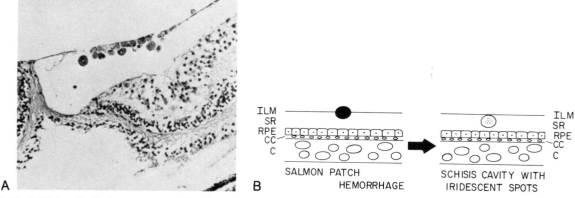

Figure 87–12. *A,* Histopathologic appearance of schisis cavity containing proteinaceous material and hemosiderin-laden macrophages (clinical iridescent spots). (From Romayananda N, Goldberg MF, Green RW: Histopathology of sickle cell retinopathy. Trans Am Acad Ophthalmol Otolaryngol 77:655, 1973.) *B,* Schematic interpretation showing salmon patch hemorrhage becoming schisis cavity. ILM, internal limiting membrane; SR, sensory retina; RPE, retinal pigment epithelium; CC, choriocapillaris; and C, choroid. (From Asdourian G, Nagpal KC, Goldbaum M, et al: Evolution of the retinal black sunburst in sickling hemoglobinopathies. Br J Ophthalmol 59:715, 1975.)

The Black Sunburst

Round or ovoid black chorioretinal scars, ranging in size from 0.5 to 2 disc diameters and characteristically located in the equatorial fundus, are called *black sunbursts* (Fig. 87–13).[47] They usually have stellate or spiculate borders caused by perivascular accumulation of pigment. They are sometimes associated with iridescent spots. Because of their peripheral location, these lesions do not produce any visual symptoms.

Fluorescein angiographic studies have shown these lesions to be areas of hypo- and hyperfluorescence, denoting changes in the retinal pigment epithelium (Fig. 87–14). Histologically,[46] these scars represent focal areas of retinal pigment epithelial hypertrophy, hyperplasia, and migration (Fig. 87–15). Occasionally, there is a distinct perivascular localization of the pigment in the sensory retina.

The pathogenesis of these scars is thought to be the result of large intraretinal hemorrhages that occur secondary to sudden arteriolar occlusions. These hemorrhages dissect to the potential space between the sensory retina and the retinal pigment epithelium and stimulate pigment production and migration, with the resultant formation of the characteristic black sunburst (Fig. 87–16).[47]

Other Nonproliferative Sickle Changes

A variety of other fundus changes have been described in patients with sickle cell disease. Areas of whitening of the peripheral retina similar to the white-without-pressure sign seen in the retinal periphery in the general population have been described (Fig. 87–17).[25, 48] Mottled brown areas of the fundus[15, 49] have also been reported in these patients (Fig. 87–18), as have angioid streaks.[50] Both of these lesions can occur independent of sickle cell disease.

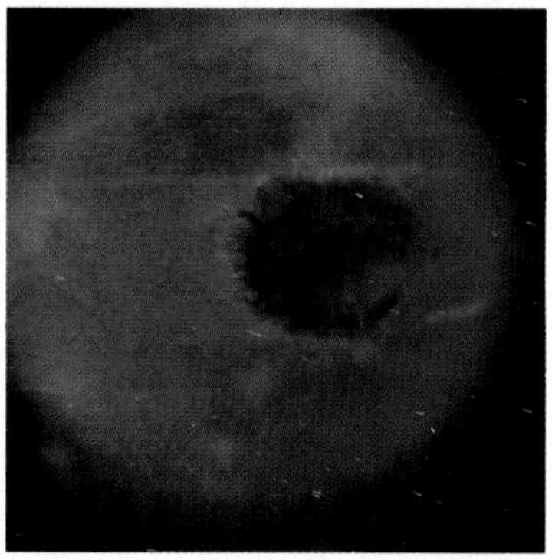

Figure 87–13. The black sunburst sign. (From Goldberg MF: Retinal vaso-occlusion in sickling hemoglobinopathies. Birth Defects 12:475, 1976.)

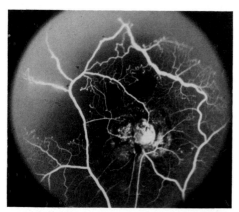

Figure 87–14. Fluorescein angiogram of black sunburst showing areas of focal hyperfluorescence and hypofluorescence. (From Asdourian G, Nagpal KC, Goldbaum M, et al: Evolution of the retinal black sunburst in sickling hemoglobinopathies. Br J Ophthalmol 59:715, 1975.)

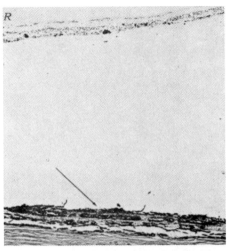

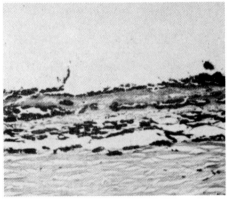

Figure 87–15. Histopathologic appearance of black sunburst showing marked proliferation of retinal pigment epithelium. (From Romayananda N, Goldberg MF, Green RW: Histopathology of sickle cell retinopathy. Trans Am Acad Ophthalmol Otolaryngol 77:657, 1973.)

PROLIFERATIVE RETINAL CHANGES

Proliferative sickle retinopathy (PSR) is the most severe ocular complication of sickle cell disease. Although neovascularization of the disc and the temporal macula have been reported,[51, 52] PSR is overwhelmingly a peripheral retinal disease.[32] PSR is more prevalent in

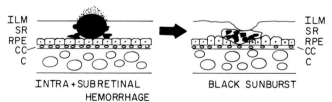

Figure 87–16. Schematic interpretation of large intraretinal hemorrhage dissecting into subretinal space and turning into a black sunburst. ILM, internal limiting membrane; SR, sensory retina; RPE, retinal pigment epithelium; CC, choriocapillaris; and C, choroid. (From Asdourian G, Nagpal KC, Goldbaum M, et al: Evolution of the retinal black sunburst in sickling hemoglobinopathies. Br J Ophthalmol 59:715, 1975.)

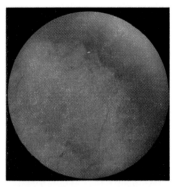

Figure 87–17. Peripheral retinal area showing the white-without-pressure sign.

patients with hemoglobin SC and hemoglobin S-thal disease than in those with homozygous hemoglobin SS disease. PSR has also been reported in patients with other hemoglobinopathies, including patients with hemoglobin AS[28] and hemoglobin AC hemoglobinopathies.[53]

The development of PSR follows a relatively orderly sequential course. On the basis of longitudinal clinical studies and observations, the development of PSR has been classified by Goldberg[20] into five stages (Fig. 87–19):

1. Peripheral arteriolar occlusions
2. Arteriolar-venular anastomoses
3. Neovascular proliferation
4. Vitreous hemorrhage
5. Retinal detachment

Stage I: Peripheral Arteriolar Occlusion

Stage I is the earliest ophthalmoscopic abnormality that can be visualized in the fundus periphery, and it can be seen even in children with no other evidence of PSR. These occlusions are arteriolar rather than venular. In actuality, venular occlusions, including central retinal vein occlusion and branch retinal vein occlusion, are very rare in patients with sickle cell disease. Con-

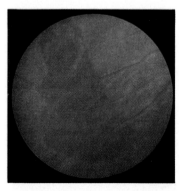

Figure 87–18. Fundus photograph showing a mottled brown area.

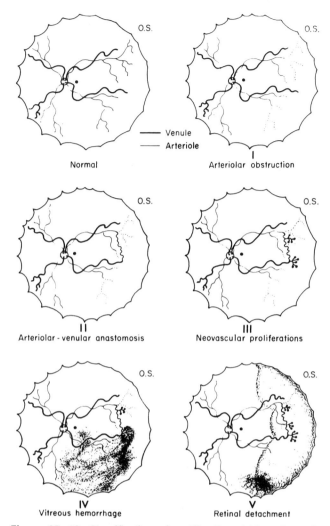

Figure 87–19. Classification of proliferative sickle retinopathy (PSR). (From Goldberg MF: Classification and pathogenesis of proliferative sickle retinopathy. Am J Ophthalmol 71:654, 1971. Published with permission from The American Journal of Ophthalmology. Copyright by The Ophthalmic Publishing Company.)

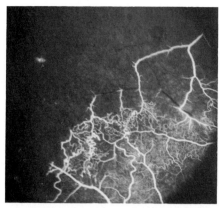

Figure 87–21. Stage I PSR; fluorescein angiography shows occluded peripheral vessels with adjacent avascular retina.

raphy clearly delineates the occluded vessels and the surrounding avascular and abnormal capillary bed (Fig. 87–21).

Stage II: Peripheral Arteriolar-Venular Anastomoses

With the arteriolar occlusions, a vascular remodeling process ensues, with some vessels remaining occluded and others demonstrating partial or complete reopening. As the blood is diverted from the occluded arterioles to the nearest venules, arteriolar-venular anastomoses develop. Anterior to these arteriolar-venular changes, the retina remains devoid of any perfusion. On fluorescein angiography there is no evidence of any leakage of dye from these anastomoses, since they do not represent true neovascularization (Fig. 87–22).

Stage III: Neovascular Proliferation

At the interface of vascular and avascular retina, new blood vessels arise from the arteriolar-venular anasto-

comitant with these arteriolar occlusions, the dependent capillary bed fails to fill and anteriorly located avascular zones become evident. The occluded arterioles can be seen as dark red lines but eventually turn into white "silver-wire" vessels (Fig. 87–20). Fluorescein angiog-

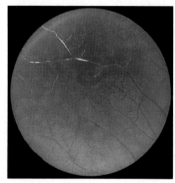

Figure 87–20. Stage I PSR; peripheral arteriolar occlusions seen as "silverwire" vessels.

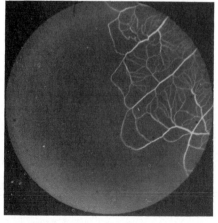

Figure 87–22. Stage II PSR; fluorescein angiography shows arteriolar-venular (A-V) anastomoses with adjacent avascular retina.

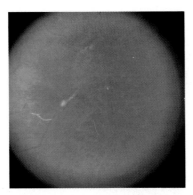

Figure 87-23. Early retinal neovascularization, which may be mistaken for microaneurysms or telangiectasia.

Stage IV: Vitreous Hemorrhage

These peripheral neovascular tufts can bleed secondary to a variety of conditions. Although bleeding can occur from minor ocular trauma, the bleeding usually happens spontaneously secondary to contraction of the vitreous, which usually shows evidence of liquefaction and partial collapse, especially close to the neovascular tufts. Vitreous traction secondary to vitreous bands and membranes can also result in vitreous hemorrhage. These bands may be the result of previous vitreous hemorrhages, which initially may be localized to the area of the sea fans and thus are asymptomatic. When the blood breaks into the center of the vitreous cavity, however, it produces visual symptoms.

Stage V: Retinal Detachment

Vitreous traction bands and membranes not only cause vitreous hemorrhage but also can produce traction on the sea fan and adjacent retina, resulting in traction retinal detachment or traction retinoschisis. Localized traction detachments may remain stationary and asymptomatic or may progress posteriorly. Traction on the retina can also cause full-thickness retinal breaks, which eventually lead to total rhegmatogenous retinal detachment.

PSR may progress rapidly in some patients, with the sea fans quickly increasing in number and size. In a majority of patients, however, PSR appears to progress slowly, and severe visual dysfunction is relatively uncommon. This may be due to the tendency of the neovascular tufts to involute or undergo autoinfarction,[54] thus effectively curing the condition (Fig. 87–26). Involution may occur because of strangulation of the neovascular tufts by fibroglial tissue, whereas autoinfarction is thought to be secondary to a spontaneous occlusion of the arteriolar feeding vessel. With total lack of perfusion, the propensity for vitreous hemorrhage is eliminated, and the patient's prognosis for vision becomes good unless a retinal detachment or macular infarction develops.

Because PSR is progressive and is the major cause of visual morbidity in these patients (12 percent of eyes

moses and grow peripherally into the preequatorial ischemic retina. The growth of these new blood vessels is thought to be in response to a vasoformative factor that is speculated to be present in the peripheral avascular and ischemic retina. These neovascular fronds initially are small and lie flat on the surface of the retina. They may be mistaken for microaneurysms or telangiectasia and are difficult to detect ophthalmoscopically (Fig. 87–23). With time, these neovascular tufts grow, acquire a characteristic fan-shaped appearance resembling the marine invertebrate *Gorgonia flabellum,* and are known as *sea fan neovascularization* (Fig. 87–24).[18]

Small sea fans usually have a single feeding arteriole and a draining venule. As they grow in size and number, however, they acquire additional feeding and draining vessels, at which time it may be very difficult to distinguish the major feeding and draining vessels. Fluorescein angiography shows leakage of dye from these neovascular tufts, with a cloud of the fluorescein usually accumulating in front of the tufts and in the vitreous cavity (Fig. 87–25).

With time, these neovascular tufts not only grow in number and size but also acquire an envelope of white glial and fibrotic tissue. The vitreous gel becomes adherent to these fronds, and with vitreous collapse they can be pulled into the vitreous cavity and appear as elevated neovascular tissue.

Figure 87-24. A, Fluorescein angiography of characteristic sea fan neovascularization. B, The sea fan neovascularization shows evidence of leakage of dye. Inferior to the neovascularization, A-V anastomosis is seen with early neovascularization.

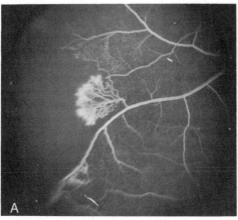
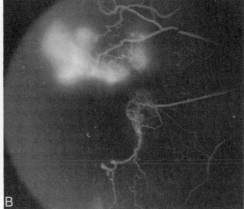

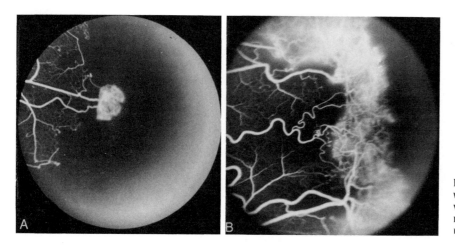

Figure 87–25. A, Sea fan neovascularization with single feeder vessel and two draining venules. B, Sea fan neovascularization with multiple feeder arterioles and draining venules.

showing evidence of visual disability), especially in young persons, obliteration of the neovascular tissue is a desirable objective and should be accomplished even before a major vitreous hemorrhage has occurred.[55]

TREATMENT OF PSR

The aim of therapy is to eliminate existing neovascularization, thus eliminating its complications.[56] Therapy eventually should be aimed at preventing the development of these neovascular fronds.

Modalities used to treat peripheral neovascularization have included diathermy,[57] cryotherapy,[58–60] xenon arc photocoagulation, and argon laser photocoagulation.[61–69]

Although diathermy treatment has been successful in obliterating neovascular tufts and their feeder vessels,[57] this therapy is seldom used today because of the high

incidence of complications accompanying this procedure, including anterior uveitis, retinal hemorrhages, and anterior segment ischemia.

Cryotherapy, both single freeze-thaw and triple freeze-thaw therapy has been used to treat retinal neovascularization in sickle cell disease.[58, 59] Cryotherapy is used to treat peripheral retinal neovascularization in the presence of vitreous hemorrhage when the neovascular tufts cannot be well visualized. Fluorescein angiography or fluorescein angioscopy is performed prior to treatment to localize the areas of peripheral leakage, which are then treated with cryotherapy. Because of the high rate of complications accompanying triple freeze-thaw cryotherapy, this modality is not used or recommended. Hanscom[60] has used cryotherapy to treat the peripheral ischemic retina rather than the neovascularization directly and has reported complete regression of neovascularization with no major complications.

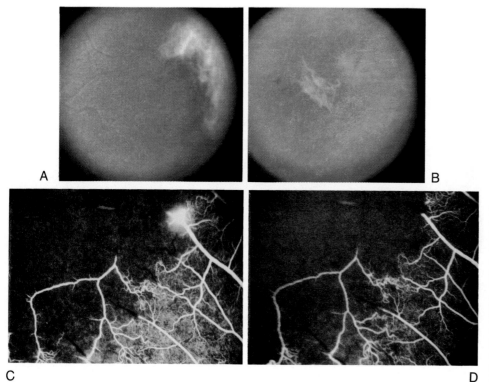

Figure 87–26. A and B, Color photographs of autoinfarcted sea fan neovascularization. C, A perfused, leaking sea fan neovascularization. D, Same area several days later shows lack of perfusion. (C and D, From Nagpal KC, Patrianakos D, Asdourian GK, et al: Spontaneous regression [autoinfarction] of proliferative sickle retinopathy. Am J Ophthalmol 80:886, 1975. Published with permission from The American Journal of Ophthalmology. Copyright by The Ophthalmic Publishing Company.)

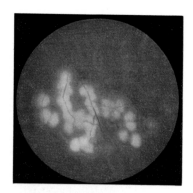

Figure 87–27. Color photograph showing feeder vessel photocoagulation. Both feeder arterioles and draining venules have been photocoagulated. The neovascular tuft is not treated.

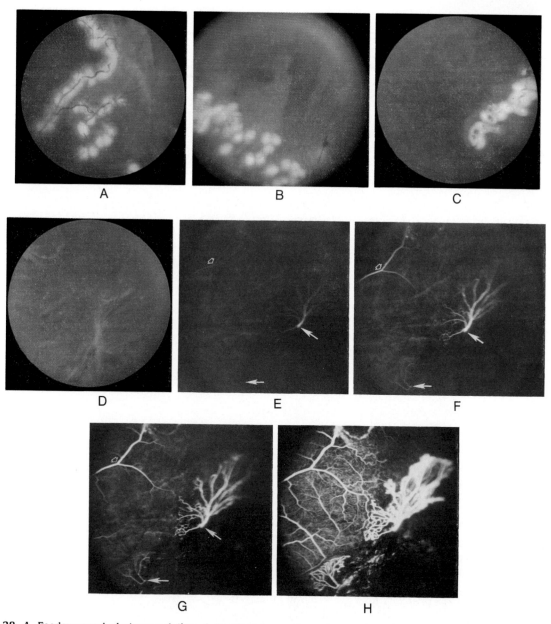

Figure 87–28. A, Feeder vessel photocoagulation. A localized hemorrhage is noted adjacent to the sea fan neovascularization. B, Feeder vessel photocoagulation. Anteriorly located triangular gray areas represent areas of choroidal ischemia. C, Feeder vessel photocoagulation. Heavy treatment has resulted in breaks in Bruch's membrane (dark areas in the center of photocoagulation spots). D, Same patient as in C. Choroidal neovascularization has occurred at site of break in Bruch's membrane. E–H, Same patient as in C. Rapid-sequence fluorescein angiography shows choroidal neovascularization occurring following heavy photocoagulation, which resulted in breaks in Bruch's membrane. (E, From Galinos SO, Asdourian GK, Woolf MB, et al: Choroido-vitreal neovascularization after argon laser photocoagulation neovascularization. Arch Ophthalmol 93:524, 1975. Copyright 1975, American Medical Association.)

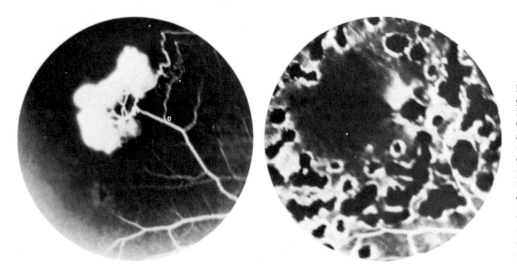

Figure 87–29. Fluorescein angiogram demonstrating a leaking sea fan neovascularization. Complete regression of lesion after scatter photocoagulation. (From Rednam KR, Jampol LM, Goldberg MF: Scatter retinal photocoagulation for proliferative sickle cell retinopathy. Am J Ophthalmol 93:594, 1982. Published with permission from The American Journal of Ophthalmology. Copyright by The Ophthalmic Publishing Company.)

Photocoagulation is the more commonly used mode of treatment for the peripheral neovascularization in sickle cell disease. The neovascular tufts can be directly treated with photocoagulation if the neovascularization is flat on the retina. Another commonly used technique is the feeder vessel treatment, whereby the feeder vessel to the neovascularization is directly photocoagulated until the blood flow in the arteriole is obliterated; then the draining vein is photocoagulated (Fig. 87–27). Both xenon arc and argon laser photocoagulation have been used in these techniques.

A prospective randomized clinical trial of feeder vessel photocoagulation for PSR was recently completed[63–65] using xenon arc photocoagulation (with the use of the O'Malley Log II xenon arc photocoagulator) and laser photocoagulation (using the Coherent Radiation Model 800 blue-green argon laser). Intense photocoagulation spots were placed on the feeding arteriole and the draining venules from each neovascularization. All neovascular tissue was treated. These studies showed that feeder vessel photocoagulation, both with xenon arc photocoagulation and with argon laser photocoagulation, was effective in preventing vitreous hemorrhage and reducing visual loss. However, feeder vessel photocoagulation has several disadvantages. The treating ophthalmologist should have considerable skill and experience when using the feeder vessel technique because very intense burns are required to obliterate the vessels. With such intense burns, breaks in Bruch's membrane can occur with subsequent choroidal hemorrhages, choroidal ischemia, and choroidal neovascularization (Fig. 87–28).[70–75] This latter complication is very common, especially after xenon arc photocoagulation, and can cause further vitreous hemorrhages and visual loss. Other complications include retinal tears and macular fibrosis.[76]

Because of the complications of feeder vessel photocoagulation, recent studies have been described in which the peripheral nonperfused ischemic retina has been photocoagulated in the hope of eliminating the stimulus for neovascularization, which is thought to be present in these peripheral ischemic retinas. These scatter photocoagulation techniques can be either localized[66]—i.e., confined to the area anterior to perfused neovascular fronds (Fig. 87–29)—or circumferential (Fig. 87–30),[67–69] in which 360-degree peripheral circumferential retinal scattered photocoagulation can be used. Both of these techniques show evidence of neovascularization regression, with minimal complications when compared with those of the feeder vessel photocoagulation techniques. At the present time, it is not known whether the localized scatter photocoagulation or the circumferential 360-degree scatter photocoagulation is the more appropriate form of treatment. The rationale of 360-degree scatter photocoagulation is to eliminate existing neovascularization and to prevent the formation of any neovascularization in the peripheral retina.

At present, scatter photocoagulation treatment seems to be best. If after scatter treatment there is no evidence

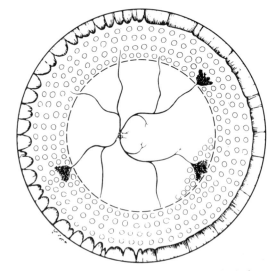

Figure 87–30. Fundus drawing illustrating the technique of peripheral circumferential retinal scatter photocoagulation. (From Creuss AF, Stephens RF, Magargal LE, et al: Peripheral circumferential retinal scatter photocoagulation for treatment of proliferative sickle retinopathy. Published courtesy of Ophthalmology [1983;90:273].)

of regression or only partial regression in which the patient continues to have problems, feeder vessel techniques may then be used to completely eliminate these neovascular fronds.

Unfortunately, patients will still experience nonclearing vitreal hemorrhages, as well as retinal detachment, as a complication of PSR. In these circumstances, scleral buckling or vitrectomy procedures, or both, are recommended to treat the problem.[77, 78] However, these procedures are fraught with many problems in sickle cell patients. Both ocular and systemic serious complications can occur with these treatment modalities. Ocular complications include anterior segment ischemia,[79] as well as intraoperative hemorrhages with secondary glaucoma. Systemic complications include thromboembolic complications such as pulmonary or cerebral embolism or thrombosis. Patients who need vitreoretinal surgery should be evaluated by experienced medical personnel to decrease the systemic complications of surgery.

REFERENCES

1. Goldberg MF: Retinal vaso-occlusion in sickling hemoglobinopathies. Birth Defects 12:475, 1976.
2. Goldberg MF: The value of fluorescein angiography in sickle cell retinopathy. Doc Ophthalmol 9:587, 1976.
3. Lieb WA, Geeraets WJ, Guerry D: Sickle cell retinopathy. Ocular and systemic manifestations of sickle cell disease. Acta Ophthalmol Suppl 58:1, 1959.
4. Paton D: Conjunctival sign of sickle cell disease. Arch Ophthalmol 66:90, 1961.
5. Paton D: Conjunctival sign of sickle cell disease. Further observations. Arch Ophthalmol 68:627, 1962.
6. Comer PB, Fred HL: Diagnosis of sickle-cell disease by ophthalmoscopic inspection of the conjunctiva. N Engl J Med 271:544, 1964.
7. Serjeant GR, Serjeant BE, Condon PI: The conjunctival sign in sickle cell anemia. JAMA 219:1428, 1972.
8. Goodman G, von Sallmann L, Holland MG: Ocular manifestations of sickle cell disease. Arch Ophthalmol 58:655, 1957.
9. Nagpal KC, Asdourian GK, Goldbaum MH, et al: The conjunctival sickling sign, hemoglobin S, and irreversibly sickled erythrocytes. Arch Ophthalmol 95:808, 1977.
10. Galinos S, Rabb MF, Goldberg MF, et al: Hemoglobin SC disease and iris atrophy. Am J Ophthalmol 75:421, 1973.
11. Chambers J, Puglisi J, Kernitsky R, et al: Iris atrophy in hemoglobin SC disease. Am J Ophthalmol 77:247, 1974.
12. Condon PI, Serjeant GR, Ikeda M: Unusual chorioretinal degeneration in sickle cell disease. Possible sequelae of posterior ciliary occlusion. Br J Ophthalmol 57:81, 1973.
13. Dizon RV, Jampol LM, Goldberg MF, et al: Choroidal occlusive disease in sickle cell hemoglobinopathies. Surg Ophthalmol 23:297, 1979.
14. Goldbaum MH, Jampol LM, Goldberg MF: The disc sign in sickling hemoglobinopathies. Arch Ophthalmol 96:1597, 1978.
15. Condon PI, Serjeant GR: Ocular findings in homozygous sickle cell anemia in Jamaica. Am J Ophthalmol 73:533, 1972.
16. Condon PI, Serjeant DR: Ocular findings in hemoglobin SC disease in Jamaica. Am J Ophthalmol 74:921, 1972.
17. Condon PI, Serjeant DR: Ocular findings in sickle cell thalassemia in Jamaica. Am J Ophthalmol 74:1105, 1972.
18. Welch RB, Goldberg MF: Sickle cell hemoglobin and its relation to fundus abnormality. Arch Ophthalmol 75:353, 1966.
19. Goldberg MF: Sickle cell retinopathy. In Duane TD, Jaeger EA (eds): Clinical Ophthalmology, vol. 3, Chap. 17. Philadelphia, JB Lippincott, 1979.
20. Goldberg MF: Classification and pathogenesis of proliferative sickle retinopathy. Am J Ophthalmol 71:649, 1971.
21. Goldberg MF: Natural history of untreated proliferative sickle retinopathy. Arch Ophthalmol 85:428, 1971.
22. Okun E: Development of sickle cell retinopathy. Doc Ophthalmol 26:574, 1969.
23. Raichand M, Goldberg MF, Nagpal KC, et al: Evolution of neovascularization in sickle cell retinopathy. A prospective fluorescein angiographic study. Arch Ophthalmol 95:1543, 1977.
24. Goldberg MF, Charache S, Acacio I: Ophthalmologic manifestations of sickle cell thalassemia. Arch Intern Med 128:33, 1971.
25. Condon PI, Serjeant GR: The progression of sickle cell eye disease in Jamaica. Doc Ophthalmol 39:203, 1975.
26. Condon PI, Gray R, Serjeant GR: Ocular findings in children with sickle cell hemoglobin C disease in Jamaica. Br J Ophthalmol 58:644, 1974.
27. Nagpal KC, Goldberg MF, Rabb MF: Ocular manifestations of sickle hemoglobinopathies. Surv Ophthalmol 21:391, 1977.
28. Nagpal KC, Asdourian GK, Patrianakos D, et al: Proliferative retinopathy in sickle cell trait. Arch Intern Med 137:325, 1977.
29. Condon PI, Serjeant GR: Ocular findings in elderly cases of homozygous sickle cell disease in Jamaica. Br J Ophthalmol 60:361, 1976.
30. Condon PI, Serjeant GR: Behavior of untreated proliferative sickle retinopathy. Br J Ophthalmol 64:404, 1980.
31. Talbot JF, Bird AC, Serjeant GR, et al: Sickle cell retinopathy in young children in Jamaica. Br J Ophthalmol 66:149, 1982.
32. Goldberg MF: Retinal neovascularization in sickle cell retinopathy. Trans Am Acad Ophthalmol Otolaryngol 83:409, 1977.
33. Kabakow B, van Weimokly SS, Lyons HA: Bilateral central artery occlusion. Arch Ophthalmol 54:670, 1955.
34. Conrad WC, Penner R: Sickle cell trait and central retinal artery occlusion. Am J Ophthalmol 63:465, 1967.
35. Knapp JE: Isolated macular infarction in sickle cell (SS) disease. Am J Ophthalmol 73:857, 1972.
36. Acacio I, Goldberg MF: Peripapillary and macular vessel occlusions in sickle cell anemia. Am J Ophthalmol 75:861, 1973.
37. Ryan SJ: Occlusion of macular capillaries in sickle cell hemoglobin C disease. Am J Ophthalmol 77:459, 1974.
38. Asdourian GK, Goldberg MF, Rabb MF: Macular infarction in sickle cell B+ thalassemia. Retina 2:155, 1982.
39. Jampol LM, Condon P, Dizon-Moore R, et al: Salmon-patch hemorrhages after central retinal artery occlusion in sickle cell disease. Arch Ophthalmol 99:237, 1981.
40. Stevens TS, Busse B, Lee C, et al: Sickling hemoglobinopathies: Macular and perimacular vascular abnormalities. Arch Ophthalmol 92:455, 1974.
41. Asdourian GK, Nagpal KC, Busse B, et al: Macular and perimacular vascular remodeling in sickling hemoglobinopathies. Br J Ophthalmol 60:431, 1976.
42. Marsh RJ, Ford SM, Rabb MF: Macular vasculature, visual acuity, and irreversibly sickled cells in homozygous sickle cell disease. Br J Ophthalmol 66:155, 1982.
43. Goldbaum MH: Retinal depression sign indicating a small retinal infarct. Am J Ophthalmol 86:45, 1978.
44. Kaplan GR, van Houten PA, Goldberg MF, et al: Computer assisted area analysis of macular ischemia in sickle cell retinopathy. Invest Ophthalmol Vis Sci 28(Suppl):111, 1987.
45. Gagliano DA, Goldberg MF: The evolution of salmon-patch hemorrhages in sickle cell retinopathy. Arch Ophthalmol 107:1814, 1989.
46. Romayananda N, Goldberg MF, Green RW: Histopathology of sickle cell retinopathy. Trans Am Acad Ophthalmol Otolaryngol 77:652, 1973.
47. Asdourian G, Nagpal KC, Goldbaum M, et al: Evolution of the retinal black sunburst in sickling hemoglobinopathies. Br J Ophthalmol 59:710, 1975.
48. Nagpal KC, Huamonte F, Constantaras A, et al: Migratory white-without-pressure retinal lesions. Arch Ophthalmol 94:576, 1976.
49. Nagpal KC, Goldberg MF, Asdourian GK, et al: Dark-without-pressure fundus lesions. Br J Ophthalmol 59:476, 1975.
50. Nagpal KC, Asdourian G, Goldbaum M, et al: Angioid streaks and sickle hemoglobinopathies. Br J Ophthalmol 60:31, 1976.
51. Frank RN, Cronin MA: Posterior pole neovascularization in a patient with hemoglobin SC disease. Am J Ophthalmol 88:680, 1979.
52. Ober RR, Michels RG: Optic disk neovascularization in hemoglobin SC disease. Am J Ophthalmol 85:711, 1978.

53. Moschandreou M, Galinos SO, Valenzuela R, et al: Retinopathy in hemoglobin C trait (AC hemoglobinopathy). Am J Ophthalmol 77:465, 1974.
54. Nagpal KC, Patrianakos D, Asdourian GK, et al: Spontaneous regression (autoinfarction) of proliferative sickle retinopathy. Am J Ophthalmol 80:885, 1975.
55. Stephens RF: Proliferative sickle cell retinopathy: The disease and a review of its management. Ophthalmic Surg 19:222, 1987.
56. Goldberg MF: Treatment of proliferative sickle retinopathy. Trans Am Acad Ophthalmol Otolaryngol 75:532, 1971.
57. Condon PI, Serjeant GR: Photocoagulation and diathermy in the treatment of proliferative sickle retinopathy. Br J Ophthalmol 58:650, 1974.
58. Lee C, Woolf MB, Galinos SO, et al: Cryotherapy of proliferative sickle retinopathy. Part I. Single freeze-thaw cycle. Ann Ophthalmol 7:1299, 1975.
59. Goldbaum MH, Asdourian GK, Nagpal KC, et al: Cryotherapy of proliferative sickle retinopathy. Read before the Association for Research in Vision and Ophthalmology, Sarasota, FL, April 1975.
60. Hanscom TA: Indirect treatment of peripheral retinal neovascularization. Am J Ophthalmol 93:88, 1982.
61. Goldberg MF, Acacio I: Argon laser photocoagulation of proliferative sickle retinopathy. Arch Ophthalmol 90:35, 1973.
62. Condon PI, Serjeant GR: Photocoagulation in proliferative sickle retinopathy: Results of a 5-year study. Br J Ophthalmol 64:832, 1980.
63. Jampol LM, Condon P, Farber M: A randomized clinical trial of feeder vessel photocoagulation of proliferative sickle cell retinopathy. I. Preliminary results. Ophthalmology 90:540, 1983.
64. Condon P, Jampol LM, Farber MD, et al: A randomized clinical trial of feeder vessel coagulation of proliferative sickle cell retinopathy. II. Update and analysis of risk factors. Ophthalmology 91:1496, 1984.
65. Jacobson MS, Gagliano DA, Cohen SB, et al: A randomized clinical trial of feeder vessel photocoagulation of sickle cell retinopathy. A long-term follow-up. Ophthalmology 98:581, 1991.
66. Rednam KR, Jampol LM, Goldberg MF: Scatter retinal photocoagulation for proliferative sickle cell retinopathy. Am J Ophthalmol 93:594, 1982.
67. Creuss AF, Stephens RF, Magargal LE, et al: Peripheral circumferential retinal scatter photocoagulation for treatment of proliferative sickle retinopathy. Ophthalmology 90:272, 1983.
68. Jampol LM, Farber M, Rabb MF, et al: An update on techniques of photocoagulation treatment of proliferative sickle cell retinopathy. Eye 5:260, 1991.
69. Kimmel AS, Magargal LE, Stephen RF, et al: Peripheral circumferential retinal scatter photocoagulation for the treatment of proliferative sickle retinopathy. An update. Ophthalmology 93:1429, 1986.
70. Goldbaum MH, Galinos SO, Apple D, et al: Acute choroidal ischemia as a complication of photocoagulation. Arch Ophthalmol 94:1025, 1976.
71. Condon PI, Jampol LM, Ford SM, et al: Choroidal neovascularization induced by photocoagulation in sickle cell disease. Br J Ophthalmol 65:192, 1981.
72. Dizen-Moore RV, Jampol LM, Goldberg MF: Chorioretinal and choriovitreal neovascularization: Their presence after photocoagulation of proliferative sickle cell retinopathy. Arch Ophthalmol 99:842, 1980.
73. Carney MD, Paylor RR, Cunha-Vaz JG, et al: Iatrogenic choroidal neovascularization in sickle cell retinopathy. Ophthalmology 93:1163, 1986.
74. Condon PI, Hayes RJ, Serjeant GR: Retinal and choroidal neovascularization in sickle cell disease. Trans Ophthalmol Soc UK 100:434, 1980.
75. Galinos SO, Asdourian GK, Woolf MB, et al: Choroido-vitreal neovascularization after argon laser photocoagulation. Arch Ophthalmol 93:524, 1975.
76. Jampol LM, Goldberg MF: Retinal breaks after photocoagulation of proliferative sickle cell retinopathy. Arch Ophthalmol 98:676, 1980.
77. Goldbaum MH, Peyman GA, Nagpal KC: Vitrectomy in sickling retinopathy: Report of five cases. Ophthalmic Surg 7:92, 1976.
78. Jampol LM, Green JL, Goldberg MF, et al: An update on vitrectomy surgery and retinal detachment repair in sickle cell disease. Arch Ophthalmol 100:591, 1982.
79. Ryan SJ Jr, Goldberg MF: Anterior segment ischemia following scleral buckling in sickle cell hemoglobinopathy. Am J Ophthalmol 72:35, 1971.

Chapter 88

■

Behçet's Disease

BISHARA M. FARIS and C. STEPHEN FOSTER

Behçet's disease is named after the Turkish dermatologist Dr. Hulusi Behçet (1889 to 1948), who in 1937 described the characteristic triad of symptoms: recurrent hypopyon-iritis and oral and genital ulcerations.[1]

The disorder is an immune complex disease with occlusive vasculitis as its main pathologic feature. It affects many organs, and symptoms recur on average every 1 to 2 mo. The disease is most prevalent in the Middle and Far East. An increasing number of cases, however, have been reported in Europe and North America. Owing to the growing international recognition and importance of this entity, five international congresses have been held to discuss new clinical and laboratory developments. The most recent of these was in 1989 in Rochester, Minnesota. This chapter covers primarily the ophthalmic aspects of the disease. The reader is strongly encouraged also to read Chapter 253, which is devoted to the systemic and immunologic manifestations of the disease.

EPIDEMIOLOGY

As already noted, Behçet's disease occurs worldwide but is found predominantly in the Middle and Far East.[2–5] Its highest prevalence, 7 to 8.5 cases/100,000 population, is in Japan. More than 20 percent of Japanese cases of uveitis are secondary to Behçet's disease.[6] In the United States, the prevalence is 4 cases/1 million population,[2] and Behçet's disease represents 0.2 to 0.4 percent of cases of uveitis in this country.[7]

Reports, mainly from the Middle and Far East, have shown a preponderance of males, with an overall male: female ratio of 2.3 : 1.[7] The complete type (see later discussion) of Behçet's disease is more frequent in males; the incomplete type has the same frequency in both sexes. A recent report, however, shows a reversal of the male : female ratio to 0.77 : 1.[8] In North America and Great Britain, there is a slight preponderance of the disease in males or a nearly even distribution of the disease in males and females.[9, 11]

The mean age of onset is 25 to 35 yr worldwide, with a range of 2 mo to 72 yr. More cases of Behçet's disease in children have been reported recently.[12]

ETIOLOGIC AND IMMUNOPATHOLOGIC CONSIDERATIONS

The cause of Behçet's disease remains unknown; the original viral theory has not been confirmed. Many environmental factors[13] have been implicated but not proved. Data incriminating herpes simplex virus or streptococcal species, or both, have emerged from multiple laboratories. There is no consistent inheritance pattern, but histocompatibility antigen studies have shown an association with the HLA-B5 phenotype and its subtype HLA-Bw51, suggesting a genetic influence on disease susceptibility. This association was found in Japan[6, 14] and in Turkey, but not in whites living in the United States and England.[15, 16] The high prevalence of the disease in Japan and the Eastern Mediterranean countries can be explained by the spread of the susceptibility gene, linked to the HLA-B5 phenotype, on the Silk Route by the Turks. More specific associations between HLA type and clinical manifestations of the disease have been noted: HLA-B12 is associated with the mucocutaneous type, HLA-B27 is associated with the arthritic type, and HLA-B5 is associated with the ocular type.[17] Such specific associations could not be confirmed in the Turkish populations.[18]

Few reports have correlated the changes seen in T cells with disturbances found in Behçet's disease,[19] but current evidence suggests that during active attacks, T cells are activated (up-regulation of CD25 of the interleukin (IL) 2 receptor glycoprotein), class II (HLA-DR) expression on T cells is depressed, and both helper (CD4) and suppressor-cytotoxic (CD8) T cells have cytophilic IgA bound to their surfaces. Natural killer cells are increased in number and activity, and cytokines IL1, IL6, and tumor necrosis factor are elevated in the circulation. Levels of soluble IL2 receptors and immunoglobulins A, E, and M are increased. Circulating immune complexes (including IgA-containing immune complexes), as determined by C1q binding or Raji cell assays, are also present, and elevated levels of the inhibitor to tissue plasminogen activator have been reported. Blood viscosity is increased during active disease, and the vascular endothelium shows impaired prostaglandin I_2 synthesis.

Taken together, these bits and pieces of data suggest that Behçet's disease develops in the genetically predisposed individual who encounters some environmental trigger, the most notable contenders being microbes. Resultant dysregulation of immune responses may result in suppressor-cell impairment, helper T-cell activation, and cytokine synthesis dysregulation, with immune complex formation, neutrophil and natural killer–cell activation, and vasculitis. The sometimes favorable response to cyclosporine, an "anti–T-cell drug," is taken as evidence for a causal relationship between T cells and Behçet's disease, but alterations in B-lymphocyte functions also have been described, and it is important to remember that few diseases are pure T-cell or pure B-cell disorders.

The tissue damage in Behçet's disease is caused by the associated vasculitis and the immune complex deposition within the blood vessel wall, together with the activation of the complement system.[20, 21]

CLINICAL MANIFESTATIONS AND DIAGNOSTIC CRITERIA

The diagnosis of Behçet's disease is based on clinical findings rather than on specific laboratory test results. High levels of serum proteins, circulating immune complexes, acute-phase reactants such as α_1-acid glycoprotein and properdin Factor B, and other complement-reactive proteins may be found in the acute phase.[20] Circulating autoantibodies such as antinuclear antibody may be present. None of these laboratory findings alone can confirm the diagnosis, nor are they found in all cases of classic Behçet's disease.

The disease has a variety of clinical manifestations that do not occur simultaneously. There are periods of remission followed by exacerbation. Many clinical criteria have been used since Behçet's first report of this entity in 1937; those most commonly accepted are those set by the Behçet's Disease Research Committee of Japan (Table 88–1),[22] or by O'Duffy (Table 88–2).

Four types of Behçet's disease have been identified: (1) complete, (2) incomplete, (3) suspect, and (4) possible (see Tables 88–1 and 88–2). Clinicians and investigators have come to realize that greater weight should be given to ocular manifestations in the diagnosis of Behçet's disease. At present, the incomplete type may be diagnosed based on two of the following criteria: oral, dermal, ocular, or genital involvement, plus two minor criteria (e.g., arthritis, gastrointestinal lesions, vascular lesions, central nervous system involvement) or ocular involvement only and two minor criteria. Since the diagnosis is made solely on clinical findings, a reliable history and physical examination, as well as consultations among specialists (dermatologist, neurologist, and others) are essential to avoid errors in diagnosis.

The variations in the diagnostic criteria used account for some of the discrepancies in the results of epidemiologic, etiologic, and genetic studies.

Table 88–1. DIAGNOSTIC CRITERIA FOR BEHÇET'S DISEASE

Major Criteria*

Oral aphthous ulceration
Skin lesions
    Erythema nodosum–like eruptions
    Subcutaneous thrombophlebitis
    Cutaneous hypersensitivity
Ocular lesions
    Recurrent hypopyon iritis or iridocyclitis
    Chorioretinitis
Genital aphthous ulcerations

Minor Criteria

Arthritic symptoms and signs (arthralgia, swelling, redness in
    large joints)
Gastrointestinal lesions (appendicitis-like pains, melena,
    diarrhea, and so on)
Epididymitis
Vascular lesions (obliterative vasculitis, occlusions,
    aneurysms)
Central nervous system involvement
    Brain stem syndrome
    Meningoencephalomyelitic syndrome
    Psychiatric symptoms

Types of Behçet's Disease

Complete: All four major symptoms appear in the clinical
    course
Incomplete:
    Three of four major symptoms appear in the clinical course
    Recurrent hypopyon-iritis or typical chorioretinitis and one
        other major symptom appear in the clinical course
Suspect: Two major criteria appear in the clinical course
Possible: One major criterion appears in the clinical course

From Behçet's Disease Research Committee: Clinical Research Section Recommendation. Jpn Ophthalmol 18:291, 1974.
*Major criteria are common manifestations of the disease but not necessarily the most severe.

OCULAR BEHÇET'S DISEASE

Ocular involvement, frequently termed *ocular Behçet's disease*, has serious implications in that legal blindness usually ensues within 4 yr unless the patient is treated with immunosuppressive drugs.[22] The reported frequency of ocular involvement in cases of Behçet's disease is 83 to 95 percent in males and 67 to 73 percent in females.[28] Ocular symptoms usually follow the buccal and genital lesions by 3 to 4 yr.[29] The initial ocular manifestations can be unilateral, but progression to bilateral involvement is the rule in at least two thirds of cases.[9] Recurrence is common and the recurrent attacks of inflammation usually result in severe, permanent compromise of vision unless effective treatment is instituted.

All eye structures can be affected by the central histopathologic feature of this vasculitic disease, which is a nongranulomatous inflammation with necrotizing obliterative vasculitis. Clinically, ocular findings may be present in the anterior or posterior segment, or more commonly, in both.

Clinical Manifestations

ANTERIOR SEGMENT

The classic finding in ocular Behçet's disease is iridocyclitis with hypopyon, which is present in 19 to 31 percent of cases (Fig. 88–1A).[9, 30] The patient complains of periorbital pain, redness, photophobia, and blurred vision. Slit-lamp biomicroscopy shows conjunctival and ciliary injection (Fig. 88–1B) with aqueous flare and cells. Fine keratic precipitates are present on the corneal endothelium. The hypopyon may change position with head movement and can form and disappear rapidly. A more common presentation is iridocyclitis without hypopyon, which is found in two thirds of cases.[30]

The attack lasts for 2 to 3 wk and then subsides. Recurrences are the rule, with subsequent iris atrophy and posterior synechiae formation (Fig. 88–1C).

In our experience in the Middle East,[31] hypopyon formation is not common, probably because of the early and aggressive treatment with local and systemic steroids. Similar findings were reported from the United States[9] and recently from Turkey.[32] Other less frequent findings[30] are episcleritis (Fig. 88–1D), subconjunctival hemorrhage, and keratitis.

POSTERIOR SEGMENT

Vitreous cellular infiltration (vitritis) is always present during the acute phase. The classic fundus finding is retinal vasculitis[9] affecting both arteries and veins in the posterior pole (Fig. 88–2A).

Ophthalmoscopy shows venous and capillary dilation with engorgement. There is patchy perivascular sheathing with inflammatory exudates surrounding retinal hemorrhages (Fig. 88–2B). Yellow-white exudates may form deep in the retina (Fig. 88–2C). Retinal edema is present in 10 to 20 percent of cases, especially in the macula.[9] Severe vasculitis leads to thrombosis of vessels with secondary ischemic retinal changes. Branch or central retinal vein (or artery) occlusions may be present (Fig. 88–2D).[33] In severe cases, infarction of large segments of the retina may be found. Venous occlusions in

Table 88–2. DIAGNOSTIC CRITERIA FOR BEHÇET'S DISEASE (O'DUFFY)

Major Findings

    Aphthous stomatitis
    Genital ulcers
    Uveitis
    Dermal vasculitis
    Arthritis

Minor Findings

    Central nervous system involvement
    Colitis
    Phlebitis
    Large vessel arteritis

Diagnosis

    Oral or genital ulceration
        plus
    Two other major findings

From Behçet's Disease Research Committee: Clinical Research Section Recommendations. Jpn J Ophthalmol 18:291, 1974.

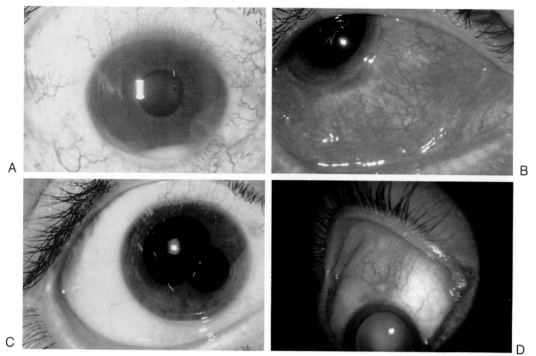

Figure 88–1. Anterior segment findings. *A,* Iridocyclitis with hypopyon. *B,* Iridocyclitis without hypopyon and with subconjunctival hemorrhage. *C,* Iris atrophy with posterior synechiae. *D,* Episcleritis.

the retina cause tissue hypoxia, which stimulates the growth of new vessels. Because of their thin and fragile walls, these new vessels bleed into the vitreous cavity and subsequently fibrose. Retinal detachment is not commonly seen.

The optic nerve may be involved, with papillitis in the acute phase seen in at least one fourth of cases.[9]

Papilledema is not frequent. Progressive optic atrophy may occur as a result of microvasculitis of the arterioles feeding the optic nerve.

Patients with ocular Behçet's disease have periods of remission and exacerbation. Each attack damages the eye. In the chronic stage, slit-lamp biomicroscopy shows few cells in the anterior chamber. The iris shows patchy

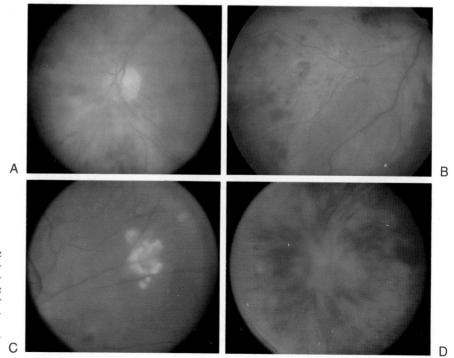

Figure 88–2. Fundus findings in the acute phase of ocular Behçet's disease. *A,* Vitreous haze, vasculitis with retinal vessel engorgement, and retinal hemorrhages in the posterior pole. *B,* Patchy, perivascular sheathing with surrounding retinal hemorrhages involving inferotemporal vessels. *C,* Yellow and white exudates deep in the retina. *D,* Central retinal vein occlusion.

areas of atrophy and posterior synechiae. The lens may become cataractous. The vitreous has floating pigmented cells and flare caused by vascular incompetence. The fundus has narrowed and occluded "silver-wired" vessels (Fig. 88–3A). Arteriolar attenuation is usually striking. The optic nerve is pale and atrophic.

Fluorescein leakage from retinal vessels may be seen before there are obvious ophthalmoscopic signs of vasculitis. We believe that fundus fluorescein angiography is mandatory in the study and longitudinal care of patients with ocular Behçet's disease in order to monitor the extent of damage to the vasculature of the retina and optic nerve.[34, 35] During acute inflammation, there is dilatation of retinal capillaries, with dye leakage on angiography, especially in the radial peripapillary area. Affected vessels in the retina and optic nerve leak the dye profusely in early transit (Fig. 88–4A). Their walls stain in late transit. The dye accumulates in areas of retinal infiltrates and in the edematous retina (Fig. 88–4B–D). There is common loss of a clearly defined capillary-free zone (Fig. 88–4E).

When central retinal vein occlusion exists, there is delayed filling and emptying of the involved segments. Leakage from the dilated vessels is present in late transit (Fig. 88–4F and G). Months later, repeat angiograms may show areas of collateral circulation, capillary nonperfusion, intraretinal microvascular formation, and neovascularization. At sites of retinal pigment epithelial changes, window defects are present (Fig. 88–4H). Together with slit-lamp examination, fluorescein angiography is used to evaluate the response to medical treatment. Decreased fluorescein leakage indicates a favorable response to therapy.

Bilaterality is present in 76 to 90 per cent of cases.[30, 36, 37] The second eye is generally affected within 1 yr of disease onset in the first eye, but disease in the second eye may not occur for as long as 7 yr. The severity of inflammation in each eye varies, however, and is frequently quite asymmetric.[9]

NEUROOPHTHALMIC FINDINGS

Approximately 10 percent of patients with neuro-Behçet's disease show ocular involvement. Conversely, perhaps up to 30 percent of patients with ocular Behçet's disease have neuro-Behçet's disease. This is an important relationship and one that the ophthalmologist must clearly understand, given the fact that it is the central nervous system manifestations of Behçet's disease that usually cause fatalities. The following neuroophthalmic changes have been noted in Behçet's disease:[38] (1) palsies of cranial nerves VI and VII caused by brain stem involvement—such palsies are usually transient; (2) central scotomas due to papillitis and visual field defects;[39] and (3) papilledema[40–43] resulting from pseudotumor cerebri caused by thrombosis of the intradural venous sinuses.

Ocular Complications and Differential Diagnosis

In the Middle and Far East, ocular complications are more frequent in males than in females.[30] They occur following chronic recurrences, usually within 1 to 4 yr after the onset of the systemic manifestations.

Cataract formation is the most frequent anterior segment complication, occurring in up to 36 percent of cases in one series.[30] It is caused by the recurrent inflammation or the adverse effects of steroids.

Secondary glaucoma, caused by posterior and peripheral synechiae, was seen in 11 percent of cases in one series of 28 patients.[30] Hyphema is rare.

Posterior segment complications included optic atrophy in 15 percent of cases in one series and macular degeneration in 13 percent of patients in another study (see Fig. 88–3A).[30] Retinal breaks (Fig. 88–5), rhegmatogenous retinal detachment, and retinal neovascularization are infrequent.

Posterior segment changes may resemble those seen in sarcoidosis, viral retinitis, polyarteritis nodosa, systemic lupus erythematosus, Whipple's disease, Crohn's disease, and relapsing polychondritis.

Ocular Histopathologic Features[30, 45]

The ocular histopathologic changes are basically identical to those occurring in other organs—i.e., necrotizing, leukocytoclastic obliterative vasculitis that is probably immune complex–mediated and affects both arteries and veins of all sizes. The pericorneal and episcleral vessels show inflammatory cell infiltration. During the acute inflammation, the iris has neutrophils in its stroma and around its vessels, and later, monocytes, lymphocytes, and mast cells are present. Following many recurrences, atrophy and fibrosis of the iris with posterior synechiae formation are seen.

During acute inflammation, the ciliary body and choroid show diffuse infiltration with neutrophils. During remission, infiltration with lymphocytes and plasma cells is seen. In the late, chronic stages, there is proliferation of collagen fibers, sometimes with formation of a cyclitic membrane thickening of the choroid and sometimes hypotony and phthisis bulbi.

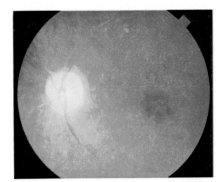

Figure 88–3. Fundus findings in the chronic phase of ocular Behçet's disease. Optic atrophy, narrowed vessels with "silver-wiring," and macular pigmentary degeneration.

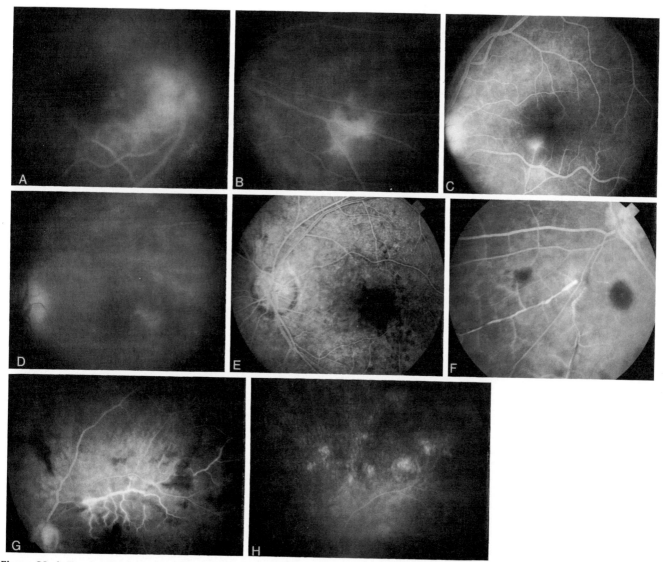

Figure 88–4. Fundus fluorescein angiograms. *A,* Leakage from the nerve head and peripapillary area in acute papillitis. *B,* Staining of the retina in area of infiltrates seen in Figure 88–2C. *C,* Leakage from an area of focal vasculitis in macular edema. *D,* Petaloid staining of the retina in chronic macular edema. *E,* Loss of well-defined capillary-free zone in the zone in the macular area. *F,* Angiogram in acute vasculitis with venous occlusion. *G,* Staining of the blood vessel wall in late transit (same eye as in *F*). *H,* Retinal pigment epithelium window defects.

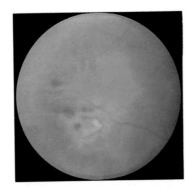

Figure 88–5. Retinal break with shallow retinal detachment.

Of all ocular tissues, the retina is damaged the most in ocular Behçet's disease. During the acute inflammation, there is severe vasculitis with marked infiltration of leukocytes in and around blood vessels and into retinal tissues. The retinal vessels have thickened basement membranes; their endothelial cells are swollen, neutrophils marginate, and thrombus formation begins. Veins are sometimes more affected than are arteries. During remission, few lymphocytes and plasma cells are found in and around the vessel walls. There is localized loss of rods and cones in areas of prior involvement, and fibrosis is present in the inner nuclear layer. Retinal pigment epithelium destruction is minimal. In more advanced cases, there is fibrosis of the blood vessel wall and sometimes complete vascular obliteration.

The optic nerve vessels are affected by the angiitic process in the acute phase, and the nerve tissue itself is often infiltrated by inflammatory cells. Optic atrophy is present in the chronic stage, secondary to the angiitic ischemia and optic neuritis.

Treatment

The initiation of treatment is based on a definite diagnosis of Behçet's disease. The appropriate medications for effectively treating Behçet's disease have *potential* serious adverse side effects, and expert knowledge of immunosuppressants is an absolute prerequisite for individuals treating these patients. Immunosuppressive agents are *clearly* the class of drug required for the effective treatment of patients with ocular Behçet's disease.

To be effective, treatment must be started early. The goal is to suppress inflammation, reduce the frequency and severity of recurrences, and halt any involvement of the retina. The choice of medications is determined by the severity of the disease. In general, treatment of the ocular form of the disease must be more aggressive when the following conditions are present: multiple recurrences of uveitis; complete Behçet's disease, especially with neurologic and vascular involvement; male sex;[30] patient origin in the Mediterranean area or Far East;[30] and retinal and bilateral involvement.

The most commonly used antiinflammatory drugs are corticosteroids, cytotoxic agents, cyclosporine, and col-

chicine. A complete discussion of these drugs, their indications, potential side effects, dosage, and monitoring requirements is presented in Chapter 253.

CORTICOSTEROIDS

Introduced in the 1950s, corticosteroids were the first immunosuppressants to be used in the treatment of Behçet's disease. Systemic corticosteroids have a rapid and definite antiinflammatory effect in all phases of ocular Behçet's disease, but especially in the acute phase. From our experience in the 1960s, however, these drugs failed to prevent visual deterioration[31, 32] and the ultimate tragedy of blindness from the consequences of ocular Behçet's disease. This was the experience of other investigators as well.[9, 30, 46] Still, oral or intravenous steroid therapy, or both, forms an important component in the plan of care for the patient with Behçet's disease. In acute anterior segment inflammation, topical corticosteroids, with or without periocular corticosteroids, are indicated. In posterior segment inflammation, systemic corticosteroids (1 to 1.5 mg/kg of prednisone/day) are used in combination with immunosuppressive drugs, and then the steroids are gradually tapered. The advantage of this regimen is to obtain benefit from the immediate corticosteroid antiinflammatory action while waiting for the full effect of the cytotoxic drug's action, which usually takes from 3 to 6 wk. In select chronic cases, maintenance doses (15 to 30 mg/day) of prednisone may be required in combination with immunosuppressive drugs to control the uveitis. This combination lowers the prevalence of adverse effects from either drug.[47]

CYTOTOXIC AGENTS

The use of cytotoxic drugs in inflammatory and immune-mediated ocular diseases has been reviewed in Chapter 253. Chlorambucil, cyclophosphamide, and azathioprine are currently used in the treatment of ocular Behçet's disease.

Chlorambucil. The mode of action of this slow-acting alkylating agent is the same as that of cyclophosphamide (see further on). It was the first cytotoxic drug to be tried in ocular Behçet's disease and is still the most commonly used. Disappointment with corticosteroids in patients with ocular Behçet's disease in Lebanon led us to try chlorambucil in 1970.[48] Long remissions were obtained. Subsequently, these results were confirmed worldwide, and our recent experience enjoyed a 70 percent success rate in achieving total control of blinding ocular inflammation.[9]

A favorable response may take 1 to 3 mo to become evident. Subsequently, the drug dosage is reduced, and a maintenance dose is given for 1 to 2 yr, depending on the symptoms, ocular findings, and bone marrow tolerance. In refractory cases, dosages of up to 22 mg/day may be indicated.

Cyclophosphamide. This fast-acting alkylating agent is superior to corticosteroids in controlling uveitis in Behçet's disease.[9] Cyclophosphamide has been used successfully in cases refractory to chlorambucil[9] and is given intravenously in severe cases of vasculitis. In both of our patients treated with intravenous cyclophosphamide, disease was finally controlled after treatment failure with multiple other agents, and studies from Turkey, France, and Iran have demonstrated the safety and efficacy of intravenous pulse cyclophosphamide (1 g/sq m every 4 wk) in the treatment of patients with Behçet's disease.

Azathioprine. Earlier reports of treatment with this agent gave inconclusive results.[9, 54] Recently, azathioprine given orally (2.5 mg/kg/day) decreased recurrences of ocular Behçet's disease.[36] Our results with azathioprine have been less spectacular.

CYCLOSPORINE

Favorable results have been reported using cyclosporine in ocular Behçet's disease.[62–64] The dose employed, however (10 mg/kg/day), was associated with renal toxicity, and this dose is no longer recommended. Given in combination with bromocriptine (2.5 mg 3 to 4 times/day) in an effort to reduce the severity of nephrotoxicity, Cyclosporine A, at a dose of 5 to 7 mg/kg/day, has been distinctly inferior to chlorambucil, cyclophosphamide, and probably azathioprine in the treatment of ocular Behçet's disease.[9] Reports from Japan, Italy, and Saudi Arabia confirm these findings and further demonstrate the high relapse rate following cyclosporine withdrawal, unlike the permanent cures effected with chlorambucil.

COLCHICINE

Colchicine has a mild antiinflammatory effect. It interferes with neutrophil migration and function. Colchicine can be used in combination with other drugs in treating all forms of ocular Behçet's disease.[9, 66, 67] It may allow the disease to be controlled using lower doses of immunosuppressive drugs.

In summary, the best therapeutic results are obtained with a combination of drugs.[9] Treatment requires long-term care (1 to 4 yr) with drugs that have many potentially serious adverse effects. However, if untreated, or treated only with steroids and colchicine, ocular Behçet's disease progresses to bilateral blindness in a very high percentage of patients. The seriousness of the situation should be fully discussed with the patient and informed written consent obtained prior to starting treatment. Treatment *must* be managed by an individual who is, by virtue of training and experience, truly expert in the use of systemic chemotherapeutic drugs, in the early recognition of their side effects, and in treatment of these side effects.

EYE SURGERY

Surgery is sometimes indicated in eyes afflicted with Behçet's disease, but surgical trauma may precipitate a recurrence of the inflammation.

Surgery is indicated whenever visual improvement can be expected *and* the eye has been free of inflammation for a minimum of 3 mo. Operating on eyes with cataract and uveitis has its special problems. This subject has been comprehensively reviewed by Foster and associates.[69]

Earlier reports using intracapsular cataract techniques during remission of ocular Behçet's disease showed a 60 percent improvement in final visual acuity.[30, 70] Although the immediate postoperative inflammation was more intense in 25 percent of cases, the frequency of subsequent recurrences was the same for the preoperative and postoperative periods.[30] Our results with extracapsular cataract surgery with or without lens implantation is considerably more successful today.[9]

Our recommendations for successful cataract surgery and for minimizing postoperative uveitis are as follows: Uveitis should be inactive for at least 3 mo preoperatively, systemic and topical steroids should be used prophylactically for 1 wk preoperatively and continued postoperatively, immunosuppressive drugs should be continued, complete removal of cortical material should take place, and a one-piece polymethyl methacrylate posterior chamber intraocular lens should be used *if* the patient and surgeon understand the special nature of this surgery, its risks, and the prognosis for success.

Laser photocoagulation for retinal neovascularization is sometimes indicated in patients with retinal hypoxia from Behçet's vasculopathy. Laser surgery does not induce postoperative inflammation.

One of the authors (BF) has operated on two eyes with rhegmatogenous retinal detachment in the quiescent stage of Behçet's disease (see Fig. 88–5). Scleral buckling has been performed without complications. Topical and systemic steroids were given preoperatively as well as postoperatively.

In conclusion, surgical intervention in eyes with inactive Behçet's uveitis is well tolerated, with no provocation of the inflammation *provided* that inflammation is totally controlled preoperatively.

Prognosis for Vision

The natural history of ocular Behçet's disease in countries of highest prevalence (Japan, Turkey) is very impressive, and the visual prognosis is poor. Legal blindness was present in more than 50 percent of cases within 4 yr.[48, 49, 52] Reports from North America are more favorable, with a prevalence of legal blindness of 25 percent.[9, 37, 76] One possible explanation for this discrepancy is a genetic predisposition for severe Behçet's disease in the Middle and Far East. Also, immunosuppressive agents gave long-lasting remissions and improved the visual prognosis in North America,[9] as well as in countries of high prevalence.[36, 49]

Flash electroretinogram and pattern visually evoked cortical potential studies on patients with Behçet's disease with posterior segment involvement were reported recently.[77] A decrease in amplitude of pattern visually evoked cortical potential was noted early in the disease, even when visual acuity and flash electroretinogram results were normal. This finding may serve as a criterion for monitoring fundus changes and visual prognosis in ocular Behçet's disease.

REFERENCES

1. Behçet H: Uber rezidivierende, aphthose, durch ein Virus verursachte Geschwere am Mund, am Auge und an den Genitalien. Dermatol Wochenschr 36:1152, 1937.
2. O'Duffy JD: Behçet's disease. In Kelly WN, Harris ED Jr, Ruddy S, Sledge CB (eds): Textbook of Rheumatology. Philadelphia, WB Saunders, 1985, pp 1174–1178.
3. Chamberlain MA: Behçet's syndrome in 32 patients in Yorkshire. Ann Rheum Dis 36:491, 1977.
4. Sulheim O, Dalgaard JB, Anderson SR: Behçet's syndrome: Report of case with complete autopsy performed. Acta Pathol Microbiol Scand 45:145, 1959.
5. Cooper DA, Penny R: Behçet's syndrome: Clinical, immunological, and therapeutic evaluation of 17 patients. Med J Aust 4:585, 1974.
6. Mishima S, Masuda K, Izawa Y, et al: Behçet's disease in Japan: Ophthalmologic aspects. Trans Am Ophthalmol Soc 77:225, 1979.
7. Chajek T, Fainaru M: Behçet's disease: Report of 41 cases and a review of the literature. Medicine 54:179, 1975.
8. Aoki K, Fujioka K, Katsumata H, et al: Epidemiological studies on Behçet's disease in the Hokkaido district. Jpn J Clin Ophthalmol 25:2239, 1971.
9. Baer JC, Raizman MB, Foster CS: Ocular Behçet's disease in the United States: Clinical presentation and visual outcome in 29 patients. In Masahiko U, Shigeaki O, Koki A (eds): Proceedings of the Fifth International Symposium on the Immunology and Immunopathology of the Eye, Tokyo, 13–15 March 1990. New York, Elsevier Science, 1990, p 383.
10. O'Duffy JD, Carney JA, Deodhar S: Behçet's disease: Report of 10 cases, 3 with new manifestations. Ann Intern Med 75:561, 1971.
11. O'Duffy JD, Goldstein NP: Neurologic involvement in seven patients with Behçet's disease. Am J Med 61:170, 1976.
12. Ammann AJ, Johnson A, Fyfe GA, et al: Behçet's syndrome. J Pediatr 107:41, 1985.
13. Cengiz K: Serum zinc, copper, and magnesium in Behçet's disease. [Abstract 22] Royal Society of Medicine International Conference on Behçet's Disease, London, September 5 and 6, 1985.
14. Raizman MB, Foster CS: Plasma exchange in the therapy of Behçet's disease. Graefes Arch Clin Exp Ophthalmol 227:360, 1989.
15. Ohno S, Char DH, Kimura SJ, O'Connor GR: Studies on HLA antigens in American patients with Behçet's disease. Jpn J Ophthalmol 22:58, 1978.
16. O'Duffy JD, Taswell HF, Elveback LR: HLA antigens in Behçet's disease. J Rheumatol 3:1, 1976.
17. Lehner T, Barnes CG: Criteria for diagnosis and classification of Behçet's syndrome. In Lehner T, Barnes CG (eds): Behçet's Syndrome: Clinical and Immunological Features. Proceedings of a Conference Sponsored by Royal Society of Medicine, February 1979. London, Academic Press, 1979, pp 1–9.
18. Muttuoglu AU, Yazici H, Yrudakul S, et al: Behçet's disease: Lack of correlation of clinical manifestations with HLA antigens. Tissue Antigens 17:226, 1981.
19. Valesini G, Pivetti-Pezzi P, Mastrandrea F, et al: Evaluation of T cell subsets in Behçet's syndrome using anti–T cell monoclonal antibodies. Clin Exp Immunol 60:55, 1985.
20. Levinsky RJ, Lehner T: Circulating, soluble immune complexes in recurrent oral ulcerations and Behçet's syndrome. Clin Exp Immunol 32:193, 1978.
21. Burton-Kee JE, Mobray JF, Lehner T: Different cross-reacting circulating immune complexes in Behçet's syndrome and recurrent oral ulcers. J Lab Clin Med 97:559, 1981.
22. Behçet's Disease Research Committee: Clinical Research Section Recommendation. Jpn J Ophthalmol 18:291, 1974.
23. Strachan RW, Wigzell FW: Polyarthritis in Behçet's multiple symptom complex. Ann Rheum Dis 22:26, 1963.
24. Muftuoglu U, Yurdakul S, Yazici H, et al: Vascular involvement in Behçet's disease: A review of 129 cases. In Lehner T, Barnes CG (eds): Recent Advances in Behçet's Disease. London, Royal Society of Medicine Services, 1986, pp 255–260.
25. Kalbian VV, Challis MT: Behçet's disease: Report of twelve cases with three manifesting as papilledema. Am J Med 19:823, 1970.
26. Bietti GB, Bruna R: An ophthalmic report on Behçet's disease. In International Symposium on Behçet's Disease, Rome, 1965. Basel, S Karger, 1966, p 77.
27. Inaba G: Clinical features of neuro-Behçet's syndrome. In Lehner T, Barnes CG (eds): Recent Advances in Behçet's Disease. London, Royal Society of Medicine Services, 1986, pp 235–246.
28. Masuda K, Inaba G, Mizushima H, et al: A nation-wide survey of Behçet's disease in Japan. 2. Clinical Survey. Jpn J Ophthalmol 19:278, 1975.
29. Yazici H, Pazarli H, Yurdakal S, et al: The time of onset of eye involvement in Behçet's syndrome. Behçet's Disease Fifth International Conference. [Abstracts] Rochester, MN, September 14–15, 1989.
30. Mishima S, Masuda S, Izawa Y, et al: Behçet's disease in Japan: Ophthalmologic aspects. Trans Am Ophthalmol Soc 77:225, 1979.
31. Mamo JG, Baghdasarian A: Behçet's disease: A report of 28 cases. Arch Ophthalmol 71:38, 1964.
32. Pazarli H, Ozyazgen Y, Aktunc T: Clinical observations on hypopyon attacks of Behçet's disease in Turkey. Behçet's Disease Fifth International Conference. [Abstracts] Rochester, MN, September 14–15, 1979.
33. Bonamour G, Grange JD, Bonnet M: Retinal vein involvement in Behçet's disease. In Dilsen N, Konice M, Ovul C (eds): Behçet's Disease. Proceedings of an International Symposium on Behçet's Disease, Istanbul, September 29–30, 1977. Amsterdam-Oxford, Excerpta Medica, 1979, pp 142–144.
34. Matsuo N, Ojima M, Kumashiro O, et al: Fluorescein angiographic disorders of the retina and the optic disc in Behçet's disease. In Inaba G (ed): Behçet's Disease: Pathogenetic Mechanism and Clinical Future. Proceedings of the International Conference on Behçet's Disease. Tokyo, October 23–24, 1981. Tokyo, University of Tokyo Press, 1982, pp 161–170.
35. Sanders MD: Ophthalmic features of Behçet's disease. In Lehner T, Barnes CG (eds): Behçet's Syndrome: Clinical and Immunological Features. Proceedings of a Conference Sponsored by the Royal Society of Medicine, February 1979. London, Academic Press, 1979, pp 183–189.
36. Yazici H, Pazarli H, Barnes C, et al: A controlled trial of azathioprine in Behçet's syndrome. N Engl J Med 322:281, 1990.
37. Michelson JB, Dhisari FV: Behçet's disease. Surv Ophthalmol 26:190, 1982.
38. Anaba G: Clinical features of neuro-Behçet's syndrome. In Lehner T, Barnes CG (eds): Recent Advances in Behçet's Disease. London, Royal Society of Medicine Services, 1986, pp 235–246.
39. James DG, Spiteri MA: Behçet's disease. Ophthalmology 89:1279, 1982.
40. Bank I, Weart C: Dural sinus thrombosis in Behçet's disease. Arthritis Rheum 27:816, 1984.
41. Pamir MN, Kansu T, Ervengi A, Zileli T: Papilledema in Behçet's syndrome. Arch Neurol 38:643, 1981.
42. Wechsler B, Bousser MG, Du LTH, et al: Central venous sinus thrombosis in Behçet's disease. [Letter] Mayo Clin Proc 60:891, 1985.
43. Kansu T: Optic nerve involvement in Behçet's disease. Behçet's Disease Fifth International Conference. [Abstracts] Rochester, MN, September 14–15, 1989.
44. Aktunc T, Bahcecioglu H, Ozyazgan Y, et al: The relationship of the posterior vitreous with the macula in Behçet's uveitis. Behçet's Disease Fifth International Conference. [Abstracts] Rochester, MN, September 14–15, 1989.
45. Fenton Rh, Easton HA: Behçet's syndrome: A histopathologic study of the eye. Arch Ophthalmol 72:71, 1984.
46. Chajek T, Fainaru M: Behçet's disease. Report of 41 cases and a review of the literature. Medicine 54:179, 1975.
47. Santamaria J: Steroidal agents: The systemic and ocular complications. Ocular Inflammation Ther 1:19, 1988.
48. Mamo JG, Azzam SA: Treatment of Behçet's disease with chlorambucil. Arch Ophthalmol 84:446, 1970.
49. Benezra D, Cohen E: Treatment and visual prognosis in Behçet's disease. Br J Ophthalmol 70:589, 1986.

50. Bietti GB, Cerulli L, Pivetti-Pezzi P: Behçet's disease and immunosuppressive treatment. Mod Probl Ophthalmol 16:314, 1976.
51. O'Duffy JD, Robertson DM, Goldstein NP: Chlorambucil in the treatment of uveitis and meningoencephalitis of Behçet's disease. Am J Med 76:75, 1984.
52. Pezzi PP, Gasparri V, De Liso P, et al: Prognosis in Behçet's disease. Ann Ophthalmol 17:20, 1985.
53. Tabbara KF: Chlorambucil in Behçet's disease: A reappraisal. Ophthalmology 90:906, 1983.
54. Nussenblatt RB, Palestine AG: Cyclosporine: Immunology, pharmacology, and therapeutic uses. Surv Ophthalmol 31:159, 1986.
55. Rokover Y, Adar H, Tal I, et al: Behçet's disease: Long-term follow up of three children and review of the literature. Pediatrics 83:986, 1989.
56. Matteson EL, O'Duffy JD: Treatment of Behçet's disease with chlorambucil. Behçet's Disease Fifth International Conference. [Abstracts] Rochester, MN, September 14–15, 1989.
57. Wong VG: Immunosuppressive agents in ophthalmology. Surv Ophthalmol 13:290, 1969.
58. Shand FL, Liew FY: Differential sensitivity to cyclophosphamide of helper T cells for humoral responses and suppressor T cells for delayed-type hypersensitivity. Eur J Immunol 10:480, 1980.
59. Tabor DR, Kiel DP, Jacobs RF: Cyclophosphamide-sensitive activity of suppressor T cells during treponemal infection. Immunology 62:127, 1987.
60. Fraunfelder FT, Meyer SM: Ocular toxicity of antineoplastic agents. Ophthalmology 90:1, 1983.
61. Trenn G, Taffs R, Hohman R, et al: Biochemical characterization of the inhibitory effect of CsA on cytolytic T lymphocyte effector functions. J Immunol 142:3796, 1989.
62. Nussenblatt RB, Palestine AG, Chan CC, et al: Effectiveness of cyclosporine therapy for Behçet's disease. Arthritis Rheum 28:672, 1985.
63. Masuda K, Nakajima A: A double-masked study of cyclosporine treatment in Behçet's disease. In Schindler R (ed): Cyclosporine in Autoimmune Diseases. Berlin, Springer-Verlag, 1985, pp 162–164.
64. BenEzra D, Brodsky M, Peer J, et al: Cyclosporine (CyA) versus conventional therapy in Behçet's disease: Preliminary observations of a masked study. In Schindler R (ed): Cyclosporine in Autoimmune Diseases. Berlin, Springer-Verlag, 1985, pp 158–161.
65. Matsumura N, Mizushima Y: Leukocyte movement and colchicine treatment in Behçet's disease. Lancet 2:813, 1975.
66. Jijikata K, Masuda K: Visual prognosis in Behçet's disease: Effects of cyclophosphamide and colchicine. Jpn J Ophthalmol 22:506, 1978.
67. Raynor A, Askari AD: Behçet's disease and treatment with colchicine. J Am Acad Dermatol 2:396, 1980.
68. Wizemann AJS, Wizemann V: Therapeutic effects of short-term plasma exchange in endogenous uveitis. Am J Ophthalmol 97:565, 1984.
69. Foster CS, Fong LP, Singh G: Cataract surgery and intraocular lens implantation in patients with uveitis. Ophthalmology 96:281, 1988.
70. Mimura Y: Surgical results of complicated cataract in Behçet's disease. In Report of the Behçet's Disease Research Committee. Japan, Ministry of Health and Welfare, 1976, pp 152–159.
71. Diamond JG, Kaplan HJ: Lensectomy and vitrectomy for complicated cataract secondary to uveitis. Arch Ophthalmol 96:1798, 1978.
72. Nobe JR, Kokoris N, Diddie KR, et al: Lensectomy-vitrectomy in chronic uveitis. Retina 3:71, 1983.
73. Girard LJ, Rodriguez J, Mailman ML, et al: Cataract and uveitis management by pars plana lensectomy and vitrectomy by ultrasonic fragmentation. Retina 5:107, 1985.
74. Flynn HW Jr, Davis JL, Culbertson WW: Pars plana lensectomy and vitrectomy for complicated cataracts in juvenile rheumatoid arthritis. Ophthalmology 95:1114, 1988.
75. Yazici H, Tuzun YU, Pazarli H, et al: Influence of age of onset and patient's sex on the prevalence and severity of manifestations of Behçet's syndrome. Ann Rheum Dis 43:783, 1984.
76. O'Duffy JD, Matheson EL: Treatment of Behçet's disease with chlorambucil. Behçet's Disease Fifth International Conference. [Abstracts] Rochester, MN, September 14–15, 1989.
77. Cruz RD, Adachi-Usami E, Kakisu Y: Flash electroretinograms and pattern visually evoked cortical potentials in Behçet's disease. Jpn J Ophthalmol 34:142, 1990.

Chapter 89

■

Traumatic Retinopathy

MARK W. BALLES

Blunt or nonpenetrating ocular trauma may be associated with chorioretinal injury. Ocular damage may be due to direct injury to the globe or to distant orbital or systemic trauma acting indirectly to produce chorioretinal abnormalities.

DIRECT OCULAR INJURY

Choroidal Rupture

A choroidal rupture is a tear in the choroid, Bruch's membrane, and retinal pigment epithelium (RPE)[1] and was first described by von Graefe in 1854.[2] Choroidal ruptures may occur anteriorly, at which point they are usually parallel to the ora serrata, or posteriorly, at which point they are usually crescentic and oriented around the optic nerve (Fig. 89–1). Hemorrhage, which may be subretinal, retinal, or preretinal, may obscure the choroidal rupture acutely (Fig. 89–2). As the hemorrhage clears, the site of the choroidal rupture may be identified.

Vision may be decreased acutely because of associated hemorrhage, commotio retinae, or pigment epithelial contusion. Vision may return to normal; however, if the fovea is involved it often remains poor. Because of damage to Bruch's membrane, patients are at risk for the development of choroidal neovascularization months or years following their initial injury.[3] Laser photocoagulation may be beneficial in treating these membranes.[4] Chorioretinal anastomoses have also been described following choroidal rupture.[5]

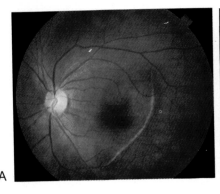

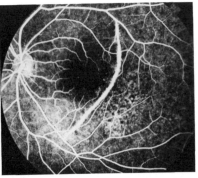

Figure 89–1. A, Choroidal rupture in a 25-year-old man with 20/20 vision who was previously struck in the left eye. B, Angiography shows deep hyperfluorescence in the region of the choroidal rupture. Late frames showed scleral staining without leakage.

Commotio Retinae

First described in 1873,[6] commotio retinae (Berlin's edema) occurs after blunt injury to the eye and is characterized by acute decrease in vision and a gray-white discoloration of the outer retina. This condition may affect the macula or the peripheral retina (Fig. 89–3). The retinal whitening may be accompanied by retinal, subretinal, or preretinal hemorrhage and choroidal rupture.[3] Vision may be restored as the retinal whitening resolves; however, in other cases, central vision loss may be permanent and associated with pigmentary changes and migration or macular hole formation.[7] The peripheral pigmentary changes that may occur following commotio retinae may mimic retinitis pigmentosa.

Fluorescein angiography typically shows no alteration in retinal vascular permeability.[8, 9] Experimentally produced commotio retinae in owl monkeys has shown disruption of the photoreceptor outer segments and acute damage to the photoreceptor cells.[10] This was followed by pigment migration to the ganglion cell layer and, in severe injuries, thinning of the outer plexiform and outer nuclear layers with loss of the photoreceptor outer segments. No evidence of intracellular or extracellular retinal edema was seen in this model, which appears clinically identical to human patients with this condition.

The visual prognosis is good in extrafoveal or mild injuries. Permanent vision loss may occur if there is damage in the fovea. There is no treatment with proven benefit for this condition.

Contusion Necrosis of the RPE and Serous Macular Detachment

Blunt ocular trauma may also cause contusion injury to the RPE, with cream-colored discoloration at the RPE level and patchy staining seen on fluorescein angiography.[11] Leakage through the pigment epithelium may cause serous retinal elevation.[3] The mechanism is unknown; however, some experimental evidence suggests rupture of the RPE cell membranes with associated intracellular edema and damage to the photoreceptor outer segments.[12, 13]

Macular Hole

Because the fovea is especially thin, possessing no inner retinal layers or blood supply, it may be vulnerable to hole formation following blunt trauma. Presumed mechanisms include contusion necrosis, subfoveal hemorrhage, and vitreous traction. Macular holes may be seen in association with commotio retinae, subretinal hemorrhage caused by choroidal rupture, or whiplash separation of the vitreous from the retina.[3] Vision is usually 20/100 to 20/400 following development of a full-thickness macular hole.

Chorioretinitis Sclopetaria

Trauma to the retina and choroid caused by transmitted shock waves from a high-velocity projectile pene-

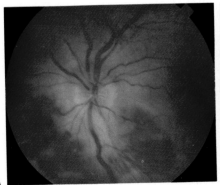

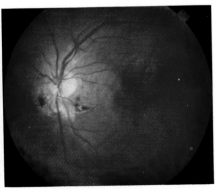

Figure 89–2. A, Choroidal rupture. Acutely after injury, retinal and subretinal hemorrhage and commotio retinae obscure the peripapillary choroidal rupture from view. B, The same patient, 2 mo later. After clearing of the hemorrhage, the peripapillary, concentric choroidal rupture can now be seen.

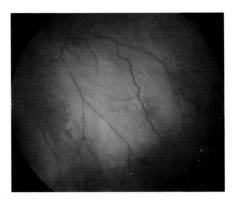

Figure 89–3. Commotio retinae in the extramacular retina. The retinal whitening affects the outer retina and is seen in this patient in association with retinal hemorrhage. One month later, the retinal whitening had resolved with some pigment migration into the neurosensory retina.

trating the orbit but not the globe was described by Goldzieher in 1901 as chorioretinitis sclopetaria.[14] The concussive force of the injury causes rupture of the retina and choroid with associated hemorrhage (Fig. 89–4).

Both the posterior pole and the peripheral retina may be involved, with marked choroidal and retinal hemorrhages associated with tears in these layers. The sclera remains intact, and vitreous hemorrhage may be present. Retinal detachment rarely occurs, and the lesion heals with the formation of a white fibrous scar and associated pigment migration and clumping.[15] The visual prognosis is usually poor because of the initial severity of the injury. Vitrectomy may be used to remove nonclearing vitreous hemorrhage;[16] however, surgery is not usually required.

Traumatic Retinal Tears, Dialysis, and Detachment

Blunt trauma to the eye can cause retinal tears, dialysis, and retinal detachment. Traumatic retinal detachments account for approximately 15 percent of all detachments and tend to occur in a much younger patient population than do nontraumatic detachments. Traumatic detachment is more common in males with a ratio of almost 4 : 1 compared with a similar incidence between the sexes for nontraumatic detachments.[17, 18]

Retinal dialysis is the most common type of retinal break associated with traumatic retinal detachment. It occurs most commonly in the inferotemporal quadrant (31 percent of detachments) followed by the superonasal quadrant (22 percent of detachments). In the same series, giant retinal tears accounted for 16 percent of detachments, retinal flap tears accounted for 11 percent of detachments, and tears in an area of lattice accounted for 8 percent of detachments.[18] Avulsion of the anterior vitreous base in association with detachment always indicates a history of ocular trauma.

Retinal tears associated with ocular trauma may be treated with cryotherapy or photocoagulation. Traumatic retinal detachments can be treated using scleral buckling or vitrectomy techniques.

Optic Nerve Evulsion

Evulsion of the optic nerve is uncommon and is usually associated with profound loss of vision. Cases usually involve severe orbital trauma;[19, 20] however, other cases of partial evulsion have been reported following seemingly minor trauma.[21, 22] Fundus examination shows

Figure 89–4. A, Chorioretinitis sclopetaria. This 16-year-old boy noted decreased vision after being shot with a BB gun from 4 ft away. Vision was 8/200. Note the entry wound in the left lower lid just above the inferior orbital rim. Subconjunctival hemorrhage is also visible. B, Fundus photographs of the inferonasal quadrant in this patient showing the acute appearance of choroidal and retinal rupture with preretinal hemorrhage in chorioretinitis sclopetaria. The sclera remained intact. C, The computed tomography scan shows the location of the BB at the orbital apex. Note that the globe appears intact, without the "flat tire" sign seen in perforating injuries. D, Seven months later, the patient's vision has improved to 20/70. The retina has remained attached without surgical intervention, and a white scar with pigment proliferation and intraretinal pigment migration along its margins is present in the inferonasal quadrant.

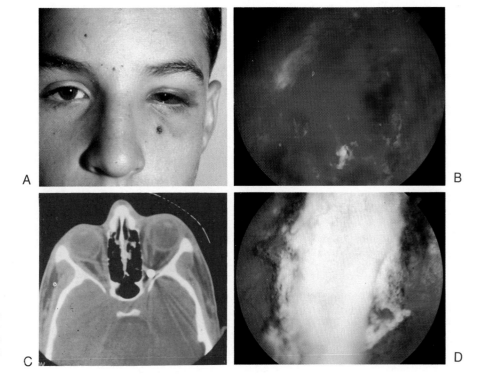

total or partial lack of the optic disc with associated hemorrhage. Partial evulsion may mimic optic nerve pit in appearance. Serous macular detachment has been reported following partial evulsion injury.[21]

Fluorescein angiography may demonstrate normal, partial, or a lack of retinal vascular filling. Computed tomography or magnetic resonance imaging usually demonstrates an intact nerve sheath.[16]

Presumed mechanisms of injury include extreme rotation and anterior globe displacement, a sudden marked increase in intraocular pressure rupturing the lamina cribosa,[19] and contrecoup injury as the markedly retropulsed globe returns to its normal position more rapidly than the more firmly anchored optic nerve is able to.[21, 22]

INDIRECT OCULAR INJURY

Purtscher's Retinopathy

Purtscher described patches of retinal whitening, retinal hemorrhages, and disc edema in a patient with a compression injury to the head in 1912.[23] Patients may experience loss of vision in one or both eyes with similar retinal abnormalities following severe compression injury to the chest.[24]

The characteristic retinal findings in Purtscher's retinopathy are multiple patches of superficial retinal whitening and retinal hemorrhages surrounding the optic nerve. The disc may appear normal initially, but an afferent pupillary defect may be present, and later optic disc edema followed by atrophy may develop. Fluorescein angiography may show leakage of dye in the region of the white retinal patches, retinal and disc edema, venous staining, and areas of capillary nonperfusion.[25]

Several theories have been advanced to explain the pathogenesis of Purtscher's retinopathy. Retinal vascular injury with endothelial damage,[24, 25] complement-induced granulocyte aggregation,[26] air embolism associated with crushing chest injuries,[25] and fat embolism associated with long bone fractures[27] have all been proposed as possible mechanisms. Patients with acute pancreatitis may have associated fat emboli, and present with a Purtscher-like retinopathy.[28] The complement system is also activated in acute pancreatitis, as well as in severe trauma,[16] which leads support to the theory of retinal intravascular clotting as the mechanism of Purtscher's retinopathy.

Terson's Syndrome

Terson's syndrome is the term used to describe the association of retinal and vitreous hemorrhage with subarachnoid and subdural hemorrhage, first described by Terson in 1900.[29] Approximately 20 percent of patients with spontaneous or posttraumatic subarachnoid hemorrhage will present with intraocular hemorrhage.[30] These hemorrhages are typically between the internal limiting membrane and the retina and may occasionally break into the vitreous cavity. The blood usually clears spontaneously; however, in cases of nonclearing vitreous hemorrhage, vitrectomy may be beneficial.[31]

The mechanism of intraocular hemorrhage in Terson's syndrome is thought to be due to bleeding from epipapillary and peripapillary capillaries that are ruptured secondary to a sudden increase in venous pressure.[29]

Valsalva's Retinopathy

Duane first used the term *Valsalva's hemorrhagic retinopathy* in 1972[32] to describe the retinal hemorrhages observed in association with heavy lifting, coughing, vomiting, or straining at stool.

Patients may note a sudden decrease in vision associated with these Valsalva maneuvers. Typical fundus findings include a well-circumscribed, round or dumbbell-shaped, subinternal limiting membrane or intraretinal hemorrhage in or near the fovea. There may be associated vitreous hemorrhage or dissection of blood beneath the retina. The blood is initially bright red, with a prominent light reflex on the surface, but may turn yellow after several days or weeks (Fig. 89–5). A fluid level may develop early, with settling of red blood cells.[3] The visual prognosis is good; most patients return to normal vision.

The presumed mechanism of retinal hemorrhage is rupture of superficial retinal capillaries due to a sudden increase in retinal venous pressure following the rapid increase in intrathoracic or intraabdominal pressure associated with a Valsalva maneuver, such as coughing or vomiting, as previously noted.

Shaken Baby Syndrome

Shaken baby syndrome presents as retinal hemorrhages and cotton-wool spots[3, 33] in an abused infant who may have sustained violent shaking, direct eye, head, or chest trauma, or choking. Papilledema and vitreous

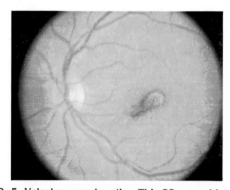

Figure 89–5. Valsalva maculopathy. This 22-year-old man noted decreased vision and a central scotoma immediately after a coughing episode 3 wk prior to presentation. Visual acuity was 20/50. Note the bilobed appearance of the preretinal hemorrhage, now yellow because of hemolysis. Along the inferior margin of the hemorrhage, blood can be seen breaking through the internal limiting membrane and extending into the vitreous cavity inferiorly. One month later, the hemorrhage had almost completely resolved, and vision had improved to 20/25.

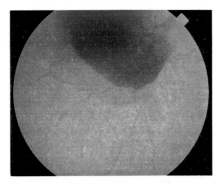

Figure 89–6. Shaken baby syndrome. This 1-month-old child was hospitalized in the neonatal intensive care unit with subarachnoid and subdural hemorrhages due to child abuse. The fundus photograph of the right eye taken at that time demonstrates a large, bean-shaped macular subinternal limiting membrane hemorrhage. A glistening light reflex is present on its surface, and white, intraretinal patches are seen in the macula temporal to the hemorrhage. Similar findings were present in the fellow eye.

hemorrhage may occur in association, along with subdural or subarachnoid hemorrhage or cerebral contusion. Ocular injury may be present in up to 30 to 40 percent of abused children.[33-35] Retinal manifestations are most common (Fig. 89–6) and may appear similar to Terson's syndrome, Purtscher's retinopathy, or central retinal vein occlusion.[3] The prognosis is poor, with children suffering from the sequelae of their intracranial injuries as well as ocular visual loss, which may be secondary to macular scarring, vitreous hemorrhage, or retinal detachment,[36] or from amblyopia. Retinal reattachment surgery or vitrectomy for nonclearing vitreous hemorrhage may be beneficial.[16]

REFERENCES

1. Aguilar JP, Green WR: Choroidal rupture. A histopathologic study of 47 cases. Retina 4:269–275, 1984.
2. von Graefe A: Zwei Falle von Ruptur der Choroidia. Graefes Arch Clin Exp Ophthalmol 1:402, 1854.
3. Gass JDM: Stereoscopic Atlas of Macular Diseases: Diagnosis and Treatment, 3rd ed. St Louis, CV Mosby, 1987, pp 170, 552–565.
4. Fuller B, Gitter KA: Traumatic choroidal rupture with late serous detachment of the macula: Report of successful argon laser treatment. Arch Ophthalmol 89:354–355, 1973.
5. Goldberg MF: Choroidoretinal vascular anastomoses after blunt trauma to the eye. Am J Ophthalmol 82:892–895, 1976.
6. Berlin R: Zur sogenannten Commotio Retinae. Klin Monatsbl Augenheilkd 1:42–78, 1873.
7. Duke-Elder S (ed): System of Ophthalmology, vol. 14, part 1. St Louis, CV Mosby, 1972, p 165. (macular hole following commotio retinae)
8. Pulido JS, Blair NP: The blood-retinal barrier in Berlin's edema. Retina 7:233–236, 1987.
9. Hart JCD, Frank HJ: Retinal opacification after blunt nonperforating concussional injuries to the globe: A clinical and retinal fluorescein angiographic study. Trans Ophthalmol Soc UK 95:94–100, 1975.
10. Sipperley JO, Quigley HA, Gass JD: Traumatic retinopathy in primates: The explanation of commotio retinae. Arch Ophthalmol 96:2267–2273, 1978.
11. Friberg TR: Traumatic retinal pigment epithelial edema. Am J Ophthalmol 88:18–21, 1979.
12. Blight R, Hart JCD: Histological changes in the internal retinal layers produced by concussive injuries to the globe: An experimental study. Trans Ophthalmol Soc UK 98:270–280, 1978.
13. Blight R, Hart JCD: Structural changes in the outer retinal layers following blunt mechanical non-perforating trauma to the globe: An experimental study. Br J Ophthalmol 61:573–587, 1977.
14. Goldzieher W: Beitrag zur Pathologie der orbitalen Schussverletzungen. Z Augenheilkd 6:277, 1901.
15. Richards RD, West CE, Meisels AA: Chorioretinitis sclopetaria. Am J Ophthalmol 66:852–860, 1968.
16. Williams DF, Mieler WF, Williams GA: Posterior segment manifestations of ocular trauma. Retina 10:S35–S44, 1990.
17. Cox MS, Schepens CL, Freeman HM: Retinal detachment due to ocular contusion. Arch Ophthalmol 76:678–685, 1966.
18. Goffstein R, Burton TC: Differentiating traumatic from nontraumatic retinal detachment. Ophthalmology 89:361–368, 1982.
19. Lister W: Some concussive changes met with in military practise. Br J Ophthalmol 8:305, 1924.
20. Caiger H: Ocular injuries resulting from the war. Trans Ophthalmol Soc UK 61:54–73, 1941.
21. Delaney WV, Geiss M: Partial evulsion of the optic nerve. Ann Ophthalmol 20:371–372, 1988.
22. Chow AY, Goldberg MF, Frenkel M: Evulsion of the optic nerve in association with basketball injuries. Ann Ophthalmol 72:969–971, 1971.
23. Purtscher O: Angiopathia retinae traumatica. Lymphorrhagien des Augengrundes. Graefes Arch Clin Exp Ophthalmol 82:347–371, 1912.
24. Kellen JS: Purtscher's retinopathy related to chest compression by safety belts: Fluorescein angiographic findings. Am J Ophthalmol 74:278–283, 1972.
25. Burton TC: Unilateral Purtscher's retinopathy. Ophthalmology 87:1096–1105, 1980.
26. Jacob HS, Craddock PR, Hammerschmidt DE, Moldow CF: Complement-induced granulocyte aggregation. An unsuspected mechanism of disease. N Engl J Med 302:789–794, 1980.
27. Urbanek J: Uber Fettembolie des Auges. Graefes Arch Clin Exp Ophthalmol 131:147–173, 1934.
28. Inkeles DM, Walsh JB: Retinal fat emboli as a sequela to acute pancreatitis. Am J Ophthalmol 80:935–938, 1975.
29. Terson A: De l'hemorragie dans le corps vitre au cours de l'hemorragie cerebrale. Clin Ophthalmol 6:309, 1900.
30. Shaw HE Jr, Landers MB III, Sydnor CF: The significance of intraocular hemorrhages due to subarachnoid hemorrhage. Ann Ophthalmol 9:1403–1405, 1977.
31. Clarkson JG, Flynn HW Jr, Daily MJ: Vitrectomy in Terson's syndrome. Am J Ophthalmol 90:549–552, 1980.
32. Duane TD: Valsalva hemorrhagic retinopathy. Trans Am Ophthalmol Soc 70:298–313, 1972.
33. Harley RD: Ocular manifestations of child abuse. J Pediatr Ophthalmol Strabismus 17:5–13, 1980.
34. Friendly DS: Ocular manifestation of the physical child abuse. Trans Am Acad Ophthalmol Otolaryngol 75:318–332, 1971.
35. Jensen AD: Ocular clues to child abuse. J Pediatr Ophthalmol 8:270, 1971.
36. Harcourt B, Hopkins D: Permanent chorioretinal lesions in childhood of suspected origin. Trans Ophthalmol Soc UK 93:199–205, 1973.

Chapter 90

■

Photic Retinopathy

MONICA A. DE LA PAZ and DONALD J. D'AMICO

LIGHT DAMAGE AND THE EYE

Visible light is radiation that spans a region of the electromagnetic spectrum from 400 to 700 nm. Higher wavelengths extend into the infrared region, and lower wavelengths continue into the ultraviolet (UV) range. The damaging effects of light on the eye have been recognized for centuries. According to Plato, Socrates advised that a solar eclipse should be observed only by looking at its reflection in water.[1] Galileo injured his eye while looking at the sun through his telescope.[1] It has been suggested that the blindness of Saul of Tarsus was from solar retinopathy.[2]

Three recognized mechanisms of light injury include thermal, mechanical, and photochemical damage.[3–6] Thermal damage results from extensive light absorption in the retinal pigment epithelium (RPE) and surrounding structures, which causes a local temperature elevation. The end result is coagulation of retinal proteins and tissue disruption. An example of a cause of thermal injury is clinical laser photocoagulation.

Mechanical light damage results when the retinal power density of the absorbed light is high enough to cause sonic transients, gaseous formation, or shock waves that mechanically disrupt retinal tissue. The injury may be due to ionizing effects that strip electrons from molecules in the target tissue, producing a collection of ions and electrons known as *plasma*.[4] Tissue damage is the result of rapid plasma expansion and tissue stress. An example of a cause of mechanical light damage is the Q-switched or mode-locked neodymium-ytrrium-aluminum-garnet (Nd.YAG) laser burns set at nanosecond to picosecond durations.

Photochemical injury is a form of light damage that is a consequence of certain biochemical reactions, resulting in the degeneration of retinal tissues when there is no temperature elevation. The pathologic condition is primarily localized to the photoreceptors, and light exposures are longer than those for thermal or mechanical damage. The outer segments are most sensitive, and slow recovery is possible if the damage does not destroy the inner segments of the photoreceptors.[7] Although the exact mechanism is unknown, it is most likely due to tissue oxidation induced by free radical formation resulting in lipid peroxidation.[3, 5] Experimental evidence in the rat supports this mechanism.[8] The end result is an inhibition of metabolic homeostasis resulting from disruption of cellular membranes.[5] It has also been suggested that liberation of toxic photoproducts secondary to chronic bleaching from light exposure may be involved.[8] Environmental and near-UV light have been implicated in this form of damage.[9, 10] Solar retinopathy

and photic retinopathy from the operating microscope are examples of causes of photochemical injury.

Boettner and Wolter[11] measured the spectral transmittance of light in humans. They found that the maximal total transmittance of the eye is approximately 84 percent and is obtained in the region of the spectrum from 650 to 840 nm. The transmittance of ocular media falls rapidly in the 400- to 440-nm range, primarily because of absorption by the lens. Ham and Mueller[12] found that the retinal sensitivity increased in the blue-wavelength region of the visible spectrum. Although the retinal sensitivity increases in this wavelength range, the number of photons reaching the retina is reduced dramatically by the absorption and scattering of the lens.[87] The eye has other protective mechanisms against photochemical damage, including pupillary constriction, photosensitivity with eye closure, light absorption by melanin in the retinal pigment epithelium, and antioxidants such as superoxide dismutase, catalase, peroxidase, and vitamin E.[13]

SOLAR RETINOPATHY

Solar retinopathy is a well-recognized clinical entity of retinal damage caused by direct or indirect viewing of the sun. Synonymous terms include *foveomacular retinitis*, *eclipse retinopathy*, and *solar retinitis*.

The first clinical description of retinal damage in association with the viewing of an eclipse was by Saint-Yves in 1722.[1] There have subsequently been numerous reports of clusters of cases of photic retinopathy resulting from viewing an eclipse.[1, 15–17] Affected individuals present with decreased vision after observing an eclipse without wearing appropriate protective eyewear.

Foveomacular retinitis was originally described as a distinct clinical syndrome of unknown cause consisting of bilateral decreased vision and foveal lesions in young military personnel.[18–21] In many instances, however, a history of sun gazing was subsequently elicited.[22, 23, 84, 86] Many of these patients were diagnosed with psychiatric disorders.[22] In some cases, there was an association with drug use or an attempt to manipulate a change to noncombat duty or discharge.[22] Other cases occur in military personnel who have followed the flight of airplanes near the sun.[18, 24]

Photic retinopathy has also been described in association with direct sun gazing by sunbathers[6] and patients with psychotic disorders,[25] as part of religious rituals,[24] and in association with the use of drugs such as lysergic acid diethylamide (LSD).[22, 26, 27] The appearance and clinical course in each instance is identical.

Various factors have been implicated in determining the severity of the retinal lesion. Increasing length of exposure is a risk factor.[6] However, severe lesions have been described in individuals with minimal exposure, and vice versa. It has been suggested but not proved that increasing fundus pigmentation may protect against photic damage.[1, 17] Patients with uncorrected high refractive errors may be protected when compared with emmetropes because the damaging light is inadequately focused on the retina.[1] In the presence of amblyopia or strabismus, the dominant eye is more susceptible to damage.[17] Younger patients may be at increased risk because the transmissibility of the lens to damaging visible blue and UV light decreases with age.[11] LSD induces mydriasis and cycloplegia, which make the drug abuser more susceptible to severe retinal burn because of inhibition of the usual protective effects of miosis and ciliary spasm.[22] An increased risk of retinal damage has been associated with the use of certain drugs that photosensitize the eye.[6] Examples include tetracycline and psoralen. In addition, it has also been suggested that certain geophysical factors such as a reduction in the ozone layer and the distance of the sun from the earth are risk factors.[6]

Prior to 1970, the cause was believed to be due to thermal damage produced by the absorption of infrared rays by the RPE.[15] Studies in rhesus monkeys subsequently demonstrated that similar lesions can be produced by exposure to blue light at powers too low to generate a temperature elevation in the retina, providing evidence for a photochemical mechanism of damage.[28] It is postulated that the principal mechanism of photochemical damage is from retinal irradiance by high-energy wavelengths, including short wavelength–visible blue light and lower levels of UVA or near-UV radiation (320 to 400 nm).[6]

Symptoms of solar retinopathy usually develop within 1 to 4 hr after exposure and include decreased vision, metamorphopsia, micropsia, and central or paracentral scotomata of 1 to 7 degrees. Patients may also present with chromatopsia, photophobia, after image, and frontal or temporal headache with orbital or retroorbital pain. Acutely, vision usually ranges from 20/40 to 20/100 but may be worse. There is no correlation between the severity of the fundus lesion and the visual acuity.[16]

The fundus examination is variable. Although usually bilateral, unilateral cases are not uncommon. The typical lesion is a small yellow spot with a surrounding gray zone in the foveolar or parafoveolar area within the first few days after exposure. In mild cases, however, little or no change can be noted. The foveal reflex may be lacking but becomes more distinct as the lesion resolves. After several days, the yellow spot becomes reddish with a halo of surrounding pigmentary change. By 10 to 14 days, this lesion fades and is usually replaced by a red, well-circumscribed, faceted lamellar hole or depression (Fig. 90–1A). The oval lamellar depression, which has a diameter of 100 to 200 μ, is believed to be permanent and is highly suggestive of a previous episode of sun gazing.[6, 29] There may be a larger area of foveal or parafoveal mottling of the RPE.[6] Several lesions may be present, suggestive of multiple episodes of sun gazing. Similar lesions have been produced by blunt trauma[23] and whiplash injury.[30]

Fluorescein angiography is often normal in the early and late stages of the disease. In some patients, focal areas of staining corresponding to the macular lesions are noted.[85] Leakage of fluorescein is rare but has been described in the acute stages.[31] Days to weeks later, the only finding may be small spots of hyperfluorescence caused by changes in the RPE (Fig. 90–1B). It has been postulated that the presence of xanthophyll in the fovea may be responsible for the difficulty in demonstrating minor retinal pigment epithelial changes in many patients.[29]

Visual acuity usually improves to 20/20 to 20/40 by 6 mo.[17] Kerr[19] found that patients with acute visual acuities of less than 20/200 had a worse prognosis for recovery of visual function. Even with improvement in visual acuity, there may be residual metamorphopsia or paracentral or central scotomata. MacFaul[32] suggests that the best prognostic guide for recovery is the rate of return of visual acuity and the behavior of the scotoma within the first month after injury.

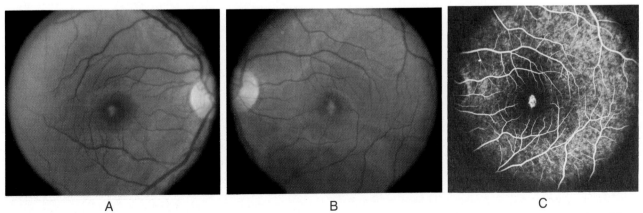

A   B   C

Figure 90–1. A and B, Fundus photographs of a 27-year-old man with a history of sun gazing 1 yr prior to presentation. Bilateral reddish-yellow foveal lesions are present. C, Fluorescein angiography of the left eye of the same patient. Focal staining in the arteriovenous phase corresponds to the site of the lesion in the fundus photograph. No late leakage is present. (A and B, courtesy of Mark W. Balles, M.D.)

Tso[31] has studied the histopathologic features of lesions in patients who gazed at the sun for 1 hr prior to enucleation for uveal melanoma. Approximately 2 days after sun gazing, most of the injury involved the RPE. Necrosis, pigment granule irregularity, and focal detachments of the retinal pigment epithelium were described. In one patient who demonstrated early leakage on fluorescein angiography, a focal detachment of the sensory retina was found at the site of the lesion. The photoreceptors were intact. The RPE adjacent to the lesion lost its apical pigment granules and extended along Bruch's membrane beneath the detached RPE. After 48 hr to 5 days, there is photoreceptor destruction. Much of this damage is reversible and may explain the ability of many patients to recover good visual function after sun gazing.[29]

Oral corticosteroids have been used in the treatment of acute lesions associated with severe visual loss.[17, 19, 22] However, no beneficial effect has been clearly demonstrated, primarily because lesions tend to spontaneously improve without treatment. Appropriate protective measures when viewing an eclipse and education about the hazards of direct sun gazing are of utmost importance in the prevention of this disease.

PHOTIC RETINOPATHY FROM OPHTHALMIC INSTRUMENTS

The potentially damaging effect of light from ophthalmic instruments has been recognized since 1973, when Tso demonstrated a characteristic retinopathy in rhesus monkeys after exposure to the light of an indirect ophthalmoscope for 1 hr.[33] In 1983, McDonald and Irvine[34] described a characteristic macular lesion in a group of patients who had undergone recent cataract extraction and intraocular lens placement. They noted that the lesion resembled the light-induced lesion in rhesus monkeys described by Tso. A clear cause-and-effect relationship was established by Robertson and Feldman in 1986,[35] when they demonstrated that a 60-min exposure to light from an operating microscope can cause a retinal lesion in humans. The exact incidence is unknown. In a review of 135 consecutive patients who had undergone cataract extraction, retinal changes suggestive of photic retinopathy were found in 10 patients (7.4 percent).[36]

Subsequently, there have been numerous reports in the literature of retinal lesions caused by the light from ophthalmic instruments. Most cases pertain to the operating microscope.[34–45] Other implicated ophthalmic instruments include the indirect ophthalmoscope,[5, 46–49] the fiberoptic endoilluminator used in vitrectomies,[50, 51] the direct ophthalmoscope,[47] and the slit lamp.[52] Experimental ophthalmic light–induced retinal lesions from light sources other than the operating microscope have been described in animal studies but have not been described in humans. Of significance is the fact that the retinal irradiance of the operating room microscope is up to 10 times higher than that of the indirect ophthalmoscope.[39]

Studies in pseudophakic rhesus monkeys demonstrate that the threshold exposure with the high-intensity setting of the coaxial illumination of the Zeiss OpMi-6 30W operating microscope for an ophthalmoscopically visible lesion is between 4 and 7.5 min.[53] Irreversible retinal lesions induced by the indirect ophthalmoscope require approximately 15 min of exposure.[47] Retinal damage is noted after 40 min of exposure to the slit lamp[52] and after 1 hr of exposure to the direct ophthalmoscope.[47]

Photic retinopathy by the operating microscope is believed to be caused by photochemical damage from the focusing of high-intensity coaxial light on the retina.[34, 53, 54] Much of the damage may be due to short-wavelength blue light and UV light.[53, 56] The filtering of shorter-wavelength light lessens the degree of retinal damage.[43] It has also been suggested that infrared light may be involved because much of the irradiance produced by ophthalmic instruments has a wavelength greater than 700 nm.[57]

The most significant risk factor in the development of photic retinopathy from the operating microscope is a prolonged operating time. Khwarg and associates[36] found that the mean operating time in affected patients was significantly higher at 124 min, compared with 73 min in unaffected patients. No significant difference in the rate of retinopathy in patients with and without intraocular lenses has been shown. Lack of UV filters in intraocular lenses and operating room microscopes is a contributing factor.[43, 52, 58, 59] Photic retinopathy in a phakic patient who underwent refractive surgery has been described, indicating that the presence of the crystalline lens does not adequately protect the retina.[38] Failure to constrict the pupil intraoperatively after cataract extraction has been suggested to increase the risk of damage.[42]

The intensity of the light beam is also an important factor. Berler and Peyser[54] found that increased intensity of the operating microscope is associated with decreased postoperative visual acuity in patients who have undergone cataract surgery. The risk of light damage from fiberoptic endoilluminators may be higher with increasing proximity to the retina, such as in membrane peeling procedures.[51]

In addition, higher temperatures are associated with photic damage. Retinal damage is potentiated by elevated body temperature.[47, 49] Rinkoff and colleagues[60] demonstrated that a hypothermic infusion fluid during vitreous surgery reduced the risk of retinal light damage induced by the fiberoptic probe.

In most instances, patients are asymptomatic, and a suggestive lesion is noted postoperatively on biomicroscopic examination. When symptomatic, patients may note decreased vision or paracentral scotoma, usually on the first or second postoperative day. Vision usually returns to normal after several months. In some cases, a paracentral scotoma may persist.

The retinal lesion consists of an oval area of a light yellow to white deep retinal lesion with a size varying from 0.8 to 2.5 disc diameters. The shape of the lesion resembles the illuminating source.[37] Halogen-fiberoptic illuminating sources produce round or irregular oval lesions with the long axis vertically oriented, whereas tungsten sources produce round or horizontal oval lesions. Most lesions are not centered on the fovea but assume a parafoveal location. The distance from the foveal center usually ranges from 0 to 2.5 disc diameters. One study found the lesions to be usually located inferior to the fovea,[36] and another study found a tendency for lesions to be in the temporal macula.[37] Rarely, they are located outside the arcades. The size and shape may also be related to the eye position during surgery, the duration of exposure, and the focusing of the microscope. Lesions inferior to the fovea may represent the use of a superior bridle suture to infraduct the globe.[36] Mottled pigmentation of the lesion occurs over the next few weeks. In the late stages, the lesion changes to a sharply outlined area of retinal pigment epithelial atrophy (Fig. 90–2A). Occasionally, multiple parafoveal satellite lesions may be present.

Fluorescein angiography demonstrates intense staining of the acute lesion. Irregular window defects corresponding to the retinal pigment epithelial changes are noted in the presence of late-stage lesions (Fig. 90–2B). Leakage is not a characteristic finding.

The histopathologic appearance of a human eye exposed to unfiltered light from an operating microscope for 60 min prior to enucleation at 72 hr for uveal melanoma demonstrated extensive changes in the retina and RPE.[58] There was localized necrosis, loss of apical villi, and extrusion of pigment granules of the RPE. Extensive photoreceptor outer segment disruption was found. Near the margins of the lesion, the RPE appeared to be migrating under the injured pigment epithelium, suggesting an attempt to repair the damage. Studies in the rhesus monkey after prolonged exposure to the indirect ophthalmoscope demonstrate similar acute findings, which are followed by the formation of a plaque of spindle cells between Bruch's membrane and the RPE at the site of the lesion by 3 mo.[49] There is a tendency of the photoreceptor outer segments to regenerate, although some irregularity can persist.

As in the case of solar retinopathy, prevention is of great importance. UV protective intraocular lenses, which were introduced in 1978, have been shown to decrease the risk of photic retinopathy in animals.[61] Currently, the majority of implanted intraocular lenses protect against UV light. It is also recommended that filtration to cut off wavelengths less than 450 nm be incorporated into the operating microscope illumination system.[62] Glass fiberoptic bundles automatically provide very good UV light absorption, perhaps making further filtration unnecessary.[63] The avoidance of intense illumination by reducing the brightness as much as possible is recommended.[89] Oblique illumination during wound closure may help to place the intense image of the beam in the retinal periphery.[63] Various measures to defocus the illumination beam on the retina by placing an air bubble in the anterior chamber do not prevent photic retinopathy.[36] Pupil constriction and the use of corneal covers and eclipse filters to limit retinal illumination during prolonged operations is also recommended. It has been suggested that interference filters be used to block wavelengths greater than 700 nm to reduce total light exposure without interfering with image quality,[3] that vitreoretinal surgeons avoid warming infusion fluids to greater than room temperature,[60] and that low wavelengths be filtered as much as possible.[50]

It has been postulated but not proved that chronic cystoid macular edema after cataract surgery is caused by photic damage from the operating microscope.[39, 64, 65, 88] Kraff and coworkers[66] conducted a prospective randomized study to assess the effect of UV filtration in intraocular lenses on the angiographic evidence of cystoid macular edema in patients who underwent cataract surgery. The use of intraocular lenses with UV filters resulted in a statistically significant decrease in the incidence of cystoid macular edema. However, in a prospective randomized study of patients undergoing extracapsular cataract extraction and intraocular lens insertion, Jampol and associates[67] found that the presence of UV filter on the operating microscope made no difference in the angiographic incidence of cystoid macular edema or the visual outcome.

WELDING ARC MACULOPATHY

Unprotected exposure to a welding arc results in a form of photic retinopathy.[29, 68–70] Photochemical damage by wavelengths at the blue end of the visible spectrum, rather than thermal damage, is believed to be the mechanism of injury.[71] Patients usually present with decreased vision after welding without goggles. The biomicroscopic examination and course resembles those of solar retinopathy.[29]

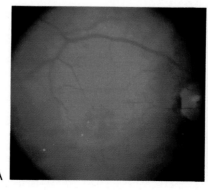 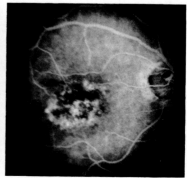

Figure 90–2. A, Fundus photograph of a 67-year-old man 2 yr after cataract extraction. Visual acuity is 20/50. There is an area of depigmentation near the fovea consistent with photic maculopathy. B, Fluorescein angiography of the same patient demonstrates mottled hyperfluorescence in the fovea corresponding to the retinal pigment epithelial changes.

A   B

ACCIDENTAL LASER BURNS

Retinal damage from accidental exposure to a laser can result in immediate loss of vision.[72-77] Clinically, the lesion may resemble that of clinical laser photocoagulation. Damage occurs by a thermal or mechanical mechanism, depending on the type of laser. A retinal scar subsequently develops. Although vision may improve, a paracentral or central scotoma may persist.

PHOTOTOXICITY AND THE AGING MACULA

The relationship of light damage to age-related macular degeneration has been suggested but remains unproved.[3, 13, 78-80] The cumulative effect of repeated mild photic insult during life may increase the susceptibility of the aging macula to degenerative changes.

Light activates destructive oxidizing reactions in the retina, resulting in the initiation of free-radical reactions and peroxidation of lipids in the photoreceptor membranes.[55] This has been demonstrated in the rat retina.[8] Rod outer segment membranes are particularly susceptible to peroxidative damage because they contain extremely high levels of polyunsaturated fatty acids.[81]

Experimental evidence suggests that the susceptibility of human retinal tissue from the posterior pole to peroxidative damage increases with age and that the susceptibility of the posterior pole is distinctly higher than that of the retinal periphery.[82] Whether this is related to chronic light exposure or some other factor resulting in dysfunction of the normal protective mechanisms against oxidative damage is a subject of current investigation.

It has been postulated that antioxidants such as ascorbate and vitamin E protect the retina from light damage by terminating destructive free-radical–mediated reactions.[13, 83] Epidemiologic studies are currently in progress to determine whether supplemental antioxidants in the diet retard the progression of disease in patients with age-related macular degeneration. The identification of an environmental factor such as chronic light exposure or an antioxidant vitamin deficiency may provide a basis for a program of preventive medicine.

REFERENCES

1. Duke-Elder SS: Radiational injuries. In System of Ophthalmology, vol. 14, part 2. St Louis, CV Mosby, 1972, p 888.
2. Manchester PT, Manchester PT: The blindness of Saint Paul. Arch Ophthalmol 88:316–321, 1972.
3. Mainster MA, Ham WT, DeLori FC: Potential retinal hazards. Instrument and environmental light sources. Ophthalmology 90:927–932, 1983.
4. Mainster MA: The spectra, classification, and rationale of ultraviolet-protective intraocular lenses. Am J Ophthalmol 102:727–732, 1986.
5. Tso MOM, Woodford BJ: Effect of photic injury on the retinal tissues. Ophthalmology 90:952–963, 1983.
6. Yanuzzi LA, Fisher YL, Krueger A, Slakter J: Solar retinopathy: A photobiological and geophysical analysis. Trans Am Ophthalmol Soc 85:120–154, 1987.
7. Lanum J: The damaging effects of light on the retina. Empirical

findings. Theoretical and practical implications. Surv Ophthalmol 22:221–249, 1978.
8. Wiegand RD, Giusto NM, Rapp LM, Anderson RE: Evidence for rod outer segment lipid peroxidation following illumination of the rat retina. Invest Ophthalmol Vis Sci 24:1433–1435, 1983.
9. Rapp LM, Tolman BL, Dhindsa HS: Separate mechanisms for retinal damage by ultraviolet-A and mid-visible light. Invest Ophthalmol Vis Sci 31:1186–1193, 1990.
10. Zigman S: Effects of near-ultraviolet radiation on the lens and retina. Doc Ophthalmol 55:375–391, 1983.
11. Boettner EA, Wolter JR: Transmission of the ocular media. Invest Ophthalmol 1:776–783, 1962.
12. Ham WT, Mueller HA: Retinal sensitivity to damage from short wavelength light. Nature 260:153–155, 1976.
13. Mainster MA: Light and macular degeneration: A biophysical and clinical perspective. Eye 1:304–310, 1987.
14. Agarwal LP, Malik SRK: Solar retinitis. Br J Ophthalmol 43:366–370, 1959.
15. Cordes FC: Eclipse retinopathy. Am J Ophthalmol 31:101–102, 1948.
16. Dhir SP, Gupta A, Jain IS: Eclipse retinopathy. Br J Ophthalmol 65:42–45, 1981.
17. Penner R, McNair JN: Eclipse blindness. Am J Ophthalmol 61:1452–1457, 1966.
18. Cordes FC: A type of foveo-macular retinitis observed in the US Navy. Am J Ophthalmol 27:803–816, 1944.
19. Kerr LM, Little HL: Foveomacular retinitis. Arch Ophthalmol 76:498–504, 1966.
20. Kuming BS: Foveomacular retinitis. Br J Ophthalmol 70:816–818, 1986.
21. Marlor RL, Blaise BR, Preston FR, Bowden DG: Foveomacular retinitis, an important problem in military medicine: Epidemiology. Invest Ophthalmol 12:5–16, 1973.
22. Ewald RA: Sun gazing associated with the use of LSD. Ann Ophthalmol 3:15–17, 1971.
23. Grey RHB: Foveo-macular retinitis, solar retinopathy, and trauma. Br J Ophthalmol 62:543–546, 1978.
24. Rosen E: Solar retinitis. Br J Ophthalmol 32:23–35, 1948.
25. Anaclerio A, Wicker HC: Self-induced solar retinopathy by patients in a psychiatric hospital. Am J Ophthalmol 69:731–736, 1970.
26. Fuller DG: Severe solar maculopathy associated with the use of lysergic acid diethylamide (LSD). Am J Ophthalmol 81:413–416, 1976.
27. Schatz H, Mendelblatt F: Solar retinopathy from sun-gazing under the influence of LSD. Br J Ophthalmol 57:270–273, 1973.
28. Ham WT, Ruffolo JJ, Mueller HA, et al: Histologic analysis of photochemical lesions produced in rhesus retina by short-wavelength light. Invest Ophthalmol Vis Sci 17:1029–1035, 1978.
29. Gass JDM: Stereoscopic Atlas of Macular Diseases, 3rd ed, vol. 2. St Louis, CV Mosby, 1987, pp 570–579.
30. Kelley JS, Hoover RE, George T: Whiplash maculopathy. Arch Ophthalmol 96:834–835, 1978.
31. Tso MOM, LaPiana FG: The human fovea after sungazing. Trans Am Acad Ophthalmol Otolaryngol 79:OP788–795, 1975.
32. MacFaul PA: Visual prognosis after solar retinopathy. Br J Ophthalmol 53:534–541, 1969.
33. Tso MOM: Photic maculopathy in rhesus monkey. A light and electron microscopic study. Invest Ophthalmol 12:17–34, 1973.
34. McDonald HR, Irvine AR: Light-induced maculopathy from the operating microscope in extracapsular cataract extraction and intraocular lens implantation. Ophthalmology 90:945–951, 1983.
35. Robertson DM, Feldman RB: Photic retinopathy from the operating room microscope. Am J Ophthalmol 101:561–569, 1986.
36. Khwarg SG, Linstone FA, Daniels SA, et al: Incidence, risk factors, and morphology in operating microscope light retinopathy. Am J Ophthalmol 103:255–263, 1987.
37. Boldrey EE, Ho BT, Griffith RD: Retinal burns occurring at cataract extraction. Ophthalmology 91:1297–1302, 1984.
38. Brod RD, Barron BA, Suelflow JA, et al: Phototoxic retinal damage during refractive surgery. Am J Ophthalmol 102:121–123, 1986.
39. Calkins JL, Hochheimer BF: Retinal light exposure from operation microscope. Arch Ophthalmol 97:2363–2367, 1979.
40. Irvine AR, Wood I, Morris BW: Retinal damage from the

illumination of the operating microscope. An experimental study in pseudophakic monkeys. Arch Ophthalmol 102:1358–1365, 1984.

41. Johnson RN, Schatz H, McDonald HR: Photic maculopathy: Early angiographic and ophthalmoscopic findings and late development of choroidal folds. Arch Ophthalmol 105:1633–1634, 1987.

42. Khwarg SG, Geoghegan M, Hanscom TA: Light-induced maculopathy from the operating microscope. Am J Ophthalmol 98:628–630, 1984.

43. Parver LM, Auker CR, Fine BS: Observations on monkey eyes exposed to light from an operating microscope. Ophthalmology 90:964–972, 1983.

44. Robertson DM, McLaren JW: Photic retinopathy from the operating room microscope. Study with filters. Arch Ophthalmol 107:373–375, 1989.

45. Ross WH: Light-induced maculopathy. Am J Ophthalmol 98:488–493, 1984.

46. Borges J, Li Z-Y, Tso MOM: Effect of repeated photic exposures on the monkey macula. Arch Ophthalmol 108:727–733, 1990.

47. Friedman E, Kuwabara T: The retinal pigment epithelium. IV. The damaging effects of radiant energy. Arch Ophthalmol 80:265–279, 1968.

48. Tso MOM, Wallow IHL, Powell JO, Zimmerman LE: Recovery of the rod and cone cells after photic injury. Trans Am Acad Ophthalmol Otolaryngol 76:1247–1262, 1972.

49. Tso MOM, Fine BS, Zimmerman LE: Photic maculopathy produced by the indirect ophthalmoscope. Am J Ophthalmol 73:686–699, 1972.

50. Meyers SM, Bonner RF: Yellow filter to decrease the risk of light damage to the retina during vitrectomy. Am J Ophthalmol 94:677, 1982.

51. Meyers SM, Bonner RF: Retinal irradiance from vitrectomy endoilluminators. Am J Ophthalmol 94:26–29, 1982.

52. Hochheimer BF, D'Anna SA, Calkins JL: Retinal damage from light. Am J Ophthalmol 88:1039–1044, 1979.

53. Irvine AR, Wood I, Morris BW: Retinal damage from the illumination of the operating microscope: An experimental study in pseudophakic monkeys. Trans Am Ophthalmol Soc 82:239–260, 1984.

54. Berler DK, Peyser R: Light intensity and visual acuity following cataract surgery. Ophthalmology 90:933–936, 1983.

55. Noell WK, Walker VS, Kang BS, Berman S: Retinal damage by light in rats. Invest Ophthalmol 5:450–473, 1966.

56. Ham WT, Mueller HA, Ruffolo JJ, et al: Action spectrum for retinal injury from near-ultraviolet radiation in the aphakic monkey. Am J Ophthalmol 93:299–306, 1982.

57. Michels M, Dawson WW, Feldman RB, Jarolem K: Infrared. An unseen and unnecessary hazard in ophthalmic devices. Ophthalmology 94:143–148, 1987.

58. Green WR, Robertson DM: Pathologic findings of photic retinopathy in the human eye. Am J Ophthalmol 112:520–527, 1991.

59. Werner JS, Hardenbergh FE: Spectral sensitivity of the pseudophakic eye. Arch Ophthalmol 101:758–763, 1983.

60. Rinkoff FJ, Machemer R, Hida T, Chandler D: Temperature-dependent light damage to the retina. Am J Ophthalmol 102:452–462, 1986.

61. Peyman GA, Zak R, Sloane H: Ultraviolet-absorbing pseudophakos. An efficacy study. J Am Intraocul Implant Soc 9:161, 1983.

62. Keates RH, Armstrong PF: Use of a short-wavelength filter in an operating microscope. Ophthalmic Surg 16:40–41, 1985.

63. McIntyre DJ: Phototoxicity. The eclipse filter. Ophthalmology 92:361–365, 1985.

64. Henry MM, Henry LM, Henry LM: A possible cause of chronic cyclic maculopathy. Ann Ophthalmol 9:455–457, 1977.

65. Mannis MJ, Becker B: Retinal light exposure and cystoid macular edema. Arch Ophthalmol 98:1133, 1980.

66. Kraff MC, Sanders DR, Jampol LM, Lieberman HL: Effect of an ultraviolet-filtering intraocular lens on cystoid macular edema. Ophthalmology 92:366–369, 1985.

67. Jampol LM, Kraff MC, Sanders DR, et al: Near-UV radiation from the operating microscope and pseudophakic cystoid macular edema. Arch Ophthalmol 103:28–30, 1985.

68. Romanchuk KG, Pollak V, Schneider RJ: Retinal burn from a welding arc. Can J Ophthalmol 13:120–122, 1978.

69. Uniat L, Olk RJ, Hanish SJ: Welding arc maculopathy. Am J Ophthalmol 102:394–395, 1986.

70. Wurdemann HV: The formation of a hole in the macula. Light burn from exposure to electric welding. Am J Ophthalmol 19:457–459, 1936.

71. Naidoff MA, Sliney DH: Retinal injury from a welding arc. Am J Ophthalmol 77:663–668, 1974.

72. Boldrey EE, Little HL, Flocks M, et al: Retinal injury due to industrial laser burns. Ophthalmology 88:101–107, 1981.

73. Curtin TL, Boyden DG: Reflected laser beam causing accidental burn of retina. Am J Ophthalmol 65:188–189, 1968.

74. Fowler BJ: Accidental industrial laser burn of macula. Ann Ophthalmol 15:481–483, 1983.

75. Jacobson JH, McClean JM: Accidental laser retinal burns. Arch Ophthalmol 74:882, 1965.

76. Rathky AS: Accidental laser burn of the macula. Arch Ophthalmol 74:346–348, 1965.

77. Zweng HC: Accidental Q-switched laser lesion of human macula. Arch Ophthalmol 78:596–599, 1967.

78. Pryor WA: The free radical theory of aging revisited: A critique and a specific disease-specific theory. In Butler RN, Sprott RL, Schneider EL (eds): Modern Biological Theories of Aging. New York, Raven Press, 1987, pp 42–63.

79. Tso MOM: Pathogenetic factors of aging macular degeneration. Ophthalmology 92:628–635, 1985.

80. Young RW: Solar radiation and age-related macular degeneration. Surv Ophthalmol 32:252–269, 1988.

81. Fliesler SJ, Anderson RE: Chemistry and metabolism of lipids in the vertebrate retina. Prog Lipid Res 22:79, 1983.

82. De La Paz MA, Anderson RE: Regional and age-dependent variation of the human retina to oxidative damage. Invest Ophthalmol Vis Sci, in press.

83. Li Z-Y, Tso MOM, Woodford BJ, et al: Amelioration of photic injury in rat retina by ascorbic acid. ARVO abstracts. Invest Ophthalmol Vis Sci 25(Suppl):90, 1984.

84. Ewald RA: Sun gazing as the cause of foveomacular retinitis. Am J Ophthalmol 70:491–497, 1970.

85. Freedman J, Gombos GM: Fluorescein fundus angiography in self-induced solar retinopathy. Can J Ophthalmol 6:124–127, 1971.

86. Gladstone GJ, Tasman W: Solar retinitis after minimal exposure. Arch Ophthalmol 96:1368–1369, 1978.

87. Ham WT, Mueller HA, Ruffolo JJ, Clarke AM: Sensitivity of the retina to radiation damage as a function of wavelength. Photochem Photobiol 29:735, 1979.

88. Hochheimer BF: A possible cause of chronic cyclic maculopathy: The operating microscope. Ann Ophthalmol 13:153–155, 1981.

89. Sliney DH: Eye protective techniques for bright lights. Ophthalmology 90:937–944, 1983.

Chapter 91

■

Radiation Retinopathy

SHIZUO MUKAI, DAVID R. GUYER, and
EVANGELOS S. GRAGOUDAS

Radiation retinopathy is a slowly progressive, delayed-onset disease of retinal blood vessels that occurs secondary to ionizing radiation treatment. Alteration in the structure and permeability of retinal and optic nerve blood vessels usually develops months to years after exposure to radiation. Ophthalmoscopic and fluorescein angiographic findings characteristic of radiation retinopathy include macular edema, disc edema, capillary nonperfusion, cotton-wool spots, capillary telangiectasia, microaneurysms, retinal hemorrhages, intraretinal exudation, disc pallor, optic atrophy, neovascularization of the disc or retina, and perivascular sheathing. Clinically, these signs are often identical to the findings seen in diabetic retinopathy. To establish the diagnosis of radiation retinopathy, one must carefully interview the patient to elicit a history of radiotherapy or radiation exposure, and medical records should be thoroughly reviewed to determine whether the eye was included in the radiation field. Patients with radiation retinopathy usually lose vision from macular edema, macular hemorrhages, macular exudates, perifoveal capillary nonperfusion, disc edema, or optic atrophy. In 1933, Stallard was the first to describe radiation retinopathy in patients who had been treated with radon seeds for retinoblastoma and retinal capillary hemangioma.[1] Many reports describing radiation retinopathy have followed.[2–39]

CLINICAL FEATURES

Macular edema is an early sign of radiation retinopathy. Microvascular changes, including microaneurysms and telangiectasia, are also seen, followed by cotton-wool spots and patches of capillary nonperfusion (Fig. 91–1). Retinal hemorrhages, hard exudates, and perivascular sheathing also appear (Figs. 91–2 and 91–3).

Extensive retinal vascular occlusion can lead to neovascularization of the retina, disc, and iris and may lead to vitreous hemorrhage and neovascular glaucoma (Fig. 91–4). In addition to the microangiopathic changes, central retinal artery occlusion[27] and central retinal vein occlusion have also been described in radiation retinopathy.[28] Subretinal neovascularization has also been observed.[29] Late fundus changes include retinal pigment epithelial atrophy and, in some cases, a generalized retinal pigment epithelial disturbance in a salt-and-pepper pattern. Fluorescein angiography clearly demonstrates the vascular changes described.

Optic nerve damage from radiation is characterized by disc edema, hemorrhages, cotton-wool spots, and hard exudates (Fig. 91–5). Fluorescein angiography may show telangiectasia and nonperfusion of the optic nerve head and peripapillary retinal capillaries. Disc edema may remain for several months. Eventually it resolves or is replaced with optic atrophy (Fig. 91–6).[2]

We studied radiation retinopathy in 335 patients with choroidal melanoma who were treated with proton beam irradiation. The choroidal melanomas were less than 15 mm in diameter, less than 5 mm in height, and within 4 disc diameters of the macula or disc. Proton beam radiation, 70 Gy, was delivered in five fractions. In all these cases, the macula and the optic nerve received high doses of radiation because of the tumor location. Two hundred eighteen patients met the criteria for the radiation maculopathy study,[2] whereas 223 patients met the criteria for the radiation papillopathy study.[3] Eighty-nine percent of the eligible patients experienced radiation maculopathy and 67 percent experienced radiation papillopathy.

The earliest and most common macular finding was macular edema, which was present in 61 percent of the patients at 1 yr and in 87 percent of the patients at 3 yr after radiation treatment. Microvascular changes con-

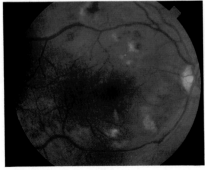
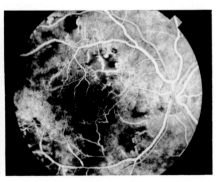

Figure 91–1. A, Fundus photograph of an eye with choroidal melanoma treated with proton beam irradiation. Cotton-wool spots, retinal hemorrhages, microaneurysms, and telangiectasia are seen. B, Fluorescein angiogram of the same eye highlighting the microvascular changes, including capillary nonperfusion, microaneurysms, and telangiectasia.

A
B

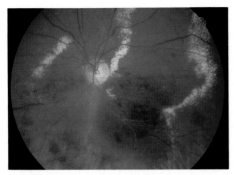

Figure 91–2. Radiation retinopathy in an eye with proton beam–irradiated choroidal melanoma. Extensive exudation, retinal hemorrhages, vascular occlusion, and macular edema are seen.

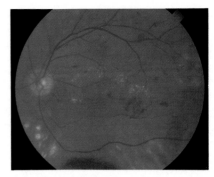

Figure 91–4. Neovascularization of the disc after proton beam irradiation for choroidal melanoma.

sisting of telangiectasia and microaneurysms were the next macular changes to appear. They occurred in 40 percent of patients at 1 yr and in 76 percent of the patients at 3 yr after irradiation. Intraretinal hemorrhages, hard exudates, nerve fiber layer infarcts, and capillary nonperfusion seen by fluorescein angiography developed more slowly, being present in 70, 55, 48, and 64 percent of the patients at 3 yr, respectively. The least common vascular lesion was vascular sheathing; only one third of the patients had vascular sheathing at 3 yr following irradiation. Lesions occurred more frequently with higher radiation doses.[2]

Nerve fiber layer infarcts showed the highest frequency of resolution. Two thirds of these lesions had resolved at the last available follow-up examination. Macular edema, in contrast, persisted in 95 percent of the patients. Capillary nonperfusion, microaneurysms, and telangiectasia rarely resolved spontaneously.[2]

The most common optic nerve lesion was disc pallor, which was seen in 63 percent of the cases at 5 yr. There was no definite peak in the annual rate, which reached a plateau at 12 mo. Disc edema, hemorrhages, and nerve fiber layer infarcts were seen in 35, 43, and 41 percent of the cases, respectively, peaking at approximately 24 mo. Hard exudates were seen in 34 percent of the eyes; their annual rate reached a plateau at 12 mo and remained constant. The least common finding was neovascularization of the disc, which was present in only 7 percent of the cases at 5 yr. As expected, the

disc changes were more prominent when the disc received the full dose of radiation (70 Gy). There was an age effect for three of the findings. Older patients were more likely to experience disc hemorrhage and nerve fiber layer infarcts but were less likely to experience nerve pallor.[3]

Brown and associates studied 36 patients with radiation exposure to the eye.[4] Twenty patients received cobalt plaque treatment (brachytherapy) for treatment of intraocular tumors, and 16 patients received external beam irradiation (teletherapy). In the group that received brachytherapy, hard exudates and intraretinal hemorrhages were the two most common findings, being seen in 85 and 65 percent of the patients, respectively. Retinal telangiectasia was seen in 35 percent of the patients, whereas 30 percent had cotton-wool spots, and 20 percent had vascular sheathing. In the group that received external beam irradiation, intraretinal hemorrhages and microaneurysms were the most common findings, being present in 88 and 81 percent of the patients, respectively. Hard exudates, retinal telangiectasia, and cotton-wool spots were seen in 38 percent of the patients. Twenty-five percent of patients had vascular sheathing. The main difference in the two groups was in the frequency of hard exudates. Brown and associates postulated that the higher frequency of hard exudates seen in brachytherapy patients might be due to some intrinsic factor released from the tumor that causes enhanced vascular leakage.[4]

Neovascularization was significantly more common in the external beam–treated group; there were two cases of disc neovascularization, five cases of retinal neovascularization, and four cases of neovascular glaucoma. Only one patient in the brachytherapy group had neovascularization. The higher frequency of neovascularization in the external beam group is thought to be secondary to the larger area of retina that was treated by the radiation.[4]

The vascular changes in radiation retinopathy usually became apparent several months after treatment, and in some eyes not until a few years following irradiation. In Brown and associates' study, the average time of onset for radiation retinopathy in the brachytherapy group was 14.6 mo, with a range of 4 to 32 mo; for the external beam group, it was 18.7 mo, with a range of 7 to 36 mo.[4]

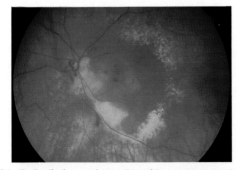

Figure 91–3. Radiation retinopathy with severe macular edema and exudation. Vascular sheathing is seen at the inferotemporal arcade.

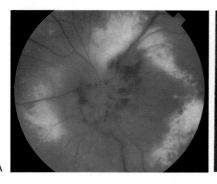
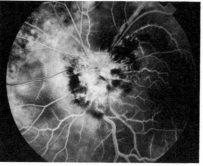

Figure 91–5. A, Radiation papillopathy with severe disc edema, hemorrhages, and exudation. B, Fluorescein angiogram of the same disc showing telangiectasia of the optic nerve vessels, as well as capillary nonperfusion of the surrounding retinal vessels.

The threshold for radiation retinopathy depends on the total dose delivered, the volume of retina irradiated, and the fractionation scheme. In general, greater total dose results in more severe radiation retinopathy. A higher fraction dose also results in more pronounced radiation retinopathy. The usual daily fractions used in radiotherapy are between 2 and 3 Gy, and they are often administered over a course of 1 to 2 mo for a total of 35 to 72 Gy. When patients receiving 2-Gy fractions were compared with those receiving 2.5-Gy fractions, radiation damage to the optic nerve was seen in 22 percent of the patients receiving 2.5-Gy fractions compared with 12.5 percent of the patients receiving 2-Gy fractions.[12]

In one report, retinal vascular changes were seen after as little as 15 Gy of external beam radiation.[21] The usual dose at which radiation retinopathy develops is between 30 and 35 Gy. Fifty percent of the patients who received 60 Gy to the eye experienced retinal damage, and 85 to 95 percent of the patients experienced retinopathy after 70 to 80 Gy.[30] In another report, all patients who received greater than 45 to 50 Gy external beam irradiation for sinus cancer showed retinal changes but no visual loss.[31] Mild decreases in vision were noted after 65 Gy, and severe visual loss was noted after 68 Gy of radiation. In most studies, the prevalence of radiation retinopathy increased with a longer interval before the follow-up examination.

PATHOLOGIC FEATURES

The histopathologic features of radiation retinopathy are vascular damage of the retinal vessels, consisting of occlusion of the retinal and optic nerve head arterioles with thickening of the vessel walls by fibrillar and hyaline material. Capillary damage is prominent. Larger vessels may show vessel wall proliferation. Intraretinal exudation, cystic changes of the outer plexiform and inner nuclear layers, and ganglion cell loss are also seen. In general, there is preferential damage to the inner retinal layers reflecting the damage to the retinal vessels.[32–36] The photoreceptors are relatively resistant to radiation damage.

The onset and course of radiation retinopathy have been studied in animals. Irvine and Wood irradiated monkey eyes with 30 Gy and followed them for subsequent changes.[37] The earliest histopathologic findings showed focal loss of capillary endothelial cells and

pericytes. These areas became confluent, and nerve fiber layer infarcts appeared. As the cotton-wool spots faded, larger areas of capillary nonperfusion developed. The earlier changes were observed in the deeper small retinal vessels. The larger retinal vessels were involved later. Intraretinal neovascularization was seen in this model, but there was no disc neovascularization. Rubeosis iridis and neovascular glaucoma appeared 30 to 42 mo following irradiation.

DIFFERENTIAL DIAGNOSIS

Clinically, the retinal vascular changes seen in radiation retinopathy can be identical to those seen in diabetic retinopathy, although severe fibrovascular proliferation is much less common in radiation retinopathy. The retinal findings may mimic multiple branch vein or artery occlusions or retinal telangiectasia. The diagnosis of radiation retinopathy and papillopathy is greatly aided by a history of radiation exposure to the eye. Medical records should be carefully reviewed to determine whether the eye was included in the radiation field and, if so, the estimated dose received by the eye. Radiation damage to the visual system is anticipated when the eyes are included in the radiation field. Radiation retinopathy is common after treatment of intraocular tumors and is occasionally seen following orbital radiation of thyroid disease or pseudotumor. Intracranial radiation, paranasal sinus radiation therapy, and irradiation of skin tumors of the face and eyelids can all expose the eye to radiation.

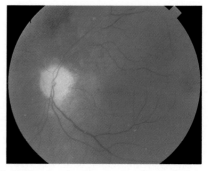

Figure 91–6. Optic atrophy in an eye with choroidal melanoma treated with proton beam irradiation. Vascular sheathing is also seen.

TREATMENT

Visual loss from ischemic maculopathy secondary to capillary nonperfusion is not reversible with any treatment. Cystoid macular edema may benefit from a macular grid treatment, but the effectiveness of this modality has not been established in a randomized trial. If there are localized capillary changes causing exudative retinopathy, focal treatment to these areas may dry up the macula.[18] In many patients, the maculopathy after radiation progresses from a leaking and exudative phase to an occlusive phase, and focal grid photocoagulation might serve only as a temporary measure. Panretinal photocoagulation appears to be beneficial in reducing neovascularization of the disc and the retina and may prevent the development or progression of neovascular glaucoma.[38]

PROGNOSIS

Radiation retinopathy is a delayed-onset, slowly progressive disease leading to visual loss from central macular capillary nonperfusion, macular edema, macular hemorrhages, macular exudation, disc edema, and optic atrophy. In the late stages, visual loss from vitreous hemorrhage, neovascular glaucoma, or retinal detachment may develop. There are three reported situations that can exacerbate the microangiopathy seen in radiation retinopathy. Patients with preexisting diabetic retinopathy appear to have a lower threshold for the development of radiation retinopathy.[4,7] Certain chemotherapeutic agents such as 5-fluorouracil appear to predispose an irradiated eye to radiation retinopathy even if the chemotherapy is not administered concomitantly.[13] Simultaneous use of hyperbaric oxygen and radiation was also seen to exacerbate radiation retinopathy.[39] Interestingly, hyperbaric oxygen has been proposed as a treatment for radiation retinopathy, and the role of hyperbaric oxygen in the pathogenesis and therapy of radiation retinopathy still needs to be elucidated.

REFERENCES

1. Stallard HB: Radiant energy as (a) a pathogenic and (b) a therapeutic agent in ophthalmic disorders. Br J Ophthalmol 6(Suppl):1–126, 1933.
2. Guyer DR, Mukai S, Eagan KM, et al: Radiation maculopathy following proton beam irradiation for choroidal melanoma. Ophthalmology 99:1278–1285, 1992.
3. Mukai S, Guyer DR, Eagan KM, et al: Radiation papillopathy after proton irradiation of choroidal melanoma. Ophthalmology 98(Suppl):116, 1991.
4. Brown GC, Shields JA, Sanborn G, et al: Radiation retinopathy. Ophthalmology 89:1494–1501, 1982.
5. Brown GC, Shields JA, Sanborn G, et al: Radiation retinopathy. Trans Pa Acad Ophthalmol Otolaryngol 34:144–150, 1981.
6. Tomsak RL, Smith JL: Radiation retinopathy in a patient with lung carcinoma metastatic to brain. Ann Ophthalmol 12:619–622, 1980.
7. Wara WM, Irvine AR, Neger RE, et al: Radiation retinopathy. Int J Radiat Oncol Biol Phys 5:81–83, 1979.
8. Bagan SM, Hollenhurst RW: Radiation retinopathy after irradiation of intracranial lesions. Am J Ophthalmol 88:694–697, 1979.
9. Egbert PR, Donaldson SS, Moazed K, Rosenthal AR: Visual results and ocular complications following radiotherapy for retinoblastoma. Arch Ophthalmol 96:1826–1830, 1978.
10. Rotman M, Long RS, Packer S, et al: Radiation therapy of choroidal melanoma. Trans Ophthalmol Soc UK 97:431–435, 1977.
11. Char DH, Lonn LI, Margolis LW: Complications of cobalt plaque therapy of choroidal melanomas. Am J Ophthalmol 84:536–541, 1977.
12. Harris JR, Levene MB: Visual complications following irradiation for pituitary adenomas and craniopharyngiomas. Radiology 120:167–171, 1976.
13. Chan RC, Schukovsky LJ: Effects of irradiation on the eye. Radiology 120:673–675, 1976.
14. Lommatzsch P: Treatment of choroidal melanomas with (^{106}Ru/^{106}Rh) beta-ray applicators. Surv Ophthalmol 19:85–100, 1974.
15. MacFaul PA, Bedford MA: Ocular complications after therapeutic irradiation. Br J Ophthalmol 54:237–247, 1970.
16. Bedford MA, Bedotto C, MacFaul PA: Radiation retinopathy after the application of cobalt plaque. Br J Ophthalmol 54:505–509, 1970.
17. Hayreh SS: Post-radiation retinopathy. A fluorescence fundus angiographic study. Br J Ophthalmol 54:705–714, 1970.
18. Gass JDM: A fluorescein angiographic study of macular dysfunction secondary to retinal vascular disease. VI. X-ray irradiation, carotid artery occlusion, collagen vascular disease, and vitritis. Arch Ophthalmol 80:606–617, 1968.
19. Chee PHY: Radiation retinopathy. Am J Ophthalmol 66:860–865, 1968.
20. Stallard HB: Radiotherapy for malignant melanoma of the choroid. Br J Ophthalmol 50:147–155, 1966.
21. Perrers-Taylor M, Brinkley D, Reynolds T: Choroido-retinal damage as a complication of radiotherapy. Acta Radiol Ther Phys Biol 3:431–440, 1965.
22. Rosengren B: Two cases of atrophy of the optic nerve after previous roentgen treatment of the chiasmal region and the optic nerves. Acta Ophthalmol 36:874–877, 1958.
23. Cibis PA, Noell WK, Eichel B: Ocular effects produced by high-intensity x-radiation. Arch Ophthalmol 53:651–663, 1955.
24. Flick JJ: Ocular lesions following the atomic bombing of Hiroshima and Nagasaki. Am J Ophthalmol 31:137–154, 1948.
25. Stallard HB: Radiotherapy of malignant intra-ocular neoplasms. Br J Ophthalmol 32:618–639, 1948.
26. Moore RF: Presidential address. Trans Ophthalmol Soc UK 55:3–26, 1935.
27. Cogan DG: Lesions of the eye from radiant energy. JAMA 142:145–151, 1950.
28. Shukovsky LJ, Fletcher GH: Retinal and optic nerve complications in a high-dose irradiation technique of ethmoid sinus and nasal cavity. Radiation 104:629–634, 1972.
29. Boozalis GT, Schachat AP, Green WR: Subretinal neovascularization from the retina in radiation retinopathy. Retina 7:156–161, 1987.
30. Merriam GR, Szechter A, Focht EF: The effects of ionizing radiation on the eye. Front Radiat Ther Oncol 6:346–385, 1972.
31. Nakissa N, Rubin P, Strohl R, Keys H: Ocular and orbital complications following paranasal sinus malignancies and review of literature. Cancer 51:980–986, 1983.
32. Seddon JM, Gragoudas ES, Albert DM, et al: Ciliary body and choroidal melanomas treated by proton beam irradiation. Histopathologic study of eyes. Arch Ophthalmol 101:1402–1408, 1983.
33. Ferry AP, Blair CJ, Gragoudas CS, Volk SC: Pathologic examination of ciliary body melanoma treated with proton beam irradiation. Arch Ophthalmol 103:1849–1853, 1985.
34. Kincaid MC, Folberg R, Torczynski E, et al: Complications after proton beam therapy for uveal malignant melanoma. A clinical and histopathologic study of 5 cases. Ophthalmology 95:982–991, 1988.
35. Zinn KM, Stein-Pokorny K, Jakobiec FA, et al: Proton beam–irradiated epithelioid melanoma of the ciliary body. Ophthalmology 88:1315–1321, 1981.
36. Saornil MA, Egan KM, Gragoudas ES, et al: Histopathology of uveal melanomas treated by proton beam irradiation: A comparison study. Arch Ophthalmol 110:1112–1118, 1992.
37. Irvine AR, Wood IS: Radiation retinopathy as an experimental model for ischemic proliferative retinopathy and rubeosis iridis. Am J Ophthalmol 103:790–797, 1987.
38. Chandhuri PR, Austin DJ, Rosenthal AR: Treatment of radiation retinopathy. Br J Ophthalmol 65:623–625, 1981.
39. Stanford MR: Retinopathy after irradiation and hyperbaric oxygen. J R Soc Med 77:1041–1043, 1984.

Chapter 92

Retinal Toxicity of Systemic Drugs

DAVID V. WEINBERG and DONALD J. D'AMICO

It is important for ophthalmologists to have a knowledge of common drugs with the potential for retinal toxicity for at least two reasons: First, ophthalmologists are frequently called upon by medical colleagues to evaluate patients taking medications with known toxic potential, such as hydroxychloroquine and thioridazine. A knowledge of the toxic properties of these drugs will guide the appropriate evaluation and recommendations. Second, when confronted with an unusual retinopathy, an index of suspicion may prompt appropriate questioning, leading to an otherwise overlooked diagnosis. This may protect the patient from unnecessary and fruitless diagnostic procedures and from future exposure to the offending drug.

CHLOROQUINE AND HYDROXYCHLOROQUINE

Chloroquine and hydroxychloroquine are related drugs in the quinoline family. Although the therapeutic and toxic doses differ, the clinical indications for use and manifestations of retinal toxicity of the two drugs are essentially identical, so they are discussed together.

History

Chloroquine was first popularized for prophylaxis against and treatment of malaria, and it was widely used during World War I. At the doses and durations of therapy used for antimalarial purposes, chloroquine-related retinopathy was unknown.

Later, chloroquine and hydroxychloroquine were recognized as effective for the treatment of certain connective tissue diseases, most notably rheumatoid arthritis and lupus erythematosus. The higher daily dosages and the prolonged duration of therapy for these chronic diseases led to cumulative doses in excess of those used in antimalarial therapy. A case of an unusual pigmentary retinopathy reported in 1957 was attributed to systemic lupus erythematosus[1] but was probably the first reported case of chloroquine retinopathy. In the same year, Goldman and Preston reported two patients who experienced unspecified "severe fundal changes" and visual field constriction attributed to chloroquine.[2] Hobbs and associates gave the first description of the retinal findings in three cases of retinopathy attributed to chloroquine.[3] Hydroxychloroquine has largely replaced chloroquine for the treatment of connective tissue diseases, but it can produce a retinopathy identical to that of chloroquine.

Clinical Findings

The ocular toxicity of these drugs is not limited to the retina. Reversible corneal opacities have been reported to occur in up to two thirds of patients taking chloroquine.[4–6] Abnormalities of motility, accommodation, and the crystalline lens have all been attributed to chloroquine. These extraretinal manifestations of toxicity seem to be much more frequent with chloroquine than with hydroxychloroquine.[6]

Patients' subjective complaints attributed to chloroquine retinopathy usually relate to central or paracentral scotomas. Other symptoms reported include photophobia, nyctalopia, and photopsias. Patients with definite retinopathy may be asymptomatic.[6, 7]

The earliest fundus findings are usually in the macula and begin with irregularity of the macular pigmentation and loss of the foveal reflex.[7, 8] The presence of mild macular abnormalities without significant functional abnormalities has been termed *premaculopathy* or *preretinopathy* by some authors.[6, 9] These early stages of maculopathy are indistinguishable from the changes that frequently occur with aging. The fact that many patients on chloroquine or hydroxychloroquine therapy are elderly makes these early findings nonspecific and emphasizes the value of examination and photography prior to the institution of therapy.

With time, the pigmentary irregularity progresses, tending to be more prominent in the inferior macula.[10] A central zone of irregular hyperpigmentation may become surrounded by a concentric zone of hypopigmentation, usually horizontally oval,[10] resulting in the classic appearance of bull's-eye maculopathy (Fig. 92–1). The presence of macular edema was described by some early observers[4, 11] but has not been well characterized or documented. If the process progresses, the end-stage fundus may assume an appearance indistinguishable from that of retinitis pigmentosa, with peripheral pigmentary irregularity and bone spicule formation, vascular attenuation, and optic disc pallor.[8, 12]

Fluorescein angiography highlights the pigment changes in the fundus of patients with retinopathy, leading to the advocacy of its use for diagnosis.[13] Cruess and colleagues compared the sensitivity of color photographs and fluorescein angiography. They found that if the photographs showed a normal fundus, angiography

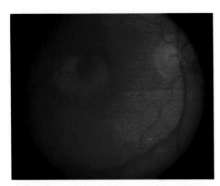

Figure 92–1. Bull's-eye maculopathy typical of chloroquine and hydroxychloroquine toxicity. There is a zone of depigmentation surrounding the fovea. The zone is typically horizontally oval and more prominent inferiorly.

did not contribute any additional sensitivity. If the history and fundus appearance are highly suggestive of chloroquine retinopathy, fluorescein angiography is unlikely to provide any additional information. Fluorescein angiography may be useful if the fundus is abnormal, but diagnoses other than chloroquine retinopathy are being considered.[14]

The fundus changes and functional defects have been reported to regress or return to normal following the discontinuation of therapy. Conversely, there are well-documented cases of progression of retinopathy and visual deficits following discontinuation of therapy. The earliest changes of maculopathy are the most likely to improve. More advanced retinopathy never returns to normal and may be more likely to progress following discontinuation of the drug.[5, 8, 12, 15–17]

Tests for Retinopathy

Since the fundus appearance of early retinopathy is nonspecific and may not be noticed until after permanent damage has occurred and since patients with retinopathy may be asymptomatic, it would be desirable to have a reliable test to detect the earliest stages of retinal toxicity and monitor injury and recovery. The literature in this area is very confusing, controversial, and even contradictory. Much of this confusion has been due to a lack of standardization of the testing procedures and to the lack of consensus as to the definition of which constellation of signs and symptoms defines the earliest stages of retinopathy. Some investigators have relied mostly on functional tests to define toxic effects, whereas others have emphasized the fundus findings.

The test that has been most advocated and used is measurement of the central visual field using Goldmann perimetry or other standard methods. Small paracentral scotomas very close to (within 10 degrees) but usually sparing fixation are consistent findings in early maculopathy and tend to be more common superior to than inferior to fixation, which is consistent with the predominance of pigment changes inferior to the fovea.[10] Con-

striction of the peripheral field occurs[18] but is less specific. Rarely, peripheral field loss may predominate.[19] Careful evaluation of central fields with small test objects is recommended and detects abnormalities before they become symptomatic.[7] Red test objects seem to improve the sensitivity significantly.[9] Amsler grid testing has been advocated as a quick, effective alternative for screening central visual fields of patients at risk.[20–22] As the maculopathy progresses, the central visual field defects enlarge and multiply. Patients become more symptomatic and central visual acuity suffers. The central defects enlarge further and may break through to the periphery, especially the superotemporal periphery.

Retinal threshold profile, a technique related to visual field testing, has been shown to be a very sensitive test for the early effects of these drugs. Carr and coworkers in 1966[23] used different-colored stimuli to determine the subjective threshold retinal sensitivity at a horizontal series of points across the macula. Even at doses thought to be less than the toxic threshold, nearly all patients taking chloroquine had elevated thresholds compared with controls. Furthermore, the degree of change in retinal threshold seemed to be dose-related. Although the findings of this study were promising, they were based on a relatively small number of patients.

Much attention has been given to electrodiagnostic testing in the early diagnosis of chloroquine and hydroxychloroquine retinopathy. Abnormalities in the electroretinogram are common in more advanced retinopathy[7, 8, 12] but are inconsistent in treated patients without retinopathy or with early retinopathy.[12, 24–26]

The light : dark, or Arden, ratio as measured by electooculography may be reduced in patients taking chloroquine or hydroxychloroquine.[7, 9, 27–29] Henkind and associates found a greater incidence of a reduced electrooculogram (EOG) in patients with chloroquine retinopathy than in those taking chloroquine who did not have retinopathy.[7] Arden and Kolb found the average EOG to be lower in patients taking chloroquine or hydroxychloroquine, even at low cumulative doses, but not in patients with rheumatoid disease who were not taking these drugs.[27] The issue is complicated by reports of reduced EOGs in patients with untreated rheumatoid disease.[29, 30] Initiation of treatment may cause an initial elevation of the light : dark ratio followed by a reduction.[31] If electrooculography is to be used in monitoring patients, it is best to perform a pretreatment baseline study and consider discontinuation of the drug if the ratio falls significantly.[6, 32, 33] Unfortunately, the definition of a "significant" fall has not been well established. The current body of evidence does not strongly support the usefulness of electrooculography as a screening test for early retinal toxicity.[6, 29]

Simple tests of color vision, such as the Hardy-Rand-Rittler plates, have been favored by some investigators as an effective screening test for early retinopathy,[8, 34] but they generally have not been found reliable.[6, 8, 17, 35, 36] Poor performance on these tests is probably the result of central scotomas, which are more effectively detected by central visual field testing.

Incidence

Widely varying incidence figures have been reported in the literature, mainly because of differing definitions of retinopathy and differing drug dosages in the population at risk. If the most subtle macular changes are defined as chloroquine retinopathy, incidences up to 50 percent have been reported.[7, 16] These studies failed to use controls to account for the age-related changes that occur in the untreated population. Based on a review of the reported cases of retinopathy, Bernstein estimated an incidence of 10 percent in unmonitored patients taking chloroquine and 3 to 4 percent in unmonitored patients taking hydroxychloroquine. Regular monitoring of such patients can significantly reduce the incidence of significant retinopathy.[6]

Despite the heterogeneity of the statistics in the literature, two trends are consistent. The incidence of retinopathy increases with both the dose and the duration of treatment.[6, 7, 12, 16, 25, 37, 38] For chloroquine, a daily dose of 250 mg or less, a cumulative dose of less than 100 g, and duration of treatment less than 1 yr have each been associated with a very low incidence of retinopathy.[6, 25, 38, 39] For hydroxychloroquine, 400 mg/day or less has been associated with a low risk of retinopathy.[37]

There is evidence that the most important factor in the safety of therapy is the daily dose. If the daily dose is kept at less than a safe threshold, it seems that there is no limit to the safe duration or total cumulative dose. The safe dose has been reported to be 3.5 mg/kg/day for chloroquine and 6.5 mg/kg/day for hydroxychloroquine.[40, 41] These dosages are based on lean body weight. For smaller patients, the usual doses of 250 mg/day for chloroquine and 400 mg/day for hydroxychloroquine may be excessive.[40]

A rational plan for following patients taking chloroquine or hydroxychloroquine would ideally include baseline examination and central visual field, as well as baseline photographs. The minimal effective dose should be used at or less than the recommended daily milligrams per kilogram dose. Semiannual examination, including questioning for symptoms of visual changes, repeated central visual field testing, and ophthalmoscopy, should reveal the rare cases of maculopathy at an early stage.

Mechanism of Injury

Chloroquine's affinity for pigmented structures, especially in the eye, may account for some of its toxic properties. Chloroquine and its principal metabolite have been found in the pigmented ocular structures at concentrations many times greater than in any other tissue in the body.[35, 42] With more prolonged exposure, the drug accumulates in the retina as well.[42] The drug is retained in the pigmented structures long after its discontinuation. The kinetics of chloroquine metabolism are complicated, with the half-life increasing as the dosage is increased.[43] In patients with retinopathy, traces of chloroquine have been found in plasma, erythrocytes, and urine 5 yr or more after discontinuation.[35]

Pathologic studies of patients with chloroquine retinopathy are few and are limited to cases with advanced retinopathy.[44–47] Consistent findings include degeneration of the outer retina, particularly the photoreceptors and the outer nuclear layer, with relative sparing of the photoreceptors in the fovea. Pigment migration into the retina is seen. Pathologic changes in the ganglion cells have also been a consistent finding. Sclerosis of the retinal arterioles is variable.

Clues to the primary site of injury of chloroquine are found in animal studies. Ganglion cells show the first morphologic changes following exposure to chloroquine. Rosenthal and coworkers gave monkeys the equivalent of triple the daily human dose by intramuscular injection.[42] Membranous cytoplasmic bodies were seen in the ganglion cells within 1 wk of the onset of treatment. These bodies were later seen in the other neural cells of the retina and their presence was reversible for up to 6 mo of therapy.

Continued exposure resulted in progressive degeneration of the ganglion cells and photoreceptor cell bodies and nuclei. Outer segments were affected later in the course. The most severe changes tended to be perifoveal, with relative foveal sparing. Abnormalities of the pigment epithelium and choroid were seen only after degeneration of the ganglion cells and photoreceptors was established. All of the observations described were made prior to any detectable abnormalities in the fundus or on the electroretinogram.

Ganglion cell changes were also the earliest findings in rats,[48, 49] cats, and dogs[49] given chloroquine.

PHENOTHIAZINES

The phenothiazines are a subclass of drugs also known as antipsychotics or neuroleptics. The chemical backbone of all phenothiazines consists of the same polycyclic structure. The substitution of different groups at two positions on this structure alters the potency, therapeutic effects, and side effects of the drug.[50] Like the quinolines, the phenothiazines have a distinct affinity for pigmented structures,[51–54] possibly accounting for a disposition toward ocular toxicity; however, the mechanism of injury has not been elucidated.

An unacceptably high incidence of pigmentary retinopathy and visual disturbance forced the withdrawal of a phenothiazine known as NP 207, released for limited clinical use in 1955.[55–57] The toxic effect was clearly dose-related and at higher doses was seen in the majority of the patients.[56] Among phenothiazines in clinical use today, thioridazine, a drug closely related to NP 207, has been most clearly established as a cause of retinopathy.

Thioridazine

The popularity of thioridazine has grown because many of the side effects associated with other phenothiazines tend to be less frequent and less severe with this drug. After its introduction in the late 1950s, it was used at doses of up to several grams per day—very high by today's standards. Reports rapidly appeared of a subacute form of retinal toxicity.[58, 59] These and later reports described a very characteristic clinical course[58–64] that was strikingly similar to that associated with NP 207. After 2 wk or more of high-dose therapy, patients complain of a variety of visual symptoms, including blurring, nyctalopia, and the experience of a brown discoloration of vision. The visual loss may be mild to profound. Initially, the fundus may appear normal, but within a week or two characteristic fundus changes evolve. The earliest finding is a granularity of the postequatorial fundus (Fig. 92–2). Transient edema of the disc and retina after the appearance of pigmentary changes has been described. If the drug is withdrawn at the onset of symptoms, patients usually report improvement of symptoms within weeks, often to baseline levels. In contrast to the usual symptomatic improvement, the fundus changes usually progress.[65, 66] The pigmentation becomes more coarse over time and may eventually coalesce in patches to form large plaques of hyperpigmentation. Areas of depigmentation and loss of choriocapillaris may also develop eventually (Fig. 92–3). Rarely, symptoms may develop without the appearance of retinopathy.[67]

A very characteristic variation of the pigment change has been described as nummular retinopathy and is seen in patients taking somewhat lower doses of thioridazine for longer periods.[68–70] These patients are less likely to be symptomatic. The fundus picture consists of multiple, large, round areas of depigmentation and atrophy posterior to the equator, with relative sparing of the macula (Fig. 92–4). Over time, the areas of atrophy may enlarge and become confluent.

Fluorescein angiography demonstrates changes in the retinal pigment that are more severe than evident clinically, as well as loss of choriocapillaris within areas of depigmentation.[65, 70]

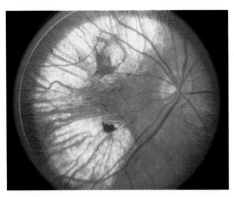

Figure 92–3. Advanced thioridazine retinopathy with large areas of atrophy of the retinal pigment epithelium and choriocapillaris.

Visual field changes in patients with thioridazine retinopathy are nonspecific, but most characteristically show irregular paracentral scotomas or ring scotomas.[61, 64, 65] Electrooculographic ratios and electroretinographic amplitudes (both photopic and scotopic) are variably reduced, and dark adaptation is abnormal.[64, 70] No studies have been performed to determine whether any of these tests are of value in detecting early retinopathy or predicting the course of established retinopathy.

The risk of retinopathy appears to be dose-related, particularly with respect to the daily dose. De Margerie reported 31 patients receiving daily doses of 800 mg or more. No cases of pigmentary retinopathy were seen among 17 patients taking doses less than 1000 mg daily for up to 26 mo. Of those taking 1000 mg or more/day, 10 of 14 patients were judged to have some degree of retinopathy.[71] Applebaum reported no cases of retinopathy among 77 patients taking 100 to 600 mg daily for up to 14 mo.[72] Hagopian and colleagues examined 164 patients taking thioridazine and found 5 cases of retinopathy. All of the affected patients were among 8 patients receiving doses of 1800 mg/day or more.[62] The manufacturer's current recommendation is that the dose be titrated to the minimal effective dose of 300 mg/day or less, with an absolute maximum of 800 mg/day. Cases of retinopathy among patients treated within these guidelines are very rare.[70, 73, 74]

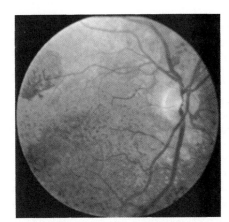

Figure 92–2. Coarse pigment granularity and formation of larger pigmented plaques are seen in this patient following high doses of thioridazine. Large areas of atrophy of the retinal pigment epithelium and choriocapillaris eventually developed despite discontinuation of the drug. (From Davidorf FH: Thioridazine pigmentary retinopathy. Arch Ophthalmol 90:251–255, 1973. Copyright 1973, American Medical Association.)

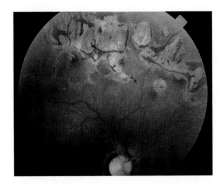

Figure 92–4. Thioridazine retinopathy associated with chronic use (nummular retinopathy). Round areas of depigmentation develop posterior to the equator. In contrast to the more acute form of toxicity, the macula is usually spared. (Courtesy of Lee M. Jampol, M.D.)

Chlorpromazine

Chlorpromazine is one of the oldest phenothiazines in clinical use. Ocular and adnexal abnormalities include pigmentation of the conjunctiva and sun-exposed skin and characteristic changes of the cornea and lens.[75–77] Rare cases of retinopathy have been alternately described as round, depigmented spots in the posterior pole[75] and as pigmentary clumping. In contrast to the pigmentary changes of thioridazine, the pigment clumping of chlorpromazine is finer and more reversible.[78]

METHANOL

Unlike most of the other substances discussed in this section, ocular toxicity of methanol occurs in conjunction with severe systemic toxicity. Methanol shares, to a lesser extent, the intoxicating properties of ethanol, is inexpensive, and has been used as a substitute when ethanol was not available. Poisoning usually occurs after the ingestion of solutions intentionally denatured or unintentionally tainted with methanol. Regulation of alcoholic beverages has eliminated some of the large-scale outbreaks of poisoning; however, methanol is still used in many solvents and other readily available products that may be consumed accidentally or intentionally.

Although drinking is the most common route of ingestion, toxicity can occur by inhalation of vapors or skin contact. Following the ingestion of methanol, patients experience a period of intoxication. This is followed by a latent period of about 24 hr (it can be as brief as 6 hr and as long as 72 hr), after which generalized toxicity begins to become apparent.[79–81] This is marked by a metabolic acidosis, often severe, accompanied by a depressed level of consciousness, progressing variably to stupor, coma, and death.[80] The toxic dose is highly variable from individual to individual. Blindness and death have occurred following ingestion of 1 oz or less, whereas some individuals may be unaffected by much larger doses.[80]

Affected patients frequently complain of visual impairment, usually described as a white clouding of the vision.[81] Presenting loss of vision can be mild to profound. Fundus findings are present in the vast majority of patients with symptomatic loss of vision. Edema of the disc and peripapillary retina is the first finding. The retinal edema may spread outward from the disc, especially along the major vascular arcades, and may be accompanied by dilatation of the retinal vessels.[79, 81, 82] The fundus findings may be indistinguishable from changes caused by increased intracranial pressure (papilledema). Severe retinal findings have a poor prognosis in terms of both survival and ultimate visual acuity.[81] Patients who survive often show improvement in vision; however, if vision has not returned to normal by the sixth day, improvement is unlikely and may actually continue to worsen.[81] In more severely affected patients, optic atrophy and excavation become apparent in 1 to 2 mo.[82, 83]

Other ocular findings in affected patients include nystagmus and dilated, poorly reactive pupils. Patients with fixed, dilated pupils usually do not survive.[80] The characteristic visual field deficit resulting from methanol toxicity is a central or centrocecal scotoma.[79, 81, 82]

The diagnosis of methanol poisoning is based on history, characteristic symptoms, physical examination, and laboratory findings, including an anion gap acidosis. Medical treatment includes respiratory support, treatment of metabolic acidosis, dialysis, and possible therapeutic use of ethanol as a competitive inhibitor of the metabolism of methanol.

Histopathologic findings in the eyes of patients dying of methanol poisoning have been inconsistent.[79, 81–85] Drastic interspecies differences have confounded efforts to determine the pathophysiologic features of methanol toxicity using animal models. Nonprimates are unsuitable for most studies because they do not demonstrate acidosis, and retinal toxicity is inconsistently induced.[86, 87] Monkeys reproduce the human findings well,[87–89] but despite numerous monkey experiments, many aspects of methanol toxicity are unsettled. Visual loss in methanol intoxication was for many years attributed to retinal injury from methanol itself, from one of its metabolites (such as formaldehyde), or from the acidosis.[90] The most recent evidence indicates that the primary site of injury is the optic nerve and that the clinical findings can be explained based on axoplasmic stasis and secondary swelling of the optic disc and retina.[89, 91]

CANTHAXANTHINE

Canthaxanthine is a naturally occurring non–provitamin A carotenoid. When taken orally, it causes a bronzing of the skin. It is this property that has led to its use as a medical treatment for vitiligo and some photosensitive dermatoses; it is also used as an artificial tanning agent.[92, 93] The unique and very characteristic appearance of canthaxanthine retinopathy was first reported in 1982.[94] Patients with canthaxanthine retinopathy are usually asymptomatic but may complain of metamorphopsia or mildly decreased vision.[94, 95] There is a collection of highly refractile yellow deposits in the innermost layers of the retina. They are distributed predominantly in a ring surrounding the fovea (Fig. 92–5). Crystalline retinopathy was found in 22 of 53 (41 percent) patients with cumulative doses from 7.5 to 178 g of canthaxanthine.[92] A cumulative dose of 30 to 40 g has produced retinopathy in about 50 percent of patients.[92, 96] At doses greater than 60 g, 55 to 100 percent of patients have demonstrated retinopathy.[92, 97] Other factors that seem related to the development of retinopathy include increasing age, ocular hypertension, and concurrent macular disease. Ingestion of other carotenoids in combination with canthaxanthine may have a synergistic effect on the development of retinopathy.[95, 96] Photographic study has shown that following cessation of the drug, the number of visible retinal deposits decreases slowly over several years.[98]

Static perimetry of the central 10-degree field has shown reduced sensitivity in patients with retinopathy

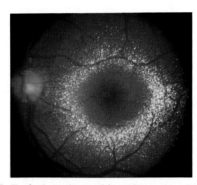

Figure 92–5. Typical canthaxanthin retinopathy with large yellow inner retinal crystals distributed in a prominent ring around the fovea. (Courtesy of Paul Arrigg, M.D.)

but not in patients taking canthaxanthine without retinopathy.[99] The reduced sensitivity in patients with retinopathy returned to normal after cessation of the drug.[99] Electroretinographic and electrooculographic testing has not revealed any consistent abnormalities.[96, 97]

Histologic examination was performed on the eyes of one 72-year-old woman with clinically apparent canthaxanthine retinopathy. Birefringent crystals were found throughout the nerve fiber layer of the retina, even in areas in which crystals were not seen clinically. The crystals were greatest in number and size in the typical, clinically apparent paracentral location. Chemical and spectroscopic analyses confirmed the presence of canthaxanthine in the retina.[93]

NIACIN

A small subset of patients taking high doses of niacin (nicotinic acid, vitamin B_6) for the purpose of lowering serum cholesterol levels have experienced an unusual, partially or fully reversible maculopathy.[100, 101] All reported cases have been in men taking a minimum of 1.5 g of niacin daily. Symptoms begin weeks to months after initiation of the drug and include metamorphopsia, blurring, central scotomas, or halos. Visual acuity is usually only mildly affected but may be as low as 20/80. Central visual changes are usually demonstrable by Amsler grid testing.

The remarkable fundus finding is a bilateral maculopathy that mimics cystoid macular edema (Fig. 92–6). The cysts in this condition have been described as smaller than in true cystoid macular edema from other causes.[101] Early frames of the fluorescein angiogram may demonstrate increased choroidal transmittance in the area of the cysts, but in contrast to true cystoid macular edema, there is no accumulation of fluorescein.

One patient had subjective blurring of his vision with 20/20 acuity and a normal eye examination. His vision subjectively returned to normal days after discontinuation of niacin, suggesting that symptoms may precede any objective findings.

Both the subjective and the objective changes tend to be most severe in the morning. On cessation of the

drug, there is prompt improvement, but subtle functional and physical abnormalities may persist. Repeated challenge with high doses of niacin caused the condition to recur in an affected patient.[100]

Screening of 15 patients taking high-dose niacin revealed no cases of drug-related maculopathy in asymptomatic patients.[101]

TAMOXIFEN

Tamoxifen is an estrogen antagonist used in the therapy of certain types of breast carcinoma. Retinopathy was first described in patients on prolonged, high-dose (>180 mg/day) therapy.[102, 103] Duration of treatment ranged from 17 to 27 mo, and the cumulative dose ranged from 90 to 230 g. A symptomatic decrease in vision was noted by four of five patients. Visual acuity at the time of diagnosis ranged from 20/20 to 20/100. Characteristic fundus findings were small, white refractile deposits of the sensory retina concentrated posteriorly, especially in the perimacular area, and an associated variable degree of pigment irregularity (Fig. 92–7). Fluorescein angiography demonstrated macular edema in most cases. White, whorl-like subepithelial corneal deposits have also been described secondary to tamoxifen therapy.[102, 104]

At lower, more conventional doses (20 to 40 mg/day), one study found no cases of tamoxifen retinopathy in 19 patients after 3 to 48 mo of treatment.[105] Another group reported 2 cases of probable asymptomatic retinopathy in 17 patients taking 20 to 30 mg/day for 7 to 25 mos.[106]

Pathologic examination of the eyes of one patient with clinical retinopathy showed the lesions to be limited to the nerve fiber and inner plexiform layers of the retina. Based on the location and electron microscopic findings, the lesions were believed to be the products of axonal degeneration.[104]

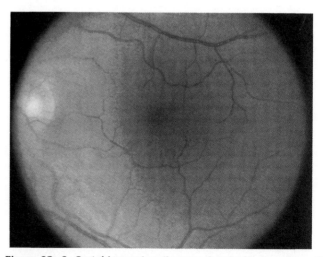

Figure 92–6. Cystoid maculopathy associated with ingestion of high doses of nicotinic acid. (From Millay RH, Klein ML, Illingworth DR: Niacin maculopathy. Published courtesy of Ophthalmology [1988;95:930–936].)

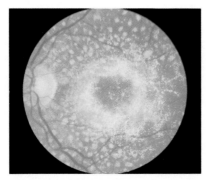

Figure 92–7. Fine refractile intraretinal crystals, as well as granular deposits at the level of the pigment epithelium associated with high-dose tamoxifen chemotherapy for breast cancer. Cystoid macular edema was seen by fluorescein angiography. (From McKeown CA, Swartz M, Blom J, Maggiano JM: Tamoxifen retinopathy. Br J Ophthalmol 65:177–179, 1981.)

METHOXYFLURANE

Methoxyflurane is an inhalation anesthetic agent. Two metabolites of methoxyflurane, fluoride and oxalic acid, are known nephrotoxins, and renal failure is a recognized rare complication of methoxyflurane anesthesia.

Two cases of crystalline retinopathy following methoxyflurane anesthesia have been reported. One of these patients also suffered renal failure attributed to prolonged methoxyflurane anesthesia. Three years later, fundus examination showed yellow-white punctate lesions in the posterior pole and midperiphery of both eyes, mimicking fundus albipunctatus. At autopsy, this patient had widespread calcium oxalate crystal deposition throughout the body, including the retinal pigment epithelium and retina. The other patient also had a history of prolonged methoxyflurane anesthesia and similar fundus findings, but histologic examination was not performed.[107, 108]

An additional case of crystalline retinopathy was found in a patient with renal failure and a history of illicit methoxyflurane abuse. Fundus examination showed cotton-wool spots and a striking pattern of large retinal crystals, distributed predominantly along retinal arteries but also at the level of the pigment epithelium. Renal biopsy confirmed the presence of oxalate crystals in the kidney.[109] The fundus appearance in this case was similar to that described in primary hyperoxaluria.[110]

REFERENCES

1. Cambiaggi A: Unusual ocular lesions in a case of systemic lupus erythematosus. Arch Ophthalmol 57:451, 1957.
2. Goldman L, Preston RH: Reactions to chloroquine observed during the treatment of various dermatologic disorders. Am J Trop Med Hyg 6:654, 1957.
3. Hobbs HE, Sorsby A, Freedman A: Retinopathy following chloroquine therapy. Lancet 2:478, 1959.
4. Hobbs HE, Eadie SP, Somerville F: Ocular lesions after treatment with chloroquine. Br J Ophthalmol 45:284, 1961.
5. Henkind P, Rothfield NF: Ocular abnormalities in patients treated with synthetic antimalarial drugs. N Engl J Med 269:433, 1963.
6. Bernstein HN: Ophthalmic considerations and testing in patients receiving long-term antimalarial therapy. Am J Med 75:25, 1983.
7. Henkind P, Carr RE, Siegel IM: Early chloroquine retinopathy: Clinical and functional findings. Arch Ophthalmol 71:157, 1964.
8. Okun E, Gouras P, Bernstein H, Von Sallmann L: Chloroquine retinopathy: A report of eight cases with ERG and dark-adaptation findings. Arch Ophthalmol 69:59, 1963.
9. Percival SPB, Behrman J: Ophthalmological safety of chloroquine. Br J Ophthalmol 53:101, 1969.
10. Hart WM, Burde RM, Johnston GP, et al: Static perimetry in chloroquine retinopathy, perifoveal patterns of visual field depression. Arch Ophthalmol 102:377, 1984.
11. Ellsworth RJ, Zeller RW: Chloroquine (Aralen)-induced retinal damage. Arch Ophthalmol 66:269, 1961.
12. Nylander U: Ocular damage in chloroquine therapy. Acta Ophthalmol 44:335, 1966.
13. Kearns TP, Hollenhorst RW: Chloroquine retinopathy: Evaluation by fluorescein fundus angiography. Arch Ophthalmol 76:378, 1966.
14. Cruess AF, Schachat AP, Nicholl J, et al: Chloroquine retinopathy: Is fluorescein angiography necessary? Ophthalmology 92:1127, 1985.
15. Burns RP: Delayed onset of chloroquine retinopathy. N Engl J Med 275:693, 1966.
16. Carr RE, Henkind P, Rothfeld N, et al: Ocular toxicity of antimalarial drugs, long-term follow-up. Am J Ophthalmol 66:738, 1968.
17. Brinkley JR, Dubois EL, Ryan SJ: Long-term course of chloroquine retinopathy after cessation of medication. Am J Ophthalmol 88:1, 1979.
18. Tobin DR, Krohel GB, Rynes RI: Hydroxychloroquine: Seven-year experience. Arch Ophthalmol 100:81, 1982.
19. Lowes M: Peripheral visual field restriction in chloroquine retinopathy: Report of a case. Acta Ophthalmol 54:819, 1976.
20. Easterbrook M: The use of Amsler grids in early chloroquine retinopathy. Ophthalmology 91:1368, 1984.
21. Easterbrook M: The sensitivity of Amsler grid testing in early chloroquine retinopathy. Trans Ophthalmol Soc UK 104:204, 1985.
22. Wolfe KA, Sadun AA, Kitridou RC: The detection of hydroxychloroquine maculopathy with threshold Amsler grid testing. Invest Ophthalmol Vis Sci 31(Suppl):136, 1990.
23. Carr RE, Gouras P, Gunkel RD: Chloroquine retinopathy, early detection by retinal threshold test. Arch Ophthalmol 75:171, 1966.
24. Schmidt B, Müller-Limmroth W: Electroretinographic examination following the application of chloroquine. Acta Ophthalmol 70(Suppl):245, 1961.
25. Voipio H: Incidence of chloroquine retinopathy. Acta Ophthalmol 44:349, 1966.
26. Sassaman FW, Cassidy JT, Alpern M, et al: Electroretinography in patients with connective tissue disease treated with hydroxychloroquine. Am J Ophthalmol 70:515, 1970.
27. Arden GB, Kolb H: Antimalarial therapy and early retinal changes in patients with rheumatoid arthritis. Br Med J 29:270, 1966.
28. Reijmer CN, Tijssen JGP, Kok GA, et al: Interpretation of the electro-oculogram of patients taking chloroquine. Doc Ophthalmol 48:273, 1979.
29. Pinkers A, Broekhuyse RM: The EOG in rheumatoid arthritis. Acta Ophthalmol 61:831, 1983.
30. Graniewski-Wijnands HS, Van Lith GHM, Vijfvinkel-Bruinenga S: Ophthalmological examination of patients taking chloroquine. Doc Ophthalmol 48:231, 1979.
31. Heckenlively JR, Martin D, Levy J: Chloroquine retinopathy. Am J Ophthalmol 89:150, 1980.
32. Van Lith GHM, Mak GTM, Wijnands H: Clinical importance of the electro-oculogram with special reference to the chloroquine retinopathy. Bibl Ophthalmol 85:2, 1976.
33. Van Lith GHM: Electro-ophthalmology and side-effects of drugs. Doc Ophthalmol 44:19, 1977.
34. Nozik RA, Weinstock FJ, Vignos PJ: Ocular complications of chloroquine, a series and case presentation with a simple method for early detection of retinopathy. Am J Ophthalmol 58:774, 1969.
35. Bernstein H, Zvaifler N, Rubin M, et al: The ocular deposition of chloroquine. Invest Ophthalmol 2:384, 1963.

36. Shearer RV, Dubois EL: Ocular changes induced by long-term hydroxychloroquine (Plaquenil) therapy. Am J Ophthalmol 64:245, 1967.
37. Scherbel AL, Mackenzie AH, Nousek JE, et al: Ocular lesions in rheumatoid arthritis and related disorders with particular reference to retinopathy. A study of 741 patients treated with and without chloroquine drugs. N Engl J Med 273:360, 1965.
38. Bernstein HN: Chloroquine ocular toxicity. Surv Ophthalmol 12:415, 1967.
39. Marks JS: Chloroquine retinopathy: Is there a safe daily dose? Ann Rheum Dis 41:52, 1982.
40. Mackenzie AH: Dose refinements in long-term therapy of rheumatoid arthritis with antimalarials. Am J Med 75:40, 1983.
41. Johnson MW, Vine AK: Hydroxychloroquine therapy in massive total doses without retinal toxicity. Am J Ophthalmol 104:139, 1987.
42. Rosenthal RA, Kolb H, Bergsma D, et al: Chloroquine retinopathy in the rhesus monkey. Invest Ophthalmol Vis Sci 17:1158, 1978.
43. Frisk-Holmberg M, Bergkvist Y, Domeij-Nyberg B, et al: Chloroquine serum concentration and side-effects: Evidence for dose-dependent kinetics. Clin Pharmacol Ther 25:347, 1979.
44. Monahan RH, Horns RC: The pathology of chloroquine in the eye. Trans Am Acad Ophthalmol Otolaryngol 68:40, 1964.
45. Wetterholm DH, Winter FC: Histopathology of chloroquine retinal toxicity. Arch Ophthalmol 71:116, 1964.
46. Ramsey MS, Fine BS: Chloroquine toxicity in the human eye: Histopathologic observations by electron microscopy. Am J Ophthalmol 73:229, 1972.
47. Bernstein HN, Ginsberg J: The pathology of chloroquine retinopathy. Arch Ophthalmol 71:238, 1964.
48. Ivanina TA, Zueva MN, Lebedeva AI, et al: Ultrastructural alterations in cat and rat retina and pigment epithelium induced by chloroquine. Graefes Arch Clin Exp Ophthalmol 220:32, 1983.
49. Gregory MH, Rutty DA, Wood RD: Differences in the retinotoxic action of chloroquine and phenothiazine derivatives. J Pathol 102:139, 1970.
50. Boet DJ: Toxic effects of phenothiazines on the eye. Doc Ophthalmol 28:1, 1970.
51. Potts AM: The concentration of phenothiazines in the eye of experimental animals. Invest Ophthalmol 1:522, 1962.
52. Potts AM: Further studies concerning the accumulation of polycyclic compounds on uveal melanin. Invest Ophthalmol 3:399, 1964.
53. Potts AM: The reaction of uveal pigment in vitro with polycyclic compounds. Invest Ophthalmol 3:405, 1964.
54. Kimbrough BO, Campbell RJ: Thioridazine levels in the human eye. Arch Ophthalmol 99:2188, 1981.
55. Verrey F: Dégénérescence pigmentaire de la rétine d'origine médicamenteuse. Ophthalmologica 131:296, 1956.
56. Goar EL, Fletcher MC: Toxic chorioretinopathy following the use of NP 207. Trans Am Ophthalmol Soc 54:129, 1956.
57. Burian HM, Fletcher MC: Visual functions in patients with retinal pigmentary degeneration following the use of NP 207. Arch Ophthalmol 60:612, 1958.
58. May RH, Selymes P, Weekley RD, et al: Thioridazine therapy: Results and complications. J Nerv Ment Dis 130:230, 1960.
59. Weekley RD, Potts AM, Reboton J, et al: Pigmentary retinopathy in patients receiving high doses of a new phenothiazine. Arch Ophthalmol 64:65, 1960.
60. Scott AW: Retinal pigmentation in a patient receiving thioridazine. Arch Ophthalmol 70:775, 1963.
61. Connell MM, Poley BJ, McFarlane JR: Chorioretinopathy associated with thioridazine therapy. Arch Ophthalmol 71:816, 1964.
62. Hagopian V, Stratton DB, Busiek RD: Five cases of pigmentary retinopathy associated with thioridazine administration. Am J Psychiatry 123:97, 1966.
63. Finn R: Pigmentary retinopathy associated with thioridazine: Report of a case with a maximum daily dose of 1400 mgm. Am J Psychiatry 120:913, 1964.
64. Davidorf FH: Thioridazine pigmentary retinopathy. Arch Ophthalmol 90:251, 1973.
65. Cameron ME, Lawrence JM, Olrich JG: Thioridazine (Melleril) retinopathy. Br J Ophthalmol 56:131, 1972.
66. Leinfelder PJ, Burian HM: Mellaril intoxication of retina with full restitution of function. Invest Ophthalmol 3:466, 1964.
67. Morrison SB: Transient visual symptoms associated with Mellaril medication. Am J Psychiatry 116:1032, 1960.
68. Meredith TA, Aaberg TM, Willerson WD: Progressive chorioretinopathy after receiving thioridazine. Arch Ophthalmol 96:1172, 1978.
69. Miller FA, Bunt-Milam AH, Kalina RE: Clinical ultrastructural study of thioridazine retinopathy. Ophthalmology 89:1478, 1982.
70. Kozy D, Doft BH, Lipkowitz J: Nummular thioridazine retinopathy. Retina 4:253, 1984.
71. De Margerie J: Ocular changes produced by a phenothiazine drug: Thioridazine. Trans Can Ophthalmol Soc 25:160, 1962.
72. Applebaum A: An ophthalmoscopic study of patients under treatment with thioridazine. Arch Ophthalmol 69:578, 1963.
73. Heshe J, Englestoft FH, Kirk L: Retinabeskadigelse opstået under thioridazinbehandling. Nord Psykiatr Tidsskr 3:442, 1961.
74. Reboton J, Weekley RD, Bylenga ND, May RH: Pigmentary retinopathy and iridocycloplegia in psychiatric patients. J Neuropsychiatry 3:311, 1962.
75. Zelickson AS, Zeller HC: A new and unusual reaction to chlorpromazine. JAMA 188:144, 1964.
76. DeLong SL, Poley BJ, McFarlane JR: Ocular changes associated with long-term chlorpromazine therapy. Arch Ophthalmol 73:611, 1965.
77. Siddall JR: The ocular toxic findings with prolonged and high-dosage chlorpromazine intake. Arch Ophthalmol 74:460, 1965.
78. Siddall JR: Ocular and toxic changes associated with chlorpromazine and thioridazine. Can J Ophthalmol 190:190, 1966.
79. Krohlman GM, Pidde WJ: Acute methyl alcohol poisoning. Can J Ophthalmol 3:270, 1968.
80. Bennett IL, Carey FH, Mitchell GL, et al: Acute methyl alcohol poisoning: A review based on experiences in an outbreak of 323 cases. Medicine 32:431, 1953.
81. Benton CD, Calhoun FP: The ocular effects of methyl alcohol poisoning: Report of a catastrophe involving three hundred and twenty persons. Trans Am Acad Ophthalmol Otolaryngol 56:875, 1952.
82. McGregor IS: A study in the histopathological changes in the retina and late changes in the visual field in acute methyl alcohol poisoning. Br J Ophthalmol 27:523, 1943.
83. Benton CD, Calhoun FP: The ocular effects of methyl alcohol poisoning: Report of a catastrophe involving 320 persons. Am J Ophthalmol 36:1677, 1953.
84. Fink WH: The ocular pathology of methanol poisoning. Am J Ophthalmol 26:802, 1943.
85. Röe O: The ganglion cells of the retina in cases of methanol poisoning in human beings and experimental animals. Acta Ophthalmol 26:169, 1948.
86. Potts AM, Praglin J, Farkas I, et al: Studies on the visual toxicity of methanol. VIII. Additional observations on methanol poisoning in the primate test object. Am J Ophthalmol 40:76, 1955.
87. Gilger AP, Potts AM: Studies on the visual toxicity of methanol. V. The role of acidosis in experimental methanol poisoning. Am J Ophthalmol 39:63, 1954.
88. Martin-Amat G, Tephly TR, McMartin KE, et al: Methyl alcohol poisoning. II. Development of a model for ocular toxicity in methyl alcohol poisoning using the rhesus monkey. Arch Ophthalmol 95:1847, 1977.
89. Hayreh MS, Hayreh SS, Baumbach GL, et al: Methyl alcohol poisoning. III. Ocular toxicity. Arch Ophthalmol 95:1851, 1977.
90. Potts AM, Johnson LV: Studies on the visual toxicity of methanol. I. The effect of methanol and its degradation products on retinal metabolism. Am J Ophthalmol 35:107, 1952.
91. Baumbach GL, Cancilla PA, Martin-Amat G, et al: Methyl alcohol poisoning. IV. Alterations of the morphological findings of the retina and optic nerve. Arch Ophthalmol 95:1859, 1977.
92. Ros AM, Leyon H, Wennersten G: Crystalline retinopathy in patients taking an oral drug containing canthaxanthine. Photodermatol 2:183, 1985.
93. Daiker B, Schiedt K, Adnet JJ, et al: Canthaxanthin retinopathy. An investigation by light and electron microscopy and physio-

chemical analysis. Graefes Arch Clin Exp Ophthalmol 225:189, 1987.

94. Cortin P, Corriveau LA, Rousseau AP, et al: Maculopathie en paillettes d'or. Can J Ophthalmol 17:103, 1982.

95. Cortin P, Boudreault G, Rousseau AP, et al: La Rétinopathie à la canthaxanthine. 2. Facteurs prédisposants. Can J Ophthalmol 19:215, 1984.

96. Boudreault G, Cortin P, Corriveau LA, et al: La rétinopathie à la canthaxanthine. 1. Etude clinique de 51 consommateurs. Can J Ophthalmol 18:325, 1983.

97. Metge P, Mandirac-Bonnefoy C, Bellaube P: Thésaurismose rétinienne à la canthaxanthine. Bull Mem Soc Fr Ophthalmol 95:547, 1984.

98. Harnois C, Samson J, Malenfant M, et al: Canthaxanthin retinopathy. Anatomic and functional reversibility. Arch Ophthalmol 107:538, 1989.

99. Harnois C, Cortin P, Samson J, et al: Static perimetry in canthaxanthin maculopathy. Arch Ophthalmol 106:58, 1988.

100. Gass JDM: Nicotinic acid maculopathy. Am J Ophthalmol 76:500, 1973.

101. Millay RH, Klein ML, Illingworth DR: Niacin maculopathy. Ophthalmology 95:930, 1988.

102. Kaiser-Kupfer MI, Lippman ME: Tamoxifen retinopathy. Cancer Treat Rep 62:315, 1978.

103. McKeown CA, Swartz M, Blom J, et al: Tamoxifen retinopathy. Br J Ophthalmol 65:177, 1981.

104. Kaiser-Kupfer MI, Kupfer C, Rodrigues MM: Tamoxifen retinopathy: A clinicopathologic report. Ophthalmology 88:89, 1981.

105. Beck M, Mills PV: Ocular assessment of patients with tamoxifen. Cancer Treat Rep 63:1833, 1979.

106. Vinding T, Nielsen NV: Retinopathy caused by treatment with tamoxifen at low dosage. Acta Ophthalmol 61:45, 1983.

107. Bullock JD, Albert DM: Flecked retina. Appearance secondary to oxalate crystals from methoxyflurane anesthesia. Arch Ophthalmol 93:26, 1975.

108. Albert DM, Bullock JD, Lahav M, et al: Flecked retina secondary to oxalate crystals from methoxyflurane anesthesia: Clinical and experimental studies. Trans Am Acad Ophthalmol Otolaryngol 79:OP817, 1975.

109. Novak MA, Roth AS, Levine MR: Calcium oxalate retinopathy associated with methoxyflurane abuse. Retina 8:230, 1988.

110. Meredith TA, Wright JD, Gammon JA, et al: Ocular involvement in primary hyperoxaluria. Arch Ophthalmol 102:584, 1984.

Chapter 93

■

Lattice Degeneration of the Retina

ROBERT HAIMOVICI and DON H. NICHOLSON

Lattice degeneration of the retina (equatorial degeneration, pigmentary degeneration, snail track degeneration, retinal erosion) is the most commonly recognized vitreoretinal abnormality of the peripheral fundus known to predispose to rhegmatogenous retinal detachment. Approximately 30 percent of patients with retinal detachment also have lattice degeneration.

EPIDEMIOLOGY

Lattice degeneration is a common disorder that is present in approximately 7 to 8 percent of the general population in clinical series.[1, 2] In autopsy series, the proportion is slightly higher—10.7 to 16.4 percent.[3, 4] This condition is bilateral in 42 to 45 percent of cases.[1, 4] Men and women appear to be equally affected, and no racial predilection has been noted. Patients with lattice degeneration more frequently have myopia than the population in general.[3]

CLINICAL FEATURES

Ophthalmoscopically, the lattice lesion is a sharply outlined, round or oval, often elongated area of retinal thinning or irregularity (Fig. 93–1 and Table 93–1). It is best seen with binocular indirect ophthalmoscopy and

scleral depression. Vitreous liquefaction overlying the retinal thinning and vitreous attachment to its edges, although consistently present, may be difficult to visualize without contact lens biomicroscopy. The majority of lesions are circumferential and are most frequently

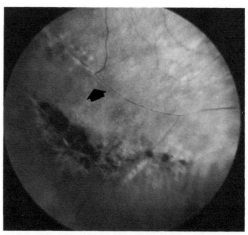

Figure 93–1. Clinical appearance of lattice degeneration. Two parallel rows, the upper (arrow) paravascular in orientation without pigmentation, shows surface white dots and vascular sheathing. The lower pigmented patch of lattice shows a prominent interlacing pattern of white lines, representing hyalinized blood vessels.

Table 93–1. HISTOPATHOLOGY OF LATTICE DEGENERATION

Circumscribed retinal thinning
Absent internal limiting membrane
Overlying vitreous liquefaction
Increased vitreoretinal adherence to borders
Retinal capillary obliteration
Retinal pigment epithelial pigment loss, hyperplasia, and pigment migration
Glial proliferation on vitreous face (late)

located slightly posterior to the midpoint between the ora serrata and the equator.[1] Two or more lesions may be parallel and overlap one another. Oblique lesions and radial paravascular lesions may also be seen. Patches of lattice degeneration vary in length from a fraction of a disc diameter to more than 12 disc diameters.[3] The width of most lesions is between one quarter and two thirds of a disc diameter, with an average of one half of a disc diameter. Lattice lesions are most commonly found in the 11 o'clock to 1 o'clock and the 5 o'clock to 7 o'clock meridians, and the inferotemporal quadrant is most commonly involved. Variable clinical features include abnormal retinal or choroidal pigmentation, yellow-white surface flecks, reddish patches, and branching white lines. Both abnormal pigmentation and superficial yellow-white flecks are seen in approximately 80 percent of patients with lattice degeneration.[1] Branching white lines, which represent occluded or sheathed retinal blood vessels, are seen in 17 percent of patients. These white lines were once felt to be pathognomonic of this disorder, and the term *lattice degeneration* is derived from the interlacing pattern of these white vessels, even though they are now known to be present in just a fraction of lesions. The focal reddish areas within lattice lesions are zones of retinal thinning. Atrophic retinal holes may result from progressive retinal thinning and are present in about 25 percent of eyes with lattice degeneration.[3, 5] Traction retinal tears are less common, occurring in 1.0 to 2.4 percent of eyes with lattice degeneration.[3, 5]

FLUORESCEIN ANGIOGRAPHY

Fluorescein angiography of early lattice lesions may show a near-normal retinal circulation.[6] Later, there may be poor or no perfusion of retinal vessels within the area of degeneration, as well as leakage from the underlying choriocapillaris. Retinal vessels proximal to lattice lesions have been reported to show delayed filling, microaneurysms, extravasation of fluorescein, or formation of arteriovenous shunts.[7]

HISTOLOGIC FEATURES

Light microscopy reveals the lack of internal limiting membrane, retinal thinning, overlying vitreous liquefaction, vitreous condensation, and exaggerated vitreoretinal adherence at the borders of these lesions (Table 93–2).[8] Although retinal thinning results from loss of inner layers initially, in advanced lesions all retinal layers are affected. Retinal pigment epithelial abnormalities, occurring in 92 percent of lesions, include focal loss of pigmentation, hyperplasia, and pigment migration into the retina, particularly around retinal vessels.[3] Trypsin digestion preparations reveal loss of capillaries, decreased numbers of endothelial cells, and obliteration of vessels within the area of degeneration. Irregular clumps of PAS-positive material correspond to the gray-white particles at the margin or within lattice lesions. In advanced lesions, glial proliferation at the interface between liquid and formed vitreous may be seen (Fig. 93–2).[8]

ELECTRON MICROSCOPY

The internal limiting lamina is consistently lacking over areas of lattice degeneration.[3, 9] Glial cell processes may remodel the retinal surface and extend into the vitreous cavity. Scanning electron microscopy shows that individual glial cells at the edge of lattice lesions may extend onto the vitreous surface as a proliferative membrane.[10]

CLINICAL COURSE

Most lattice lesions are present by the beginning of the second decade of life.[1, 3] There is no age-related trend in morphologic characteristics or location of lattice lesions. The degree of vitreoretinal adhesion and the prevalence of pigmentary changes, white lines, retinal holes, posterior vitreous detachment, and retinal tears increase with time. Despite these tendencies to progression, the majority of lattice lesions remain unchanged for long periods, and the age of the patient cannot be correlated with the appearance of the lesion.[2] Atrophic retinal holes and traction retinal tears, the two factors associated with the risk of retinal detachment, do increase with time. Byer observed new atrophic holes in 12.7 percent of patients who were followed for many years.[5] Sixty-five percent of these retinal holes appeared before the age of 35 yr. Traction retinal tears in lattice

Table 93–2. FEATURES OF LATTICE DEGENERATION

Clinical Features
Sharply outlined, round, oval, or elongated area of retinal thinning or irregularity

Variable Features
Branching white lines
Reddish patches
Yellow-white surface flecks
Retinal or choroidal pigmentation

Topography
Orientation
Circumferential > oblique > radial
Location
Between ora serrata and equator
11:00 to 1:00 and 5:00 to 7:00 meridians and inferotemporal quadrants most common

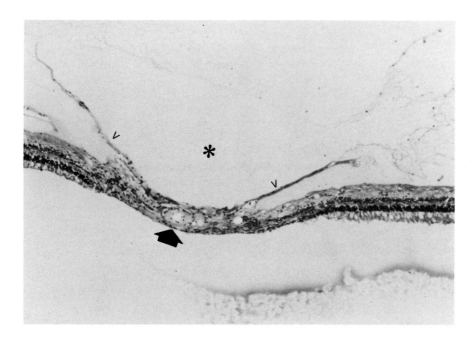

Figure 93–2. Histopathologic appearance of lattice degeneration. Cross-sectional view with anterior border to the left. Separation of sensory retina from pigment epithelium is fixation artifact. V indicates condensed sheets of vitreous collagen firmly adherent to anterior and posterior borders. The *asterisk* represents an overlying pool of liquefied vitreous. The *arrow* shows a thick-walled, hyalinized blood vessel.

degeneration are produced when posterior vitreous detachment occurs because of the strong adherence of condensed vitreous at the junction of healthy retina and the thinned zone of lattice (Fig. 93–3).

The prevalence of lattice degeneration was found by Karlin and Curtin to increase with increasing axial length among a population of patients with myopia.[19] Celorio and Pruett,[20] however, found the prevalence higher in moderate (6 to 9D) myopia with an axial length of 26 to 27 mm than in high (> 24D) myopia with an axial length greater than 32 mm.

HEREDITY

The genetics of lattice degeneration have not been resolved. The prevalence of lattice degeneration in first-degree relatives of patients with this condition is about 23 percent or three times as high as in the general population. These data were thought to adhere most closely to a polygenic or multifactorial mode of inheritance.[11] Autosomal dominant inheritance has been postulated and supported by reports of pedigrees with familial retinal detachment often associated with lattice degeneration.[2] These pedigrees, however, may not represent the same group of patients as those without a high incidence of retinal detachment. Still others feel that the inheritance pattern is recessive but that it exhibits pseudodominance.[12]

PATHOGENESIS

The pathogenesis of lattice degeneration is still speculative. Localized vitreoretinal traction,[13] a primary retinal vasculopathy,[10] and a localized anomaly of the internal limiting membrane[9] have all been suggested.

LATTICE DEGENERATION AND RETINAL DETACHMENT

The association between lattice degeneration and retinal detachment is well known. Approximately 30 percent of patients who present with a retinal detachment will have lattice degeneration on examination.[3, 5, 14, 15] Because the prevalence of this condition is high in the general population, the risk of development of a retinal detachment in any single patient with lattice degeneration has been estimated at only 0.3 to 0.5 percent (Table 93–3).[2]

Atrophic Round Holes

Byer[21] observed subclinical retinal detachment caused by atrophic round holes in 6.7 percent of eyes with lattice degeneration that were followed for many years. Unequivocal progression of these subclinical detachments, however, occurs very rarely in nonfellow eyes. Only 2 of 11 patients with subclinical detachment showed slight enlargement of the detachment, and none progressed to frank clinical detachment in Byer's series.

When retinal detachment is produced by round atrophic holes, it is unrelated to posterior vitreous detachment and almost always occurs in patients 30 yr of age or younger (Fig. 93–4). These detachments may display multiple "high water mark" demarcation lines (suggesting insidious progression) and have a good prognosis for successful surgical repair.[16]

Traction Tears

In eyes with lattice degeneration, strong vitreoretinal adhesions at the edges of lattice lead to tears along the posterior border or at the end of lattice after posterior

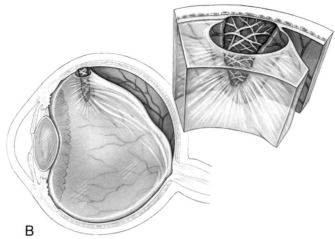

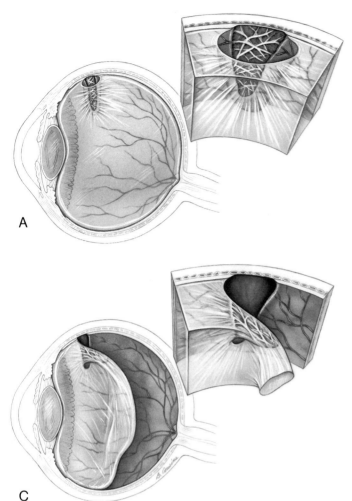

Figure 93–3. Pathogenesis of traction tears in lattice degeneration. *A,* Vitreous condensations adhere firmly to the borders of a superior circumferential patch of lattice degeneration. *B,* Posterior vitreous separation. The force of gravity increases traction transmitted along sheets of vitreous condensation. *C,* A traction tear begins as the retina rips along the line of vitreoretinal adhesion. The tear will assume the typical horseshoe configuration as the anterior vector of traction force increases following the posterior rip, creating radial extensions toward the ora serrata at each end of the patch of lattice degeneration.

vitreous detachment (Fig. 93–5; see also Fig. 93–3). Traction retinal tears also occur in ophthalmoscopically normal areas of retina in eyes with lattice degeneration. Traction tears and the detachments they produce occur at the time of posterior vitreous separation, generally after 40 yr of age. Of 423 nonfellow phakic eyes with lattice degeneration followed by Byer for an average of 11 yr, new traction tears were noted in only 5 eyes (1 percent). Davis' observations in patients with traction tears in general suggest that the greatest risk for progression to retinal detachment occurs within the first 6 wk after a new symptomatic traction tear appears.[28]

Burton[18] found that myopia and lattice degeneration are both risk factors for the development of retinal detachment. The lifetime risk of retinal detachment for an emmetropic patient without lattice degeneration is 0.3 percent, as compared with 2.2 percent for a patient with high myopia. The emmetropic patient with lattice degeneration has a lifetime risk of 1.7 percent for retinal detachment as compared with the 35.9 percent lifetime risk in the highly myopic eye with lattice degeneration. He concluded, therefore, that high myopia and lattice degeneration together are more strongly correlated with retinal detachment than is either alone.

MANAGEMENT OF LATTICE DEGENERATION

Background

Since the 1940s, various therapeutic modalities have been proposed for the prophylaxis of retinal detachment in patients with lattice degeneration. Studies supporting the use of penetrating diathermy, and more recently cryotherapy and photocoagulation, are found throughout the literature. Enthusiasm for prophylactic treatment of lattice degeneration has waned with a clearer understanding of the natural history of this disorder.

Table 93–3. RISK FACTORS FOR LATTICE-ASSOCIATED RETINAL DETACHMENT (IN ORDER OF INCREASING SIGNIFICANCE)

Atrophic round holes
Fellow eye of retinal detachment
High myopia
Traction retinal tear (symptomatic)

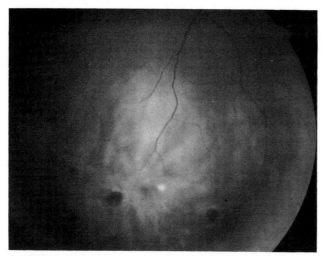

Figure 93–4. Atrophic round holes in lattice degeneration causing inferior detachment in a 29-year-old myopic patient.

The inherently low incidence of retinal detachment associated with lattice degeneration and the frequent origin of tears in ophthalmoscopically normal retina have tempered the enthusiasm for prophylactic treatment.

Nonfellow Phakic Eyes

LATTICE DEGENERATION WITHOUT RETINAL BREAKS

Byer's long-term natural history study reports a 1 percent risk of retinal detachment in patients with lattice degeneration, with or without atrophic holes.[21] Prophylactic therapy is not indicated for this group.

LATTICE DEGENERATION WITH ATROPHIC HOLES

Although subclinical retinal detachment is frequent among patients with atrophic round holes in lattice degeneration, the incidence of clinical or progressive subclinical detachment is only about 2 percent.[21] Symptoms from these detachments, however, may be insidious. Murakami-Nagasako and Ohba found that 75 percent of patients with this type of detachment did not seek care until central vision was impaired.[22] Inferior detachments from atrophic holes in lattice degeneration have an excellent prognosis for successful surgical repair by scleral buckling.[17]

Prophylactic therapy is not indicated for atrophic holes in lattice degeneration. If subclinical detachment caused by atrophic holes is present, treatment is indicated only if the patient cannot be followed at regular intervals on a long-term basis.

LATTICE DEGENERATION WITH RETINAL TEARS

Traction retinal tears in eyes with lattice degeneration may occur in ophthalmoscopically normal retina or along the posterior and lateral borders of lattice (see Figs. 93–

3 and 93–5). Traction tears *without* acute symptoms are treated in (1) fellow eyes of patients with retinal detachment, (2) patients with a strong family history of retinal detachment, and (3) aphakic eyes. Asymptomatic traction tears in patients with lattice degeneration do not otherwise require treatment.

Prophylactic treatment is generally recommended for acute *symptomatic* tears in both phakic and aphakic eyes. These eyes have a relatively high risk of progression to retinal detachment.

Fellow Eye in Lattice Retinal Detachment

The overall rate of retinal detachment in untreated fellow eyes of patients with lattice degeneration and lattice-associated retinal detachment in the first eye is approximately 5.1 percent.[23] In patients with myopia and lattice degeneration, it may be as high as 24.6 percent.[24] Folk and associates reduced the overall rate of retinal detachment in the fellow eye to 1.8 percent over a 7-yr period with prophylactic treatment.[23] However, they found no beneficial effect in subgroups with greater than six clock hr of lattice degeneration and 6 D or more of myopia. This study concludes that prophylactic treatment of 100 fellow eyes would be necessary to prevent three retinal detachments.[23] Since lattice-associated retinal detachment has a good chance of successful reattachment with conventional surgery, and since new tears are notoriously frequent in ophthalmoscopically normal retina,[2, 14] controversy continues concerning the benefit of prophylactic therapy in asymptomatic fellow eyes.

PAVING STONE DEGENERATION OF THE RETINA

Paving stone degeneration of the retina (cobblestone degeneration) is a common and distinctive condition

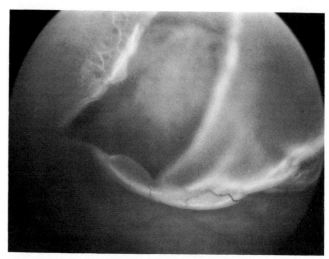

Figure 93–5. Large traction tear in lattice degeneration. Bullous detachment is to the right of the tear (posterior) and lattice degeneration is elevated in the flap to the left (anterior).

that was found in 27 percent of patients in a large autopsy study.[25] Small, rounded, yellow-white areas, often with pigmented margins, are located between the ora serrata and the equator. Prominent underlying choroidal vessels are characteristic. Histopathologically, the retina is thinned by loss of outer retinal layers and fusion of sensory retina with retinal pigment epithelium. The choriocapillaris may be attenuated or lacking. The vitreous is normal overlying these foci. Paving stone degeneration does not predispose to retinal detachment. The strong adherence between the attenuated retina and the underlying choroid may actually deflect or delimit detachment of the sensory retina. Rarely, secondary retinal breaks do occur, as detached retina tears away from the adhesion.[25]

SNOWFLAKE DEGENERATION OF THE RETINA

Snowflake degeneration is an uncommon and usually familial retinal finding that may be seen in families at high risk for retinal detachment. Hirose and colleagues have described a pedigree with progressive cataract, vitreous degeneration, and peripheral retinal findings of probable autosomal dominant inheritance.[26] Progressive retinal findings described in this family were extensive white with pressure, snowflake degeneration, sheathing of retinal vessels, and increased pigmentation and disappearance of retinal vessels. Five of 15 patients studied experienced a retinal detachment. In another family, Robertson and associates reported white or yellow-white granule-like deposits in the peripheral retina that were not associated with vitreous degeneration or retinal detachment.[27]

REFERENCES

1. Byer NE: Clinical study of lattice degeneration of the retina. Trans Am Acad Ophthalmol Otolaryngol 69:1064, 1965.
2. Byer NE: Lattice degeneration of the retina. Surv Ophthalmol 23:213, 1978.
3. Straatsma BR, Zeegen PD, Foos RY, et al: Lattice degeneration of the retina. Trans Am Acad Ophthalmol Otolaryngol 78:OP87, 1974.
4. Foos RY, Simons KB: Vitreous in lattice degeneration of retina. Ophthalmology 91:452, 1984.
5. Byer NE: Changes in and prognosis of lattice degeneration of the retina. Trans Am Acad Ophthalmol Otolaryngol 78:OP114, 1974.
6. Tolentino FI, Lapus JV, Novalis G, et al: Fluorescein angiography of the degenerative lesions of the peripheral fundus and rhegmatogenous retinal detachment. Int Ophthalmol Clin 16:13, 1976.
7. Sato K, Tsunakawa N, Inaba K, Yanagisawa Y: Fluorescein angiography on retinal detachment and lattice degeneration. Part I. Equatorial degeneration with idiopathic retinal detachment. Acta Soc Ophthalmol Jpn 75:635, 1971.
8. Straatsma BR, Allen RA: Lattice degeneration of the retina. Trans Am Acad Ophthalmol Otolaryngol 66:600, 1962.
9. Streeten BW, Bert M: The retinal surface in lattice degeneration of the retina. Am J Ophthalmol 74:1201, 1972.
10. Robinson MR, Streeten BW: The surface morphology of retinal breaks and lattice retinal degeneration: A scanning electron microscopic study. Ophthalmology 93:237, 1986.
11. Murakami F, Ohba N: Genetics of lattice degeneration of the retina. Ophthalmologica 185:136, 1982.
12. Falls HF: The genetics of lattice degeneration. In Kimura SJ, Caygill WM (eds): Retinal Diseases: Symposium on Differential Diagnostic Problems of Posterior Uveitis. Philadelphia, Lea & Febiger, 1966, p 162.
13. Tolentino FI, Schepens CL, Freeman HM: Vitreoretinal Disorders: Diagnosis and Management. Philadelphia, WB Saunders, 1976, p 340.
14. Dumas J, Schepens CL: Chorioretinal lesions predisposing to retinal breaks. Am J Ophthalmol 61:620, 1966.
15. Morse PH: Lattice degeneration of the retina and retinal detachment. Am J Ophthalmol 78:930, 1974.
16. Tillery WV, Lucier AC: Round atrophic holes in lattice degeneration—An important cause of phakic retinal detachment. Trans Am Acad Ophthalmol Otolaryngol 81:509, 1976.
17. Yoshino Y, Ideta H, Ishikawa M, Inone S: Relations between onset, age and refraction in rhegmatogenous retinal detachment with lattice degeneration. Acta Soc Ophthalmol Jpn 92:377, 1988.
18. Burton TC: The influence of refractive error and lattice degeneration on the incidence of retinal detachment. Trans Am Ophthalmol Soc 87:143, 1990.
19. Karlin DB, Curtin BJ: Peripheral chorioretinal lesions and axial length of the myopic eye. Am J Ophthalmol 81:625, 1976.
20. Celorio JM, Pruett RC: Prevalence of lattice degeneration and its relation to axial length in severe myopia. Am J Ophthalmol 111:20, 1991.
21. Byer NE: Long-term natural history of lattice degeneration of the retina. Ophthalmology 96:1396, 1989.
22. Murakami-Nagasako F, Ohba N: Phakic retinal detachment associated with atrophic hole of lattice degeneration of the retina. Graefes Arch Clin Exp Ophthalmol 220:175, 1983.
23. Folk JC, Arrindell EL, Klugman MR: The fellow eye of patients with phakic lattice retinal detachment. Ophthalmology 96:72, 1989.
24. Folk JC, Burton TC: Bilateral phakic retinal detachment. Ophthalmology 89:815, 1982.
25. O'Malley P, Allen RA, Straatsma BR, O'Malley CC: Paving-stone degeneration of the retina. Arch Ophthalmol 73:169, 1965.
26. Hirose T, Lee KY, Schepens CL: Snowflake degeneration in hereditary vitreoretinal degeneration. Am J Ophthalmol 77:143, 1974.
27. Robertson DM, Link TP, Rostvold JA: Snowflake degeneration of the retina. Ophthalmology 89:1513, 1982.
28. Davis MD: The natural history of retinal breaks without detachment. Trans Am Ophthalmol Soc 71:343, 1973.

Chapter 94

■

Retinal Breaks

ARNOLD J. KROLL and SAMIR C. PATEL

A retinal break is a full-thickness discontinuity of retinal tissue, usually located in the fundus periphery or midperiphery and only occasionally more posteriorly. Its clinical significance is that it may provide access for fluid vitreous to enter the subretinal space, creating a primary retinal detachment. The relationship between retinal breaks and primary retinal detachment has led to the term *rhegmatogenous retinal detachment* from the Greek word *rhegma,* which means a rent. Secondary retinal detachment, caused by subretinal transudation from tumors or from degenerative or inflammatory lesions, occurs without retinal breaks and is outside the scope of this discussion.

Retinal breaks were first described in 1853,[1] and their important relationship to retinal detachment was noted as early as 1870.[2] It was not until 1921, however, that Gonin conclusively established that retinal breaks cause retinal detachments by demonstrating that closing a retinal break can reattach a detached retina.[3]

Normally, the retina is kept in its attached state by a variety of mechanical, physical, and metabolic forces,[4] including intraocular pressure, osmotic pressure from choroidal extracellular protein,[5] the possible adhesive effect of the interphotoreceptor matrix,[6] and the pumping effect of the retinal pigment epithelium.[4]

Forces acting to detach the retina include vitreoretinal traction and intraocular fluid currents.[7] When a retinal break is present and the forces acting to detach the retina exceed those keeping it attached, fluid vitreous enters the subretinal space through the retinal break and a retinal detachment ensues.

The clinician looks for findings that may increase the risk of a retinal break and a subsequent retinal detachment, including (1) presence of a symptomatic posterior vitreous detachment; (2) vitreoretinal traction on the retina, especially on the flap of a retinal horseshoe tear; (3) lattice degeneration of the retina; (4) cystic retinal tufts; (5) high myopia; (6) a history of retinal detachment in the fellow eye; (7) a family history of retinal detachment; (8) a history of previous cataract surgery; and (9) trauma to the globe. Indeed, combinations of these risk factors further increase the likelihood of retinal detachment.

There are three types of retinal breaks: tears, holes, and dialyses. A retinal tear is a full-thickness rent in retinal tissue caused by vitreoretinal traction. A retinal hole is a round or oval full-thickness discontinuity of retina caused by atrophy and is not related to vitreous traction. A retinal dialysis is a full-thickness disinsertion of the retina at the ora serrata that is often, but not always, associated with blunt trauma to the globe.

Macular breaks are a different clinical entity and are discussed in Chapters 67 and 68.

RETINAL TEARS

Posterior Vitreous Detachment

In young individuals, the vitreous gel uniformly fills the vitreous cavity and consists of hyaluronic acid, water, soluble salts and proteins, and an insoluble meshwork of fine collagen fibrils.[8] The vitreous gel is also strongly adherent to the pars plana and peripheral retina in an irregular band extending 360 degrees around the fundus periphery and called the *vitreous base.* It is much less strongly adherent to the disc and macula. In late middle age (even sooner in individuals with high myopia), as well as in vitreous inflammation and cases of trauma (nonsurgical or surgical), the vitreous gel liquefies (syneresis) and eventually collapses, causing a posterior vitreous detachment.[9, 10] At the time of posterior vitreous detachment, the collapsed vitreous gel is usually at least partially freed from the posterior pole but remains suspended 360 degrees from the strongly adherent vitreous base. The patient may experience floaters because of newly visible condensations of the vitreous on the elevated, newly mobile posterior hyaloid. These condensations had been previously attached to the disc and to a lesser extent to the macula. Floaters may be accompanied by vitreous hemorrhage, causing many more floaters, when the detaching posterior hyaloid ruptures disc capillaries or tears the retina. The patient may experience photopsia (flashes of light) from tugging of the newly mobile vitreous on the peripheral retina, especially during saccadic eye movements. The patient sees photopsias more easily in the dark.

If a posterior vitreous detachment does not tear the retina, it requires no treatment. However, the patient should be warned that delayed tearing of the retina can occur and that similar symptoms could occur at any time in the fellow eye. If new symptoms appear in either eye, prompt reexamination should be performed.

Vitreoretinal Adhesion

At the time of posterior vitreous detachment or shortly thereafter, tractional forces are transmitted to physiologic and pathologic areas of strong vitreoretinal adhesion. These areas include the vitreous base, margins of lattice retinal degeneration, cystic retinal tufts, and paravascular retina. When the tractional forces at these sites exceed the tensile strength of the retina, the retina tears.

VITREOUS BASE

Vitreoretinal adhesion occurs normally in all eyes at the vitreous base, which is an approximately 4-mm circumferential band of vitreous condensation strongly attached to the pars plana and peripheral retina. Retinal tears commonly occur at the posterior margin of the vitreous base,[11] especially in aphakic eyes.

LATTICE DEGENERATION OF THE RETINA

Lattice degeneration of the retina was first clearly described in 1928.[12] It is found in 8 percent of all eyes and is the major fundus lesion leading to retinal tears and retinal detachment.[13] Indeed, it is the cause of up to 30 percent of retinal detachments.[14] It is commonly associated with myopia.[15–17] It typically consists of equatorially oriented patches of criss-crossing white lines (Fig. 94–1), but there are many variations, including pigmentation, radial orientation, reddish coloration, and a frosted appearance lacking white lines, known as snail track degeneration (Fig. 94–2). Histopathologically, the retina is thinned, the overlying vitreous is liquefied, and there is strong vitreous adhesion at its margins.[13] This strong vitreous adhesion is the factor that can cause tearing of the retina at the posterior or lateral margin of a lattice lesion when there is a posterior vitreous detachment[18] and, indeed, most retinal detachments associated with lattice degeneration are caused by these kinds of retinal tears.[19, 20]

CYSTIC RETINAL TUFTS

Cystic retinal tufts are congenital, small, focal nodular projections of retinal tissue, usually located posterior to the vitreous base and found in 5 percent of autopsied eyes.[11, 21] Clinically, they are discrete white lesions, with or without underlying pigment clumping, that are strongly attached to vitreous strands. Vitreous traction

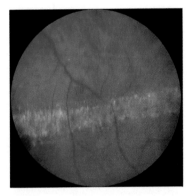

Figure 94–2. Snail track degeneration. Generally acknowledged to be a form of lattice degeneration, this lesion has a frosted appearance of yellow-white flecks and lacks the characteristic criss-crossing white lines.

associated with posterior vitreous detachment can cause retinal horseshoe tears or operculated retinal tears at the site of cystic retinal tufts and can account for up to 10 percent of primary retinal detachments.[21, 22] Cystic retinal tufts are more comprehensively discussed in Chapter 95.

PARAVASCULAR VITREORETINAL ADHESIONS

Paravascular vitreoretinal adhesions occur on or adjacent to retinal blood vessels. They are rarely detectable clinically before the occurrence of a posterior vitreous detachment.[23] They can cause avulsion of peripheral retinal veins without retinal break formation,[24] or they can cause full-thickness retinal horseshoe tears[25] and vitreous hemorrhage.[26] These lesions are more commonly associated with recurrent hemorrhage than with retinal breaks and retinal detachment.

Types of Retinal Tears

The most common form of tearing of the retina is the flap tear or horseshoe tear (Fig. 94–3). It is caused by localized vitreous traction that breaks the retina, elevating a flap of retina and forming the typical horseshoe-shaped tear with the flap of the tear hinged anteriorly. If the tear interrupts a retinal vessel, there will be retinal and vitreous hemorrhage. By tugging the flap in the direction of the vitreous, persisting vitreous traction on the flap of the tear (Fig. 94–4) can encourage elevation of the tear by subretinal fluid, causing a retinal detachment (Fig. 94–5). If the peripheral vitreous traction is extremely strong, it may exceed the tensile strength of the flap of the horseshoe tear, causing operculation of the tear (Fig. 94–6). This may actually be clinically beneficial because it relieves the vitreous traction on the tear, making a retinal detachment less likely. On occasion, vitreoretinal traction may simultaneously cause a horseshoe tear and an operculated tear just posterior to the horseshoe tear (Fig. 94–7).[27] Presumably, the mechanical advantage of the more posterior vitreoretinal

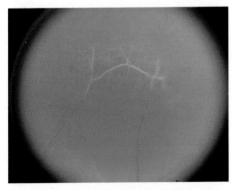

Figure 94–1. Lattice retinal degeneration. Clinical appearance in detached retina. The oval, equatorially oriented patch of thinned retina has criss-crossing white lines (sclerotic vessels) and pigment clumping.

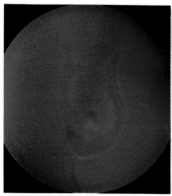

Figure 94–3. Retinal horseshoe tear (flap tear). Localized vitreoretinal traction has exceeded the tensile strength of the retina, tearing it. The vitreoretinal traction elevated the flap of the tear, producing the characteristic curving horseshoe shape. Flecks of hemorrhage on the margins and flap of the tear indicate interruption of small retinal vessels.

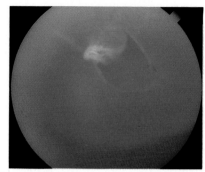

Figure 94–5. Retinal horseshoe tear causing retinal detachment. Focal vitreoretinal traction is seen pulling the flap of the tear up and to the left. Fluid vitreous has seeped through the tear into the subretinal space, elevating the retina into a bullous detachment.

adhesion exerts stronger traction, operculating the posterior tear.

Giant retinal tears (Fig. 94–8) have been defined as circumferential retinal breaks of 90 degrees or more.[28] The formation of a giant retinal tear is similar to the formation of a retinal horseshoe tear in that both frequently occur at the posterior margin of the vitreous base. However, they differ in that the vitreoretinal adhesion that produces a horseshoe tear is localized, whereas the vitreoretinal adhesion that produces a giant retinal tear extends over an area of 90 degrees or more.[29] It is almost as if the entire anterior edge of a giant retinal tear is the equivalent of the flap of a retinal horseshoe tear! Once a tear greater than 90 degrees occurs, the posterior edge of the tear, which is not attached to the vitreous, becomes independently mobile and can curl on itself (Fig. 94–8).[30]

It is essential to distinguish between a giant retinal tear as described and a retinal dialysis of 90 degrees or more. In a retinal dialysis, the posterior edge of the break remains attached to the vitreous base, splinting it and preventing it from curling on itself.[31] Giant retinal dialyses have a much better prognosis than do giant retinal tears because of this splinting action of the vitreous base on the posterior edge of the tear (see Retinal Dialyses.)

Management of Retinal Tears

For purposes of treatment, retinal tears can be conveniently classified as symptomatic or asymptomatic.

SYMPTOMATIC RETINAL TEARS

The incidence of retinal tears in acute posterior vitreous detachment approaches 15 percent.[10, 18, 32–34] Therefore, the clinician is obliged to carefully evaluate the patient who presents with photopsia and floaters, the symptoms of a posterior vitreous detachment. Unfortunately, clinical history alone cannot distinguish a patient with a posterior vitreous detachment causing a retinal tear from a patient with a posterior vitreous detachment

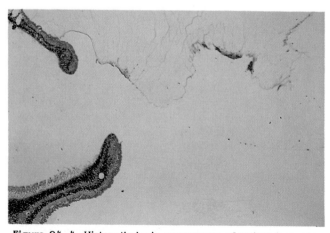

Figure 94–4. Histopathologic appearance of retinal horseshoe tear. The vitreous is adherent to the flap of the tear, exerting traction on it. The posterior edge of the tear is artifactually elevated. PAS stain.

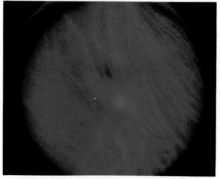

Figure 94–6. Operculated retinal tear. Vitreoretinal traction has exceeded the tensile strength of the flap of the tear, freeing it completely from the underlying retina. The resulting free operculum is suspended over the tear from the posterior hyaloid of the retracting vitreous. Persistence of vitreous traction makes it more likely that a retinal detachment will be caused by a horseshoe tear rather than by an operculated tear.

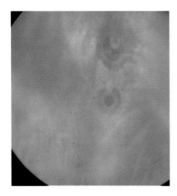

Figure 94–7. Simultaneous formation of horseshoe tear and operculated tear (eye bank eye). The more posterior operculated tear was produced by stronger vitreoretinal traction than was on the flap of the horseshoe tear.

and no retinal tear. Only careful examination of the fundus with indirect ophthalmoscopy and scleral depression of the fundus periphery, including slit-lamp biomicroscopy, can make this determination.

When a posterior vitreous detachment produces an acute symptomatic retinal horseshoe tear, a retinal detachment ensues in 25 to 90 percent of cases.[35–37] However, prophylactic treatment can decrease the incidence of retinal detachment to as little as 5 percent.[38–45] This is a strong case for prophylactic treatment of symptomatic retinal horseshoe tears. Indeed, symptomatic retinal horseshoe tears should be treated even in eyes with less risk, such as in patients with phakic, nonmyopic eyes and no history of retinal detachment in the fellow eye or no family history of retinal detachment, because of the frequency of retinal detachment even in these eyes.

Acute symptomatic operculated retinal tears, in which the flap of the tear has torn free and become suspended on the posterior hyaloid overlying the retinal break (see Fig. 94–6), usually have no residual vitreous traction on the break and have little risk of subsequent retinal

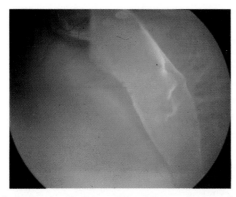

Figure 94–8. Giant retinal tear. When vitreoretinal traction at the posterior border of the vitreous base is not localized, as in a retinal horseshoe tear, but extends for 90 degrees or more, a giant retinal tear may form. The posterior edge of the tear, to which vitreous is not attached, may roll up on itself, permitting the examiner to look directly at the rolled posterior surface of the retina.

detachment.[37, 46] Conservative management is advised in most cases, unless they are acute, large, superiorly located, associated with vitreous hemorrhage,[46] or occur in a patient with high myopia or aphakia, or in the fellow eye of a patient with a history of retinal detachment. In addition, careful examination of the break with slit-lamp biomicroscopy is indicated to rule out persistent vitreoretinal traction on the margins of the break because this is associated with an increased incidence of retinal detachment.[47] Prophylactic treatment is indicated for such breaks. The management of giant retinal tears is outside the scope of this discussion and is covered in Chapters 97 and 100.

ASYMPTOMATIC RETINAL TEARS

In general, asymptomatic retinal tears are much less likely to lead to retinal detachment than are symptomatic retinal tears.[48, 49] Therefore, asymptomatic retinal tears—both horseshoe and operculated—can be managed conservatively in patients with no history of retinal detachment in the fellow eye, no history of aphakia, and no positive family history, even if the tear has a superior location.[48, 49] One exception may be in a patient about to have cataract surgery because of the increased incidence of subsequent retinal detachment. However, there is a high risk of retinal detachment in patients with asymptomatic retinal tears and a history of retinal detachment in the fellow eye, and the tear should be treated.[50, 51]

The value of prophylactic treatment of asymptomatic retinal horseshoe tears in aphakic eyes is uncertain.[52] Old retinal tears, especially those with a preexisting posterior vitreous detachment, have a much better prognosis than do fresh tears and can be managed conservatively.[50] Asymptomatic retinal horseshoe tears in patients with high myopia and no other risk factors have not been conclusively studied.

TECHNIQUES OF PROPHYLACTIC TREATMENT

The goal of prophylactic treatment of retinal tears is to establish an adhesion between the outer retina and the underlying pigment epithelium—Bruch's membrane. This adhesion should be strong and complete enough so that subretinal fluid is denied access to the subretinal space, preventing retinal detachment. At the present time, three modalities of treatment—laser photocoagulation, cryopexy, and diathermy—are used to accomplish this goal. All three modalities create the chorioretinal adhesion by means of thermal injury. However, each modality has its own actual and theoretical advantages and disadvantages. There is no convincing evidence that one modality creates a stronger adhesion than another.[53]

Laser photocoagulation lesions can be very accurately placed with the desired spot size and intensity under the surgeon's visual control, using only topical anesthesia and either a slit-lamp or indirect ophthalmoscope delivery system. No conjunctival incision is required. There is minimal thermal injury to the choroid and no injury to the sclera. There is no scattering of pigment epithelial cells into the vitreous. The disadvantages of laser photocoagulation are that it requires relatively clear media, a cooperative patient, and a newly introduced indirect ophthalmoscope delivery system in order to reach the very anterior retina. In addition, laser photocoagulation is of limited use in the presence of significant elevation of the retina, because excessively high power is required to obtain a photocoagulation lesion.

Cryopexy can be accurately placed under indirect ophthalmoscopic control, does not alter the sclera, and can be used transconjunctivally. It is best for equatorial anterior lesions that do not require a conjunctival incision. It can be used in the presence of greater amounts of vitreous hemorrhage than can laser photocoagulation because laser energy must traverse the opaque vitreous and cryotreatment does not. Its disadvantages are that it requires more anesthesia than does photocoagulation, usually subconjunctival lidocaine; it cannot reach posterior to the conjunctival cul-de-sac without a conjunctival incision; it scatters loose pigment epithelial cells into the vitreous,[54] which theoretically may increase the risk of proliferative vitreoretinopathy; and it may cause breakdown of the blood-aqueous barrier, resulting in cystoid macular edema and exudative detachments.[55]

Diathermy, either under scleral flaps alone or under scleral flaps in conjunction with scleral buckling, requires more extensive surgery than do the other two modalities. Its primary limitation is that it weakens and shrinks the sclera, requiring scleral dissection. In addition, the surgeon must look directly at the sclera rather than at the retina when diathermy is applied, limiting visual control. Its theoretical advantage is that it does not scatter pigment epithelial cells into the vitreous.[54] It is currently being used much less than are the other two modalities.

The authors recommend laser photocoagulation for posterior tears and for anterior tears that can be adequately surrounded by laser treatment. We recommend cryopexy for most anterior tears because it is important to treat retinal horseshoe tears adequately between the anterior margin of the tear and the ora serrata to prevent delayed anterior extension of the retinal tear through the areas of treatment to reach untreated retina. This could permit later formation of retinal detachment despite treatment.[43, 56, 57] If adequate treatment with laser between the retinal tear and the ora serrata cannot be obtained, transconjunctival cryopexy of this area can be added.

It has been the experience of one of us (AJK), in a series of 216 symptomatic retinal horseshoe tears, that transconjunctival cryopexy resulted in the posttreatment operculation of the flap of the tear, releasing traction on the tear in 27 eyes—approximately 1 of 8 (unpublished data). When the flap does not operculate but does extend further anteriorly because of persistent vitreoretinal traction, there may be a small amount of vitreous hemorrhage from the anterior extension of the tear. However, adequate previous anterior cryotreatment does not permit retinal detachment because the

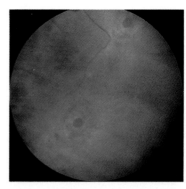

Figure 94–9. Retinal holes. Round atrophic retinal holes may be found in lattice degeneration or without other apparent pathologic condition. They are not caused by vitreous traction.

anterior extension of the tear does not reach untreated retina. We do not use scleral buckling in the management of retinal tears unless there is significant retinal detachment at the time of treatment.

In using laser photocoagulation or cryopexy, we recommend two rows of medium-intensity laser or one row of medium-intensity cryotherapy at the margins surrounding the tear and, in the case of a horseshoe tear, extending treatment to the ora serrata. It is not necessary, and is possibly harmful, to treat the bared pigment epithelium within the tear.

RETINAL HOLES

Retinal holes are round or oval atrophic full-thickness discontinuities of retinal tissue, usually located in the fundus periphery or midperiphery (Fig. 94–9) and only occasionally in the macula. They are distinguished from retinal tears in that they do not form as a result of vitreoretinal traction and therefore have no associated flap or free operculum. They are found in 2.3 percent of autopsied eyes and are most commonly associated with lattice degeneration of the retina (Fig. 94–10).[58]

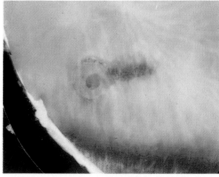

Figure 94–10. Pigmented lattice retinal degeneration with associated retinal hole and localized retinal detachment (eye bank eye). The retina has been opacified by formalin. The localized retinal detachment surrounding the hole has a pigmented demarcation line, suggesting that the retinal detachment has remained the same size for some time.

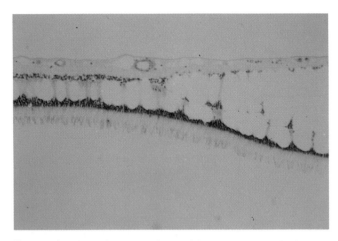

Figure 94–11. Peripheral retinoschisis. Retinoschisis is formed when peripheral cystoid spaces coalesce to produce an internal splitting of the retina. PAS stain.

Other associated conditions include myopia,[59] chorioretinitis,[60] congenital meridional folds,[61] zonular traction tufts,[11] and degenerative retinoschisis (Fig. 94–11).[62]

Lattice Degeneration of the Retina

A significant percentage of all retinal detachments are caused by retinal holes in lattice degeneration.[20] Although the majority of retinal detachments associated with lattice degeneration are caused by retinal tears, 30 to 45 percent are caused by atrophic holes within the lattice.[10, 19] Nevertheless, Byer followed a large series of phakic eyes with lattice degeneration and no history of retinal detachment in the fellow eye for up to 25 yr and noted only a 2 percent incidence of progressive retinal detachment from atrophic retinal holes in the lattice. This seeming discrepancy is explained by the high prevalence of atrophic retinal holes in lattice degeneration in the general population.[63] Byer recommended that prophylactic treatment in phakic nonfellow eyes should be discontinued.

Unlike the clinical situation with posterior vitreous detachment and retinal horseshoe tears, retinal holes in lattice degeneration in the presence of symptomatic posterior vitreous detachment are not necessarily associated with imminent danger of a retinal detachment. The retinal holes without a flap or free operculum are not caused by the posterior vitreous detachment, and a retinal detachment need not ensue. Conversely, in the presence of an acute posterior vitreous detachment and atrophic holes in lattice degeneration, careful slit-lamp biomicroscopy should be performed to evaluate vitreous traction on the margins of the lattice lesions.[7, 64] Treatment may be considered if vitreous traction is found.[60]

Degenerative Retinoschisis

Degenerative retinoschisis occurs when the cysts of peripheral cystoid degeneration coalesce, with resultant lamellar splitting of the retina. Clinically, it is characterized by a smooth, convex elevation of the inner layer of the schisis cavity in the peripheral fundus. A degenerative retinoschisis usually has yellow flecks on its surface and is commonly seen after the fifth decade of life in the inferotemporal quadrant.

Retinal holes are more commonly seen in the outer layer rather than in the inner layer of retinoschisis and are of variable size and number (Fig. 94–12).[65] Byer followed 123 patients (218 eyes) with asymptomatic degenerative retinoschisis for up to 21 yr. Twenty-four outer layer holes were present or had developed by the end of the study. Fifty-eight percent of these patients experienced localized retinal detachments. They were followed for approximately 6 yr, and during this time none experienced symptomatic clinical retinal detachment. Byer concluded that no treatment was indicated for outer layer holes in retinoschisis unless they were causing symptomatic progressive retinal detachment.[66] However, in selected patients, some authors have shown a more frequent rate of progressive retinal detachment.[67, 68] Other authors treat outer layer holes if they are close to the macula.[69]

RETINAL DIALYSES

Retinal dialyses are full-thickness disinsertions of the retina at the ora serrata. Histologically, they are a separation of the sensory retina from the nonpigmented ciliary epithelium of the pars plana. They were first described in 1882,[70] cause 8 to 17 percent of all retinal detachments, and are the most common type of retinal break, causing retinal detachments in patients under 20 yr of age.[71] Dialyses may be idiopathic or traumatic in origin.

Idiopathic Retinal Dialyses

Idiopathic retinal dialyses are commonly found in the inferotemporal quadrant,[72] usually in young individuals, and they characteristically lead to a slowly progressive retinal detachment.[73] Posterior vitreous detachment is

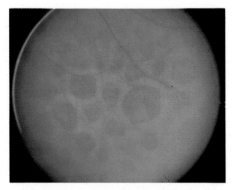

Figure 94–12. Multiple round retinal holes in the outer layer of degenerative retinoschisis. Such holes may be single or multiple and of variable size. They occur much more frequently in the outer layer than in the inner layer of retinoschisis.

rarely found in these patients.[74] There often is involvement of both eyes, a strong family history,[75] and no history of blunt trauma to the eye.

Traumatic Retinal Dialyses

In a large series of retinal dialyses, 37 percent were attributable to trauma.[71] It has been found that blunt anteroposterior trauma to the globe, which causes rapid equatorial stretching of the globe, can acutely distort the relatively immobile vitreous base, disinserting the retina at the ora serrata.[76] In contrast to the typical inferotemporal location of idiopathic dialyses, traumatic dialyses are most often found in the superonasal quadrant[77, 78] but may also be inferotemporal. They may or may not be associated with a disinsertion of the vitreous base, which appears as an irregular, round, movable cord of translucent tissue suspended over the ora serrata, adherent at each end to the attached vitreous base at its margins. Retinal dialyses may also complicate perforating injuries of the globe, as well as pars plana vitrectomy surgery near the pars plana instrumentation sites.[79]

Management

It is characteristic of retinal dialyses that the vitreous base usually remains intact and adheres to the posterior edge of the dialysis, splinting it.[31] This immobilizes the posterior edge of the dialysis to some degree, making it easy to "close" the break with scleral depression using indirect ophthalmoscopy. Indeed, a small retinal dialysis may not be visible when scleral depression takes place directly under it. It may only become visible when it is opened by scleral depression to one side of it.

These characteristics of retinal dialyses, and their far peripheral location, make them surprisingly easy to close with scleral buckling surgery. They usually have a good prognosis even when quite large.

In the operating room, dialyses are completely surrounded by cryopexy under indirect ophthalmoscopic control. The margins are localized and the entire break is buckled, including a small margin of unbroken ora serrata on either side. The treated break tends to flatten easily on the buckling as long as the buckling is not too high. A high buckling can cause a "fish mouth" opening of the break. A low buckling can best be accomplished by not draining subretinal fluid and using a segmental soft buckling material such as silicone sponge or preferably Miragel (a hydrophic acrylate explant),[80] with closely spaced mattress sutures. Cryopexy, rather than diathermy, is the preferred treatment modality because cryopexy tends to soften the eye, similar to tonography, whereas diathermy causes scleral contraction and tends to harden the eye.

After tightening the mattress sutures overlying the explant, the central retinal artery should be carefully monitored so as not to exceed the systolic blood pressure. Systemic acetazolamide, osmotic agents, and paracentesis of the anterior chamber can all help control increased intraoperative tension. Most often, however, simple patience on the part of the surgeon is all that is required because the eye will gradually soften.

REFERENCES

1. Coccius A: Über die Anwendung des Augen-Spiegels nebst Angabe eines neuen Instruments. Leipzig, Immanuel Muller, 1853, p 131.
2. de Wecker L, de Jaiger E: Traite des maladie du fond l'oeil et atlas d'ophthalmoscopie. Paris, A. Delahaye, 1870, p 151.
3. Gonin J: Le traitment de decollement retinien. Ann d'Ocul 158:175, 1921.
4. Ryan AJ (ed): Retina, vol. 3. St Louis, CV Mosby, 1989, pp 76–87.
5. Pederson JE, Tsuboi S, Toris CB: Extravascular albumin concentration of the uvea. Invest Ophthalmol Vis Sci 28(Suppl 1):69, 1987.
6. Shirakawa H, Ishiguro SI, Itoh Y, et al: Are sugars involved in the binding of rhodopsin-membranes by retinal pigment epithelium? Invest Ophthalmol Vis Sci 28:628, 1987.
7. Machemer R: Importance of fluid absorption, traction, intraocular currents and chorioretinal scars in the therapy of rhegmatogenous retinal detachments. XLI Edward M Jackson Memorial Lecture. Am J Ophthalmol 98:681, 1984.
8. Eisner G: Clinical anatomy of the vitreous. In Jakobiec FA (ed): Ocular Anatomy, Embryology and Teratology. Philadelphia, Harper & Row, 1982, p 391.
9. Sebag J: Aging of the vitreous. Eye 1:254, 1987.
10. Foos RY, Wheeler NC: Vitreoretinal juncture: Synchysis senilis and posterior vitreous detachment. Ophthalmology 96:783, 1983.
11. Foos RY: Vitreous base, retinal tufts and retinal tears: Pathogenetic relationships. In Pruett RC, Regan CDJ (eds): Retina Congress. New York, Appleton-Century-Crofts, 1974, pp 259–280.
12. Rehsteiner K: Ophthalmoskopische Untersuchungen über Veranderungen der Fundusperipherie in myopen and senilen Augen. Arch Ophthalmol 120:282, 1928.
13. Byer NE: Lattice degeneration of the retina. Surv Ophthalmol 23:213, 1979.
14. Straatsma BR, Allen RA: Lattice degeneration of the retina. Trans Am Acad Ophthalmol Otolaryngol 66:600, 1962.
15. Schepens CL, Bahn GC: Examination of the ora serrata: Its importance in retinal detachment. Arch Ophthalmol 44:677, 1950.
16. Cambiaggi A: Recherches sur le role des alterations myopiques chorioretinienne dans la pathogenie de decollement de la retine. Ophthalmologica 156:124, 1968.
17. Karlin DB, Curtin BJ: Axial length measurements and peripheral fundus changes in the myopic eye. In Pruett RC, Regan CDJ (eds): Retina Congress. New York, Appleton-Century-Crofts, 1974, p 629.
18. Tasman WS: Posterior vitreous detachment and peripheral retinal breaks. Trans Am Acad Ophthalmol Otolaryngol 72:217, 1968.
19. Byer NE: Changes in and prognosis of lattice degeneration of the retina. Trans Am Acad Ophthalmol Otolaryngol 78:114, 1974.
20. Benson WE, Morse PH: The prognosis of retinal detachment due to lattice degeneration. Ann Ophthalmol 10:1197, 1978.
21. Byer NE: Cystic retinal tufts and their relationship to retinal detachment. Arch Ophthalmol 99:1788, 1981.
22. Murakami-Nagasko F, Ohba N: Phakic retinal detachment associated with cystic retinal tuft. Graefes Arch Clin Exp Ophthalmol 219:188, 1982.
23. Spencer LM, Foos RY: Paravascular vitreoretinal attachments. Role in retinal tears. Arch Ophthalmol 84:557, 1970.
24. Vine AK: Avulsed retinal veins without retinal breaks. Am J Ophthalmol 98:723, 1984.
25. Okun E: Gross and microscopic pathology in autopsy eyes. Part III. Retinal breaks without detachment. Am J Ophthalmol 51:369, 1961.
26. Jaffe N: Complications of acute posterior vitreous detachment. Arch Ophthalmol 79:568, 1968.
27. Cibis PA: Vitreoretinal pathology and surgery in retinal detachment. St Louis, CV Mosby, 1985, pp 59–65.

28. Freeman HM: Treatment of giant retinal tears. *In* McPherson A (ed): New and controversial aspects of retinal detachment. New York, Harper & Row, 1968, pp 391–399.

29. Leaver PK, Lean JS: Management of giant retinal tears using vitrectomy and silicone oil fluid exchange. A preliminary report. Trans Ophthalmol Soc UK 101:189, 1981.

30. Scott JD: Treatment of massive vitreous retraction. Trans Ophthalmol Soc UK 95:429, 1975.

31. Chignell AH: Retinal Detachment Surgery. Berlin and Heidelberg, Springer-Verlag, 1988, p 59.

32. Lindner B: Acute posterior vitreous detachment and its retinal complications. Acta Ophthalmol 87(Suppl):1, 1966.

33. Boldrey EE: Risk of retinal tears in patients with vitreous floaters. Am J Ophthalmol 96:783, 1983.

34. Tabotabo MM, Karp LA, Benson WE: Posterior vitreous detachment. Ann Ophthalmol 12:59, 1980.

35. Davis MD: Natural history of retinal breaks. Arch Ophthalmol 92:183, 1974.

36. Colyear BH Jr, Pischel DK: Clinical tears in the retina without detachment. Am J Ophthalmol 41:773, 1956.

37. Neumann E, Hyams S: Conservative management of retinal breaks. A follow-up study of subsequent retinal detachment. Br J Ophthalmol 56:482, 1972.

38. Chignell AH, Shilling J: Prophylaxis of retinal detachment. Br J Ophthalmol 57:291, 1973.

39. Colyear BH Jr, Pischel DK: Preventive treatment of retinal detachment by means of light coagulation. Trans Pac Coast Oto-ophthalmol Soc 41:193, 1960.

40. Morse PH, Scheie HG: Prophylactic cryoretinopexy of retinal breaks. Arch Ophthalmol 92:204, 1974.

41. Nadel AJ, Geiser RG: The treatment of acute horseshoe retinal tears by transconjunctival cryopexy. Ann Ophthalmol 7:1568, 1975.

42. Pollak A, Oliver M: Argon laser photocoagulation of symptomatic flap tears and retinal breaks of fellow eyes. Br J Ophthalmol 65:469, 1981.

43. Robertson DM, Norton EWD: Long-term follow-up of treated retinal breaks. Am J Ophthalmol 75:395, 1973.

44. Sollner F: Über de prophylaktische Behandlung der Ablatio retinae durch Lichtcoagulation. Ber Zusammenkunft Dtsch Ophthalmol Ges 66:327, 1964.

45. Tasman WS, Joegers KR: A retrospective study of xenon photocoagulation and cryotherapy in the treatment of retinal breaks. *In* Pruett RC, Regan CDJ (eds): Retina Congress. New York, Appleton-Century-Crofts, 1972, pp 557–564.

46. Benson WE: Prophylactic therapy of retinal breaks. Surv Ophthalmol 22:41, 1977.

47. Davis MD: The natural history of retinal breaks without detachment. Trans Am Ophthalmol Soc 71:343, 1973.

48. Byer NE: Prognosis of asymptomatic retinal breaks. Arch Ophthalmol 85:669, 1971.

49. Byer NE: The natural history of asymptomatic retinal breaks. Ophthalmology 89:1033, 1982.

50. Neumann E, Hyams S, Barkai S, et al: The natural history of retinal holes with special reference to the development of retinal detachment and the time factor involved. Isr J Med Sci 8:1424, 1972.

51. Davis MD, Segal PP, McCormick A: The natural course followed by the fellow eye in patients with rhegmatogenous retinal detachment. *In* Pruett RC, Regan CDJ (eds): Retina Congress. New York, Appleton-Century-Crofts, 1974, p 643.

52. Michels RG, Wilkinson CP, Rice TA: Retinal Detachment. St Louis, CV Mosby, 1990, p 1075.

53. Verdaguer JT, Vaisman M: Treatment of symptomatic retinal breaks. Am J Ophthalmol 87:783, 1979.

54. Campochiaro PA, Kaden IH, Vidaurri-Leal J, Glaser BM: Cryotherapy enhances intravitreal dispersion of viable retinal pigment cells. Arch Ophthalmol 103:434, 1985.

55. Ackerman AL, Topilow HW: A reduced incidence of cystoid macula edema following retinal detachment surgery using diathermy. Ophthalmology 92:1092, 1985.

56. Benson WE, Morse PH, Nantawan P: Late complications following cryotherapy of lattice degeneration. Am J Ophthalmol 84:515, 1977.

57. Delaney WV Jr: Retinal tear extension through the cryosurgical scar. Br J Ophthalmol 55:205, 1971.

58. Foos RY: Retinal holes. Am J Ophthalmol 86:354, 1978.

59. Hyams SW, Neumann E: Peripheral retina in myopia: With particular reference to retinal breaks. Br J Ophthalmol 53:300, 1969.

60. Straatsma BR, Zeegan PD, Foos RY, et al: Lattice degeneration of the retina. Trans Am Acad Ophthalmol Otolaryngol 78:87, 1974.

61. Byer NE: Clinical study of retinal breaks. Trans Am Acad Ophthalmol Otolaryngol 71:461, 1967.

62. Straatsma BR, Foos RY: Typical and reticular degenerative retinoschisis. XXVI Francis I. Proctor Memorial Lecture. Am J Ophthalmol 75:551, 1973.

63. Byer NE: Long-term natural history of lattice degeneration of the retina. Ophthalmology 96:1396, 1989.

64. Michels RG, Wilkinson CP, Rice TA: Retinal Detachment. St Louis, CV Mosby, 1990, p 1081.

65. Foos RY: Senile retinoschisis. Trans Am Acad Ophthalmol Otolaryngol 74:33, 1970.

66. Byer NE: Long-term natural history study of senile retinoschisis with implications for management. Ophthalmology 93:1127, 1986.

67. Dobbie JG: Cryotherapy in the management of senile retinoschisis. Trans Am Acad Ophthalmol Otolaryngol 73:1047, 1969.

68. Hagler WS, Woldoff HD: Retinal detachment in relation to senile retinoschisis. Trans Am Acad Ophthalmol Otolaryngol 77:OP99, 1973.

69. Sulonen JM, Wells CG, Barricks ME, et al: Degenerative retinoschisis with giant outer layer breaks and retinal detachment. Am J Ophthalmol 99:114, 1985.

70. Leber T: Über die Entstehung der Netzhautablosung. Ber Vers Ophthalmol 14:18, 1882.

71. Hagler WS: Retinal dialysis: A statistical and genetic study to determine pathogenetic factors. Trans Am Ophthalmol Soc 38:687, 1980.

72. Chignell AH: Retinal dialysis. Br J Ophthalmol 57:572, 1973.

73. Kinyoun JK, Knobloch WH: Idiopathic retinal dialysis. Retina 4:9, 1984.

74. Tolentino FI, Schepens CL, Freeman HM: Vitreoretinal Disorders. Diagnosis and Management. Philadelphia, WB Saunders, 1976, p 384.

75. Francois J: Role of heredity in retinal detachment. *In* McPherson A (ed): New and Controversial Aspects of Retinal Detachment. New York, Harper & Row, 1968, p 101.

76. Cox MS, Schepens CL, Freeman HM: Retinal detachment due to ocular contusion. Arch Ophthalmol 76:678, 1966.

77. Hagler WS, North AW: Retinal dialysis and retinal detachment. Arch Ophthalmol 79:376, 1968.

78. Zion VM, Burton TC: Retinal dialysis. Arch Ophthalmol 98:1971, 1980.

79. Carter VB, Michels RG, Glaser BM, De Bustros S: Iatrogenic retinal breaks complicating pars plana vitrectomy. Ophthalmology 97:848, 1990.

80. Tolentino FI, Refojo MF, Schepens CL: A hydrophilic acrylate implant for scleral buckling: Technique and clinical experience. Retina 1:281, 1981.

Chapter 95

Cystic Retinal Tuft and Miscellaneous Peripheral Retinal Findings

NORMAN E. BYER

This chapter discusses a wide variety of peripheral retinal findings, not discussed in other chapters, that frequently must come within the purview of clinicians examining the retina and must be well understood in order to arrive at correct diagnostic and prognostic conclusions (Tables 95–1 and 95–2). The entities are discussed under the headings of developmental abnormalities, significant normal variations, and miscellaneous peripheral degenerations and findings. By far the most important entity to be discussed is cystic retinal tuft, which continues to be very poorly understood by most ophthalmologists and, strangely, is seldom discussed even by retina specialists even though it is second in importance only to lattice degeneration as a visible peripheral retinal lesion that is a precursor to retinal detachment.

DEVELOPMENTAL ABNORMALITIES

Cystic Retinal Tuft

Cystic retinal tuft is a congenital peripheral vitreoretinal abnormality consisting primarily of glial tissue. This designation was applied in 1967[1] to a lesion that was probably first described by Vogt in 1936,[2] who presented numerous beautiful drawings. Later publications probably discussing the same entity referred to it as granular patch and floaters;[3] globular masses and spheres;[4] granular patches, globules, and floaters;[5] and rosette-like formations.[6] It has been thoroughly described histologically by Foos.[7]

Histologically,[7] it consists of a microcystic, elevated, peripheral retinal lesion of 0.1 to 1.0 mm in diameter. Pigment is often found in the base, and trophic changes may be present in the immediately adjacent retina. Vitreous condensations frequently are visible at the surface of the lesion. Degenerative changes in the outer retinal layers (including the pigment epithelium) are usually present, and the larger tufts consistently show a lack of photoreceptor elements. Neuronal elements usually are replaced by microcysts and proliferating glial cells, and a cap of glial cells with dense cytoplasm is a consistent finding on the surface of the lesion. Electron microscopy shows the vitreoretinal junction to be characterized by deep crypt and microcyst formation, with extensive penetration of vitreous. The proliferating glial cell processes around the microcysts are tightly packed and have extremely dense cytoplasm. Cystic retinal tufts may be avulsed by vitreous traction with or without posterior vitreous detachment. Topographically, lesions are found in the retrobasal zone and are distributed equally in all quadrants of the retina. They are found in the eyes of newborn infants and are represented equally in all age groups. Foos[7] documented in autopsied eyes that cystic retinal tufts can be causally related to tractional retinal tears. In a large autopsy series,[8] he found that operculated tears resulting from this lesion accounted for 36 percent of postoral vitreoretinal tractional tears and that they occurred in the extrabasal zone (i.e., posterior to the vitreous base). In autopsied eyes, as contrasted with clinical studies, the tears seen

Table 95–1. PREVALENCE OF CYSTIC RETINAL TUFT AND MISCELLANEOUS PERIPHERAL RETINAL FINDINGS

Lesion or Finding	Prevalence in Adult Population (%)	Association of Lesion With Later Retinal Detachment	Proportion of Detachments Accounted for By This Lesion
Cystic retinal tuft	5	0.28%	10%
Noncystic retinal tuft	33	0	0
Zonular traction tuft	15	Very rare	Nil
Meridional fold	26	Very rare	Nil
Enclosed ora bay	6	Very rare	Nil
Peripheral cystoid degeneration	100	0	0
Paving stone degeneration	22	0	0
Pearl of the ora serrata	20	0	0
Pars plana cyst	18	0	0
White with pressure	Common	0	0

Table 95–2. MANAGEMENT OF CYSTIC RETINAL TUFT AND MISCELLANEOUS PERIPHERAL RETINAL FINDINGS

Lesion or Finding	Need for Prophylactic Treatment
Cystic retinal tuft	0
Noncystic retinal tuft	0
Zonular traction tuft	0
Meridional fold	0
Enclosed ora bay	0
Peripheral cystoid degeneration	0
Paving stone degeneration	0
Pearl of the ora serrata	0
Pars plana cyst	0
White with pressure	0

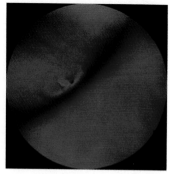

Figure 95–2. Cystic retinal tuft in a 27-year-old woman, with a small atrophic retinal hole and a small localized area of subretinal fluid. (From Byer NE: The Peripheral Retina in Profile—A Stereoscopic Atlas. Torrance, CA, Criterion Press, 1952, p. 23.)

are primarily tractional tears with free opercula, caused by vitreoretinal avulsion. They begin to appear in an age group 2 decades younger than the age group in which posterior vitreous detachment begins to occur. The prevalence of cystic retinal tufts in autopsy series is 5 percent, with a bilaterality rate of 6 percent.

Clinically,[9] the lesion is seen as a tiny discrete mound, sharply circumscribed, rounded or ovoid, characteristically chalky white (Figs. 95–1 and 95–2; see Figs. 95–4 and 95–5), and occasionally with pigment adjacent to the lesion. On examination with scleral indentation, it is slightly or moderately elevated, with a broad base and borders that gradually slope and merge with the adjacent retina. The lesion may sometimes be mistaken for a small elevated flap of retina, but because of its chalky-white appearance, it does not show the translucency of a retinal flap. Generally the lesion is found in the region of the equator, is approximately 0.1 to 0.5 disc diameter, and may show mirror symmetry with similar lesions in the fellow eye.

In two clinical series of retinal detachments caused by cystic retinal tuft, the predominant break was a tear with attached flap in 93 percent[9] and 66 percent[10] of cases, respectively. These two studies also concluded that cystic retinal tuft probably is associated with 10 percent of retinal detachments in general. This makes it the second most important peripheral retinal degeneration in this regard next to lattice degeneration, which is

associated with approximately 30 percent of detachments.

There are three types of retinal breaks caused by cystic retinal tuft (Figs. 95–2 to 95–5).[9, 11] The most important and most frequent is a tractional tear following posterior vitreous detachment (Figs. 95–4 and 95–5). Tractional tears with attached flap may also occur in persons as young as 20 yr old, as the result of a localized, asymptomatic form of vitreous detachment without a posterior vitreous detachment. These tears may later become avulsed as tears with free opercula, and such tears with free opercula also may occur after generalized posterior vitreous detachment because the cystic retinal tuft represents such a small localized lesion against which vitreous traction is exerted. Similarly, a prophylactically treated tractional tear that later shows an avulsed free operculum generally confirms that the initial lesion was a cystic retinal tuft.

Because cystic retinal tuft is present in 5 percent of individuals in autopsy studies,[12] it can be calculated that the risk of retinal detachment is only about 0.28 percent (or 1 in 357 persons with cystic retinal tuft). Therefore, it is obvious that prophylactic treatment of such lesions is not to be recommended.

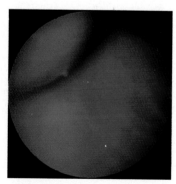

Figure 95–1. Cystic retinal tuft in a 48-year-old woman. (From Byer NE: The Peripheral Retina in Profile—A Stereoscopic Atlas. Torrance, CA, Criterion Press, 1952, p. 21.)

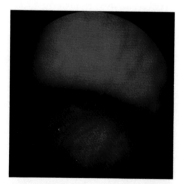

Figure 95–3. Cystic retinal tuft in a 26-year-old man, in whom the flap of a small retinal tear (which had been observed for 6 yr without change) has now been avulsed as a free operculum. (From Byer NE: The Peripheral Retina in Profile—A Stereoscopic Atlas. Torrance, CA, Criterion Press, 1952, p. 25.)

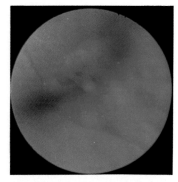

Figure 95–4. Cystic retinal tuft in a 68-year-old woman with acute symptomatic retinal tear, following posterior vitreous detachment. Note the chalky-white lesion on the apex of the flap. (From Byer NE: The Peripheral Retina in Profile—A Stereoscopic Atlas. Torrance, CA, Criterion Press, 1952, p. 35.)

Noncystic Retinal Tuft[1, 7, 12]

Noncystic retinal tuft is a thin, slightly elevated wisp of retinal tissue, less than 0.1 mm in diameter at its base. Internally it contains Müller cell processes. It is usually found in clusters within the vitreous base and without associated cystic or pigmentary changes. It may degenerate, producing tiny floating spherical fragments that probably represent decapitation of tufts by avulsion. Noncystic retinal tufts appear initially in the latter part of the first decade of life and occur in about one third of adults. They are most prevalent nasally and are not associated with retinal detachment.

Zonular Traction Tuft

Zonular traction tuft is a developmental abnormality[1, 13] in which there is a posterior displacement of zonular attachments to the peripheral retina, resulting in an abnormal tuft of tissue drawn from the surrounding retinal surface toward the ciliary body at an acute angle, the anterior tip of which is either pointed or bulbous. It is associated with trophic changes of adjacent retinal cystoid spaces, thinning, and occasionally full-thickness retinal holes. Tractional changes may be seen in slightly

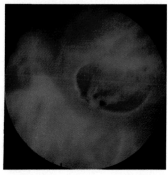

Figure 95–5. Cystic retinal tuft in a 58-year-old woman with a large acute symptomatic retinal tear, following posterior vitreous detachment. (From Byer NE: The Peripheral Retina in Profile—A Stereoscopic Atlas. Torrance, CA, Criterion Press, 1952, p. 34.)

elevated retinal folds radiating posteriorly from the base, and rarely by rupturing of the tuft, or a full-thickness retinal tear. Microscopically,[13] the tuft contains neuroglial cells and at the base often shows cystic degeneration with neuroglial replacement of neuronal elements. There may be marked retinal thinning, full-thickness holes, and proliferation of pigment epithelium.

Zonular traction tufts are statistically more frequent in males and are found in 15 percent of autopsied cases, being bilateral in 15 percent of cases.[13] Eighty-one percent of these traction tufts are found in the nasal quadrants, and they are most prevalent in the inferonasal quadrant. However, they occur independently of meridional complexes, which are also predominantly found on the nasal side. The bases of 4 percent of tufts have associated full-thickness retinal holes.

In a large autopsy study of postoral retinal tears, Foos[8] found that zonular traction tufts accounted for 6 percent of tears, which were either flap tears (if the tufts were partially avulsed) or tears with free opercula (if the tufts were completely avulsed). Retinal tears, if present, are almost always found within the vitreous base (i.e., intrabasal) and can be recognized clinically by careful examination of the flap of the tear or by the elongated shape of the operculum. Retinal detachment is uncommon from this cause and is usually localized. Prophylactic treatment of zonular traction tuft is not indicated.

SIGNIFICANT NORMAL VARIATIONS

Meridional Fold

A meridional fold is a radially oriented, linear elevation of the peripheral retina that is aligned with a dentate process of the ora serrata (81 percent of cases) or with an ora bay (19 percent of cases).[14] It represents a normal developmental variation that originates at the ora serrata and extends posteriorly for 0.6 to 6.0 mm (average 1.5 disc diameters). In about 14 percent of cases, there is a small focus of retinal thinning just posterior to the fold and rarely a true full-thickness retinal break.[11, 14, 15] Meridional folds occur in 26 percent of persons and are bilateral in 55 percent of cases, affecting 20 percent of eyes. They are found equally in all age groups and are statistically more prevalent among males.[14] There is a strong predilection for location at or just above the nasal horizontal meridian (Fig. 95–6).

Meridional folds have no clinical significance except for rare retinal breaks located near their posterior end, but they are very useful as retinal landmarks to help an examiner locate a previously seen retinal pathologic condition.

Enclosed Ora Bays

An enclosed ora bay is a developmental abnormality in which an island of nonpigmented pars plana epithe-

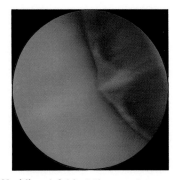

Figure 95–6. Meridional fold at the nasal ora serrata, near the horizontal meridian. (From Byer NE: The Peripheral Retina in Profile—A Stereoscopic Atlas. Torrance, CA, Criterion Press, 1952, p. 14.)

lium becomes isolated from the rest of the pars plana and is completely or nearly completely surrounded by peripheral retinal tissue (Fig. 95–7). Conversely, it may be considered a localized absence of neuroretinal epithelium. Microscopically, the area anterior to the lesion shows cystic degeneration and disorganization of neural elements. The underlying pigment epithelium is usually hyperplastic and sometimes is seen to have migrated into adjacent retina.

Enclosed ora bays, or partially enclosed bays, are found in 6 percent of autopsied eyes[12] and are almost equally distributed between nasal and temporal clock hour positions, usually near the horizontal meridian.[16] They exist as single lesions in 80 percent of involved eyes.[17] About 73 percent of enclosed ora bays are associated with meridional complexes located in the same clock hour positions. A meridional fold can be seen immediately anterior or posterior to 20 percent of enclosed ora bays.[16] It has also been found that 16 percent of enclosed or partially enclosed ora bays may each have an associated retinal tear, meridionally aligned with and posterior to it, following a posterior vitreous detachment.[17] There is no association between the presence of enclosed ora bays and either the size of the globe or the presence of peripheral retinal excavations.

The primary clinical importance of enclosed ora bays is the necessity to differentiate them from true peripheral retinal breaks. This can be confusing, but it is made

much easier by noting the following ophthalmoscopic characteristics of enclosed ora bays:

1. Enclosed ora bays are very frequently aligned with meridional complexes or meridional folds.

2. During scleral indentation, the borders of an enclosed ora bay are seen to be gradually sloping, with a gradual transition from the appearance inside the lesion to that of the normal retina outside. In the case of a true retinal break, this border should be sharp and show an abrupt change in appearance.

3. The color and texture of the tissue inside the enclosed ora bay should correspond exactly to the color and texture of the adjacent pars plana. This can be confirmed by quickly alternating the field of view from the enclosed ora bay to the pars plana and back again.

Because they can be easily identified ophthalmoscopically, enclosed ora bays are also very useful as retinal landmarks, in conjunction with which other, more subtle, previously recorded lesions, such as tiny retinal breaks, can be found again more easily.

MISCELLANEOUS PERIPHERAL DEGENERATIONS AND FINDINGS

Peripheral Cystoid Degeneration

Peripheral cystoid degeneration is a process that is characterized by clusters of many tiny intraretinal spaces located just posterior to the ora serrata and usually aligned with dentate processes.[18] Histologically,[19] two types of this degenerative process have been described, designated as typical (involving the middle retinal layers) and reticular (involving the superficial layers of the retina), but these two forms are not distinguishable on clinical examination. The clusters of cystoid units tend to have their broad bases located against the ora serrata and extend posteriorly in a variety of shapes, such as trapezoid, fan-shaped, or club-shaped. The process extends by contiguity both posteriorly and circumferentially and may eventually form a band of varying width completely or partially encircling the eye at the ora serrata. Involvement tends to be more prominent temporally than nasally and superiorly than inferiorly. It has been seen histologically in a child as young as 6 days of age, and by the age of 8 yr it is present in all eyes.[18] There is a progressive increase in severity up to the seventh decade of life.

The extent of peripheral cystoid degeneration is unrelated to the axial length of the eye. It also occurs independently of lattice degeneration, paving stone degeneration, and pars plana cysts, both in incidence and in extent of involvement. Study of autopsied eyes[19] suggests that peripheral cystoid degeneration has a causal relationship to senile retinoschisis. Posterior vitreous detachment, even when it extends more anterior than the posterior limits of peripheral cystoid degeneration, does not show any apparent increased deleterious effects on these areas, and retina involved with peripheral cystoid degeneration does not appear to be more friable or more subject to retinal tears.

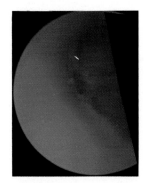

Figure 95–7. Enclosed ora bay.

Clinically, areas of peripheral cystoid degeneration may frequently be identified, but in many cases, it goes unrecognized because of its ophthalmoscopic subtlety. On scleral indentation, small, smoothly elevated, sometimes stippled areas of the inner retinal surface of these lesions can frequently be observed in the far anterior retinal periphery. It is sometimes difficult to differentiate these from early small lesions of senile retinoschisis, in relation to which peripheral cystoid degeneration appears to be a preceding formative pathologic stage.

Paving Stone Degeneration of the Retina

Paving stone degeneration is characterized by prominent, discrete, rounded, yellow-white lesions between the ora serrata and the equator, numbering from one to several dozen (Fig. 95–8).[20] They vary in size from 0.1 to 1.5 mm in diameter, but multiple adjacent lesions may coalesce into much larger lesions. The distinctive yellow-white color is caused by the relatively unobstructed view of the inner surface of the sclera, which may also show several large choroidal vessels superimposed on it. Lesions frequently have prominent pigment borders, and pigmented septa may intersect adjacent lesions.

Histologically,[20] lesions show sharply circumscribed outer retinal thinning caused by loss of rods and cones and the outer limiting lamina and also involving variable degrees of loss of the outer plexiform and outer nuclear layers. The pigment epithelial layer is abruptly absent, and the inner layer of Bruch's membrane is altered. There is also variable loss of the choriocapillaris, which in the larger lesions is completely absent. The overlying vitreous is unchanged in the involved areas. Lesions show no apparent increase in glial cells and are not associated with the presence of inflammatory cells.

Paving stone lesions appear in about 22 percent of adults and are bilateral in 38 percent of involved patients.[20] They tend to be bilaterally symmetric and become more extensive with increasing age, especially among males. Lesions are most prevalent in the inferotemporal quadrant but are also very common in the inferonasal quadrant, with more than 50 percent of lesions being seen between the 5 o'clock and the 7

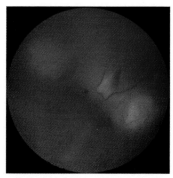

Figure 95–9. Paving stone degeneration, showing "pseudoholes" in the area of retinal detachment. (From Byer NE: The Peripheral Retina in Profile—A Stereoscopic Atlas. Torrance, CA, Criterion Press, 1952, p. 138.)

o'clock meridians. The area of the nasal horizontal meridian tends to be spared. Although not statistically proved, there is suggestive evidence that highly myopic eyes may have more extensive involvement.

Clinically, paving stone degeneration presents no threat to vision and never requires prophylactic treatment. When found in eyes in which later retinal detachment occurs, the paving stone lesions generally provide an effective barrier to extension of the detachment. However, occasionally the retina may detach over these lesions and then present circumscribed reddish areas corresponding to the location of the paving stone lesions, which are caused by the extreme retinal thinning; this may cause these areas to appear as "pseudoholes" (Fig. 95–9).[11] Rarely, the detaching retina may also cause secondary, irregular tractional tears in the region of the paving stone lesions.[20]

Pearl of the Ora Serrata

Pearl of the ora serrata is a fitting discriptive term for a very interesting and distinctive lesion seen in the far anterior periphery of the retina and always located beneath a dentate process, either in line with or slightly anterior to the ora serrata.[21] On ophthalmoscopic examination, this lesion makes itself immediately and strikingly apparent as a small glistening, bright yellow or opalescent sphere (Fig. 95–10).

Histologically,[21] these lesions appear to be drusen-like structures on the inner surface of Bruch's membrane and may be analogous to giant drusen of the retina. In their early stages they appear as homogeneous, eosinophilic-staining projections from Bruch's membrane beneath the pigment epithelium. Later, as they enlarge, they appear dark because of the intact pigment epithelium that covers their surface. Still later, this pigmented covering is lost, revealing the typical appearance. Examples have been seen of a still later stage in which the pearl loses its attachment to Bruch's membrane and floats freely within one of the spaces of peripheral cystoid degeneration. Chemical analysis with various histologic stains indicates they have a predominantly acid carbohydrate composition. There is no evidence of lipid content.

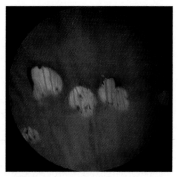

Figure 95–8. Paving stone degeneration.

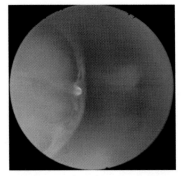

Figure 95–10. Pearl of ora serrata located at a dentate process of the ora serrata. (From Byer NE: The Peripheral Retina in Profile—A Stereoscopic Atlas. Torrance, CA, Criterion Press, 1952, p. 127.)

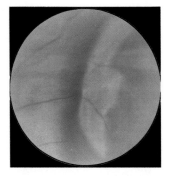

Figure 95–12. White-with-pressure phenomenon. (From Byer NE: The Peripheral Retina in Profile—A Stereoscopic Atlas. Torrance, CA, Criterion Press, 1952, p. 135.)

Clinically, they are found in 20 percent of individuals[21] in all age groups and may occur in any quadrant of the eye. They tend to be bilaterally symmetric and increase significantly in incidence with advancing age. They have no known association with ocular disease but are very useful as easily found retinal landmarks to orient the position of other less obvious but important retinal findings.

Pars Plana Cysts

Pars plana cysts are smooth cystic lesions of variable size lying adjacent and just anterior to the ora serrata. They conform to the individual ora bays and are more prevalent on the temporal side of the eye. They may be single or multiple and are unilateral in two thirds of cases.[22] Clinically, they usually may be seen only with indirect ophthalmoscopy and are best visualized with scleral indentation, by which they appear as ovoid, smoothly convex, turgid-appearing lesions in uniform, parallel, radial alignment immediately anterior to the ora serrata (Fig. 95–11). Microscopically, they sometimes seem to arise from vacuoles within nonpigmented epithelial cells but more often as a separation of the nonpigmented from the pigmented cell layer of the pars plana epithelium. The cysts contain basophilic granular

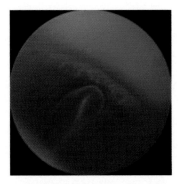

Figure 95–11. Cyst of the pars plana in a 54-year-old woman. (From Byer NE: The Peripheral Retina in Profile—A Stereoscopic Atlas. Torrance, CA, Criterion Press, 1952, p. 148.)

material. In larger cysts, attachments of zonular fibers to the inner cyst wall may be seen.

The cause of pars plana cysts is not known. Although various factors have been suggested, these lesions probably should be considered to be the result of aging and degenerative changes.[23] As possible mechanisms of formation, there is some suggestion that tractional forces exerted by the zonular fibers or the pars plana portion of the vitreous base may play some role.[23]

In two autopsy series pars plana cysts have been reported in 16 percent[22] and 18 percent[23] of cases, respectively. They usually appear after age 40 yr, and the prevalence increases steadily with increasing age.[22, 23] Pars plana cysts have not been shown to have a statistical association with any other ocular pathologic condition, and they have a uniformly good prognosis.

White-With-Pressure Sign

The term *white with pressure* was coined by Okamura[24] to describe a very interesting fundus appearance that is produced in some eyes during indirect ophthalmoscopy when the technique of scleral indentation is employed. The reason or reasons for this phenomenon have never been satisfactorily explained. The unusual appearance consists of a change in color of the fundus from the customary orange-red, characteristic of the retina and choroid and with good visibility of the choroidal vascular pattern, to an opaque yellow-orange or yellow-white with loss of visibility of the choroidal pattern. The area involved in this change has distinct boundaries that are altogether variable in configuration but that tend to have a "geographic" outline (Fig. 95–12), beyond which there is an abrupt transition back to the normal appearance. The white-with-pressure appearance occurs only in certain predetermined but wholly unpredictable areas and not everywhere the sclera is indented. The size of the involved area varies greatly. The white-with-pressure sign may be found over a wide age range and frequently among patients younger than 20 yr of age. It may be seen in any area of the fundus and usually is found in a narrow band immediately posterior to and parallel with the ora serrata. It is often seen in the equatorial region but may also be seen quite posterior to this area. It occasionally can be found adjacent to other fundus abnormalities, such as lattice degeneration, cystic retinal tufts, and retinal breaks, but is not confined to lesions involving the vitreoretinal interface. It can also be located adjacent to lesions involving deep structures, such as congenital hypertrophy of the pigment epithelium.

Scleral indentation itself has several unique characteristics that tend to markedly change the color of the ocular fundus but are unrelated to the white-with-pressure phenomenon. Some of these effects were illustrated by drawings in the early literature on this subject by Schepens[25] and are strikingly visible in actual stereoscopic fundus photographs.[11] One of these characteristics of scleral indentation is the fact that a posteriorly convex band of dusky shadow is uniformly produced just posterior to the point of maximal indentation. This then provides a dark background against which any retinal abnormality tends to stand out in sharp contrast and can therefore be seen much more clearly. In addition, various retinal lesions tend to assume an immediately increased whitened appearance in the indented area. This is often true in lesions of lattice degeneration and also in the presence of a subclinical, low-lying retinal detachment. This characteristic combination of dark background shadow and increased whitening of superimposed retinal lesions greatly enhances the clinician's ability to discern details of these lesions and also provides marked improvement in the quality of fundus photography possible in such areas.[11]

This type of whitening, however, is not the same as, and must be differentiated from, the classic phenomenon known as white with pressure. This entity is definitely not correlated with any other retinal pathologic condition and has not been shown to be a clinical precursor of any retinal disease. White with pressure has been reported as one step among various retinal fundus changes that precede the development of giant retinal breaks in the fellow eyes of such patients.[26] It must be emphasized, however, that the white-with-pressure finding is of no help in predicting the initial occurrence in eyes of patients who will later develop giant retinal breaks.

In senile retinoschisis, a similar color change is occasionally produced and is seen arising from the outer layer during scleral indentation, but it is not known whether the cause is the same as that of the classic phenomenon. In senile retinoschisis, it is obvious that the color change is produced at the level of the deep retina, the outer limiting lamina, or Bruch's membrane.

A typical white-with-pressure sign is a clinically interesting curiosity but is of no diagnostic or prognostic significance. It is frequently observed in the eyes of healthy young individuals who have no history of ocular disease. As a particular patient with this finding is observed over a period of years, it sometimes happens that the phenomenon disappears entirely from an area in which it was previously seen and drawn, or it may migrate to a new area several clock hours away. This is inconsistent with the concept that it may represent actual pathologic structural changes within the retina, which has been alleged.[27, 28]

REFERENCES

1. Foos RY, Allen RA: Retinal tears and lesser lesions of the peripheral retina in autopsy eyes. Am J Ophthalmol 64:643–655, 1967.
2. Vogt A: Die operative Therapie und die Pathogenese der Netzhautablösung. Stuttgart, Germany, Ferdinand Enke Verlag, 1936, pp 213–239.
3. Teng CC, Katzin HM: An anatomic study of the peripheral retina: I. Nonpigmented epithelial cell proliferation and hole formation. Am J Ophthalmol 34:1237–1248, 1951.
4. Okun E: Gross and microscopic pathology in autopsy eyes. III. Retinal breaks without detachment. Am J Ophthalmol 51:369–391, 1961.
5. Rutnin U, Schepens CL: Fundus appearance in normal eyes. II. The standard peripheral fundus and developmental variations. Am J Ophthalmol 64:840–852, 1967.
6. Daicker B: Anatomie und Pathologie der menschlichen retinoziliaren Fundus-peripherie. New York, S Karger, 1972, pp 107–118.
7. Foos RY: Vitreous base, retinal tufts, and retinal tears: Pathogenic relationships. In Pruett RC, Regan CDJ (eds): Retina Congress. New York, Appleton-Century-Crofts, 1972, pp 259–279.
8. Foos RY: Postoral peripheral retinal tears. Ann Ophthalmol 6:679–687, 1974.
9. Byer NE: Cystic retinal tufts and their relationship to retinal detachment. Arch Ophthalmol 99:1788–1790, 1981.
10. Murakami-Nagasako F, Ohba N: Phakic retinal detachment associated with cystic retinal tuft. Graefes Arch Clin Exp Ophthalmol 219:188–192, 1982.
11. Byer NE: The Peripheral Retina in Profile—A Stereoscopic Atlas. Torrance, CA, Criterion, 1982.
12. Straatsma BR, Foos RY, Feman SS: Degenerative diseases of the peripheral retina. In Tasman W, Jaeger EA (eds): Duane's Clinical Ophthalmology, rev ed. Philadelphia, JB Lippincott, 1989, pp 1–29.
13. Foos RY: Zonular traction tufts of the peripheral retina in cadaver eyes. Arch Ophthalmol 82:620–632, 1969.
14. Spencer LM, Foos RY, Straatsma BR: Meridional folds and meridional complexes of the peripheral retina. Trans Am Acad Ophthalmol Otolaryngol 73:204–217, 1969.
15. Schepens CL: Discussion of Spencer LM, Foos RY, Straatsma BR: Meridional folds and meridional complexes of the peripheral retina. Trans Am Acad Ophthalmol Otolaryngol 73:217–221, 1969.
16. Spencer LM, Foos RY, Straatsma BR: Meridional folds, meridional complexes, and associated abnormalities of the peripheral retina. Am J Ophthalmol 70:697–714, 1970.
17. Spencer LM, Foos RY, Straatsma BR: Enclosed bays of the ora serrata—Relationship to retinal tears. Arch Ophthalmol 83:421–425, 1970.
18. O'Malley PF, Allen RA: Peripheral cystoid degeneration of the retina. Arch Ophthalmol 77:769–776, 1967.
19. Foos RY: Senile retinoschisis—Relationship to cystoid degeneration. Trans Am Acad Ophthalmol Otolaryngol 74:33–50, 1970.
20. O'Malley PF, Allen RA, Straatsma BR, O'Malley CC: Paving-stone degeneration of the retina. Arch Ophthalmol 73:169–182, 1965.
21. Lonn LI, Smith TR: Ora serrata pearls. Arch Ophthalmol 77:809–813, 1967.
22. Okun E: Gross and microscopic pathology in autopsy eyes. Part I. Introduction and long posterior ciliary nerves. Am J Ophthalmol 50:424–429, 1960.
23. Allen RA, Miller DH, Straatsma BR: Cysts of the posterior ciliary body (pars plana). Arch Ophthalmol 66:302–313, 1961.
24. Schepens CL: Retinal Detachment. Philadelphia, WB Saunders, 1983, p 157.
25. Schepens CL: Subclinical retinal detachments. Arch Ophthalmol 47:593–606, 1952.
26. Freeman HM: Fellow eyes of giant retinal breaks. Trans Am Ophthalmol Soc 76:344–382, 1978.
27. Watzke RC: The ophthalmic sign "white-with-pressure." Arch Ophthalmol 66:812–823, 1961.
28. Watzke RC: White with pressure: An experimental and histologic study. In Blodi FC (ed): Current Concepts in Ophthalmology, St Louis, CV Mosby, 1974, pp 344–352.

Chapter 96

∎

Retinoschisis

TATSUO HIROSE

Retinoschisis is splitting (*schisis*) of the neural retinal layer, which is embryologically derived from the inner layer of the optic cup.[1] Although retinoschisis resembles retinal detachment in that both show retinal elevation in the ocular fundus, the latter is an actual separation of the neural retinal layer from the pigment epithelium.

Retinoschisis can be classified into three categories: acquired (senile, degenerative), congenital (juvenile, hereditary, developmental), and secondary, in which splitting of the neural retina occurs as a result of, or in association with, primary fundus disease or trauma.

ACQUIRED RETINOSCHISIS

The most common type of retinoschisis is acquired retinoschisis, which is found in 4 to 22 percent of the normal population older than 40 yr of age[2–4] and usually affects both sexes equally. Previously called senile retinoschisis,[1] it usually affects persons older than 50 yr. Although rare, this type of retinoschisis can be found in patients in their 20s and 30s, making it more appropriately termed *acquired* rather than senile.[5] Splitting in acquired retinoschisis occurs in the outer plexiform layer,[6] or occasionally in the inner nuclear layer,[7] as a result of confluence of the area of cystoid degeneration. Histologically, two types of acquired retinoschisis are seen, one relatively flat, which is called *reticular cystoid degeneration,* and the other bullous.[8] However, clinical distinctions between the two are not always easy to make; the two types are often seen in the same eye. Since retinoschisis starts from the extreme peripheral fundus near the ora serrata, usually in a lower temporal quadrant, patients commonly have no visual symptoms except in the most advanced stages of the disease.

Clinical Features

Ophthalmoscopically, early acquired retinoschisis appears as a flat, smooth, retinal elevation that is best appreciated when the area is viewed tangentially with a binocular indirect ophthalmoscope on scleral depression. The elevated retina, which represents an inner layer of the retinoschisis, always contains retinal blood vessels, some of which appear white in the periphery as though they were occluded (Fig. 96–1). A number of small, shiny, yellow-white dots, resembling snowflakes, are observed on the elevated retinal surface. These dots may represent the footsteps of the pillars of the Müller cells.

Retinoschisis usually remains stationary over many years; a spontaneous collapse may occur but this is rare.[9, 10] In some cases, retinoschisis expands in three directions: toward the posterior pole, circumferentially along the ora serrata, and toward the vitreous cavity, increasing the height of the elevation. In an advanced stage, retinoschisis forms a large, fixed, ballooning elevation of the inner layer that looks almost transparent. The surface is smooth and does not undulate (Fig. 96–2). The presence of an outer layer of retinoschisis is demonstrated by a white-with-pressure sign on indirect ophthalmoscopy with scleral depression. The outer layer often shows multiple, reddish, round spots that resemble clusters of fish or frog eggs (Fig. 96–3). The inner layer also has a pitted appearance on its back, which is best appreciated by slit-lamp examination with retroillumination. Cases in which retinoschisis reaches the macula are rare. Concomitant age-related macular degeneration may be found because of the advanced age of patients. A break or breaks may be found in one or both layers of retinoschisis (Fig. 96–4). The outer layer break tends to be single, larger, and more frequently found than the inner layer break, which tends to be small.

Retinal detachment may develop in the eye with acquired retinoschisis as a complication of the retinoschisis or as a result of a full-thickness retinal break located in the area unaffected by retinoschisis. The inner layer break(s) alone does not cause retinal detachment. A break or breaks in the outer layer alone or in both layers may lead to retinal detachment (Figs. 96–5 and 96–6). When the retinoschisis is limited to the area anterior to the equator, usually no field defect is detected. If the retinoschisis extends posterior to the equator, it usually causes a field defect that is an absolute scotoma with its edge of different isopters very sharp or steep. The visual field defect is usually seen in the superonasal quadrant, corresponding to the retinoschisis located in the inferotemporal quadrant.

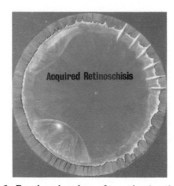

Figure 96–1. Fundus drawing of acquired retinoschisis.

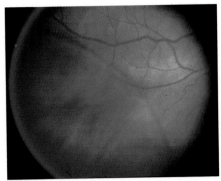

Figure 96–2. Fundus photograph of relatively advanced stage of acquired retinoschisis.

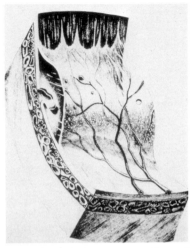

Figure 96–4. Drawing of the cross section of the eye with retinoschisis showing breaks in the outer and inner layers.

Retinoschisis may be misdiagnosed as a retinal detachment; conversely, a long-standing inferior retinal detachment can be mistaken for retinoschisis. In retinal detachment, the detached retina is less transparent, undulates, or is mobile, forming large folds or multiple minute folds called *shagreen;* subretinal fluid may shift with a change in position of the patient's head. In retinoschisis, the surface is smooth and the height of the elevation stays the same regardless of the patient's head position. If a horseshoe tear or a break with an operculum is found in the elevated portion of the retina, the elevation is probably retinal detachment rather than retinoschisis, because a horseshoe tear or an operculum with a break rarely forms in the inner layer of retinoschisis. One application of photocoagulation to the bare pigment epithelium through the detached retina causes no reaction or a very faint gray-yellow reaction; the same application to the intact outer layer of retinoschisis causes a white coagulation mark. These clinical features, which may help differentiate retinal detachment from retinoschisis, are listed in Table 96–1.

However, these criteria are not absolute—exceptions exist. For instance, photocoagulation may not show a white mark on the outer layer of retinoschisis if the layer is atrophic or extensively degenerated. The field defect in retinal detachment usually shows some slope at the edge, but in long-standing retinal detachment, the border of the field defect may be sharp and the

defect absolute, resembling the field defect in retinoschisis.

Natural History

Acquired retinoschisis generally remains stable without causing any visual impairment. Spontaneous flattening of the retinoschisis does occur, although it is rare, as mentioned previously. In a small percentage of patients, the retinoschisis does progress. Among 245 eyes with uncomplicated retinoschisis followed for 1 mo to 15 yr without treatment, 33 eyes (13.5 percent) showed progression from 1 mo to 10 yr. In these eyes, the

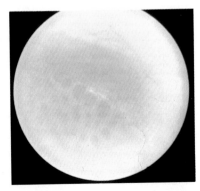

Figure 96–3. Fundus photograph of the outer layer of acquired retinoschisis showing multiple pits giving a fish or frog egg appearance.

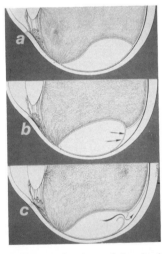

Figure 96–5. Probable mechanism of developing full-thickness retinal detachment from the outer layer break without inner layer break in retinoschisis. *a,* Ballooning retinoschisis. *b,* Outer layer and surrounding full-thickness retina are lifted or elevated. The detached outer layer becomes thin and stretched (*arrows*). *c,* Outer layer breaks at or near the edge of retinoschisis driving the fluid (*arrow*) into the subretinal space. There is no communication between the vitreous cavity and the subretinal space. Retinal detachment remains localized.

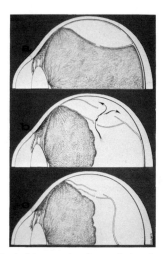

Figure 96–6. Probable mechanism of development of retinal detachment from the breaks in both layers of retinoschisis. *a*, Retinoschisis with breaks in both layers without retinal detachment. The vitreous gel may be in contact with the inner layer break. *b*, When the liquid vitreous is in contact with the inner layer break, a full-thickness retinal detachment can result. *c*, Retinal detachment can become quite extensive, sometimes total, because the vitreous cavity and subretinal space are connected by the breaks in both layers of retinoschisis (*arrows*).

retinoschisis expanded or formed a new break in one or both layers of the retinoschisis. The progression is usually slow, with significant expansion taking months or years. Figure 96–7 illustrates how retinoschisis located in the inferotemporal periphery in 13 eyes extended over a long observation period. Figure 96–8 illustrates the extension of retinoschisis in nine eyes in which the condition started in the superotemporal quadrant. The speed of progression varies from patient to patient; even the fastest growing progression reaching inside the major vascular arcade from the equator took 7 yr.

Management

The management of acquired retinoschisis requires bilateral fundus drawings and visual field plotting. The extent of retinoschisis should be marked in relation to the adjacent fundus landmarks, such as branches of

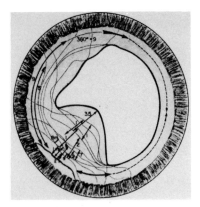

Figure 96–7. Composite drawing of the extent of progressive retinoschisis in 13 eyes on the initial and the last examinations. Retinoschisis started in the inferotemporal quadrant. *Numbers* next to *arrows* indicate the follow-up periods in years except for one number (8) followed by *m* (months). *Arrows* indicate the extent of progression.

retinal vessels or vortex ampulla. A good initial fundus drawing helps the examiner determine whether the retinoschisis expanded at the follow-up visit. Fundus photograph localization is not useful in the early stage of retinoschisis because of its peripheral location and the small degree of elevation of the lesion. If the retinoschisis is relatively flat without any break and is limited to the area anterior to the equator, examination is repeated in a year. In such a case, retinoschisis is probably a finding incidental to the reason for the ocular examination. If the retinoschisis has a break or breaks in one of the layers or is already extended posterior to the equator, reexamination is recommended in 3 to 6 mo, depending on the severity of the lesions; examination should take place sooner if the patient notices symptoms such as floaters or visual disturbances. If there is no change in the retinoschisis at the second visit, the schedule of annual examinations should be continued until otherwise indicated. Indications for treatment of acquired retinoschisis are controversial.

The method of treatment is more controversial. Be-

Table 96–1. DIFFERENTIATING RETINAL DETACHMENT AND RETINOSCHISIS

Characteristic	Retinal Detachment	Retinoschisis
Transparency	Little	Much
Mobility	Mobile	Immobile
Surface	Folds	Smooth
Fluid shift	Often present	Absent
Horseshoe tear, break with operculum	Common	Rare
Reaction to photocoagulation	Absent or faint	Whiten, rarely absent
Field defect	Sloping border	Sharp border

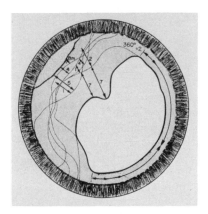

Figure 96–8. Composite drawing of the extent of progressive retinoschisis that started in the superotemporal quadrant in nine eyes. *Arrows* indicate the extent of progression. *Numbers* next to *arrows* indicate the follow-up periods in years except for one number (8) followed by *m* (months).

cause the incidence of acquired retinoschisis is relatively high among the normal population and visual disturbances caused by retinoschisis or complications thereof are relatively rare, and because treatment is not always effective or can be met with serious complications, one has to be cautious in treating these patients. After following 218 eyes with retinoschisis for an average of 9.1 yr, Byer did not find a single eye with subjectively impaired vision either from extension of retinoschisis or from development of retinal detachment, although he found the original retinoschisis had expanded in 3.2 to 6.4 percent of patients or had formed new breaks in 6.4 percent of eyes that were followed.[11] From this observation, he concluded that no treatment is needed unless retinoschisis is associated with a symptomatic progressive retinal detachment, which he did not observe in his patients.[11]

The study statistics vary depending on the patient population. A study performed in a normal population or in patients seeking refraction from a primary care ophthalmologist would result in a different conclusion from a study of patients examined by tertiary-care retinal specialists. Patients who experience serious complications of retinoschisis may not remain in the care of their primary physician, possibly biasing these statistics; conversely, patients who display early acquired retinoschisis diagnosed by the tertiary-care physician may have other conditions or symptoms unrelated to the retinoschisis. However, it is unknown whether the presence of other retinal or vitreous abnormalities, such as age-related macular degeneration, affects the natural course of retinoschisis. Statistics are helpful in the overall view of the nature of retinoschisis; however, each case requires individual management.

It is well known that extensive retinal detachment and very posteriorly extended retinoschisis cause irreparable visual field defects whether or not patients have visual complaints. It is generally true that uncomplicated retinoschisis is asymptomatic even when it balloons or extends posteriorly in the fundus. Patients often experience symptoms when retinal detachment develops; however, they may be unaware of symptoms despite the presence of retinal detachment. This typically is seen in those detachments associated with dialysis in young individuals. This type of retinal detachment is usually located in the inferotemporal quadrant; the affected patients are often asymptomatic, and they do not seek medical care until detachment extends close to the macula. Multiple subretinal demarcation lines and secondary retinal cysts, often found in dialysis, indicate that the retinal detachment is long-standing. In a case such as this, we should not confuse retinal detachment in young dialysis patients with uncomplicated acquired retinoschisis. The cause of retinal dialysis in young patients is not known. Most dialysis in young patients probably is unrelated to retinoschisis. However, evidence suggests that some dialysis in young patients is due to breaks in both layers of acquired retinoschisis that occurred in these individuals.[12–14] As shown in Figure 96–9, the dialysis may not be a single full-thickness retinal break formed at the ora serrata. Careful

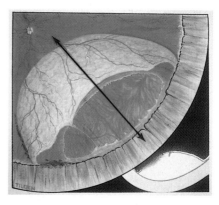

Figure 96–9. Fundus drawing of retinal detachment in a young dialysis patient. The dialysis of the retina probably represents breaks in both layers of retinoschisis formed at the ora serrata, as shown in the schema of the cross-sectional view through the *arrow*, drawn in the right lower corner.

examination reveals that the dialysis is composed of two breaks in two retinal layers, strongly suggesting that this dialysis, or break at the ora serrata, represents breaks in both layers of the retinoschisis. Because of the extensive and highly elevated retinal detachment, one cannot judge at which point the retinoschisis ends and the retinal detachment starts. However, it is obvious in this case that the retinal detachment was caused by breaks at the ora serrata in acquired retinoschisis. No one would question the necessity of operating on such a retinal detachment, which probably originated from retinoschisis, although this detachment may be asymptomatic.

A case in which an asymptomatic full-thickness retinal detachment developed as a result of a large outer layer break and small, multiple inner layer breaks also was reported.[15] This eye was operated upon successfully before the detachment extended to the macula.[15] Therefore, the retinal detachment that develops as a complication of acquired retinoschisis is not always symptomatic. Furthermore, although quite rare, acquired retinoschisis does extend to the posterior pole.[16, 18] Some authors challenged this by stating that these cases may not be actual retinoschisis involving the macula but rather retinal detachment in the macula caused by the posteriorly located outer layer break.[19] However, it is highly unlikely that the outer layer breaks were missed by these authors. Retinoschisis that has encroached upon the posterior pole is well documented during the course of observation and should be considered a potential candidate for treatment, although it may be asymptomatic. Retinoschisis already may have extended quite posteriorly in the fundus with a large field defect at the time of initial examination. Such a case may be watched closely without immediate treatment, particularly if the patient does not have symptoms, since the speed with which the retinoschisis extended thus far is uncertain. Fundus photographs, in addition to the drawing and visual fields, are helpful in follow-up. If the retinoschisis progresses further, treatment should be considered.

The presence of a break or breaks in an outer layer

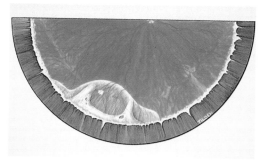

Figure 96–10. Fundus drawing of retinal detachment with three outer layer breaks. The detachment is limited to the area affected by retinoschisis.

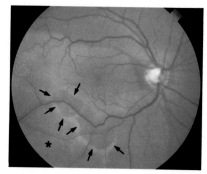

Figure 96–12. Fundus photograph of full-thickness retinal detachment in the posterior pole caused by outer layer breaks (*arrows*). The posterior edge of the breaks is not entirely clear. The outer layer in the area located anterior to the breaks is still attached to the pigment epithelium and has a fish egg appearance (*asterisk*).

or in both the outer and the inner layers without significant retinal detachment is considered a subclinical detachment and should be managed as such. Some breaks will develop extensive retinal detachment, impairing vision, and others will not. An outer layer break alone rarely causes full-thickness retinal detachment, particularly if the break is round and trophic in nature, even though it can be large or multiple. Retinal detachment can be limited within the area of retinoschisis; this is actually a detachment of the outer layer of retinoschisis from the pigment epithelium (Figs. 96–10 and 96–11).[5, 11] Full-thickness retinal detachment or a retinal detachment that extended outside the area of retinoschisis was observed in 16 percent of eyes with breaks only in an outer layer and in 77 percent of eyes with breaks in both layers.[18] Retinal detachment caused by an outer layer break or breaks alone usually is located near the break within the area of retinoschisis and spreads slightly beyond the retinoschisis, thus creating detachment of the full-thickness retina. The retinal detachment is usually shallow and stays localized (Fig. 96–12).

Retinal detachment caused by breaks in both outer and inner layers of retinoschisis often becomes extensive, sometimes total (Fig. 96–13). Therefore, retinoschisis with breaks in both layers without retinal detachment causes more attention to be given to prophylactic

treatment than does one involving an outer layer break alone. When breaks are present in both layers of retinoschisis, multiple superior and posterior inner layer breaks are accompanied by retinal detachment more frequently than one or a few inferiorly and anteriorly located inner layer breaks (Table 96–2 and Fig. 96–14). Multiple outer layer breaks combined with inner layer breaks tend to develop retinal detachment more frequently than does a single outer layer break (Table 96–3). Size, location, and number of breaks; presence or absence of a full-thickness break outside the retinoschisis; and whether or not the retinoschisis is progressive are factors taken into consideration in treatment to prevent retinal detachment. Furthermore, the presence of cataract or glaucoma, for which pilocarpine drops are needed, may impair the fundus view. It would be better, therefore, if breaks are treated before cataract surgery or glaucoma treatment. The status of the fellow eye and the patient's age and general medical condition may also be considered. To determine treatment, one must always weigh the treatment risks against those of observation. It also should be remembered that the field defect produced by disruption of the neural network of the retina cannot be improved by reattaching two disrupted

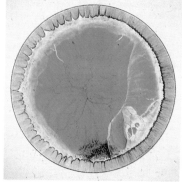

Figure 96–11. Fundus drawing of retinal detachment with six breaks formed in the outer layer of retinoschisis. The detachment is limited to the area affected with retinoschisis.

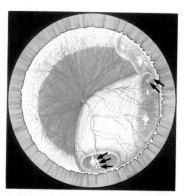

Figure 96–13. Fundus drawing of full-thickness retinal detachment caused by the breaks in the outer layer at the 6 and 2:30 o'clock meridians, with rolled edges and five small breaks in the inner layer (*arrows*).

Table 96–2. INNER LAYER BREAKS AND DETACHMENTS IN 78 EYES

Inner Layer Breaks	Detachment (%)	No detachment (%)	Total (%)
Number			
1	16 (67)	8 (33)	24 (100)
2–4	30 (75)	10 (25)	40 (100)
≥5	14 (100)	0 (0)	14 (100)
Total	60	18	78
Location			
Superonasal	1 (33)	2 (67)	3 (100)
Superotemporal	37 (84)	7 (16)	44 (100)
Inferotemporal	22 (71)	9 (29)	31 (100)
Inferonasal	0 (0)	0 (0)	0
Total	60	18	78
Ora–equator	22 (67)	11 (33)	33 (100)
Equator–midway	37 (84)	7 (16)	44 (100)
Midway–posterior pole	1 (100)	0 (0)	1 (100)
Total	60	18	78

Table 96–3. OUTER LAYER BREAKS AND RETINAL DETACHMENTS IN 78 EYES

Outer Layer Breaks (Number)	Detachment (%)	No detachment (%)	Total (%)
1	27 (68)	13 (32)	40 (100)
2–4	26 (87)	4 (13)	30 (100)
≥5	7 (88)	1 (12)	8 (100)
Total	60	18	78

retinal layers. Therefore, treatment is directed toward preventing further progression of retinoschisis or retinal detachment.

There are two modes of treatment. The first is demarcation of the advancing edge of retinoschisis by photocoagulation or cryoapplications, or a combination of the two. This method requires destruction of the normal retina at the edge of the retinoschisis, which already may be far advanced at the time of treatment. Therefore, the treatment further increases the field defect. The second mode is an attempt to collapse the inner layer by applying photocoagulation[16] or cryotherapy,[17] or both, to the entire outer layer with or without drainage of fluid from the cavity of the retinoschisis. The theories behind this method are that, because the cellular elements of the retina are responsible for secretion of fluid into the retinoschisis cavity, their destruction by photocoagulation or cryotherapy explains the collapse of the retinoschisis,[20] or that the diffusion barrier present at the retinal pigment epithelium level

is disrupted by photocoagulation or cryotherapy, causing the fluid in the retinoschisis cavity to diffuse into the choroid.[21] In the past, treatment with strong xenon photocoagulation caused the formation of the outer layer break and subsequent retinal detachment.[16, 18] Mild, contiguously applied laser coagulation appears much safer. The fluid in the retinoschisis cavity is usually very thick, making its complete removal through one perforation in the sclera difficult. The inner layer collapses in the area of the perforation site as the fluid is drained, but the fluid tends to be trapped in the area of retinoschisis away from the perforation. However, it is not essential to remove every drop of schisis fluid; the fluid either can be absorbed slowly or remains without increasing in volume after the treatment.

The full-thickness retinal detachment caused by a break or breaks of the outer layer without a break in the inner layer presents unique clinical features. The retinoschisis usually is highly elevated before the formation of the outer layer break, which usually consists of a tear at the edge of the retinoschisis (Fig. 96–15) or multiple circular trophic holes (see Fig. 96–12). The break can be seen easily if it is a tear with an edge that may be rolled; it sometimes is difficult to detect because the contrast between the bare pigment epithelium and the attached outer layer can be poor. Sometimes it is impossible to detect the posterior edge of a break that leads to a full-thickness retinal detachment (see Fig. 96–12). The retinal detachment is usually shallow and often involves the macula (see Fig. 96–12). Five such cases in which the treatment was successful were described by Sulonen and associates.[22] If the outer layer surrounding the tear is still attached or is only slightly elevated from the pigment epithelium, laser photocoagulation or cryo-

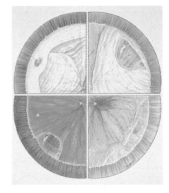

Figure 96–14. Fundus drawing with breaks in both layers of retinoschisis located superiorly, producing full-thickness retinal detachment (*upper left and right*), whereas inferiorly located breaks did not (*lower left and right*).

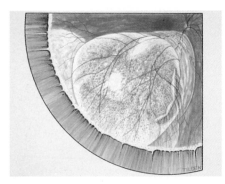

Figure 96–15. Fundus drawing of ballooning retinoschisis with a large outer break with rolled edges causing shallow full-thickness retinal detachment posteriorly.

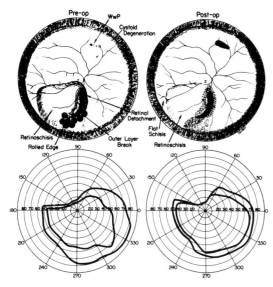

Figure 96–16. Fundus drawing of the same eye as in Figure 96–15 showing before photocoagulation and cryoapplication around the outer layer break (*upper left*). After treatment, full-thickness retinal detachment disappeared. Retinoschisis remains the same (*upper right*). Visual fields before (*left*) and after (*right*) treatment are shown at bottom of figure.

therapy, or both, applied around the outer layer break may effectively close it, resulting in the spontaneous reattachment of the full-thickness retina (Fig. 96–16). This treatment is least invasive ocularly, but it probably will not prevent a new break from forming, with subsequent recurrent retinal detachment and a highly elevated retinoschisis. The outer layer break still may open with persistent retinal detachment.[19] The scleral buckling procedure, whereby the buckle is applied to close the outer layer break with drainage of subretinal fluid and fluid from the retinoschisis cavity through the perforation made from the sclera and choroid, results in retinal reattachment and almost complete collapse of the retinoschisis (Fig. 96–17). The perforation for fluid drainage

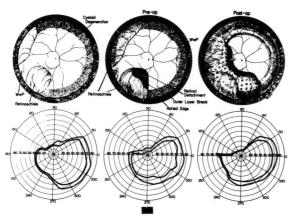

Figure 96–17. Fundus drawing of the eye with retinoschisis (*upper left*). Several months later, the same eye developed a large outer layer break at the posterior edge of the retinoschisis, causing full-thickness retinal detachment posteriorly (*upper middle*). After scleral buckling, the retina was reattached. A small pocket of fluid in the retinoschisis cavity remained in the periphery on the buckle (*upper right*). Visual fields on each occasion are shown at the bottom of figure.

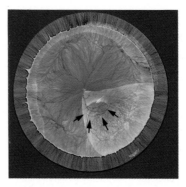

Figure 96–18. Fundus drawing of the retinoschisis with outer layer break (*arrows*) and full-thickness retinal detachment in the posterior pole. No inner layer break is found. The outer layer of retinoschisis, which is not detached from the pigment epithelium, shows a fish egg appearance.

is made through the existing break in the outer layer. The outer layer break can be large and often is located posteriorly. The application of a large buckle posteriorly tends to form the retinal fold and distort the macula, and the surgery can be quite invasive. The better approach is to ablate the entire outer layer with laser coagulation alone or a combination of laser and cryotherapy and drain the fluid and the subretinal space.[19]

One such case is shown in Figures 96–18 to 96–21. The patient was a 54-year-old man with a 2-mo history of visual disturbance in his left eye. The best-corrected vision was 20/70. The fundus of this eye showed extensive retinoschisis in the entire inferotemporal quadrant (see Fig. 96–18). The break in the outer layer (see Fig. 96–18) was located on the posterior edge of the retinoschisis in the area of the inferior major arcade of vessels. A shallow retinal detachment was observed posterior to the break involving the macula. The outer layer break was not easily recognizable (see Fig. 96–19). Only the anterior edge of the break was visible; the posterior edge was not. It was also nearly impossible to determine at which point the retinoschisis ended and the full-thickness retinal detachment began. The white laser coagulation marks on the attached outer layer delineate the anterior edge of the outer layer break (see Fig. 96–20). The laser applied directly to the outer layer break did not whiten because only the bare pigment epithelium

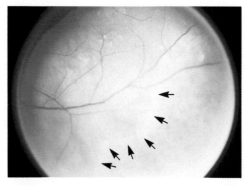

Figure 96–19. Fundus photograph of the area of the outer layer break in the same eye as seen in Figure 96–18. The *arrows* indicate the anterior edge of the break.

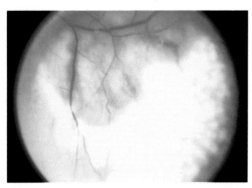

Figure 96–20. Fundus photograph of the same area as seen in Figure 96–19, immediately after photocoagulation. The anterior edge of the outer layer is well delineated by the photocoagulation mark.

was exposed. The entire area of retinoschisis was treated contiguously with laser coagulation except in the periphery, at which point cryotherapy was applied because of the easy accessibility of the peripheral retina by cryoprobe (see Fig. 96–21). After the treatment, the retinoschisis collapsed and the retina reattached. The vision improved to 20/40, and the fundus was stable without signs of retinoschisis for 10 yr after treatment.

Recently, another treatment approach was intro-

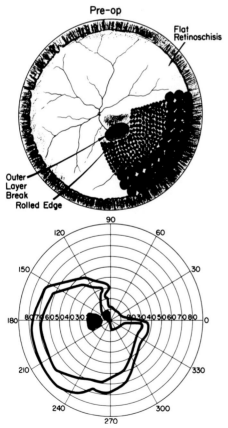

Figure 96–21. Fundus drawing showing the area treated with photocoagulation (*small black circles*) and with cryopexy (*large black circles*). The retina is detached posteriorly. The visual field is shown at the bottom of the figure.

duced[23]—namely, closed vitrectomy followed by internal drainage of subretinal and retinoschisis fluid through the intentional break created in the inner layer. As the fluid is drained internally, the gas is injected into the vitreous. The results appeared encouraging except for the formation or advancement of the cataract, which often resulted after uncomplicated closed vitrectomy. The retinal detachment caused by the breaks in both the outer and the inner layers can become quite extensive (see Fig. 96–13) or total, obviously because of the free communication between the vitreous cavity and the subretinal space through the breaks in both layers of retinoschisis (see Fig. 96–6). The goal of treatment in such cases is to reattach the retina by closing all outer layer breaks, which may be difficult to recognize because only a portion of the break may be visible. The scleral buckling procedure is usually effective in closing the outer layer breaks. A full-thickness retinal break may coexist and should also be closed. When the entire edge of the outer layer break is not well visualized, the surgeon must determine the size and contour of the break from the visible portion and ascertain that the buckle is large enough to be effective. If the initial scleral buckling procedure fails and the retina again becomes detached, or if the retina temporarily attaches but becomes detached later, it is usually difficult to find the original outer layer break postoperatively. As long as one detects and surgically closes all the breaks in the outer layer and the full-thickness retina, the results are relatively favorable.[24]

Several cases of retinal detachment were treated by cryopexy with simultaneous external subretinal fluid drainage and intraocular gas injection without a buckling procedure, which also led to favorable results.[15]

There are different methods to treat the retinal detachment associated with retinoschisis. Accumulation of more data from cases treated by different methods with long-term follow-up is needed to determine the best method in each case.

CONGENITAL RETINOSCHISIS

In congenital retinoschisis, retinal splitting usually occurs in the nerve fiber layer.[25] The disease is usually transmitted by an X-linked recessive trait and is nearly always found in males, with the mother being an obligatory carrier. Rare cases of an autosomal type have been reported.[26–28] The retinal abnormality in these patients is probably present at birth; thus, it may be called congenital.[29] In this chapter, we describe the most common X-linked recessive type.

Clinical Features

Since congenital retinoschisis frequently affects the macula or often causes vitreous hemorrhage, the initial symptoms are poor vision, strabismus, or nystagmus. The macular abnormalities vary. However, microcystic elevation or fine radiating folds from the fovea, or a

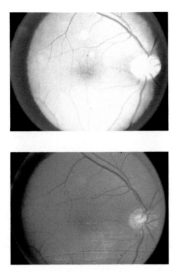

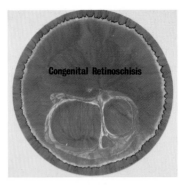

Figure 96–24. Fundus drawing of congenital retinoschisis with large inner layer breaks.

Figure 96–22. *Top,* Fundus photograph of the macula in congenital retinoschisis showing a fine radiating fold from the fovea, which becomes more distinct with monochromatic photograph (*bottom*).

combination of both, are characteristic (Fig. 96–22).[29] Fluorescein angiography shows no dye leakage into these cystoid spaces, which is distinctly different from the microcystoid macular edema. In some cases, the retina is elevated extensively, almost occupying the entire posterior pole that is surrounded by the major vascular arcade (Fig. 96–23). The macular abnormality can be very subtle, with the superficial radiating fold barely detectable by careful slit-lamp examination. The use of red-free light usually helps detect the change (see Fig. 96–22). In some cases, pigment mottling may be the only change, and in other cases, the absence of a foveal reflex is the only obvious macular abnormality. The macula may be displaced by vitreoretinal traction, or it may show a punched-out lesion of thinning of the pigment epithelium and atrophy of the choriocapillaris, which may lead to misdiagnosis of a congenital toxoplasmosis lesion.

The macular abnormality may be the only fundus finding in congenital retinoschisis. The most characteristic lesion outside of the macula is the ballooning elevation of the inner layer with a large oval hole or holes usually in the lower fundus (Fig. 96–24). In congenital retinoschisis, the inner layer breaks are larger and encountered more frequently than are the outer layer breaks, in contrast with acquired retinoschisis in which the opposite is true. This difference probably occurs because the splitting occurs in the nerve fiber layers, the superficial layers of the retina in congenital retinoschisis,[25] as compared with acquired retinoschisis in which the splitting occurs in the deeper retinal layer of the outer plexiform[6] or the inner nuclear layers.[7]

The retinal blood vessels usually run in the inner layer or occasionally bridge the inner and outer layers. In some cases, the inner layer is so elevated that it can be seen behind the lens on slit-lamp examination (Fig. 96–25). The inner layer holes can become quite large, almost as large as the retinoschisis itself, and the retinal vessels and the attached flimsy retinal tissue bridge these holes. In some cases, the inner layer is missing and the retinal vessels may float free in the vitreous cavity, a condition Mann called a congenital vascular veil.[30] White, fine dendritic figures of probable vascular origin are often seen in the peripheral fundus in which the inner layer is not highly elevated. Retinoschisis in the periphery may be indistinct and may be detected as a very low elevation of the inner layer only by viewing the fundus tangentially with a binocular indirect ophthalmoscope with scleral depression. Ophthalmoscopy without scleral depression often fails to detect very

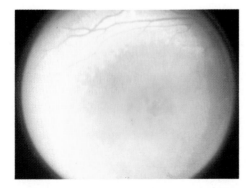

Figure 96–23. Fundus photograph of the posterior pole of congenital retinoschisis showing huge blister-like elevation of the retina reaching the major vascular arcade.

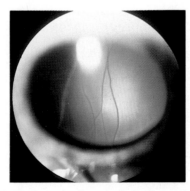

Figure 96–25. Photograph of congenital retinoschisis with highly elevated inner layer visible behind the lens.

shallow retinoschisis in the periphery. Beside the vascular veil, which is actually the inner layer of the retinoschisis, translucent membranes without vessels often are seen floating free in the vitreous cavity, a part of the membrane attached to the inner layer, or to the retina outside of the retinoschisis. The membrane may attach to the optic nerve or the macula, causing pseudopapillitis, dragging the retinal vessels near the disc, or causing macular displacement. Hemorrhage, which can be the first symptom within the retinoschisis cavity or vitreous, is relatively common. The anterior limit of retinoschisis usually does not extend to the ora serrata. In the late stage of congenital retinoschisis, the entire inner layer is missing, and the retinal vessels are invisible. The outer layer degenerates, and multiple pigment clumps appear (Fig. 96–26). Male patients with pigmentation and no visible retinal vessels in the lower half of the fundus should be suspected of having congenital retinoschisis until it is proved otherwise.

The electroretinogram (ERG) in congenital retinoschisis is very characteristic and diagnostic.[31] Because of the polymorphous fundus appearance in congenital retinoschisis, diagnosis from the fundus examination may be difficult. In such a case, the ERG may help in the diagnosis. The ERG in congenital retinoschisis is characterized by a disproportional decrease of the b-wave amplitude compared with that of the a-wave. In the early stage of the disease or in mild cases, only a decrease of the b-wave amplitudes, along with the oscillatory potential and no change in the a-wave, is observed. The b:a wave amplitude ratio is especially reduced (Fig. 96–27B). Normal ERG tracings are shown in Figure 96–27A for comparison. This electroretinographic finding is observed even in cases in which the visible fundus abnormality is limited to the macula. Since the ERG is a mass response, an abnormal ERG signifies that the retina outside the macula is diffusely affected, even in cases in which the visible abnormality is limited to the macula. When the disease progresses and the receptor degenerates, the a-wave amplitude also becomes smaller. However, the b-wave amplitude reduction is always greater; therefore, a low b:a wave amplitude ratio is always maintained (Fig. 96–27C). When the retinoschisis is far advanced and the fundus

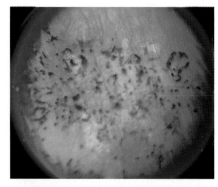

Figure 96–26. Fundus photograph of advanced congenital retinoschisis showing extensive pigmentation and loss of retinal vessels in the inferior fundus.

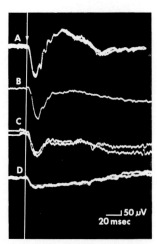

⎯⎯⏋50 μV
20 msec

Figure 96–27. Electroretinogram (ERG) in congenital retinoschisis recorded with a relatively bright single flash of light under dark adaptation. A, Normal ERG shows b : a wave amplitude ratio larger than 1 with good oscillatory potential. B, ERG in an eye with only the macula involved with no peripheral retinoschisis showing selective depression of b-wave amplitude without depression of the a-wave. Oscillatory potential also is diminished. C, ERG in an eye whose retina is extensively involved in the macula as well as in the periphery showing that both the b- and the a-waves are depressed, but the b-wave depression is more prominent. D, ERG in far-advanced retinoschisis. ERG shows only a small negative wave (a-wave) with complete loss of the b-wave.

shows extensive pigment clumping, and when the retinal vessels are absent from the lower half or the more extended area of the fundus, the b-wave of the ERG may be entirely absent, leaving only a small a-wave or P III component (Fig. 96–27D).[32] With further progression of the disease, the a-wave also disappears, making the ERG completely nonrecordable.

The clinical picture in the end-stage of congenital retinoschisis is not too different from that of retinitis pigmentosa: extensive pigmentation with narrow retinal vessels and a nonrecordable ERG with complete night blindness.[31] If the small a-wave is recordable with complete loss of the b-wave in the eye with pigmentary retinal degeneration, congenital retinoschisis should be suspected. The small b:a wave ratio in congenital retinoschisis indicates that the inner neural retinal layer is more involved than the receptor or Müller cells, which are impaired if we consider that the b-wave is generated by those cells.[33] Dark adaptation,[31] the absolute thresholds for both rods and cones,[34] is only slightly impaired in the early stage of congenital retinoschisis or in a mild case when the ERG b-wave is already significantly depressed. This dissociation of electrophysiologic findings and the psychophysical results were interpreted by Peachey and coworkers,[34] who indicated that in congenital retinoschisis the pathologic condition starts with the Müller cells, whereas the sensory neural pathways are by and large operating with limited dysfunction, at least in the early stage of disease. A characteristic low electroretinographic b:a wave amplitude ratio in congenital retinoschisis is not observed in acquired retinoschisis, in which the ERG is either normal or subnormal, depending on the extent of the area involved without preferential depression of the b-wave amplitude. This indicates that acquired retinoschisis is not a diffuse retinal degeneration like congenital retinoschisis.

Female heterozygote carriers have normal ophthalmoscopic and electroretinographic findings, but some abnormalities have been reported to show wrinkling of the internal limiting membrane around the fovea[35] or peripheral retinal alterations similar to those found in affected males.[36] With the use of restriction fragment length polymorphisms as genetic markers, linkage was demonstrated between polymorphic markers on the short arm of the X chromosome in the Xp22 region and the retinoschisis locus.[37, 38] Based on linkage data, the retinoschisis gene appeared to lie close to DNA probes 99.6 and D2. A DNA-based diagnosis appears to help identify heterozygous carriers of congenital retinoschisis and also serves in the early diagnosis of affected infants, along with ophthalmoscopic and electrophysiologic methods.[38]

In addition to genetic methods, psychophysical testing has been reported to be helpful in detecting heterozygous carriers. The method uses the impairment of the cone system to detect flicker as rods dark-adapt in normal individuals; conversely, if the dark-adapted rods are exposed to dim light, cone function improves. These normal rod-cone interactions are lacking in heterozygous carriers.[39]

Management

Congenital retinoschisis is typically stable, and slow progression may alternate with spontaneous remission or collapsing of retinoschisis. Rapid progression of the disease is likely to occur during the first decade of life. By age 20 yr, most cases, with few exceptions, stabilize in terms of the size of the retinoschisis.[29] Management of congenital retinoschisis requires careful fundus examination with binocular indirect ophthalmoscopy, scleral depression, and large fundus drawing. Examination under general anesthesia is often necessary for infants and small children. Visual field plotting is important but often unsatisfactory in the case of infants or young children. We examine patients at intervals of every 3 mo to 1 yr, and at least once a year as long as no new signs and symptoms appear.

Because of the nonprogressive nature of congenital retinoschisis in most patients, no treatment is indicated unless complications arise that impair or threaten vision. Attempting to collapse the retinoschisis with photocoagulation is an unsatisfactory approach because of frequent complications of new break formation in the outer layer followed by retinal detachment.[40] Vitrectomy in uncomplicated congenital retinoschisis is met with technical difficulty in removing the cortical vitreous strongly adherent to the retinal surface, and attempting to collapse the inner layer with air-fluid exchange after internal fluid drainage in the schisis cavity is unsatisfactory. A fresh vitreous hemorrhage is best treated conservatively with bedrest alone and the use of bilateral patches. If the vitreous clears, the possible source of bleeding should be sought. Sources of vitreous hemorrhage may

be neovascular tufts or stretched retinal vessels crossing a large inner layer break or those bridging the inner and outer layers. Closing the offending vessels with laser should be attempted when there is a recurrence of vitreous hemorrhage. If the vitreous does not clear within 1 wk, it is often impractical to continue bedrest. The child may return to normal activity, including attending school, but must avoid vigorous physical exercise and be followed with periodic examinations. The vitreous usually clears several months after a vitreous hemorrhage. Vitrectomy is rarely necessary in eyes with significant vitreous hemorrhage in congenital retinoschisis.

Retinal detachment has been considered a relatively rare complication in congenital retinoschisis.[41] However, it does occur and is not entirely rare in patients in whom the vitreoretinal pathologic condition is extensive. In one family, three boys who were affected with congenital retinoschisis all experienced retinal detachment.

Three types of retinal detachment are found in eyes with congenital retinoschisis. The first is retinal detachment caused by breaks in both layers of retinoschisis (Fig. 96–28). The second type is caused by a full-thickness retinal break that develops outside the retinoschisis; this type of retinal detachment does not appear to be related directly to the retinoschisis, but the formation of the full-thickness retinal break may be related to the vitreoretinal pathologic condition involved in the eye with retinoschisis. The third type is a tractional retinal detachment, which is similar to that of proliferative diabetic retinopathy in its fundus appearance and probably also in its mechanism of detachment—namely, that the fibrovascular proliferative tissues grow in front of the disc, contract, and detach the retina (Fig. 96–29). The retinal detachment thus created showed a tabletop detachment, with the highest elevation of the retina at its point of adhesion to the fibrovascular membrane. Detachment of the retina becomes shallow in the periphery. The retina may stay attached in the extreme periphery. The full-thickness retinal detachment caused

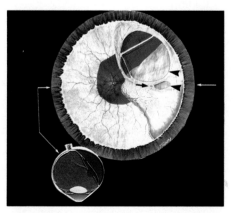

Figure 96–28. Fundus drawing of congenital retinoschisis with breaks in the inner (*arrowheads*) and the outer layers (*black arrow*), causing full-thickness retinal detachment. Schema of cross section through the horizontal line (*white arrow*) is also shown.

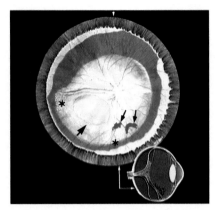

Figure 96–29. Fundus drawing of traction retinal detachment in congenital retinoschisis with fibrovascular tissues from the disc. A large inner layer break is present (*large arrow*), but there is no outer layer break. Blood in the vitreous (*small arrows*) and the dendritic figures characteristic of congenital retinoschisis are seen at the 6:00 and 8:30 o'clock meridians (*asterisks*). Schema of the cross section on vertical line (*white arrow*) is shown at lower right of figure.

by an outer layer break alone without a break in the inner layer seen in acquired retinoschisis has not been observed in congenital retinoschisis. The goal of treatment in retinal detachment is to close all outer layer and full-thickness breaks. In traction retinal detachment, vitrectomy is performed to reattach the retina. The result of surgery is reasonably favorable considering the complexity of this type of retinal detachment. Comparisons of clinical features between acquired and congenital retinoschisis are listed in Table 96–4.

GOLDMANN–FAVRE DISEASE

One special type of congenital retinoschisis is Goldmann-Favre disease. It is a syndrome that consists of congenital retinoschisis indistinguishable ophthalmoscopically from the X-linked recessive type, pigmenta-

tion in the fundus, complete night blindness, or loss of the scotopic b-wave of the ERG.[42, 43] The disease is transmitted by autosomal recessive inheritance. Favre reported two young patients afflicted with this condition. Because the disease affects the vitreous, retina, and retinal pigment epithelium, it is also called vitreotaperetinal degeneration.[44]

The fundus appearance of congenital retinoschisis of X-linked recessive inheritance is polymorphous and complex. Because Goldmann-Favre disease apparently affects the retinal pigment epithelium in its early stage, in addition to the presence of the congenital retinoschisis, the clinical findings of this disease are complex and sometimes misleading. Diffuse pigmentary retinal degeneration associated with rhegmatogenous retinal detachment[45] or a macular cyst[46] with no congenital retinoschisis should not be considered Goldmann-Favre disease. The absence of typical peripheral retinoschisis makes the diagnosis of Goldmann-Favre disease more difficult because the visible abnormality in the fundus is limited to the macula, which may not show any typical findings of retinoschisis. The fundus findings in Goldmann-Favre disease probably vary, depending on the severity and stage of the disease, just as in X-linked retinoschisis.

The electrophysiologic tests, particularly the ERG and the electrooculogram (EOG), are helpful in diagnosis. Although the original two case reports of this disease describe nonrecordable ERGs, stimulus light used at that time was just dim enough to elicit the scotopic b-wave for normal individuals. With stronger stimulus light, the ERG is recordable in patients with Goldmann-Favre disease. It is characterized by reduction of both the b- and the a-waves, but the reduction of the b-wave is more prominent than that of the a-wave and as a result the b:a wave amplitude ratio is reduced similar to the ERG in X-linked retinoschisis. Besides the decrease of the a-wave amplitude, its implicit time is prolonged in all cases, as is that of the b-wave. As a result, the ERG recorded with bright stimulus light shows a peculiar shape with small a- and b-

Table 96–4. COMPARISON BETWEEN ACQUIRED AND CONGENITAL RETINOSCHISIS

Characteristic	Acquired	Congenital
Location of splitting in the retina	Outer plexiform layer or inner nuclear layer	Nerve fiber layer
Age	Usually over 50 yr	Usually 1 to 5 yr
Bilaterally	Very common (75–90%)	Virtually always (98%)
Hereditary	Occurs without heredity; rarely autosomal recessive or incomplete dominance	X-linked recessive; rarely autosomal
Subjective complaints	Rarely present in early stage	Poor vision, strabismus, nystagmus
Macula	Rarely affected	Usually affected, characteristic
Location of retinoschisis	Most commonly inferotemporal, contiguous to ora serrata	Inferior half, anterior edge located posterior to ora serrata
Breaks	Outer layer breaks large, more frequent (25%) than inner layer breaks (16%)	Inner layer breaks large and more frequent (44%) than outer layer breaks (16%)
Vitreous membranes	Usually absent	Common (50%)
Vitreous hemorrhage	Rare	Common (40%)
Retinal detachment	Rhegmatogenous	Rhegmatogenous or traction
Associated with other anomalies	None	Filtration angle anomalies, night blindness; negative (−) type ERG
Attempt to collapse retinoschisis	Often successful	Usually unsuccessful and controversial

waves, the latter more depressed than the former and the bottom of the a-wave having a round appearance rather than the normal spiky or pointed trough.[47] Furthermore, the ERG recorded under light adaptation does not differ much from that recorded in dark adaptation in Goldmann-Favre disease.[48] The EOG is abnormal in Goldmann-Favre disease.[47] The EOG in congenital retinoschisis is normal and becomes abnormal only in a very advanced stage of disease.[31] Difficulty in diagnosing the disease from the fundus findings has already been mentioned. The fundus appearance recently described as "a new clinical entity" and called *enhanced S cone syndrome* resembles that of Goldmann-Favre disease.[49, 50] There is a unique electrophysiologic feature in the enhanced S cone syndrome, whereby the ERG recorded with bright white stimulus flash under light adaptation is not different from that obtained with dark adaptation despite greatly reduced 30-Hz flicker responses. Furthermore, there is an enhanced b-wave recorded with blue stimulation. These unique electroretinographic findings are observed in patients with Goldmann-Favre disease.[51] Whether the enhanced S cone syndrome is nothing but the new ERG finding in the disease of Goldmann-Favre or includes wider clinical entities than Goldmann-Favre disease is not known at this time.

OTHER TYPES OF RETINOSCHISIS

Splitting neural layers of the retina or retinoschisis can be found in association with specific disease. In such cases, the retinoschisis usually is considered a complication of the original diseases, although cause-and-result relationships between the two or a mechanism by which the retinoschisis develops is not entirely clear in some cases. Conditions in which retinoschisis may develop include proliferative diabetic retinopathy,[5] regressed retinopathy of prematurity,[5] peripheral uveitis,[52] trauma,[53] tumors, phakomatosis,[54] occlusive vascular diseases, long-standing retinal detachment (retinal cyst), and optic pit.[55] Although retinoschisis develops in the eyes afflicted with these conditions, a retinal detachment also may occur. In such a situation, it is often difficult to make a distinction between retinoschisis and long-standing retinal detachment when one is confronted with each clinical case. For instance, one often sees the peripheral retina elevated in young adults with regressed retinopathy of prematurity. The elevated retina shows signs of vitreoretinal traction or a break or breaks. Occasionally, two adjacent retinal vessels are pulled into the vitreous with the thin retina attached to them, but there is a defect or a large break in the retina bridging these two vessels. If the elevation does not progress during the course of observation, despite the presence of a break, this retinal elevation may be retinoschisis rather than retinal detachment.

One peculiar type of retinoschisis is seen in conjunction with an optic pit that displays retinal elevation in the posterior pole.[55] The finding that this elevation is retinoschisis rather than a sensory retinal detachment is appreciated by stereofundus photographs. The inner layers are transparent, and through them circumscribed detachment of the outer layers is seen. The outer layer detachment is round and does not communicate with the disc. The elevation of the inner layers is oval and much more extensive, communicating with the optic nerve pit. This retinoschisis in the macula does not share the clinical features of retinoschisis elsewhere in the fundus in that it does not cause absolute scotoma, and vision improves when the inner layer is flattened. Lincoff and colleagues[55] speculate that this low elevation of the inner layer may not disrupt the neural network of the retina, but long, obliquely oriented Henle's fibers take a vertical course when the inner layer is elevated.

Retinoschisis also is noted in battered babies who show no evidence of ocular trauma. The fundus shows blood-filled retinal cysts that are often large and multiple concentrated in the posterior pole.[53] The splitting of the neural layer of the retina is considered to occur as a result of violent shaking. Subsequently, the blood migrates from the retina into the vitreous, leaving the retinal scar and markedly narrow retinal arteries. The selective reduction of the ERG b-wave amplitude with good preservation of the a-wave clearly indicates impairment of the diffuse lesions in the neural retinal layer.

REFERENCES

1. Shea M, Schepens CL, von Pirquet SR: Retinoschisis. I. Senile type. Arch Ophthalmol 63:1, 1960.
2. Foos RY, Spencer IM, Straatsma BR: Trophic degeneration of the peripheral retina. *In* Symposium on Retina and Retinal Detachment Surgery. Transactions of the New Orleans Academy of Ophthalmology. St Louis, CV Mosby, 1969, pp 90–102.
3. Byer NE: Clinical study of senile retinoschisis. Arch Ophthalmol 79:36, 1968.
4. Rutnin U, Schepens CL: Fundus appearance in normal eyes. III. Peripheral degenerations. Am J Ophthalmol 64:1040, 1967.
5. Schepens CL: Retinal Detachment and Allied Diseases, vol. 2. Philadelphia, WB Saunders, 1983.
6. Zimmerman LE, Spencer WH: The pathologic anatomy of retinoschisis. Arch Ophthalmol 63:10, 1960.
7. Gottinger W: Senile Retinoschisis. (Smith JWB, trans.) New York, George Thieme Publishers, PSG Publishing, 1978.
8. Foos RY: Senile retinoschisis, relationship with cystoid degeneration. Trans Am Acad Ophthalmol Otolaryngol 74:33, 1970.
9. Byer NE: Spontaneous regression of senile retinoschisis. Arch Ophthalmol 88:207, 1972.
10. Adams ST: Spontaneous collapse at senile retinoschisis. Can J Ophthalmol 7:240, 1972.
11. Byer NE: Long-term natural history study of senile retinoschisis with implications for management. Ophthalmology 93:1127, 1986.
12. Duke-Elder WS: The relation between peripheral retinal cysts and dialysis. Br J Ophthalmol 33:388, 1949.
13. Leffertstra LJ: Disinsertions at the ora serrata. Report of 200 cases. Ophthalmologica 119:1, 1950.
14. Hruby K: Zur Pathogenese der Cysten-Ablatio. Graefes Arch Clin Exp Ophthalmol 166:451, 1964.
15. Ambler JS, Meyers SM, Zogana H, Gutman F: The management of retinal detachment complicating degenerative retinoschisis. Am J Ophthalmol 107:171, 1989.
16. Okun E, Cibis PA: The role of photocoagulation in management of retinoschisis. Arch Ophthalmol 72:309, 1964.
17. Dobbie JG: Cryotherapy in the management of senile retinoschisis. Trans Am Acad Ophthalmol Otolaryngol 73:1047, 1969.

18. Hirose T, Marcil G, Schepens CL, Freeman HM: Acquired retinoschisis: observations and treatment. *In* Pruett RC, Regan CDJ (eds): Retina Congress. New York, Appleton-Century-Crofts, 1972, pp 489–504.
19. Ambler JS, Gass JDM, Gutman FA: Symptomatic retinoschisis—Detachment involving the macula. Am J Ophthalmol 112:8, 1991.
20. Richards JSF, Harris GS: Retinoschisis treated by photocoagulation. Can J Ophthalmol 2:199, 1967.
21. Straatsma BR, Foos RY: Typical and reticular degenerative retinoschisis. Am J Ophthalmol 75:551, 1973.
22. Sulonen JM, Wells CG, Barricks ME, et al: Degenerative retinoschisis with giant outer layer breaks and retinal detachment. Am J Ophthalmol 99:114, 1985.
23. Sneed SR, Blodi CF, Folk JC, et al: Pars plana vitrectomy in the management of retinal detachments associated with degenerative retinoschisis. Ophthalmology 97:470, 1990.
24. Hagler WS, Waldoff HS: Retinal detachment in relation to senile retinoschisis. Trans Am Acad Ophthalmol Otolaryngol 77:99, 1973.
25. Condon GP, Brownstein S, Wang N-S, et al: Congenital hereditary (juvenile X-linked) retinoschisis. Histopathologic and ultrastructural findings in three eyes. Arch Ophthalmol 104:576, 1986.
26. Cibis PA: Retinoschisis—Retinal cysts. Trans Am Ophthalmol Soc 63:417, 1965.
27. Lewis RA, Lee GB, Martony CL, et al: Familial foveal retinoschisis. Arch Ophthalmol 95:1190, 1977.
28. Yassur Y, Nissenkorn I, Ben-Sira I, et al: Autosomal dominant inheritance of retinoschisis. Am J Ophthalmol 94:338, 1982.
29. Kraushaur MF, Schepens CL, Kaplan JA, Freeman HM: Congenital retinoschisis. *In* Bellows JG (ed): Contemporary Ophthalmology Honoring Sir Stuart Duke-Elder. Baltimore, Williams & Wilkins, 1972, pp 265–290.
30. Mann I, Macrae A: Congenital vascular veils in the vitreous. Br J Ophthalmol 22:1, 1938.
31. Hirose T, Wolfe E, Hara A: Electrophysiological and psychophysical studies in congenital retinoschisis of X-linked recessive inheritance. Doc Ophthalmol Proc Series 13:173, 1977.
32. Granit R: Sensory Mechanisms of the Retina With an Appendix on Electroretinography. London, Geoffrey Cumberlege, Oxford University Press, 1947, p 270.
33. Dowling JE: Organization of vertebrate retinas. Invest Ophthalmol 9:655, 1970.
34. Peachey NS, Fishman GA, Derlack DJ, Brigell MG: Psychophysical and electroretinographic findings in X-linked juvenile retinoschisis. Arch Ophthalmol 105:513, 1987.
35. Wu G, Cotlier E, Brodie S: A carrier state of X-linked juvenile retinoschisis. Ophthalmic Pediatr Genet 5:13, 1985.
36. Kaplan J, Pelet A, Hentati H, et al: Contribution to carrier detection and genetic counselling of X-linked retinoschisis. J Med Genet 28:383, 1991.
37. Alitalo T, Karna J, Forsias H, et al: X-linked retinoschisis is closely linked to DXS41 and DXS16 but not DXS85. Clin Genet 32:192, 1987.
38. Dahl N, Petterson U: Use of linked DNA probes for carrier detection and diagnosis of X-linked juvenile retinoschisis. Arch Ophthalmol 106:1414, 1988.
39. Arden GB, Gorin MB, Polkinghome PJ, et al: Detection of the carrier state of X-linked retinoschisis. Am J Ophthalmol 105:590, 1988.
40. Brockhurst RJ: Photocoagulation in congenital retinoschisis. Arch Ophthalmol 84:158, 1970.
41. Deutman AF: The hereditary dystrophies of the posterior pole of the eye. Springfield, IL, Charles C Thomas, 1971.
42. Goldmann H: Alterations degeneratives. *In* Busacca A, Goldmann H, Schiff-Wertheimer S (eds): Biomicroscopie du Corps Vitre et du Fond de l'Oeil. Rapports presentes a la Societ Francaise d'Ophthalmologie. Paris, Masson, 1957, p 164.
43. Favre M: A propos de deux cas de degenerescene hyaloideoretinienne. Ophthalmologica 135:604, 1958.
44. Ricci A: Clinique et transmission genetique des differentes formes de degenerescences vitreo-retiniennes. Ophthalmologica 139:338, 1960.
45. Francois J, Van Oye R: Degenerescence hyaloideo-tapetoretinienne de Goldmann-Favre. Ann Ocul (Paris) 200:664, 1967.
46. MacVicar JE, Wilbrandt HR: Hereditary retinoschisis and early hemeralopia: A report of two cases. Arch Ophthalmol 83:629, 1970.
47. Hirose T, Schepens CL, Brockhurst RJ, et al: Congenital retinoschisis with night blindness in two girls. Ann Ophthalmol 12:848, 1980.
48. Fishman GA, Jampol LM, Goldberg MF: Diagnostic features of the Favre-Goldmann syndrome. Br J Ophthalmol 60:345, 1976.
49. Jacobson SG, Marmor MF, Kemp CM, Knighton RW: SWS (blue) cone hypersensitivity in a newly identified retinal degeneration. Invest Ophthalmol Vis Sci 31:827, 1990.
50. Marmor MF, Jacobson SG, Foerster MH, et al: Diagnostic clinical findings of a new syndrome with night blindness, maculopathy and enhanced S cone sensitivity. Am J Ophthalmol 110:124, 1990.
51. Jacobson SG, Roman AJ, Roman MI, et al: Relative enhanced S cone function in Goldmann-Favre syndrome. Am J Ophthalmol 111:446, 1991.
52. Brockhurst RJ: Retinoschisis complication of peripheral uveitis. Arch Ophthalmol 99:1998, 1981.
53. Greenwald MJ, Weiss A, Oesterle CS, Friendly DS: Traumatic retinoschisis in battered babies. Ophthalmology 93:618, 1986.
54. Schachat AP, Glaser BM: Retinal hamartoma, acquired retinoschisis and retinal hole. Am J Ophthalmol 99:604, 1985.
55. Lincoff H, Lopez R, Kreissig I, et al: Retinoschisis associated with optic nerve pits. Arch Ophthalmol 106:61, 1988.

Chapter 97

▪

Retinal Detachment

LUCY H. Y. YOUNG and DONALD J. D'AMICO

Retinal detachment occurs when fluid accumulates between the sensory retina and the retinal pigment epithelium. It is different from conditions such as retinoschisis and choroidal detachment, in which the retina is elevated but not separated from the underlying pigment epithelium.

Retinal detachments are often classified into three major groups, depending on their underlying pathogenetic mechanism. The most common type is the *rhegmatogenous* detachment, in which fluid from the vitreous cavity enters the potential subretinal space through a break in the retina and dissects the retina from the retinal pigment epithelium (Fig. 97–1). The second most common type is the *tractional* retinal detachment

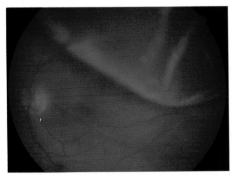

Figure 97–1. Superotemporal rhegmatogenous retinal detachment with macular involvement caused by a peripheral flap tear.

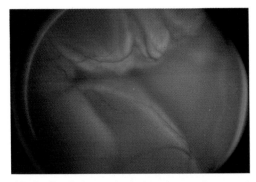

Figure 97–3. Exudative retinal detachment in a patient with inflammatory uveal effusion. (Courtesy of Robert J. Brockhurst, M.D.)

and includes detachments caused by vitreoretinal fibro-proliferative membranes that mechanically pull the retina away from the underlying retinal pigment epithelium (Fig. 97–2). The detached retina is typically smooth and is concave toward the anterior segment, unlike the rhegmatogenous detachments in which the retina is characteristically corrugated or bullous and is convex toward the pupil. In addition, tractional retinal detachment is usually more confined and rarely extends to the ora serrata. In some cases, retinal tears result from increasing vitreoretinal traction, thus resulting in a combined tractional-rhegmatogenous detachment. The third type is the *secondary* or *exudative* retinal detachment (Fig. 97–3). This group includes retinal detachments caused by retinal or choroidal conditions that disturb the retinal pigment epithelium or blood-retinal barrier, allowing fluid to build up in the subretinal space. A characteristic finding associated with this type of detachment is the presence of "shifting fluid," which explains the varying location of the detachment as the patient is examined in different positions.

It is absolutely crucial to distinguish among different types of retinal detachment, as the management of each type is quite different. An exudative detachment, e.g., will usually resolve without surgery if the underlying condition can be treated. In tractional retinal detachment, the treatment of choice is to release the vitreoretinal traction, which is usually performed with vitrectomy and membrane dissection, whereas in rhegmatogenous retinal detachment, all breaks have to be

identified and treated in order to successfully reattach the retina. Ocular conditions such as retinoschisis and choroidal detachment may be mistaken for rhegmatogenous retinal detachment and must be differentiated.

The remainder of this chapter describes some of the conditions that predispose to retinal detachment.

RHEGMATOGENOUS RETINAL DETACHMENT

Posterior Vitreous Detachment

Rhegmatogenous detachment often results from retinal breaks caused by posterior vitreous detachment. The latter is commonly found in elderly patients, and especially in those with aphakia. In an autopsy study, posterior vitreous detachment was present in 63 percent of patients older than 70 yr.[1] The incidence of posterior vitreous detachment is much higher in aphakic eyes.[2] It is also found at an earlier age in myopic eyes.[3] The normal aging process that the vitreous gel undergoes is often accelerated by trauma, cataract surgery, yttrium-aluminum-garnet (YAG) capsulotomy, intraocular inflammation, diabetes, vitreous hemorrhage, and certain hereditary conditions. Approximately 10 to 15 percent of all patients with acute, symptomatic posterior vitreous detachment have at least one retinal break.[4–8] The incidence of breaks is higher in myopic eyes. In patients with acute posterior vitreous detachment and vitreous hemorrhage, the incidence of retinal tears increases to 70 percent.[4–8]

Peripheral Fundus Lesions

Peripheral lesions that predispose to retinal detachment include enclosed oral bays, meridional folds, cystic retinal tufts, and lattice degeneration. Retinal breaks associated with peripheral cystic retinal tufts may account for up to 10 percent of rhegmatogenous detachments.[9]

Although lattice degeneration is a common finding and is the leading fundus lesion that predisposes to retinal breaks, only 22 to 30 percent of retinal detach-

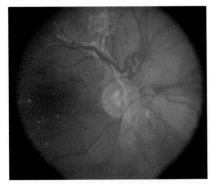

Figure 97–2. Severe proliferative diabetic retinopathy with tractional retinal detachment nasal to the disc.

ments are associated with lattice degeneration.[10, 11] The risk of lattice degeneration developing into retinal detachment is estimated to be approximately 0.3 to 0.5 percent.[10, 12] In both autopsy and clinical studies, small atrophic round holes are seen within the lattice lesions in about 25 percent of eyes with lattice degeneration.[10, 13] Although atrophic holes rarely develop into retinal detachment, except in young patients with myopia, they account for 30 to 45 percent of retinal detachments caused by lattice degeneration.[10, 11, 14–16] The remaining 55 to 70 percent of detachments are caused by tears posterior to or at the edge of a lattice bed.[10, 11] Interestingly, 70 percent of patients with retinal detachment caused by atrophic holes in the lattice lesion have myopia and are younger than 40 yr of age.[11, 15] This finding is in contrast to patients with retinal detachments caused by tears at the edge of lattice lesions; 90 percent of these individuals are 50 yr of age or older and only 43 percent of the detachments are associated with myopia.[11]

Myopia

Patients with myopia are at a much higher risk of experiencing rhegmatogenous retinal detachment.[17–19] The lifetime incidence of retinal detachment among patients with myopia is estimated to be 0.7 to 6 percent, compared with an incidence of 0.06 percent for patients with emmetropia.[19] More than a third of retinal detachments are found to occur in myopic eyes.[17, 19, 20] Myopia is present in at least one third of patients with retinal detachment. It predisposes to retinal detachment for a combination of reasons, including premature and higher rates of posterior vitreous detachment, increased incidence of lattice degeneration, and possibly thinner peripheral retina.[21–24]

Senile Retinoschisis

There are two types of degenerative or senile retinoschisis: reticular and typical forms. The reticular form is more frequently associated with outer layer holes, which are necessary for the development of rhegmatogenous retinal detachment. In an autopsy study, 23 percent of eyes with senile retinoschisis had outer layer holes.[25] Byer found outer layer holes in 16 percent of 218 eyes with retinoschisis in a long-term follow-up study.[26] The reported incidence of retinal detachment with outer layer holes and retinoschisis varies considerably. In Byer's study, 58 percent of eyes with outer layer breaks had a localized detachment.[26] Natural history studies have shown that this type of localized detachment rarely progresses to symptomatic rhegmatogenous retinal detachments.[26, 27] In addition, studies have shown that posterior extension of retinoschisis into the macula is also rare.[28, 29]

Cataract Extraction

Cataract extraction is a major cause of retinal detachment. Up to 40 percent of retinal detachments occur in aphakic and pseudophakic eyes.[30–33] The incidence of retinal detachment is 2 to 5 percent after intracapsular cataract extraction and 0 to 1.4 percent after extracapsular cataract extraction.[34–39] However, the incidence may approach 20 percent with vitreous loss. Although extracapsular cataract extraction is safer, capsulotomy (surgical or YAG) that is frequently required at a later time is associated with an approximately threefold increased incidence of retinal detachment.[38, 40–42]

The incidence of postoperative detachment is substantially increased in myopic eyes. Most reports suggest that the incidence is approximately 6 percent, and the rate goes up with high myopia.[36, 43–47] One study showed that the incidence of detachment was as high as 40 percent for eyes with myopia greater than 10 D.[48]

Several reports indicate that at least 50 percent of detachments occur within the first year after cataract surgery, and thereafter the incidence remains higher than in phakic eyes.[20, 39, 49–54] Two studies have indicated an annual incidence of later detachments of approximately 1 percent.[55, 56]

The clinical features of pseudophakic or aphakic retinal detachments are different from detachments in phakic eyes. Detachments following cataract extraction typically have small flap tears along the posterior margin of the vitreous base. They are usually more extensive and often involve the macula. Multiple breaks are found in more than 50 percent of retinal detachments following cataract extraction.[20]

Retinal detachment is also a well-known complication of congenital cataract extraction. However, the interval between surgery and the development of retinal detachment is much longer in children (20 to 30 yr) than in adults (50 percent occur within the first year after surgery).[57–61] The incidence of retinal detachment following surgery for congenital cataract is not well established. One review in the literature reported incidences ranging from 2 to 8 percent and another reported incidences of 5 to 25 percent.[62, 63] A more recent study looked at patients who had cataract extraction using newer surgical techniques and found that only 1.5 percent of the patients experienced later retinal detachment. However, the incidence is probably higher because the mean follow-up period in this study was only 5.5 yr.[64]

An important fact to remember when dealing with retinal detachments following congenital cataract extraction is that 70 percent of these patients will experience detachment in the fellow eye, and therefore they require careful follow-up.[60]

Other Ocular Surgery

The development of later retinal detachments is also associated with surgical procedures such as penetrating keratoplasty and pars plana vitrectomy. Following keratoplasty, detachments have been reported to occur in between 2.4 and 3.6 percent of cases, but this complication is essentially confined to eyes that have undergone combined cataract extraction or have suffered vitreous loss.[65, 66] Detachment is quite rare after keratoplasty in phakic eyes. As to pars plana vitrectomy, later detachments occur between 3 and 6 percent of the time and are usually due to breaks located posterior to pars plana sclerotomies, probably caused by traction on the vitreous base or by the introduction of instruments such as scissors.[67–72]

Inadvertent Scleral Perforation

Inadvertent perforation of the sclera may occur during retinal reattachment surgery, strabismus surgery, retrobulbar-peribulbar injection of an anesthetic agent, and placement of a bridal suture through the superior rectus muscle. Fortunately, these are rare complications. Scleral perforation is frequently accompanied by a retinal break and subsequent vitreoretinal changes, leading to rhegmatogenous retinal detachment.

Trauma

Retinal detachment is a frequent complication of ocular trauma. Studies have shown that up to a third of retinal detachments may be attributed to trauma.[73, 74] In children and young adults, ocular contusion is the leading cause of retinal detachment.[75] Traumatic detachments typically occur in males, and boxers are at much higher risk.[75–77] The majority of traumatic detachments are caused by blunt trauma.[74, 78, 79]

Retinal dialyses constitute 75 percent of retinal breaks found after blunt trauma, and in eyes with traumatic detachments retinal dialyses are present in up to 85 percent of cases.[75, 76, 78, 80–82] Detachments following penetrating injuries are usually characterized by the presence of transvitreal fibroproliferative membranes.

Intraocular Inflammation-Infection

Intraocular inflammatory and infectious conditions are often complicated by retinal detachments caused by vitreoretinal traction from posterior vitreous detachment. In patients with the acute retinal necrosis syndrome, rhegmatogenous retinal detachment occurs in 50 to 75 percent of afflicted eyes.[83, 84] Retinal breaks are usually found within or adjacent to areas of necrosis. Exudative detachments may also occur during the acute phase of this condition.

Rhegmatogenous retinal detachment is also a common complication in patients with cytomegalovirus retinitis; however, it is less frequent when compared with acute retinal necrosis syndrome.[85–87] In four studies reviewed, with a total of 169 eyes, 16 percent had rhegmatogenous retinal detachment.[88–91]

Ocular toxocariasis, toxoplasmosis, and pars planitis are also known to be associated with an increased incidence of retinal detachment from vitreoretinal changes initiated during the acute phase of inflammation.[92–95] Both traction and rhegmatogenous retinal detachments have been reported. Hagler and coworkers analyzed 100 cases of ocular toxocariasis and found

retinal detachments in 11 percent.[95] Friedmann and Knox found rhegmatogenous retinal detachments in 5 percent of 63 patients with ocular toxoplasmosis.[92] Smith and colleagues reported rhegmatogenous retinal detachments in 5.5 percent of 182 eyes with pars planitis.[93]

Colobomas of the Choroid and Retina

Retinal detachments associated with colobomas of the choroid and retina can be caused by retinal breaks within or outside the coloboma. The incidence of undetected breaks is high.[96, 97] Retinal detachment may also result as a complication of lens colobomas and is usually due to giant tears.[98]

Wagner-Jansen-Stickler Syndrome

There is a wide range of familial vitreoretinal disorders associated with retinal detachment. The Wagner-Jansen-Stickler Syndrome (also known as Wagner's or Stickler's syndrome) is associated with eyes having an optically empty vitreous cavity and lattice retinal degeneration. The frequency of retinal detachment varies among pedigrees. Hirose and coworkers reported retinal detachment in 47 percent of 79 eyes diagnosed as having Wagner's syndrome; 42 percent of these patients had bilateral detachments.[99]

Goldmann-Favre Syndrome

Goldmann-Favre vitreoretinal degeneration is an autosomal recessive condition characterized by a combination of cataract, optically empty vitreous cavity, peripheral pigmentary retinal changes, peripheral and macular retinoschisis, and lattice degeneration. Rhegmatogeneous retinal detachment is a complication of this rare entity.

X-linked Juvenile Retinoschisis

In X-linked juvenile retinoschisis, the retinal splitting occurs within the nerve fiber layer. In the periphery, the inner layer may be elevated, simulating a retinal detachment. Holes in the inner layer are common but do not cause detachment. However, the rarer outer layer holes can result in retinal detachment. True retinal detachment associated with juvenile retinoschisis is rare.[100]

Marfan's Syndrome

The ocular features of Marfan's syndrome are characterized by axial myopia, ectopia lentis, and retinal detachment. Retinal detachment in this disorder is related to a combination of factors, including axial length, lens subluxation, and aphakia.[101, 102] In one study, detachment occurred in 9 percent of phakic eyes and 19 percent of aphakic eyes.[101] Retinal detachment was found only in aphakic eyes or in eyes with subluxed lenses. The rate of vitreous loss is high during lens removal in these patients, thus putting them at higher risk for the development of retinal detachment.[103] Maumenee analyzed a group of 160 patients with Marfan's syndrome and found that rhegmatogenous retinal detachment did not occur in eyes with normal axial length.[102]

Homocystinuria and the Ehlers-Danlos Syndrome

Homocystinuria is also characterized by ectopia lentis. The incidence of retinal detachment is similar to that associated with Marfan's syndrome. In the Ehlers-Danlos syndrome, both myopia and retinal detachment are associated with this autosomal dominant condition, but the prevalence of retinal detachment is low.[104]

TRACTIONAL RETINAL DETACHMENT

Proliferative Diabetic Retinopathy

Diabetes mellitus is the most common systemic disease associated with retinal detachment. Proliferative diabetic retinopathy is characterized by neovascular proliferations arising from the retinal vessels, typically in the posterior pole. As the process of vitreous detachment proceeds in such an eye, the vitreous remains attached to the areas of neovascularization, resulting in vitreous hemorrhage and traction retinal detachment. If the fovea is elevated, a loss of central vision will result. Retinal breaks may develop with continued vitreoretinal traction, resulting in a combined tractional-rhegmatogenous detachment.

Sickle Cell Retinopathy

Of the sickling disorders (hemoglobins AS, SS, SC, S-thallassemia), proliferative retinopathy is most commonly found in patients with hemoglobin SC or hemoglobin S-thallassemia disease. In contrast to diabetic retinopathy, retinal arteriolar occlusion in sickle cell retinopathy is more prominent in the peripheral retina. Peripheral fibrovascular proliferation occurs on the posterior vitreous surface, which causes vitreoretinal traction that results in vitreous hemorrhage or tractional retinal detachment. With continued traction, breaks may develop adjacent to the neovascular fronds, causing a combined tractional-rhegmatogenous detachment. Retinal breaks may also develop at the edge of laser scars.[105] In one study, 8.7 percent of 46 eyes treated with argon laser for proliferative sickle cell retinopathy experienced retinal breaks.[105]

Retinopathy of Prematurity

Retinopathy of prematurity, or retrolental fibroplasia, is a proliferative vitreoretinopathy that commonly causes retinal detachment in newborns and young adults. Retinal detachment occurs as a result of tractional forces caused by the neovascular proliferation, and its presentation can range from a mild peripheral tractional retinal detachment to total tractional detachment. Retinal detachments that develop shortly after birth are usually due to mechanical traction or exudation from the retinal vessels in the active stage of proliferation. Those that develop later in life are usually of the rhegmatogenous type associated with the cicatricial stage.[106]

Familial Exudative Vitreoretinopathy

Familial exudative vitreoretinopathy is a dominantly inherited condition and is associated with a wide spectrum of retinal changes. Retinal detachment is not an uncommon complication of this condition, and it is usually tractional or exudative.[107]

EXUDATIVE RETINAL DETACHMENT

Choroidal Tumors

Choroidal lesions such as uveal melanoma, metastatic carcinoma, and hemangioma are frequently associated with exudative retinal detachment. In these conditions, it is postulated that leakage of proteinaceous fluid occurs from the neoplasm, and this fluid accumulates under the retina. Treatment of the neoplasm by irradiation, photocoagulation, or cryotherapy may permit resorption of the subretinal fluid.

Harada's Disease

Patients with Harada's disease may experience rapid loss of vision in one or both eyes because of extensive bullous serous retinal detachment.[108–110] The serous detachment in this disease is caused by a diffuse choroiditis, and it typically shifts with positioning of the patient.

Posterior Scleritis

Posterior scleritis is an inflammation of the posterior sclera with associated vascular leakage, and it is often difficult to diagnose. Only 50 percent of patients with posterior scleritis have a history of rheumatoid arthritis. Fundus changes vary, depending on the intensity of inflammation and may include exudative retinal detachment, choroidal detachments, a subretinal mass, chorioretinal folds, disc edema, and cystoid macular edema.[111, 112]

Idiopathic Central Serous Chorioretinopathy

Multiple foci of serous detachment of the retina may occur in eyes with central serous chorioretinopathy. An extensive bullous retinal detachment may develop when these foci coalesce.[113-115] Patients with this atypical presentation may be mistakenly thought to have other types of retinal detachment, but fluorescein angiography is usually helpful in making the correct diagnosis.

Idiopathic Uveal Effusion Syndrome

This syndrome usually presents in healthy middle-aged men as an insidious, progressive, often bilateral serous detachment of the choroid, ciliary body, and retina. There is striking shifting of the subretinal fluid, which this is attributed to its high protein content.[116-118]

Nanophthalmos

Exudative retinal detachments may result from compression of the vortex veins by the thickened sclera in nanophthalmic eyes.[119] The treatment of choice in this condition is decompression of the vortex veins.

Malignant Hypertension

Patients with malignant hypertension may experience exudative detachment of the retina caused by ischemic infarction of the underlying retinal pigment epithelium.[120, 121]

Toxemia of Pregnancy

Serous retinal detachment may occur in patients with toxemia of pregnancy, usually shortly before or immediately after childbirth.[122] Although the incidence is low, patients with severe toxemia may experience total serous retinal detachment.[123]

Disseminated Intravascular Coagulopathy

Disseminated intravascular coagulation is a widespread process that results in the formation of thrombi in the small vessels throughout the body. Bilateral serous detachment of the retina is one of the many ocular manifestations associated with this condition.[124]

Collagen Vascular Disease

Collagen vascular disease may be complicated by serous retinal detachment caused by fibrinoid necrosis of the choroidal vessels and subsequent ischemic infarction of the overlying retinal pigment epithelium.

Retinal Telangiectasis

The abnormal vessels leak in retinal telangiectasis, resulting in the accumulation of exudate in and under the retina. There is a wide spectrum of clinical findings, ranging from minimal retinal vascular malformation to massive areas of telangiectasis and extensive exudative retinal detachment.

MISCELLANEOUS CONDITIONS

The pathophysiology of retinal detachment in some of the congenital malformations is unknown and therefore they are discussed separately.

Optic Nerve Pit

Serous detachment of the macula associated with optic nerve pit has been reported by many authors, but the source of subretinal fluid remains unclear.[125] Brown and coworkers reviewed 75 eyes with congenital pits of the optic nerve head and found that less than 20 percent of small pits (i.e., <0.25 disc diameter in size) were associated with retinal detachment. However, the incidence of detachment approached 90 percent in eyes with pits larger than 0.4 disc diameter.[126] Spontaneous reattachment occurs in more than 25 percent of patients with optic nerve pits, but it may take months to years, after which time cystic degeneration of the macula may have taken place.

Morning Glory Syndrome

The most frequent complication associated with morning glory syndrome is retinal detachment. In three reports, a third of patients with this disc anomaly were found to have detachment of the posterior pole.[127-129] Many pathogenic mechanisms have been suggested to explain the origin of the subretinal fluid, but the pathophysiology of retinal detachment associated with this malformation has yet to be established.[128, 130, 131]

REFERENCES

1. Foos RY, Wheeler NC: Vitreoretinal juncture: Synchisis senilis and posterior vitreous detachment. Ophthalmology 89:1502, 1982.
2. Heller MD, Straatsma BR, Foos RY: Detachment of the posterior vitreous in phakic and aphakic eyes. Mod Probl Ophthalmol 10:23, 1972.
3. Goldmann H: The diagnostic value of biomicroscopy of the posterior parts of the eye. Br J Ophthalmol 45:449, 1961.
4. Jaffe N: Complications of acute posterior vitreous detachment. Arch Ophthalmol 79:568, 1968.
5. Tasman WS: Posterior vitreous detachment and peripheral retinal breaks. Trans Am Acad Ophthalmol Otolaryngol 72:217, 1968.

6. Lindner B: Acute posterior vitreous detachment. Am J Ophthalmol 80:44, 1975.
7. Tabotabo MD, Karp LA, Benson WE: Posterior vitreous detachment. Ann Ophthalmol 12:59, 1980.
8. Boldrey EE: Risk of retinal tears in patients with vitreous floaters. Am J Ophthalmol 96:783, 1983.
9. Byer NE: Cystic retinal tufts and their relationship to retinal detachment. Arch Ophthalmol 99:1788, 1981.
10. Byer NE: Changes in and prognosis of lattice degeneration of the retina. Trans Am Acad Ophthalmol Otolaryngol 78:114, 1974.
11. Benson WE, Morse PH: The prognosis of retinal detachment due to lattice degeneration. Ann Ophthalmol 10:1197, 1978.
12. Byer NE: Lattice degeneration of the retina. Surv Ophthalmol 23:213, 1979.
13. Straatsma BR, Zeegen PD, Foos RY, et al: Lattice degeneration of the retina. Trans Am Acad Ophthalmol Otolaryngol 78:OP87, 1974.
14. Morse PH: Lattice degeneration of the retina and retinal detachment. Am J Ophthalmol 78:930, 1974.
15. Tillery WV, Lucier AC: Round atrophic holes in lattice degeneration—An important cause of phakic retinal detachment. Trans Am Acad Ophthalmol Otolaryngol 81:509, 1976.
16. Murakami-Nagasako F, Ohba N: Phakic retinal detachment with atrophic hole of lattice degeneration of the retina. Graefes Arch Clin Exp Ophthalmol 220:175, 1983.
17. Schepens CL, Marden D: Data on the natural history of retinal detachment. Further characterization of certain unilateral non-traumatic cases. Am J Ophthalmol 61:213, 1966.
18. Ruben M, Razpurohit P: Distribution of myopia in aphakic retinal detachments. Br J Ophthalmol 60:517, 1976.
19. Curtin BJ: The Myopias. Philadelphia, Harper & Row, 1985, p 337.
20. Ashrafzadeh MT, Schepens CI, Elzeneinaj IH, et al: Aphakic and phakic retinal detachment. Arch Ophthalmol 89:476, 1973.
21. Byer N: Clinical study of lattice degeneration of the retina. Trans Am Acad Ophthalmol Otolaryngol 69:1064, 1965.
22. Hyams SW, Neumann E, Friedman Z: Myopia-Apakia. II. Vitreous and peripheral retina. Br J Ophthalmol 59:483, 1975.
23. Karlin DB, Curtin BJ: Peripheral chorioretinal lesions and axial length of the myopic eye. Am J Ophthalmol 81:625, 1976.
24. Takahashi M, Jalkh A, Hoskins J, et al: Biomicroscopic evaluation and photography of liquified vitreous in some vitreoretinal disorders. Arch Ophthalmol 99:1555, 1981.
25. Straastma BR, Foos RY: Typical and reticular degenerative retinoschisis. XXVI Francis L. Proctor Memorial Lecture. Am J Ophthalmol 75:551, 1973.
26. Byer NE: A long-term natural history of senile retinoschisis with implications for management. Ophthalmology 93:1127, 1986.
27. Byer NE: The natural history of senile retinoschisis. Trans Am Acad Ophthalmol Otolaryngol 81:458, 1976.
28. Okun E, Cibis PA: The role of photocoagulation in the management of retinoschisis. Arch Ophthalmol 72:309, 1964.
29. Brockhurst RJ: Discussion of Dobbie JG: Cryotherapy in the management of senile retinoschisis. Trans Am Acad Ophthalmol Otolaryngol 73:1060, 1969.
30. Schepens CL: Retinal detachment and aphakia. Arch Ophthalmol 45:1, 1951.
31. Norton EWD: Retinal detachment in aphakia. Am J Ophthalmol 58:111, 1964.
32. Hagler WS, Pollard ZF, Janett WH, Donnelly EH: Results of surgery for ocular Toxocara canis. Ophthalmology 88:1081, 1981.
33. Haimann MH, Burton TC, Brown CK: Epidemiology of retinal detachment. Arch Ophthalmol 100:289, 1982.
34. Scheie HG, Morse PH, Aminlari A: Incidence of retinal detachment following cataract extraction. Arch Ophthalmol 89:293, 1973.
35. Clayman HM, Jaffe NS, Light DS: Intraocular lenses, axial length, and retinal detachment. Am J Ophthalmol 92:778, 1981.
36. Percival SPB, Anand V, Das SK: Prevalence of aphakic retinal detachment. Br J Ophthalmol 67:43, 1983.
37. Seward HC, Doran RML: Posterior capsulotomy and retinal detachment following extracapsular lens surgery. Br J Ophthalmol 68:379, 1984.
38. Coonan P, Fung WE, Webster RG, et al: The incidence of retinal detachment following extracapsular cataract extraction. A ten-year study. Ophthalmology 92:1096, 1985.
39. Smith PW, Stark WJ, Maumenee AE, et al: Retinal detachment after extracapsular cataract extraction with posterior chamber intraocular lens. Ophthalmology 94:495, 1987.
40. McPherson AR, O'Malley RE, Bravo J: Retinal detachment following late posterior capsulotomy. Am J Ophthalmol 95:593, 1983.
41. Winslow RL, Taylor BC: Retinal complications following YAG laser capsulotomy. Ophthalmology 92:785, 1985.
42. Ober RR, Wilkinson CP, Fiore JV, Maggrano JM: Rhegmatogenous retinal detachment after neodymium-YAG laser capsulotomy in phakic and pseudophakic eyes. Am J Ophthalmol 101:81, 1986.
43. Hyams SW, Bialik M, Neumann E: Myopia-aphakia. 1. Prevalence of retinal detachment. Br J Ophthalmol 59:480, 1975.
44. Praeger DL: Five years' follow-up in the surgical management of cataracts in high myopia treated with Kelman phacoemulsification technique. Ophthalmology 86:2024, 1979.
45. Jaffe NS, Clayman HM, Jaffe MS: Retinal detachment in myopic eyes after intracapsular and extracapsular cataract extraction. Am J Ophthalmol 97:48, 1984.
46. Goldberg MF: Clear lens extraction for axial myopia an appraisal. Ophthalmology 94:571, 1987.
47. Lusky M, Weinberger D, Ben-Sira I: The prevalence of retinal detachment in aphakic high-myopic patients. Ophthalmic Surg 18:444, 1987.
48. Ruben M, Rajpurohit P: Distribution of myopia in aphakic retinal detachments. Br J Ophthalmol 60:517, 1976.
49. Wilkinson CP, Anderson LS, Little JH: Retinal detachment following phacoemulsification. Ophthalmology 85:151, 1978.
50. Hurite FG, Sorr EM, Everett WG: The incidence of retinal detachment following phacoemulsification. Ophthalmology 86:2004, 1979.
51. Hagler WS: Pseudophakic retinal detachment. Trans Am Ophthalmol Soc 80:45, 1982.
52. Ho PC, Tolentino FI: Pseudophakic retinal detachment. Surgical success rate with various types of IOLs. Ophthalmology 91:847, 1984.
53. Wilkinson CP: Pseudophakic retinal detachments. Retina 5:1, 1985.
54. Cousins S, Bonuik I, Okun E, et al: Pseudophakic retinal detachments in the presence of various IOL types. Ophthalmology 93:1198, 1986.
55. Meredith TA, Maumenee AE: A review of one thousand cases of intracapsular cataract extractions. I. Complications. Ophthalmic Surg 10:32, 1979.
56. Folk JC, Burton TC: Bilateral aphakic retinal detachment. Retina 3:1, 1983.
57. Kanski JJ, Elkington AR, Daniel R: Retinal detachment after congenital cataract surgery. Br J Ophthalmol 58:92, 1974.
58. Taylor BC, Tasman WS: Retinal detachment following congenital cataract surgery. Tex Med 70:83, 1974.
59. Toyofuku H, Hirose T, Schepens CL: Retinal detachment following congenital cataract surgery. Arch Ophthalmol 98:669, 1980.
60. Jagger JD, Cooling RJ, Fison LG, et al: Management of retinal detachment following congenital cataract surgery. Trans Ophthalmol Soc UK 103:103, 1983.
61. McLeod D: Congenital cataract surgery: A retinal surgeon's viewpoint. Aust NE J Ophthalmol 14:79, 1986.
62. Francois J: Late results of congenital cataract surgery. Ophthalmology 86:1586, 1979.
63. Ryan SJ, Blanton FM, von Noorden GK: Surgery of congenital cataract. Am J Ophthalmol 60:583, 1965.
64. Chrousos GA, Parks MM, O'Neill JF: Incidence of chronic glaucoma, retinal detachment and secondary membrane surgery in pediatric aphakic patients. Ophthalmology 91:1238, 1986.
65. Forstot SL, Bender PS, Fitzgerald C, Kaufman HE: The incidence of RD after penetrating keratoplasty. Am J Ophthalmol 80:102, 1975.
66. Musch DC, Meyer RF, Sugar A, Vine AK: Retinal detachment following penetrating keratoplasty. Arch Ophthalmol 104:1617, 1986.
67. Michels RG: Vitrectomy for macular pucker. Ophthalmology 91:1384, 1984.

68. McDonald HR, Verre WP, Aaberg TM: Surgical management of idiopathic epiretinal membranes. Ophthalmology 93:978, 1986.
69. Margherio RR, Cox MS Jr, Trese MT, et al: Removal of epimacular membranes. Ophthalmology 92:1075, 1985.
70. Isernhagen RD, Smiddy WE, Michels RG, et al: Vitrectomy for nondiabetic vitreous hemorrhage not associated with vascular disease. Retina 8:81, 1988.
71. Smiddy WE, Isernhagen RD, Michels RG, et al: Vitrectomy for nondiabetic vitreous hemorrhage: Retinal and choroidal vascular disorders. Retina 8:88, 1988.
72. Oyakawa RT, Schachat AP, Michels RG, et al: Complications of vitreous surgery for diabetic retinopathy. 1. Intraoperative complications. Ophthalmology 90:517, 1983.
73. Tulloh CG: Trauma in retinal detachment. Br J Ophthalmol 52:317, 1968.
74. Malbran E, Dodds R, Hulsbris R: Traumatic retinal detachment. Mod Probl Ophthalmol 10:479, 1972.
75. Cox MS, Schepens CL, Freeman HM: Retinal detachment due to ocular contusion. Arch Ophthalmol 76:678, 1966.
76. Ross WH: Traumatic retinal dialyses. Arch Ophthalmol 99:1371, 1981.
77. Maguire JI, Benson WE: Retinal injury and detachment in boxers. JAMA 255:2451, 1986.
78. Dumas JJ: Retinal detachment following contusion of the eye. Int Ophthalmol Clin 7:19, 1967.
79. Goffstein R, Burton TC: Differentiating traumatic from nontraumatic retinal detachment. Ophthalmology 89:361, 1982.
80. Tasman W: Peripheral retinal changes following blunt trauma. Trans Am Ophthalmol Soc 70:190, 1972.
81. Holmes Sellors PJ, Mooney D: Fundus changes after traumatic hyphaema. Br J Ophthalmol 57:600, 1973.
82. Eagling EM: Ocular damage after blunt trauma to the eye. Its relationship to the nature of the injury. Br J Ophthalmol 58:126, 1974.
83. Clarkson JG, Blumenkranz MS, Culbertson WW, et al: Retinal detachment following the acute retinal necrosis syndrome. Ophthalmology 91:1665, 1984.
84. Kreiger AE: Discussion of Clarkson JG, Blumenkranz MS, Culbertson WW, et al: Retinal detachment following the acute retinal necrosis syndrome. Ophthalmology 91:1665, 1984.
85. Meredith TA, Aaberg TM, Reeser FH: Rhegmatogenous retinal detachment complicating cytomegalovirus retinitis. Am J Ophthalmol 87:793, 1979.
86. Freeman WR, Henderly DE, Wan WL, et al: Prevalence, pathophysiology, and treatment of rhegmatogenous retinal detachment in treated cytomegalovirus retinitis. Am J Ophthalmol 103:527, 1987.
87. Teich SA, Orellana J, Freidman AH: Prevalence, pathophysiology and treatment of rhegmatogenous retinal detachment in treated cytomegalovirus retinitis. Am J Ophthalmol 104:312, 1987.
88. Henderly DE, Freeman WR, Causey DM, Rao NA: Cytomegalovirus retinitis and response to therapy with ganciclovir. Ophthalmology 94:425, 1987.
89. Holland GN, Sidikaro Y, Kreiger AE, et al: Treatment of cytomegalovirus retinopathy with ganciclovir. Ophthalmology 94:815, 1987.
90. Jabs DA, Newman C, DeBustros S, Polk BF: Treatment of cytomegalovirus retinitis with ganciclovir. Ophthalmology 94:824, 1987.
91. Orellana J, Teich SA, Friedman AH, et al: Combined short- and long-term therapy for the treatment of cytomegalovirus retinitis using ganciclovir (BWB759U). Ophthalmology 94:831, 1987.
92. Friedmann CT, Knox DL: Variations in recurrent active toxoplasmic retinochoroiditis. Arch Ophthalmol 81:481, 1969.
93. Smith RE, Godfrey WA, Kimura SJ: Chronic cyclitis. 1. Course and visual prognosis. Trans Am Acad Ophthalmol Otolaryngol 77:760, 1973.
94. Hagler WS, Jarrett WH, Chang M: Rhegmatogenous retinal detachment following chorioretinal inflammatory disease. Am J Ophthalmol 86:373, 1978.
95. Hagler WS, Pollard ZF, Jarrett WH, Donnelly EH: Results of surgery for ocular Toxocara canis. Ophthalmology 88:1081, 1981.
96. Jesberg DO, Schepens CL: Retinal detachment associated with coloboma of the choroid. Arch Ophthalmol 65:163, 1961.
97. Wang K, Hilton GF: Retinal detachment associated with coloboma of the choroid. Trans Am Ophthalmol Soc 83:49, 1985.
98. Hovland KR, Schepens CL, Freeman HM: Developmental giant retinal tears associated with lens coloboma. Arch Ophthalmol 80:325, 1968.
99. Hirose T, Lee KY, Schepens CL: Wagner's hereditary vitreoretinal degeneration and retinal detachment. Arch Ophthalmol 89:176, 1973.
100. Deutman AF: In Archer D (ed): Krill's Hereditary and Choroidal Diseases, vol. 2: Clinical Characteristics. New York, Harper & Row, 1977, p 1043.
101. Cross HE, Jensen AD: Ocular manifestations in the Marfan syndrome and homocystinuria. Am J Ophthalmol 75:405, 1973.
102. Maumenee IH: The eye in the Marfan syndrome. Trans Am Ophthalmol Soc 79:684, 1981.
103. Jarrett WH II: Dislocation of the lens: A study of 166 hospitalized cases. Arch Ophthalmol 78:289, 1967.
104. Beighton P: Serious ophthalmological complications in the Ehlers-Danlos syndrome. Br J Ophthalmol 54:263, 1970.
105. Jampol LM, Goldberg MF: Retinal breaks after photocoagulation of proliferative sickle cell retinopathy. Arch Ophthalmol 98:676, 1980.
106. Tasman W: Late complications of retrolental fibroplasia. Ophthalmology 86:1724, 1979.
107. Miyakubo H, Hashimoto K, Miyakubo S: Retinal vascular pattern in familial exudative vitreoretinopathy. Ophthalmology 91:1524, 1984.
108. Ohno S, Char DH, Kimura SJ, O'Connor GR: Vogt-Koyanagi-Harada syndrome. Am J Ophthalmol 83:735, 1977.
109. Perry HD, Font RL: Clinical and histopathologic observations in severe Vogt-Koyanagi-Harada syndrome. Am J Ophthalmol 83:242, 1977.
110. Snyder DA, Tessler HH: Vogt-Koyanagi-Harada syndrome. Am J Ophthalmol 90:69, 1980.
111. Cleary PE, Watson PG, McGill JI, Hamilton AM: Visual loss due to posterior segment disease in scleritis. Trans Ophthalmol Soc UK 95:297, 1975.
112. Benson WE, Shields JA, Tasman W, et al: Posterior scleritis. Arch Ophthalmol 97:1482, 1979.
113. Gass JDM: Bullous retinal detachment: An unusual manifestation of idiopathic central serous choroidopathy. Am J Ophthalmol 75:810, 1973.
114. O'Connor PR: Multifocal serous choroidopathy. Ann Ophthalmol 7:237, 1975.
115. Benson WE, Shields JA, Annesley WH Jr, et al: Idiopathic central serous retinopathy with bullous retinal detachment. Ann Ophthalmol 12:920, 1980.
116. Brockhurst RJ, Lain KW: Uveal effusion. II. Report of a case with analysis of subretinal fluid. Arch Ophthalmol 90:399, 1973.
117. Wilson RS, Hanna C, Morris MD: Idiopathic chorioretinal effusion: An analysis of extracellular fluids. Ann Ophthalmol 9:647, 1977.
118. Gass JDM, Jallow S: Idiopathic serous detachment of the choroid, ciliary body, and retina (uveal effusion syndrome). Ophthalmology 89:1018, 1982.
119. Brockhurst RJ: Nanophthalmos with uveal effusion. A new clinical entity. Arch Ophthalmol 93:1289, 1975.
120. Klien BA: Ischemic infarcts of the choroid (Elschnig spots): A cause of retinal separation in hypertensive disease with renal insufficiency: A clinical and histopathological study. Am J Ophthalmol 66:1069, 1968.
121. Stropes LL, Luft FC: Hypertensive crisis with bilateral bullous retinal detachment. JAMA 238:1948, 1977.
122. Fastenberg DM, Fetkenhour CL, Choromokos E, Shoch DE: Choroidal vascular changes in toxemia of pregnancy. Am J Ophthalmol 89:362, 1980.
123. Oliver M, Uchenick D: Bilateral exudative retinal detachment in eclampsia without hypertensive retinopathy. Am J Ophthalmol 90:792, 1980.
124. Cogan DG: Ocular involvement in disseminated intravascular coagulopathy. Arch Ophthalmol 93:1, 1975.
125. Apple DJ, Rabb MF, Walsh PM: Congenital anomalies of the optic disc. Surv Ophthalmol 27:3, 1982.

126. Brown GC, Shields JA, Goldberg RE: Congenital pits of the optic nerve head. II. Clinical studies in humans. Ophthalmology 87:51, 1980.

127. Steinkuller PG: The morning glory disk anomaly: Case report and literature review. J Pediatr Ophthalmol Strabismus 17:81, 1980.

128. Chang S, Haik BJ, Ellsworth RM, et al: Treatment of total retinal detachment in morning glory syndrome. Am J Ophthalmol 97:596, 1984.

129. Haik BG, Greenstein SH, Smith ME, et al: Retinal detachment in the morning glory anomaly. Ophthalmology 91:1638, 1984.

130. von Fricken MA, Dhungel R: Retinal detachment in the morning glory syndrome: Pathogenesis and management. Retina 4:97, 1984.

131. Irvine AR, Crawford JB, Sullivan JH: The pathogenesis of retinal detachment with morning glory disc and optic pit. Retina 6:146, 1986.

Chapter 98

■

Scleral Buckling Surgery

GARY D. HAYNIE and DONALD J. D'AMICO

The diagnosis and management of retinal detachment has evolved dramatically in this century. Formerly a frequent cause of irreparable visual loss, rhegmatogenous retinal detachment (detachment caused by one or more holes or breaks in the retina) is currently treated with increasing success by a variety of surgical techniques. Scleral buckling surgery for rhegmatogenous retinal detachment may be thought of as a subset of the more comprehensive discipline of vitreoretinal surgery; any modern discussion of scleral buckling surgery must therefore remain mindful of the many powerful vitreoretinal techniques available today, including vitrectomy, intraocular tamponades, endolaser treatment, and retinotomy. Nevertheless, a focused approach to the topic of scleral buckling surgery is justified for several reasons: It is a surgical approach of continuing success for a large group of patients with retinal detachment; it represents an extremely important chapter in the history of vitreoretinal surgery; and it illuminates certain questions regarding the mechanisms of retinal detachment.

This chapter examines scleral buckling surgery for retinal detachment. The reader is also advised to consult Chapters 94, 97, 100, and 101 for a more complete understanding of this topic.

HISTORICAL PERSPECTIVE

Prior to the introduction of the ophthalmoscope, retinal detachment was known only from histopathologic observations and glimpses into living eyes. From one observer such a glimpse yielded the description "amaurotic cat's eye," representing the change in the pupillary reflex in the presence of a partially detached retina.[1] Without the aid of optical instruments, others saw a white, vascularized membrane.[2]

The Helmholtz ophthalmoscope was introduced in 1851. The key element in this instrument was a partially reflecting mirror composed of a stack of glass plates that were set at an angle to reflect the rays from an adjacent bright light source into the subject's eye. Aided by a focusing lens or lenses, the examiner viewed the subject's eye by looking directly through the obliquely oriented glass plates at the unreflected retinal image.[3] The value of this instrument in making the interior of the eye accessible to examiners is revealed in the flurry of published observations that appeared in the first few years following its invention.[4-7] Many technical improvements followed the original instrument, including a concave mirror with central viewing hole (as in modern head mirrors), changeable lenses of multiple powers arranged on a disc, and a variety of adaptations to enable a binocular view.[8] However, the most revolutionary subsequent development in the visualization of the ocular fundus was the binocular, indirect ophthalmoscope, introduced by Schepens in 1951, in a form very similar to that of modern indirect ophthalmoscopes.[9]

The value of the history of retinal detachment surgery is that it shows us the stepwise recognition of principles, each of which allowed a new subset of patients to be treated successfully. The most important of these insights was the recognition of the role of retinal breaks in the pathogenesis of retinal detachment. Retinal breaks had been noted by Coccius and others in the first few years following the invention of the ophthalmoscope, but the primary role of breaks in retinal detachment was not understood. Leber was closest to the correct theory; he observed the formation of breaks in eyes with vitreous bands and assigned a role to them in the development of detachments in eyes with vitreous traction.[10]

Gonin's ignipuncture technique, first described in 1921,[11] was revolutionary because it was directed at the retinal breaks. These breaks were localized in an exacting manner on the day prior to surgery, and their positions were confirmed on the day of surgery. At surgery, the sclera was incised over the break (or breaks), and a Paquelin cautery instrument was inserted to a depth of 3 to 4 mm for a period of 2 to 3 sec.[12] Initially, this procedure was not greeted with enthusiasm, but eventually it achieved wide acclaim. It is significant because it showed retinal detachment could be cured, although only by attention to the retinal break.

The success of ignipuncture, although modest by modern standards, stimulated a search for methods to close the retinal break by stimulating chorioretinal adhesion around it, with less tissue destruction than with ignipuncture. One of the earliest of these methods was chemical cautery, in which potassium hydroxide was introduced suprachoroidally via trephined scleral holes.[13, 14] Electrolysis was briefly advocated by some.[15] However, the predominant technique for inducing chorioretinal adhesion soon became diathermy, favored for its convenience and versatility. Diathermy through full-thickness sclera caused scleral shrinkage and necrosis; this could be avoided by applying the diathermy via pins that penetrated the sclera and simultaneously created channels for the drainage of subretinal fluid.[16–19] Scleral necrosis could also be avoided by applying the diathermy in a partial-thickness scleral bed.[20] This practice continues today in scleral buckling using implants; the diathermy is applied in the partial-thickness bed created to receive the implant.

Cryotherapy was used for chorioretinal adhesion briefly in the 1930s[21, 22] but was not widely favored because it was not felt to create an adhesion as strong as that of diathermy, and its delivery was less convenient (i.e., solid carbon dioxide held against the sclera).[21] In 1961, intracapsular cataract extraction using a probe cooled to subfreezing temperatures was described.[23] Shortly thereafter, this form of cryotherapy was applied to retinal detachment surgery by Lincoff and associates.[24] It facilitated the development of explant buckling surgery because cryotherapy could be administered through full-thickness sclera, eliminating the need for lamellar scleral dissection. Following technical modifications of the cryotherapy device, cryoretinopexy became the predominant method of chorioretinal adhesion.

The impact of focused sunlight on the retina was noted in patients with solar retinopathy shortly after the introduction of the ophthalmoscope and was soon reproduced experimentally.[25] Meyer-Schwickerath designed instruments using sunlight and artificial light sources to induce retinal photocoagulation, the utility of which was reduced by technologic limitations. Then, in the late 1950s, the xenon arc photocoagulator was introduced, and a practical—although cumbersome—means of inducing chorioretinal adhesion by photocoagulation was available.[145] The first laser came into existence in 1960; experimental photocoagulation began within a year. By the early 1970s, the argon laser had succeeded the xenon arc as the light source for photocoagulation.[25] Although laser photocoagulation is not the principal means of inducing chorioretinal adhesion in routine scleral buckling, it is commonly applied to retinal breaks without detachment or after reattachment by other methods.

Modern scleral buckling techniques are the direct intellectual descendants of scleral resection. Taking into account the causative role of myopia in some retinal detachments, shortening of the eye by full-thickness scleral resection was proposed early in this century.[26]

The most notable step in the subsequent evolution of this procedure was the advent of partial-thickness scleral resection around 1950.[27] In the basic approach, a superficial scleral defect was created. When the margins of this defect were sutured together, the inner scleral layer buckled inward. With little delay, investigators noted that inward buckling of the sclera improved the chances for successful reattachment by closing the retinal break (through the apposition of choroid against retina) and relieving the effects of vitreoretinal traction (by the inward displacement of choroid).

Recognizing the value of scleral indentation, Custodis initiated the use of episcleral explants, initially made of polyvinyl alcohol.[28, 29] Scleral buckling was brought to the United States in 1951 by Schepens and coworkers, who adopted polyethylene tubing, typically placed in a partial-thickness scleral bed in which diathermy had been applied.[20] The use of silicone rubber for buckling appliances was advanced by Schepens and colleagues[30] and advocated by Lincoff and associates.[31] The technique practiced by most surgeons today uses cryotherapy followed by the episcleral attachment of a silicone rubber element, without lamellar dissection.

Injections of air into the vitreous were undertaken as early as 1911,[32] and the value of an intravitreal bubble in closing retinal breaks was appreciated as early as 1938.[33] This technique was abandoned until the late 1960s, however, when it was rediscovered by Norton and coworkers.[34] Now intravitreal bubbles are in common use, employing recently discovered long-acting gases, as well as air.

Relief of vitreoretinal traction by modification of the vitreous itself is a relatively recent development that has revolutionized the approach to retinal detachment. The techniques for vitreous surgery evolved at the Bascom Palmer Institute in Miami in the hands of Kasner and Machemer. In 1962, Kasner treated a ruptured globe with vitreous prolapse by repeatedly engaging the vitreous with a sponge, withdrawing it gently through the wound, and cutting it with scissors. Subsequently, this fairly bold maneuver was repeated on other patients, demonstrating that removal of vitreous could safely be undertaken.[35, 36] In 1970, Machemer and Parel and colleagues designed an instrument for vitreous removal whose name expressed the multiple functions performed by a single probe: VISC, for vitreous-infusion-suction-cutting. Later, illumination was provided by an optional fiberoptic sleeve, which further increased the diameter of the already bulky probe.[37, 38] The greatest subsequent technologic improvement has been the separation of the multiple functions into separate units, each with its own site of entry through the pars plana: (1) infusion, (2) illumination, and (3) aspiration-cutting.[39] As one might expect, the size and weight of the instruments have been greatly reduced.

MECHANISMS OF ATTACHMENT OF THE NORMAL RETINA

The forces maintaining the position of the retina within the eye are complex and only partially understood. Undoubtedly, multiple factors are involved, of which the following have been investigated: hydrostatic pressure, acid mucopolysaccharide in the subretinal space, and photoreceptor—retinal pigment epithelium (RPE) interaction. Naturally, maintenance of normal retinal attachment may fail in the presence of the abnormal tractional forces associated with a variety of pathologic conditions.

Hydrostatic pressure may be important as a mechanism of retinal attachment in the normal eye. The term *hydrostatic pressure* implies a pressure gradient across a barrier. In this case, it is hypothesized that the pressure within the vitreous is higher than in the subretinal space, applying an outwardly directed force to the retina. Presumably, the pressure gradient is maintained by the physiologic removal of subretinal fluid. Indeed, fluid confined to the subretinal space is removed relatively rapidly. This observation has been made in clinical cases following repair of retinal detachment, in which residual subretinal fluid remote from any open retinal break resorbs spontaneously. Controversy surrounds the source of the gradient. Theories include (1) passive diffusion of water across the RPE resulting from the elevated colloid osmotic pressure generated by the high concentration of protein in choroidal tissue fluid and (2) active pumping by the RPE.[40] In any event, this mechanism (a hydrostatic pressure gradient) requires that the retina be relatively impermeable to water, a feature of the retina for which there is some experimental evidence.[41] If the retina is held in place by fluid pressure in the vitreous cavity, it follows that retinal breaks lead to detachment by equalizing the pressure in the preretinal and subretinal compartments. This is supported by the observation that most retinal detachments are associated with retinal breaks. It seems unlikely, however, that hydrostatic pressure is the sole force involved in retinal attachment because the vast majority of retinal breaks are not associated with detachment.

The presence of viscoelastic substance between the photoreceptors and RPE cells has been demonstrated biomechanically and shown to contribute to chorioretinal adhesion.[42] Histochemically, the substance has been identified as acid mucopolysaccharide.[43]

The existence of molecular interaction between photoreceptors and RPE cells, which promotes adhesion, is suggested by studies showing that chorioretinal adhesion is reduced minutes after death or enucleation.[44, 45] The interdigitating RPE projections contain actin filaments, lining the plasma membrane,[46] which may promote adhesion by inducing and maintaining close conformation to the overlying photoreceptors. It is plausible that acid mucopolysaccharide and direct cell-to-cell interactions prevent detachment in some patients with retinal breaks and limit the size of detachment in others.

In many pathologic conditions, such as lattice degeneration of the peripheral retina, epiretinal membrane formation and fibrous ingrowth after penetrating trauma, and proliferative retinopathies such as occur in association with diabetes and sickle cell disease, there is an abnormal tractional pull exerted on the retina that enhances the tendency for the retina to detach, either with or without retinal breaks. It is commonly observed that retinal detachment is more likely to occur if retinal breaks are associated with ongoing traction in the area of the retinal break.

CLINICAL PRESENTATION OF RHEGMATOGENOUS RETINAL DETACHMENT

Patients with retinal detachment may present with a variety of complaints ranging from no symptoms to severe visual loss. Many patients will present with an established foveal detachment and will understandably have a reduction in central acuity. In other patients, a progressive scotoma corresponding to the area of peripheral detachment may be the presenting feature, and confrontation finger counting fields may often indicate the affected area prior to definitive ophthalmoscopic examination. Other patients will notice flashing lights or vitreous floaters, or both, resulting from traction on the retina, vitreous detachment, vitreous hemorrhage, or a combination. Peripheral detachments may be "subclinical" and detected only by careful indirect ophthalmoscopic examination with scleral depression. (For the management of peripheral retinal breaks without detachment see Chap. 94).

Although the clinical entities that result in retinal detachment are many, it is possible to highlight a few typical presentations and to emphasize the characteristic features of each. Primary prognostic importance for visual recovery resides in the presence or absence of foveal detachment, although a great many other preoperative factors correlate with prognosis for successful reattachment. Many phakic patients will present with a single flap or horseshoe retinal break and a contiguous retinal detachment of variable extent. Patients with lattice degeneration may have multiple tears, either round or horseshoe-shaped, in association with lattice lesions or in other areas of the eye. Aphakic or pseudophakic patients often present with retinal detachments with multiple minute retinal breaks that are located just posterior to the ora serrata. Blunt and penetrating trauma may cause rhegmatogenous retinal detachment in many ways, of which the creation of an inferotemporal retinal dialysis or disinsertion at the ora serrata is noteworthy. Certain eyes develop retinal detachment from giant retinal breaks, which are defined as retinal breaks larger than 90 degrees.

GOALS OF SURGERY FOR RETINAL DETACHMENT

The purpose of surgery for retinal detachment is the preservation or restoration of visual acuity and visual field by prevention or repair of a detachment involving the macula and peripheral retina. Macular function is given the higher priority, and the function of the peripheral retina may be sacrificed if required. Fortunately, in the most common forms of rhegmatogenous retinal detachment, the scleral buckling operation in-

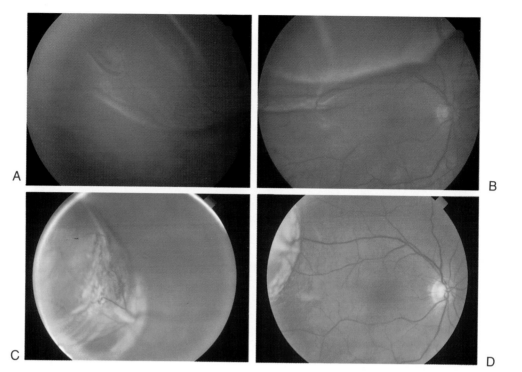

Figure 98–1. Retinal detachment with horseshoe break repaired with scleral buckling. *A,* Right eye with superotemporal detachment and horseshoe break posterior to the equator. *B,* Posterior pole of the same eye showing foveal detachment; visual acuity is 20/400. *C,* Postoperative photograph 4 mo after scleral buckle; the retinal break is reattached on a high radial buckle, and cryopexy scar is evident. *D,* Posterior pole of the same eye showing retinal reattachment; visual acuity is 20/25.

volves the extreme retinal periphery; this portion of the retina is nonvisual.

The surgical objectives of scleral buckling are (1) closure of all retinal breaks and (2) relief of inward traction on the retina (in particular, traction on retinal breaks). In certain cases, the surgeon must address an additional objective, the elimination of subretinal fluid, although this generally occurs spontaneously if the two primary objectives are achieved.

At surgery, the closing of retinal breaks is accomplished by indenting the sclera with an external appliance; this accounts for the descriptive term *scleral buckling* that is applied to this procedure (Fig. 98–1). Temporary closure of retinal breaks may also be achieved by internally applied tamponades using air, long-acting gas (commonly sulfur hexafluoride, perfluoroethane, or perfluoropropane), or silicone oil.

Permanent closure of retinal breaks is provided by creating a chorioretinal scar around the retinal break by the application of retinopexy (cryotherapy, photocoagulation, or diathermy). The development of this chorioretinal scar usually requires contact of the retinal break to the RPE, which is typically provided by the indentation of the sclera with external buckling material. Buckling of the sclera is also effective in reducing or eliminating traction on retinal breaks and other areas of the retinal periphery, and this is important not only for permitting contact of existing breaks with the RPE but also for prevention of new retinal breaks and recurrent detachment. Although certain circumstances require drainage of the subretinal fluid (as discussed further on), closure of the breaks without drainage usually results in elimination of subretinal fluid because of the action of the factors previously discussed. In a small number of operations, retinal breaks are not actually closed at the time of surgery. In these nondrainage

operations, cryotherapy is typically performed, followed by placement of a scleral buckle under the break or breaks. The subretinal fluid gradually resorbs, with closure of the retinal break in the postoperative period. The mechanism of resorption of subretinal fluid in the presence of an open retinal break is unknown but may relate to rapid passage of subretinal fluid across the RPE induced by cryotherapy and to apposition of the break against the vitreous body induced by the scleral buckle.

CLINICAL EXAMINATION AND RETINAL DRAWING

In all patients with retinal detachment, the history is followed by a comprehensive ophthalmic examination, including measurement of visual acuity and intraocular pressure. Although the intraocular pressure is usually reduced in rhegmatogenous retinal detachment, normal or elevated pressure will occur in some patients.

The essential task in the preoperative evaluation is identification of all the retinal breaks. This is best accomplished with the patient in the recumbent position, ensuring adequate room darkness and maximal pupil dilatation. The location and extent of the associated detachment are noted, and other features that have important implications for surgical technique are detailed, including epiretinal or subretinal membranes, star folds, vitreous hemorrhage, macular abnormalities, choroidal detachment, and vitreous traction. A fundus drawing is made, typically using the fundus chart originally described by Amsler and Dubois.[47] This format was proposed in the days of ignipuncture, whose success depended on exacting preoperative localization. Even though modern techniques facilitate intraoperative localization, preparation of the drawing preoperatively makes it possible to thoroughly survey the retina without the pressure and distractions of the operating room.

Hospitalization prior to the day of surgery is usually not necessary. In the past, it was held that surgical success could be promoted by ocular rest enforced by bilateral patching. Retinal detachments that settled with bedrest were known to have a favorable prognosis, no doubt reflecting the absence of substantial vitreous traction and proliferative vitreoretinopathy. In fact, although it is prudent to discourage strenuous exertion in those patients presenting with the fovea still attached, preoperative activity probably has little bearing on overall surgical outcome.

SURGICAL TECHNIQUE

Anesthesia

In most cases, local anesthesia is the preferred mode of anesthesia for retinal detachment surgery. The advantages of retrobulbar anesthesia include reduced operating time, decreased postoperative nausea, unaltered gas kinetics for air or gas tamponades that may be injected into the eye, rapid postoperative positioning in the alert patient, and decreased risk of cardiovascular morbidity and death. This risk should be carefully assessed preoperatively; it is determined chiefly by indicators of myocardial performance. In particular, congestive heart failure and recent myocardial infarction (within 6 mo) have been shown to increase the morbidity of general anesthesia, but other indicators of myocardial compromise, such as angina or arrhythmia, are also adverse findings. Age is an acknowledged risk factor.[48] Since adequate positive-pressure ventilation may be hard to achieve in patients with emphysema, this, too, is a relative contraindication to general anesthesia. The disadvantages of local anesthesia include its unsuitability for children and for patients who are uncooperative, claustrophobic, or extremely anxious. It may also be inappropriate for complex procedures expected to last longer than about 2 hr.

If local anesthesia is to be used, it is generally advisable to select an agent or mixture of agents with a prolonged duration of action. A recommended mixture is a 7 : 3 combination of 0.5 percent bupivicaine and 2 percent lidocaine (to which hyaluronidase, 150 units/10 ml, may be added), in which the long-acting bupivicaine is the major constituent. If additional anesthetic is required intraoperatively, it can usually be injected into the intraconal space with an olive-tip cannula. If the globe is closed, and only conjunctival anesthesia is required, it is generally sufficient to apply tetracaine topically. A retrobulbar cannula for repeated administration of anesthetic has been described.[49]

Use of general anesthesia avoids the procedural risks attached to local (i.e., retrobulbar) anesthesia, namely, globe perforation, retrobulbar hemorrhage, and injection into the optic nerve dura (potentially causing retinal vascular occlusion or brain stem respiratory suppression). More importantly, general anesthesia avoids two specific problems of local anesthesia: patient discomfort during the relatively protracted period of immobility necessitated by the surgery and the loss of local anesthetic effect before the end of the procedure.

If general anesthesia is chosen, two technical points must be noted. First, cholinesterase inhibitors, such as topical echothiophate iodide, must be withdrawn 6 wk prior to surgery or there may be prolongation of the effect of intravenous succinylcholine. Second, nitrous oxide must be discontinued 20 min prior to instillation of any gas into the eye. Because it is exceedingly soluble, nitrous oxide easily diffuses in and out of gas-filled spaces, such as may occur in the eye if an intravitreal air or gas bubble is injected for tamponade or for replacement of intraocular volume lost after drainage of subretinal fluid. In a patient receiving nitrous oxide by inhalation, this causes marked elevation of intraocular pressure intraoperatively, with loss of the gas volume postoperatively as the soluble nitrous oxide is discharged in the exhaled gases.

Surgical Opening

The circumcorneal conjunctival incision (peritomy) may be made at the limbus or up to 4 mm posterior to it. The advantages of placing the incision at the limbus are compelling: It is technically simpler and faster than a more posterior incision, it places the surgical opening at a greater distance from any underlying buckling material, and Tenon's capsule remains attached to the overlying conjunctiva so that together the two layers can easily be replaced over the buckle. The incision is made by tenting up the conjunctiva near the limbus with forceps so that it can be incised at the limbus with scissors (Fig. 98–2). The incision is continued for the full 360 degrees in most cases; relaxing incisions at the 3 and 9 o'clock positions are to be avoided, as they may compromise the closure and lead to exposure and infection of buckling materials.

Blunt scissors are inserted in the quadrants between the rectus muscles, and Tenon's capsule is bluntly dissected from the underlying sclera, taking care to avoid damage to the vortex veins found just posterior to the equator. Each rectus muscle is then isolated with a

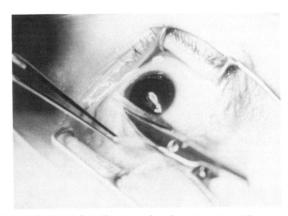

Figure 98–2. Conjunctival opening for scleral buckling surgery.

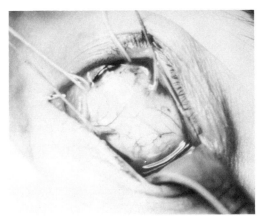

Figure 98–3. Exposure provided by rectus sutures and retractor.

muscle hook, followed by a 2–0 cotton suture passed under the insertion. These traction sutures permit rotation of the globe and exposure of the quadrants (Fig. 98–3). It is important to inspect the globe for scleral thinning at the outset of the procedure.

Localization of Retinal Breaks

The chances for a successful outcome following retinal detachment surgery are greatly reduced if localization of the retinal breaks is not accurate and thorough. In the operating room, the surgeon should carefully reexamine the retina, compare the findings with the preoperative fundus drawing, and note any additional breaks not discovered preoperatively. Localization is performed by indenting the sclera overlying the break while viewing the retina by indirect ophthalmoscopy. The operative assistant should facilitate this procedure by stabilizing the eye using the rectus muscle traction sutures. When the scleral indenter is in a position corresponding to the retinal break, the position is marked on the sclera by increasing the pressure on the marking end of the instrument. The temporary mark is then augmented with dye or cautery. Localization can also be performed by indenting with a blunt diathermy probe and marking with a light diathermy burn. When the breaks are large, both the anterior and the posterior margins should be marked.

There are two main pitfalls to avoid in retinal break localization. First, the examiner must avoid indenting the sclera with the shaft rather than the end of the indenter, because this will cause the mark to be placed too far posteriorly. Second, when the retina is highly elevated, the area of RPE that is visible through the break is posterior to the site on which the break will fall when the retina is flat. The surgeon must avoid marking the sclera too posteriorly. This error will be easier to avoid as experience is gained.

Chorioretinal Adhesion

After localization of the breaks, chorioretinal adhesion is stimulated by retinopexy. The methods available

for retinopexy—each has its adherents—include cryotherapy, diathermy, and photocoagulation. Cryotherapy is the method preferred by most retinal surgeons for routine scleral buckling surgery. It may be applied easily under precise indirect ophthalmoscopic visualization across full-thickness sclera, unlike diathermy, which may be applied only to a partial-thickness scleral bed and therefore requires scleral dissection. Major vessels, such as the long ciliary arteries or vortex veins, are not occluded by cryotherapy, as they may be by diathermy.[50] Unlike diathermy,[51] cryotherapy does not cause tissue necrosis, an appreciable benefit when operating on thin sclera. Its most important disadvantage relative to diathermy is that it causes a greater disruption of the blood-retinal barrier and an increased mobilization of RPE cells,[52, 53] both of which are factors of presumed importance in the development of proliferative vitreoretinopathy. Laser photocoagulation has the advantage of causing less disruption of the blood-retinal barrier than does cryotherapy. Photocoagulation has been used primarily in the outpatient treatment of retinal breaks without detachment, although endolaser treatment during vitrectomy is an increasingly useful modality. Recently introduced indirect ophthalmoscopic laser systems may offer a valuable option to cryotherapy for certain routine scleral buckling operations. However, indirect ophthalmoscopic laser treatment of retinal breaks at scleral buckling surgery requires clear visualization through the media and contact of the retinal break with the RPE; these features are not always present at surgery.

Intraoperatively, cryotherapy is applied around each break, avoiding the exposed RPE within the break, to minimize the risk of preretinal proliferation. This is accomplished by indenting the sclera with the cryoprobe under indirect ophthalmoscopic visualization (Fig. 98–4). The probe is then activated until whitening of the retina is noted. Retinal whitening may not be achieved when the retina is highly elevated. In this case, vague dulling of the underlying RPE may serve as the endpoint of treatment. There is evidence that freezing the RPE alone, although not ideal, is sufficient to create an adequate chorioretinal bond. Using overlapping applications, cryotherapy is applied in a 2- to 3-mm-wide

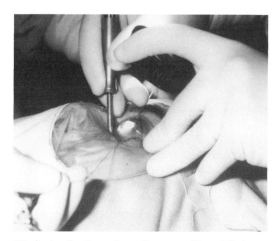

Figure 98–4. Application of cryotherapy with ophthalmoscopic visualization.

area around each lesion. It is useful to note whether the break can be closed by scleral indentation during cryotherapy. If so, buckling alone will probably be sufficient to close the break without the need for drainage of subretinal fluid.[54]

Certain technical considerations must be observed during cryotherapy. The sclera must be indented with the tip (not the shaft) of the probe. Failure to adhere to this precaution will lead to freezing of tissues posterior to the desired site. Furthermore, the shaft must be covered by an insulating sheath. After each application, the probe must be held in place against the sclera for a few seconds to allow thawing of the frozen tissue. If the probe is moved while it is still adherent to the underlying ice ball, scleral or choroidal rupture may occur. When repositioning the probe, care must be taken to avoid incorporating the lid between probe and sclera. Finally, the probe should be applied to the tissue firmly; this may promote faster freezing by locally reducing choroidal blood flow and preventing the conduction of heat from the surrounding tissue into the cryotherapy site.[55]

Securing the Scleral Buckle

Numerous materials have been used in the recent past for scleral buckling. Today, all the buckling appliances in common use are made of silicone rubber, including cylinders of silicone sponge that are round or oval in cross section. They are often split lengthwise to achieve indenting of the sclera without unnecessary bulk. Solid silicone buckling material is supplied in multiple widths and contours. These solid silicone pieces typically have a groove to accept a thin overlying encircling band, which is also of solid silicone.

There are two predominant methods of buckling. Explants are sutured externally to the sclera, and intrascleral implants are placed in the intrascleral bed created by scleral dissection for the purpose of diathermy. The use of explants eliminates the need for intrascleral dissection with its increased risk of globe perforation, rupture, and intrusion of buckling material and greater technical difficulty at reoperation. Although explants present a slightly greater risk of infection and extrusion, the numerous advantages of the explant technique have made it the method used by a majority of surgeons. Explant buckling is the focus of this discussion.

Buckling appliances are sutured to the eye using 4–0 or 5–0 nylon, Dacron, or Supramid sutures on a curved spatula needle.[55] The eye is immobilized by the assistant, using the rectus muscle traction sutures. Tenon's capsule is retracted using a Schepens retractor. The surgeon stabilizes the globe further by grasping the insertion of the nearest rectus muscle with forceps (Fig. 98–5). The needle penetrates the sclera to one half of its thickness. It is then advanced 2 to 3 mm in the interlamellar plane before reemerging through the superficial sclera. The needle is not allowed to rotate in the needle holder because this will allow the sharp edges of the spatula tip to partially or completely divide the thin overlying scleral bite. It is not necessary to take extraordinarily

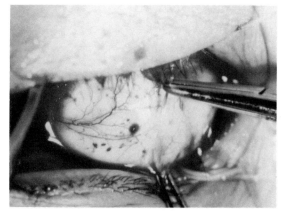

Figure 98–5. Placement of intrascleral suture (for circumferential buckle) in relation to methylene blue pen mark on the sclera.

deep or long bites; the buckle must be anchored only until it is enveloped by fibrosis, which takes place in a few weeks. The usual suture configuration is the mattress suture. In most cases, the separation of the scleral bites is 2 mm greater than the width of the explant (Figs. 98–6 and 98–7). The variation of this distance largely determines the depth of the buckling.

As a general rule, the buckling appliance must be sufficiently large to support the break (or breaks) with a margin of a least 1 to 2 mm. The buckle should be of the minimal height necessary to accomplish the two fundamental objectives—i.e., close the break and relieve vitreoretinal traction.

The length and configuration of the explant is determined by the character of the retinal breaks. Radially oriented explants are most useful for posterior breaks and horseshoe breaks in which radially oriented folds cause "fish mouthing" of the break that is not likely to be resolved by a circumferential buckle. Segmental circumferential buckles are most appropriate for dialyses, wide retinal breaks, and closely grouped breaks. Encircling bands are used when multiple breaks are present or when breaks are suspected but cannot be localized. Because they can effectively relieve traction

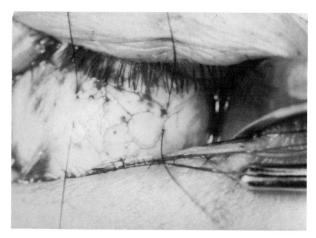

Figure 98–6. Suture in place; width is 2 to 3 mm greater than the intended buckling material.

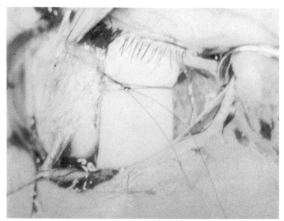

Figure 98–7. Buckling element is passed under rectus and suture is temporarily tied.

at the vitreous base, encircling bands are also useful in proliferative vitreoretinopathy.

If drainage of subretinal fluid is to be undertaken, it should be carried out before tightening the buckling sutures. If no drainage is planned, funduscopic reevaluation at this time should show the break to be in contact with or very close to the underlying RPE and surrounded on all sides by indentation of the eye wall.

Drainage of Subretinal Fluid

Drainage is not indicated in all buckling procedures. If buckling alone brings the break into contact with (or close to) the underlying RPE, as it will in many detachments, drainage is not necessary. However, drainage is probably performed in most retinal detachment operations for a combination of reasons, including (1) to provide intraoperative contact between the retinal break and the buckled eye wall for development of retinopexy-induced adhesion, (2) to verify buckle positioning when the location of the breaks on the buckle has not been unequivocally demonstrated (as when there are multiple, widely separated breaks or when localization was tentative), (3) to reduce the intraocular volume to accommodate the indentation of the buckling material or the injection of intraocular air or other tamponade, and (4) to relieve concern that the subretinal fluid resorption may not occur spontaneously. This final consideration is especially applicable in high myopia, in which fluid resorption may be delayed by underlying choroidal abnormalities, and certain inferior detachments, in which subretinal fluid accumulation may be promoted by gravity. In long-standing retinal detachment, suggested by RPE demarcation lines or atrophy of the detached retina, the subretinal fluid may be very viscous, which also leads to a delay in resorption. Drainage should also be considered in highly elevated detachments and detachments complicated by preretinal membranes.

Certain guidelines may be helpful in selecting the drainage site. The site should be relatively avascular. If circumstances permit, this can be achieved by locating the site immediately above or below one of the horizontal rectus muscles (preferably lateral, for ease of exposure), in which the underlying choroidal vessels are smallest. The site should be located away from the break under an area of high retinal elevation to ensure evacuation of subretinal fluid, rather than preretinal fluid or formed vitreous. Fixed folds constitute a nearly ideal site for drainage, since the relative rigidity of the folds prevents retinal incarceration. It is best to drain in the bed of the buckle because an inadvertent retinal perforation will automatically be supported without need to revise the buckle.

The draining sclerotomy is usually a radial incision 3 to 4 mm in length. The buckling material is passed through the sutures in the area of the drainage site, which are loosened to permit movement of the buckling material posteriorly and away from the intended incision in the bed of the buckle. Scleral lamellae are carefully divided until exposed choroid bulges slightly between the lips of the sclerotomy. The exposed choroid is then transilluminated to reveal any large vessels in the drainage site. Diathermy may be applied to the exposed choroid with a blunt probe. The choroid is then penetrated by a 30-gauge needle 2 to 3 mm into the drainage site. It is usually necessary to indent the opposite side of the globe to accelerate the fluid discharge. Great care is given to maintaining the intraocular pressure at a normal level, both by avoiding undue tension on the recti and by inserting cotton-tipped applicators between the globe and the orbital rim to compensate for the removal of subretinal fluid. When sufficient drainage is completed, the securing mattress suture of the scleral buckle suture should be tightened to prevent retinal prolapse and hypotony. If the drainage site is outside the bed of the scleral buckle, a mattress suture should be pre-placed in the lips of the incision. This suture is tightened following completion of subretinal fluid drainage and prior to any globe or buckle manipulation.

Adjusting Intraocular Volume

Tightening of the sutures around the explant causes the intraocular pressure to rise because of displacement of intraocular volume as the sclera is indented. During and after tying of the sutures, the intraocular pressure may be monitored by palpation of the globe and Schiøtz tonometry. Of greatest importance, however, is the fundus examination to ensure that the central retinal artery remains patent. If the intraocular pressure rises above systolic pressure, occluding the central retinal artery, measures to reduce the pressure must be performed promptly. In phakic eyes or in eyes with a posterior chamber intraocular lens (IOL), paracentesis may be performed. Anterior chamber paracentesis is somewhat more hazardous in aphakic eyes (in which vitreous may be drawn forward and incarcerated in the paracentesis wound) or eyes with an anterior chamber IOL (in which reducing the anterior chamber volume may bring the IOL into contact with the corneal epithelium).[56] In these eyes, it may be necessary to loosen one or more sutures to relieve the elevated pressure. Usually, the simple expedient of tying the sutures slowly, leaving time for pressure equilibrium between each, prevents the untoward rise in pressure.

If the eye is too soft after the sutures are tied, the intraocular volume must be augmented with air or gas. Injections of either are made 4 mm posterior to the limbus using a 30-gauge needle directed toward the optic nerve. Balanced saline solution may also be used, but air and gas are preferred, because they have the advantage of being a tamponade for closure of retinal breaks. The injection of intraocular gas is discussed in greater detail in the section on Pneumatic Retinopexy.

Closure

After all buckling sutures are cut, the conjunctiva and Tenon's capsule are brought forward. Using 5–0 or 6–0 absorbable gut suture, the leading edge of Tenon's capsule is secured at the level of the muscle insertions using one suture at each side of the four rectus muscle insertions. These maneuvers are facilitated by leaving the rectus traction sutures in place until the closure of Tenon's capsule is completed. Tightening sutures are placed in the free margin of the conjunctiva at the 3 and 9 o'clock positions, and any other conjunctival defects are repaired with sutures as required. Topical antibiotic ointment and cycloplegic drops are applied, and the eye is covered with sterile gauze and a metal shield.

Postoperative Care

Usually, the patient may be discharged on the first postoperative day, and many surgeons have moved to perform scleral buckling surgery on an outpatient basis. There is no standard practice regarding postoperative medications. For most phakic cases, topical scopolamine, 0.25 percent, and topical antibiotics three or four times daily will be sufficient, adding topical steroids for some or all patients according to the surgeon's judgment. The use of topical steroids must be weighed against the risk of interfering with the healing of the conjunctival closure, and many surgeons find it preferable to omit steroids unless a specific indication is present, such as a preexisting corneal graft. If gas has been injected, the patient will require specific instructions regarding head position and restriction from plane travel. Activity restriction is also highly variable among surgeons but probably has little bearing on the outcome in the majority of cases.

ALTERNATIVES TO SCLERAL BUCKLING

Vitrectomy

The use of vitrectomy in the management of retinal detachment is discussed in detail in Chapter 100.

Pneumatic Retinopexy

The use of intravitreal gas to treat retinal detachment was described in 1938[33] in the era when the first successful techniques for treating retinal detachment were being pioneered. In the 1960s, the use of intravitreal gas as an adjunct in the repair of retinal detachment was rediscovered.[34] It has been proposed that retinal breaks may be closed with intravitreal gas alone, avoiding the complications associated with scleral buckling and subretinal fluid drainage.[57, 58]

In this procedure, as in all treatments for retinal detachment, the basic aims of the surgery remain closure of all retinal breaks and relief of traction on the retina, especially traction on retinal breaks. The closure of retinal breaks is achieved temporarily by the intravitreal bubble, which prevents transmission of fluid through the break by virtue of its surface tension; permanent closure is provided by cryopexy, as in routine buckling surgery. It is important to recognize that the role of the bubble does not include "pushing" the retina into place, since, naturally, the subretinal fluid is incompressible. The elimination of subretinal fluid, which is necessary for a successful outcome, is accomplished by the natural forces previously mentioned, which remove fluid from the subretinal space when no open retinal breaks are present. Pneumatic retinopexy is ineffective in achieving one of the fundamental goals—i.e., relief of traction,[59] and the success of the procedure requires that a given retina not have substantial traction, particularly in the area of the retinal break. Since the description of pneumatic retinopexy in the English literature, proliferative vitreoretinopathy of grades C and D has been considered a contraindication.[58]

Because its resorption is relatively rapid, air is not typically used for pneumatic retinopexy without scleral buckling. The three inert gases commonly used are sulfur hexafluoride (SF_6), perfluoroethane (C_2F_6), and perfluoropropane (C_3F_8), all of which expand over 1 to 2 days by absorption of nitrogen and oxygen from blood or surrounding tissues and remain in the eye longer than air (Table 98–1). In the eye, pure SF_6 expands in volume 2.5 times and has a half-life of about 5 days; C_2F_6 expands 3.3 times and has a half-life of 10 days; C_3F_8 expands 4 times and is half-resorbed in 35 days.[60–62] Only small quantities of the pure forms of these gases should be used to avoid occlusion of the central retinal artery from progressive intravitreal expansion. The gases can be made nonexpansile by mixing with air. For SF_6, the nonexpansile concentration is 18 percent;[62] for C_3F_8, it is 12 percent.[63]

As pioneered by Hilton and associates,[58, 64] pneumatic retinopexy is indicated for single retinal breaks or small groups of breaks confined to 1 clock hour, located in the superior 8 clock hours of the fundus. Established contraindications are proliferative vitreoretinopathy of grade C or worse, glaucoma, and inability to maintain the necessary head positioning. After retrobulbar anesthesia, the retina around the break is treated with cryotherapy, firmly applying the cryoprobe in order to reduce the intraocular pressure. A Honan balloon or

Table 98–1. PROPERTIES OF THE PRINCIPAL GASES USED IN PNEUMATIC RETINOPEXY

Gas	Half-life of Gas After Intraocular Injection	Intraocular Expansion of Pure Gas	Nonexpansile Concentration
Sulfur hexafluoride (SF_6)	5 days	2.5 times	18%
Perfluoroethane (C_2F_6)	10 days	3.3 times	—
Perfluoropropane (C_3F_8)	35 days	4 times	12%

other device may then be used to further soften the eye. The eye is prepared with povidone-iodine solution. Using a 30-gauge needle inserted 4 mm posterior to the limbus, 0.3 ml of pure, filtered C_3F_8 or 0.6 ml SF_6 is injected. Central retinal artery perfusion is monitored, but paracentesis is rarely necessary. The head is positioned so that the bubble is in contact with the break. This posture is maintained 16 hr/day for 5 days; at night the patient sleeps on his or her side.[65]

In a randomized trial comparing pneumatic retinopexy against scleral buckling, the rates of prolonged reattachment were 73 and 82 percent, respectively.[66] Even though these rates are similar, pneumatic retinopexy has not been uniformly embraced. The reason for this may derive from the fact that in most hands, the rate of anatomic success after pneumatic retinopexy has been variable, ranging from 63 to 83 percent,[67–69] whereas most surgeons expect a much higher anatomic success rate—about 95 percent—for scleral buckling in these relatively simple retinal detachments.[70, 71] In one retrospective study of retinal detachments that would have been candidates for pneumatic retinopexy but were treated with scleral buckling, the rate of anatomic success was 96 percent.[69] In addition, retinopexy is sometimes complicated by new retinal breaks, possibly because of reorientation of tractional forces as vitreous is displaced by the intraocular bubble.

For the present, it seems reasonable to conclude that pneumatic retinopexy is a valuable technique whose most promising application is in patients with suitable detachments and contraindications to the anesthesia required for scleral buckling surgery. In addition, variations of the pneumatic retinopexy technique are extremely useful in the management of recurrent retinal detachment after scleral buckling surgery—particularly in combination with indirect ophthalmoscopic laser retinopexy—and in the management of untreated retinal breaks with retinal detachment following vitrectomy.

Lincoff Balloon

Introduced by Lincoff and coworkers in 1979,[72] the Lincoff balloon technique uses cryotherapy followed by an inflatable balloon to indent the sclera in an outpatient procedure. The balloon is inserted against the sclera via a small conjunctival incision, and verification of positioning is obtained by indirect ophthalmoscopy immediately after inflation of the balloon. Subretinal fluid is not drained in this procedure but is absorbed spontaneously, and the balloon is subsequently removed. This procedure addresses all the goals of scleral buckling surgery, including relief of retinal traction, while the buckle is inflated. However, despite the conceptual attractiveness of the balloon buckle, its use has remained limited. Applicable detachments are restricted to those with a single break or a group of closely spaced breaks without proliferative vitreoretinopathy. Although this method is acknowledged to have fewer complications than standard buckling, the initial success rate is lower.[73–75] Most significantly, the procedure requires a higher degree of patient motivation and continuing surgical manipulation than does scleral buckling, and these requirements have proved inconvenient to both the patient and the surgeon.

Photocoagulation-Cryotherapy

For certain retinal detachments, demarcation by laser photocoagulation or cryotherapy is sufficient. This approach is usually reserved for small peripheral detachments around a single break with minimal subretinal fluid and is most commonly considered in patients in whom anesthesia presents substantial risk.

SPECIAL CIRCUMSTANCES

Unseen Retinal Breaks

In a fraction of rhegmatogenous detachments (10 percent or less), no retinal break is visualized.[76, 77] It seems reasonable to assume that in most cases the break is not seen because it is small; in addition, varying degrees of media opacity undoubtedly contribute to the concealment of the break. Naturally, care must be taken to ensure that the retinal detachment is not exudative. When no break has been visualized, the retinal detachment may be considered rhegmatogenous only in the absence of conditions predisposing to exudative detachment, such as central serous choroidopathy, uveitis, eclampsia, or tumor, as well as clinical features suggestive of exudative detachment, such as shifting subretinal fluid.[76] Fluorescein angiography may be useful to exclude central serous choroidopathy, which may present with bullous retinal detachment. Senile retinoschisis requires careful discrimination by indirect ophthalmoscopy, and this differentiation may be aided by examination of the fellow eye. X-linked retinoschisis has been mistaken for retinal detachment and unneeded surgery has been offered; in this disease, the family history, examination of the fellow eye, and characteristic macular changes should secure the correct diagnosis. In presumed rhegmatogenous retinal detachment without a confirmed break, the preoperative search for the break may be aided by the guidelines proposed by Lincoff and Gieser,[78] in which the distribution of subretinal fluid indicates the probable location of the break. Even if the break is still not identified, these guidelines may suggest which part of the retina to treat with retinopexy.

Detachments involving fewer than three quadrants may be repaired by segmental circumferential buckling after cryotherapy has been applied in the involved quadrants just posterior to the ora serrata. For detachments of three or four quadrants, scleral buckling for 360 degrees is recommended. Drainage of subretinal fluid should be performed routinely when the break has not been localized.

In the absence of significant proliferative vitreoretinopathy, vitrectomy does not improve the outcome,[79] although it may reveal the unseen break. Unfortunately, failure to find the break is often associated with other adverse factors, such as increased extent and duration, greater likelihood of macular detachment, and proliferative vitreoretinopathy. Therefore, the rate of surgical reattachment is reduced somewhat, typically to around 75 to 85 percent.[76, 77]

Macular Break

Most macular breaks do not lead to retinal detachment. Detachment due to a macular break is uncommon except in a few clinical situations: myopia, aphakia, and blunt trauma.[80] Even when a macular break is present, peripheral breaks, if there are any, must be treated before the macular break is treated. Usually, this cures the retinal detachment. If it does not, or if no peripheral breaks are seen, it will be necessary to treat the macular break directly.

Formerly, the treatment involved buckling the macula by various means, including a metal clip[81, 82] or scleral buckling elements secured by a variety of techniques.[83] Naturally, a hazard was posed by the thin sclera of myopic patients. In 1982, effective treatment was demonstrated using pars plana vitrectomy and intraocular

gas.[84] Since then, the injection of intraocular gas on an outpatient basis without vitrectomy has been employed in treating retinal detachment caused by macular holes,[85, 86] with a success rate approximating that of vitrectomy.[87]

Prior to instillation of gas, the eye must be softened. This has been achieved in a variety of ways: (1) external pressure (Honan balloon) combined with osmotic agents,[88, 89] (2) anterior chamber paracentesis,[90, 91] (3) removal of liquid vitreous,[92] and (4) drainage of subretinal fluid.[91] The rate of permanent reattachment after one procedure falls in the range of 70 to 90 percent for all these techniques.[93] It is not clear that adjuvant photocoagulation is necessary, and some investigators have reported good results without it.[89, 91, 92]

For most retinal detachments due to a macular hole, it will be sufficient to inject a long-acting gas such as SF_6 via the pars plana after reducing the intraocular volume by anterior chamber paracentesis, osmotic agents, and external pressure. If vitreomacular strands are noted on examination, or if redetachment occurs following simple gas injection, vitrectomy with gas-fluid exchange and endolaser treatment may be undertaken. Rarely, silicone oil may be required (Fig. 98–8).

Giant Break

For the simplest giant breaks, the surgical approach may vary little from that for routine retinal breaks. If there is no associated retinal detachment, prophylactic cryotherapy or photocoagulation may be successful. If a shallow detachment is present, a standard scleral buckling procedure may be sufficient.

Regrettably, most giant retinal tears are complicated by inward rolling of the posterior margin, and it is this feature that distinguishes giant retinal tears and defines the essential tasks in their management: the unrolling of the flap and stabilization of the unrolled retina while chorioretinal scarring takes place. This inrolling may be further complicated by reduced mobility caused by proliferation of membranes on the retina. Vitrectomy is typically required in these cases for many reasons,

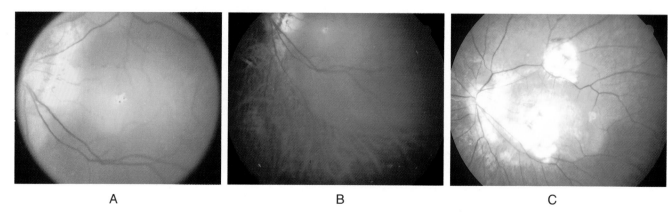

| A | B | C |

Figure 98–8. Retinal detachment due to macular break in a patient with high myopia and posterior staphyloma. A, Left eye with retinal detachment due to macular break; visual acuity is at the counting fingers level at 1 ft. B, Detachment is confined to the posterior pole and does not extend to the periphery. C, Postoperative appearance after vitrectomy with endodrainage of subretinal fluid, endolaser, and silicone oil tamponade; the retina is attached and visual acuity is unchanged at the counting fingers level at 1 ft.

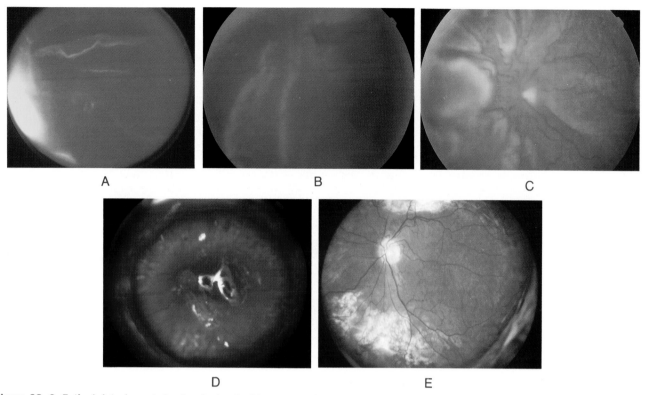

Figure 98–9. Retinal detachment due to giant retinal break. *A,* Wide-angle photograph displays total retinal detachment with superior giant break from the 10 to the 2 o'clock positions in the left eye. *B,* Preoperative photograph from another patient with a total retinal detachment due to a giant break from the 12 to the 6 o'clock positions in the left eye. *C,* Posterior pole of same eye as in *B;* visual acuity is at the hand motions level. *D,* Postoperative photograph 2 days after surgery from same patient; an encircling scleral buckle, cryopexy, vitrectomy, and prone fluid-air exchange were performed, and the reattached retina is seen through perfluoropropane gas tamponade. *E,* Posterior pole of the same eye 4 mo later; visual acuity is 20/200.

including removal of membranes, removal of the vitreous gel, manipulation of the retina into position against the RPE, endolaser treatment, and placement of intraocular tamponade.

There are numerous techniques for the repair of retinal detachment with giant breaks, and the full armamentarium of vitreoretinal surgery has been employed in this condition (Fig. 98–9). In cases in which the giant break is to be supported by a scleral buckle and secured by the development of a chorioretinal scar after cryotherapy, it is common to perform the cryotherapy prior to the vitrectomy so that the RPE cells dislodged by cryotherapy can be removed during vitrectomy.[94] It has been shown that membranes observed in proliferative vitreoretinopathy may originate from these cells,[95] and their removal from the eye may reduce the rate of glial proliferation and recurrent retinal detachment. A scleral buckle has been commonly used in the past but may be unnecessary in cases in which vitrectomy techniques have successfully relieved all traction. In cases in which a scleral buckle is desired, it is most convenient to put the buckling sutures and explant in place around the eye early in the procedure. A broad buckle will be required to incorporate all aspects of the tear on the buckle, and a fully encircling buckle is used most commonly.

Vitrectomy is then performed, during which sufficient formed vitreous is removed to admit a large gas bubble.

The vitreous overlying the rolled retinal flap must be removed.[96] Most importantly, any membranes restricting the mobility of the flap must be removed. The mobilized posterior flap of the giant break may then be unrolled by a variety of techniques, including air-fluid exchange (prone or supine),[96] fluid-silicone exchange, or direct manipulation with vitrectomy instruments, tacks,[97, 98] or sutures.[94] The reattached retina is held in position by the instillation of air, long-acting gas, or silicone oil.

The use of heavier-than-water liquid perfluorocarbons has revolutionized manipulation of the mobilized flap of giant retinal breaks.[99] In this technique, a perfluorocarbon fluid is continuously introduced on the surface of the disc. The retina is gradually unrolled against the RPE as subretinal fluid is expressed anteriorly and removed from the eye. This technique may be performed with or without scleral buckling and with a variety of retinopexy options. After the retina is completely reattached, the perfluorocarbon fluid is removed from the eye and exchanged for tamponade with gas or silicone oil. If necessary, photocoagulation of the flap margins may be performed intraoperatively by indirect laser ophthalmoscopy or postoperatively by slit-lamp guidance.

Prior to the development of vitrectomy, the prognosis for rolled giant tears was very poor.[100, 101] With continued technical improvement, the rate of success has increased and is currently as high as 90 percent.[94, 99]

Proliferative Vitreoretinopathy

The most common cause of failure of retinal detachment surgery is proliferative vitreoretinopathy, which complicates about 10 percent of operations.[102, 103] Preretinal membranous proliferation is sometimes present preoperatively but is more often seen after retinal detachment surgery. Risk factors for the postoperative development of proliferative vitreoretinopathy include preexisting proliferative vitreoretinopathy, previous procedures (especially vitrectomy and cryotherapy), giant breaks, vitreous hemorrhage, and choroidal detachment.[103–105] Retinal detachments of longer duration are more likely to exhibit proliferative vitreoretinopathy;[106] indeed, advanced proliferative vitreoretinopathy is the end-stage of an untreated retinal detachment. Membranous proliferations are typically found on the posterior aspect of the detached vitreous gel, creating a membrane parallel to the iris, whose contraction causes traction, detachment, and tears in the peripheral retina. Membranes on one or both surfaces of the retina commonly cause the retina to be thrown into folds (Fig. 98–10). Membranes may also invest the ciliary body, causing hypotony as well as anterior traction on the retina to which they are connected. There is excellent evidence that at least some of the cells in these contracting membranes are derived from RPE cells.[95]

The surgical repair of the retinal detachment complicated by proliferative vitreoretinopathy should make use of the simplest possible procedure that accomplishes the basic aims stated earlier: closure of retinal breaks, relief of retinal traction, and elimination of subretinal fluid (Fig. 98–11). Typical surgery includes a broad, high

encircling buckle.[102, 107, 108] In addition, a pars plana vitrectomy is performed,[102, 103, 107–110] in which the lens and central gel are removed along with any transvitreal membranes, epiretinal membranes, and condensed gel and membranes at the vitreous base (especially inferiorly). Fluid-gas exchange is performed, during which subretinal fluid is drained via a posterior break or through a peripheral break with a subretinal extrusion cannula. This is followed by extensive endolaser treatment to all retinal breaks and the placement of a tamponade with long-acting gas or silicone oil. Although the prognosis for these eyes was once dismal, reattachment can now be achieved in the majority of cases.[107, 108, 110, 111] In some patients, flattening of the retina cannot be accomplished by these techniques and requires incision of the retina (retinotomy), with an anatomic success rate on the order of 40 to 60 percent.[112–114] Novel methods employed to inhibit proliferative vitreoretinopathy include cytotoxic agents,[115–120] colchicine administration,[119, 121] and steroids,[122] but as yet there is no practical application of these in the management of proliferative vitreoretinopathy.

COMPLICATIONS (Table 98–2)

Intraoperative

Scleral perforation during placement of scleral sutures may lead to (1) perforation of the retina, (2) choroidal bleeding, or (3) premature release of subretinal fluid. If the retina is perforated, the site must be treated with cryotherapy and supported on the buckle, modifying the

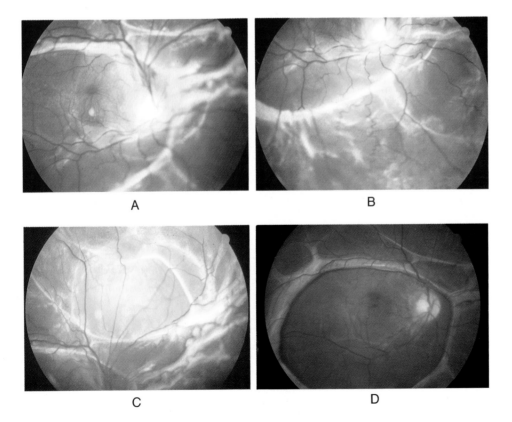

A

B

C

D

Figure 98–10. Retinal detachment with preoperative subretinal membranes. *A,* Preoperative appearance of rhegmatogenous detachment with peripheral retinal break in the right eye and extensive subretinal strands encircling the macula and extending to the periphery. *B,* Inferior view of the same eye displaying subretinal strands with overlying retinal vessels. *C,* Superior view of the same eye with similar subretinal strands. *D,* Postoperative photograph 2 mo after scleral buckle procedure (without vitrectomy or membrane manipulation) to close the retinal break; the macula has reattached despite residual tight folds caused by subretinal membranes.

Figure 98-11. Retinal detachment associated with proliferative vitreoretinopathy. *A*, Wide-angle photograph of right eye with total retinal detachment with prominent star fold temporally and numerous inferior folds. *B*, Preoperative photograph from another patient with total retinal detachment in the left eye with extensive retinal folds caused by preretinal membranes. Visual acuity is at the hand motions level. *C*, Postoperative photograph 3 mo after scleral buckle, vitrectomy, membrane removal, endodrainage, endolaser, and perfluoropropane gas tamponade. The nasal portion of an encircling buckle is seen, and the retina is reattached. *D*, Posterior pole of the same eye showing subretinal pigment fallout under the macula and the endolaser scar around the drainage retinotomy superior to the disc. Visual acuity is 20/50.

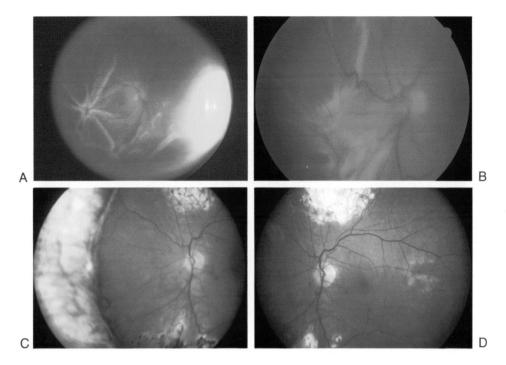

buckling element if necessary. Choroidal bleeding should be managed by increasing the intraocular pressure and possibly applying external pressure at the perforation site to retard the bleeding. It is essential to reposition the eye to elevate the fovea and inhibit migration of blood into the subfoveal space (Fig. 98-12*A*). If subretinal fluid is released prematurely by scleral perforation, hypotony may ensue, rendering additional suture placement difficult. In extreme hypotony, augmentation of intraocular volume with saline solution may be necessary so that the operation may be continued.

The most hazardous operative step is drainage of subretinal fluid. Drainage may result in multiple complications: retinal perforation, retinal incarceration, vitreous loss, vitreous hemorrhage, and choroidal hemorrhage. The first three are treated, in part, by scleral buckling, and the preference for placing the drainage site in the bed of the intended buckle is apparent. With an incarceration, it is usually not technically possible to release the retina. The visual prognosis may not be adversely affected if there are no folds involving the macula. Loss of vitreous during drainage may lead to vitreoretinal traction or subretinal vitreous deposition, preventing retinal reattachment.

As mentioned earlier, elevation of the intraocular pressure during buckling, if not recognized, may lead to retinal vascular occlusion, resulting in permanent ischemic damage.

Table 98-2. COMPLICATIONS OF SCLERAL BUCKLING SURGERY

Intraoperative Complications

Retinal perforation
Choroidal hemorrhage
Premature release of subretinal fluid
Vitreous loss
Vitreous hemorrhage
Retinal incarceration
Retinal vascular occlusion

Postoperative Complications

Angle-closure glaucoma
Anterior segment ischemia
Endophthalmitis
Cystoid macular edema
Epiretinal membrane
Choroidal detachment
Infection or extrusion of buckling element
Abnormal ocular alignment
Myopic shift
Proliferative vitreoretinopathy
Persistent or recurrent retinal detachment
Macular distortion caused by misplaced buckle
Lid abnormalities

Postoperative

Angle-closure glaucoma may result from a change in the orientation of the ciliary body resulting from choroidal effusion, particularly in association with a tight encircling buckle. Pupillary block is usually not present. The elevated intraocular pressure can usually be managed medically; rarely, it may be necessary to drain the choroidal fluid.

Anterior segment ischemia is typically manifested by corneal edema, fibrinous reaction in the aqueous, and elevated intraocular pressure. There is experimental evidence that anterior segment ischemia may be caused by obstruction of anterior or posterior ciliary arteries[50] or of venous drainage from the choroid.[123] Mild cases may be successfully managed with steroids; severe cases may require prompt loosening or removal of the buckling element.

Endophthalmitis is uncommon in this largely extra-

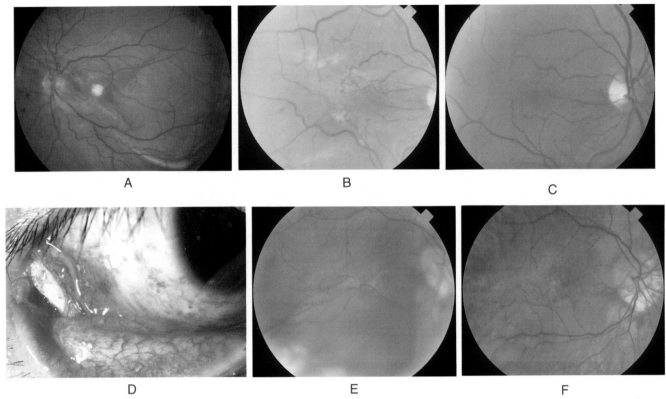

Figure 98–12. Complications of scleral buckling. *A,* Submacular hemorrhage after drainage of subretinal fluid; the visual acuity is 3/200, and the trail of blood from the temporal periphery is seen. *B,* Epiretinal membrane in the macula; visual acuity is 20/200. *C,* Same eye 9 mo after vitrectomy and membrane peeling; visual acuity is 20/40. *D,* Extrusion of scleral buckling element in the temporal aspect of the right eye. *E,* Macular distortion after scleral buckling for peripheral break with unintended macular indentation caused by misplaced inferotemporal radial element in the right eye; the retina is attached and visual acuity is 3/200. *F,* Postoperative appearance 3 mo after removal of the posterior aspect of the radial buckle; the macular distortion is relieved, and visual acuity is 20/70.

ocular surgery but has grave prognostic significance. Pain, anterior chamber reaction (especially hypopyon), and diminution or loss of the red reflex, all in rapid evolution, point to this diagnosis. Management will require vitreous biopsy, intravitreal antibiotics, and possibly vitrectomy.

Cystoid macular edema is a common transient finding following retinal detachment surgery. Most patients will not require treatment. In patients who do not recover with observation for 3 to 6 mo, topical or oral antiinflammatory medications, oral acetazolamide, and vitrectomy may be considered, based on the specific findings.

Epiretinal membrane in the macula (macular pucker) occurs in 8 to 17 percent of cases following surgery,[124, 125] but only the minority of cases require surgical removal of the membrane (Fig. 98–12*B* and *C*). Epiretinal membranes may be present preoperatively, and their occurrence is probably increased in cases with substantial vitreous hemorrhage, large breaks, or excessive retinopexy.

Choroidal detachment is common and usually remits without intervention. If there are compelling circumstances, such as angle-closure glaucoma or protracted contact between elevated choroid and retina from opposite sides of the globe, drainage may be necessary, with volume augmentation via paracentesis or intravitreal injection.

Infection or extrusion of the buckling element usually presents with hyperemia, chemosis, and possibly subconjunctival hemorrhage within the first few months following surgery (Fig. 98–12*D*). A few cases can be resolved by medical management alone—i.e., obtaining cultures and treating with topical and systemic antibiotics; however, most will require removal of the buckling element. Attempts to cover a sterile but exposed buckling element are usually unsuccessful because of epithelial ingrowth around the element, which prevents conjunctival closure.

Diplopia may occur in the early postoperative period, induced by alteration of the extraocular muscles or decompensation of a preexisting phoria. Most cases resolve spontaneously within a few months. Prisms may be given as a first resort for chronic cases. Rarely, surgical therapy is required and may include alteration or removal of the buckling element, as well as muscle surgery.

Many patients experience a change in the refractive error in the buckled eye. Most commonly, this change is a myopic shift of 1 to 2 Ds.[126] In particular, patients with attached maculas and excellent vision preoperatively need to be warned of refractive change with surgery, as they may be unduly concerned in the immediate postoperative period. Permanent refraction is usually performed 3 to 4 mo after surgery.

Persistent or recurrent retinal detachment is best understood in light of the goals of surgery, namely, identification and closure of all breaks, relief of vitreo-retinal traction, and elimination of subretinal fluid. If all breaks are observed to be closed on the scleral buckle, residual fluid may be left to resorb, and this process may take a variable time. Occasionally, a transient increase in subretinal fluid may occur in the early postoperative period because of exudation from the choroid, but observation over the subsequent several days will confirm subretinal fluid resorption. However, worrisome signs include a continued increase in the amount of subretinal fluid or the reopening of retinal breaks previously closed. If postoperative redetachment is due to a break that is not fully supported on the buckle, it may be sufficient to inject air or gas to close the break, followed by photocoagulation. This approach is difficult with inferior breaks for which modification of the buckle may be required. Late postoperative redetachment is usually due to new breaks or the development of proliferative vitreoretinopathy. Management typically includes revision of the scleral buckle or vitrectomy.

In addition to persistent retinal detachment, incorrect placement of the buckling appliance may lead to distortion of the macula (Fig. 98–12E and F), requiring revision of the buckle.

PROGNOSIS

The surgical outcome of retinal detachment surgery must be discussed in terms of two separate criteria: (1) complete reattachment of the retina, usually referred to as *anatomic success,* and (2) visual acuity, often called *functional success.* Overall, retinal detachment surgery is successful in reattaching the retina (i.e., anatomic success) in more than 90 percent of cases.

One subset of patients with retinal detachment achieves nearly 100 percent anatomic success after one operation. This includes patients with retinal dialysis;[127] round, atrophic holes associated with lattice degeneration;[128] and retinal detachments in which pigment demarcation lines are present.[129] Routine horseshoe-shaped flap-tears fare only slightly worse, anatomic success being achieved after the first surgical attempt in 90 to 95 percent of cases.[70, 128]

Aphakia and pseudophakia confer a moderate reduction in the rate of reattachment. Patients with anterior chamber IOLs have a lower probability of reattachment after one procedure (about 60 to 70 percent) than do patients with posterior chamber IOLs (>80 percent).[130, 131] Traditionally, aphakia has been associated with a significant reduction in anatomic success. In recent years, rates of 85 to 95 percent have been achieved.[77, 132]

Certain clinical phenomena are associated with a greatly reduced chance of success. Proliferative vitreoretinopathy is the most common such finding; the estimates of anatomic success in the presence of proliferative vitreoretinopathy vary from less than 50 percent to more than 75 percent,[107, 108, 110, 133, 135] although the success rate continues to improve. For giant breaks, in which success formerly was achieved in only about 50 percent of cases with one operation,[96, 101, 135] improved techniques

have led to greater success, with rates of reattachment as high as 90 percent.[94, 99, 136] Preoperative choroidal detachment has a very unfavorable impact on reattachment, with success in 50 percent of cases or less.[137, 138]

Even if the retina is fully reattached, restoration of visual acuity is not guaranteed. Most authors agree that *functional success* depends in part on preoperative visual acuity and patient age. The chances of restoring good vision decline with advancing age.[139, 140] In general, 85 to 90 percent of patients with preoperative acuity of 20/30 or better will achieve postoperative acuity of 20/30 or better.[70, 141, 142]

A major determinant of postoperative visual acuity is the status of the macula. Macular detachment of any duration, even 1 day, results in reduced postoperative acuity. For the first few weeks of macular detachment, recovery of vision does not seem to correlate with duration of detachment. However, after an interval of about 4 to 8 wk, an additional decrement in the odds of recovering good vision is noted.[140, 142, 143] Overall, 40 to 50 percent of patients with macular detachment achieve acuity of 20/50 or better postoperatively.[139, 140, 142, 143]

Friberg has noted that in macular detachments, visual acuity as measured by the potential acuity meter is an excellent predictor of postoperative acuity, perhaps more predictive than the duration of foveal detachment.[144]

CONCLUSIONS

When treating rhegmatogenous retinal detachment, the surgeon must keep in mind at all times that the principle objectives are to close the retinal break and to relieve all vitreoretinal traction. The surgeon must also ensure the removal of subretinal fluid, although in most cases in which the first two objectives are accomplished, subretinal fluid will spontaneously resolve. These lessons are illustrated in the historical development of retinal detachment repair, in which the ignipuncture technique of Gonin drew attention to the break itself, and scleral shortening revealed the value of scleral indenting for closing the break and relieving vitreoretinal traction. Even though some detachments could be treated successfully by methods such as ignipuncture and surface diathermy, it was the introduction of scleral buckling surgery in the 1950s and 1960s that raised the likelihood of a successful surgical outcome from less than 50 percent to 75 percent or more. The wide variety of techniques subsumed under the term *vitrectomy* have once again revolutionized the repair of retinal detachment, enabling retina surgeons to treat complicated detachments—as in giant retinal tears and proliferative vitreoretinopathy—with high rates of success.

REFERENCES

1. Beer GJ: Lehre von den Augenkrankheiten, als Leitfaden zu seinen offentlichen Vorlesungen entworfen, vol. 2. Vienna, Heubner & Volke, 1817, pp 495–498.
2. Duke-Elder S: Diseases of the Retina, System of Ophthalmology, vol. 10. St Louis, CV Mosby, 1967, p 816.
3. Helmholtz H: Beschreibung eines Augen-spiegels zur Untersu-

chung der Netzhaut im Lebenden Auge. Berlin, A Foerstner'sche Verlagsbuchhandlung, 1851.

4. Coccius A: Ueber die Anwendung des Augenspiegels nebst Angabe eines neuen Instruments. Leipzig, Immanuel Muller, 1853, p 125.

5. van Trigt AC: Der Augenspiegel; seine Anwendung und Modification. Lahr, Geiger, 1854.

6. Arlt F: Die Krankheiten des Auges, fuer praktische Aerzte, vol. 2. Prague, FA Credner, 1858–1859, pp 159–160.

7. von Graefe A: Notiz ueber die Abloesungen der Netzhaut von der Chorioidea. Albrecht v. Graefes Arch Ophthal 1:362–371, 1854.

8. Michels RG, Wilkinson CP, Rice, TA: Retinal Detachment. St Louis, CV Mosby, 1990, pp 248–251.

9. Schepens CL: Progress in detachment surgery. Trans Am Acad Ophthalmol Otolaryngol 55:607–615, 1951.

10. Leber T: Ueber die Entstehung der Netzhautabloesung. Ber Deutsch Ophth Gesellsch 35:120–124, 1908.

11. Gonin J: Le traitement du décollement rétinien. Ann d'oculist (Parel) 158:175–194, 1921.

12. Gonin J: The treatment of detached retina by searing the retinal tears. Arch Ophthalmol 4:621–625, 1930.

13. Guist G: Eine neue Ablatiooperation. Ztschr f Augenheilkd 74:232–242, 1931.

14. Lindner K: Ein Beitrag zur Entstehung und Behandlung der idiopathischen und der traumatischen Netzhautabhebung. Albrecht v. Graefes Arch Ophthal 127:177–295, 1931.

15. Michels RG, Wilkinson CP, Rice TA: Retinal Detachment. St Louis, CV Mosby, 1990, pp 261–262.

16. Safar K: Behandlung der Netzhautabhebung mit Elektroden fuer multiple diathermische Stichelung. Ber Deutsch Ophth Gesellsch 49:119–134, 1932.

17. Walker CB: Retinal detachment: Technical observations and new devices for treatment, with a specially arranged diathermy unit for general ophthalmic service. Am J Ophthalmol 17:1–17, 1934.

18. Weve H: Zur Behandlung der Netzhautabloesung mittels Diathermie. Abhandlungen aus der Augenheilkunde und ihren Grenzgebieten (Beihefte zur Zeitschrift fuer Augenheilkunde), vol. 14. Berlin, S Karger, 1932, p 9.

19. Pischell DK: Diathermy operation for retinal detachment: Comparative results of different types of electrodes. Trans Am Ophthalmol Soc 42:543–567, 1944.

20. Schepens CL, Okamura ID, Brockhurst RJ: The scleral buckling procedures. I. Surgical techniques and management. Arch Ophthalmol 58:797–811, 1957.

21. Bietti GB: Corioretiniti adhesive da crioapplicazioni episcleral. Acta XIV Conc Ophthalmol (Madrid), vol. 2, 1933, p 12.

22. Deutschmann R: Ueber zwei Verfahren bei Behandlung der Netzhautabloesung (eines davon der Diathermie scheinbar entgegengesetzt) nebst Bemerkungen zur Genese des Netzhautrisses und seines Verhaeltnisses zur Entstehung der Abloesung. Klin Monatsbl Augenheilkd 91:450–456, 1933.

23. Krwawicz T: Intracapsular extraction of intumescent cataract by application of low temperature. Br J Ophthalmol 45:279–283, 1961.

24. Lincoff HA, McLean JM, Nano H: Cryosurgical treatment of retinal detachment. Trans Am Acad Ophthalmol Otolaryngol 68:412–432, 1964.

25. Michels RG, Wilkinson CP, Rice TA: Retinal Detachment. St Louis, CV Mosby, 1990, pp 294–297.

26. Mueller L: Eine neue operative Behandlung der Netzhautabhebung. Klin Monatsbl Augenheilkd 41:459–462, 1903.

27. Shapland CD: Scleral resection—Lamellar. Trans Ophthalmol Soc UK 71:29–51, 1951.

28. Custodis E: Beobachtungen bei der diathermischen Behandlung der Netzhautabloesung und ein Hinweis zur Therapie der Amotio retinae. Ber Deutsch Ophth Gesellsch 57:227–230, 1951.

29. Custodis E: Bedeutet die Plombenaufnaehung auf die Sklera einen Fortschritt in der operativen Behandlung der Netzhautabloesung? Ber Deutsch Ophth Gesellsch 58:102–105, 1953.

30. Schepens CL, Okamura ID, Brockhurst RJ, Regan CDJ: The scleral buckling procedures. V. Synthetic sutures and silicone implants. Arch Ophthalmol 64:868–881, 1960.

31. Lincoff HA, Baras I, McLean J: Modifications to the Custodis

32. Ohm J: Ueber die Behandlung der Netzhautabloesung durch operative Entleerung der subretinalen Fluessigkeit and Einspritzung von Luft in der Glaskoerper. Albrecht v. Graefes Arch Ophthal 79:442–450, 1911.

33. Rosengren B: Ueber die Behandlung der Netzhautabloesung mittelst Diathermie und Luftinjektion in den Glaskoerper. Acta Ophthalmol 16:3–42, 1938.

34. Norton EWD, Aaberg T, Fung W, Curtin VT: Giant retinal tears. I. Clinical management with intravitreal air. Trans Am Ophthalmol Soc 67:374–393, 1969.

35. Kasner D: Vitrectomy: A new approach to management of vitreous. Highlights Ophthalmol 11:304–329, 1969.

36. Kasner D, Miller GR, Taylor WH, et al: Surgical treatment of amyloidosis of the retina. Trans Am Acad Ophthalmol Otolaryngol 72:410–418, 1968.

37. Machemer R, Parel JM, Buettner H: A new concept for vitreous surgery. I. Instrumentation. Am J Ophthalmol 73:1–7, 1972.

38. Parel JM, Machemer R, Aumayr W: A new concept for vitreous surgery. 4. Improvements in instrumentation and illumination. Am J Ophthalmol 77:6–12, 1974.

39. Michels RG, Wilkinson CP, Rice TA: Retinal Detachment. St Louis, CV Mosby, 1990, p 306.

40. Bill A: Blood circulation and fluid dynamics in the eye. Physiol Rev 55:383–417, 1975.

41. Orr G, Goodnight R, Lean JS: Relative permeability of retina and retinal pigment epithelium to the diffusion of tritiated water from vitreous to choroid. Arch Ophthalmol 104:1678–1680, 1986.

42. DeGuillebon H, Zauberman H: Experimental retinal detachment: Biophysical aspects of retinal peeling and stretching. Arch Ophthalmol 87:545–548, 1972.

43. Zimmerman LE, Eastham AB: Acid mucopolysaccharide in the retinal pigment epithelial and visual cell layer of the developing mouse eye. Am J Ophthalmol 47:488–499, 1959.

44. Kain HL: A new model for examining chorioretinal adhesion experimentally. Arch Ophthalmol 102:608–611, 1984.

45. Zauberman H, deGuillebon H: Retinal traction in vivo and postmortem. Arch Ophthalmol 87:549–554, 1972.

46. Burnside B, Laties AM: Actin filaments in apical projections of the primate pigmented epithelial cell. Invest Ophthalmol Vis Sci 15:570–575, 1976.

47. Amsler M, Dubois H: Topographie ophtalmoscopique et décollement rétinien. Ann d'Oculist (Paris) 165:667–675, 1928.

48. Goldman L, Caldera DL, Nussbaum SR, et al: Multifactorial index of cardiac risk in noncardiac surgical procedures. N Engl J Med 297:845–850, 1977.

49. Mein CE, Woodcock MG: Local anesthesia for vitreoretinal surgery. Retina 10:47–49, 1990.

50. Freeman HM, Hawkins WR, Schepens CL: Anterior segment necrosis: An experimental study. Arch Ophthalmol 75:644–650, 1966.

51. Schwartz A, Rathbun E: Scleral strength impairment and recovery after diathermy. Arch Ophthalmol 93:1173–1177, 1975.

52. Campochiaro PA, Kaden IH, Vidaurri-Leal J, Glaser BM: Cryotherapy enhances intravitreal dispersion of viable retinal pigment epithelial cells. Arch Ophthalmol 103:434–436, 1985.

53. Hilton GF: Subretinal pigment migration: Effects of cryosurgical retinal reattachment. Arch Ophthalmol 91:445–450, 1974.

54. O'Connor PR: Cryosurgical probing of retinal tears. Am J Ophthalmol 78:411–414, 1974.

55. Benson WE: Retinal Detachment. Diagnosis and Management. Philadelphia, JB Lippincott, 1988, pp 121–124.

56. Benson WE: Retinal Detachment. Diagnosis and Management. Philadelphia, JB Lippincott, 1988, p 146.

57. Dominquez DA: Cirugia precoz y ambulatoria del desprendimiento de retina. Arch Soc Esp Oftal 48:47–54, 1985.

58. Hilton GF, Grizzard WS: Pneumatic retinopexy: A two-step outpatient operation without conjunctival incision. Ophthalmology 93:626–641, 1986.

59. Kreissig I: Bisherige Erfahrungen mit SF$_6$-Gas in der Ablatio-Chirurgie. Ber Deutsch Ophth Gesellsch 76:553–560, 1979.

60. Lincoff A, Haft D, Liggett P, Reifer C: Intravitreal expansion of perflourocarbon bubbles. Arch Ophthalmol 98:1646, 1980.

61. Lincoff H, Coleman J, Kreissig I, et al: The perfluorocarbon

procedure for retinal detachment. Arch Ophthalmol 73:160–163, 1965.

gases in the treatment of retinal detachment. Ophthalmology 90:546–551, 1983.
62. Abrams GW, Edelhauser HF, Aaberg TM, Hamilton LH: Dynamics of intravitreal sulfur hexafluoride gas. Invest Ophthalmol Vis Sci 13:863, 1974.
63. Peters MA, Abrams GW, Hamilton LH, et al: The nonexpansile, equilibrated concentration of perfluoropropane gas in the eye. Am J Ophthalmol 100:831–839, 1985.
64. Hilton GF, Kelly NE, Salzano TC, et al: Pneumatic retinopexy: A collaborative report of the first 100 cases. Ophthalmology 94:307–314, 1987.
65. Tornambe PE, Hilton GF, Kelly NF, et al: Expanded indications for pneumatic retinopexy. Ophthalmology 95:597–600, 1988.
66. Tornambe PE, Hilton GF, The Retinal Detachment Study Group: Pneumatic retinopexy: A multicenter randomized controlled clinical trial comparing pneumatic retinopexy with scleral buckling. Ophthalmology 96:772–784, 1989.
67. Algvere P, Hallnas K, Palmqvist B-M: Success and complications of pneumatic retinopexy. Am J Ophthalmol 106:400–404, 1988.
68. Chen JC, Robertson JE, Coonan P, et al: Results and complications of pneumatic retinopexy. Ophthalmology 95:601–608, 1988.
69. McAllister IL, Meyers SM, Zegarra H, et al: Comparison of pneumatic retinopexy with alternative surgical techniques. Ophthalmology 95:877–883, 1988.
70. Hilton GF, McLean EB, Chuang EL: Retinal Detachment. San Francisco, American Academy of Ophthalmology, 1989, pp 155–159.
71. McPherson AR: Discussion of Hilton GF, Kelly NE, Salzano TC, et al: Pneumatic retinopexy: A collaborative report of the first 100 cases. Ophthalmology 94:312–314, 1987.
72. Lincoff H, Kreissig I, Hahn YS: A temporary balloon buckle for the treatment of small retinal detachments. Ophthalmology 86:586–592, 1979.
73. Lincoff H, Kreissig I: Results with a temporary balloon buckle for the repair of retinal detachment. Am J Ophthalmol 92:245–251, 1981.
74. Lincoff H, Kreissig I, Farber M: Results of 100 aphakic detachments treated with a temporary balloon buckle: A case against routine encircling operations. Br J Ophthalmol 69:798–804, 1985.
75. Schoch LH, Olk RJ, Arribas NP, et al: The Lincoff temporary balloon buckle. Am J Ophthalmol 101:646–649, 1986.
76. Griffith RD, Ryan EA, Hilton GF: Primary retinal detachments without apparent breaks. Am J Ophthalmol 81:420–427, 1976.
77. Norton EWD: Retinal detachment in aphakia. Trans Am Ophthalmol Soc 61:770–789, 1963.
78. Lincoff H, Gieser R: Finding the retinal hole. Arch Ophthalmol 85:565–569, 1971.
79. Wong D, Billington BM, Chignell AH: Pars plana vitrectomy for retinal detachment with unseen retinal holes. Graefes Arch Clin Exp Ophthalmol 225:269–271, 1987.
80. Margherio RR, Schepens CL: Macular breaks. 1. Diagnosis, etiology, and observations. Am J Ophthalmol 74:219–232, 1972.
81. Kloeti R: Eine Operationsmethode fuer maculalochbedingte Netzhautabloesungen. Ophthalmologica 148:42–56, 1964.
82. Kloeti R: Silver clip for central retinal detachments with macular hole. Mod Probl Ophthalmol 12:330–336, 1974.
83. Theodossiadis GP: Treatment of retinal detachment due to macular holes without chorioretinal lesions. A seven-year follow-up study. Trans Ophthalmol Soc UK 102:198–202, 1982.
84. Gonvers M, Machemer R: A new approach to treating retinal detachment with macular hole. Am J Ophthalmol 94:468–472, 1982.
85. Kreissig I, Stanowsky A, Lincoff H, Richard G: The treatment of difficult retinal detachments with an expanding gas bubble without vitrectomy. Graefes Arch Clin Exp Ophthalmol 224:51–54, 1986.
86. Lincoff H, Kreissig I, Brodie S, Wilcox L: Expanding gas bubbles for the repair of tears in the posterior pole. Graefes Arch Clin Exp Ophthalmol 219:193–197, 1982.
87. Kuriyama S, Matsumura M, Harada T, et al: Surgical techniques and reattachment rates in retinal detachment due to macular hole. Arch Ophthalmol 108:1559–1561, 1990.
88. Menchini U, Scialdone A, Visconti C, Brancato R: Pneumoretinopexy in the treatment of retinal detachment with macular hole. Int Ophthalmol 12:213–215, 1988.

89. Rashed O, Sheta S: Evaluation of the functional results after different techniques for treatment of retinal detachment due to macular holes. Graefes Arch Clin Exp Ophthalmol 227:508–512, 1989.
90. Blodi CF, Folk JC: Treatment of macular hole retinal detachments with intravitreal gas. Am J Ophthalmol 98:811, 1984.
91. Miyake Y: A simplified method of treating retinal detachment with macular hole. Arch Ophthalmol 104:1234–1236, 1986.
92. Blankenship GW, Ibanez-Langlois S: Treatment of myopic macular hole and detachment: Intravitreal gas exchange. Ophthalmology 94:333–336, 1987.
93. Garcia-Arumi J, Correa CA, Corcostegui B: Comparative study of different techniques of intraocular gas tamponade in the treatment of retinal detachment due to macular hole. Ophthalmologica 201:83–91, 1990.
94. Michels RG, Rice TA, Blankenship G: Surgical techniques for selected giant retinal tears. Retina 3:139–153, 1983.
95. Machemer R: Proliferative vitreoretinopathy (PVR): A personal account of its pathogenesis and treatment. Proctor Lecture. Invest Ophthalmol Vis Sci 29:1771–1783, 1988.
96. Machemer R, Allen AW: Retinal tears 180° and greater. Arch Ophthalmol 94:1340–1346, 1976.
97. Abrams GW, Williams GA, Neuwirth J, McDonald HR: Clinical results of titanium retinal tacks with pneumatic insertion. Am J Ophthalmol 102:13–19, 1986.
98. DeJuan E Jr, McCuen BW, Machemer R: Mechanical retinal fixation using tacks. Ophthalmology 94:337–340, 1987.
99. Chang S, Lincoff H, Zimmerman NJ, Fuchs W: Giant retinal tears: Surgical techniques and results using perfluorocarbon liquids. Arch Ophthalmol 107:761–766, 1989.
100. Schepens CL, Freeman HM: Current management of giant retinal breaks. Trans Am Acad Ophthalmol Otolaryngol 71:474–487, 1967.
101. Kanski JJ: Giant retinal tears. Am J Ophthalmol 79:846–852, 1975.
102. Michels RG: Surgery of retinal detachment with proliferative vitreoretinopathy. Retina 4:63–83, 1984.
103. Cowley M, Conway BP, Campochiaro PA, et al: Clinical risk factors for proliferative vitreoretinopathy. Arch Ophthalmol 107:1147–1151, 1989.
104. Bonnet M: Clinical factors predisposing to massive proliferative vitreoretinopathy in rhegmatogenous retinal detachment. Ophthalmologica 188:148–152, 1984.
105. Bonnet M: The development of severe proliferative vitreoretinopathy after retinal detachment surgery. Grade B: A determining risk factor. Graefes Arch Clin Exp Ophthalmol 226:201–205, 1988.
106. Ho PC, Yoshida A, Schepens CL, et al: Severe proliferative vitreoretinopathy and retinal detachment. 1. Initial clinical findings. Ophthalmology 91:1531–1537, 1984.
107. Fisher YL, Shakin JL, Slakter JS, et al: Perfluoropropane gas, modified panretinal photocoagulation, and vitrectomy in the management of severe proliferative vitreoretinopathy. Arch Ophthalmol 106:1255–1260, 1988.
108. Lewis H, Aaberg TM, Abrams GW: Causes of failure after initial vitreoretinal surgery for severe proliferative vitreoretinopathy. Am J Ophthalmol 111:8–14, 1991.
109. Lewis H, Aaberg TM: Causes of failure after repeat vitreoretinal surgery for recurrent proliferative vitreoretinopathy. Am J Ophthalmol 111:15–19, 1991.
110. Aaberg TM: Management of anterior and posterior vitreoretinopathy. XLV Edward Jackson Memorial Lecture. Am J Ophthalmol 106:519–532, 1988.
111. Hanneken AM, Michels RG: Vitrectomy and scleral buckling methods for proliferative vitreoretinopathy. Ophthalmology 95:865–869, 1988.
112. Han DP, Lewis MT, Kuhn EM, et al: Relaxing retinotomies and retinectomies: Surgical results and predictors of visual outcome. Arch Ophthalmol 108:694–697, 1990.
113. Iverson DA, Ward TG, Blumenkranz MS: Indications and results of relaxing retinotomy. Ophthalmology 97:1298–1304, 1990.
114. Machemer R, McCuen BW, deJuan E Jr: Relaxing retinotomies and retinectomies. Am J Ophthalmol 102:7–12, 1986.
115. Blumenkranz MS, Ophir A, Claflin AJ, Hajek A: Fluorouracil for the treatment of massive periretinal proliferation. Am J Ophthalmol 94:458–467, 1982.

116. Blumenkranz M, Hernandez E, Ophir A, Norton EWD: 5-Fluorouracil: New applications in complicated retinal detachment for an established antimetabolite. Ophthalmology 91:122–130, 1984.
117. Kirmani M, Santana M, Sorgente N, et al: Antiproliferative drugs in the treatment of experimental proliferative vitreoretinopathy: Control by daunomycin. Retina 3:269–272, 1983.
118. Stern WH, Lewis GP, Erickson PA, et al: Fluorouracil therapy for proliferative vitreoretinopathy after vitrectomy. Am J Ophthalmol 96:33–42, 1983.
119. Verdoorn C, de Lavalette VWR, Dalma-Weizhausz J, et al: Cellular migration, proliferation, and contraction: An in vitro approach to a clinical problem—Proliferative vitreoretinopathy. Arch Ophthalmol 104:1216–1219, 1986.
120. Wiedemann P, Lemmen K, Schmiedl R, Heimann K: Intraocular daunorubicin for the treatment and prophylaxis of traumatic proliferative vitreoretinopathy. Am J Ophthalmol 104:10–14, 1987.
121. Lemor M, deBustros S, Glaser BM: Low-dose colchicine inhibits astrocyte, fibroblast, and retinal pigment epithelial cell migration and proliferation. Arch Ophthalmol 104:1223–1225, 1986.
122. Chandler DB, Hida T, Sheta S, et al: Improvement in efficacy of corticosteroid therapy in an animal model of proliferative vitreoretinopathy by pretreatment. Graefes Arch Clin Exp Ophthalmol 225:259–265, 1987.
123. Hayreh SS, Baines JAB: Occlusion of the vortex veins: An experimental study. Br J Ophthalmol 57:217–238, 1973.
124. Lobes LA Jr, Burton TC: The incidence of macular pucker after retinal detachment surgery. Am J Ophthalmol 85:72–77, 1978.
125. Meredith TA, Reeser FH, Topping TM, Aaberg TA: Cystoid macular edema after retinal detachment surgery. Ophthalmology 87:1090–1095, 1980.
126. Rubin ML: The induction of refractive errors by retinal detachment surgery. Trans Am Ophthalmol Soc 73:452–490, 1975.
127. Hagler WS, North AW: Retinal dialyses and retinal detachment. Arch Ophthalmol 79:376–388, 1968.
128. Benson WE, Morse PH: The prognosis of retinal detachment due to lattice degeneration. Ann Ophthalmol 10:1197–1200, 1978.
129. Benson WE, Nantawan P, Morse PH: Characteristics and prognosis of retinal detachments with demarcation lines. Am J Ophthalmol 84:641–644, 1977.
130. Ho PC, Tolentino FI: Pseudophakic retinal detachment: Surgical success rate with various types of IOLs. Ophthalmology 91:847–852, 1984.
131. Cousins S, Boniuk I, Okun E, et al: Pseudophakic retinal detachments in the presence of various IOL types. Ophthalmology 93:1198–1208, 1986.
132. O'Connor PR: External buckling without drainage for selected detachments in aphakic eyes. Am J Ophthalmol 82:358–364, 1976.
133. De Bustros S, Michels R: Surgical treatment of retinal detachments complicated by proliferative vitreoretinopathy. Am J Ophthalmol 98:694–699, 1984.
134. Sternberg P Jr, Machemer R: Results of conventional vitreous surgery for proliferative vitreoretinopathy. Am J Ophthalmol 100:141–146, 1985.
135. Freeman HM, Schepens CL, Couvillion GC: Current management of giant retinal breaks. Part II. Trans Am Acad Ophthalmol Otolaryngol 74:59–74, 1970.
136. Vidaurri-Leal J, de Bustros S, Michels RG: Surgical treatment of giant retinal tears with inverted posterior retinal flaps. Am J Ophthalmol 98:463–466, 1984.
137. Gottlieb F: Combined choroidal and retinal detachment. Arch Ophthalmol 88:481–486, 1972.
138. Seelenfreund MH, Kraushar MF, Schepens CL, Freilich DB: Choroidal detachment associated with primary retinal detachment. Arch Ophthalmol 91:254–258, 1974.
139. Tani P, Robertson DM, Langworthy A: Prognosis for central vision and anatomic reattachment in rhegmatogenous retinal detachment with macula detached. Am J Ophthalmol 92:611–620, 1981.
140. McPherson AR, O'Malley RE, Butner RW, Beltangady SS: Visual acuity after surgery for retinal detachment with macular involvement. Ann Ophthalmol 14:639–645, 1982.
141. Burton TC: Recovery of visual acuity after retinal detachment involving the macula. Trans Am Ophthalmol Soc 80:475–497, 1982.
142. Grupposo SS: Visual acuity following surgery for retinal detachment. Arch Ophthalmol 93:327–330, 1975.
143. Davidorf FH, Havener WH, Lang JR: Macular vision following retinal detachment surgery. Ophthalmic Surg 6(4):74–81, 1975.
144. Friberg TR, Eller AW: Prediction of visual recovery following scleral buckling of macula–off retinal detachments. Am J Ophthalmol 114:715–722, 1992.
145. Meyer-Schwickerath G: Light Coagulation. St Louis, CV Mosby, 1960, pp 17–20.

Chapter 99

■

Proliferative Vitreoretinopathy

JOHN S. LEAN

DEFINITION

Proliferative vitreoretinopathy (PVR) is defined as the growth and contraction of cellular membranes within the vitreous cavity and on both surfaces of the retina following rhegmatogenous retinal detachment.[1] This process is extremely important, as these membranes exert traction and may cause recurrent detachment by reopening otherwise successfully treated retinal breaks, create new retinal breaks, and distort or obscure the macula. PVR is the primary cause of visual failure following surgical therapy for rhegmatogenous retinal detachment.

PATHOBIOLOGY

Origin of PVR Membranes

Membranes occurring in PVR (PVR membranes) are composed of cells originating from the retinal glia[2] and retinal pigment epithelium (RPE), inflammatory macrophages, and collagen.[3] Continued dispersal and proliferation of RPE cells from the exposed pigment epithelium, combined with glial cell proliferation, ultimately results in a contracted collagenous membrane that covers both surfaces of the retina and the exposed vitreous matrix and produces the characteristic funnel-shaped retinal detachment of advanced PVR.

Glial Cell Component

The glial component comprises extensions of Müller cells and astrocytes[4] that form membranes on both surfaces of the retina. These membranes originate directly from the sustentacular glia and develop as a result of damage to the retinal surface;[5] they are also stimulated by platelet-derived growth factor (PDGF)[6] and proliferating RPE cells.[7, 8] PDGF is released by platelet aggregation in blood clots.[9]

RPE Cell Component

RPE cells are dispersed by three mechanisms into the vitreous cavity following retinal detachment:

1. During initial retinal tear formation, some RPE cells remain adherent to the retina and are avulsed from the pigment epithelium.[3]
2. After retinal separation, some RPE cells elongate in a vertical direction and are eventually "pinched off" of Bruch's membrane and form motile RPE macrophages.[10]
3. RPE cells are released by cryotherapy and scleral depression during the course of surgery for retinal detachment repair.[11]

RPE cells occur as three cell types in periretinal and vitreal membranes:[3] (1) pigment epithelial macrophages that form clumps rather than membranes but that may stimulate membrane formation,[12] (2) RPE cells with retained epithelial morphologic characteristics, and (3) RPE cells that have undergone epithelial-mesenchymal transformation into fibroblast-like cells. This transformation occurs in vivo when isolated RPE cells are not in contact with Bruch's membrane or when they are exposed to intravitreal fluid.[13] A similar transformation occurs in vitro when RPE cells are exposed to vitreous collagen[14] or fibrin.[15]

Macrophage Component

Macrophages in periretinal membranes[16] are derived from circulating blood monocytes that enter the vitreous from ciliary,[17] retinal,[10] and choroidal[18] circulation and from free RPE cells that transform into macrophage-like cells.[9]

Collagen Component

The stroma of PVR membranes is composed mainly of types I, II, and III collagen.[19] Type II collagen is a major component of normal vitreous, but RPE cells in vitro are also capable of synthesizing this type of collagen.[20] Therefore, its presence in PVR membranes may result from the development of membranes in areas of residual vitreous attachment or may represent newly secreted material. Types I and III collagen are not found in the normal retina or vitreous and therefore are presumably synthesized by cells within the membranes.

Glial cells are capable of synthesizing type I collagen,[21] and RPE cells in culture can synthesize both type I and type III collagen.[20]

Stimuli for Growth of PVR Membranes

Conditioned media from RPE cell cultures[22] and glial cell cultures,[23] and vitreous macrophages,[24] bovine retinal extracts,[25] and human subretinal fluid from chronic retinal detachment[26] all stimulate RPE proliferation in vitro. It is probable that local cellular production of growth factors is responsible for these mitogenic effects. The evidence for growth control by local autocrine or paracrine mechanisms is well established in analogous biologic systems such as wound healing, in which, e.g., PDGF is synthesized by fibroblasts and then leads to their further proliferation.[27] With relevance to PVR, it has been shown that (1) PDGF-like proteins[28] are present in the conditioned media of RPE cells and are released by activated macrophages;[12] (2) RPE cells in culture produce transforming growth factor-β (TGF-β),[29] and vitreous aspirates from eyes with PVR have more than three times the amount of TGF-β found in eyes with uncomplicated retinal detachment.[30] TGF-β has multiple actions, including stimulation of fibrosis in wound healing[31] and synthesis of collagen and fibronectin by RPE cells.[32] The synthesis of growth factors by the cellular component of PVR membranes may explain the characteristic tendency of this disease to gather momentum once initiated and to recur after surgical intervention. However, the contribution of growth factors to the proliferation of cells in PVR is complex because the response of cells to growth factors is not necessarily growth but depends on a variety of other factors, such as the underlying matrix, contact with other cells, the presence of other growth factors, and the presence of specific receptors.[33]

Although breakdown of the blood-ocular barrier (e.g., by cryotherapy) causes stimulation of cell proliferation,[34] it is unlikely that this is the source of growth factors because the concentration in plasma is either very low or nonexistent. For example, PDGF stimulates proliferation of RPE cells,[35] but its plasma level is approximately 1 ng/ml, less than that required to evoke proliferation. Presumably, disruption of the blood-ocular barrier is a general stimulus that evokes cellular production of growth factors.

Mechanism of Contraction in PVR

Transformed, fibroblast-like RPE cells are characteristically motile and move by extending lamellipodia covered with coated pits, which adhere to surrounding surfaces and then retract.[36] In vitreous, this cycle of extension and retraction leads to the gathering up of collagen fibers in the vicinity of the cell and thus to progressive contraction of the gel.[37] The ability of RPE cells to "reel in" collagen fibers in this way is prodigious, with as much as 5 mm of fiber accumulating beneath a single cell in a 24-hr period. It is for this reason that vitreous contraction can be severe, despite its relative hypocellularity.[38] On the surface of the retina on which RPE cells are entrapped in areas of residual vitreous, or when they encounter collagen produced by other RPE or glial cells, a similar process may produce contraction of the retina, although these membranes, at least initially, are generally more cellular.[39] In contrast, glial cells are only weakly contractile.[12] However, these cells create strong attachment points for RPE cells in PVR membranes and transmit contractile forces generated by the RPE component to the underlying retina.[40]

The generation of contraction by RPE cells depends on the presence of fibronectin (an extracellular matrix protein that mediates the adhesion of cells to one another and to structural proteins such as collagen)[41] and does not occur in serum-free media or in the presence of a peptide that specifically blocks cell binding to fibronectin.[42] A high concentration of fibronectin is typically found in the vitreous of eyes with PVR.[43] It is derived mainly from serum and results from cryotherapy[44] and associated breakdown of the blood-retinal barrier,[45] but RPE cells in culture also produce fibronectin,[20] and this additional source may further increase their ability to generate traction.[46] The amount of fibronectin within periretinal membranes may also have surgical consequences: Early membranes contain large amounts of fibronectin and are correspondingly difficult to peel from the retinal surface; later membranes, however, have much less fibronectin, and this coincides with their easier surgical removal.[47] Fibronectin also directly stimulates RPE motility.[48] Since, as we have previously noted, contraction is a result of cell movement, fibronectin therefore both facilitates and provokes contraction in PVR. PDGF also stimulates RPE motility and contraction,[49] and PVR occurs more frequently when retinal detachment is complicated by vitreous hemorrhage.[50, 51] Finally, activated macrophages produce fibronectin and interleukin-1,[12] which is found in the subretinal fluid of eyes with PVR[52] and stimulates the migration of RPE cells.[53]

CLINICAL DIAGNOSIS AND CLASSIFICATION

The widely used classification of PVR published by the Retina Society[1] has been revised.[54] The major changes are separate description and grading of PVR membranes in the anterior and posterior retina and elimination of the width of the retinal funnel as a component of the classification. The revised system of diagnosis and classification is further described in the remainder of this section (Table 99-1).

In the earliest manifestation of PVR, clumps of RPE cells and a protein flare are present in the vitreous (grade A). This is followed by the development of PVR membranes, which are initially almost transparent but cause distortion of the retina (grade B). These membranes subsequently become opaque and produce sev-

Table 99–1. CLASSIFICATION OF PROLIFERATIVE VITREORETINOPATHY (PVR)*

Grade	Type of Contraction	Location of PVR†	Summary of Clinical Signs
A	—	—	RPE clumps in vitreous and on retina, protein flare
B	—	—	Surface wrinkling, rolled edge of tears, vascular tortuosity
C			Full-thickness retinal folds
	1	Posterior	Star fold
	2	Posterior	Confluent irregular folds in posterior retina; remainder of retina drawn posteriorly; optic disc may not be visible
	3	Posterior	Subretinal "napkin ring" or irregular elevation of retina
	4	Anterior	Irregular folds in anterior retina; series of radial folds more posteriorly; irregular circumferential retinal fold in coronal plane
	5	Anterior	Smooth circumferential retinal fold in coronal plane
	6	Anterior	Circumferential fold of retina at insertion of posterior hyaloid pulled forward; trough of peripheral retina; ciliary processes under traction with possible hypotony; iris may be retracted

*Modified from The Retina Society Terminology Committee: The classification of retinal detachment with proliferative vitreoretinopathy. Ophthalmology 90:121–25, 1983; and Lean JS, Stern WH, Irvine AR, et al: Classification of proliferative vitreoretinopathy used in the silicone study. Ophthalmology 96:765–71, 1989.
†Anterior or posterior to retina equator.

eral characteristic patterns of contraction (grade C), in either the posterior or the anterior retina. In the posterior retina, defined as posterior to the retinal equator, these patterns of contraction consist of (1) star fold, which represents the contraction of a single focus of PVR (type 1) (see Fig. 99–1A); (2) irregular fixed folds, indicating multiple epicenters of contraction (type 2) (Fig. 99–1B); or (3) an elevated fold without visible preretinal membrane—either an annulus around the disc ("napkin ring") or an extended linear fold ("washing line") (type 3) (Fig. 99–1C). In the anterior retina, the patterns of contraction consist of (4) a series of radial folds at the insertion of the posterior hyaloid—contraction in a circumferential direction creates an irregular equatorial fold (type 4) (Fig. 99–1D); (5) contraction of the posterior hyaloid creating a smooth circumferential equatorial fold (type 5) (Fig. 99–1E); and (6) anterior displacement of the peripheral retina as the result of PVR occurring on the surface of the residual basal

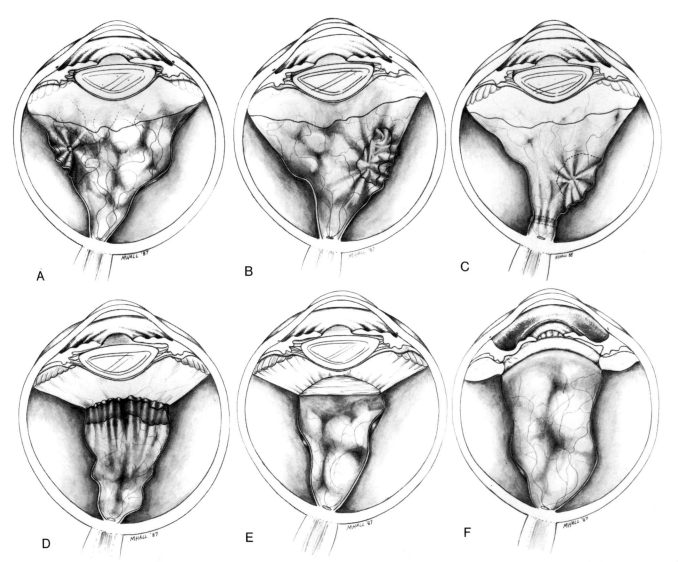

Figure 99–1. Types of grade C proliferative vitreoretinopathy (PVR) (see text). *A,* Type 1. Regular folds radiate ("star fold") from a focal area of PVR; traction is exerted centripetally toward the area of PVR. *B,* Type 2. Irregular folds are present in the posterior retina. The retina is contracted in an anteroposterior direction, which flattens its normally bullous convex curvature, and in a circumferential direction, which creates a series of radial folds in the anterior retina. Traction is exerted on the remainder of the retina, pulling it in both a posterior direction and a circumferential direction. Traction in a perpendicular direction pulls the retina toward the center of the vitreous cavity, narrowing the funnel of retinal detachment over the optic disc. *C,* Type 3. Subretinal membrane creates an annular constriction around the disc ("napkin ring") or irregular folds more anteriorly. In the napkin ring configuration, traction in a circumferential direction gathers the posterior retina together anterior to the optic disc. With irregular folds, traction is mainly perpendicular to the retinal surface, elevating the retina toward the center of the vitreous cavity. *D,* Type 4. Irregular folds are present in the retina immediately behind the vitreous base, and the adjacent posterior hyaloid is contracted. Contraction of the retina in a circumferential direction causes radial folds posterior to the area of PVR. The anterior retina within the vitreous base is stretched inward to form a fold in the coronal plane because circumferential contraction exerted along the concavity of the retina produces a secondary traction vector perpendicular to the retinal surface, toward the center of the vitreous cavity. *E,* Type 5. The posterior hyaloid is contracted. The anterior retina is pulled in a perpendicular direction toward the center of the vitreous cavity. Radial folds are also formed as a result of contraction in a circumferential direction. *F,* Type 6. The anterior retina is pulled forward as a result of contraction in an anteroposterior direction of the posterior hyaloid, the anterior hyaloid, and the vitreous base that remain after vitrectomy. The underlying retina forms a trough within the vitreous base.

vitreous remaining after vitrectomy. The basal vitreous is contracted in an anteroposterior direction. Since the anterior portion of the vitreous base is anchored to the pars plana, the peripheral retina is pulled forward, forming a trough in the extreme retinal periphery (type 6) (Fig. 99–1*F*).

PVR, grades B and C, are further illustrated in Figure 99–2.

SURGICAL MANAGEMENT

Cases of PVR can be divided into those in which surgery can be expected to result in the sustained closure of all retinal breaks and those in which recurrent traction can be anticipated to cause postoperative rhegmatogenous detachment despite operative closure of all breaks. The features that distinguish these two groups of cases

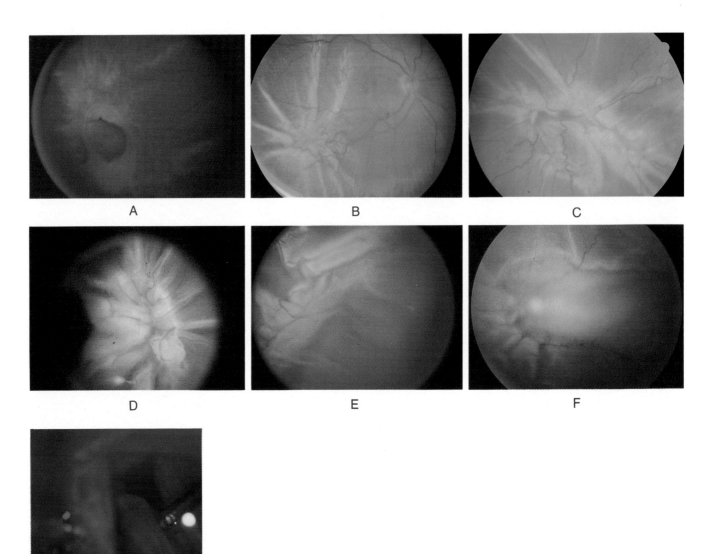

A

B

C

D

E

F

G

Figure 99–2. Photographic illustration of types of PVR. *A*, Grade B. The posterior lip of a large tear is rolled inward by PVR localized at its edge. *B*, Grade C, type 1. A single epicenter of PVR creates a star fold in the posterior retina. *C*, Grade C, type 2. Diffuse PVR in the posterior retina. *D*, Grade C, type 3. Subretinal PVR closes the funnel of retinal detachment anterior to the disc. *E*, Grade C, type 4. PVR at the retinal equator produces a circumferential fold immediately behind the insertion of the posterior hyaloid (left side of photograph); peripheral retina within the vitreous base is stretched inward (right side of photograph). *F*, Grade C, type 5. Contraction of the posterior hyaloid (located more posteriorly than usual in this case, as indicated by the line of pigment immediately behind its insertion inferiorly) creates a circumferential fold in the coronal plane. *G*, Grade C, type 6. An operative photography showing a trough of retina anteriorly (immediately to the left of the vitrectomy probe), covered by an opaque PVR membrane.

are not well understood. However, eyes with mild PVR, a single or adjacent group of breaks, or predominantly posterior PVR usually fall into the first category; eyes with severe PVR, multiple breaks, and extensive vitreous base contraction are more likely to be in the second category.

Selection of Surgical Procedure

The following case examples are given to illustrate the general principles involved in selecting the appropriate surgical procedure for retinal detachment complicated by PVR. A detailed description of these procedures is beyond the scope of this chapter.

CASE 1

The retinal detachment in this case (Fig. 99–3A) is due to a single large horseshoe tear with a rolled posterior edge (grade B PVR; see Table 99–1) in the lower temporal quadrant. A focus of PVR in the posterior retina produces a star fold (grade C, type 1) and exerts traction on the tear. An area of more remote PVR, which is not affecting the tear, is present for 2 clock hours of the retinal circumference at and immediately behind the insertion of the posterior hyaloid (grade C, type 4).

Such a detachment is treated by buckling the tear using a radial element and by draining subretinal fluid to approximate the tear to the buckle. Removal of the star fold is generally not necessary because the radial buckle reverses traction vectors exerted on the tear and compresses it onto the buckle.[55] It would also be prudent to encircle the eye, for two reasons. The star fold will continue to exert traction on the break, and with time the height of an unsupported buckle can decrease. Under these circumstances, the traction exerted on the break might overcome the tensile strength of the chorioretinal reaction around it and the break might reopen. Supporting the break with an encircling band will prevent this. A second reason for encircling the eye is that the area of PVR adjacent to the insertion of the posterior hyaloid will create a shallow traction detachment. The retina will eventually

become atrophic in this area and the combination of persistent traction and attenuated retina may eventually create a break, with resultant recurrent detachment. Encirclement relieves this traction vector and allows the retina to remain attached and thus preempts the sequence of events just described. The postoperative result is shown in Figure 99–3B–D.

CASE 2

The retinal detachment in this case is illustrated in Figure 99–4A. Three horseshoe tears are present approximately 1 clock hour apart in the lower temporal quadrant. The eye has been treated previously by vitrectomy and the tears have occurred as a result of traction on the posterior hyaloid by residual vitreous incarcerated in the adjacent sclerotomy.[56] PVR has also occurred on the residual vitreous matrix adjacent to the tears, creating localized anterior loop traction (grade C, type 6). The combination of mechanical incarceration of residual hyaloid in the adjacent sclerotomy and localized PVR has led to gross elevation of the tears from the RPE.

It might be possible to treat this detachment simply by buckling the tears using a segmental explant supported by an encircling strap (the strap is needed for the same reasons as in Case 1). This treatment may fail, however, because persistent traction on the breaks causes redetachment of the anterior portion of the breaks, leading to an "end run" of fluid, similar to that occurring when a buckle is placed too posteriorly. A better approach would be to combine buckling with the direct removal of traction, using vitrectomy, visualizing the anterior dissection by means of coaxial illumination and deep scleral indentation.[57] The postoperative result is depicted in Figure 99–4B.

CASE 3

The retinal detachment in this eye (Fig. 99–5A), which has previously undergone vitrectomy, is caused by four horseshoe tears in the lower temporal quadrant. In addition, considerable PVR is present. The insertion of the residual posterior hyaloid membrane is opacified, and its contraction has led to a series of radial retinal pleats (grade C, type 4) for 5 clock hours of the retinal circumference, extending

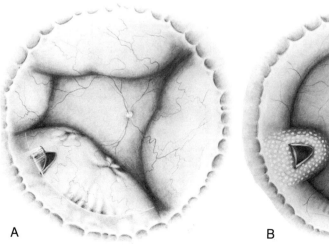
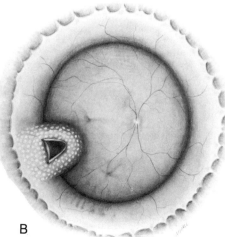

Figure 99–3. Case 1 (see text). A, Preoperative appearance. PVR is present in the inferotemporal quadrant. The large horseshoe tear has rolled edges (grade B PVR). Two star folds in the posterior retina (grade C PVR), radial folds between the 7:30 and the 6:30 meridians, and opacification of the posterior hyaloid in the anterior retina (grade C PVR) are present. B, Postoperative result. The horseshoe tear is closed with a radial buckle and is surrounded by chorioretinal reaction. The eye has been encircled to maintain the height of the radial buckle. The star-shaped folds and radial folds are almost invisible.

A   B

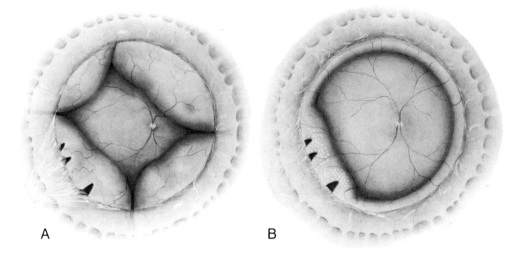

Figure 99–4. Case 2 (see text). *A,* Preoperative appearance. A vitrectomy has been performed previously. PVR associated with vitreous incarcerated in the lower temporal sclerotomy has caused opacification and contraction of the adjacent basal vitreous (grade C PVR) and resulted in three horseshoe tears. *B,* Postoperative result. Traction has been relieved (1) directly by transecting and trimming the incarcerated vitreous and resecting the anterior flaps of the horseshoe tears and (2) indirectly by supporting the tears with a segmental buckle.

Figure 99–5. Case 3 (see text). *A,* Preoperative appearance. A vitrectomy has been performed previously. PVR involves both inferior retinal quadrants. Several star folds are present in the posterior retina. PVR is present on the residual vitreous and immediately behind the insertion of the posterior hyaloid and has contracted the anterior retina in a circumferential direction. *B,* Postoperative appearance after additional basal vitrectomy, scleral buckle, laser photocoagulation, and gas tamponade. Residual anterior PVR has resulted in persistent anterior detachment, but this has been successfully "walled off" by the scleral buckle and laser photocoagulation. *C,* Postoperative appearance after additional basal vitrectomy, scleral buckle, laser photocoagulation, and silicone oil injection. Residual anterior PVR has "broken through" the barrier of laser photocoagulation, but recurrent detachment is limited by the presence of the silicone bubble in the vitreous cavity. *D,* Postoperative appearance after additional basal vitrectomy, anterior retinectomy, laser photocoagulation, and gas tamponade. Anterior PVR has been completely resected and the posterior edge of the retinectomy sealed with laser treatment.

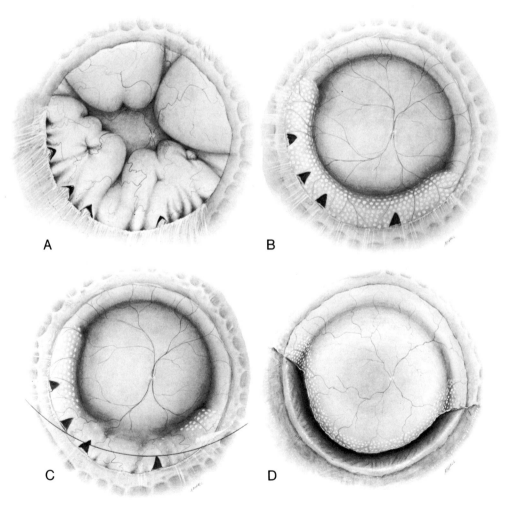

from the 9 o'clock to the 4 o'clock meridians. Within this zone of the retinal circumference, between the 8 o'clock and the 5 o'clock meridians, PVR spreads behind the equator, resulting in a diffuse area of contraction (grade C, type 2) and anterior to the equator, producing opacification of the residual vitreous matrix together with anterior displacement of the insertion of the remnant of the posterior hyaloid membrane (grade C, type 6). It is unlikely that a high buckling element will permanently close the breaks. Even with dissection of the anterior loop and associated membranes, relief of traction will probably be incomplete and there will be a high risk of postoperative recurrence. Treatment must be designed, therefore, with the presumption that permanent closure of the breaks by a combination of vitrectomy, buckling, and sealing of the break is unlikely to be successful.

Three alternative treatment techniques are available:

1. The breaks can be closed by internal tamponade until a barrier of laser treatment can be applied to wall off recurrent detachment in the retinal periphery. Either air, combined with a relatively insoluble gas (generally perfluoropropane) to prolong its presence in the vitreous cavity, or temporary installation of silicone oil is used for internal tamponade (Fig. 99–5B).

2. Recurrent retinal detachment can be confined by a permanent bubble of silicone oil in the vitreous cavity. Provided that silicone does not pass through a break, the extent of recurrent detachment is limited to the volume of aqueous surrounding the silicone bubble (Fig. 99–5C).

3. The breaks, together with the associated vitreous base, can be resected using an anterior retinectomy. Repositioning of the resulting giant tear is facilitated by the temporary injection of perfluorocarbon liquid into the vitreous cavity (Fig. 99–5D).[58]

RESULTS OF SURGICAL PROCEDURES FOR PVR

Experience with the surgical management of PVR indicates that results are strongly dependent on the severity of the disease and also that the anteroposterior location of PVR is important in determining treatment strategies and their likely outcomes. Thus, posterior PVR is easily visualized, can often be completely removed, and is frequently relatively remote from retinal breaks. Permanent closure of breaks with a scleral buckle alone or in combination with vitrectomy is therefore likely to be successful. In contrast, anterior PVR may be more difficult to visualize, is difficult or impossible to completely excise, and is usually associated with retinal breaks, either preexisting or iatrogenic. Permanent closure of breaks with scleral buckling and vitrectomy is less certain, even with prolonged internal tamponade using a relatively insoluble gas mixture or silicone oil, and retinectomy may be required. The prognosis with these procedures is correspondingly more pessimistic. The results in published series, therefore, indicate as much the mixture of cases included as the success of a particular procedure.

Scleral Buckling

In two large series, scleral buckling alone was successful in 34 percent[59] and 47 percent[60] of cases, respectively.

Vitrectomy

Vitrectomy combined with endolaser photocoagulation,[61] prolonged tamponade with gas,[62, 63] and more extensive dissection of anterior PVR[64] results in a higher proportion of cases with anatomic success. Successful results in several series ranged from 53 percent[65] to 80 percent[66] to 90 percent,[67] although additional surgery for initial failure was required to achieve these results in 19 percent, 50 percent, and 45 percent of these cases, respectively.

Vitrectomy Combined With Silicone Oil

At least in the United States, this technique has generally been employed only following initial failure with gas tamponade. Not surprisingly, therefore, results have generally been poorer than with gas tamponade. Eventual reattachment posterior to the encircling buckle was reported in 66 percent[68] and 65 percent[69] of cases in two series, although additional surgery for recurrent detachment was required in 23 percent and 37 percent of cases, respectively. There is some evidence that late redetachment may occur with silicone oil,[70] and a randomized trial is currently being conducted in the United States to assess the relative risks and benefits of silicone oil and gas tamponade in eyes with comparable degrees of PVR.[71]

Retinectomy

This procedure has been used by most surgeons only after alternative methods of relieving retinal traction have failed, although its use to permanently isolate the posterior retina from traction in the vitreous base has been described.[72] Using this technique, reattachment was achieved in 58 percent[73] and 83 percent[74] of cases in two series and was compatible with good visual acuity.

COMPLICATIONS OF SURGICAL PROCEDURES FOR PVR

Scleral Buckling

Placement of the high, broad encircling buckles traditionally used in PVR surgery is frequently complicated by choroidal effusion presumably caused by disturbance of the vortex veins, secondary either to compression by the buckle or to tearing of the vessel wall during dissection to expose the sclera. Usually the effusion reabsorbs spontaneously without complications, although by prolonging postoperative breakdown of the blood-ocular barrier it may contribute to recurrent PVR. Occasionally, however, a massive choroidal hemorrhage occurs, and in these cases the visual potential is usually lost. Disturbance of ocular motility is also common. In eyes with good return of visual acuity, diplopia is occasionally troublesome; more commonly sensory confusion is experienced, in which a blurred eccentric image from the eye with PVR is superimposed on a sharp foveal image from the fellow eye. More rarely, the buckle can become infected, particularly as complete conjunctival coverage may be difficult to achieve if the conjunctiva is grossly scarred. Ocular perforation during suturing of the buckle can also occur. This is particularly likely to happen if scleral dissection and diathermy have been employed at an earlier procedure. Because of the numerous problems associated with scleral buckling, there is an increasing tendency among retinal surgeons treating PVR to avoid manipulating the scleral buckle whenever possible and, instead, to manage the detachment entirely "from the inside."

Vitrectomy

Retinal breaks posterior to the sclerotomy "entry sites" are a potential complication of any vitrectomy procedure. They usually occur indirectly when instruments put traction on the posterior hyaloid,[56] but in surgery for PVR in which the retina is drawn forward over the pars plana, holes can be made directly through the retina. Such peripheral holes can be difficult to close because of persistent traction in the vitreous base. The posterior retinotomy used for endodrainage may also be a source of subsequent PVR.[75] In phakic eyes, transient cataract occurs because of the prolonged gas bubble in the vitreous cavity; less commonly, the gas bubble leads to either corneal decompensation or glaucoma in aphakic eyes.

Silicone Oil

Silicone oil can result in a number of complications, which are summarized in this section. However, details of their prevention and management are beyond the scope of this chapter and for further information the reader is directed to the references that are cited and particularly to a recent review article.[76]

Cataract is probably inevitable[77] in eyes permanently filled with silicone oil, but there is some evidence that cataract may not develop if silicone oil remains in the eye only temporarily.[78] In eyes with reasonably good visual potential, subsequent cataract extraction can be performed, often with good results.[76] When permanent tamponade with silicone is required, an intracapsular cataract extraction combined with an inferior peripheral iridectomy (see later) is preferred, since extracapsular extraction is often complicated by late migration of silicone into the anterior chamber. In eyes from which the silicone can be removed, subsequent extracapsular extraction with placement of an intraocular lens is ideal.

Glaucoma can result from pupillary block by the anterior surface of the silicone bubble or from the accumulation and subsequent fibrosis of multiple small droplets in the anterior chamber angle. Pupillary-block glaucoma is most commonly prevented by an inferior iridectomy,[79] although this has a tendency to close with time.[80] Droplet formation may be reduced by the use of more purified silicone of higher viscosity.[81]

Keratopathy occurs if the anterior chamber is filled with silicone. This complication is unusual in eyes with normal aqueous production and a patent inferior peripheral iridectomy,[82] but it is common in eyes with severe hypotony.[83]

Retinal toxicity from permanent placement of silicone oil has been suggested by several authors,[84–86] but remains unproved. It has also been proposed that silicone may stimulate PVR membranes by loculating growth factors in the preretinal space.[87] Although these membranes may lead to retinal breaks,[88] their clinical effect is, in fact, minimized by the presence of the silicone bubble.

Because of its potential complications, silicone oil is generally removed from eyes in which it is considered safe to do so once the process of PVR has become quiescent. However, this step should be taken with considerable caution for the following reasons: (1) In an aphakic eye with a functioning iridectomy, complications of silicone oil may not develop. (2) If complications do develop, they can usually be managed and the preexisting level of vision preserved. (3) Silicone oil removal is rarely, if ever, complete. The small bubbles of silicone in the trabecular meshwork persist and thus the potential for development of fibrosis in the anterior chamber angle still exists. (4) Silicone removal is associated with a considerable risk of retinal detachment. In one study of the complications of prophylactic silicone oil removal, the retina redetached in 25 percent of cases.[89] The authors of this study concluded that ". . . silicone oil should be removed only in carefully selected cases . . . patients with no significant vitreoretinal traction and those most likely to develop sight threatening anterior segment complications remain the obvious candidates."

PREVENTION OF PVR

Although dispersal of RPE cells into the vitreous cavity occurs in all eyes with retinal detachment, PVR develops in only a minority of cases. Detachments at particular risk of provoking severe PVR include those with any of the following characteristics:

1. Giant, large, or multiple breaks: One study found that the risk of severe PVR increased 10-fold if the tears exposed an area of more than 3 disc diameters of RPE.[90] This increased risk reflects not only the increased spread of RPE into the vitreous cavity but also the greater difficulty of closing such retinal breaks. Eyes with the combination of open retinal breaks and RPE that has been "activated" by cryotherapy are particularly prone to the development of PVR.[91]

2. Choroidal detachment:[60] Under these circumstances, there is breakdown of the blood-ocular barrier and therefore increased stimulation of RPE proliferation and contraction.

3. Vitreous hemorrhage:[51, 52] PDGF liberated by the breakdown of platelets is a powerful mitogen for both RPE and glial cells.

4. PVR, grades B[51] and C[90]: Retinal detachment surgery further increases the magnitude of stimuli that led to the development of these earlier grades of PVR.

5. Incomplete vitreous detachment:[51] The presence of vitreous on the retinal surface stimulates the formation of contractile PVR membranes by encouraging the fibroblastic transformation of RPE cells. Furthermore, failure of the vitreous to separate completely to the posterior border of the vitreous base (particularly inferiorly) allows PVR to develop, in association with vitreous, more posteriorly than usual, creating a more difficult surgical problem with a correspondingly worse prognosis.[92]

In eyes with high-risk characteristics, it is usually possible to preempt the development of PVR by prompt reattachment of the retina.[91] The precise procedure selected depends on the particular anatomic situation encountered and is beyond the scope of this chapter. However, in an eye with inferior PVR in which the detachment stems from a superior break and in which there is shallow surrounding subretinal fluid, a scleral buckle without drainage of subretinal fluid may be appropriate. In contrast, a break highly elevated on a balloon of subretinal fluid is best treated by primary drainage of subretinal fluid, air injection, cryotherapy and a low-profile buckle (DACB).[92] For eyes with vitreous hemorrhage, choroidal detachment, multiple breaks in various anteroposterior locations, or degenerative vitreous, a vitrectomy with internal closure of retinal breaks, either alone or in combination with a scleral buckle, may offer the best option, although a multivariant analysis has suggested that this procedure, per se, may predispose to PVR.[93]

CONCLUSIONS

PVR occurs following rhegmatogenous retinal detachment when ectopic RPE and glial cells proliferate and form contractile membranes on the retinal and vitreal surfaces. The clinical diagnosis of the established disease depends on the presence of characteristic patterns of retinal distortion or white or pigmented membranes on the retinal surface or within the vitreous. Surgical management is guided by an assessment (usually made at the time of operation) of the likelihood that the disease will recur postoperatively, thereby leading to recurrent rhegmatogenous detachment. If such recurrence is unlikely, the goal of the surgery is to seal all retina breaks. If recurrence is likely, the aim of surgery is to limit either the spread of subretinal fluid (by means of laser coagulation) or its volume (by instillation of silicone oil); alternatively, the break or breaks and associated contracted retina are removed by basal retinectomy.

Overall anatomic results of surgery for PVR have improved during the 1980s. However, to achieve these results, in many cases multiple procedures have been performed, and these additional procedures increase ocular morbidity and have a high economic and social cost. Visual results have been disappointing, but continued improvements in diagnosis and therapy may be expected to improve the visual prognosis. The challenge for the future lies in preventing PVR by identifying and appropriately managing those eyes at high risk for this condition, as well as in determining the most effective method of treating those eyes in which PVR is already established.

REFERENCES

1. The Retina Society Terminology Committee: The classification of retinal detachment with proliferative vitreoretinopathy. Ophthalmology 90:121, 1983.
2. Laqua H, Machemer R: Glial cell proliferation in retinal detachment (massive periretinal proliferation). Am J Ophthalmol 80:602, 1975.
3. Machemer R, Laqua H: Pigment epithelium proliferation in retinal detachment (massive periretinal proliferation). Am J Ophthalmol 80:1, 1975.
4. McLeod D, Hiscott PS, Grierson I: Age-related cellular proliferation at the vitreoretinal juncture. Eye 1:263, 1987.
5. Foos RY, Gloor BP: Vitreoretinal juncture; healing of experimental wounds. Graefes Arch Clin Exp Ophthalmol 196:213, 1975.
6. Harvey AK, Roberge F, Hjelmeland LM: Chemotaxis of rat retinal glia to growth factors found in repairing wounds. Invest Ophthalmol Vis Sci 28:1092, 1987.
7. Peters MA, Burke JM, Clowry M, et al: Development of traction retinal detachment following intravitreal injections of retinal Müller and pigment epithelial cells. Graefes Arch Clin Exp Ophthalmol 224:554, 1986.
8. Rowen SL, Glaser BM: Retinal pigment epithelial cells release a chemoattractant for astrocytes. Arch Ophthalmol 103:704, 1985.
9. Ross R, Raines EW, Bowen-Pope DF: The biology of platelet-derived growth factor. Cell 46:155, 1986.
10. Johnson NF, Foulds WS: Observations on the retinal pigment epithelium and retinal macrophages in experimental retinal detachment. Br J Ophthalmol 61:564, 1977.
11. Singh AK, Michels RG, Glaser BM: Scleral indentation following cryotherapy and repeat cryotherapy enhance release of viable retinal pigment epithelial cells. Retina 6:176, 1986.
12. Gilbert C, Hiscott P, Unger W, et al: Inflammation and the formation of epiretinal membranes. Eye 2:S140, 1988.
13. Lean JS, Noorily SW, Crisp AF, et al: Response of the RPE monolayer to retinal hole formation. In Heimann K, Wiedemann P (eds): Proliferative Vitreoretinopathy. Heidelberg, Kaden, 1989.
14. Vidaurri-Leal J, Hohman R, Glaser BM: Effect of vitreous on morphologic characteristics of retinal pigment epithelial cells: A new approach to the study of proliferative vitreoretinopathy. Arch Ophthalmol 102:1220, 1984.
15. Vidaurri-Leal JS, Glaser BM: Effect of fibrin on morphologic characteristics of retinal pigment epithelial cells. Arch Ophthalmol 102:1376, 1984.
16. Newsome DA, Rodrigues MM, Machemer R: Human massive periretinal proliferation. In vitro characteristics of cellular components. Arch Ophthalmol 99:873, 1981.
17. Cleary PE, Ryan SJ: Histology of wound, vitreous, and retina in experimental posterior penetrating eye injury in the rhesus monkey. Am J Ophthalmol 88:221, 1979.
18. Grierson I, Forrester JV: Vitreous haemorrhage and vitreal membranes. Trans Ophthalmol Soc UK 100:140, 1980.
19. Jerdan JA, Pepose JS, Michels RG, et al: Proliferative vitreoretinopathy membranes. An immunohistochemical study. Ophthalmology 96:801, 1989.
20. Campochiaro PA, Jerdan JA, Glaser BM: The extracellular matrix

of human retinal pigment epithelial cells in vivo and its synthesis in vitro. Invest Ophthalmol Vis Sci 27:1615, 1986.

21. Burke JM, Kower HS: Collagen synthesis by rabbit neural retina in vitro and in vivo. Exp Eye Res 31:213, 1980.

22. Bryan JA III, Compochiaro PA: A retinal pigment epithelial cell–derived growth factor(s). Arch Ophthalmol 104:422, 1986.

23. Burke JM, Foster SJ: Induction of DNA synthesis by co-culture of retinal glia and pigment epithelium. Invest Ophthalmol Vis Sci 26:636, 1985.

24. Burke JM, Twining SS: Vitreous macrophage elicitation: Generation of stimulants for pigment epithelium in vitro. Invest Ophthalmol Vis Sci 28:1100, 1987.

25. Campochiaro PA, Glaser BM: A retina-derived stimulator(s) of retinal pigment epithelial cell and astrocyte proliferation. Exp Eye Res 43:449, 1986.

26. Hackett SF, Conway BP, Campochiaro PA: Subretinal fluid stimulation of RPE migration and proliferation is dependent upon certain features of the detachment. Arch Ophthalmol 107:391, 1989.

27. Sporn MB, Roberts AB: Introduction: Autocrine, paracrine and endocrine mechanisms of growth control. Cancer Surv 4:627, 1985.

28. Campochiaro PA, Sugg R, Grotendorst G, et al: Retinal pigment epithelial cells produce PDGF-like proteins and secrete them into their media. Invest Ophthalmol Vis Sci 29(Suppl):305, 1988.

29. Connor T, Roberts A, Sporn M, et al: RPE cells synthesize and release transforming growth factor-beta, a modulator of endothelial cell growth and wound healing. Invest Ophthalmol Vis Sci 29(Suppl):307, 1988.

30. Connor TB Jr, Roberts AB, Sporn MB, et al: Correlation of fibrosis and transforming growth factor-beta type 2 levels in the eye. J Clin Invest 83:1661, 1989.

31. Mustoe TA, Pierce GF, Thomason A, et al: Accelerated healing of incisional wounds in rats induced by transforming growth factor-β. Science 237:1333, 1987.

32. Sporn MB, Roberts AB, Wakefield LM, et al: Some recent advances in the chemistry and biology of transforming growth factor-beta. J Cell Biol 105:1039, 1987.

33. Burke JM: Cell interactions in proliferative vitreoretinopathy: Do growth factors play a role? In Heimann K, Wiedemann P (eds): Proliferative Vitreoretinopathy. Heidelberg, Kaden, 1989.

34. Campochiaro PA, Bryan JA III, Conway BP, et al: Intravitreal chemotactic and mitogenic activity: Implication of blood-retinal barrier breakdown. Arch Ophthalmol 104:1685, 1986.

35. Bryan JA III, Campochiaro PA: Platelet-derived growth factor facilitates but is not required for human RPE growth in vitro. Invest Ophthalmol Vis Sci 27(Suppl):305, 1986.

36. Glaser BM, Lemor M: Pathobiology of proliferative vitreoretinopathy. In Glaser BM, Michels RG (eds): Surgical Retina. St Louis, CV Mosby, 1989.

37. Glaser BM, Cardin A, Biscoe B: Proliferative vitreoretinopathy. The mechanism of development of vitreoretinal traction. Ophthalmology 94:327, 1987.

38. Blumenkranz MS, Hartzer M: Contractile mechanisms in proliferative vitreoretinopathy (PVR). Invest Ophthalmol Vis Sci 27(Suppl):188, 1986.

39. Hiscott PS, Grierson I, McLeod D: Retinal pigment epithelial cells in epiretinal membranes: An immunohistochemical study. Br J Ophthalmol 68:708, 1984.

40. Hiscott PS, Grierson I, Trombetta CJ, et al: Retinal and epiretinal glia—An immunohistochemical study. Br J Ophthalmol 68:698, 1984.

41. Yamada KM: Cell surface interactions with extracellular materials. Ann Rev Biochem 52:761, 1983.

42. Avery RL, Glaser BM: Inhibition of retinal pigment epithelial cell attachment by a synthetic peptide derived from the cell-binding domain of fibronectin. Arch Ophthalmol 104:1220, 1986.

43. Campochiaro PA, Jerdan JA, Glaser BM, et al: Vitreous aspirates from patients with proliferative vitreoretinopathy stimulate retinal pigment epithelial cell migration. Arch Ophthalmol 103:1402, 1985.

44. Csaky K, Hillenius J, Liggett P, et al: Effects of laser and cryotherapy on vitreal fibronectin (FN) concentrations in rabbits. Invest Ophthalmol Vis Sci 28(Suppl):209, 1987.

45. Jaccoma EH, Conway BP, Campochiaro PA: Cryotherapy causes extensive breakdown of the blood-retinal barrier: A comparison with argon laser photocoagulation. Arch Ophthalmol 103:1728, 1985.

46. Grierson I, Boulton M, Hiscott P, et al: Human retinal pigment epithelial cells in the vitreous of the owl monkey. Exp Eye Res 43:491, 1986.

47. Morino I, Hiscott P, McKechnie N, et al: Variation in epiretinal membrane components with clinical duration of the proliferative tissue. Br J Ophthalmol 74:393, 1990.

48. Campochiaro PA, Jerdan JA, Glaser BM: Serum contains chemoattractants for human retinal pigment epithelial cells. Arch Ophthalmol 102:1830, 1984.

49. Campochiaro PA, Glaser BM: Platelet-derived growth factor is chemotactic for human retinal pigment epithelial cells. Arch Ophthalmol 103:576, 1985.

50. Bonnet M: The development of severe proliferative vitreoretinopathy after retinal detachment surgery. Grade B: A determining risk factor. Graefes Arch Clin Exp Ophthalmol 226:201, 1988.

51. Yoshizumi MO, Kreiger AE, Sharp DM: Risk factors associated with the development of massive periretinal proliferation. In Ryan SJ, Dawson AK, Little HL (eds): Retinal Diseases. Orlando, Grune & Stratton, 1984.

52. Davis JL, Jalkh AE, Roberge F, et al: Subretinal fluid from human retinal detachment contains interleukin 1. Invest Ophthalmol Vis Sci 29(Suppl):396, 1988.

53. Kirchhof B, Kirchhof E, Sorgente N, et al: Interleukin 1 stimulates migration but not proliferation of pigment epithelial cells in vitro. Invest Ophthalmol Vis Sci 28(Suppl):208, 1987.

54. Lean JS, Stern WH, Irvine AR, et al: Classification of proliferative vitreoretinopathy used in the silicone study. Ophthalmology 96:765, 1989.

55. Michels RG, Thompson JT, Rice TA, et al: Effect of scleral buckling on vector forces caused by epiretinal membranes. Am J Ophthalmol 102:449, 1986.

56. Carter JB, Michels RG, Glaser BM, et al: Iatrogenic retinal breaks complicating pars plana vitrectomy. Ophthalmology 97:848, 1990.

57. Rosen PH, Wong HC, McLeod D: Indentation microsurgery: Internal searching for retinal breaks. Eye 3:277, 1989.

58. Chang S, Ozmert E, Zimmerman NJ: Intraoperative perfluorocarbon liquids in the management of proliferative vitreoretinopathy. Am J Ophthalmol 106:668, 1988.

59. Grizzard WS, Hilton GF: Scleral buckling for retinal detachments complicated by periretinal proliferation. Arch Ophthalmol 100:419, 1982.

60. Yoshida A, Ho PC, Schepens CL, et al: Severe proliferative vitreoretinopathy and retinal detachment. II. Surgical results with scleral buckling. Ophthalmology 91:1538, 1984.

61. Parke DW, Aaberg TM: Intraocular argon laser photocoagulation in the management of severe proliferative vitreoretinopathy. Am J Ophthalmol 97:434, 1984.

62. Chang S, Coleman J, Lincoff H, et al: Perfluoropropane gas in the management of proliferative vitreoretinopathy. Am J Ophthalmol 98:180, 1984.

63. Blumenkranz M, Gardner T, Blankenship G: Fluid gas exchange and photocoagulation after vitrectomy: Indications, technique and results. Arch Ophthalmol 104:291, 1986.

64. Aaberg TM: Management of anterior and posterior proliferative vitreoretinopathy. XLV Edward Jackson Memorial Lecture. Am J Ophthalmol 106:519, 1988.

65. Lewis H, Aaberg TM: Anterior proliferative vitreoretinopathy. Am J Ophthalmol 105:277, 1988.

66. Hanneken AM, Michels RG: Vitrectomy and scleral buckling methods for proliferative vitreoretinopathy. Ophthalmology 95:869, 1988.

67. DeJuan E Jr, McCuen BW II: Management of anterior vitreous traction in proliferative vitreoretinopathy. Retina 9:258, 1989.

68. McCuen BW II, Landers MB III, Machemer R: The use of silicone oil following failed vitrectomy for retinal detachment with advanced proliferative vitreoretinopathy. Ophthalmology 92:1029, 1985.

69. Cox MS, Trese MT, Murphy PL: Silicone oil for advanced proliferative vitreoretinopathy. Ophthalmology 93:646, 1986.

70. Sell CH, McCuen BW II, Landers MB III, et al: Long-term

results of successful vitrectomy with silicone oil for advanced proliferative vitreoretinopathy. Am J Ophthalmol 103:24, 1987.

71. The Silicone Study Group: Proliferative vitreoretinopathy. Am J Ophthalmol 99:593, 1985.

72. Haut J, Larricart JP, van Effenterre G, et al: Some of the most important properties of silicone oil to explain its action. Ophthalmologica 191:150, 1985.

73. Morse LS, McCuen BW II, Machemer R: Relaxing retinotomies. Analysis of anatomic and visual results. Ophthalmology 97:642, 1990.

74. Iverson DA, Ward TG, Blumenkranz MS: Indications and results of relaxing retinotomy. Ophthalmology 97:1298, 1990.

75. McDonald HR, Lewis H, Aaberg TM, et al: Complications of endodrainage retinotomies created during vitreous surgery for complicated retinal detachment. Ophthalmology 96:358, 1989.

76. Leaver PK: Complications of intraocular silicone oil. In Glaser BM, Michels RG (eds): Surgical Retina. St Louis, CV Mosby, 1989.

77. Billington BM, Leaver PK: Vitrectomy and fluid/silicone-oil exchange for giant retinal tears: Results at 18 months. Graefes Arch Clin Exp Ophthalmol 224:7, 1986.

78. Casswell AG, Gregor ZJ: Silicone oil removal I. The effect on the complications of silicone oil. Br J Ophthalmol 71:893, 1987.

79. Ando F: Intraocular hypertension resulting from pupillary block by silicone oil. Am J Ophthalmol 99:87, 1985.

80. Laganowski HC, Leaver PK: Silicone oil in the aphakic eye: The influence of a six o'clock peripheral iridectomy. Eye 3:338, 1989.

81. Gabel VP: Polydimethylsiloxane and the factors influencing its intraocular biocompatibility. In Heimann K, Wiedemann P (eds): Proliferative Vitreoretinopathy. Heidelberg, Kaden, 1989.

82. Beekhuis WH, Ando F, Zivojnovic R, et al: Basal iridectomy at 6 o'clock in the aphakic eye treated with silicone oil: Prevention of keratopathy and secondary glaucoma. Br J Ophthalmol 71:197, 1987.

83. McCuen BW II, de Juan E Jr, Landers MB III, et al: Silicone oil in vitreoretinal surgery. Part 2: Results and complications. Retina 5:198, 1985.

84. Refojo MF, Chung H, Ueno N, et al: Solubility of retinol in intraocular silicone oil. Invest Ophthalmol Vis Sci 28(Suppl):210, 1987.

85. Gonvers M, Hornung JP, de Courten C: The effect of liquid silicone on the rabbit retina: Histologic and ultrastructural study. Arch Ophthalmol 104:1057, 1986.

86. Gray RH, Cringle SJ, Constable IJ: Fluorescein angiographic findings in three patients with long-term intravitreal liquid silicone. Br J Ophthalmol 73:991, 1989.

87. Lambrou FH, Burke JM, Aaberg TM: Effect of silicone oil on experimental traction retinal detachment. Arch Ophthalmol 105:1269, 1987.

88. Glaser BM, de Bustros S, Michels RG: Postoperative retinal breaks occurring after intravitreal silicone oil injection. Retinal 4:246, 1984.

89. Casswell AG, Gregor ZJ: Silicone oil removal. II. Operative and postoperative complications. Br J Ophthalmol 71:898, 1987.

90. Bonnet M: Clinical factors predisposing to massive proliferative vitreoretinopathy in rhegmatogenous retinal detachment. Ophthalmologica 188:148, 1984.

91. Leaver PK: Retinal detachment—When to refer? Identifying the complicated case. Eye 3:754, 1989.

92. Gilbert C, McLeod D: D-ACE surgical sequence for selected bullous retinal detachments. Br J Ophthalmol 69:733, 1985.

93. Cowley M, Conway BP, Campochiaro PA, et al: Clinical risk factors for proliferative vitreoretinopathy. Arch Ophthalmol 107:1147, 1989.

Chapter 100

▪

Vitreoretinal Surgery: Principles and Applications

DONALD J. D'AMICO

The development of vitreoretinal surgery may be traced from the first ophthalmoscopic visualization of the retina in patients, through the development of scleral buckling surgery, and culminating in the complex maneuvers performed within the eye in modern vitreoretinal surgery. The historical aspects of this continuing evolution are summarized in Chapter 98.

This chapter presents the principles and primary applications of vitreoretinal surgery. The applications of vitreoretinal surgery are extensive, and the broad categories are summarized in Table 100–1. The themes in this chapter overlap many others in this text, and the reader will wish to consult the companion chapters for detailed information regarding visual results and other specific information in each area of application. In particular, Chapters 56, 57, 74, 97 to 99, and 101 to 103 will be of interest.

INSTRUMENTATION AND SURGICAL SETTING

Rapid developments in instrumentation for vitreoretinal surgery have led to increasing sophistication in surgical technique.[1-19] Many systems have been introduced and may be roughly divided into three-port systems (either 20- or 19-gauge) and single-port systems, combining vitreous cutting, aspiration, illumination, and infusion in a single instrument (combined-function instruments). In addition, systems have included the use of a hand-held irrigating contact lens for visualization,[20] a sutured retaining ring with floating lenses of various types,[21] a temporary keratoprosthesis for patients with opacification of the cornea,[22, 23] and a wide-angle lens,[24] as well as systems that require no contact lens at all.[25]

The basic instrumentation available to the vitreoret-

Table 100–1. APPLICATIONS OF VITREORETINAL SURGERY

Removal of vitreous opacity
Removal of foreign body or dislocated lens, intraocular lens, or vitreous
Repair of retinal detachment or retinal distortion
  Relief of transvitreal and surface retinal traction
  Creation of chorioretinal adhesion and closure of retinal breaks
  Mobilization and repositioning of the retina
Control of neovascularization of the retina and iris
Diagnostic vitrectomy and retinal biopsy
Removal of inflammatory products or vitreous structural scaffold
Miscellaneous applications
  Ciliary body ablation or valve implantation for glaucoma
  Evacuation of choroidal or subretinal hemorrhage
  Adjunct to eye wall resection of choroidal melanoma
  Removal of choroidal neovascular membranes

inal surgeon is listed in Table 100–2. The diversity of these systems is further increased by various combinations of functions, e.g., illuminated forceps, irrigating light pipes, and so on.[26–51]

Anesthesia for vitreoretinal procedures may be provided by retrobulbar injection of anesthetic (with intravenous sedation as well) or by general anesthesia. The choice of anesthesia is a function of the patient, the surgeon, and the anticipated duration of the procedure. Advantages of local anesthesia are many[52] and include decreased cardiovascular risk and morbidity, rapid recovery from anesthesia, unaltered gas kinetics in eyes with intraocular tamponades,[53] better postoperative patient cooperation for positioning with tamponades or other maneuvers, and shortened operating times. For these reasons, local anesthesia appears preferable for the majority of vitreoretinal procedures, but general anesthesia is also widely used and is required for pediatric and other uncooperative or anxious patients.

The conjunctival incisions required for a vitreoretinal procedure range from a single incision, to permit the introduction of a combined-function instrument, to a 360-degree peritomy. Rectus muscles may be isolated if desired for fixation or in anticipation of an associated scleral buckling procedure. In other cases, and with preexisting scleral buckles that are to remain undisturbed, rectus muscle sutures are not placed.

Maintenance of ocular volume with removal of vitreous is provided by continuous infusion of fluid. The composition of infusion fluids has advanced considerably since the 1970s, and the addition of glutathione and other constituents to the basic balanced saline formulation has resulted in prolonged clarity of the lens and preservation of the corneal endothelium.[54–57] In addition, 3 ml of 50 percent glucose may be added to the 500-ml bottle of infusion fluid if the lens is to be preserved during vitreoretinal surgery for complications of proliferative diabetic retinopathy.[58] Epinephrine may be added for prolongation of pupillary dilatation.[59] Enlargement of the pupil may also be accomplished by excising iris with the vitrectomy instrument or by stretching the pupil with sutures or tacks.[51] Although some surgeons

routinely add antibiotics to the infusion solution,[60] the possibility of retinal toxicity resulting from a dosage error almost certainly exceeds the risks of endophthalmitis after vitrectomy, particularly in nontraumatic cases.[61–63]

The infusion cannula is of variable length, with 2.5-mm cannulas used in eyes destined to remain phakic, and 4.0-mm cannulas used in pseudophakic or aphakic eyes. The cannula is secured in position by a pre-placed mattress suture (5–0 Dacron or similar suture material) in the inferotemporal quadrant 4.0 mm posterior to the limbus in phakic eyes and 3.0 or 3.5 mm posterior to

Table 100–2. INSTRUMENTATION FOR VITREORETINAL SURGERY

Vitrectomy systems	Photocoagulation
Three-port systems (20- or 19-gauge) with a separate port for infusion, illumination, and vitrectomy instrument	Endophotocoagulation
	Endolaser
	Argon green and blue-green
Combined-function instruments (vitrectomy, infusion, and illumination)	Diode 810 nm
	Endoxenon
Visualization	Indirect ophthalmoscopic photocoagulation
Hand-held irrigating contact lens	Argon green and blue-green
Floating of sutured contact lens	Diode 810 nm
Wide-angle lens	Transscleral laser photocoagulation
Keratoprosthesis	Nd.YAG systems
Operating microscope for anterior maneuvers	Diode 810 nm
Illumination	Cryotherapy
Fiberoptic light pipe	Transscleral
Fiberoptic light sleeve for other instruments	Transvitreal
	Diathermy
Fiberoptic light cannula	Transvitreal
Illumination collars for other ports	Bipolar unimanual
	Bipolar bimanual
Illumination from operating microscope	In combination with other instruments
Infusion	Transscleral
Infusion cannula	Scleral buckling elements
Infusion sleeves for other instruments	Silicone sponges
	Solid silicone plates
Air pump–silicone oil pump	Silicone bands
Instruments	Tamponades
Scissors (many types, manual or automated)	Air
	Long-acting gases
Forceps (many types, manual or automated)	Sulfur hexafluoride
	Perfluoroethane
Picks	Perfluoropropane
Ultrasonic needles for lens removal	Silicone oil
	Liquid perfluorochemicals
Aspiration catheters, fluted vacuum needles	Cyanoacrylate glue
	Tacks (retina and iris)
Magnets (intraocular, extraocular)	Sutures (retina and iris)
	Giant tear table
Ancillary intravitreal drugs and agents	
Epinephrine	
Antibiotics, antiviral agents	
Antiinflammatory agents	
Antiproliferative agents	
Tissue plasminogen activator	
Hyaluronic acid	
Thrombin	

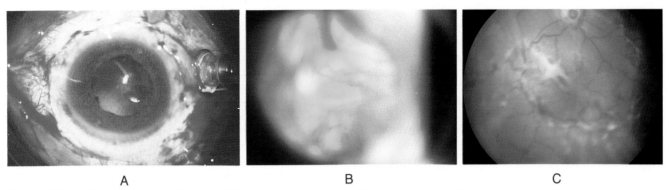

Figure 100–1. *A,* Infusion cannula sutured 3 mm posterior to the limbus in an aphakic eye. *B,* Total retinal detachment with proliferative vitreoretinopathy following penetrating trauma, displaying synechiae of the retina to the iris; an anterior chamber infusion needle was used initially in this case. Visual acuity is at the light perception level. *C,* Postoperative appearance following vitrectomy, scleral buckle, retinotomy, endolaser, and perfluoropropane gas tamponade. An epimacular membrane is seen, the retina is attached, and visual acuity is at the hand motions level.

the limbus in pseudophakic or aphakic eyes (Fig. 100–1A). It should be noted that special situations may call for the use of additional care in the establishment of a safe infusion cannula, such as preexisting choroidal detachment, endophthalmitis, or anterior proliferative vitreoretinopathy (Fig. 100–1B and C). In these circumstances, special techniques may be required, such as longer cannulas (6.0 mm), infusion needles, infusion sleeves around the light pipe or other instruments, combined-function vitrectomy instruments with infusion, or limbal infusion. These special maneuvers may be required only temporarily at the beginning of the case in order to ensure that the infusion cannula is properly placed with the internal tip of the cannula in the vitreous. Failure to correctly place the internal tip of the cannula not only endangers the lens and retina but also may result in the creation of progressive choroidal detachment with obliteration of surgical access to the vitreous.

The sclerotomy incisions in the standard three-port vitrectomy technique are typically placed at the 10 and 2 o'clock positions at the same distance from the limbus as the infusion cannula. However, if the circumstances of the case (such as an adhesion of the retina to the posterior iris) indicate the unsuitability of these locations, other sites may be chosen. At the conclusion of the procedure, sclerotomies are closed with 7–0 Vicryl or 8–0 nylon suture.

REMOVAL OF VITREOUS OPACITY

Opacification of the vitreous by blood, amyloid, dense membranes such as those occurring in persistent hyperplastic primary vitreous, severe asteroid hyalosis, and other substances may reduce vision as a consequence of their interference with the clarity of the ocular media. Removal of the opacity may be accomplished by vitrectomy, and visual restoration may be anticipated if no abnormalities are present in the underlying retina. The most common indication for removal of vitreous opacity

is the removal of blood in patients with proliferative diabetic retinopathy.[64–71] In this circumstance, the hemorrhage will clear spontaneously over several weeks to months in many patients and vitrectomy may not be required. In the past, vitreous hemorrhage in proliferative diabetic retinopathy was classified on the basis of its duration, with surgery being offered for hemorrhages that did not clear with observation alone after 3 to 6 mo. However, other factors may influence the need for earlier or later vitrectomy. In particular, the presence of untreated severe proliferative retinopathy, rubeosis, neovascular glaucoma, or visual need in a patient with only one eye may suggest earlier intervention.[66–74] The presence of extrafoveal traction retinal detachment is not an indication for earlier surgery,[75] but foveal detachment or a rhegmatogenous detachment in association with vitreous hemorrhage requires prompt intervention.[76–85]

In the eye of a diabetic patient, in particular, care is taken to avoid removal of the lens, as removal is associated with an increased risk of postoperative neovascularization of the iris.[86–88] Consequently, the lens is preserved unless removal is absolutely required for attainment of media clarity sufficient for the completion of the vitrectomy or for postoperative vision or photocoagulation. However, if the lens has a preexisting cataract, or if cataract develops intraoperatively, lens removal may be performed using an ultrasonic instrument (or the vitrectomy instrument itself if the lens is relatively soft) through the pars plana.[89] The addition of glucose to the infusion fluid will retard the intraoperative development of cataract in the diabetic eye,[58] and posterior opacification ("feathering") occurring during surgery will often clear postoperatively if it is minor. Recently, numerous techniques have been devised for combined lens removal, vitrectomy, and intraocular lens (IOL) implantation at the time of diabetic vitrectomy. They include performance of a conventional extracapsular extraction or phacoemulsification with posterior chamber IOL insertion followed by the pars plana vitrectomy, pars plana lens removal followed by vitrectomy and anterior chamber or posterior chamber IOL implantation, and variations of these techniques.[90–92] At the present time, the benefits of improved visual rehabilitation with an IOL (compared with aphakic glasses or a contact lens in a diabetic patient) appear to outweigh the additional surgical risks of IOL implantation in more straightforward cases such as diabetic vitreous hemorrhage alone. However, it is probable that increasing experience and sophistication with IOL implantation at the time of vitrectomy will result in wider use of these techniques, particularly in those situations in which patients have been left with unilateral aphakia in the past, such as penetrating trauma or complicated retinal detachment.

Although proliferative diabetic retinopathy remains the principal cause of vitreous hemorrhage in eyes undergoing vitrectomy, visual improvement has also been reported following vitrectomy for hemorrhage resulting from branch vein occlusion,[93, 94] trauma,[95–97] proliferative sickle retinopathy,[98, 99] Terson's syndrome,[100, 101] age-related macular degeneration,[102, 103] and media opacity from other causes such as amyloidosis,[104, 105] persistent hyperplastic primary vitreous,[106] or severe asteroid hyalosis.[107–109]

REMOVAL OF FOREIGN OR DISLOCATED MATERIALS IN THE POSTERIOR SEGMENT

Vitreoretinal surgery has had a major impact on the removal of foreign and dislocated materials in the posterior segment of the eye. Three distinct vitreoretinal surgical themes are encountered in this context: (1) removal of formed vitreous surrounding an object to be manipulated in order to avoid traction on the retina with the possible consequences of retinal break, detachment, or hemorrhage; (2) direct manipulation and removal of an intraocular foreign body (or replacement if it is a dislocated IOL); and (3) maneuvers such as membrane removal, endolaser treatment, and retinal break tamponade in order to repair any associated retinal abnormalities such as a retinal break or detachment.

Ocular trauma with an intraocular foreign body (IOFB) illustrates the utility of these approaches.[110–117] IOFBs may be broadly categorized into nonmagnetic and magnetic groups. Nonmagnetic foreign bodies require direct removal by forceps, whereas magnetic foreign bodies provide additional surgical options—removal with external or intraocular magnets. For all IOFB removal procedures using forceps, vitrectomy is first performed to mobilize the IOFB and to permit removal from the eye without traction on the retina. For midvitreal IOFBs without associated membrane formation, this may be a relatively simple aspect of the procedure; for IOFBs associated with extensive membrane formation or those embedded in the retina, the careful and complete removal of vitreous and membranes surrounding the IOFB may be exceedingly difficult. Nevertheless, it is important to mobilize the IOFB and to convert the surrounding area to a fluid environment prior to any consideration of grasping the IOFB with forceps (Fig. 100–2). Failure to perform this portion of the surgery successfully not only will result in difficulty in IOFB extraction but also may create retinal breaks, detachment, or hemorrhage as the IOFB is delivered from the eye.

With regard to magnetic foreign bodies, some surgeons prefer a magnet-assisted removal in a variety of approaches, including (1) placing a large magnet external to the limbus or pars plana and withdrawing the IOFB through an appropriately sized incision (before, after, or without a vitrectomy), (2) performing a vitrectomy to mobilize the IOFB as previously described, and using an intraocular magnetic probe instead of a forceps to remove the IOFB. Currently, forceps and intraocular magnet extractions are preferred in the great majority of cases. The disadvantages of external magnetic extraction are many, particularly if performed without prior vitrectomy, and include the possibility of additional ocular damage as the IOFB is rapidly drawn to the magnet in a relatively uncontrolled fashion.[117] Nevertheless, in certain cases in which features such as choroidal

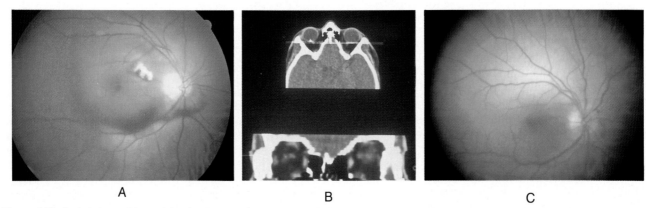

Figure 100–2. A, Intraocular steel foreign body embedded in the nasal macula of the right eye in association with vitreous hemorrhage; visual acuity is 20/200. B, Computed tomography (CT) scan documenting a single foreign body in the posterior pole of the right eye. C, Postoperative appearance 1 mo after vitrectomy and forceps removal. There is a small pigment spot at the point of impact, and visual acuity is 20/70.

hemorrhage or corneal opacity preclude the visualization required for direct manipulation of the IOFB by forceps or intraocular magnet, the external magnet has a continued role.

The third phase of vitreoretinal surgery for IOFBs includes repair of associated abnormalities in the posterior segment. In the diverse situations encountered, this may include identification and treatment of retinal breaks and retinal detachment and control and removal of intraocular hemorrhage.[118–120]

Removal or replacement of a dislocated IOL shares important similarities with the surgery for IOFBs.[121–123] In the first phase of the surgery, the formed vitreous is removed and the IOL is mobilized. If total removal from the eye is intended, in the second phase the IOL is grasped by forceps and delivered from the eye by a limbal or pars plana incision. Other techniques have been described for replacement of the mobilized IOL into the ciliary sulcus or pars plana by means of fixation sutures. In one such technique, a loop of suture is held by forceps and introduced through a pars plana incision. It is then placed around the haptic of the IOL (which is lying freely on the retina) and drawn anteriorly and tied into position; a second loop of suture through a contralateral incision is used to secure the remaining haptic anteriorly. Other techniques include transscleral fixation sutures or the placement of a different IOL in the anterior chamber. Recently, liquid perfluorochemicals have been used to float dislocated IOLs or lens fragments to the pupillary aperture, from which they may be removed.[124]

A dislocated crystalline lens (whole, fragment, or nucleus) may cause an inflammatory reaction with increased intraocular pressure.[125–127] In these situations, removal of the inciting material will typically cure the inflammation and often the glaucoma as well. Opinions differ as to the precise indications for removal of the dislocated lens and its various parts. A dislocated complete lens may be well tolerated by the eye indefinitely; it may be observed if it does not cause inflammation, pupillary block, glaucoma, visual compromise, or other problems. Conversely, a dislocated lens nucleus or large nuclear fragment (as may occur as a complication of extracapsular cataract extraction with nucleus expression or phacoemulsification) usually provokes a severe reaction, and most surgeons suggest prompt removal from the eye.[125–127] This may be performed at the time of occurrence, if possible, or at the earliest subsequent date. Other situations (small nuclear fragment, cortical fragments) are intermediate, and management includes observation, with vitrectomy performed if inflammation and its sequelae exceed a modest degree that is controllable with topical antiinflammatory or glaucoma medications. Although rare, similar considerations pertain to vitrectomy for inflammation associated with intraocular parasites such as *Cysticercus cellulosae*.[128–130] In addition, the retrieved parasitic fragments may be processed for identification after retrieval from the eye.

In a number of conditions, vitreous itself is abnormally positioned in the eye and produces ocular dysfunction. Vitreous loss may occur as a complication of cataract extraction or other surgery and may result in vitreous incarceration in the cataract wound.[131–133] In its most evident form, this vitreous incarceration is associated with an irregularity of the pupil ("peaked pupil"), intraocular inflammation, and cystoid macular edema. The pathogenesis of this syndrome is uncertain, but theories favor the adverse effects of iridovitreal contact and macular traction. Furthermore, the evaluation of any form of therapy is complicated by the fact that many cases will resolve with observation alone within the first months after cataract surgery, and certain patients will recover with antiinflammatory medications.[133] A randomized study found visual improvement with vitrectomy in patients who had persisting macular edema, with a gain of slightly more than 2 lines of visual acuity when compared with unoperated controls.[134] At the present time, vitrectomy is typically reserved for patients who have persisting macular edema 6 mo after initial surgery and whose condition has failed to improve on a regimen of antiinflammatory medications. If vitrectomy is performed, careful attention is given to removing the vitreous in the anterior chamber, on the iris surface, and in the posterior vitreous.

Corneal decompensation may occur in eyes with prolonged vitreocorneal contact.[135] Corneal pachymetry, endothelial cell counts, and visual acuity determinations are helpful in evaluating the need for removal. In vitrectomy performed for corneal touch, it is frequently possible to perform the surgery from a limbal incision, and far posterior and peripheral vitrectomy may be avoided.

VITRECTOMY FOR RETINAL DETACHMENT AND RETINAL DISTORTION

Vitreoretinal surgery has revolutionized the management of retinal detachment. In addition, it has provided the first effective surgical approach for correction of visual abnormalities caused by distortion of the retina by membranes or incarceration. The application of vitreoretinal surgery in this broad area is discussed in relation to three major themes: (1) relief of transvitreal and surface retinal traction, (2) creation of chorioretinal adhesion and closure of retinal breaks, and (3) mobilization and repositioning of the retina.

Vitrectomy for Relief of Transvitreal and Surface Retinal Traction

Traction on the retina may occur as transvitreal traction (perpendicular to the retinal surface) or surface traction (along the retinal surface), or a combination of directions. Although these distinctions are arbitrary, they assist in the understanding of the rationale for certain surgical maneuvers. For instance, transvitreal traction observed in vitreous attachment to a horseshoe retinal break may be addressed externally by scleral buckling or internally by vitrectomy, or by a combina-

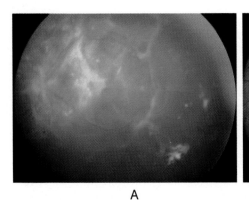

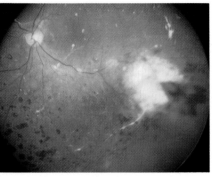

A   B

Figure 100–3. *A,* Proliferative diabetic retinopathy with combined traction–rhegmatogenous retinal detachment involving the fovea caused by a retinal break along the inferotemporal arcade in the left eye. Visual acuity is at the counting fingers level at 2 ft. *B,* Photograph showing retinal reattachment and closure of the break following vitrectomy combined with a localized, posteriorly placed scleral buckle and cryopexy along the inferotemporal arcade; visual acuity is 20/200.

tion of both maneuvers. However, surface traction, as may occur with an epiretinal membrane or a retinal incarceration, will not be relieved by externally applied buckling but will be addressed by membrane removal[136–138] in the first case and by an incision of the retina (retinotomy) in the second case.[139–142]

Transvitreal traction is a major component in the development of primary rhegmatogenous retinal detachment such as occurs in association with lattice peripheral degeneration and posterior vitreous detachment and following cataract surgery with vitreous loss.[143, 144] In these cases, it is frequently possible to completely relieve the elevation of the retinal break by scleral buckling coupled with retinopexy (photocoagulation, cryotherapy, or diathermy) to create a chorioretinal scar around the retinal break. Conceptually, this same result—relief of transvitreal traction—could be achieved with vitrectomy alone by division of the vitreous attachments to the retinal break, in association with similar retinopexy treatment. A series has been reported using vitrectomy alone as a primary procedure for primary rhegmatogenous detachment, and successful repair of the detachment was accomplished in 79 percent of cases.[145] Nevertheless, at the present time, scleral buckling procedures are preferred for straightforward cases of primary retinal detachment. This is a consequence of the continued success with scleral buckling surgery alone, as well as the comparative difficulties (particularly trauma to the lens) in performing peripheral vitrectomy in phakic eyes. In other situations, such as a posterior retinal break with vitreous traction after penetrating

trauma or in traction retinal detachment in proliferative diabetic retinopathy, vitrectomy assumes the primary role in the relief of the transvitreal component of traction.[146] This is a result of many factors, including the relatively greater ease of the surgical approach to posterior traction with vitrectomy as compared with posteriorly located scleral buckles, and the need for other maneuvers that require vitrectomy as well, such as membrane removal and the placement of intraocular tamponade with air, gas, or silicone oil.

In many cases, these two methods of transvitreal traction relief—scleral buckling and vitrectomy—are additive and are combined to achieve the necessary relief of traction (Fig. 100–3). A peripheral retinal break that cannot be supported on a scleral buckle of reasonable height will require peripheral vitrectomy for successful closure of the break, and a posterior break that does not completely settle with removal of vitreous attachments may benefit from the additional support of a scleral buckle.

Surface traction on the retina, in its purest form, can be relieved only by vitrectomy. This form of traction is caused by (1) membranes on either surface of the retina,[136–138, 147–150] (2) horizontal traction from a flat contraction of the posterior hyaloid (as may occur in macular hole formation),[151, 152] or (3) incarceration or intrinsic contracture of the retina rendering it unable to conform to the contour of the globe.[139–141] For instance, an epiretinal membrane with macular distortion requires membrane removal for relief of surface traction (Fig. 100–4). In rhegmatogenous retinal detachment associ-

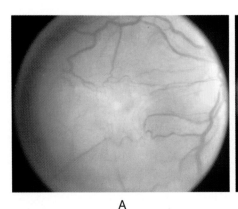

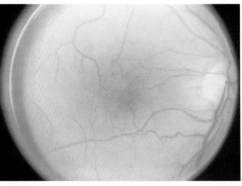

A   B

Figure 100–4. *A,* Epiretinal membrane in the right eye following peripheral cryopexy; visual acuity is 20/200. *B,* Postoperative appearance following vitrectomy with membrane peeling; visual acuity is 20/25.

Figure 100–5. *A,* Severe proliferative vitreoretinopathy in the right eye following motor vehicle accident. The disc and macula are obscured by membranes and retinal folds, and the lower border of a gas bubble from a previous surgical procedure is just visible at the top of the photograph. Visual acuity is at the light perception level. *B,* Postoperative photograph 1 mo after vitrectomy with extensive membrane peeling, pneumohydraulic reattachment, endolaser, and silicone oil tamponade. The retina is attached but distorted because of residual subretinal membranes and contracture, and visual acuity is at the hand motions level.

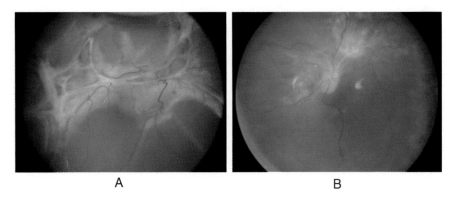

A

B

ated with proliferative vitreoretinopathy (Fig. 100–5), fixed folds in the retina are commonly caused by membranes on the anterior surface of the retina (star folds), but folds caused by subretinal membranes are also encountered in some cases. In order to relieve surface traction (particularly in areas with retinal breaks that require mobilization in order to achieve closure of the break), the removal of membranes from the retinal surface is an extremely important aspect of the procedure.[153–163] Membranes are typically engaged with bent picks or needles, but they may also be engaged with forceps, scissors, or other instruments. In order to remove membranes on the undersurface of the retina, access to the subretinal space is created by the use of one or more planned retinotomies over the membrane. Subretinal membranes are usually elastic and fortunately do not require removal except in more extreme variations.

In the patient with an impending macular hole, current understanding suggests that the hole is caused by progressive horizontal contracture of the posterior hyaloid with removal of a portion of macular retina as the curve of the posterior hyaloid is shortened to a straight chord.[151, 152] This form of surface traction requires removal of the posterior hyaloid for relief, although the precise benefits and indications for such surgery remain unknown.[164, 165] Patients with full-thickness macular holes typically have reduced visual acuity, but it has been demonstrated that a portion of the vision loss is due to the lack of retinal tissue, and a variable portion of vision loss is due to a cuff of subretinal fluid surrounding the macular hole.[166] Surgery to relieve horizontal contraction on the margin of the macular hole may result in reattachment of this critical macular retina. Although visual results are highly variable and unpredictable, visual improvement has been demonstrated following this procedure.[166] In patients with retinal incarceration with the macula tightly drawn toward the incarceration site (Fig. 100–6), relaxing retinotomy will mobilize the retina; subsequently the retinotomy is closed by retinopexy and intraocular tamponade.[139–141, 167–169] It should be noted that an older and alternative approach to retinal incarceration or contracture is available in a procedure called scleral shortening.[170] In this procedure, the scleral eye wall under the shortened retina is thinned by lamellar scleral dissection, creating a bed of thinned sclera. Subsequently, the eye wall is shortened by suturing together the full-thickness sclera at the opposite sides of the bed, concealing the thinned sclera from view and creating an indentation in the eye that resembles a scleral buckle. Although this procedure is conceptually related to the discussion of surface traction, it is seldom

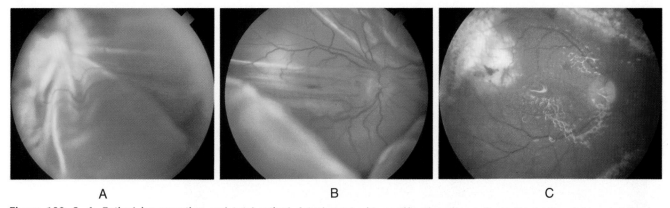

A

B

C

Figure 100–6. *A,* Retinal incarceration and total retinal detachment with proliferative vitreoretinopathy in the right eye following penetrating trauma. The incarceration site in the temporal equator is shown, with detached folds emanating from the site. *B,* Posterior pole of the same eye, showing tight folds extending temporally toward the incarceration site. Visual acuity is at the hand motions level. *C,* Appearance 2 mo after vitrectomy with extensive retinotomy, endolaser, and silicone oil tamponade. The retina is reattached and the macular folds are relieved. The retinotomy may be seen temporally, there is a reflex over the macula due to silicone oil, and visual acuity is at the counting fingers level at 1 ft.

performed at present, because of the technical difficulties of the scleral shortening procedure and the development of more effective retinotomy techniques.

In the majority of situations in which retinal traction is encountered, both transvitreal and surface traction are present in various combinations in different areas of the retina. In vitreoretinal surgery for proliferative vitreoretinopathy, e.g., membranes on both surfaces of the retina must be removed completely in order to relieve surface traction and mobilize the retina. In the same procedure, vitreous attachments to the retina are divided, and a scleral buckle is frequently placed to relieve transvitreal traction in the far peripheral retina. Retinotomy is currently reserved as a last resort for the relief of surface traction and is used in situations in which traction is unrelieved despite technically complete membrane removal or in situations in which the retina is incarcerated or contracted.[139–141, 167–169] Conceptually, it is possible to consider a more liberal use of retinotomy, in which membranes producing surface traction would be divided with the underlying retina rather than removed, but the additional problems engendered by the creation of the large retinotomies have limited enthusiasm for this approach.

Similar considerations are encountered in surgery for traction detachment of the fovea in proliferative diabetic retinopathy (Fig. 100–7). The strong attachment of the posterior hyaloid to the neovascular proliferations arising from the retinal vessels creates a complex array of transvitreal and surface traction.[79] These forces may be approached surgically in a number of ways. In one approach, the transvitreal traction is addressed by dividing the vitreous, which is typically detached at the equator, and carrying this division in an equatorial fashion around the globe.[171] This results in a separation of the vitreous base from the posterior pole. Subsequently, the posterior hyaloid with its attached membranous and neovascular proliferations is divided with vertically oriented scissors, carefully cutting around the neovascular stalks, which are the points of strongest attachment of the posterior hyaloid. This has the result of mobilizing the posterior retina and allowing the previously closely contracted points to separate. In a second surgical approach (en bloc excision), the transvitreal traction provided by the preexisting anteroposterior vitreous is used to provide continued tension on the posterior hyaloid.[172, 173] By making an opening in the equatorial detached vitreous, a flat scissors may be introduced approaching the posterior pole in the plane of the intended separation between the posterior hyaloid and the retina. This approach necessitates cutting across all neovascular stalks, with the possibility of increased bleeding, but it has the advantage that complete removal of surface tissue and traction is attained. At the conclusion of this approach, the posterior hyaloid snaps off the retina with the final cut, signaling the complete release of the transvitreal traction; the vitrectomy instrument is subsequently used to excise this tissue and residual peripheral vitreous. Additional techniques include the use of hyaluronic acid injection under the posterior hyaloid in order to more clearly define the plane of transection.[174]

Vitrectomy for Creation of Chorioretinal Adhesion and Closure of Retinal Breaks

Numerous techniques are available to the vitreoretinal surgeon for the closure of retinal breaks and the creation of chorioretinal adhesion (Table 100–3). Surgical techniques exist for the attainment of both temporary and permanent closure of retinal breaks, as well as both temporary retinal–retinal pigment epithelium (RPE) apposition and permanent chorioretinal adhesion. Lasting surgical repair of a rhegmatogenous retinal detachment depends on the natural forces that maintain retinal attachment in the absence of retinal breaks in the normal eye. Consequently, the permanent closure of retinal breaks is desired in order to permit the maintenance of retinal attachment. Permanent closure of retinal breaks is provided most commonly by the creation of a chorioretinal scar around the retinal break by the application of retinopexy (photocoagulation, cryotherapy, or diathermy). Permanent closure combined with chorioretinal adhesion of a retinal break in attached retina has also been achieved with cyanoacrylate glue.[175–177] In a conceptually related but distinct function, glue or another substance yet to be identified might also provide closure of a retinal break in detached as well as attached retina by reconstituting the retinal integrity across the break (retinoplasty).[178]

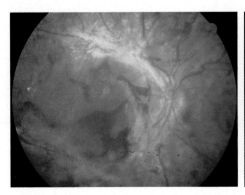

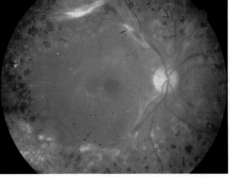

A

B

Figure 100–7. *A,* Proliferative diabetic retinopathy with traction detachment involving the fovea of the right eye. Visual acuity is 20/125. *B,* Postoperative appearance 1 yr following vitrectomy with segmentation of the posterior vitreous face, with reattachment of the retina and visual acuity of 20/40.

Table 100–3. MODALITIES FOR CREATION OF PERMANENT CHORIORETINAL ADHESION, TEMPORARY RETINAL–RETINAL PIGMENT EPITHELIUM APPOSITION, AND CLOSURE OF RETINAL BREAKS*

Permanent Chorioretinal Adhesion	Permanent Closure of Retinal Breaks
Retinopexy	Retinopexy
Photocoagulation	Photocoagulation
Laser	Laser
(Xenon)	(Xenon)
Cryotherapy	Cryotherapy
Diathermy	Diathermy
Glue	(Glue)
(Tacks)	(Silicone oil)
(Sutures)	

Temporary Retinal–Retinal Pigment Epithelium Apposition	Temporary Closure of Retinal Breaks
Air	*Immediate*
Long-acting gases	Air
Silicone oil	Long-acting gases
Liquid perfluorochemicals	Silicone oil
Photocoagulation	Liquid perfluorochemicals
Diathermy	Scleral buckling elements
Tacks	(Glue)
Sutures	*Delayed*
Scleral buckling elements	Expanding gas tamponades
	Postoperative positioning with preexisting gas or oil tamponade

*Modalities without parentheses are widely employed, and modalities in parentheses are either infrequently employed or remain experimental for a given use. See text for details.

Retinal breaks may also be closed temporarily, and temporary closure of a retinal break is extremely useful. It may permit the reattachment of the retina by natural forces, allowing the development or placement of retinopexy for permanent retinal break closure. Temporary closure of a retinal break may be either immediate or delayed. Immediate temporary closure is provided by placing an air, gas, or silicone oil bubble across the retinal break.[179–193] Delayed temporary closure is provided by expanding gas tamponade or postoperative positioning with any intraocular tamponade.[191–193] Silicone oil provides a long-acting tamponade, but its effectiveness for permanent internal closure of retinal breaks may be questioned; because the oil bubble floats on the residual aqueous fluid in the eye, it undergoes oscillatory movement with changing eye position and may permit intermittent opening of a retinal break in a ball-valve fashion. Consequently, silicone oil is most useful for temporary closure of retinal breaks, with permanent closure provided by associated retinopexy. The use of indentation by scleral buckling is also a means of closure of a retinal break in certain cases. Although scleral buckling has numerous important functions (including the relief of transvitreal traction), it is hypothesized that part of its efficacy relates to the induced contact of the vitreous body across the retinal break. Studies have documented a relative barrier to the passage of tritiated water across a retinal break in contact with formed vitreous.[194]

Temporary retinal-RPE apposition, i.e., contact between the retina and the RPE induced by means other than the closure of retinal breaks, is also extremely useful. In the short term, the retina may be held in apposition to the RPE by the flotation effect of air, gas, or silicone oil; by the compressive effect of liquid perfluorochemicals;[195–197] by a coagulum induced by heavy endophotocoagulation or transvitreal diathermy; or by retinal tacks[48, 49] and sutures.[50] This contact may provide the opportunity for placement of retinopexy in the desired location (such as at the margins of a retinal break after unfolding the posterior flap of a giant retinal break). In addition, temporary retinal-RPE apposition may be used to hold the retina in position while the retinopexy-related permanent chorioretinal adhesion develops.

There are many specific techniques available for the creation of chorioretinal adhesion and closure of retinal breaks, and these techniques are further enriched by numerous instrumental options within each modality. For instance, photocoagulation may be applied with endolaser probes with argon green or diode 810-nm wavelengths. In addition, these lasers may also be applied by indirect ophthalmoscopic delivery systems in the operating room, or advantage may be made of temporary retinal-RPE apposition created at vitrectomy with gas, oil, or other means to provide photocoagulation with slit-lamp or indirect ophthalmoscopic laser systems in the early postoperative period.[43, 187] Similarly, cryotherapy may be applied at surgery with transscleral or transvitreal probes. Diathermy for inducement of a chorioretinal scar is most typically applied by use of transscleral probes, usually in a bed of sclera thinned by lamellar dissection. The transvitreal diathermy probe is usually reserved for hemostasis, as it produces substantial inner retinal destruction with relatively little chorioretinal scar inducement. The use of glues for permanent chorioretinal adhesion has been successfully demonstrated in a small number of cases.[175–177] Sutures are of limited use for permanent chorioretinal adhesion but may have a role in temporary retinal-RPE apposition or for manipulating the detached retina into position in certain giant retinal tear procedures.[50, 198]

The use of various intraocular tamponades to close retinal breaks, provide retinal-RPE apposition, and manipulate the retina is an extremely powerful aspect of vitreous surgery, which is discussed in detail in Chapter 101. The substances used may be divided simply into four categories for conceptualization: air, long-acting gases (commonly including sulfur hexafluoride, perfluoroethane, and perfluoropropane), silicone oil, and liquid perfluorochemicals. These tamponades are variously used to accomplish three principal functions: (1) temporary closure of retinal breaks, (2) maintenance of retinal-RPE apposition, and (3) manipulation of the detached retina. The tamponades can be conveniently discussed with regard to these functions.

Closure of retinal breaks by air, long-acting gases, and silicone oil has already been discussed. The closure attained by the tamponade will be limited to its duration, and consequently, for air and the long-acting gases, the closure will be temporary and dependent on the resorption time of the tamponade, with air being the shortest and perfluoropropane the longest. The long-acting gases, if injected in pure form, will expand postoperatively and may be used to provide delayed temporary closure of a retinal break.

Retinal-RPE apposition may also be achieved by the use of intraocular tamponades. Air, gases, and silicone oil provide flotation of the retina in aqueous media and can be used to provide contact of the retina with the RPE. In combination with the removal of subretinal fluid, these materials are also capable of manipulating the detached retina in several extremely useful fashions. In the technique of pneumohydraulic retinal reattachment, a posterior retinal break is selected or created with the vitrectomy instrument or diathermy (drainage retinotomy) following removal of the vitreous and membranes restricting retina mobility.[178] Air is continuously introduced anterior to the detached retina (typically provided by connecting the infusion cannula to an air pump) while an aspiration cannula removes the preretinal fluid and subsequently the subretinal fluid through the posterior break or retinotomy, as the air bubble enlarges and descends. If transvitreal and surface traction are effectively relieved, with this technique, it is possible to completely reattach the retina in the air-filled eye. Retinopexy (commonly endolaser treatment, but cryotherapy may also be used) is then applied to reattached retinal breaks and to any retinotomy created for drainage (Fig. 100–8). This technique may also be used to evaluate the completeness of traction relief, as failure of the retina to completely reattach is signaled by the passage of air into the subretinal space. In this circumstance, additional traction-relieving measures are necessary (additional membrane removal, scleral buckling, retinotomy), or the procedure will fail to reattach the retina. In a further refinement of pneumohydraulic reattachment, a preexisting peripheral break is used instead of creating a posterior retinotomy, with aspiration of posterior subretinal fluid provided by a fine tube extended through the peripheral break and under the posterior retina.[29] For reasons of cost and convenience, air is most commonly used for this procedure, with the introduction of any long-acting gas or silicone oil made into the air-filled eye at the conclusion of the procedure. However, some surgeons prefer to perform a silicone oil infusion with subretinal fluid drainage in a related fashion, eliminating a step in cases in which silicone oil is the intended final tamponade.[162, 199]

Liquid perfluorochemicals are also used to create temporary retinal-RPE apposition and to manipulate the detached retina, with the mechanics governed by the fact that these liquids are heavier than water.[195–197, 200–203] Consequently, liquid perfluorochemical introduced on the surface of the detached retina will compress the posterior retina against the RPE and express the subretinal and preretinal fluid anteriorly and peripherally. With continuous introduction of the perfluorochemical and with continuous removal of displaced fluid through a peripheral break, the retina may be completely reattached. The use of liquid perfluorochemicals in this fashion achieves its most dramatic effectiveness in the manipulation of giant retinal breaks.[200, 201] After removal of the vitreous and mobilizing of the retina in this situation, the posteriorly curled flap of a giant break as large as 360 degrees may be unfolded anteriorly and reattached, permitting endophotocoagulation around the reattached giant break. The liquid perfluorochemicals are not used as long-term tamponades and are exchanged for long-acting gas or silicone oil at the end of the procedure.

Vitrectomy for Mobilizing and Repositioning the Retina

Several of the powerful techniques for positioning the retina at vitrectomy with intraocular tamponades have already been discussed in the previous section. The ability to reattach the retina intraoperatively, particularly with pneumohydraulic retinal reattachment under air, permits immediate endolaser photocoagulation to the reattached retina and is a cornerstone of modern vitreoretinal surgery for retinal detachment.[42, 45–47] In certain circumstances, surgery may be performed under fluid, air, or other tamponade introduced progressively in order to assess the completeness of relief of traction. At vitrectomy, the detached retina may be grasped with forceps, aspiration catheters, or other instruments, and directly manipulated, usually to position the flap of a giant retinal break or retinotomy (Fig. 100–9).[50, 198] Another method of repositioning the flap of a giant retinal break involves the performance of an air-fluid

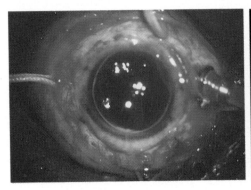

A

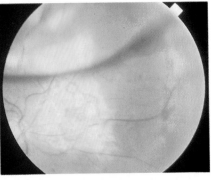

B

Figure 100–8. *A*, Surgical appearance of the air-filled aphakic eye during diabetic vitrectomy. Continued infusion of air is provided by connecting the infusion cannula to an air pump. *B*, Postoperative photograph 3 wk after vitrectomy with pneumohydraulic retinal reattachment and perfluoropropane tamponade. The receding gas tamponade reveals continued retinal reattachment and endolaser treatment nasal to the disc around previous drainage retinotomy site.

Figure 100–9. *A,* Total retinal detachment in association with dual giant retinal breaks and proliferative vitreoretinopathy in the right eye. The posterior pole is bounded by giant breaks superiorly and inferiorly, and visual acuity is at the hand motions level. *B,* Wide-angle photograph of the same eye showing a giant break from the 9 to the 1 o'clock positions, a giant break with a rolled posterior edge from the 2:30 to the 5:30 clock positions, and large breaks inferiorly with isolated peripheral attachments. *C,* Postoperative photograph 5 mo following vitrectomy with 360-degree retinotomy, supine fluid-air exchange with direct retinal manipulation, endolaser, and perfluoropropane gas tamponade. The posterior island of the retina is reattached, and visual acuity is 20/80. *D,* Photograph 1 yr postoperatively, displaying healed 360-degree retinotomy and continued retinal attachment.

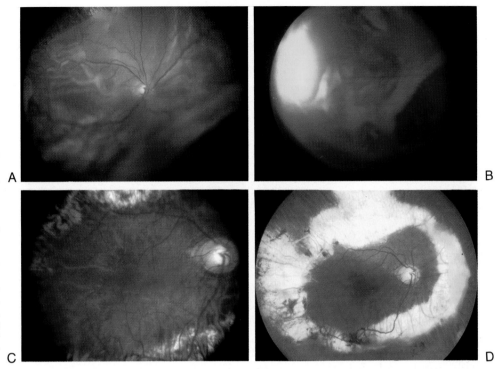

exchange with the patient in the prone position, often with the use of a special operating table for patient inversion.[204–207] In this technique, a vitrectomy is performed with mobilization of the retina, and a scleral buckle may also be placed (Fig. 100–10). The patient is turned prone (intraoperatively or postoperatively), and air is slowly injected in front of the optic disc while fluid is collected with a drainage needle from the retrolental space or from the limbus in aphakic eyes. This maneuver may be preceded by cryotherapy to the bed of the preplaced buckle or followed by photocoagulation, cryotherapy, or diathermy and instillation of long-acting gas or silicone oil for tamponade. In another technique of giant retinal break repair, sutures may be passed through the flap and used to drag the flap into position, for securing later by retinopexy.[50, 198] Hyaluronic acid has also been used in the past to mobilize the flap of a giant

retinal tear,[208] but the liquid perfluorochemicals are superior for this maneuver. Hyaluronic acid is still useful to lubricate and release the suction holding a large posterior flap folded flat against the attached retina in an air-filled eye. Retinal tacks have also been used to hold a flap in position temporarily,[48, 49] but they are little used at the present time because of the development of liquid perfluorochemical and other techniques.

VITRECTOMY FOR CONTROL OF NEOVASCULARIZATION OF THE RETINA AND IRIS

Neovascularization of the retina and iris has many causes but is primarily associated with proliferative diabetic retinopathy, proliferative sickle retinopathy,

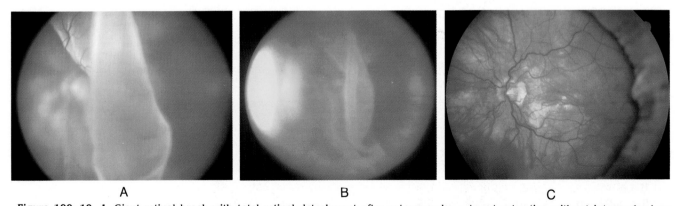

Figure 100–10. *A,* Giant retinal break with total retinal detachment after extracapsular cataract extraction without intraocular lens implantation in the left eye. The break involves 6 clock hours from the 11 to the 5 o'clock positions and is not associated with proliferative vitreoretinopathy. Visual acuity is at the hand motions level. *B,* Wide-angle photograph of same eye showing temporal giant break. *C,* Postoperative appearance following vitrectomy, scleral buckling, cryopexy, and prone fluid-air exchange. The retina is reattached on an encircling buckle, and visual acuity is 20/100.

and retinal vein occlusion. In these conditions, retinal ablation by photocoagulation or other means is the primary method of controlling the neovascularization at the present time.[209, 210] However, hemorrhage in the vitreous or anterior chamber, or both, is a frequent accompaniment of the neovascularization and may prevent visualization of the retina for ablation by photocoagulation. In this circumstance, vitrectomy may be performed in order to clear the media and permit retinal ablation by endolaser photocoagulation, indirect ophthalmoscopic laser photocoagulation, or transscleral cryotherapy, or a combination of all three modalities for maximal retinal ablation.[211, 212] Cataract, if present, may also be removed at the same procedure, and in advanced cases a filtration valve may be placed.[213] An alternative form of treatment in this circumstance of neovascularization of the retina or iris in association with media opacity is the performance of transscleral cryotherapy alone without visualization.[214] However, the lack of precision in this procedure and the failure to provide visual restoration restrict the usefulness of this procedure primarily to patients who cannot tolerate vitrectomy.

In addition to permitting retinal ablation for control of neovascularization, removal of the vitreous structure is frequently associated with regression of established retinal neovascularization in certain cases of proliferative diabetic retinopathy.[66, 67] The exact mechanism of this regression is unknown, but it is probably related to the removal of the posterior hyaloid and the structural support formerly provided to the developing proliferations.

When encountered at the time of diabetic vitrectomy, active neovascularization of the retina and iris may be treated directly with intraocular diathermy. This may be performed as a prelude to transection across a neovascular proliferation or, more commonly, to control bleeding from neovascular tissue that does not subside after a temporary increase in the intraocular pressure by prompt elevation of the infusion fluid bottle height.

Finally, highly elevated retinal neovascularization may be directly excised with scissors or the vitrectomy instrument itself, achieving removal rather than regression of the proliferation in certain cases (Fig. 100–11).

DIAGNOSTIC VITRECTOMY AND RETINAL BIOPSY

The vitreous and retina may be involved in a variety of infectious, inflammatory, or neoplastic processes,[215]

including bacterial endophthalmitis,[61, 62, 216–218] fungal endophthalmitis,[219] subretinal abscess,[220] viral retinitis,[221–223] parasitic infestations,[128–130] large cell non-Hodgkin's lymphoma (Fig. 100–12),[224, 225] and vitreous inflammation as a consequence of retinal inflammatory disease.[226–228] In most cases, the vitreous will be infiltrated with cells and inflammatory debris, and the performance of a diagnostic vitrectomy[215, 229] may establish the precise diagnosis following microscopic examination, culture results, and serologic and other test results from the excised vitreous biopsy specimen (Table 100–4). For a discussion of vitreous biopsy and culture in the setting of endophthalmitis, consult Chapter 102. The removal of intravitreal C. cellulosae with identification of the parasite by pathologic techniques has already been mentioned.[128–130] In cases of large cell non-Hodgkin's lymphoma, the diagnosis may go unsuspected for a long time unless examination of a vitreous biopsy specimen is performed.

In addition to vitreous biopsy, recent advances in technique have made possible the performance of retinal biopsy in either detached or attached retina.[230–233] This technique has been applied to difficult cases of presumed necrotizing retinitis caused by viruses and to intraretinal lesions from other causes such as neoplasms. The retrieval of a retinal biopsy specimen may permit selection of appropriate therapy and has been of great importance in evaluation of opportunistic retinitis in AIDS.

REMOVAL OF INFLAMMATORY PRODUCTS OR VITREOUS STRUCTURAL SCAFFOLD

In many diseases, the vitreous is markedly altered by the presence of inflammatory cells and products, either as a direct consequence of infection of the vitreous, as in endophthalmitis, or as a secondary consequence of retinal or other ocular inflammatory disease, as in many types of uveitis, notably pars planitis.[226–228] Removal of the vitreous body may be associated with a corresponding reduction of the inflammatory burden in the eye and result in improvement in ocular function and disease control. In this regard, vitrectomy has been used in a manner analogous to steroid therapy in order to reduce the destructive effects of ocular inflammation.[234]

In other conditions, such as proliferative vitreoretinopathy or following penetrating trauma, the vitreous structure itself provides the scaffold on which cells proliferate and membranes subsequently develop. Consequently, removal of the vitreous structure prior to

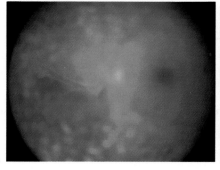
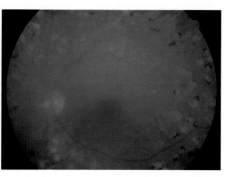

Figure 100–11. A, Proliferative diabetic retinopathy with highly elevated neovascular stalk arising from the disc in the left eye. The stalk almost reached the lens and caused repeated symptomatic vitreous hemorrhage despite extensive panretinal photocoagulation. B, Postoperative photograph after vitrectomy with direct removal of neovascularization.

Table 100–4. APPLICATIONS OF VITREOUS AND RETINAL BIOPSY

Culture
    Bacterial
    Fungal
    Viral
Microscopic examination
    Microbiologic stains
    Histologic stains
    Transmission electron microscopy
    Cytopathologic studies
    Cell surface markers
    Immunocytochemical stains
Diagnostic ELISA* and serologic tests
Polymerase chain reaction

*ELISA, enzyme-linked immunosorbent assay.

cellular organization may forestall the development of extensive membranes with associated retinal traction and detachment, although the exact indications and timing for vitreous removal after penetrating trauma are unknown. Early vitrectomy (within the first 3 days after the trauma) has been compared with intermediate vitrectomy (after 3 days but within 2 wk) and late vitrectomy (after 2 wk).[235] Compared with the latter two techniques, early vitrectomy may have the advantages of removal of inflammatory products of trauma and prevention of structural support of the formed vitreous for proliferation of cellular membranes but may have the disadvantages of an increased risk of surgical hemorrhage, an increased risk of retinal breaks because of continued attachment of the posterior vitreous to the retina, and performance of surgery on some eyes that might recover satisfactorily without any surgical intervention.[114–117]

It must be noted that the efficacy of both of these possible benefits of vitrectomy—removal of inflammatory products and removal of the vitreous scaffold—remains somewhat unpredictable in the various clinical situations for which they have been advanced, and prospective randomized trials in patients have not proved their efficacy. Nevertheless, the theoretical considerations underlying these ideas are supported by numerous retrospective clinical series and experimental studies in animals.

MISCELLANEOUS APPLICATIONS

Vitreoretinal surgery has established applications in the management of glaucoma,[213] choroidal hemorrhage,[120] and subretinal hemorrhage.[118, 119, 236, 237] It is used as a part of eye wall resection for the removal of choroidal melanomas.[238] Recently, a vitreoretinal approach has been used to remove subretinal neovascular membranes in association with age-related macular degeneration,[239, 240] presumed ocular histoplasmosis syndrome,[241] and other diseases. Although the visual results in certain cases of presumed ocular histoplasmosis syndrome have been encouraging,[241] the visual results in patients with age-related macular degeneration were poor but have improved in later series.[240]

Transvitreal destruction of the ciliary body has been performed with endolaser photocoagulation in an attempt to control glaucoma associated with neovascularization of the iris.[242] This procedure developed as a possible improvement to variable control with transscleral cryotherapy or diathermy, but it has been largely supplanted by the development of transscleral laser delivery systems for ciliary body ablation.[243]

Choroidal hemorrhage may occur spontaneously or as a result of ocular trauma or surgery.[118, 120, 244] If the hemorrhage is excessive or associated with angle-closure, glaucoma, retinal detachment, retinoretinal adhesion, an IOFB, and so on, surgical intervention by a variety of techniques may be required if there is to be any possibility of salvaging the eye. In the past, surgical options were limited to (1) observation with medical therapy for pressure and inflammation control or (2) the performance of scleral incisions in an attempt to allow for drainage of choroidal hemorrhage. In recent years, vitrectomy approaches with continued preretinal infusion of air at elevated pressure in association with scleral incisions have permitted increased and controlled drainage of choroidal hemorrhage and have correspondingly improved the results in these difficult cases.

Subretinal hemorrhage may occur with a variety of conditions, such as age-related macular degeneration, or as a result of surgical drainage of rhegmatogenous retinal detachment. If the subretinal hemorrhage involves the fovea, a reduction in visual acuity usually will occur. Vitrectomy, coupled with retinotomy, has been used to evacuate these hemorrhages in the acute stage,[118, 119, 236, 237, 239] but the appropriate timing and relative efficacy of these procedures are still unclear.

COMPLICATIONS OF VITREORETINAL SURGERY

The avoidance and management of complications are important in every field of therapy, but they are extraordinarily important in vitreoretinal surgery.[18, 19, 58, 60, 61, 64–71, 82–88, 183, 191, 199, 244–256] This is a result of the many intraocular and extraocular tissues that may be disrupted, as well as of the serious consequences of many of the conditions managed by vitreoretinal surgery. The major complications of vitreoretinal surgery are listed in Table 100–5 (Figs. 100–13 to 100–16).

Retinal detachment may result from the creation of retinal breaks in attached retina, or from failure to close preexisting retinal breaks in the repair of retinal detachment.[245–248] Retinal breaks are most frequently created during extensive membrane removal or during excision of the posterior hyaloid in surgery for traction retinal detachment in proliferative diabetic retinopathy.[66, 76–85, 172, 173] The creation of retinal breaks in these circumstances is occasionally unavoidable and is usually of less concern than the failure to relieve existing traction. In any event, a retinal break in an area of traction will inevitably lead to retinal detachment and requires treatment in the form of additional membrane removal, retinopexy, and tamponade, with perhaps scleral buckling and relaxing retinotomy in addition. Retinal breaks may also be created in the periphery resulting from the introduction of the vitreoretinal instrumentation. A

Table 100–5. COMPLICATIONS OF VITREORETINAL SURGERY

Retinal breaks	Neovascularization of the iris
Retinal detachment	Glaucoma
Vitreous hemorrhage	Neovascularization of the iris
Choroidal hemorrhage	Expanding gas tamponades
Subretinal hemorrhage	Pupillary block with
Choroidal detachment	tamponades
Cataract	Angle closure
Dislocation of existing	Emulsification of silicone oil
intraocular lens	Ghost cell formation
Corneal decompensation	Fibrin formation
Corneal epithelial defects or	Ciliary body rotation with
ulceration	buckling
Hypotony	Postoperative steroid
Fibrovascular ingrowth at	administration
sclerotomy	Anterior hyaloid fibrovascular
Endophthalmitis	proliferation
Lid abnormalities	Scleral buckle infection or
Ptosis	extrusion
Lash loss after misplaced	Strabismus
cryotherapy	Anterior segment necrosis
Epiphora	Retinal vascular occlusion
	Optic atrophy

careful examination of the internal aspect of each sclerotomy site at the conclusion of the procedure will identify these breaks and provide the opportunity for management with retinopexy, tamponade, and possibly scleral buckling.[249] Routine scleral buckling (in the absence of retinal breaks) at the conclusion of the procedure is not currently advocated for most vitreoretinal procedures but is arguably of benefit following procedures for removal of an IOFB. Retinal detachment occurring in the early postoperative period may occasionally be managed by an air-fluid exchange with additional photocoagulation to the reattached retina.[187] In other circumstances, recurrent retinal detachment may require additional vitreoretinal surgery with the highest priority given to the identification and closure of open retinal breaks.

Vitreous hemorrhage may occur intraoperatively and usually can be managed by elevation of the infusion bottle height to occlude the bleeding vessel, often in association with diathermy to the vessel. Thrombin has been used for the control of intraoperative hemorrhage at the time of diabetic vitrectomy,[251, 252] but concern over the increased postoperative inflammation observed and possible stimulation of recurrent membranes with

thrombin has limited the attractiveness of this technique. Hyaluronic acid has also been applied to the surface of the retina at the conclusion of vitrectomy in order to prevent postoperative bleeding, but a controlled study indicated no long-term benefit from this maneuver.[257] Postoperative vitreous hemorrhage most commonly occurs after procedures for proliferative diabetic retinopathy, and in this circumstance, management includes observation, with careful ultrasonographic examination to exclude the coexistence of retinal detachment, which would be an indication for prompt intervention. Hemorrhages clear more slowly in the phakic eye than in the pseudophakic or aphakic eye, but many postoperative vitreous hemorrhages will clear with observation alone if given sufficient time. An outpatient air-fluid exchange may also be performed in order to lavage the vitreous cavity, but this represents some additional risk over observation alone.[187] Hemorrhages that do not clear after 3 mo of observation are usually treated with repeat vitrectomy with attention to identifying and treating the site of bleeding intraoperatively.[211] This site may be located in the neovascular proliferations on the iris or retina, or it may be present in fibrovascular ingrowth at the internal aspect of the sclerotomy sites.[250] Photocoagulation or diathermy is added as required.

Neovascularization of the iris and neovascular glaucoma are dreaded complications that typically result after failed vitrectomy for proliferative diabetic retinopathy in association with postoperative retinal detachment.[18, 19, 66–73, 76–80, 82–88, 245–249] Unless prompt intervention can repair the retinal detachment, the eye is usually lost. Iris neovascularization, with or without neovascular glaucoma, can also result from retinal detachment from any cause and may regress following repair of the retinal detachment.[72] In addition, patients with attached retinae, but with severe ischemia in association with proliferative diabetic retinopathy, central retinal vein occlusion, and other diseases, may experience iris neovascularization and neovascular glaucoma. Vitrectomy may be required in order to perform retinal ablation by photocoagulation or cryotherapy, and postoperative retinal ablation may also be helpful in inducing regression of iris neovascularization.[209, 210] In advanced cases, filtration surgery (often with various prosthetic valves)[213] or cyclodestructive procedures (with laser, cryotherapy, and so on)[242, 243] may be performed in an attempt to salvage the eye.

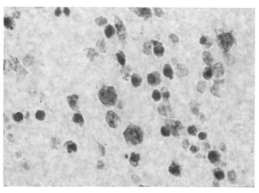

A   B

Figure 100–12. A, Fundus photograph displaying inferior vitreous opacification in a 37-year-old woman with unexplained vitreous cellular infiltrates bilaterally. B, Vitreous biopsy reveals large-cell non-Hodgkin's lymphoma (reticulum cell sarcoma).

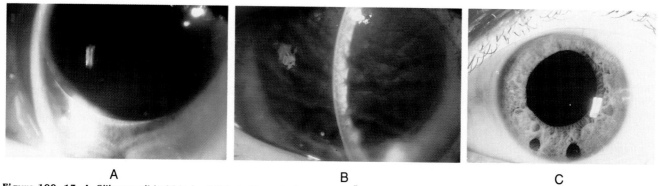

Figure 100–13. *A*, Silicone oil bubble is visible in the anterior chamber and in contact with the endothelium. *B*, Same eye 4 mo later with corneal decompensation and edema. *C*, Inferior peripheral iridectomies used to prevent silicone oil from entering the anterior chamber.

Glaucoma may result from many other mechanisms following vitrectomy.[245, 247, 248, 253–255, 258] Certainly the most common causes of intraocular pressure rise following vitrectomy relate to the use of the various intraocular tamponades. Expanding concentrations of sulfur hexafluoride, perfluoroethane, or perfluoropropane may produce very high pressures with loss of light perception.[183, 254] Particular care must be given in the early postoperative period, as prompt removal of a volume of gas from the eye will reduce the pressure and may restore vision. Pupillary block may also be produced by an intraocular tamponade of any kind; patients with silicone oil in particular require an inferior peripheral iridectomy in order to prevent this complication and to permit aqueous to enter the anterior chamber and preserve corneal clarity.[258] Angle closure may be produced by peripheral anterior synechiae, particularly in eyes with intraocular tamponade and inappropriate supine posturing, or as a result of postoperative mydriatic administration. Fibrin formation, occasionally extreme after vitrectomy for proliferative diabetic retinopathy, may produce pupillary block as well as retinal traction and detachment.[259, 260] In this circumstance, the use of

intraocular tissue plasminogen activator may be helpful in clearing the fibrin; in addition, chilled infusion solutions have also been advocated for prevention of this complication. Recurrent or residual intraocular hemorrhage may result in red blood cell debris or ghost cells with a glaucoma that may respond to medication or may require vitreous washout for control.[253–255] Silicone oil, particularly 1000-centistoke oil, may emulsify over time and produce an intraocular pressure rise, requiring removal.[85, 156, 159, 160, 190, 191, 199] An associated scleral buckle may also produce glaucoma by many means, including the anterior rotation of the ciliary body with tight encircling elements. Finally, postoperative steroid medications are frequently used and may cause a pressure rise in sensitive individuals.

Hypotony may also occur following vitreoretinal surgery. In many cases, the hypotony is a result of failure to reattach the retina, and additional surgery may be effective in restoring the intraocular pressure. However, in other cases, the goal of macular or total retinal reattachment has been achieved, but hypotony is an unwanted accompaniment. This circumstance is notable after surgery for proliferative vitreoretinopa-

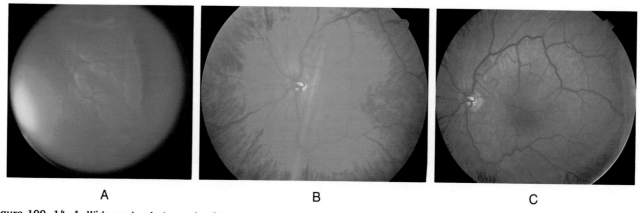

Figure 100–14. *A*, Wide-angle photograph of total retinal detachment caused by two large retinal breaks in the left eye. The breaks extend from the 11 to the 1:30 o'clock positions and from the 1:30 to the 4 o'clock positions, with a small intervening attachment at the 1:30 o'clock position. Visual acuity is 3/200. *B*, Postoperative photograph 4 wk following vitrectomy, scleral buckle, and prone fluid-air exchange. Posterior slippage of the temporal flap may be seen, with a resulting vertical fold through the macula. Visual acuity is 20/70. *C*, Six months later, the macular fold has flattened, but the fovea is inferiorly displaced and there is biomicroscopic evidence of cystoid macular edema. Visual acuity is 20/600.

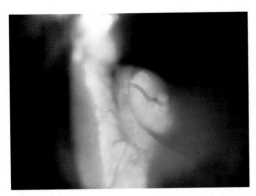

Figure 100–15. Rubeosis and total retinal detachment with retina organized to the iris after failed vitrectomy for traumatic retinal detachment.

thy.[156, 159, 160, 162, 191, 199] It is possibly more common in the subgroup managed with intraocular tamponade with silicone oil. The causes of postoperative hypotony after vitreoretinal surgery include ciliary body detachment, damage, traction, or distortion from the extensive anterior surgery required in these cases but may also include residual retinal detachment or possible generalized ocular dysfunction resulting from numerous surgical procedures. Interestingly, animal studies have demonstrated that large retinotomies do not seem to inherently result in hypotony in otherwise normal eyes,[142] but clinical observations in patients undergoing large retinotomies are inconclusive because of the severity of disease in eyes requiring large retinotomies and the coexistence of other ocular complications that may result in hypotony.[139–141]

Cataract following vitreoretinal surgery results from accidental mechanical injury to the lens or from the untoward physiologic effects of infusion solutions or intraocular tamponades.[54–57, 161, 183, 191, 245–248] Vitreoretinal procedures for removal of epiretinal membrane in the macula (performed in an older patient population) accelerate the development of nuclear sclerotic cataract, perhaps as a consequence of the greater vulnerability of the aged lens to chemical and mechanical trauma.[136–138] The formation of intraoperative cataract in the diabetic

patient may be forestalled by the addition of supplemental glucose to the infusion solution,[58] and minor opacities may clear spontaneously in the postoperative period.[245] Similarly, cataract is produced by prolonged contact of the lens with air or gas, but this may be minimized by prone positioning in the postoperative period in order to bathe the posterior lens in the residual fluid meniscus. Silicone oil will inevitably produce cataract after prolonged contact with the lens (3 mo or longer). It is therefore unsuitable for prolonged tamponade in phakic patients, unless additional lens surgery is planned or unless the life expectancy of the patient is limited, as in the repair of retinal detachment associated with cytomegalovirus retinitis in AIDS patients.[222, 261] In the AIDS patient, the benefits of retaining the lens and phakic vision may outweigh the long-term development of silicone oil cataract, but this situation may change as the life expectancy of this population increases with advances in therapy.

Corneal decompensation may also be the result of mechanical trauma or of contact with infusion solutions or tamponades in a manner similar to that described for the lens. The use of an inferior iridectomy preserves corneal clarity by preventing silicone oil from entering the anterior chamber and contacting the corneal endothelial surface.[258] Diabetic patients have an abnormal corneal surface and are particularly prone to persisting epithelial defects and corneal ulceration. Preservation of corneal clarity and integrity during vitreoretinal surgery is an extremely important aspect of the procedure. Measures to minimize corneal epithelial edema or defects include (1) keeping the cornea moist by closing the lids or covering it with a moistened piece of sponge or other material whenever possible during the procedure, (2) limiting the flow of fluid under the irrigating contact lens (possibly using hyaluronic acid instead of lens infusion fluid), and (3) refraining from removing edematous epithelium if it continues to provide an adequate surgical view. Treatment of a corneal epithelial defect or ulceration in the postoperative period requires specific and immediate care.

Endophthalmitis is an extremely rare complication of vitrectomy.[60, 61] The development of a postoperative

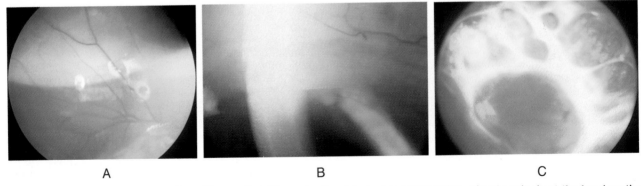

A   B   C

Figure 100–16. *A,* Subretinal emulsified silicone oil visible under the detached superior retina. Visual acuity is at the hand motions level. *B,* Anterior chamber photograph of superior meniscus of emulsified silicone oil. This patient had acute elevation of intraocular pressure, requiring silicone oil removal *C,* Recurrent membranes under silicone oil tamponade after vitreoretinal surgery for retinal detachment with the acute retinal necrosis syndrome in the right eye. The retina is detached, and visual acuity is at the light perception level.

fibrin reaction, particularly in aphakic diabetic eyes with extensive retinopexy and intraocular tamponade, may cause alarm in the postoperative period and may require vitreous biopsy for culture to rule out an infectious cause. A postoperative fibrin reaction will often clear with treatment with topical steroids over 1 to 2 wk, but it may be rapidly dissolved by intracameral injection of tissue plasminogen activator.[259, 260]

Anterior hyaloid fibrovascular proliferation is a striking complication of vitreoretinal surgery for proliferative diabetic retinopathy.[262] In this situation, the appearance of fibrovascular ingrowth along the anterior hyaloid and posterior surface of the lens signals the need for immediate intervention if the eye is to be salvaged, as the fibrovascular proliferation will continue relentlessly in most cases to produce retinal detachment and loss of the eye. At the present time, intervention consists of lens removal, additional vitrectomy, and extensive peripheral retinal ablation.

Choroidal hemorrhage is a potential accompaniment to any ocular procedure, particularly in older or myopic patients and in association with hypotony. Fortunately, it is relatively rare at vitrectomy for most indications, probably because of the closed system and controlled intraocular pressure. However, vitreoretinal surgery for ocular trauma may result in massive choroidal hemorrhage, particularly if a foreign body is embedded in the choroid. Choroidal hemorrhage may be addressed with vitrectomy, as discussed previously.[110, 114–120]

Choroidal detachment may be the result of unintended placement of the infusion cannula tip under the choroid, or it may occur in association with scleral buckling procedures or inflammatory hypotony. The careful placement of the infusion cannula will prevent infusion fluid from detaching the choroid. If this complication is recognized promptly, the replacement of the cannula into the vitreous, coupled with continued infusion of saline solution or air and a scleral incision over the choroidal detachment, may permit drainage of the choroidal detachment and allow the surgery to continue. Postoperative choroidal detachment is usually associated with encircling or high scleral buckles.

Retinal vascular occlusion may be produced by extreme elevation of intraocular pressure by any means, and this is most likely to occur with expanding intraocular tamponades, pupillary block with tamponades, or extensive scleral buckling procedures. If unrelieved, this will result in permanent optic atrophy. Rapid reduction of intraocular pressure may restore vascular perfusion. Permanent vascular occlusion may be produced by inaccurately placed photocoagulation or diathermy to a major retinal vessel. Optic atrophy—a final consequence of uncontrolled glaucoma or unrelieved retinal vascular occlusion—may also result from the placement of transvitreal diathermy on neovascular proliferations on the surface of the optic disc. This problem is more likely to occur with the use of separate diathermy clips as compared with unimanual bipolar diathermy probes.

Associated scleral buckling procedures are capable of producing many of the same complications already described; the complications of scleral buckling are discussed in Chapter 98. In association with vitrectomy, therefore, the placement or alteration of buckling material or manipulation of the extraocular muscles may produce strabismus, anterior segment necrosis, or postoperative infection or extrusion of scleral buckling materials.

REFERENCES

1. Kasner D, Miller GR, Taylor WH, et al: Surgical treatment of amyloidosis of the vitreous. Trans Am Acad Ophthalmol Otolaryngol 72:410–418, 1968.
2. Machemer R, Buettner H, Norton EWD, Parel JM: Vitrectomy: A pars plana approach. Trans Am Acad Ophthalmol Otolaryngol 75:813–820, 1971.
3. Machemer R, Buettner H, Parel JM: A new concept for vitreous surgery. 1. Instrumentation. Am J Ophthalmol 73:1–7, 1972.
4. Machemer R: A new concept for vitreous surgery. 2. Surgical technique and complications. Am J Ophthalmol 74:1022–1033, 1972.
5. Machemer R, Norton EWD: A new concept for vitreous surgery. 3. Indications and results. Am J Ophthalmol 74:1034–1056, 1972.
6. O'Malley C, Heintz RM: Vitrectomy via the pars plana: A new instrument system. Trans Pac Coast Otoophthalmol Soc 53:121–137, 1972.
7. Parel J-M, Machemer R, Aumayr W: A new concept for vitreous surgery. 4. Improvements in instrumentation and illumination. Am J Ophthalmol 77:6–12, 1974.
8. Kloti R: Vitrektomie. I: Ein neues instrument für die hintere Vitrektomie. Graefes Arch Clin Exp Ophthalmol 187:161–170, 1973.
9. Parel J-M, Machemer R, Aumayr W: A new concept for vitreous surgery. 5. An automated operating microscope. Am J Ophthalmol 77:161–168, 1977.
10. Machemer R: A new concept for vitreous surgery. 6. Anesthesia and improvements in surgical techniques. Arch Ophthalmol 92:402–406, 1974.
11. Machemer R: A new concept for vitreous surgery. 7. Two instrument techniques in pars plana vitrectomy. Arch Ophthalmol 92:407–412, 1974.
12. Aaberg TM, Machemer R: Vitreous band surgery: Instrumentation and technique. Arch Ophthalmol 87:542–544, 1972.
13. Charles S, Wang C: A linear suction control for the vitreous cutter (ocutome). Arch Ophthalmol 99:1613, 1981.
14. Schepens CL: Clinical and research aspects of subtotal open sky vitrectomy. XXXVII Edward Jackson Memorial Lecture. Am J Ophthalmol 91:143–171, 1981.
15. Tolentino FI, Banko A, Schepens CL, et al: Vitreous surgery. XII. New instrumentation for vitrectomy. Arch Ophthalmol 93:667–672, 1975.
16. Douvas NG: The cataract roto-extractor. Trans Am Acad Ophthalmol Otolaryngol 77:792–800, 1972.
17. Machemer R, Hickingbotham D: The three-port microcannular system for closed vitrectomy. Am J Ophthalmol 100:590–592, 1985.
18. Michels RG, Ryan SJ: Results and complications of 100 consecutive cases of pars plana vitrectomy. Am J Ophthalmol 80:24–29, 1975.
19. Peyman GA, Huamonte FU, Goldberg MF: One hundred consecutive pars plana vitrectomies using the vitrophage. Am J Ophthalmol 81:263–271, 1976.
20. Parel J-M, Machemer R: Steam-sterilizable fundus contact lenses. Arch Ophthalmol 99:151, 1981.
21. De Juan E, Landers MB III, Hickingbotham D: An improved contact-lens holder for vitreous surgery. Am J Ophthalmol 99:213, 1985.
22. Landers MB, Foulks GN, Landers DM, et al: Temporary keratoprosthesis for use during pars plana vitrectomy. Am J Ophthalmol 91:615–619, 1981.
23. Eckardt C: A new temporary keratoprosthesis for pars plana vitrectomy. Retina 7:34–37, 1987.
24. Spitznas M, Reiner J: A stereoscopic diagonal inverter (SDI) for wide-angle vitreous surgery. Graefes Arch Clin Exp Ophthalmol 225:9–12, 1987.

25. Spitznas M: A binocular indirect ophthalmomicroscope (BIOM) for non-contact wide-angle vitreous surgery. Graefes Arch Clin Exp Ophthalmol 225:13–15, 1987.
26. Charles S, Wang C: A motorized gas injector for vitreous surgery. Arch Ophthalmol 99:1398, 1981.
27. Hueneke RL, Aaberg TM: Instrumentation for continuous fluid-air exchange during vitreous surgery. Am J Ophthalmol 96:547–548, 1983.
28. Zivojnovic R, Vijfvinkel GJ: A modified flute needle. Am J Ophthalmol 96:548–549, 1983.
29. Flynn HW Jr, Blumenkranz MS, Parel J-M, Lee WG: Cannulated subretinal fluid aspirator for vitreoretinal surgery. Am J Ophthalmol 103:106–108, 1987.
30. Charles S, Wang C: Pneumatic intraocular microscissors. Arch Ophthalmol 99:1251, 1981.
31. Charles S, White J, Dennison C, Eichenbaum D: Bimanual bipolar intraocular diathermy. Am J Ophthalmol 81:101–102, 1976.
32. Machemer R: Transvitreal radiofrequency diathermy. Am J Ophthalmol 83:282, 1977.
33. Schepens CL, Delori F, Rogers FJ, Constable IJ: Optimized underwater diathermy for vitreous surgery. Ophthalmic Surg 6:82–89, 1975.
34. Parel J-M, O'Grady GE, Machemer R: A bipolar coaxial microprobe for safe transvitreal diathermy. Arch Ophthalmol 99:494–497, 1981.
35. Machemer R, Parel J-M, Hickingbotham D, Nose I: Membrane peeler cutter; automated vitreous scissors and hooked needle. Arch Ophthalmol 99:152–153, 1981.
36. Coleman DJ, Orcutt D: A lighted irrigator for vitrectomy. Am J Ophthalmol 95:565–566, 1983.
37. Gonvers M: A new silicone oil pump. Am J Ophthalmol 99:210, 1985.
38. Olk RJ, Escoffery RF: Modified vitreoretinal pics and spatulas. Am J Ophthalmol 99:608–609, 1985.
39. Rappazzo JA, Michels RG: New system of intraocular instruments. I. Guillotine intraocular forceps. Arch Ophthalmol 101:814–815, 1983.
40. Crock GW, Janakiraman P, Reddy P: Intraocular magnet of Parel. Br J Ophthalmol 70:879–885, 1986.
41. Charles S: Endophotocoagulation. Retina 1:117–120, 1981.
42. Parke DW II, Aaberg TM: Intraocular argon laser photocoagulation in the management of severe proliferative vitreoretinopathy. Am J Ophthalmol 97:434–443, 1984.
43. Friberg TR, Eller AW: Pneumatic repair of primary and secondary retinal detachments using a binocular indirect ophthalmoscope laser delivery system. Ophthalmology 95:187–193, 1988.
44. Mizuno K, Takaku Y: Dual delivery system for argon laser photocoagulation: Improved techniques of the binocular indirect argon laser photocoagulator. Arch Ophthalmol 101:648–652, 1983.
45. Peyman GA, Salzano TC, Green JL Jr: Argon endolaser. Arch Ophthalmol 99:2037–2038, 1981.
46. Fleischman JA, Swartz M, Dixon JA: Argon laser endophotocoagulation: An intraoperative trans–pars plana technique. Arch Ophthalmol 99:1610–1612, 1981.
47. Landers MB III, Trese MT, Stefansson E, Bessler M: Argon laser intraocular photocoagulation. Ophthalmology 89:785–788, 1982.
48. Ando F, Kondo J: A plastic tack for the treatment of retinal detachment with giant tear. Am J Ophthalmol 95:260–261, 1983.
49. Abrams GW, Williams GA, Neuwirth J, McDonald HR: Clinical results of titanium retinal tacks with pneumatic insertion. Am J Ophthalmol 102:13–19, 1986.
50. Federman JL, Shakin JL, Lanning KC: The microsurgical management of giant retinal tears with trans-scleral sutures. Ophthalmology 89:832–839, 1982.
51. Eckardt C: Pupillary stretching: A new procedure in vitreous surgery. Retina 5:235–238, 1985.
52. Chin GN, Almquist HT: Bupivacaine and lidocaine retrobulbar anesthesia: A double-blind clinical study. Ophthalmology 90:369–372, 1983.
53. Wolf GL, Capuano C, Hartung J: Effect of nitrous oxide on gas bubble volume in the anterior chamber. Arch Ophthalmol 103:418–419, 1985.
54. Edelhauser HF, Van Horn DL, Schultz RO, Hyndiuk RA: Comparative toxicity of intraocular irrigating solutions on the corneal epithelium. Am J Ophthalmol 81:473–481, 1976.
55. Benson WE, Diamond JG, Tasman W: Intraocular irrigating solutions for pars plana vitrectomy: A prospective, randomized, double-blind study. Arch Ophthalmol 99:1013–1015, 1981.
56. Christianson JM, Kollarits CR, Fukui H, et al: Intraocular irrigating solutions and lens clarity. Am J Ophthalmol 82:594–597, 1976.
57. Rosenfeld SI, Waltman SR, Olk RJ, Gordon M: Comparison of intraocular irrigating solutions in pars plana vitrectomy. Ophthalmology 93:109–115, 1986.
58. Haimann MH, Abrams GW: Prevention of lens opacification during diabetic vitrectomy. Ophthalmology 91:116–121, 1984.
59. Jaffe NS: Cataract Surgery and Its Complications. St Louis, CV Mosby, 1984, p 74.
60. Ho PC, Tolentino F: Bacterial endophthalmitis after closed vitrectomy. Arch Ophthalmol 102:207–210, 1984.
61. Kattan HM, Flynn HW Jr, Pflugfelder SC, et al: Nosocomial endophthalmitis survey. Current incidence of infection after intraocular surgery. Ophthalmology 98:227–238, 1991.
62. Levin MR, D'Amico DJ: Diagnosis and management of traumatic endophthalmitis. In Shingleton B, Hersh P, Kenyon K (eds): Ocular Trauma. St Louis, Mosby–Year Book, 1991, pp 242–252.
63. Blankenship GW: Endophthalmitis after pars plana vitrectomy. Am J Ophthalmol 84:815–817, 1977.
64. Michels RG, Rice TA, Rice EF: Vitrectomy for diabetic vitreous hemorrhage. Am J Ophthalmol 95:12–21, 1983.
65. Peyman GA, Huamonte FU, Goldberg MF, et al: Four hundred consecutive pars plana vitrectomies using the vitrophage. Arch Ophthalmol 96:45–50, 1978.
66. Blankenship G: Pars plana vitrectomy for diabetic retinopathy: A report of eight years' experience. Mod Probl Ophthalmol 20:376–386, 1979.
67. Machemer R, Blankenship G: Vitrectomy for proliferative diabetic retinopathy associated with vitreous hemorrhage. Ophthalmology 88:643–646, 1981.
68. Diabetic Retinopathy Vitrectomy Study Research Group: Early vitrectomy for severe vitreous hemorrhage in diabetic retinopathy: Two-year results of a randomized trial. Diabetic Retinopathy Vitrectomy Study Report 2. Arch Ophthalmol 103:1644–1652, 1985.
69. Diabetic Retinopathy Vitrectomy Study Research Group: Early vitrectomy for severe vitreous hemorrhage in diabetic retinopathy: Four-year results of a randomized trial. Diabetic Retinopathy Vitrectomy Study Report 5. Arch Ophthalmol 108:958–964, 1990.
70. Thompson JT, de Bustros S, Michels RG, Rice TA: Results and prognostic factors in vitrectomy for diabetic vitreous hemorrhage. Arch Ophthalmol 105:191–195, 1987.
71. Mandelcorn MS, Blankenship G, Machemer R: Pars plana vitrectomy for the management of severe diabetic retinopathy. Am J Ophthalmol 81:561–570, 1976.
72. Blankenship G: Preoperative iris rubeosis and diabetic vitrectomy results. Ophthalmology 87:176–182, 1980.
73. Scuderi J, Blumenkranz M, Blankenship G: Regression of diabetic rubeosis iridis following successful surgical reattachment of the retina by vitrectomy. Retina 2:193–196, 1982.
74. Ramsay RC, Knobloch WH, Cantrill HL: Timing of vitrectomy for active proliferative diabetic retinopathy. Ophthalmology 93:283–289, 1986.
75. D'Amico DJ: Diabetic traction retinal detachments threatening the fovea and panretinal argon laser photocoagulation. Semin Ophthalmol 6:11–18, 1991.
76. Michels RG: Vitrectomy for complications of diabetic retinopathy. Arch Ophthalmol 96:237–246, 1978.
77. Rice TA, Michels RG, Rice EF: Vitrectomy for diabetic traction retinal detachment involving the macula. Am J Ophthalmol 95:22–33, 1985.
78. Hutton WL, Bernstein I, Fuller D: Diabetic traction retinal detachment: Factors influencing final visual acuity. Ophthalmology 87:1071–1077, 1980.
79. Michels RG: Proliferative diabetic retinopathy: Pathophysiology of extraretinal complications and principles of vitreous surgery. Retina 1:1–17, 1981.

80. Aaberg TM: Pars plana vitrectomy for diabetic traction retinal detachment. Ophthalmology 88:639–642, 1981.
81. Charles S, Flinn CE: The natural history of diabetic extramacular traction retinal detachment. Arch Ophthalmol 99:66–68, 1981.
82. Tolentino FI, Freeman HM, Tolentino FL: Closed vitrectomy in the management of diabetic traction retinal detachment. Ophthalmology 87:1078–1089, 1980.
83. Thompson JT, deBustros S, Michels RG, Rice TA: Results and prognostic factors in vitrectomy for diabetic traction retinal detachment of the macula. Arch Ophthalmol 105:497–502, 1987.
84. Barrie T, Feretis E, Leaver P, McLeod D: Closed microsurgery for diabetic traction macular detachment. Br J Ophthalmol 66:754–758, 1982.
85. Heimann K, Dahl B, Dimopoulos S, Lemmen KD: Pars plana vitrectomy and silicone oil injection in proliferative diabetic retinopathy. Graefes Arch Clin Exp Ophthalmol 227:152–156, 1989.
86. Blankenship G, Cortez R, Machemer R: The lens and pars plana vitrectomy for diabetic retinopathy complications. Arch Ophthalmol 97:1263–1267, 1979.
87. Rice TA, Michels RG, Maguire MG, Rice EF: The effect of lensectomy on the incidence of iris neovascularization and neovascular glaucoma after vitrectomy for diabetic retinopathy. Am J Ophthalmol 95:1–11, 1983.
88. Blankenship GW: The lens influence on diabetic vitrectomy results: Report of a prospective randomized study. Arch Ophthalmol 98:2196–2198, 1980.
89. Benson WE, Blankenship GW, Machemer R: Pars plana lens removal with vitrectomy. Am J Ophthalmol 84:150–152, 1977.
90. Koenig SB, Han DP, Mieler WF, et al: Combined phacoemulsification and pars plana vitrectomy. Arch Ophthalmol 108:362–364, 1990.
91. Blankenship GW, Flynn HW, Kokame GT: Posterior chamber intraocular lens insertion during pars plana lensectomy and vitrectomy for complications of proliferative diabetic retinopathy. Am J Ophthalmol 108:1–5, 1989.
92. Kokame GT, Flynn HW, Blankenship GW: Posterior chamber intraocular lens implantation during diabetic pars plana vitrectomy. Ophthalmology 96:603–610, 1989.
93. Smiddy WE, Isernhagen RD, Michels RG, et al: Vitrectomy for nondiabetic vitreous hemorrhage: Retinal and choroidal vascular disorders. Retina 8:88–95, 1988.
94. Oyakawa RT, Michels RG, Blase WP: Vitrectomy for nondiabetic vitreous hemorrhage. Am J Ophthalmol 96:517–525, 1983.
95. Coles WH, Haik GM: Vitrectomy in intraocular trauma. Arch Ophthalmol 87:621–628, 1972.
96. De Juan E, Sternberg P, Michels RG: Penetrating injuries: Types of injuries and visual results. Ophthalmology 90:1318–1322, 1983.
97. Isernhagen RD, Smiddy WE, Michels RG, et al: Vitrectomy for non-diabetic vitreous hemorrhage. Not associated with vascular disease. Retina 8:81–87, 1988.
98. Morgan CM, D'Amico DJ: Vitrectomy surgery in proliferative sickle retinopathy. Am J Ophthalmol 104:133–138, 1987.
99. Pulido JS, Flynn HW Jr, Clarkson JG, Blankenship GW: Pars plana vitrectomy in the management of complications of proliferative sickle retinopathy. Arch Ophthalmol 106:1553–1557, 1988.
100. Schultz PN, Sobol WM, Weingeist TA: Long-term visual outcome in Terson syndrome. Ophthalmology 98:1814–1819, 1991.
101. Clarkson JG, Flynn HW Jr, Daily MJ: Vitrectomy in Terson's syndrome. Am J Ophthalmol 90:549–552, 1980.
102. Krieger AE, Haidt SJ: Vitreous hemorrhage in senile macular degeneration. Retina 3:318–321, 1983.
103. Tani PM, Buettner H, Robertson DM: Massive vitreous hemorrhage and senile macular choroidal degeneration. Am J Ophthalmol 90:525–533, 1980.
104. Irvine AR, Char DH: Recurrent amyloid involvement of the vitreous body after vitrectomy. Am J Ophthalmol 82:704–708, 1976.
105. Savage DJ, Mango CA, Streeten BW: Amyloidosis of the vitreous: Fluorescein angiographic findings and association with neovascularization. Arch Ophthalmol 100:1776–1779, 1982.
106. Karr DJ, Scott WE: Visual acuity results following treatment of persistent hyperplastic primary vitreous. Arch Ophthalmol 104:662–667, 1986.
107. Feist RM, Morris RE, Witherspoon CD, et al: Vitrectomy in asteroid hyalosis. Retina 10:173–177, 1990.
108. Renaldo DP: Pars plana vitrectomy for asteroid hyalosis. Retina 1:252–254, 1981.
109. Lambrou FH Jr, Sternberg P Jr, Meredith TA, et al: Vitrectomy when asteroid hyalosis prevents laser photocoagulation. Ophthalmic Surg 20:100–102, 1989.
110. Brinton GS, Aaberg TM, Reeser FH, et al: Surgical results in ocular trauma involving the posterior segment. Am J Ophthalmol 94:271–278, 1982.
111. Michels RG: Surgical management of nonmagnetic intraocular foreign bodies. Arch Ophthalmol 93:1003–1006, 1975.
112. Slusher MM, Sarin LK, Federman JL: Management of intraretinal foreign bodies. Ophthalmology 89:369–373, 1982.
113. Hutton WL, Snyder WB, Vaiser A: Surgical removal of nonmagnetic foreign bodies. Am J Ophthalmol 80:838–843, 1975.
114. Ryan SJ, Allen AW: Pars plana vitrectomy in ocular trauma. Am J Ophthalmol 88:483–491, 1979.
115. Sternberg P, de Juan E, Michels RG: Multivariate analysis of prognostic factors in penetrating ocular injuries. Am J Ophthalmol 98:467–472, 1984.
116. Hutton WL, Fuller DG: Factors influencing final visual results in severely injured eyes. Am J Ophthalmol 97:715–722, 1984.
117. Shock JP, Adams D: Long-term visual acuity results after penetrating ocular injuries. Am J Ophthalmol 100:714–718, 1985.
118. Han DP, Mieler WF, Schwartz DM, Abrams GW: Management of traumatic hemorrhagic retinal detachment with pars plana vitrectomy. Arch Ophthalmol 108:1281–1286, 1990.
119. Wade EC, Flynn HW Jr, Olsen KR, et al: Subretinal hemorrhage management by pars plana vitrectomy and internal drainage. Arch Ophthalmol 108:973–978, 1990.
120. Lambrou FH Jr, Meredith TA, Kaplan HJ: Secondary surgical management of expulsive choroidal hemorrhage. Arch Ophthalmol 105:1195–1198, 1987.
121. Smiddy WE, Flynn HW Jr: Management of dislocated posterior chamber intraocular lenses. Ophthalmology 98:889–894, 1991.
122. Campo RV, Chung KD, Oyakawa RT: Pars plana vitrectomy in the management of dislocated posterior chamber intraocular lenses. Am J Ophthalmol 108:529–534, 1989.
123. Maguire AM, Blumenkranz MS, Ward TG, Winkelman JZ: Scleral loop fixation for posteriorly dislocated intraocular lenses: Operative technique and long-term results. Arch Ophthalmol 109:1754–1758, 1991.
124. Shapiro MJ, Resnick KI, Kim SH: Management of the dislocated crystalline lens with a perfluorocarbon liquid. Am J Ophthalmol 112:401–405, 1991.
125. Fastenberg DM, Schwartz PL, Shakin JL, Golub BM: Management of dislocated nuclear fragments after phacoemulsification. Am J Ophthalmol 112:535–539, 1991.
126. Hutton WL, Snyder WB, Vaiser A: Management of surgically dislocated intravitreal lens fragments by pars plana vitrectomy. Ophthalmology 85:175–189, 1978.
127. Blodi BA, Flynn HW Jr, Blodi CF, et al: Retained nuclei after cataract surgery. Ophthalmology 99:41–44, 1992.
128. Luger MHA, Stilma JS, Ringens PJ, van Baarlen J: In toto removal of subretinal Cysticercus cellulosae by pars plana vitrectomy. Br J Ophthalmol 75:561–563, 1991.
129. Hutton WL, Vaiser A, Snyder WB: Pars plana vitrectomy for removal of intravitreous Cysticercus. Am J Ophthalmol 81:571–573, 1976.
130. Steinmetz RL, Masket S, Sidikaro Y: The successful removal of a subretinal Cysticercus by pars plana vitrectomy. Retina 9:276–280, 1989.
131. Gass JDM, Norton EWD: Cystoid macular edema and papilledema following cataract extraction. Arch Ophthalmol 76:646–661, 1966.
132. Gass JDM, Norton EWD: Follow-up study of cystoid macular edema following cataract extraction. Trans Am Acad Ophthalmol Otolaryngol 73:665–682, 1969.
133. Bradford JD, Wilkinson CP, Bradford RH: Cystoid macular edema following extracapsular cataract extraction and posterior chamber intraocular lens implantation. Retina 8:161–164, 1988.
134. Fung WE: Vitrectomy-ACME Study Group: Vitrectomy for chronic aphakic cystoid macular edema. Results of a national, collaborative, prospective, randomized investigation. Ophthalmology 92:1102–1111, 1985.

135. Wilkinson CP, Rowsey JJ: Closed vitrectomy for the vitreous touch syndrome. Am J Ophthalmol 90:304–308, 1980.
136. Michels RG: Vitrectomy for macular pucker. Ophthalmology 91:1384–1388, 1984.
137. Margherio RR, Cox MS Jr, Trese MT, et al: Removal of epimacular membranes. Ophthalmology 92:1075–1083, 1985.
138. Pesin SR, Olk RJ, Grand MG, et al: Vitrectomy for premacular fibroplasia: Prognostic factors, long-term follow-up and time course of visual improvement. Ophthalmology 98:1109–1114, 1991.
139. Machemer R: Retinotomy. Am J Ophthalmol 92:768–774, 1981.
140. Machemer R, McCuen BW, de Juan E: Relaxing retinotomies and retinectomies. Am J Ophthalmol 102:7–12, 1986.
141. Han DP, Lewis MT, Kuhn EM, et al: Relaxing retinotomies and retinectomies: Surgical results and predictors of visual outcome. Arch Ophthalmol 108:694–697, 1990.
142. Hutchins RK, D'Amico DJ, Casey V-NJ, Morin B: Experimental retinectomy in the rabbit. Retina 10:72–77, 1990.
143. Foos RY, Simons KB: Vitreous in lattice degeneration of retina. Ophthalmology 91:452–457, 1984.
144. Javitt JC, Vitale S, Canner JK, et al: National outcomes of cataract extraction. I. Retinal detachment after inpatient surgery. Ophthalmology 98:895–902, 1991.
145. Escoffery RF, Olk RJ, Grand MG, Boniuk I: Vitrectomy without scleral buckling for primary rhegmatogenous retinal detachment. Am J Ophthalmol 99:275–281, 1985.
146. Blankenship GW: Posterior retinal holes secondary to diabetic retinopathy. Arch Ophthalmol 101:885–887, 1983.
147. Ryan SJ: The pathophysiology of proliferative vitreoretinopathy in its management. Am J Ophthalmol 100:188–193, 1985.
148. Sternberg P, Machemer R: Subretinal proliferation. Am J Ophthalmol 98:456–462, 1984.
149. Wallyn RH, Hilton GF: Subretinal fibrosis in retinal detachment. Arch Ophthalmol 97:2128–2129, 1979.
150. Van Horn DL, Aaberg TM, Machemer R, Fenzl R: Glial cell proliferation in human retinal detachment with massive periretinal proliferation. Am J Ophthalmol 84:383–393, 1977.
151. Gass JDM: Idiopathic senile macular hole: Its early stages and pathogenesis. Arch Ophthalmol 166:629–639, 1988.
152. Gass JDM, Joondeph BC: Observations concerning patients with suspected impending macular holes. Am J Ophthalmol 109:638–646, 1990.
153. Machemer R: Massive periretinal proliferation. A logical approach to therapy. Trans Am Ophthalmol Soc 75:556–586, 1977.
154. Machemer R, Aaberg TM, Freeman HM, et al: An updated classification of retinal detachment with proliferative vitreoretinopathy. Am J Ophthalmol 112:159–165, 1991.
155. Lewis H, Aaberg TM, Abrams GW, et al: Subretinal membranes in proliferative vitreoretinopathy. Ophthalmology 96:1403–1415, 1989.
156. Cox MS, Trese MT, Murphy PL: Silicone oil for advanced proliferative vitreoretinopathy. Ophthalmology 93:646–650, 1986.
157. Ratner CM, Michels RG, Auer C, Rice TA: Pars plana vitrectomy for complicated retinal detachments. Ophthalmology 90:1323–1327, 1983.
158. Sternberg P, Machemer R: Results of conventional surgery for proliferative vitreoretinopathy. Am J Ophthalmol 100:141–146, 1985.
159. Gonvers M: Temporary silicone oil tamponade in the management of retinal detachment with proliferative vitreoretinopathy. Am J Ophthalmol 100:239–245, 1985.
160. Grey RHB, Leaver PK: Silicone oil in the treatment of massive periretinal preretinal retraction. I. Results in 105 eyes. Br J Ophthalmol 63:355–360, 1979.
161. Chang S, Coleman DJ, Lincoff H, et al: Perfluoropropane gas in the management of proliferative vitreoretinopathy. Am J Ophthalmol 98:180–188, 1984.
162. Lean JS, Leaver PK, Cooling RJ, McLeod D: Management of complex retinal detachments by vitrectomy and fluid-silicone exchange. Trans Ophthalmol Soc UK 102:203–205, 1982.
163. Scott JD: The treatment of massive vitreous retraction by the separation of pre-retinal membranes using liquid silicone. Mod Probl Ophthalmol 15:285–290, 1975.
164. Smiddy WE, Michels RG, Glaser BM, de Bustros S: Vitrectomy for impending macular holes. Am J Ophthalmol 105:371–376, 1988.
165. Johnson RN, Gass JDM: Idiopathic macular holes: Observations, stages of formation, and implications for surgical intervention. Ophthalmology 95:917–924, 1988.
166. Kelly NE, Wendel RT: Vitreous surgery for idiopathic macular holes: Results of a pilot study. Arch Ophthalmol 109:654–659, 1991.
167. Haut J, Seigle P, Larricart P, Flamand M: Subtotal circular retinectomy and semicircular inferior retinotomy: Preliminary report. Ophthalmologica 191:65–74, 1985.
168. Haut J, Monin C, Larricart P, et al: Study of a new series of large relaxing retinotomies. Ophthalmologica 198:35–39, 1989.
169. Federman JL, Eagle RC Jr: Extensive peripheral retinectomy combined with posterior 360° retinotomy for retinal reattachment in advanced proliferative vitreoretinopathy cases. Ophthalmology 97:1305–1320, 1990.
170. Lindner K: Shortening of the eyeball for retinal detachment. Arch Ophthalmol 42:634–645, 1949.
171. Machemer R: Vitrectomy: A Pars Plana Approach. New York, Grune & Stratton, 1975, pp 1–131.
172. Abrams GW, Williams GA: "En bloc" excision of diabetic membranes. Am J Ophthalmol 103:302–308, 1987.
173. Williams DF, Williams GA, Hartz A, et al: Results of vitrectomy for diabetic traction retinal detachments using the en bloc excision technique. Ophthalmology 96:752–758, 1989.
174. Michels RG, Stark WJ, Stirpe M (eds): Sodium Hyaluronate in Anterior and Posterior Segment Surgery. Padova, Italy, Liviana Press, 1989.
175. Sheta SM, Hida T, McCuen BW: Cyanoacrylate tissue adhesive in the management of recurrent retinal detachment caused by macular hole. Am J Ophthalmol 109:28–32, 1990.
176. McCuen BW II, Hida T, Sheta SM: Transvitreal cyanoacrylate retinopexy in the management of complicated retinal detachment. Am J Ophthalmol 104:127–132, 1987.
177. Gilbert CE: Adhesives in retinal detachment surgery. Br J Ophthalmol 75:309–310, 1991.
178. Charles S: Vitreous Microsurgery, 2nd ed. Baltimore, Williams & Wilkins, 1987, pp 89–92, 140–141, 161.
179. Rosengren B: Results of treatment of detachment of the retina with diathermy and injection of air into the vitreous. Acta Ophthalmol 16:573–579, 1938.
180. Norton EWD: Intraocular gas in the management of selected retinal detachments. Trans Am Acad Ophthalmol Otolaryngol 77:85–98, 1973.
181. Cibis PA, Becker B, Okun E, Canaan S: The use of liquid silicone oil in retinal detachment surgery. Arch Ophthalmol 68:590–599, 1962.
182. Lincoff H, Coleman J, Kreissig I, et al: The perfluorocarbon gases in the treatment of retinal detachment. Ophthalmology 90:546–551, 1983.
183. Sabates WI, Abrams GW, Swanson DE, Norton EWD: The use of intraocular gases: The results of sulfur hexafluoride in retinal detachment surgery. Ophthalmology 88:447–454, 1981.
184. Chang S, Lincoff HA, Coleman DJ, et al: Perfluorocarbon gases in vitreous surgery. Ophthalmology 92:651–656, 1985.
185. Lincoff A, Haft D, Liggett P, Reifer C: Intravitreal expansion of perfluorocarbon bubbles. Arch Ophthalmol 98:1646, 1980.
186. Gardner TW, Norris JL, Zakov JL: A survey of intraocular gas use in North America. Arch Ophthalmol 106:1188–1189, 1988.
187. Blumenkranz M, Gardner T, Blankenship G: Fluid-gas exchange and photocoagulation after vitrectomy: Indications, technique, and results. Arch Ophthalmol 104:291–296, 1986.
188. Lincoff H, Mardirossian J, Lincoff A, et al: Intravitreal longevity of three perfluorocarbon gases. Arch Ophthalmol 98:1610–1611, 1980.
189. Peters MA, Abrams GW, Hamilton LH, et al: The nonexpansile, equilibrated concentration of perfluoropropane gas in the eye. Am J Ophthalmol 100:831–839, 1985.
190. Gabel V-P, Kampik A, Gabel CH: Silicone oil with a high specific gravity for intraocular use. Br J Ophthalmol 71:262–267, 1987.
191. Lucke KH, Foerster MH, Laqua H: Long-term results of vitrectomy and silicone oil in 500 cases of complicated retinal detachments. Am J Ophthalmol 104:624–633, 1987.

192. Hilton GF, Grizzard WS: Pneumatic retinopexy: A two-step outpatient operation without conjunctival incision. Ophthalmology 93:626–641, 1986.
193. Tornambe PE, Hilton GF, Brinton DA, et al: Pneumatic retinopexy: A two-year follow-up study of the multicenter clinical trial comparing pneumatic retinopexy with scleral buckling. Ophthalmology 98:1115–1123, 1991.
194. Foulds WS, Allan D, Moseley H, Kyle PM: Effect of intravitreal hyaluronidase on the clearance of tritiated water from the vitreous to the choroid. Br J Ophthalmol 69:529–532, 1985.
195. Chang S: Low-viscosity liquid fluorochemicals in vitreous surgery. Am J Ophthalmol 103:38–43, 1987.
196. Nabib M, Peyman GA, Clark LC: Experimental evaluation of perfluorophenanthrene as a high specific gravity vitreous substitute: A preliminary report. Ophthalmic Surg 20:286–293, 1989.
197. Flores-Aguilar M, Crapotta JA, Munguia D, et al: Perfluorooctylbromide (PFOB) as a temporary vitreous substitute. Invest Ophthalmol Vis Sci 32(Suppl):1225, 1991.
198. Michels RG, Rice TA, Blankenship G: Surgical techniques for selected giant retinal tears. Retina 3:139–153, 1983.
199. McCuen BW II, de Juan E Jr, Machemer R: Silicone oil in vitreoretinal surgery. Part I. Surgical techniques. Retina 5:189–197, 1985.
200. Chang S, Lincoff H, Zimmerman NJ, Fuchs W: Giant retinal tears: Surgical techniques and results using perfluorocarbon liquids. Arch Ophthalmol 107:761–766, 1989.
201. Glaser BM, Carter JB, Kuppermann BD, Michels RG: Perfluoro-octane in the treatment of giant retinal tears with proliferative vitreoretinopathy. Ophthalmology 98:1613–1621, 1991.
202. Chang S, Ozmert E, Zimmerman NJ: Intraoperative perfluorocarbon liquids in the management of proliferative vitreoretinopathy. Am J Ophthalmol 106:668–674, 1988.
203. Chang S, Reppucci V, Zimmerman NJ, et al: Perfluorocarbon liquids in the management of traumatic retinal detachments. Ophthalmology 96:785–792, 1989.
204. Schepens CL, Freeman HM, Thompson RF: A power-driven multipositional operating table. Arch Ophthalmol 73:671–673, 1965.
205. Trese MT: An inexpensive bed for giant retinal tear surgery. Am J Ophthalmol 93:525–527, 1982.
206. Peyman GA: A new operating table for the management of giant retinal breaks. Arch Ophthalmol 99:498–499, 1981.
207. Machemer R, Allen AW: Retinal tears 180° and greater: Management with vitrectomy and intravitreal gas. Arch Ophthalmol 94:1340–1348, 1976.
208. Fitzgerald CR: The use of Healon in a case of rolled-over retina. Retina 1:227–231, 1981.
209. Murphy RP, Egbert PR: Regression of iris neovascularization following panretinal photocoagulation. Arch Ophthalmol 97:700–702, 1979.
210. Wand M, Dueker DK, Aiello LM, Grant WM: Effects of panretinal photocoagulation on rubeosis iridis, angle neovascularization, and neovascular glaucoma. Am J Ophthalmol 86:332–339, 1978.
211. Liggett PE, Lean JS, Barlow WE, Ryan SJ: Intraoperative argon endophotocoagulation for recurrent vitreous hemorrhage after vitrectomy for diabetic retinopathy. Am J Ophthalmol 103:146–149, 1987.
212. Pavan PR, Folk JC, Weingeist TA, et al: Diabetic rubeosis and panretinal photocoagulation. A prospective, controlled, masked trial using iris fluorescein angiography. Arch Ophthalmol 101:882–884, 1983.
213. Lloyd MA, Heuer DK, Baerveldt G, et al: Combined Molteno implantation and pars plana vitrectomy for neovascular glaucoma. Ophthalmology 98:1401–1405, 1991.
214. Daily MJ, Gieser RG: Treatment of proliferative diabetic retinopathy with panretinal cryotherapy. Ophthalmic Surg 15:741–745, 1984.
215. Green WR: Diagnostic cytopathology of ocular fluid specimens. Ophthalmology 91:726–749, 1984.
216. Driebe WT, Mandelbaum S, Forster RK, et al: Pseudophakic endophthalmitis: Diagnosis and management. Ophthalmology 93:442–448, 1986.
217. Olson JC, Flynn HW, Forster RK, Culbertson WW: Results in the treatment of postoperative endophthalmitis. Ophthalmology 90:692–699, 1983.
218. Brinton GS, Topping TM, Hyndiuk RA, et al: Posttraumatic endophthalmitis. Arch Ophthalmol 102:547–550, 1984.
219. Pflugfelder SC, Flynn HW Jr, Zwickey TA, et al: Exogenous fungal endophthalmitis. Ophthalmology 95:19–30, 1988.
220. Halperin LS, Roseman RL: Successful treatment of a subretinal abscess in an intravenous drug abuser. Arch Ophthalmol 106:1651–1652, 1988.
221. D'Amico DJ, Talamo JH, Felsenstein D, et al: Ophthalmoscopic and histologic findings in BW-B759U–treated cytomegalovirus retinitis. Arch Ophthalmol 104:1788–1793, 1986.
222. Dugel PU, Liggett PE, Lee MB, et al: Repair of retinal detachment caused by cytomegalovirus retinitis in patients with the acquired immunodeficiency syndrome. Am J Ophthalmol 112:235–242, 1991.
223. Blumenkranz MS, Culbertson WW, Clarkson JG, Dix R: Treatment of the acute retinal necrosis syndrome with intravenous acyclovir. Ophthalmology 93:296–300, 1986.
224. Michels RG, Knox DL, Erozan YS, Green WR: Intraocular reticulum cell sarcoma: Diagnosis by pars plana vitrectomy. Arch Ophthalmol 93:1331–1335, 1975.
225. Case Records of the Massachusetts General Hospital: Histiocytic lymphoma of the eye. N Engl J Med 313:436–443, 1985.
226. Belmont JB, Michelson JB: Vitrectomy in uveitis associated with ankylosing spondylitis. Am J Ophthalmol 94:300–304, 1982.
227. Nobe JR, Kokoris N, Diddie KR, et al: Lensectomy-vitrectomy in chronic uveitis. Retina 3:71–76, 1983.
228. Algvere P, Alanko H, Dickhoff K, et al: Pars plana vitrectomy in the management of intraocular inflammation. Acta Ophthalmol 59:727–736, 1981.
229. Davis JL, Solomon D, Nussenblatt RB, et al: Immunocytochemical staining of vitreous cells: Indications, techniques, and results. Ophthalmology 99:250–256, 1992.
230. Freeman WR, Stern WH, Gross JG, et al: Pathologic observations made by retinal biopsy. Retina 10:195–204, 1992.
231. Chan C-C, Paelstine AG, Davis JL, et al: Role of chorioretinal biopsy in inflammatory eye disease. Ophthalmology 98:1281–1286, 1991.
232. Taylor D, Day S, Tiedemann K, et al: Chorioretinal biopsy in a patient with leukaemia. Br J Ophthalmol 65:489–493, 1981.
233. Destro M, D'Amico DJ, Gragoudas EG, et al: Retinal manifestations of neurofibromatosis: Diagnosis and management. Arch Ophthalmol 109:662–666, 1991.
234. Diamond JG, Kaplan HJ: Uveitis: Effect of vitrectomy combined with lensectomy. Ophthalmology 86:1320–1327, 1979.
235. Coleman DJ: Early vitrectomy in the management of the severely traumatized eye. Am J Ophthalmol 93:543–551, 1982.
236. Hanscom TA, Diddie KR: Early surgical drainage of macular subretinal hemorrhage. Arch Ophthalmol 105:1722–1723, 1987.
237. Vander JF, Federman JL, Greven C, et al: Surgical removal of massive subretinal hemorrhage associated with age-related macular degeneration. Ophthalmology 98:23–27, 1991.
238. Peyman GA, Rednam KVR, Juarez CP: Improvement in eyewall resection technique. Ophthalmic Surg 14:588–590, 1983.
239. De Juan E, Machemer R: Vitreous surgery for hemorrhagic and fibrous complications of age-related macular degeneration. Am J Ophthalmol 105:25–29, 1988.
240. Lambert HM, Capone A, Aaberg TM, et al: Surgical excision of subfoveal neovascular membranes in age-related macular degeneration. Am J Ophthalmol 113:257–262, 1992.
241. Thomas MA, Kaplan HJ: Surgical removal of subfoveal neovascularization in the presumed ocular histoplasmosis syndrome. Am J Ophthalmol 111:1–7, 1991.
242. Pater A, Thompson JT, Michels RG, Quigley HA: Endolaser treatment of the ciliary body for uncontrolled glaucoma. Ophthalmology 93:825–829, 1986.
243. Hampton C, Shields MB, Miller KN, Blasini M: Evaluation of a protocol for transscleral neodymium: YAG cyclophotocoagulation in one hundred patients. Ophthalmology 97:910–917, 1990.
244. Fastenberg DM, Perry HD, Donnenfeld ED, et al: Expulsive choroidal hemorrhage with scleral buckling surgery. Arch Ophthalmol 109:323, 1991.
245. Faulborn J, Conway BP, Machemer R: Surgical complications of pars plana vitreous surgery. Ophthalmology 85:116–125, 1978.
246. Oyakawa RT, Schachat AP, Michels RG, Rice TA: Complications of vitreous surgery for diabetic retinopathy. I. Intraoperative complications. Ophthalmology 90:517–521, 1983.

247. Schachat AP, Oyakawa RT, Michels RG, Rice TA: Complications of vitreous surgery for diabetic retinopathy. II. Postoperative complications. Ophthalmology 90:522–530, 1983.
248. Aaberg TM, Van Horn DL: Late complications of pars plana vitreous surgery. Ophthalmology 85:126–140, 1978.
249. Tardif YM, Schepens CL, Tolentino FI: Vitreous surgery. XIV. Complications from sclerotomy in 89 consecutive cases. Arch Ophthalmol 95:229–234, 1977.
250. Tardif YM, Schepens CL: Closed vitreous surgery. XV. Fibrovascular ingrowth from the pars plana sclerotomy. Arch Ophthalmol 95:235–239, 1977.
251. De Bustros S, Glaser BM, Johnson MA: Thrombin infusion for the control of intraocular bleeding during vitreous surgery. Arch Ophthalmol 103:837–839, 1985.
252. Thompson JT, Glaser BM, Michels RG, de Bustros S: The use of intravitreal thrombin to control hemorrhage during vitrectomy. Ophthalmology 93:279–282, 1986.
253. Campbell DG, Simmons RJ, Grant WM: Ghost cells as a cause of glaucoma. Am J Ophthalmol 81:441–450, 1976.
254. Han DP, Lewis H, Lambrou FH, et al: Mechanisms of intraocular pressure elevation after pars plana vitrectomy. Ophthalmology 96:1357–1362, 1989.
255. Campbell DJ, Simmons RJ, Tolentino FI, McMeel JW: Glaucoma occurring after closed vitrectomy. Am J Ophthalmol 83:63–69, 1977.
256. Sabates NR, Sabates FN, Sabates R, et al: Macular changes after retinal detachment surgery. Am J Ophthalmol 108:22–29, 1989.
257. Packer AJ, McCuen BW, Hutton WL, Ramsay RC: Procoagulant effects of intraocular sodium hyaluronate (Healon) after phakic diabetic vitrectomy: A prospective, randomized study. Ophthalmology 96:1491–1494, 1989.
258. Ando F: Intraocular hypertension resulting from pupillary block by silicone oil. Am J Ophthalmol 99:87–88, 1985.
259. Jaffe GJ, Abrams GW, Williams GA, Han DP: Tissue plasminogen activator for postvitrectomy fibrin formation. Ophthalmology 97:184–189, 1990.
260. Williams GA, Lambrou FH, Jaffe GA, et al: Treatment of postvitrectomy fibrin formation with intraocular tissue plasminogen activator. Arch Ophthalmol 106:1055–1058, 1988.
261. Sidikaro Y, Silver L, Holland GN, Krieger AE: Rhegmatogenous retinal detachments in patients with AIDS and necrotizing retinal infections. Ophthalmology 98:129–135, 1991.
262. Lewis H, Abrams GW, Williams GA: Anterior hyaloidal fibrovascular proliferation after diabetic vitrectomy. Am J Ophthalmol 104:607–613, 1987.

Chapter 101

■

Vitreous Substitutes

JANET R. SPARROW and STANLEY CHANG

The success of surgery for retinal detachment is dependent on attaining closure of a retinal break, relieving traction on the retina by thorough dissection of epiretinal membranes or scleral buckling, or both, and minimizing the recurrence of traction[1]. In complicated forms of retinal detachment, there has been a greater recognition of the pathoanatomic changes in vitreoretinal relationships, and advancements in the surgical instrumentation and techniques have allowed intraoperative reapproximation of the retina to a more normal position. The use of intravitreally injected gaseous and liquid materials as adjunctive agents to vitreoretinal surgery plays a vital role in facilitating retinal reattachment. These materials are used as intraoperative instruments to reestablish intraocular volume, assist in separating membranes adherent to the retina, manipulate retinal detachment, and mechanically flatten detached retina. Over the longer term, intravitreal gases and silicone oil maintain the neural retina in apposition to retinal pigment epithelium postoperatively.

This chapter discusses vitreous substitutes as adjuncts to vitreoretinal surgery and their use both intraoperatively and postoperatively in the management of complicated forms of retinal detachment requiring vitrectomy (Table 101–1). Emphasis is placed on the characteristics of a given vitreous substitute material as they are applied to solving a clinical problem. The benefits, potential drawbacks, and complications related to the use of these agents are summarized. Descriptions of surgical techniques are described when applicable to the use of these agents, but more detailed techniques relating to individual disease processes can be found elsewhere.[2–8]

INTRAOPERATIVE USE OF VITREOUS SUBSTITUTE MATERIALS

During surgery, substances are injected into the vitreous cavity for several purposes. First, the intraocular volume must be restored after drainage of subretinal fluid or vitrectomy. Intravitreally placed materials are also used for their mechanical properties to function as "soft instruments." These liquids assist in separation of

Table 101–1. COMPLICATED RETINAL DETACHMENTS

Retinal detachment associated with proliferative diabetic retinopathy
Retinal detachment complicated by proliferative vitreoretinopathy
Giant retinal tears
Retinal detachment with posterior breaks
Retinal detachment following penetrating trauma
Postvitrectomy retinal detachment
Retinal detachment associated with expulsive choroidal hemorrhage

Table 101–2. VITREOUS SUBSTITUTE MATERIALS USED INTRAOPERATIVELY

Balanced salt solution
Air and other gases
Viscoelastic fluids
Silicone liquid
Low-viscosity perfluorocarbon liquids
Silicone liquid

membranes or in hydrokinetic manipulation of the retina and complement the surgical techniques employed in membrane dissection, such as delamination and retinotomy. Retinal breaks must be closed by laser endophotocoagulation or retinal adhesives. Finally, at the end of the operation, a material of high surface tension is injected to maintain closure of the retinal break until maturation of the chorioretinal adhesion is attained. A variety of gaseous and liquid substances are currently used intraoperatively (Table 101–2).

Balanced Salt Solution

Balanced salt solution (BSS) is used as an irrigation fluid during vitrectomy and is also used to maintain normal intraocular volume and pressure after drainage of subretinal fluid during retinal detachment surgery and after drainage of choroidal detachments. BSS enriched with bicarbonate, dextrose, and glutathione appears to be better tolerated by ocular tissues, especially the corneal endothelium.[9–12] As an intravitreal irrigating solution, the enriched fluid also has the advantage of allowing the maintenance of more normal electroretinographic activity.[13]

Supplemental agents are also occasionally added to the irrigation solution for various purposes. During diabetic vitrectomy, additional glucose in the infusion fluid reduces the development of intraoperative cataract.[14] It is believed that the supplementation with glucose reduces osmotic fluid shifts in the lens resulting from hyperglycemia. Steroids and antibiotics are sometimes added to the infusion solution in endophthalmitis. Epinephrine is added to the infusion to maintain pupillary dilatation. The addition of thrombin may be useful during vitrectomy for controlling intraoperative bleeding.[15, 16]

Studies have shown that infusion fluid cooled to room temperature (22° C) reduces the risk of intraoperative photic light damage to the retina as compared with infusion solution used at body temperature.[17] Furthermore, the use of irrigation fluid at room temperature does not induce postoperative changes in the electroretinogram or the fluorescein angiogram or in retinal morphologic characteristics.[17, 18] Conversely, the value of using infusion solutions cooled to less than room temperature appears to be unclear. Thus, experimental studies have demonstrated that the use of hypothermic (7° C) infusion fluid (BSS) during vitrectomy is associated with less intraoperative bleeding and postoperative inflammation and fibrin than is observed with infusion

fluid at room temperature.[19] Nevertheless, the potential benefits of cooling infusion fluid to less than room temperature should be balanced against studies indicating that extreme intraocular hypothermia (2° C) may also be associated with prolonged reductions in electroretinographic activity, reversible lens opacities, and histologic changes in retina.[20]

Air and Other Gases

Air was the first gas to be employed in retinal surgery.[21] It is used intraoperatively during scleral buckling surgery to restore intraocular volume after drainage of subretinal fluid, to flatten "fish mouth tears" that form of radial folds, and to unroll the posterior flap of large retinal tears. Twenty-four to forty-eight hr after injection of air, only a small bubble remains. Since the effects of air bubble tamponade are seen almost immediately during retinal detachment surgery, the use of gases that disappear even more rapidly, such as the nonexpanding gas xenon, has been proposed.[22, 23] The functions of a gas bubble in promoting retinal reattachment are discussed later in this chapter.

During vitrectomy, the exchange of intravitreal fluid for air is used routinely. If profuse intraoperative bleeding occurs and the view of the retina is obscured, a fluid-air exchange can be helpful to improve visualization of the retina. The air bubble compartmentalizes the blood and may also have a temporary hemostatic effect. To neutralize refractive changes associated with intravitreal air, compensating contact lenses are used.[24–26]

Fluid-air exchange is most often used to flatten a retinal detachment intraoperatively. The high surface tension of the air-retina interface pushes the retina posteriorly as air is continuously infused into the eye. Subretinal fluid is also displaced posteriorly and must be aspirated through a posterior break or retinotomy in order to flatten the retina completely. Once the retina is reattached, endophotocoagulation is applied to the margins of the retinal breaks and retinotomy.

Viscoelastic Fluids

Viscous fluids used in vitreoretinal surgery include solutions of sodium hyaluronate, chondroitin sulfate, or hydroxypropyl methylcellulose. These materials are polymers with molecular weights ranging from approximately 30,000 to 4 million daltons. It is the viscoelastic properties of these materials that make them most useful for intraocular surgery. Thus, at zero shear rate (steady state) these materials exhibit high viscosity, whereas at high shear rates (shearing occurs when a fluid is made to flow) the polymers undergo temporary and reversible deformation (pseudoplastic behavior), with the result that the viscosity of the material decreases.[27] This behavior allows the material to be injected through small-gauge cannulas and yet ensures that the material will regain its shape after injection. Sodium hyaluronate (1 percent; Healon) appears to have the most favorable viscoelastic properties. Its molecular weight is approximately 4 million daltons, with a viscosity greater than 400,000 centistokes at near zero shear. At high shear, the viscosity decreases to approximately 110 centistokes. Sodium hyaluronate has multiple applications as an intraoperative adjunct in vitreoretinal surgery. For instance, during repair of a trauma-related corneal laceration, sodium hyaluronate can be used to reposit uveal tissue and re-form the anterior chamber. The depth of the anterior chamber is maintained throughout the surgery. In penetrating trauma associated with intraocular foreign bodies, sodium hyaluronate can be used to gently separate an embedded foreign body from the retinal surface or choroid.

The viscoelastic properties of sodium hyaluronate can also be helpful in the separation of epiretinal membranes found in proliferative diabetic retinopathy (Fig. 101–1).[28] The term *viscodissection* describes the hydraulic elevation of epiretinal membranes as the fluid is injected into the plane between retina and proliferative tissue. There are several advantages to this approach. First, the membranes are separated from the retinal surface with less trauma, and the remaining attachments can be more easily cut. Second, in proliferative diabetic retinopathy, blood can be displaced so that the planes between membranes and retina can be more easily seen. This approach, however, should be used more cautiously when the retina is atrophic and thin because iatrogenic retinal breaks may develop if too much injection force is applied.

Sodium hyaluronate has also been used to unfold the retina during repair of giant retinal tears and to manage hemorrhage.[4, 29–31] Sodium hyaluronate has a specific gravity only slightly greater than that of saline (1.0084 at 20° C[39]), and as an intraoperative tool it does not exert the force that can be obtained by using a liquid of high specific gravity. It is miscible with water and therefore does not have interfacial properties. Postoperative elevation of intraocular pressure may result if large volumes of sodium hyaluronate are left in the vitreous cavity after surgery.

Low-viscosity Perfluorocarbon Liquids

CHARACTERISTICS OF PERFLUOROCARBON LIQUIDS

Perfluorocarbon liquids have the high density and surface tension properties that make them ideal for intraoperative retinal manipulation in conjunction with vitrectomy. In addition, unlike silicone liquid, these liquids are readily available as low-viscosity fluids (2 to 3 centistokes at 25° C) and thus can be easily injected and aspirated through small-gauge microsurgical instruments. Perfluorocarbon liquids are optically clear and their indices of refraction are slightly dissimilar to saline solution; this property, together with the fact that perfluorocarbon liquids and water are immiscible and thus form separate phases when mixed, results in the perfluorocarbon liquid being seen and readily distinguished from irrigating solution or other fluids. Yet, because the refractive error of the eye is not altered, significant optical aberrations during membrane dissection are not induced, and conventional contact lenses can be used throughout surgery.

The specific gravity of perfluorocarbon liquids (ranging from 1.76 to 2) is almost twice the density of water. Thus, the force exerted by perfluorocarbon liquids against the retina is considerably greater than that exerted by an equivalent volume of silicone or fluorosilicone oil.[32] The interfacial tension of perfluorocarbon liquids with water is roughly equivalent to that of silicone oil, and the material tends to be cohesive, so that liquid remains in one large bubble. Furthermore, the surface tension, although not as pronounced as that of gas, provides some deterrence to passage of perfluorocarbon liquid through a break.

The high stability of the carbon-fluorine bond in a perfluorocarbon liquid can render the liquid virtually inert,[33] and perfluorocompounds composed solely of carbon and fluorine atoms have greater biologic inertness than do fluorocompounds containing heteroatoms such as nitrogen or oxygen. Several low-viscosity per-

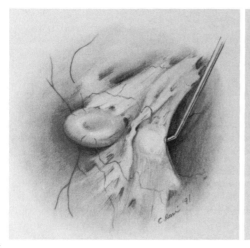
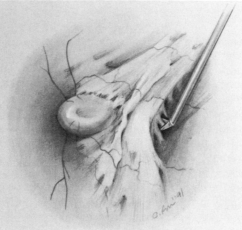

Figure 101–1. The use of sodium hyaluronate during vitreous surgery for proliferative diabetic retinopathy. *Left,* A small cannula is inserted beneath epiretinal membranes, and sodium hyaluronate is injected into the plane between the retina and the membranes to separate the fibrovascular tissue. *Right,* Horizontal cutting scissors are used to cut the remaining attachments between the retina and the epiretinal membranes.

fluorocarbon liquids have been studied for their potential intraoperative use, including perfluorotributylamine ($C_{12}F_{27}N$),[25, 34, 36, 37] perfluorodecalin ($C_{10}F_{18}$),[35-38] perflurophenanthrene ($C_{14}F_{24}$)[39, 40] perflurooethylcyclohexane (C_8F_{16}),[41] foralkyl AC-6,[42] perfluorooctylbromide,[43] and perfluoro-*n*-octane (C_8F_{18}).[35-44] The chemical structures and physical properties of some perfluorocarbon liquids commonly used for vitreoretinal surgery are presented in Figure 101–2 and Table 101–3, respectively. Of the available low-viscosity perfluorocarbon liquids, perfluoro-*n*-octane is preferred by the authors for two reasons. First, it is obtainable as a highly purified compound. Analysis of perfluoro-*n*-octane by nuclear magnetic resonance spectroscopy has shown that the compound does not contain protonated impurities (i.e., hydrogen).[44] The major impurities that could be present in perfluorocarbon liquids are hydrogen-containing and would result from the incomplete fluorination of the hydrocarbon precursor;[45] hydrogen-containing impurities are suspected of causing tissue reactivity.[46] In addition to being free of detectable impurity, this compound can also be manufactured with a uniformity of 99.9 percent; i.e., only 0.1 percent of the liquid may be a perfluorocarbon other than the principal species perfluoro-*n*-octane. Second, perfluoro-*n*-octane is a desirable liquid because it has a relatively lower boiling point and higher vapor pressure than do other perfluorocarbon liquids. Thus, small residual amounts of perfluoro-*n*-octane that remain on the retinal surface will vaporize on exposure to air during fluid-air exchange. Residual droplets of perfluorocarbon liquid, remaining following surgery, have been observed in some patients, although as surgical experience with the liquids accumulates, this occurrence is less likely. Thus far, these droplets have not been known to cause any deleterious effects. Nevertheless, whether these small droplets can affect intraocular proliferation is unknown, and because the potential long-term effects of residual perfluorocarbon liquid are uncertain, these patients are observed closely. Studies aimed at evaluating short-term (48 hr) retinal tolerance to placement of perfluoro-*n*-octane liquid intravitreally have not revealed electrophysiologic changes or morphologic evidence of toxicity.[44] Similarly, electron

Table 101–3. PHYSICAL PROPERTIES OF SOME PERFLUOROCARBON LIQUIDS

	Perfluoro-*n*-octane	Perfluoro-decalin	Perfluoro-phenanthrene
Molecular weight	438	462	624
Specific gravity	1.76	1.94	2.03
Surface tension*	14	16	16
Refractive index	1.27	1.31	1.33
Vapor pressure†	50	13.5	<1
Viscosity‡	0.8	2.7	8.03

*dyne/cm at 25°C.
†mmHg at 37°C.
‡Centistokes at 25°C.

microscopic studies of retina following intravitreal perfluoro-*n*-octane injection in pigs and rabbits for 3 and 48 hr, respectively, have shown no evidence of toxicity.[44]

INDICATIONS FOR USE AND TECHNIQUES

The use of perfluorocarbon liquids during vitreoretinal surgery evolved primarily for the treatment of retinal detachment with severe proliferative vitreoretinopathy,[35] traumatic retinal detachments,[36] and giant retinal tears.[37] Nevertheless, as the clinical efficacy and safety of this intraoperative device has been established, additional indications for use have included the management of subretinal hemorrhage, vitreous hemorrhage, dislocated human lenses and intraocular lenses,[40, 47] and retinal detachment secondary to a macular hole (Table 101–4).

The perfluorocarbon liquids are most helpful in the management of severe degrees of proliferative vitreoretinopathy (Retina Society Classification, grades C-3 or D). Following the removal of cortical vitreous and all visible posterior membranes, injection of a small amount of perfluorocarbon liquid (0.5 to 1.0 ml) over the optic disc can serve to open the funnel of the detachment and expose areas of residual traction (Fig. 101–3). The latter is revealed as persistent elevation of the retina under the perfluorocarbon liquid. The mechanical stabilization of the retina during dissection of membranes reduces the risk of iatrogenic retinal breaks. Membranes are removed from a posterior to anterior direction above the liquid, and additional perfluorocarbon liquid is added as membranes continue to be removed. Dissection of residual epiretinal membranes that

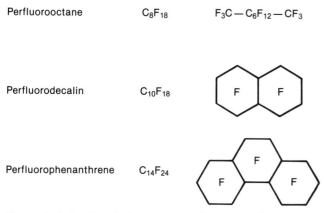

Perfluorooctane C_8F_{18} $F_3C-C_6F_{12}-CF_3$

Perfluorodecalin $C_{10}F_{18}$

Perfluorophenanthrene $C_{14}F_{24}$

Figure 101–2. Chemical structures of some perfluorocarbon liquids used in vitreoretinal surgery.

Table 101–4. INDICATIONS FOR INTRAOPERATIVE USE OF PERFLUOROCARBON LIQUIDS

Giant retinal tears
Severe proliferative vitreoretinopathy
Traumatic retinal detachment
Subretinal hemorrhage
Vitreous hemorrhage
Dislocated intraocular lens implant
Retinal detachment secondary to macular hole
Retinal detachment with subretinal gas

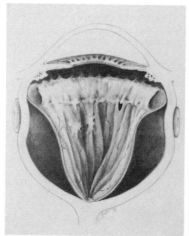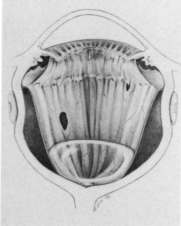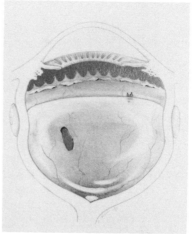

Figure 101–3. *Left,* Total retinal detachment with proliferative vitreoretinopathy. *Middle,* Perfluorocarbon liquid is injected over the optic disc to open the funnel of the detachment, and a posterior retinal break is exposed. *Right,* The perfluorocarbon liquid can be used to flatten the retinal break after the anterior traction has been relieved and the retina is completely mobile.

are exposed under the perfluorocarbon liquid can also be performed, but this should be done carefully because the development of an iatrogenic break may result in passage of the perfluorocarbon liquid into the subretinal space. As the surgery proceeds, stabilization of the posterior retina facilitates dissection of the anterior component of proliferative vitreoretinopathy.

Residual elevations of the retina under perfluorocarbon liquid may also result from subretinal membranes. These membranes may undergo sufficient flattening under perfluorocarbon liquid and may not require removal; this avoids unnecessary posterior retinotomies, which can be complicated by bleeding and reproliferation. Nevertheless, if their persistence prevents the retina from flattening under the perfluorocarbon liquid, removal can be performed later through retinotomies. Posterior retinotomy for internal drainage of subretinal fluid is not required, because the perfluorocarbon liquid displaces the subretinal fluid anteriorly through existing retinal breaks. If relaxing retinotomies (circumferential or radial) are necessary because of adherent membranes at the vitreous base, their extent can be minimized by observing the degree of flattening achieved under the perfluorocarbon liquid as the retinotomy is being performed. Retinal tacks for permanent mechanical fixation of retina can also be inserted through the perfluorocarbon liquid.

When perfluorocarbon gas is chosen for extended-term tamponade, perfluorocarbon liquid is removed by fluid-air exchange, with aspiration of liquid proceeding from an anterior to a posterior direction. If perfluorocarbon liquids with lower vapor pressure are used (e.g., perfluorodecalin, (perfluorophenanthrene) lavage with BSS is required to remove residual perfluorocarbon liquid from the retinal surface.[32] A perfluorocarbon gas-air mixture is then flushed through the vitreous cavity at the end of surgery. If silicone liquid is chosen for postoperative vitreous replacement, it can be injected directly by automated infusion as perfluorocarbon liquid

is aspirated (fluid-fluid exchange) or silicone liquid can be injected after complete fluid-air exchange.

In proliferative diabetic retinopathy, perfluorocarbon liquids have been used intraoperatively to flatten the rhegmatogenous component of a retinal detachment so that adequate endophotocoagulation can be applied.[48] Perfluorocarbon liquids do not appear to offer any advantage to the control of intraoperative bleeding in these cases; indeed, these materials should be used cautiously when significant intraocular hemorrhage exists because the liquid may not be completely removed if obscured by blood clots.

For the management of giant retinal tears (Fig. 101–4), perfluorocarbon liquid can be used to unfold the flap of the tear; the procedure minimizes retinal trauma resulting from the use of microsurgical tools. In addition, prone positioning, a requisite to management of giant tears by fluid-gas exchange,[49] is not required. Once again, posterior retinotomy to remove subretinal fluid is not necessary because the weight of the perfluorocarbon liquid forces the fluid anteriorly. The perfluorocarbon liquid serves to maintain the proper position of the tear against the retinal pigment epithelium while endophotocoagulation or transscleral cryotherapy is applied to the posterior edge of the tear through the liquid (Fig. 101–5). It is thought that intravitreal dispersion of retinal pigment epithelial cells during cryotherapy may be minimized by the perfluorocarbon liquid pressing the retinal flap against the retinal pigment epithelium, and certainly cryotherapy application is more precise and excessive treatment can be avoided. Ultimately, some cases of giant retinal tears can be managed without scleral buckling or lens removal.[37]

Retinal detachment resulting from a macular hole can be assisted by injection of a small amount of perfluorocarbon liquid over the posterior pole. The macular hole will flatten against the pigment epithelium so that endophotocoagulation can be applied. The liquid is then removed and a fluid-air exchange is performed. Diag-

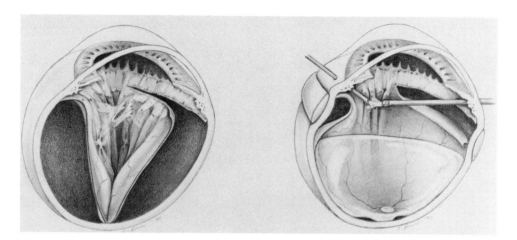

Figure 101–4. *Left,* A giant [ret]inal tear with total retinal detachment and proliferative vitreoretinopathy. *Right,* The perfluorocarbon liquid assists in flattening the retina, aids in exposing membranes within the retinal folds, and stabilizes the retina during dissection.

nostically the perfluorocarbon liquid can also be helpful in locating peripheral retinal breaks that were not seen preoperatively. Thus after vitrectomy, the perfluorocarbon liquid is injected to flatten the retina. The passage of subretinal fluid through the retinal break serves to localize the area of the break because of the difference between the refractive index of subretinal fluid and that of perfluorocarbon liquid.

Following penetrating trauma, retinal detachment is complicated by vitreous, subretinal, or choroidal hemorrhage, or a combination. After core vitrectomy is performed to remove hemorrhagic vitreous, the perfluorocarbon liquid flattens the retina without posterior retinotomy and allows the hemorrhage to be cut from the vitreous base more safely. If pooled subretinal hemorrhage is also present, the perfluorocarbon liquid can be used to displace the blood anteriorly, at which point it can be aspirated internally through a preexisting retinal break. In traumatic retinal detachments complicated by subretinal membranes or posterior proliferation

around an injury site, the perfluorocarbon liquid will help open retinal folds and allow better visualization of the site.

The management of foreign bodies is also aided by perfluorocarbon liquids. Foreign bodies such as wood or plastic can be floated anteriorly on the surface of the liquid. Metallic fragments are heavier and will sink in the liquid; however, the liquid can be used to stabilize the metal as it is grasped with forceps.

Silicone Liquid

Silicone liquid (Fig. 101–6) has been used during pars plana vitrectomy to reposition the retina, to stabilize the retina during the removal of epiretinal membranes,[50] and to unroll the flaps of retinal tears.[51] Intraoperatively, silicone liquid is introduced into the vitreous space to assist in opening retinal folds. The viscous fluid floats within the eye and as saline is aspirated, the silicone globule expands the retinal detachment so that any residual membranes can be seen and removed. (Fig. 101–7). Visualization of residual membranes is easier than when air is used, but optical reflexes are still encountered. Because of the high viscosity of silicone liquids used clinically, relatively high pressures are required for silicone injection. The high viscosity of silicone can also be problematic if removal of the liquid at the end of surgery is desired.[4] Moreover, as a liquid having a density lower than water (specific gravity of 0.97), it lacks the physical properties that, with the patient in the supine position, would provide a downward force to flatten the retina and collapse the subretinal space or unroll a retinal tear in a posterior to anterior direction. Management of the retinal flap in the presence of silicone liquid invariably requires additional bimanual manipulation of the retina to achieve correct positioning.[52] Because of its high specific gravity (1.28), fluorosilicone (see Fig. 101–6) has been advocated[53–55] as an alternative intraoperative tool. Perfluorocarbon liquids have replaced fluorosilicone liquids as intraoperative tools because of their more favorable physical properties.

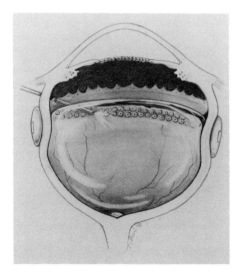

Figure 101–5. Endophotocoagulation can be applied through perfluorocarbon liquid while the perfluorocarbon liquid stabilizes the repositioned retina.

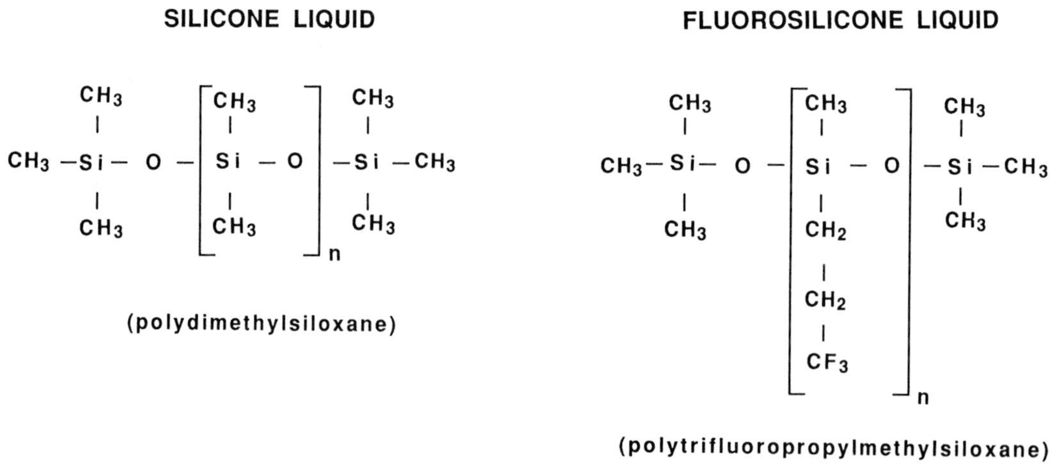

SILICONE LIQUID

$$CH_3 \enspace -Si- \enspace O \enspace - \left[Si - O \right]_n \enspace -Si -CH_3$$

(polydimethylsiloxane)

FLUOROSILICONE LIQUID

$$CH_3 -Si- \enspace O \enspace - \left[Si - O \right]_n \enspace -Si -CH_3$$

(polytrifluoropropylmethylsiloxane)

Figure 101–6. The chemical structures of silicone and fluorosilicone liquids.

THE USE OF VITREOUS SUBSTITUTES AS POSTOPERATIVE ADJUNCTS TO VITREORETINAL SURGERY

Intraocular Gas

In the United States, intraocular gases are the most commonly used agents for short-term vitreous replacement. Intraocular gases are employed for pneumatic retinopexy[3] and are used in conjunction with scleral buckling and drainage of subretinal fluid. In addition, for complicated forms of retinal detachment requiring vitrectomy, such as proliferative vitreoretinopathy or giant retinal tears, gases are used to provide internal tamponade postoperatively. A list of gases commonly employed for intraocular use is presented in Table 101–5.

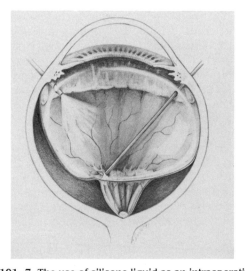

Figure 101–7. The use of silicone liquid as an intraoperative tool for management of total retinal detachment with proliferative vitreoretinopathy. After the liquid is injected into the preretinal space, the retinal folds expand and epiretinal membranes can be dissected under the silicone globule.

FUNCTIONAL ROLE OF GAS

Two properties of a gas bubble are of particular importance in the repair of retinal detachment.[56] First, the high surface tension between the gas bubble and the thin layer of aqueous covering the retina serves to tamponade (i.e., close or plug) a retinal break by blocking the flow of fluid from the vitreous cavity into the subretinal space and thus preventing accumulation of subretinal fluid. Second, since the specific gravity of air or any gas is lower than that of water, the gas bubble exerts a buoyant force that pushes the neural retina against the pigment epithelium. This force can flatten the retina by displacing subretinal fluid through the retinal breaks and into the vitreous. In flattening the retina, the relatively uniform pressure applied by the gas bubble can smooth out retinal folds on a scleral buckle or around the margins of a retinal tear. These buoyant forces must be accurately directed by careful, sustained head positioning so that the bubble is situated against the retinal break until the surrounding chorioretinal adhesion provided by diathermy or cryotherapy is established. The buoyant force provided by the gas bubble is dependent on the volume of gas used. Since a gas bubble rises to the uppermost part of the eye and the buoyant force is greatest at the apex of the arc of contact of the gas bubble with the retinal surface, and because the lower meniscus of the bubble is relatively flat and has little or no contact with the retina, intraocular gas is most useful for superior retinal breaks and is at a disadvantage when a retinal tear is located at the inferior pole. Measurements of the geometry of intraocular gas bubbles have also shown that to extend the surface of a bubble over a larger area of retina, as would

Table 101–5. GASES COMMONLY EMPLOYED FOR INTRAOCULAR USE

Xenon
Air
Sulfur hexafluoride
Perfluoroethane
Perfluoropropane

be required for inferior breaks, a disproportionately larger increase in bubble volume is required.[57-59]

Clinically used high molecular weight gases are less soluble in water than are low molecular weight blood gases; thus, following injection of a gas into the vitreous cavity, nitrogen, oxygen, and carbon dioxide, which are normally dissolved in surrounding tissue fluids, diffuse into the intravitreally injected gas, and the total gas volume increases. Gas bubble expansion continues until the partial pressures of the gases in the bubble equilibrate with that in the surrounding fluid compartments. Following an injection of pure expanding gas into the eye, the most rapid rate of volume increase occurs within the first 6 to 8 hr. Sulfur hexafluoride (SF_6) reaches its maximal expanded volume by 24 to 48 hr after injection[60] and with perfluoropropane (C_3F_8), this volume is reached after 72 to 96 hr.[61, 62] Following the expansion phase, the bubble gradually decreases in size as all of the gases diffuse out of the vitreous cavity. The decrease in the size of a gas bubble follows first-order exponential decay.[63, 64] The time that elapses before a gas bubble is reduced to 50 percent of its volume is of far greater clinical importance than the time for total dissolution of the gas because a small gas bubble in the vitreous cavity has no therapeutic value. Indeed, a gas bubble may be of therapeutic size for only 30 percent of the time it remains in the eye.[2] For the treatment of inferior retinal breaks in particular, it is of importance not only that the bubble be of sufficient volume to extend inferiorly to cover the break but also that it have sufficient longevity so that its lower meniscus does not rise too early.

CLINICAL APPLICATIONS OF INTRAOCULAR GAS

The problem of maintaining adequate gas tamponade until retinal adhesion is attained has led to the use of gases that are retained in the vitreous cavity longer than air. Indeed, with the advent of the use of sulfur hexafluoride (SF_6),[65] it became apparent that chemically inert high molecular weight gases having low water solubility and correspondingly greater intraocular longevity than air were associated with a higher rate of reattachment[66, 67] without having adverse effects on the retina.[68] Subsequently, interest was extended to perfluorocarbon gases, which have even greater expansive properties and exhibit greater persistence within the vitreous cavity. Gases in this family that have been investigated for use include perfluoromethane (CF_4)[61, 63] perfluoroethane (C_2F_6),[60, 62, 68] perfluoropropane (C_3F_8),[61-64, 69-74] octafluorocyclobutane (C_4F_8),[69, 75, 76] and perfluoro-n-butane (C_4F_{10}).[63, 77]

For gases having expansive potential, the initial rates of volume increase in the eye are probably dependent not only on the type of gas used but also on convection currents in the vitreous fluid surrounding the bubble.[70] Therefore, since the final gas volume is somewhat unpredictable and because of the potential for postoperative rise in intraocular pressure, using these gases, at gas-air mixtures of minimal or nonexpansile capability,

rather than at 100 percent concentration, is preferred. Minimally expanding, as opposed to nonexpanding, gas concentrations can be used to advantage because complete filling of the vitreous cavity with a nonexpansile gas-air mixture requires placement of the patient in the prone position with the surgeon facing the patient from below. Thus, intravitreal injection of a smaller gas volume, which undergoes a slight increase in size postoperatively, avoids the complexities and dangers associated with prone positioning.[78, 79] Minimal expansion can be achieved with gas-air concentrations of 20 to 25 percent for perfluoroethane and 17 to 20 percent for perfluoropropane. With sulfur hexafluoride, a gas concentration of 40 percent in air can be used without a rise in intraocular pressure.[80] Concentrations of approximately 16 percent for perfluoroethane, 14 percent for perfluoropropane, and 18 percent for sulfur hexafluoride are nonexpanding.[2, 62] These nonexpanding gas-air mixtures are indicated if preoperative gonioscopic examination reveals the possibility of compromised outflow, as a result of either anterior synechiae or neovascularization. Expansile mixtures are particularly to be avoided in eyes with preexisting glaucoma or synechial angle closure. To achieve the desired intraocular gas concentration at the end of surgery, intraocular air must be completely flushed from the eye by using an adequate volume of the gas-air mixture (this volume is estimated to be 25 ml)[81] (Fig. 101-8). The gas-air mixture should be prepared immediately before use so that the concentration of gas is not altered by diffusion of gas out of the plastic syringe.[82] It should also be noted that total filling of the vitreous cavity by fluid-gas exchange, with either minimally expanding or nonexpansile gas, may be desirable under some conditions, such as with an inferior retinal break, but is not always indicated. Conditions under which partial filling of the vitreous cavity may be acceptable include treatment of superior retinal breaks and the diagnosis of occult retinal breaks in the presence of retinal detachment.[83] In addition to the volume and concentration of gas injected, the presence or lack of vitreous and lens plays an important role in the rate of dissolution of the gas bubble. For instance, it has been found experimentally that the half-life of sulfur hexafluoride and perfluoropropane in phakic nonvitrectomized eyes is 2.2 to 2.7 times longer than in aphakic vitrectomized eyes.[84]

The choice of gas used for the treatment of complicated retinal detachment is an empirical decision. The preferences presented here for specific conditions of retinal detachment are for the most part based on the clinical experience of the Vitreoretinal Service at Cornell University Medical College. Factors to be considered when selecting a gas in an individual case include the type and location of the retinal problem and the duration of therapy required. In general, it is recommended that the gas chosen to manage a clinical situation should have an intraocular duration that is only as long as required for therapeutic effectiveness. Persistence of the gas at therapeutic volume is desirable until the chorioretinal adhesion resulting from photocoagulation or cryotherapy becomes maximum, approximately 8 to 11

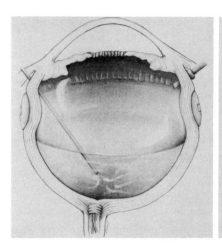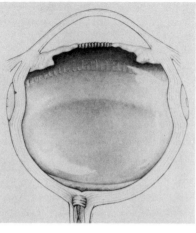

Figure 101–8. After vitrectomy, air is injected by fluid-air exchange. Fluid is aspirated as air enters through the infusion line. The air is replaced at the end of the operation with the desired gas-air mixture.

days.[85] In cases complicated by proliferative vitreoretinopathy, the aim is also to tamponade the retina until the active phase of reproliferation has passed, if possible.

Together with air, sulfur hexafluoride remains the most commonly used gas for scleral buckling procedures[66, 86] and is also frequently used for retinal detachments requiring vitreous surgery, such as those associated with proliferative diabetic retinopathy.[2, 67] Sulfur hexafluoride can also be used for superior retinal breaks above the horizontal meridian and for milder forms of proliferative vitreoretinopathy.[2] Perfluorocarbon gases with greater intravitreal longevity have proved advantageous over sulfur hexafluoride in complicated forms of retinal detachment[69, 78] such as giant retinal tears and penetrating trauma, or in highly myopic eyes with retinal detachment from macular holes. Many of these cases can be managed using perfluoroethane, which has less cataractogenic potential and allows more rapid rehabilitation of the patient, as compared with gas that is retained for a longer time, such as perfluoropropane. For instance, perfluoroethane can be used for pneumatic retinopexy and for internal tamponade of rhegmatogenous retinal detachments associated with posterior retinal breaks, proliferative diabetic retinopathy, traction retinal detachment, and penetrating trauma. For giant retinal tears not complicated by proliferative vitreoretinopathy and highly myopic eyes with retinal detachment from macular holes, perfluoroethane can provide a therapeutic volume of gas until the chorioretinal adhesion resulting from photocoagulation or cryotherapy is established. Milder forms of proliferative vitreoretinopathy may also be managed using perfluoroethane. In addition, perfluoroethane is preferred for postoperative fluid-gas exchange. Perfluoropropane gas is recommended for the management of giant retinal tears complicated by proliferative vitreoretinopathy or retinal detachments with severe forms of proliferative vitreoretinopathy (Retina Society, stages C3 and D).[70, 87–89] A major advantage to the use of perfluoropropane is that after completely filling the vitreous cavity with gas at surgery, the cavity remains more than 50 percent filled for 3 wk. Perfluoropropane is routinely used in some centers for pneumatic retinopexy[3] and for

the management of giant retinal tears,[79] but it is possible that the shorter-lasting gases, such as perfluoroethane, would be just as effective in these cases.

COMPLICATIONS OF GAS USE

Although intraocular gas bubbles have proved beneficial and are not chemically toxic,[2, 66, 68, 78, 90] some physical properties of the gas can cause complications in the eye (Table 101–6). For instance, patients with intraocular gas bubbles must be positioned with the head prone to displace the gas bubble away from the lens and cornea to avoid pupillary-block glaucoma and corneal endothelial decompensation in aphakic eyes and lens opacities in phakic eyes. The gases with greater longevity are more likely to cause these changes.[73, 78] Positioning to prevent these complications can be problematic, particularly for children and elderly, or debilitated individuals. In addition, if expanding concentrations of gas are used, careful monitoring of both the size of the gas bubble and intraocular pressure is required. Excessive bubble expansion may cause the anterior chamber to become shallow, as well as result in pupillary-block glaucoma and even central retinal artery occlusion. Intraocular pressure must be measured 6 to 8 hr following surgery,[76] preferably by using applanation tonometry, since Schiøtz tonometry can result in artificially low pressure measurements.[91–93] The incidence of elevated intraocular pressure in the immediate postoperative period ranges between 26 and 59 percent.[66, 67, 69] In most cases, increased intraocular pressure can be controlled medically by administering timolol and acetazolamide during the initial 24 hr and once complete expansion is achieved, intraocular pressure should stabilize. Difficulties in managing intraocular pressure are probably caused by compromised outflow. In patients

Table 101–6. COMPLICATIONS OF INTRAOCULAR GAS

Lens opacity
Corneal endothelial decompensation
Pupillary-block glaucoma
Expansion during air travel and nitrous oxide anesthesia
Subretinal gas

suspected of having occluded angles from neovascularization or peripheral anterior synechiae, expanding concentrations of gas should be avoided. A less frequent cause of glaucoma results from the injection of a volume of gas that, when fully expanded, exceeds the vitreous volume.[78, 87] Gas must be aspirated when this occurs.

Patients with large perfluorocarbon gas bubbles must be advised that air travel or other situations involving rapid decreases in atmospheric pressure should be avoided because a fall in atmospheric pressure can cause enlargement of the gas bubble.[94] During a rapid change in bubble size, the eye has very little time to compensate for the change by outflow of aqueous humor; thus, an elevation in intraocular pressure occurs. The greatest risk occurs during the ascent of the airplane when it may climb at rates approaching 3000 ft/min, whereas the cabin decompresses at only 300 to 500 ft/min.[94, 95] There has been some controversy concerning the volume of gas that can be tolerated during flight. Recent experimental findings concluded that volumes of intravitreal gas of up to 0.6 cc are safe,[96] although clinical experience indicates that a volume of 1.0 cc may even be tolerated.[2, 96] Nitrous oxide used for general inhalational anesthesia is also contraindicated in patients with intraocular gas who require dental work or other surgical intervention, because the high solubility of nitrous oxide (the latter is 117 times more soluble than sulfur hexafluoride) results in its rapid diffusion into the intraocular gas bubble, bubble expansion, and concomitant elevated intraocular pressure.[97, 98]

A frequent complication of a large intraocular gas bubble is the induction of lens opacities. Lens changes begin as feathery posterior subcapsular opacities or as posterior subcapsular vacuoles, most frequently in the superior portion of the lens. The opacity can be transient and disappear if a layer of fluid is maintained between the gas bubble and the posterior lens surface. By placing the patient's head in the prone position, the gas bubble should not be in contact with the posterior lens surface. Lens opacities are most likely to occur when the gas bubble occupies more than two thirds of the vitreous volume.[66, 68, 69] In addition, there is a relatively higher incidence of this complication with longer lasting gas bubbles; more than 50 percent of these patients progress to experience permanent lens opacities.

An additional drawback to the use of intraocular gas is that the scattering of light at the interface between the gas bubble and the surrounding intraocular fluid produces optical disturbances and reflections that obscure the patient's vision and make examination of the fundus and application of laser photocoagulation difficult.

Aqueous flare has been observed both by slit-lamp examination and by flaremetry following intraocular injection of gas in both humans and rabbits.[69, 70, 90, 99] In addition, anterior chamber fluorophotometry has clearly shown that there is a temporary breakdown in the blood-ocular barrier following intravitreal injection of gas in nonvitrectomized rabbits, but recovery begins to occur as early as 3 days after injection.[100, 101] Studies concerned with the effects of intravitreal gas on leakage across the blood-retinal barrier are conflicting. Thus, although vit-

reous levels of intravenously injected iodinated serum protein have been reported to be elevated,[102] other investigators conclude, on the basis of the measurement of soluble protein concentration in rabbit vitreous, that injection of perfluoropropane gas into vitreous does not provoke a measurable inflammatory response.[103] Whether these findings have implications relevant to questions concerning intravitreally injected gas and adverse effects that could contribute to an exacerbation of proliferative vitreoretinopathy is not known. Animal eyes with perfluoropropane gas bubbles have been shown to experience more severe stages of experimental traction retinal detachment than control (nonvitrectomized) eyes without gas bubbles;[104] however, in another study there was no difference in severity of experimental traction retinal detachment between gas-filled (perfluoropropane) and BSS-filled eyes.[105] Whether or not a reduction in the fluid space of gas-filled eyes and concomitant concentrating of cells contributes to this effect is not clear. Nevertheless, given the possibility that intravitreal gas could augment proliferative processes, it is frequently suggested that a gas bubble should ideally persist in the vitreous cavity for the duration of time required for the desired effect and no longer.[104]

Subretinal gas has been observed as a complication of the use of intraocular gas. Visualization of the tip of the needle during gas injection is important in order to avoid inadvertent injection of gas under the nonpigmented ciliary epithelium.[106] During pneumatic retinopexy, small bubbles of gas may travel through retinal breaks and expand in the subretinal space. This complication can be managed by closing the retinal breaks with scleral buckling and displacing the small subretinal gas bubble.[107] In some cases, vitrectomy and air-fluid exchange may be required. Subretinal gas may also develop when fluid-gas exchange is performed in eyes with large tears caused by recurrent proliferation.[108] In these eyes, vitrectomy revision is indicated.

Silicone Liquid

PROPERTIES OF SILICONE LIQUID

Silicone liquids are linear synthetic polymers made of repetitive [-Si-O-] units (see Fig. 101–6). Differences among silicone liquids are determined by the length of the polymer, which affects the viscosity, and the hydrocarbon radicals, which constitute the side groups of the polymer. Silicone liquids used clinically are generally polydimethylsiloxanes.

Silicone liquid is transparent and has a refractive index of 1.404, which being higher than that of vitreous causes the optics of an eye to change when filled with silicone. In the phakic eye, it has been estimated that if the silicone globule is in contact with the lens and the anterior surface of the globule is thus concave, a hyperopic change in refraction (to about plus 5) is induced. Since the front surface of the silicone globule is convex in an aphakic eye, the refractive power of the eye is increased such that the aphakic refractive error (hyperopia) is reduced.[6, 7] This increase in the refractive power of the eye is considered an advantage by many patients with aphakia.

Silicone liquid is lighter than water (specific gravity of 0.97); thus, a silicone globule contacts retina with an upward buoyant force. The force with which the silicone globule contacts retina is 1/30 of the pressure exerted by a gas bubble.[109] In addition, although an intravitreal gas bubble exerts forces and provides tamponade both superiorly and posteriorly,[110] a silicone globule provides little real tamponade to the posterior retina with the patient sitting upright.[111] Silicone liquid has a surface tension with water of 40 mN/m, which is less than that of a gas bubble. This surface tension combined with the buoyant force means that a silicone globule can effectively support a surgically attached retina above the horizontal meridian if it is free of traction but is insufficient to resist radially directed tractional forces on the retina.[6, 110, 112, 113] It has been suggested, however, that there are other mechanisms by which intravitreal silicone liquid can deter redetachment. For instance, the presence of the silicone globule in close proximity to the surface of the retina may impose a redirection of tractional forces so that they are aligned parallel to the retina (tangential) and are correspondingly less effective than radially transmitted traction.[6] In addition, when a large silicone globule occupies the vitreous cavity, the posterior retinal surface is covered by only a thin layer of aqueous.[110, 111] Perhaps under these conditions intraocular fluid currents are not sufficient to redetach the retina.[111, 114]

INDICATIONS AND CLINICAL CONSIDERATIONS

Silicone liquid is being used with increasing frequency when long-term or permanent support and tamponade is needed to maintain neural retina in apposition to the retinal pigment epithelium (Table 101–7). Silicone liquid is most frequently indicated for cases complicated by proliferative vitreoretinopathy,[115–126] giant retinal tears,[52, 118, 120, 123, 127–129] or retinal detachment caused by proliferative diabetic retinopathy.[111, 118, 121, 123, 130, 131] Silicone liquid has also been used after failed primary surgery in cases of severe ocular trauma.[132] Proliferative vitreoretinopathy may develop after long-term detachment, after unsuccessful reattachment surgery, or in association with perforating injuries or giant retinal tears. The use of silicone liquid in these cases is particularly indicated after the failure of previous scleral buckling, vitrectomy, membrane dissection, and intra-

Table 101–7. INDICATIONS FOR USE OF SILICONE LIQUID

Proliferative vitreoretinopathy
Giant retinal tears
Proliferative diabetic retinopathy
Traumatic retinal detachment
Retinal detachment complicated by iris neovascularization
Patient noncompliance with positioning and postoperative fluid-gas exchange
Need for air travel by patient

ocular gas injection for the treatment of proliferative vitreoretinopathy. In the United States, silicone liquid may be employed in the primary procedure if the patient, particularly a child, is unable to comply with the positioning and postoperative fluid-gas exchange required for postoperative management of gas instillation.[133] An additional complication with using gas in children is the difficulty of performing postoperative indirect ophthalmoscopic examination. Silicone liquid may also be chosen over gas in the primary procedure if the patient must travel by air. Conversely, in Europe, silicone liquid is used more frequently as part of the primary reattachment procedure for the management of giant retinal tears, proliferative diabetic retinopathy, and ocular trauma.[7, 123] As a primary vitreous substitute, silicone liquid provides extended tamponade and support of retina without the need for repeated postoperative fluid-gas exchange and is considered to prevent or limit postoperative traction rhegmatogenous detachment. Whether employed as the primary or secondary therapy, it is generally advised that silicone liquid injection be used in conjunction with one or more other surgical techniques, including extensive membrane peeling, the use of a broad scleral buckle, retinal photocoagulation or retinotomy, or a combination of these techniques.[111, 117, 131, 133–136] In conjunction with extensive relaxing retinotomies and retinectomy, the use of silicone liquid is frequently selected over gas, particularly when the need for blanketing large areas of exposed retinal pigment epithelium is a factor.[133, 137–40] The hypotony associated with retinotomy and retinectomy may also be less pronounced with the use of silicone liquid.

Iris and filtration angle neovascularization with secondary glaucoma is a serious complication of vitrectomy for proliferative diabetic retinopathy. In particular, patients with persistent retinal detachment have the greatest risk for developing iris neovascularization.[141] Intravitreal silicone liquid is considered in several reports to have value in reducing preoperative iris neovascularization or in preventing the development of iris neovascularization postoperatively.[6, 111, 130, 135, 140, 142] Indeed, there is evidence that silicone liquid acts as a diffusion-convection barrier to oxygen, an effect that is postulated to alter the stimulus for neovascularization.[143] Nevertheless, an effect on anterior segment neovascularization has not always been observed[131, 144] and may be dependent on factors such as the degree of filling.[7] The incidence of band keratopathy with silicone liquid placement is lower in cases of proliferative diabetic retinopathy than with proliferative vitreoretinopathy, an observation explained on the basis of the already elevated levels of glucose in the blood and aqueous humor.[35]

Despite the potential benefits of silicone liquid as a vitreous substitute, because of its buoyancy it rises to the superior pole of the vitreous cavity and is thus most useful when a retinal tear-detachment is located superiorly, and is less effective in the treatment of inferior lesions. Consequently, the inferior quadrants in which proliferative vitreoretinopathy (the most common obstacle to successful reattachment surgery)[145–147] also tends to be most severe,[144, 145] are usually the locus of persistent or recurrent detachments following silicone liquid injection.[119, 120, 128, 148–150] Redetachment has obvious consequences for visual function and may also secondarily precipitate lens and corneal complications by forcing the intravitreally placed silicone globule anteriorly.[151] Buckling of an inferior tear, in conjunction with intravitreally placed silicone liquid, is advocated so that the silicone globule, deformed by the buckle, will contact the tear.[148]

It is generally accepted that silicone liquid should be removed from the eye if stable anatomical reattachment has been achieved and the proliferative process is in remission. Other factors determining the time of removal are cataract formation, emulsification, and glaucoma. In some cases, the patient may not consent to the additional surgical procedure required for removal. The minimal time after which silicone liquid can be removed is considered to be 3 wk.[8] In general, it is preferred that silicone liquid be removed by 3 to 6 mo postoperatively,[134, 152, 153] and even earlier times are reported (6 wk to 3 mo postoperatively.[52, 118, 122, 128]) Twelve months has been suggested as the latest postoperative time for removal;[6] however, there are cases in which silicone liquid has remained in eyes for several years.[8] Redetachment after removal has been reported at rates of 9 to 30 percent.[6, 119, 154–157] A variety of methods have been developed for removal; these techniques employ various methods from passive drainage to special cannulae to vacuum drainage pumps.[6–8, 158, 159] Despite careful lavage, however, residual silicone liquid droplets remain in the vitreous cavity after removal.[159]

It is difficult to evaluate the benefits of intravitreal silicone liquid in terms of the visual outcome because issues such as the indications for use and optimal time of removal have not been resolved. Moreover, patients are often selected for treatment with silicone liquid after having undergone previous failed procedures, and the outlook for favorable visual outcome is inevitably poor. Poor visual acuity can also be attributed to cataract formation or to preoperative macular detachment rather than to failure of retinal reattachment. The Silicone Study, a multicenter randomized prospective clinical trial in the United States, will ultimately determine the benefits of silicone liquid versus intraocular gas in the management of proliferative vitreoretinopathy.[160, 161]

OCULAR TOLERANCE AND COMPLICATIONS

The issue of whether silicone liquid is toxic to the retina has been controversial. Histologic studies of enucleated human eyes following long-term silicone oil filling[162–165] and morphologic and histochemical analyses of experimental silicone injection in animals[166–170] have described severe sequelae, including impregnation of retinal tissue, changes in enzyme composition, lipid extraction, intraocular foreign body giant cell reaction, intracytoplasmic vacuole formation, and degenerative changes in ganglion and photoreceptor cells and the outer plexiform layer. Reports of electroretinographic studies also concluded that retinal function was reduced.[166, 168] Conversely, other studies, many of them recent, have shown no toxic effects on the retina.[171–177]

It is difficult to completely reconcile these studies because of differences in experimental design and procedures. Nevertheless, several issues should be recognized. First, intravitreal silicone oil alters the electrical conductivity of the eye; thus, electroretinographic function cannot be reliably assessed while a silicone globule is in the vitreous cavity.[174, 178–80] In addition, results from experimental work in the rabbit are probably not definitive because rabbit retina, being one third the thickness of human retina and lacking a retinal vasculature,[181] may be more susceptible to mechanical effects (e.g., the force with which the material contacts the retina) of a vitreous substitute. In clinical studies, it is not always possible to differentiate between degenerative changes arising as a result of inherent disease, preexisting retinal damage, or persistent retinal detachment on the one hand and the possible toxic effects of silicone oil on the other hand.[176] In addition, clinically used silicone liquids have not all been of the same chemical make-up, and in many cases the origins of the liquids, their purity, and their composition have not been known.[6] Indeed, there is evidence that some of the discrepancies among the clinical and experimental studies may be caused by variations in the chemical and physical properties of individual silicone liquids and by highly differing grades of purity. Two factors of importance in this regard are the proportion of short molecular chains in the liquid and the purity of the liquid. Not only may the low molecular weight constituents be capable of diffusing into surrounding tissues, thus inciting toxic or macrophage reactions, or both,[182] but they are also associated with an increase in the extent and susceptibility of silicone liquid to emulsification,[183] a factor that can contribute to the development of clinical complications such as angle-block glaucoma and keratopathy and macrophage invasion.[6] Adverse tissue reactions may also arise from the use of certain silicone liquids having high contents of hydroxyl end groups, unpolymerized monomeric dimethylsiloxane, cyclic low molecular weight siloxane units, or catalytic remnants from the polymerization process (primarily heavy metal ions).[184] In light of this, the use of purified high-viscosity liquids of homogeneous polymer length is advocated. The high-viscosity materials have less tendency to emulsify;[183, 185] indeed, polydimethylsiloxane of 5000-centistoke viscosity was shown to be significantly more resistant to emulsification than the 1000-centistoke material[185] and also to be associated with a lower incidence of glaucoma.[186]

Other complications of silicone filling, particularly those involving the anterior segment, may be related to mechanical rather than chemical factors. For instance, when silicone liquid is injected into aphakic eyes, the liquid has access to the anterior chamber, and corneal compensation is a common complication. This is thought to occur because normal access of nutrients to the corneal endothelial cells is prevented by contact between these cells and the silicone globule.[187] Animal experiments have shown that when the anterior chamber is filled with silicone liquid, within 2 to 4 wk there is a 50 percent reduction in corneal endothelial cell density.[185] The lodging of a silicone globule in the iris diaphragm also caused pupillary-block glaucoma. To reduce the risk of pupillary-block glaucoma and to keep the anterior chamber free of silicone in aphakic eyes, the use of an inferior basal iridectomy[188] and avoidance of overfilling are advocated.[109] With the iridectomy serving as a channel for passage of aqueous humor into the anterior chamber, the silicone globule can return to the vitreous cavity when the patient is prone.

All phakic eyes containing intravitreal silicone liquid will eventually develop cataracts. It is generally accepted that the cause is related to contact between the silicone globule and the posterior lens capsule and the resulting mechanical obstruction to diffusion of nutrients.[189] Consequently, either early removal of the liquid or lens extraction becomes obligatory. The incidence of cataract is most pronounced between 6 and 18 mo after surgery,[189] and opacification can develop or progress even after silicone withdrawal.[111, 122] Patients with phakic eyes should be instructed never to lie in the supine position for extended periods to avoid prolonged contact between the silicone globule and the posterior lens capsule. Some surgeons advocate lensectomy during the primary procedure in order to facilitate the surgical approach and preempt the development of cataract. Conversely, others prefer to retain the lens for protection of the anterior segment; therefore, lens extraction, with or without intraocular lens implant, remains an option at the time of silicone removal, if a cataract has formed.[6, 189]

Besides the risk of pupillary-block glaucoma in the aphakic eye, angle-block glaucoma can occur in both phakic and aphakic eyes secondary to emulsification of the liquid. As noted previously, emulsification occurs less readily with a high-viscosity liquid than with a 1000-centistoke liquid and is also minimized by the use of highly purified liquids. Although there is considerable variation from patient to patient, emulsification generally becomes a more significant factor with time, probably because proteins and phospholipids in physiologic aqueous are progressively adsorbed to the silicone globule and thereby lower the interfacial surface tension. This drop in interfacial tension, together with the accelerations induced by saccadic eye movements, are considered to be responsible for emulsification of the liquid.[110] It is assumed that droplets of emulsified silicone that reach the angle progressively obstruct the trabecular meshwork. Despite this obstruction, glaucoma may not be manifested if production of aqueous by the ciliary body is abnormally decreased or if a retinal detachment exists.[111] The pressure rise, when it occurs, is reversible once the silicone liquid is removed.[111]

Reproliferation is the major cause of failure of retinal reattachment surgery. Consequently, much interest has been paid to the issue of whether intravitreally placed silicone liquid affects the cellular proliferation associated with proliferative vitreoretinopathy. Silicone liquid has been reported by some investigators to have no effect on cellular proliferation and experimental traction retinal detachment.[121, 190, 191] Other investigators have observed more severe stages of experimental traction retinal detachment in silicone-filled eyes when compared with controls, and in in vitro proliferation assays, they have noted that samples of vitreous from silicone-filled eyes demonstrate increased mitogenic activity for retinal

pigment epithelial cells compared with fluid-filled vitreous.[105] There may be at least three issues of importance here. One issue is whether the surface of an intravitreal silicone globule can serve as a substrate on which cells attach and grow. Experiments in tissue culture have shown that fibroblasts plated at the phase boundary between silicone liquid (polydimethylsiloxane) and culture medium exhibit little ability to attach and proliferate.[46] Nevertheless, the extent to which the milieu of the vitreous cavity and adsorption of macromolecules to the intravitreally placed silicone globule induce changes in the surface of the globule that make it conducive to cell attachment is not known. Clinically, cell proliferation is observed between a silicone globule and the inner surface of the retina (perisilicone proliferation);[113] however, it is not clear that the proliferating cells are dependent on the silicone globule for attachment rather than on the inner surface of the retina. The second issue of importance is whether a silicone globule in the vitreous cavity concentrates cells and putative chemoattractants and mitogens in the residual fluid space of the vitreous cavity.[192] At least in some cases, this situation could ultimately serve to focus tractional forces. Pertinent to the third issue, that of whether intravitreal silicone liquid augments proliferative processes, is also the speculation that a breakdown in the blood-ocular barrier could affect cellular proliferation by providing a source of growth factor activity.[193–195] Recent work has revealed that silicone liquid, when placed in the vitreous cavity, does not in and of itself adversely affect the blood-aqueous barrier.[101, 196]

High Specific Gravity Liquids

To address the problem of providing tamponade and mechanical support of inferior retinal breaks, high specific gravity liquids have potential advantage. Interest in the silicone liquid has been extended to its fluorinated derivative fluorosilicone[51, 53, 54, 38, 170, 197–199] (see Fig. 101–6) as a potential long-term vitreous substitute of high specific gravity that would be useful for the treatment of inferior retinal breaks and advantageous for proliferative vitreoretinopathy, which is more severe in inferior quadrants. Nevertheless, some studies have demonstrated a pronounced inflammatory response,[38, 197] which has been suggested to be associated with the shortness of the polymer chain and with the greater difficulty encountered in purifying fluorosilicone as compared with silicone (polydimethylsiloxane) liquid.[197]

As discussed earlier, perfluorocarbon liquids of low viscosity have proved valuable for intraoperative manipulation of retinal breaks and detachment. A recent report has also described a case in which a low-viscosity perfluorocarbon liquid (perfluorophenanthrene) remained in the vitreous cavity for 3 wk postoperatively.[200] Nevertheless, as is also the case with silicone liquids, perfluorocarbon liquids of low viscosity tend to have greater susceptibility to emulsification and are thus less suitable for extended-term intraocular use.[32, 34, 40, 44] Conversely, high-viscosity perfluorocarbon liquids demonstrate resistance to emulsification. Experimental studies of both the low-viscosity[44] and the high-viscosity perfluorocarbon liquids (Chang and associates, unpublished observations) have shown that when such liquids are placed in rabbit vitreous cavity for longer than one wk, narrowing of the outer plexiform layer and the outer nuclear layer in inferior retina is progressive with time. The extent to which these changes are species-specific is not known but must be considered given that rabbit retina is notably thin and avascular and that similar changes are observed in rabbits when intravitreal silicone liquid is used.[169] In addition, placement of the high-viscosity liquid perfluoropolyether in the vitreous cavity of pigs is not associated with the morphologic retinal changes observed in rabbits (Chang and associates, unpublished observations). Nevertheless, the long-term safety of these liquids in the human eye has not been investigated.

Other Potential Methods for Postoperative Vitreous Replacement

To address the problem of providing tamponade and mechanical support of the superior and the inferior retina simultaneously, it may be possible to use liquids of low and high specific gravity in combination (Fig. 101–9). Thus, studies in rabbits aimed at evaluating the intravitreal placement of silicone liquid in combination with a high-viscosity perfluorocarbon liquid (perfluoropolyether) revealed that the two intravitreally placed liquids formed separate immiscible phases, with the denser perfluoropolyether liquid forming the lower phase and the silicone liquid forming the upper phase.[201] The slightly different refractive indices of the two liquids created a visible interface. Under conditions of an experimental model of traction retinal detachment, the retina underwent traction detachment behind the silicone globule, but retinal detachment did not extend

behind the perfluoropolyether liquid. In other experiments it was found that the extent of dispersion of a low-viscosity perfluorocarbon liquid is decreased when the latter liquid is employed in the vitreous cavity in combination with silicone liquid.[201, 202] This effect may be related to the role of the silicone globule in restricting the movement of the inferiorly situated low-viscosity liquid.

Hydrophilic polymers (hydrogels) have been suggested as promising alternatives to the use of gas or liquid materials as vitreous substitutes in some cases. Theoretically, these materials could be synthesized so that they would swell to fill the vitreous cavity at injection and provide equal support to the inferior and superior retina, yet not undergo further expansion following injection. Being homogeneous, there would be lack of liquid-liquid or gas-fluid interfaces, which otherwise create optical disturbances. Unlike intraocular gas, no special positioning of the patient would be necessary. In addition, three-dimensional polymers having mechanical strength should effectively support a surgically reattached retina. Nevertheless, hydrogel materials studied in the past (glyceryl methacrylate, poly[2-hydroxyethyl acrylate]) have proved difficult to inject, have not been tolerated by ocular tissues, or have had suboptimal optical properties.[203–205]

CONCLUSIONS

The use of vitreous substitutes has contributed significantly to the progress of vitreoretinal surgery. Advancements have been made in understanding the requirements of vitreous substitutes, with respect to the needed chemical and physical properties of the material. Nevertheless, not all aspects of the role played by vitreous substitutes in successful retinal reattachment are understood. For instance, it is speculated that a vitreous substitute can serve as a mechanical barrier to the settling of cells on the retinal surface, but definitive evidence for this is lacking. In addition, it is generally appreciated that closure of a retinal break by a vitreous substitute material is an important role; however, the potential importance of the material in providing mechanical support to retina is not clearly understood. Future investigational efforts will undoubtedly be directed toward issues such as these.

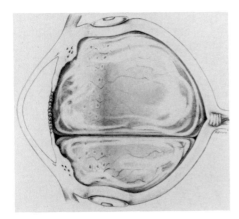

Figure 101–9. Combined use of high and low specific gravity liquids as vitreous substitutes. The two intravitreally placed liquids form two immiscible phases, with the denser perfluorocarbon liquid forming the lower phase and the silicone liquid forming the upper phase. The ratio of the volume of silicone to perfluorocarbon liquid employed is 2:1. With this volume ratio, the interface between the two liquids does not intercept the visual axis.

REFERENCES

1. Glaser BM: Surgery for proliferative vitreoretinopathy. *In* Ryan SJ (ed): Retina. St Louis, CV Mosby, 1989, p 385.
2. Chang S: Intraocular gases. *In* Ryan SJ (ed): Retina, vol. 3. St Louis, CV Mosby, 1989, p 245.
3. Hilton GF: Pneumatic retinopexy and alternative techniques. *In* Ryan SJ (ed): Retina. St Louis, CV Mosby, 1989, p 225.
4. Schepens CL: Retinal Detachment and Allied Diseases. Philadelphia, WB Saunders, 1983.
5. Scott JD: Silicone oil as an instrument. *In* Ryan SJ (ed): Retina. St Louis, CV Mosby, 1989, pp 307–315.
6. Lucke K, Laqua H: Silicone Oil in the Treatment of Complicated Retinal Detachments. Berlin, Springer-Verlag, 1990.
7. Lean JS: Use of silicone oil as an additional technique in vitreoretinal surgery. *In* Ryan SJ (ed): Retina. St Louis, CV Mosby, 1989, pp 279–292.

8. Zivojnovic R: Silicone oil in vitreoretinal surgery. Dordrecht, The Netherlands, Martinus Nijhoff/Dr W Junk, 1987.

9. Edelhauser HF, Van Horn DL, Hyndiuk RA, Schultz RO: Intraocular irrigation solutions: Their effect on the corneal endothelium. Arch Ophthalmol 93:648, 1975.

10. Edelhauser HF, Van Horn DL, Schultz RO, Hyndiuk RA: Comparative toxicity of intraocular irrigating solutions on the corneal endothelium. Am J Ophthalmol 81:473, 1976.

11. Edelhauser HF, Gonnering R, Van Horn DL: Intraocular irrigating solutions: A comparative study of BSS Plus and lactated Ringer's solution. Arch Ophthalmol 96:516, 1978.

12. Faulborn J, Conway BP, Machemer R: Surgical complications of pars plana vitreous surgery. Ophthalmology 85:116, 1978.

13. Moorhead LC, Redburn DA, Merritt J, Garcia CA: The effects of intravitreal irrigation during vitrectomy on the electroretinogram. Am J Ophthalmol 88:239, 1979.

14. Haimann MH, Abrams GW: Prevention of lens opacification during diabetic vitrectomy. Ophthalmology 91:116, 1984.

15. Blacharski PA, Charles ST: Thrombin infusion to control bleeding during vitrectomy for stage V retinopathy of prematurity. Arch Ophthalmol 105:203, 1987.

16. de Bustros S, Glaser BM, Johnson MA: Thrombin infusion for the control of intraocular bleeding during vitreous surgery. Arch Ophthalmol 103:837, 1985.

17. Rinkoff J, Machemer R, Hida T, Chandler D: Temperature-dependent light damage to the retina. Am J Ophthalmol 102:452, 1986.

18. Wolin LR, Massopust LC, Meder J: Electroretinogram and cortical evoked potentials under hypothermia. Arch Ophthalmol 72:521, 1964.

19. Jabbour NM, Schepens CL, Buzney SM: Local ocular hypothermia in experimental intraocular surgery. Ophthalmology 95:1687, 1988.

20. Zilis JD, Chandler D, Machemer R: Clinical and histologic effects of extreme intraocular hypothermia. Am J Ophthalmol 109:469, 1990.

21. Ohm J: Über die Behandlung der Netzhautablösung durch operative Entfeerung der subretinalen Flüssigkeit und Einspritzung von Luft in den Glaskörper. Graefes Arch Clin Exp Ophthalmol 79:442, 1911.

22. Lincoff H, Kreissig I: Application of xenon gas to clinical retinal detachment. Arch Ophthalmol 100:1083, 1982.

23. Lincoff A, Lincoff H, Solorzano C, Iwamoto T: Selection of xenon gas for rapidly disappearing retinal tamponade. Arch Ophthalmol 100:996, 1982.

24. Landers MB, Stefansson E, Wolbarsht ML: The optics of vitreous surgery. Am J Ophthalmol 91:611, 1981.

25. Stefansson E, McCuen BW II, McPherson SD Jr: Biconcave contact lens for examination and laser treatment of the fundus in normal and gas-filled phakic eyes. Am J Ophthalmol 98:806, 1984.

26. Stefansson E, Tiedeman J: Optics of the eye with air or silicone oil. Retina 8:10, 1988.

27. Bothner H, Wik O: Rheology of intraocular solutions. In Rosen ES (ed): Vision and Visual Health Care, vol. 2. Viscoelastic Materials. New York, Pergamon Press, 1986.

28. Michels RG, Stark WJ, Stirpe M (eds): Sodium Hyaluronate in Anterior and Posterior Segment Surgery. Padova, Italy, Liviana Press, 1989.

29. Fitzgerald CR: The use of Healon in a case of rolled-over retina. Retina 1:227, 1981.

30. Brown GC, Benson WE: Use of sodium hyaluronate for the repair of giant retinal tears. Arch Ophthalmol 107:1246, 1989.

31. Folk JC, Weingeist TA, Packer AJ: Sodium hyaluronate (Healon) in closed vitrectomy. Ophthalmic Surg 17:299, 1986.

32. Chang S: Low viscosity liquid fluorochemicals in vitreous surgery. Am J Ophthalmol 103:38, 1987.

33. Sargent JW, Seffl RJ: Properties of perfluorinated liquids. Fed Proc 29:1699, 1970.

34. Chang S, Zimmerman NJ, Iwamoto T, et al: Experimental vitreous replacement with perfluorotributylamine. Am J Ophthalmol 103:29, 1987.

35. Chang S, Ozmert E, Zimmerman NJ: Intraoperative perfluorocarbon liquids in the management of proliferative vitreoretinopathy. Am J Ophthalmol 106:668, 1988.

36. Chang S, Reppucci V, Zimmerman NJ, et al: Perfluorocarbon liquids in the management of traumatic retinal detachments. Ophthalmology 96:785, 1989.

37. Chang S, Lincoff H, Zimmerman NJ, Fuchs W: Giant retinal tears. Surgical techniques and results using perfluorocarbon liquids. Arch Ophthalmol 107:761, 1989.

38. Hammer ME, Rinder DF, Hicks EL, et al: Tolerance of perfluorocarbons, fluorosilicone and silicone liquids in the vitreous. In Freeman HM, Tolentino FI (eds): Proliferative Vitreoretinopathy. New York, Springer-Verlag, 1988, pp 156–161.

39. Nabih M, Peyman GA, Clark LC: Experimental evaluation of perfluorophenanthrene as a high specific gravity vitreous substitute: A preliminary report. Ophthalmic Surg 20:286, 1989.

40. Liu K-R, Peyman GA, Chen M-S: Use of high density vitreous substitutes in the removal of posteriorly dislocated lenses or intraocular lenses. Ophthalmic Surg 22:503, 1991.

41. Matthews GP, Ross R, Iwamoto T: Electrophysiological and histological evaluation of retinal tolerance to short-term intravitreal perfluoroethylcyclohexane liquid. Invest Ophthalmol Vis Sci 30(Suppl):439, 1990.

42. Marin J, Manzanas L, Refojo MF, Tolentino FI: Foralkyl AC-6, a perfluorocarbon liquid intravitreous tamponade agent with diminished dispersion tendency. Invest Ophthalmol Vis Sci 31(Suppl):24, 1990.

43. Flores-Aguilar M, Crapotta JA, Munguia D, et al: Perfluorooctylbromide (PFOB) as a temporary vitreous substitute. Invest Ophthalmol Vis Sci 32(Suppl):1225, 1991.

44. Chang S, Sparrow JR, Iwamoto T, et al: Experimental studies of tolerance to intravitreal perfluoro-n-octane liquid. Retina 11:367, 1991.

45. Grafstein D: Detection, estimation and removal of impurities in fluorocarbon liquids. Anal Chem 26:523, 1954.

46. Sparrow JR, Ortiz R, MacLeish PR, et al: Fibroblast behavior at aqueous interfaces with perfluorocarbon, silicone and fluorosilicone liquids. Invest Ophthalmol Vis Sci 31:638, 1990.

47. Shapiro MJ, Resnick KI, Kim SH, Weinberg A: Management of dislocated crystalline lens with a perfluorocarbon liquid. Am J Ophthalmol 112:401, 1991.

48. Mathis A, Pagot V, David J-L: The use of perfluorodecalin in diabetic vitrectomy. Fortschr Ophthalmol 88:148, 1991.

49. Freeman HM: Current management of giant retinal breaks and fellow eyes. In Ryan SJ (ed): Retina. St Louis, CV Mosby, 1989, p 431.

50. Scott JD: The treatment of massive vitreous retraction by the separation of pre-retinal membranes using liquid silicone. Mod Prob Ophthalmol 15:285, 1975.

51. Cibis PA, Becker B, Okun E, Canaan S: The use of liquid silicone in retinal detachment surgery. Arch Ophthalmol 68:46, 1962.

52. Leaver PK, Lean JS: Management of giant retinal tears using vitrectomy and silicone oil/fluid exchange. Trans Ophthalmol Soc UK 101:189, 1981.

53. Mester U, Rothe R, Zubcov A: Experimental studies with a high-density silicone oil for giant retinal tears. Ophthalmol Res 18:81, 1986.

54. Chung H, Acosta J, Refojo MJ, et al: Use of high-density fluorosilicone oil in open-sky vitrectomy. Retina 7:180, 1987.

55. Peyman GA, Smith T: Use of fluorosilicone oil to unfold a giant retinal tear. Int Ophthalmol 10:149, 1987.

56. De Juan E, McCuen B, Tiedeman J: Intraocular tamponade and surface tension. Surv Ophthalmol 30:47, 1985.

57. Parver LM, Lincoff H: Geometry of intraocular gas used in retinal surgery. Mod Probl Ophthalmol (Basel) 18:338, 1977.

58. Parver LM, Lincoff H: Mechanics of intraocular gas. Invest Ophthalmol 17:77, 1978.

59. Hilton GF, Grizzard WS: Pneumatic retinopexy: A two-step outpatient operation without conjunctival incision. Ophthalmology 93:626, 1986.

60. Abrams GW, Edelhauser HF, Aaberg TM, Hamilton LH: Dynamics of intravitreal sulfur hexafluoride gas. Invest Ophthalmol 13:863, 1974.

61. Lincoff A, Haft D, Liggett P, et al: Intravitreal expansion of perfluorocarbon bubbles. Arch Ophthalmol 98:1646, 1980.

62. Peters MA, Abrams GW, Hamilton LH: The nonexpansile, equilibrated concentration of perfluoropropane gas in the eye. Am J Ophthalmol 100:831, 1985.

63. Lincoff H, Maisel JM, Lincoff A: Intravitreal disappearance rates of four perfluorocarbon gases. Arch Ophthalmol 102:928, 1984.

64. Thompson JT: Kinetics of intraocular gases. Disappearance of air, sulfur hexafluoride and perfluoropropane after pars plana vitrectomy. Arch Ophthalmol 107:687, 1989.

65. Norton EWD: Intraocular gases in the management of selected retinal detachments. Trans Am Acad Ophthalmol Otolaryngol 77:OP85, 1973.

66. Sabates WI, Abrams GW, Swanson DE, et al: The use of intraocular gases. The results of sulfur hexafluoride gas in retinal detachment surgery. Ophthalmology 88:447, 1981.

67. Abrams GW, Swanson DE, Sabates WI: The results of sulfur hexafluoride gas in vitreous surgery. Am J Ophthalmol 94:165, 1982.

68. Fineberg E, Machemer R, Sullivan P, et al: Sulfur hexafluoride in owl monkey vitreous cavity. Am J Ophthalmol 79:67, 1975.

69. Lincoff H, Coleman J, Kreissig I, et al: The perfluorocarbon gases in the treatment of retinal detachment. Ophthalmology 90:546, 1983.

70. Chang S, Coleman JD, Lincoff H, Wilcox LM: Perfluoropropane gas in the management of proliferative vitreoretinopathy. Am J Ophthalmol 98:180, 1984.

71. Crittenden JJ, De Juan E Jr, Tiedeman J: Expansion of long-acting gas bubbles for intraocular use. Principles and practice. Arch Ophthalmol 103:831, 1985.

72. Miller B, Lean J, Miller H, et al: Intravitreal expanding gas bubble: A morphologic study in the rabbit eye. Arch Ophthalmol 102:1708, 1984.

73. Foulks GN, de Juan E, Hatchell DL: The effect of perfluoropropane on the cornea in rabbits and cats. Arch Ophthalmol 105:256, 1987.

74. Lee DA, Wilson MR, Yoshizumi MO, Hall M: The ocular effects of gases when injected into the anterior chamber of rabbit eyes. Arch Ophthalmol 109:571, 1991.

75. Vygantas CM, Peyman GA, Daily MJ, Ericson ES: Octafluorocyclobutane and other gases for vitreous replacement. Arch Ophthalmol 90:235, 1973.

76. Killey FP, Edelhauser HF, Aaberg TM: Intraocular sulfur hexafluoride and octofluorocyclobutane. Effects on intraocular pressure and vitreous volume. Arch Ophthalmol 96:511, 1978.

77. Lincoff A, Lincoff H, Iwamoto I, et al: Perfluoro-*n*-butane. A gas for a maximum duration retinal tamponade. Arch Ophthalmol 101:460, 1983.

78. Chang S, Lincoff HA, Coleman DJ, et al: Perfluorocarbon gases in vitreous surgery. Ophthalmology 92:651, 1985.

79. Hoffman ME, Sorr EM: Management of giant retinal tears without scleral buckling. Retina 6:197, 1986.

80. Machemer R, Allen AW: Retinal tears 180 degree and greater: Management with vitrectomy and intravitreal gas. Arch Ophthalmol 94:1340, 1976.

81. Williams DF, Peter MA, Abrams GW, et al: A two-stage technique for intraoperative fluid-gas exchange following pars plana vitrectomy. Arch Ophthalmol 108:1484, 1990.

82. Humayun MS, Yeo JH, Koski WS, et al: The rate of sulfur hexafluoride escape from a plastic syringe. Arch Ophthalmol 107:853, 1989.

83. Lincoff H, Kreissig I, Coleman DJ, Chang S: Use of an intraocular gas tamponade to find retinal breaks. Am J Ophthalmol 96:510, 1983.

84. Wong RF, Thompson JT: Prediction of the kinetics of disappearance of sulfur hexafluoride and perfluoropropane. Ophthalmology 95:609, 1988.

85. Bloch D, O'Connor P, Lincoff H: The mechanism of cryosurgical adhesion. III. Statistical analysis. Am J Ophthalmol 71:666, 1971.

86. Gardner TW, Norris JL, Zakov ZN: A survey of intraocular gas use in North America. Arch Ophthalmol 106:1188, 1988.

87. Bonnet M, Santamaria E, Mouche J: Intraoperative use of pure perfluoropropane gas in the management of proliferative vitreoretinopathy. Graefes Arch Clin Exp Ophthalmol 225:299, 1987.

88. Aaberg TM: Management of anterior and posterior proliferative vitreoretinopathy. Am J Ophthalmol 106:519, 1988.

89. Fisher YL, Shakin JL, Slakter JS, et al: Perfluoropropane gas, modified panretinal photocoagulation, and vitrectomy in the management of severe proliferative vitreoretinopathy. Arch Ophthalmol 106:1255, 1988.

90. Lincoff H, Mardirossian J, Lincoff A, et al: Intravitreal longevity of three perfluorocarbon gases. Arch Ophthalmol 98:1610, 1980.

91. Aronowitz JD, Brubaker RF: Effect of intraocular gas on intraocular pressure. Arch Ophthalmol 94:1191, 1976.

92. Poliner LS, Schoch LH: Intraocular pressure assessment in gas-filled eyes following vitrectomy. Arch Ophthalmol 105:200, 1987.

93. Moses RA: Schiøtz tonometry with an air bubble in the eye. Am J Ophthalmol 62:281, 1966.

94. Dieckert JP, O'Connor PS, Schacklett DE, et al: Air travel and intraocular gas. Ophthalmology 93:L642, 1986.

95. Lincoff H, Weinberger D, Reppucci V: Air travel with intraocular gas. I. The mechanisms for compensation. Arch Ophthalmol 107:902, 1989.

96. Lincoff H, Weinberger D, Stergiu P: Air travel with intraocular gas. II. Clinical considerations. Arch Ophthalmol 107:907, 1989.

97. Smith RB, Swartz M, Carl B: Effect of nitrous oxide on air in vitreous. Am J Ophthalmol 78:314, 1974.

98. Wolf GL, Capuano C, Hartung J: Nitrous oxide increases intraocular pressure after intravitreal sulfur hexafluoride injection. Anesthesiology 59:547, 1983.

99. Yamamoto K, Iwasaki T, Juzoji H, et al: Aqueous laser flaremetry following intravitreous gas injection in rabbits. Invest Ophthalmol Vis Sci 31(Suppl):439, 1990.

100. Ogura Y, Tsukada T, Negi A, et al: Integrity of the blood-ocular barrier after intravitreal gas injection. Retina 9:199, 1989.

101. Sparrow JR, Chang S, Vinals A: Evaluation of the blood-aqueous barrier following vitreous replacement with perfluoropropane gas and liquid silicone. Retina, in press.

102. Constable IJ, Swann DA: Vitreous substitution with gases. Arch Ophthalmol 93:416, 1975.

103. Wong RF, Liggett PE: Intraocular inflammation following intravitreal gas injection. Invest Ophthalmol Vis Sci31(Suppl):438, 1990.

140. Chang S, Lincoff H, Ozmert E, et al: Management of retinal detachment with moderate PVR. *In* Freeman HM, Tolentino FI (eds): Proliferative Vitreoretinopathy. New York, Springer-Verlag, 1988, p 54.

105. Lambrou FH, Burke JM, Aaberg MD: Effect of silicone oil on experimental traction retinal detachment. Arch Ophthalmol 105:1269, 1987.

106. Lincoff H, Kreissig I, Jakobiec F: The inadvertent injection of gas beneath the retina in a pseudophakic eye. Ophthalmology 93:408, 1986.

107. O'Connor PR: Intravitreous air injection and the Custodis procedure. Ophthalmol Surg 7:86, 1976.

108. Blumenkranz M, Gardner T, Blankenship G: Fluid-gas exchange and photocoagulation after vitrectomy. Arch Ophthalmol 104:291, 1986.

109. Petersen J: The physical and surgical aspects of silicone oil in the vitreous cavity. Graefes Arch Clin Exp Ophthalmol 225:452, 1987.

110. Parel J-M: Silicone oils: Physicochemical properties. *In* Ryan SJ (ed): The Retina. St Louis, CV Mosby, 1989, p 261.

111. Gonvers M: Temporary silicone oil tamponade in the treatment of complicated diabetic retinal detachments. Graefes Arch Clin Exp Ophthalmol 228:415, 1990.

112. Glaser BM, de Bustros S, Michels RG: Postoperative retinal breaks occurring after intravitreal silicone oil injection. Retina 4:246, 1984.

113. Lewis H, Burke JM, Abrams GW: Perisilicone proliferation after vitrectomy for proliferative vitreoretinopathy. Ophthalmology 95:583, 1988.

114. Machemer R: The importance of fluid absorption, traction, intraocular currents, and chorioretinal scars in the therapy of rhegmatogenous retinal detachments. Am J Ophthalmol 98:681, 1984.

115. Grey RHB, Leaver PK: Results of silicone oil injection in massive preretinal retraction. Trans Ophthalmol Soc UK 97:238, 1977.

116. Grey RHB, Leaver PK: Silicone oil in the treatment of massive preretinal retraction. I. Results in 105 eyes. Br J Ophthalmol 63:355, 1979.

117. Cairns JD, Anand N: Combined vitrectomy, intraocular micro-

surgery and liquid silicone in the treatment of proliferative vitreoretinopathy. Aust J Ophthalmol 12:133, 1984.

118. Ando F, Miyake Y, Oshima K, et al: Temporary use of intraocular silicone in the treatment of complicated retinal detachment. Graefes Arch Clin Exp Ophthalmol 224:32, 1985.

119. Cox MS, Trese MT, Murphy PL: Silicone oil for advanced proliferative vitreoretinopathy. Ophthalmology 93:636, 1986.

120. Lean JS, Leaver PK, Cooling RJ: Management of complex retinal detachments by vitrectomy and fluid/silicone exchange. Trans Ophthalmol Soc UK 102:203, 1982.

121. Lean JS, Van der Zee WAM, Ryan SJ: Experimental model of proliferative vitreoretinopathy (PVR) in the vitrectomised eye: Effect of silicone oil. Br J Ophthalmol 68:332, 1984.

122. Gonvers M: Temporary silicone oil tamponade in the management of retinal detachment with proliferative vitreoretinopathy. Am J Ophthalmol 100:239, 1985.

123. Lucke KH, Foerster MH, Laqua H: Long-term results of vitrectomy and silicone oil in 500 cases of complicated retinal detachments. Am J Ophthalmol 104:624, 1987.

124. Yeo JH, Glaser BM, Michels RG: Silicone oil in the treatment of complicated retinal detachment. Ophthalmology 94:1109, 1987.

125. Sell CH, McCuen MW, Landers MB: Long-term results of successful vitrectomy with silicone oil for advanced proliferative vitreoretinopathy. Am J Ophthalmol 103:24, 1987.

126. McCuen BW, Landers MB, Machemer R: The use of silicone oil following failed vitrectomy for retinal detachment with advanced proliferative vitreoretinopathy. Graefes Arch Clin Exp Ophthalmol 224:38, 1986.

127. Billington BM, Leaver PK: Vitrectomy and fluid/silicone-oil exchange for giant retinal tears: Results at 18 months. Graefes Arch Clin Exp Ophthalmol 224:7, 1986.

128. Leaver PK, Cooling RJ, Feretis EB: Vitrectomy and fluid/silicone-oil exchange for giant retinal tears: Results at six months. Br J Ophthalmol 68:432, 1984.

129. Glaser BM: Treatment of giant retinal tears combined with proliferative vitreoretinopathy. Ophthalmology 93:1193, 1986.

130. McLeod D: Silicone-oil injection during closed microsurgery for diabetic retinal detachment. Graefes Arch Clin Exp Ophthalmol 224:55, 1986.

131. Rinkoff JS, de Juan E Jr, McCuen BW: Silicone oil for retinal detachment with advanced proliferative vitreoretinopathy following failed vitrectomy for proliferative diabetic retinopathy. Am J Ophthalmol 101:181, 1986.

132. Antoszyk AN, McCuen BW, de Juan E Jr, et al: Silicone oil injection after failed primary vitreous surgery in severe ocular trauma. Am J Ophthalmol 107:537, 1989.

133. Iverson DA, Ward TG, Blumenkranz MS: Indications and results of relaxing retinotomy. Ophthalmology 97:1298, 1990.

134. McCuen BW, de Juan E, Machemer R: Silicone oil in vitreoretinal surgery. Part 1 Surgical techniques. Retina 5:189, 1985.

135. Heimann K, Dahl B, Dimopoulos S, et al: Pars plana vitrectomy and silicone oil injection in proliferative diabetic retinopathy. Graefes Arch Clin Exp Ophthalmol 227:152, 1989.

136. Cockerham WD, Schepens CL, Freeman HM: Silicone injection in retinal detachment. Arch Ophthalmol 83:704, 1970.

137. Abrams GW: Retinotomies and retinectomies. In Ryan SJ (ed): Retina. St Louis, CV Mosby, 1989, p 317.

138. Han DP, Lewis MT, Kuhn EM, et al: Relaxing retinotomies and retinectomies. Surgical results and predictors of visual outcome. Arch Ophthalmol 108:694, 1990.

139. Morse LS, McCuen BW, Machemer R: Relaxing retinotomies. Analysis of anatomic and visual results. Ophthalmology 97:642, 1990.

140. Federman JL, Eagle RC: Extensive peripheral retinectomy combined with posterior 360 degree retinotomy for retinal reattachment in advanced proliferative vitreoretinopathy cases. Ophthalmology 97:1305, 1990.

141. Comaratta MR, Sparrow JS, Chang S: Iris neovascularization in proliferative vitreoretinopathy. Ophthalmology 99:898, 1992.

142. Scott JD: Use of liquid silicone in vitrectomized eyes. Dev Ophthalmol 2:185, 1981.

143. De Juan E, Hardy M, Hatchell DL, Hatchell MC: The effect of

144. DeCorral LR, Peyman GA: Pars plana vitrectomy and intravitreal silicone oil injection in eyes with rubeosis iridis. Can J Ophthalmol 21:10, 1986.

145. Machemer R: Massive periretinal proliferation: A logical approach to therapy. Trans Am Ophthalmol Soc 75:556, 1977.

146. Rachal WF, Burton TC: Changing concepts of failures after retinal detachment surgery. Arch Ophthalmol 97:480, 1979.

147. Michels R: Surgery for retinal detachment with proliferative vitreoretinopathy. Retina 4:63, 1984.

148. Haut J, Larricart JP, Van Effenterre G, Pinon-Pignero FI: Some of the most important properties of silicone oil to explain its action. Ophthalmologica (Basel) 191:150, 1985.

149. Watzke RC: Silicone retinopoiesis for retinal detachment. Arch Ophthalmol 77:185, 1967.

150. Chan C, Okun E: The question of ocular tolerance to intravitreal liquid silicone. Ophthalmology 93:651, 1986.

151. McCuen BW, de Juan E, Landers MB, et al: Silicone oil in vitreoretinal surgery. Part 2. Results and complications. Retina 5:198, 1985.

152. McCuen BW, Landers MB, Machemer R: The use of silicone oil following failed vitrectomy for retinal detachment with advanced proliferative vitreoretinopathy. Ophthalmology 92:1029, 1985.

153. Hutton WL, Fuller DW, Snyder WB: Silicone oil for management of PVR: Comparison of six-month and two-year results. In Freeman HM, Tolentino FI (eds): Proliferative Vitreoretinopathy. New York, Springer-Verlag, 1988, p 166.

154. Ando F: Usefulness and limit of silicone oil in the management of complicated retinal detachment. Jpn J Ophthalmol 31:138, 1987.

155. Zilis JD, McCuen BW, de Juan E Jr, et al: Results of silicone oil removal in advanced proliferative vitreoretinopathy. Am J Ophthalmol 108:15, 1989.

156. Federman JL, Schubert HD: Complications associated with the use of silicone oil in 150 eyes after retina-vitreous surgery. Ophthalmology 95:870, 1988.

157. Casswell AG, Gregor ZJ: Silicone oil removal. II. Operative and postoperative complications. Br J Ophthalmol 71:898, 1987.

158. Fletcher ME, Peyman GA: A simplified technique for the removal of liquid silicone from vitrectomized eyes. Retina 5:168, 1985.

159. Fan RFT, Chung H, Tolentino FI, et al: Effectiveness of silicone oil removal from rabbit eyes. Graefes Arch Clin Exp Ophthalmol 225:338, 1987.

160. The Silicone Study Group: Proliferative vitreoretinopathy. Am J Ophthalmol 99:593, 1985.

161. Stern WH, Lean JS: Intraocular silicone oil versus gas in the management of PVR: A multicenter clinical study. In Freeman HM, Tolentino FI (eds): Proliferative Vitreoretinopathy. New York, Springer-Verlag, 1988, p 88.

162. Leaver PK, Grey RHB, Garner A: Complications following silicone-oil injection. Mod Probl Ophthalmol 20:290, 1979.

163. Ni C, Wang W-J, Albert DM, et al: Intravitreous silicone injection. Histopathologic findings in a human eye after 12 years. Arch Ophthalmol 101:1399, 1983.

164. Laroche L, Pavlakis C, Saraux H, Orcel L: Ocular findings following intravitreal silicone injection. Arch Ophthalmol 101:1422, 1983.

165. Parmley VC, Barishak R, Howes EL: Foreign-body giant cell reaction to liquid silicone. Am J Ophthalmol 101:680, 1986.

166. Lee PF, Donovan RH, Mukai N: Intravitreous injection of silicone: An experimental study. Ann Ophthalmol 1:15, 1969.

167. Mukai N, Lee PF, Schepens CL: Intravitreous injection of silicone: An experimental study. Ann Ophthalmol 4:273, 1972.

168. Mukai N, Lee PF, Oguri M, et al: A long-term evaluation of silicone retinopathy in monkeys. Can J Ophthalmol 10:391, 1975.

169. Gonvers M, Hornung J-P, de Courten C: The effect of liquid silicone on the rabbit retina. Histologic and ultrastructural study. Arch Ophthalmol 104:1057, 1986.

170. Refojo JF, Chung H, Cajita VN: Retinol and cholesterol in intraocular silicone and fluorosilicone oils. In: Freeman HM, Tolentino FI (eds): Proliferative Vitreoretinopathy. New York, Springer-Verlag, 1988, p 181.

intraocular silicone oil on anterior chamber oxygen pressure in cats. Arch Ophthalmol 104:1063, 1986.

171. Armaly MF: Ocular tolerance to silicones. I. Replacement of aqueous and vitreous by silicone fluids. Arch Ophthalmol 68:390, 1962.
172. Labelle P, Okun E: Ocular tolerance to liquid silicone. An experimental study. Can J Ophthalmol 7:199, 1972.
173. Ober RR, Blanks JC, Ogden TE, et al: Experimental retinal tolerance to liquid silicone. Retina 3:77, 1983.
174. Foerster MH, Esser J, Laqua H: Silicone oil and its influence on electrophysiological findings. Am J Ophthalmol 99:201, 1985.
175. Meredith TA, Lindsey DT, Edelhauser HF, Goldman AI: Electroretinographic studies following vitrectomy and intraocular silicone oil injection. Br J Ophthalmol 69:254, 1985.
176. Kirchhof B, Tavakolian U, Paulmann H: Histopathological findings in eyes after silicone oil injection. Graefes Arch Clin Exp Ophthalmol 224:34, 1986.
177. Kellner U, Lucke K, Foerster MH: Effect of intravitreal liquid silicone on optic nerve function. Am J Ophthalmol 106:293, 1988.
178. Momirov D, van Lith GHM, Zivojnovic R: Electroretinogram and electrooculogram of eyes with intravitreously injected silicone oil. Ophthalmologica (Basel) 186:183, 1983.
179. Thaler A, Jessel MR, Gnad H: The influence of intravitreously injected silicone oil on electrophysiological potentials of the eye. Doc Ophthalmol 62:41, 1986.
180. Doslak MJ: A theoretical study of the effect of silicone oil on the electroretinogram. Invest Ophthalmol Vis Sci 29:1881, 1988.
181. Prince JH: The Rabbit Eye in Research. Springfield IL, Charles C Thomas, 1964.
182. Gabel V-P, Kampik A, Burkhardt J: Analysis of intraocularly applied silicone oils of various origins. Graefes Arch Clin Exp Ophthalmol 225:160, 1987.
183. Crisp A, de Juan E, Tiedeman J: Effect of silicone oil viscosity on emulsification. Arch Ophthalmol 105:546, 1987.
184. Kreiner CF: Chemical and physical aspects of clinically applied silicones. Dev Ophthalmol 14:11, 1987.
185. Heidenkummer H-P, Kampik A, Thierfelder S: Emulsification of silicone oils with specific physicochemical characteristics. Graefes Arch Clin Exp Ophthalmol 229:88, 1991.
186. Petersen J, Ritzau-Tondrow U: Chronisches Glaukom nach Silikonölimplantation: Zwei Öle verschiedener Viskosität im Vergleich. Fortschr Ophthalmol 85:632, 1988.
187. Sternberg P, Hatchell DI, Foulks GN: The effect of silicone oil on the cornea. Arch Ophthalmol 103:90, 1985.
188. Ando F: Intraocular hypertension resulting from pupillary block by silicone oil. Am J Ophthalmol 99:87, 1985.
189. Leaver PK: Complications of intraocular silicone oil. In Ryan SJ (ed): Retina. St Louis, CV Mosby, 1989, pp 293–306.
190. Fastenberg DM, Diddie KR, Delmage M, et al: Intraocular injection of silicone oil for experimental proliferative vitreoretinopathy. Am J Ophthalmol 95:663, 1983.
191. Gonvers M, Thresher R: Temporary use of silicone oil in the treatment of proliferative vitreoretinopathy: An experimental study with a new animal model. Graefes Clin Exp Ophthalmol 221:46, 1983.
192. Charles S: Vitreous Microsurgery, 2nd ed. Baltimore, Williams & Wilkins, 1987.
193. Sen HA, Robertson TJ, Conway BP, Campochiaro PA: The role of breakdown of the blood-retinal barrier in cell-injection models of proliferative vitreoretinopathy. Arch Ophthalmol 106:1291, 1987.
194. Jaccoma EH, Conway BP, Campochiaro PA: Cryotherapy causes extensive breakdown of the blood-retinal barrier. A comparison with argon laser photocoagulation. Arch Ophthalmol 103:1728, 1985.
195. Campochiaro PA, Bryan JA, Conway BP, Jaccoma EH: Intravitreal chemotactic and mitogenic activity. Implication of blood-retinal barrier breakdown. Arch Ophthalmol 104:1685, 1986.
196. Vinals A, Gershbein A, Sparrow JR, et al: Evaluation of the blood-aqueous barrier following vitreous replacement with liquid silicone. Invest Ophthlamol Vis Sci 32(Suppl):1225, 1991.
197. Gabel V-P, Kampik A, Gabel CH: Silicone oil with high specific gravity for intraocular use. Br J Ophthalmol 71:262, 1987.
198. Tolentino RK, Cajita VN, Chung H, et al: High-density fluorosilicone oil in vitreous surgery. In Freeman HM, Tolentino FI (eds): Proliferative Vitreoretinopathy. New York, Springer-Verlag, 1988, pp 177–180.
199. Peyman GA, Smith T, Charles H: Injection of fluorosilicone oil and pars plana vitrectomy for complex retinal detachment. Can J Ophthalmol 22:276, 1987.
200. Paris CL, Peyman GA, Blinder KJ, et al: Surgical technique for managing rhegmatogenous retinal detachment following prosthokeratoplasty. Retina 11:301, 1991.
201. Sparrow JR, Jayakumar A, Berrocal M, et al: Experimental studies of the combined use of vitreous substitute materials of high and low specific gravity. Retina 12:134, 1992.
202. Soike K, Peyman GA, Conway MD: Long-term vitreous replacement with intravitreal vitreon or vitreon plus silicone. Invest Ophthalmol Vis Sci 32:1225, 1991.
203. Daniele S, Refojo MF, Schepens CL, Freeman HM: Glyceryl methacrylate hydrogel as a vitreous implant. Arch Ophthalmol 80:120, 1968.
204. Refojo MF, Zauberman H: Optical properties of gels designed for vitreous implantation. Invest Ophthalmol 12:465, 1973.
205. Chan IM, Tolentino FK, Refojo MF, et al: Vitreous substitute. Experimental studies and review. Retina 4:51, 1984.

Chapter 102

■

Postoperative Endophthalmitis

DONALD J. D'AMICO and STUART W. NOORILY

The development of infectious endophthalmitis after cataract surgery is a potentially catastrophic event. Despite prompt intervention, only 39 to 73 percent of affected eyes have visual acuity outcomes of 20/400 or better (Table 102–1).[1–5] Fortunately, the prognosis has improved considerably in recent years with refinements in diagnosis, intravitreal antibiotic therapy, and vitreous surgery. The rapid diagnosis and appropriate treatment of these cases remain a clinical challenge.

CLINICAL SETTING

Bacterial endophthalmitis occurs in a number of clinical settings. Compilation of large reported series (Table 102–2) suggests the following distribution of cases: 62 percent occur following intraocular surgery, 20 percent occur following penetrating trauma, 10 percent occur following planned or inadvertent filtering blebs, and 8 percent occur as the result of metastatic infection.[1, 2, 4–7]

Table 102–1. VISUAL RECOVERY IN TREATED ENDOPHTHALMITIS*

Authors	Culture-Negative	Culture-Positive						
		Staphylococcus epidermidis	Gram-positive†	Gram-negative‡	Fungi	Mixed	Total	
Bohigian and Olk[1]	61% (19/31)	87% (13/15)	21% (5/24)	11% (1/9)	33% (1/3)		39% (20/51)	
Diamond[2]		80% (8/10)	70% (7/10)	67% (2/3)	67% (2/3)		73% (19/26)	
Driebe et al[3]	94% (15/16)	78% (14/18)	56% (9/16)	40% (4/10)	60% (3/5)		63% (32/51)	
Puliafito et al[4]		75% (12/16)	22% (2/9)	20% (1/5)	0% (0/1)	0% (0/5)	42% (15/36)	
Rowsey et al[5]	53% (8/15)	75% (12/16)	23% (5/22)	25% (2/8)	75% (3/4)	0% (0/5)	40% (22/55)	

*Visual recovery defined as 20/400 or better visual acuity.
†Includes all gram-positive isolates except *Staphylococcus epidermidis*.
‡Total includes two miscellaneous cases in which the organism cannot be determined from the published data.

The incidence of endophthalmitis following cataract surgery was evaluated by Allen and Mangiaracine in 1964 and was found to be 0.086 percent, based on a series of 36,000 consecutive cataract operations performed at the Massachusetts Eye and Ear Infirmary.[8] A more recent evaluation of postoperative endophthalmitis was performed by Koul and coworkers, in which incidences ranging from 0.33 percent (culture-positive or unavailable) down to 0.06 percent (culture-positive) were calculated based on a review of ocular surgery performed in Sweden in 1982 to 1983, including cataract surgery and other procedures.[9] The list of possible sources of infection includes inadequate lid and conjunctival preparation, contamination by the operating room personnel, contaminated instruments or solutions, airborne contaminants, or the use of a contaminated intraocular lens (IOL).[8, 10] Entry of fluid from the conjunctival cul de sac into the eye during automated extracapsular cataract surgery has been shown to be a routine accompaniment of the procedure.[10] The routine use of subconjunctival antibiotics at the end of surgery does not completely prevent postoperative endophthalmitis; in one series of 62 culture-positive cases, 90 percent of a subgroup of patients who received subconjunctival antibiotics at the end of cataract surgery were infected with an organism sensitive to the antibiotic administered.[3] Also, the spread of infection from the anterior chamber to the vitreous appears to be impeded if the posterior capsule is intact.[11] Interestingly, one third of postoperative endophthalmitis cases reportedly follow vitreous loss or unplanned extracapsular cataract extraction. Likewise, a problem with cataract wound closure has been noted in 22 percent of cases.[3] These findings suggest that a sizable number of cases of postoperative endophthalmitis might be prevented by meticulous surgical technique.

DIAGNOSIS

The accurate diagnosis of endophthalmitis after cataract surgery requires attention to clinical symptoms and signs, as well as appropriately selected laboratory tests. The earliest symptom of endophthalmitis is usually discomfort or deep pain, although the rapid postoperative improvement in visual acuity with IOL implantation has increased the number of patients reporting a loss of vision as the initial symptom of endophthalmitis.

Signs of endophthalmitis include conjunctival hyperemia, chemosis, cells and flare in the anterior chamber, hypopyon, membrane formation on the IOL, vitritis, scattered retinal hemorrhages, loss of red reflex, and in extreme cases, corneal opacification (Figs. 102–1 and 102–2). Retinal periphlebitis may be observed as an early sign of bacterial endophthalmitis.[12] Typically, the findings of bacterial endophthalmitis have their onset within 24 to 48 hr of infection and progress rapidly. However, infection caused by less virulent organisms may delay clinical presentation from 4 to 12 days or longer. It is also important to consider the possible

Table 102–2. CLINICAL SETTING IN ENDOPHTHALMITIS

Author	Total	Postoperative	Trauma	Bleb	Metastatic
Bohigian and Olk[1]*	82	55 (67%)	16 (20%)	5 (6%)	6 (7%)
Diamond[2]†	22	16 (73%)	5 (23%)	1 (4%)	
Forster et al[6]*	140	69 (49%)	31 (22%)	25 (18%)	15 (11%)
Nelsen et al[7]*	55	42 (76%)	9 (16%)	4 (7%)	
Puliafito et al[4]*	36	24 (66%)	6 (17%)	4 (11%)	2 (6%)
Rowsey[5]†	54	34 (63%)	12 (22%)		8 (15%)
TOTAL	389	240 (62%)	79 (20%)	39 (10%)	31 (8%)

*Clinical setting reported on the basis of suspected infectious endophthalmitis.
†Clinical setting reported on the basis of culture-positive cases.

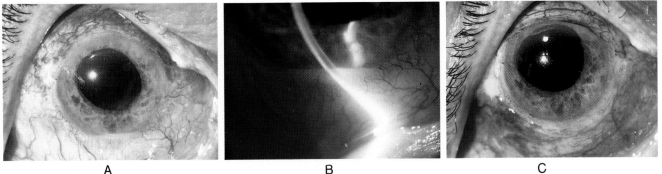

Figure 102–1. A, Postoperative endophthalmitis due to *Staphylococcus epidermidis* presenting 6 days after extracapsular cataract extraction with posterior chamber lens implantation. Visual acuity was at the hand motions level, and conjunctival hyperemia, hypopyon, and inflammatory membrane on the intraocular lens (IOL) are seen. *B,* Slit-lamp photograph of hypopyon in this patient. *C,* Visual acuity has improved to 20/500 (limited by preexisting macular degeneration) 2 wk later following vitrectomy with intravitreal administration of vancomycin (1 mg), amikacin (400 µg), and dexamethasone (200 µg). The inflammatory membrane on the IOL was removed at surgery (see text); the IOL was not removed.

masking effect of topical steroid therapy in these patients, as this may minimize the hyperemia as well as delay hypopyon formation. In some cases, perhaps as a result of traumatic wound dehiscence, metastatic infection, or infection by indolent organisms such as *Propionibacterium,* several months or years may elapse before clinical signs are apparent.[13–20]

Although pain and hypopyon constitute the classic presentation of bacterial endophthalmitis, these findings are absent in a significant percentage of patients with documented endophthalmitis,[21] particularly whom infection is caused by *Staphylococcus epidermidis.* Conversely, some patients will experience pain following cataract extraction with IOL implantation. Inflammatory reactions with symptoms and signs indistinguishable from infectious endophthalmitis have been described with phacoanaphylaxis,[22, 23] reaction to the IOL and associated materials,[24, 25] virgin silk sutures in the cataract wound,[26] and numerous other causes.[27, 28] The diagnosis of bacterial endophthalmitis must be suspected on the basis of inflammation that is out of proportion

to the clinical setting, and it is clear that there may be considerable overlap between infectious endophthalmitis and noninfectious inflammatory reactions in the postoperative cataract patient. In certain cases, ultrasound examination may be helpful in diagnosis. The combination of thickening of the retinochoroid layer and echoes in the anterior or posterior vitreous, or both, are supportive of the diagnosis of endophthalmitis.[29]

Accurate diagnosis ultimately rests with the demonstration of infectious organisms within the eye by appropriate cultures and stains. Given the rapidity with which endophthalmitis can progress to irreversible visual loss, the prompt acquisition of specimens for culture in all suspected cases is an essential element of therapy.

DIAGNOSTIC CULTURES

Approximately 64 percent of eyes with a clinical diagnosis of infectious endophthalmitis will have a positive culture result (Table 102–3).[1, 3, 5–7] The value of

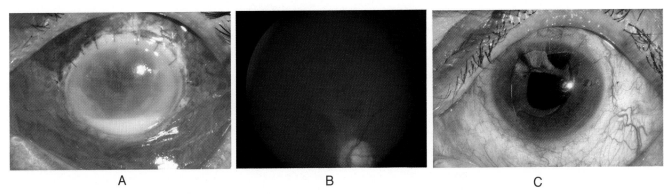

Figure 102–2. A, Postoperative endophthalmitis due to *S. epidermidis* presenting 4 days after extracapsular cataract extraction, complicated by vitreous loss, with anterior chamber lens implantation. Visual acuity is at the light perception level, and conjunctival hyperemia, mild corneal edema, hypopyon, and inflammatory membranes on the iris and both surfaces of the IOL are evident. *B,* Fundus photograph after vitrectomy documents the petechial retinal hemorrhages frequently observed in association with active endophthalmitis. *C,* Two months after vitrectomy with intravitreal administration of amikacin (400 µg), cefazolin (2.25 mg), and dexamethasone (200 µg), visual acuity has improved to 20/300. The IOL is preserved following intraoperative removal of the inflammatory membranes noted preoperatively.

Table 102–3. INCIDENCE OF A POSITIVE CULTURE RESULT IN SUSPECTED INFECTIOUS ENDOPHTHALMITIS

Bohigian and Olk[1]	62.1%	(51/82)
Driebe et al[3]*	74.7%	(62/83)
Forster et al[6]*	55.7%	(78/140)
Nelsen et al[7]	54.5%	(30/55)
Rowsey et al[5]	77.1%	(54/70)
Overall	64.0%	(275/430)

*These two series from the same institution partially overlap.

obtaining specimens for bacterial culture is twofold. Not only are cultures imperative in identifying causative organisms and directing therapy but also the presence of a negative culture result is predictive of a greatly improved visual outcome. In one series, 94 percent of culture-negative pseudophakic eyes achieved 20/400 or better visual acuity.[3]

It has been demonstrated that the vitreous is more easily infected than the anterior chamber.[30] Numerous studies have confirmed the necessity of vitreous culture in endophthalmitis, as the anterior chamber culture result is negative in the face of a positive vitreous culture result in a substantial number of cases.[3, 6, 31] Conversely, as a negative vitreous culture result may be accompanied by a positive anterior chamber culture result, both anterior chamber and vitreous cultures should be performed.[1, 3] Specimens should be cultured on blood agar at 25°C and 37°C, as well as chocolate agar, thioglycolate, and Sabouraud agar, and on an anaerobic medium such as cooked meat medium. Smears should be examined by microscopy with Gram's and Giemsa's stains. In cases of suspected fungal endophthalmitis, evaluation by Gomori's methenamine silver, and more recently Cellufluor or Calcofluor white, may allow rapid identification of fungal elements.[32] The usefulness of the Gram stain in directing therapy is limited, however, as it is inconsistent with culture results or inappropriately negative in 30 to 33 percent of cases.[5, 33] Joondeph and associates evaluated a simplified culture technique involving the direct injection of vitreous specimens into blood culture bottles; they documented a high correlation with recovery of organisms compared with the more definitive membrane filter techniques. Their simplified technique is particularly helpful in patient care settings with limited microbiologic laboratory support.[34]

The usefulness of a conjunctival specimen culture is quite limited, as it may be inappropriately negative, positive with an unrelated organism, or accurately demonstrative of the offending organism within the eye. However, because of the ease of obtaining a conjunctival specimen, culture may be carried out as a supplement to aqueous and vitreous cultures. In addition, in certain patients with blepharitis, wound dehiscence, or filtration bleb with prominent exudation, the concordance of a positive conjunctival culture with aqueous or vitreous culture lends support to the suspected route of infection and may indicate the need for external lid therapy, especially if the second eye is in jeopardy because of the presence of a filtration bleb or if the second eye is to be considered for intraocular surgery at a later date.

CULTURE RESULTS

Review of large clinical series[3–6, 35] indicates that approximately 56 to 90 percent of isolates in postoperative patients are gram-positive, 7 to 29 percent are gram-negative, and 3 to 13 percent are fungal. In general, infections involve a single organism, although an incidence of mixed gram-positive infections as high as 33 percent has been reported.[4] Of the gram-positive isolates, 30 to 50 percent are S. epidermidis, 10 to 30 percent are Staphylococcus aureus, and 15 to 30 percent are Streptococcus species. S. epidermidis is the predominant organism encountered in postoperative cases of endophthalmitis. Streptococcal species predominate in endophthalmitis associated with filtering blebs.[36] Bacillus species are primarily encountered in endophthalmitis following penetrating trauma, although cases have been reported following sepsis with this organism.[37, 38] In trauma, Bacillus has been reported to account for 26 to 46 percent of cases.[39–42]

Of the gram-negative isolates, 30 to 40 percent are Proteus species, 20 percent are Pseudomonas aeruginosa, and 20 percent are Hemophilus species. H. influenzae is the most common gram-negative isolate encountered in endophthalmitis following filtration blebs.[36]

MEDICAL THERAPY

Table 102–4 summarizes recommended drug doses, and practical guidelines for therapy are suggested in Table 102–5.

A major turning point in the development of successful therapy for endophthalmitis occurred in 1944 when von Sallmann and colleagues demonstrated that the intraocular injection of penicillin eradicated S. aureus endophthalmitis in the rabbit.[43] Intravitreal antibiotic therapy was subsequently developed further and has dramatically improved the possibility for salvaging vision in endophthalmitis.[6, 30, 44–61] The ideal antibiotic for intravitreal injection would (1) be effective against the offending organism, (2) be nontoxic to the retina and other ocular structures in bactericidal doses, (3) have an appropriate half-life within the vitreous to be effective, and (4) be injected prior to the irreversible destruction of the retina and other ocular tissues. In the interest of prompt therapy, and because of the documented inaccuracies in Gram's stain evaluation of the vitreous,[5, 33] intravitreal agents must be selected in advance of culture results, and coverage with a combination of drugs directed against gram-positive and gram-negative organisms is required. Consideration of the clinical setting (postoperative, penetrating trauma, and so on) provides some indication of the probable causative organism. Review of the most common organisms encountered after cataract extraction indicates that coverage for Staphylococci is most critical, and intravitreal cephalosporins[55] or methicillin have been widely used with success. However, the increasing emergence of methicillin-resistant Staphylococci has limited the use-

Table 102–4. POSTOPERATIVE ENDOPHTHALMITIS: SUGGESTED DOSES FOR MEDICAL THERAPY

Suspected Bacterial Cases

Intravitreal Injection*

Vancomycin, 1.0 mg *and*
Amikacin, 400 µg, *or* gentamicin, 100 µg
(Consider dexamethasone, 200–400 µg)†

Subconjunctival Injection‡

Vancomycin, 25 mg, and gentamicin, 20 mg

Topical Therapy‡

Vancomycin (25 mg/ml) q2–4 hr, staggered with
Gentamicin fortified (14 mg/ml) ~2–4 hr
Prednisolone acetate 1% q.i.d.

Systemic Therapy‡§

Vancomycin and gentamicin

Suspected Fungal Cases

Intravitreal Injection

Amphotericin B 5–10 µg

Systemic Therapy

Ketoconazole, 400–600 mg daily by oral administration *or*
Amphotericin B‖

---

*Intravitreal injections are not repeated unless repeat culture or smear demonstrates persisting organisms or profound clinical deterioration occurs despite initial injections.

†Intravitreal dexamethasone may be considered in all cases but is of particular benefit in cases with more severe inflammation; its use remains experimental.

‡Given the uncertainties regarding the importance of adjunctive subconjunctival, topical, and systemic therapy and the desire to limit systemic administration of amikacin to patients with known gentamicin-resistant organisms, amikacin is not given by these additional routes unless demanded by deterioration after initial therapy and documented bacterial resistance on culture.

§Systemic aminoglycoside therapy is usually discontinued at 72 hr if sensitivity to vancomycin is documented, and therapy is continued for 5 to 7 days.

‖There is a high incidence of side effects with systemic amphotericin B administration. Recent studies suggest that successful therapy of postoperative fungal endophthalmitis may be accomplished without the routine systemic administration of antifungal agents. In addition to these concerns, ketoconazole appears to be a safer alternative for systemic therapy for cases in which systemic therapy is desired.[96]

---

fulness of these agents.[62] Vancomycin has emerged as the intravitreal drug of choice for gram-positive coverage. In several series, 100 percent of the gram-positive organisms tested were sensitive to vancomycin.[1, 3, 36, 40, 63] Furthermore, studies in the rabbit disclose no evidence of retinal toxicity at the 1.0-mg dose recommended for intravitreal use in patients.[57, 59, 64] Although this drug is currently the drug of choice for gram-positive coverage, the recent report of vancomycin-resistant coagulase-negative *Staphylococci* indicates the need for ongoing evaluation of recommended drugs, as bacterial sensitivity and drug resistance inevitably change over time.[65]

Regarding gram-negative coverage, the aminoglycoside antibiotics continue to be effective against the majority of organisms. The retinal toxicity of these drugs has been the subject of considerable study.[46, 47, 52, 53, 61, 66–68, 69] Outer retinal toxicity consisting of alterations in the retinal pigment epithelium (RPE) and photoreceptor layers has been noted in the rabbit with a 200-µg dose of gentamicin, but a 100-µg dose has not been reported to produce toxicity in this animal.[52, 61] Higher doses of intravitreal gentamicin produced extensive disruption of

the RPE-photoreceptor layers, and full thickness retinal necrosis was seen with intravitreal doses greater than 1.0 mg. Studies in the primate suggest that a 500-µg dose does not produce retinal alterations.[58, 66] Recently, attention has been turned to the pronounced retinal toxicity observed with the inadvertent intravitreal injection of large doses (up to 40 mg) of gentamicin intended for subconjunctival injection at the end of cataract surgery.[67] The toxicity consists of a striking loss of capillaries in the retina and appears to be irreversible despite the performance of immediate vitrectomy and copious intraocular irrigation in several of these unfortunate patients. Conway and Campochiaro have documented a related situation of macular infarction in patients receiving 400 µg of intravitreal gentamicin as part of the treatment of bacterial endophthalmitis, and concerns have been raised over the safety of this dose for intravitreal use in patients.[68] Although the intravitreal injection of 100 µg of gentamicin is widely employed for gram-negative coverage, the growing occurrence of gentamicin-resistant strains in ocular infections[62, 70, 71] suggests that amikacin be considered the aminoglycoside of choice for intravitreal drug therapy as suggested by Talamo and coworkers.[60]

Steroids have increasingly been administered by systemic, periocular, and intravitreal routes in an attempt to control the ocular damage associated with endophthalmitis. Experimental studies in a rabbit model of *S. aureus* endophthalmitis demonstrated a significant decrease in inflammatory signs following treatment with antibiotics and steroids when compared with antibiotic therapy alone.[30] Another study confirmed the beneficial effects of an intravitreal injection of 400 µg of dexamethasone in experimental *Pseudomonas* endophthalmitis in the rabbit; in addition, no retinal toxicity was observed with this dose, as evaluated by light microscopy and electroretinography.[56] In a rabbit model of *S. epidermidis* endophthalmitis, an intravitreal injection of 400 µg of dexamethasone in association with intravitreal antibiotics produced superior results when compared with antibiotic therapy alone.[72] Clinical use of intravitreal steroid therapy as an adjunct to intravitreal anti-

Table 102–5. POSTOPERATIVE ENDOPHTHALMITIS: SUGGESTED GUIDELINES FOR THERAPY

1. Therapy should be prompt.
2. Vitreous and anterior chamber specimens should be obtained for culture in all suspected cases.
3. Medical therapy should be given in all cases, as suggested in Table 102–4.
4. Limited vitrectomy should be performed in selected instances, such as cases displaying loss of red reflex, failure with initial therapy, or infection associated with filtering bleb. (The benefit of vitrectomy in milder cases is unclear, and intraoperative detachments with endophthalmitis have a dismal prognosis.)
5. Intraocular lens should be retained except with infection with filamentous fungi.
6. Calcofluor white technique should be performed for evaluation of possible fungal elements on fresh vitreous specimen.
7. Surveillance should take place to detect toxicity from systemic therapy.

biotic therapy has been reported, but a randomized clinical evaluation is not available.[2, 46] Given the susceptibility of the retina to damage by endophthalmitis, as well as the documented destructive effects of endotoxin and other bacterial products,[73] intravitreal steroid therapy is increasingly recommended in the treatment of endophthalmitis, although the exact indications and dosages require further study.

In addition to intravitreal therapy, antibiotics are usually administered by topical, subconjunctival, and systemic routes for a period of 5 to 10 days. None of these extraocular routes of administration is capable of producing the levels obtained after intravitreal injection, and the importance of these adjunctive antibiotics to successful therapy is unknown, except in the obvious situation of metastatic endophthalmitis. Topical gentamicin produces antibacterial levels in the aqueous but not in the vitreous, and the aqueous level is increased in the presence of ocular inflammation.[74] Subconjunctival injection also produces significant levels in the aqueous but not in the vitreous.[75-77] Intravenous or intramuscular injection does not produce therapeutic levels in the aqueous or the vitreous.[75, 77] However, other drugs may have more favorable ocular penetration; subconjunctival injection of ceftazidime—a third-generation cephalosporin—showed significant antibacterial effect compared with subconjunctival gentamicin in a rabbit model of endophthalmitis.[78] Nevertheless, successful therapy with extraocular antibiotics alone has been documented in a series of eyes infected with S. epidermidis, although the uncertainty regarding the causative organism prior to culture diminishes the attractiveness of this approach.[79]

In any patient receiving systemic antibiotic therapy, careful attention must be given to possible systemic toxicity. Also, it must be noted that subconjunctival injection of gentamicin produces detectable serum levels,[80] and patients undergoing repeated injection, as well as those on systemic therapy, should be monitored for renal or ototoxicity resulting from aminoglycoside administration. Amphotericin B is also capable of producing renal toxicity, and in a recent series of fungal endophthalmitis cases, complications of systemic therapy were seen in every instance.[81] There has been a report of successful treatment of bacterial endophthalmitis in 15 of 16 culture-positive cases treated with intravitreal antibiotics without systemic antibiotics.[82] Although the series was admittedly biased toward more favorable cases, these findings raise important questions regarding the need for potentially toxic systemic therapy as an adjunct to intravitreal antibiotic therapy. These questions require further evaluation; at the present time, advocated treatment includes intravitreal antibiotics with adjunctive topical, periocular, and systemic therapy.

The turnover of gentamicin injected into the vitreous has been studied, and a half-life of 32 hr was found in control phakic rabbit eyes compared with 12 hr in uninflamed aphakic eyes.[51] Extrapolations of these data suggested to the authors that therapeutic vitreous levels are maintained for 24 to 48 hr after an intravitreal injection of 100 μg of gentamicin in humans. Studies in primates documented a 33-hr half-life for intravitreal gentamicin, with a 7-hr half-life for cefazolin.[83] In rabbits, the effects of inflammation, aphakia, and vitrectomy on the turnover of intravitreal cefazolin have been examined.[84] The half-life of cefazolin in the normal rabbit eye is 6.5 hr, but this half-life is prolonged to 10.4 hr if the eye is inflamed by the prior introduction of heat-killed S. epidermidis. Modest reductions in half-life were noted if the lens or vitreous was removed, particularly in eyes with coexisting inflammation. However, repeated injections into the vitreous cannot be advocated solely on the basis of maintaining vitreous levels; despite a more rapid decline in vitreous levels in the aphakic or aphakic vitrectomized eye, the threshold for retinal toxicity of these agents is not reduced.[85] This probably results from rapid accumulation of aminoglycoside in the RPE and outer retina after an intravitreal dose, and repeated injections do not appear to be relatively safer in an aphakic eye. In a clinical series, 2 of 12 patients receiving repeat injections displayed retinal atrophy and pigment clumping suggestive of drug toxicity.[35] Furthermore, in all cases, the specimen taken just prior to the second intravitreal injection was culture-negative, indicating the efficacy of a single intravitreal injection in most instances of endophthalmitis therapy.

The use of repetitive injections of combinations of vancomycin and aminoglycoside has been studied in the rabbit; although no toxicity was noted with a single set of injections, repetitive injections at intervals of 48 hr are associated with increasing degrees of retinal toxicity.[86] Other authors have, however, recommended a role for repetitive injections, but this recommendation antedates the toxicity data mentioned previously and was based on a retrospective review of cases managed through a wide variety of techniques, many without primary vitrectomy.[87] Although the relative value of primary vitrectomy versus repetitive intravitreal injections is unknown, the toxicity data suggest that a second set of intravitreal antibiotic injections should be discouraged and reserved for those cases with a persisting positive culture result 24 to 72 hr after the initial therapy. This strategy, although entailing a delay for secondary reculture results from eyes suspected of persisting infection, will minimize the unnecessary and potentially destructive antibiotic toxicity in eyes that do not require any additional therapy.

VITRECTOMY

The role of vitrectomy in endophthalmitis therapy has been examined in clinical series and experimental animals. With regard to clinical series, these studies are limited by their retrospective character, and vitrectomy is invariably offered in cases that appear more advanced on initial presentation. This understandably reduces the prognosis for the eyes receiving vitrectomy, and this bias is freely acknowledged by the various authors cited.

Driebe and associates examined 83 cases of pseudophakic endophthalmitis and provided long-term data on 50 culture-positive eyes.[3] Sixteen eyes were treated with intravitreal antibiotics alone, and 34 eyes were treated with intravitreal antibiotics with vitrectomy. In the antibiotics-only group, 94 percent achieved 20/400 or better visual acuity, compared with 50 percent attaining this acuity when vitrectomy was included in treatment. However, the authors acknowledge that vitrectomy was offered to patients with a more severe presentation or to those who did not improve with initial management with intravitreal antibiotics alone.

Puliafito and colleagues compared the visual results in endophthalmitis between cases in which vitrectomy was performed within the first 24 hr and those with later vitrectomy.[4] Improved visual results were observed with early vitrectomy. An assessment of the effectiveness of intravitreal antibiotics alone was not possible in this retrospective series, as no patients were treated in this manner. Forster and coworkers examined 34 cases of postoperative endophthalmitis and noted that 57 percent of those receiving antibiotics alone achieved 20/400 or better visual acuity, compared with 59 percent of cases also treated with vitrectomy.[6] Diamond reported 20/400 or better visual acuity in 10 of 12 culture-positive cases treated with intravitreal antibiotics and steroids only, compared with 9 of 14 cases also treated with vitrectomy.[2] However, he clearly stated that vitrectomy was offered in those cases having delay in diagnosis, nonsurgical trauma, vitreous opacities on ultrasound, or failure to respond to intravitreal drug therapy alone after 3 hr; these selection criteria inevitably worsen the prognosis for patients receiving vitrectomy.

Nevertheless, despite the admitted limitations present in the retrospective studies available, certain variables have repeatedly been found to be significant. Favorable outcomes are associated with negative culture results, less virulent organisms, prompt versus delayed therapy, good initial visual acuity, a red reflex at presentation, the absence of retinal detachment, and the absence of nonsurgical trauma.

The role of vitrectomy in endophthalmitis therapy has also been evaluated in experimental animal studies. Cottingham and Forster evaluated a rabbit model of S. epidermidis and S. aureus endophthalmitis in order to examine infection with a less virulent and a more virulent organism, respectively.[88] In their S. epidermidis subgroup, intravitreal antibiotic injection alone eradicated all infections, eliminating any possible improvement in culture results with vitrectomy. However, in their S. aureus subgroup, intravitreal antibiotics alone were curative when injections were given within the first 24 hr after infection. In eyes with more established infections treated between 25 and 31 hr and between 40 and 49 hr after infection, the addition of vitrectomy to intravitreal antibiotic therapy significantly raised the rate of success, as measured by evaluation of posttreatment culture results.

McGetrick and Peyman also examined the role of vitrectomy using an aphakic rabbit model of S. aureus endophthalmitis.[89] Three treatment regimens were examined in their study: (1) subconjunctival and intramuscular gentamicin injection, (2) intravitreal and intramuscular gentamicin, and (3) vitrectomy with intramuscular gentamicin, as well as gentamicin added in the vitreous infusion fluid. They observed that combined subconjunctival and intramuscular injections were not successful in eradicating infection, whereas the other two treatments were equally efficacious, with vitrectomy yielding somewhat greater media clarity than combined intravitreal and intramuscular antibiotics. However, the experimental design did not isolate the influence of vitrectomy in the comparison between the treatment groups. In another study of experimental endophthalmitis in the rabbit, Peyman and associates noted that rabbit eyes receiving vitrectomy in addition to intravitreal antibiotics appeared to fare worse than eyes receiving antibiotic therapy alone.[48] Talley and colleagues reexamined the role of vitrectomy in endophthalmitis, using an S. aureus model of endophthalmitis in rabbits that had previously been rendered aphakic.[90] Intravitreal antibiotics alone were as successful as intravitreal antibiotics with vitrectomy in sterilizing the eye, but media clarity was significantly improved at 14 days in the eyes receiving vitrectomy.[91]

In the setting of bacterial endophthalmitis, vitrectomy is associated with potential advantages and disadvantages. The advantages would include obtaining a vitreous sample for culture with a vitrectomy instrument, clearing of the ocular media, removing potentially toxic bacterial products and debris, removing the vitreous scaffold, reducing the number of viable organisms within the eye, and permitting ease of intravitreal drug therapy and drug circulation throughout the eye. Potential disadvantages would include the possibility of a delay associated with surgical therapy and the iatrogenic creation of retinal holes or detachments or choroidal hemorrhage, as well as other risks inherent in vitrectomy.

Nelsen and coworkers have documented a retinal detachment rate of 21 percent in eyes treated with intravitreal injections and vitrectomy versus 9 percent in eyes not receiving vitrectomy.[7] The occurrence of a retinal detachment in an eye with active endophthalmitis is indicative of a dismal prognosis at present, as salvage of useful vision in such a case has not yet been reported.

The accumulated data suggest that vitrectomy is beneficial in the restoration of media clarity. Coupled with the known advantages of obtaining definitive culture, vitrectomy therapy continues to be a mainstay of treatment. The clarification of the precise role and indications for vitrectomy in the management of aphakic bacterial endophthalmitis will require additional clinical and laboratory investigation.

SPECIAL CONSIDERATIONS

The Intraocular Lens

Postoperative endophthalmitis is now most frequently encountered in the pseudophakic eye. Infections that are in contact with a prosthesis elsewhere in the body usually require removal of the prosthesis for sterilization, but the situation in pseudophakic endophthalmitis appears to be an exception to this rule.[91] In a series of 57 cases of pseudophakic bacterial endophthalmitis, only one eye required removal of the IOL in order to eradicate intraocular Serratia marcescens. Frequently, an inflammatory membrane is present on the anterior and posterior surfaces of the IOL, and removal is most commonly performed to facilitate visualization for vitrectomy. However, it is often possible to incise and débride such lenticular membranes with a microvitreoretinal blade or a 27-gauge needle. Also, it is frequently possible to aspirate a dense hypopyon from the surface of the IOL and iris by introducing the vitrectomy instrument into the anterior chamber. These techniques will usually allow for preservation of an IOL. Given the preference of most surgeons for a "core" vitrectomy in endophthalmitis, as well as the aforementioned uncertainties regarding the role of therapeutic vitrectomy, it appears that removal of an IOL to permit far-peripheral vitrectomy or to peel inflammatory membranes from the retina is perhaps unwarranted. However, these considerations are altered in endophthalmitis resulting from filamentous fungi, as the organisms tenaciously adhere to the IOL.[3] Removal is advocated to facilitate sterilization, but information is limited in these difficult cases.

Delayed-onset Postoperative Endophthalmitis

An unusual subgroup of postoperative endophthalmitis cases caused by indolent organisms such as *Propionibacterium acnes* has recently been characterized.[13–20] Typically, these patients present with a chronic, recurring, steroid-responsive uveitis occurring months or even years following otherwise successful extracapsular cataract extraction with posterior chamber IOL implantation. Symptoms include a decrease in vision and pain. Signs include conjunctival hyperemia, keratic precipitates, a variable anterior chamber reaction that may include a hypopyon, vitritis, and possibly loss of red reflex. In addition, these eyes very typically display a white plaque within the equator of the remaining lens capsule (after extracapsular extraction); this may be mistaken for a Soemmering ring and is best visualized in a widely dilated pupil. In this syndrome, patients are often initially diagnosed with idiopathic uveitis and are often treated with topical steroids with subsequent improvement in symptoms and signs; however, after several episodes, the possibility of chronic endophthalmitis is considered and the diagnosis is established by culture of vitreous and aqueous specimens. The proper handling of the material for anaerobic culture is most critical, and cultures must be maintained for at least 14 days in order to maximize the recovery of these organisms. The most common cause of this syndrome is *P. acnes*, but *S. epidermidis*, *Propionibacterium granulosum*, *Achromobacter*, *Corynebacterium*, and fungi have also been reported.

The gram-positive *P. acnes* organisms can be demonstrated within the lens equator by histologic examination. The optimal therapy for *P. acnes* endophthalmitis is unknown; early reports suggested the simple intravitreal injection of vancomycin (to which this organism is sensitive), but recurrences are common with this therapy. Current recommendations for initial therapy include a vitrectomy with a posterior capsulectomy and intravitreal injection of vancomycin; cases that recur with this therapy are further treated with complete removal of the IOL, residual lens capsule, and equatorial material, with repeat injection of intravitreal vancomycin (and possible reimplantation of an IOL).[92] It is probable that a sizable number of "sterile" postoperative cases in the past were improperly cultured infections caused by these indolent organisms and that increasing awareness of this syndrome will refine the appropriate diagnosis and therapy.

Endophthalmitis Associated With Filtering Blebs

As a subgroup, eyes with endophthalmitis associated with filtering blebs (Fig. 102–3) have a most dismal prognosis with any available therapy, with the majority of cases deteriorating to phthisis.[36, 93] The cause of this condition is undoubtedly related to the creation of a markedly reduced tissue barrier by the filtration fistula. However, in most cases blebs are biomicroscopically intact and produce negative results on Seidel's test. This suggests that organisms penetrate an intact conjunctiva to establish infection. Streptococcal organisms are frequently encountered in these cases. The reasons for the

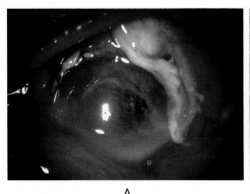
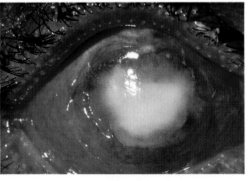

A   B

Figure 102–3. *A,* Endophthalmitis due to *Streptococcus* in an eye with a long-standing filtering bleb. Photograph displays purulent discharge, opacification of the bleb, anterior chamber cells and hypopyon, and loss of red reflex. *B,* Rapid clinical deterioration over the subsequent 2 wk despite immediate and repeated therapy including intravitreal antibiotics and vitrectomies; the eye lost all light perception.

poor results in this subgroup are not clear. It is possible that the filtration fistula dramatically alters the physiology of the antibiotics injected into the eye or permits reinfection from an extraocular nidus of bacteria. Although these possible differences are as yet unexplored and unexplained, prompt therapy—including vitrectomy, intraocular, subconjunctival, topical, and systemic antibiotics—appears warranted. The possibility that the prognosis may be improved by surgically obliterating the sclerotomy needs further study. Surgeons have been understandably reluctant to close a functioning filter, but the dismal prognosis in such cases suggests a departure from previous methods of therapy.

The Open Eye

Bacterial endophthalmitis may occur late after cataract extraction as a result of perforation of a corneal ulcer, arising either spontaneously or in association with extended contact lens wear as a correction for aphakia. There is limited information on the management of endophthalmitis in the open eye, and unique challenges are posed for successful management.[94, 95] In addition to the need for débridement and possible patch graft, glueing, or keratoplasty, the open eye frequently displays extensive choroidal detachment, with attendant difficulties in the approach to the posterior segment. Furthermore, no data are available regarding the retinal toxicity of antibiotics when injected into an eye with a greatly reduced vitreous volume. Nevertheless, an anterior approach with débridement of infected tissues, vitrectomy, and antibiotic and steroid administration by intraocular, periocular, and systemic routes in the standard dosages is currently advocated for these severe cases.

Fungal Endophthalmitis

Postoperative endophthalmitis is infrequently caused by fungi, with *Candida* species predominating in reported cases. In a series of 62 culture-positive cases, fungi were identified in 5 patients. Three of these patients achieved 20/400 or better visual acuity with therapy.[3] A well-documented epidemic of *Candida parapsilosis* endophthalmitis caused by contaminated intraocular irrigating solution has been described.[81] Intravitreal therapy with amphotericin B as well as vitrectomy is advocated, although the high incidence of complications from systemic therapy indicates the need for careful surveillance. Some experts now advocate the use of systemic ketoconazole as an alternative to amphotericin B.[96] The suggested removal of the IOL in the therapy of endophthalmitis due to filamentous fungi has been previously discussed; *Candida* endophthalmitis does not require routine IOL removal for successful sterilization, although recurrences are possible.[81] The use of Cellufluor or Calcofluor white techniques for the identification of fungal elements in a smear of fresh vitreous is a significant advance in the rapid diagnosis of fungal endophthalmitis.[32]

REFERENCES

1. Bohigian GM, Olk RJ: Factors associated with a poor visual result in endophthalmitis. Am J Ophthalmol 101:332–334, 1986.
2. Diamond JG: Intraocular management of endophthalmitis. Arch Ophthalmol 99:96–99, 1981.
3. Driebe WT Jr, Mandelbaum S, Forster RK, et al: Pseudophakic endophthalmitis: Diagnosis and management. Ophthalmology 93:442–448, 1986.
4. Puliafito CA, Baker AS, Haaf J, Foster CS: Infectious endophthalmitis. Ophthalmology 89:921–929, 1982.
5. Rowsey JJ, Newsom DL, Sexton DJ, Harms WK: Endophthalmitis: Current approaches. Ophthalmology 89:1055–1066, 1982.
6. Forster RK, Abbott RL, Gelender H: Management of infectious endophthalmitis. Ophthalmology 87:313–319, 1980.
7. Nelsen PT, Marcus DA, Bovino JA: Retinal detachment following endophthalmitis. Ophthalmology 92:1112–1117, 1985.
8. Allen HF, Mangiaracine AB: Bacterial endophthalmitis after cataract extraction. II. Incidence in 36,000 consecutive operations with special reference to preoperative topical antibiotics. Arch Ophthalmol 91:3–7, 1974.
9. Koul S, Philipson A, Philipson BT: Incidence of endophthalmitis in Sweden. Acta Ophthalmol 67:499–503, 1989.
10. Sherwood DR, Rich WJ, Jacob JS, et al: Bacterial contamination of intraocular and extraocular fluids during extracapsular cataract extraction. Eye 3:308–312, 1989.
11. Beyer TL, Vogler G, Sharma D, O'Donnell FE: Protective barrier effect of the posterior lens capsule in exogenous bacterial endophthalmitis: An experimental primate study. Invest Ophthalmol Vis Sci 25:108–112, 1984.
12. Packer AJ, Weingeist TA, Abrams GW: Retinal periphlebitis as an early sign of bacterial endophthalmitis. Am J Ophthalmol 96:66–71, 1983.
13. Jaffe GJ, Whitcher JP, Biswell R, Irvine AR: *Propionibacterium acnes* endophthalmitis seven months after extracapsular cataract extraction and intraocular lens implantation. Ophthalmic Surg 17:791–793, 1986.
14. Meisler DM, Palestine AG, Vastine DW, et al: Chronic *Proprionibacterium* endophthalmitis after extracapsular cataract extraction and intraocular lens implantation. Am J Ophthalmol 102:733–739, 1986.
15. Ormerod LD, Paton BG, Haaf J, et al: Anaerobic bacterial endophthalmitis. Ophthalmology 94:799–808, 1987.
16. Friberg TR, Kuzma PM: *Propionibacterium acnes* endophthalmitis two years after extracapsular cataract extraction. Am J Ophthalmol 109:609–610, 1990.
17. Walker J, Dangel ME, Makley TA, Opremcak EM: Postoperative *Propionibacterium granulosum* endophthalmitis. Arch Ophthalmol 108:1073–1074, 1990.
18. Zambrano W, Flynn HW, Pflugfelder SC, et al: Management options for *Propionibacterium acnes* endophthalmitis. Ophthalmology 96:1100–1105, 1989.
19. Meisler DM, Mandelbaum S: *Propionibacterium*-associated endophthalmitis after extracapsular cataract extraction: Review of reported cases. Ophthalmology 96:54–61, 1989.
20. Ficker L, Meredith TA, Wilson LA, et al: Chronic bacterial endophthalmitis. Am J Ophthalmol 103:745–748, 1987.
21. Deutsch TA, Goldberg MF: Painless endophthalmitis after cataract surgery. Ophthalmic Surg 15:837–840, 1984.
22. Apple DJ, Mamalis N, Steinmetz RL, et al: Phacoanaphylactic endophthalmitis associated with extracapsular cataract extraction and posterior chamber intraocular lens. Arch Ophthalmol 102:1528–1532, 1984.
23. McMahon MS, Weiss JS, Riedel KG, Albert DM: Clinically unsuspected phacoanaphylaxis after extracapsular cataract extraction with intraocular lens implantation. Br J Ophthalmol 69:836–840, 1985.
24. Meltzer DW: Sterile hypopyon following intraocular lens surgery. Arch Ophthalmol 98:100–104, 1980.
25. Stark WJ, Rosenblum P, Maumenee AE, Cowan CL: Postoperative inflammatory reactions to intraocular lenses sterilized with ethylene-oxide. Ophthalmology 87:385–389, 1980.
26. Soong HK, Kenyon KR: Adverse reactions to virgin silk sutures in cataract surgery. Ophthalmology 91:479–483, 1984.
27. Allen HR, Grove AS: Early acute aseptic iritis after cataract

extraction. Trans Am Acad Ophthalmol Otolaryngol 81:145–150, 1976.

28. McDonnell PJ, Green WR, Maumenee AE, Iliff WJ: Pathology of intraocular lenses in 33 eyes examined postmortem. Ophthalmology 90:386–403, 1983.
29. Chan IM, Jalkh AE, Trempe CL, Tolentino FI: Ultrasonographic findings in endophthalmitis. Ann Ophthalmol 16:778–784, 1984.
30. Maylath FR, Leopold IH: Study of experimental intraocular infections. Am J Ophthalmol 40:86–101, 1955.
31. Forster RK: Etiology and diagnosis of bacterial postoperative endophthalmitis. Ophthalmology 85:320–326, 1978.
32. Sutphin JE, Robinson NM, Wilhelmus KR, Osato MS: Improved detection of oculomycoses using induced fluorescence with Cellufluor. Ophthalmology 93:416–417, 1986.
33. Durfee K, Smith JP: Use of Gram stain to predict vitreous fluid infection. Am J Med Technol 48:525–529, 1982.
34. Joondeph B, Flynn HW, Miller DM, Joondeph HC: A new culture method for infectious endophthalmitis. Arch Ophthalmol 107:1334–1337, 1989.
35. Olson JC, Flynn HW, Forster RK, Culbertson WW: Results in the treatment of postoperative endophthalmitis. Ophthalmology 90:692–699, 1983.
36. Mandelbaum S, Forster RK, Gelender H, Culbertson WW: Late-onset endophthalmitis associated with filtering blebs. Ophthalmology 92:964–972, 1985.
37. Bouza E, Grant S, Jordan C, et al: *Bacillus cereus* endogenous panophthalmitis. Arch Ophthalmol 97:498–499, 1979.
38. Grossniklaus H, Bruner WE, Frank KE, Purnell EW: *Bacillus cereus* endophthalmitis appearing as acute glaucoma in a drug addict. Am J Ophthalmol 100:334–335, 1985.
39. Levin MR, D'Amico DJ: Diagnosis and Management of Traumatic Endophthalmitis. *In* Shingleton B, Hersh P, Kenyon K (eds): Ocular Trauma. St Louis, Mosby–Year Book, 1991, pp 242–252.
40. Affeldt JC, Flynn HW, Forster RK, et al: Microbial endophthalmitis resulting from ocular trauma. Ophthalmology 94:407–413, 1987.
41. Brinton GS, Topping TM, Hyndiuk RA, et al: Posttraumatic endophthalmitis. Arch Ophthalmol 102:547–550, 1984.
42. Schemmer GB, Driebe WT: Posttraumatic *Bacillus cereus* endophthalmitis. Arch Ophthalmol 105:342–344, 1987.
43. von Sallmann L, Meyer K, DiGrandi J: Experimental study on penicillin treatment of ectogenous infection of vitreous. Arch Ophthalmol 32:179–189, 1944.
44. Duguid JP, Ginsberg M, Fraser IC, et al: Experimental observation on the intravitreal use of penicillin and other drugs. Br J Ophthalmol 31:193–211, 1947.
45. Sorsby A, Ungar J: Intravitreal injection of penicillin. Study of the levels of concentration reached and therapeutic efficacy. Br J Ophthalmol 32:857–864, 1948.
46. Peyman GA, Herbst R: Bacterial endophthalmitis: Treatment with intraocular injection of gentamicin and dexamethasone. Arch Ophthalmol 91:416–418, 1974.
47. Peyman GA, May DR, Ericson ES, Apple D: Intraocular injection of gentamicin: Toxic effects and clearance. Arch Ophthalmol 92:42–47, 1974.
48. Peyman GA, Paque JT, Meisels HI, Bennett TO: Postoperative endophthalmitis: A comparison of methods for treatment and prophylaxis with gentamicin. Ophthalmic Surg 6:45–55, 1975.
49. Forster RK: Endophthalmitis: Diagnostic cultures and visual results. Arch Ophthalmol 92:387–392, 1974.
50. Forster RK, Zachary IG, Cottingham AJ, Norton EWD: Further observation on the diagnosis, cause, and treatment of endophthalmitis. Am J Ophthalmol 81:52–56, 1976.
51. Cobo LM, Forster RK: The clearance of intravitreal gentamicin. Am J Ophthalmol 92:59–62, 1981.
52. D'Amico DJ, Libert J, Kenyon KR, et al: Retinal toxicity of intravitreal gentamicin: An electron microscopic study. Invest Ophthalmol Vis Sci 25:564–572, 1984.
53. D'Amico DJ, Caspers-Velu L, Libert J, et al: Comparative toxicity of intravitreal aminoglycoside antibiotics. Am J Ophthalmol 100:264–275, 1985.
54. Fett DR, Silverman CA, Yoshizumi MO: Moxalactam retinal toxicity. Arch Ophthalmol 102:435–438, 1984.
55. Fisher JP, Civiletto SE, Forster RK: Toxicity, efficacy, and clearance of intravitreally injected cefazolin. Arch Ophthalmol 100:650–652, 1982.
56. Graham RO, Peyman GA: Intravitreal injection of dexamethasone: Treatment of experimentally induced endophthalmitis. Arch Ophthalmol 92:149–154, 1974.
57. Homer P, Peyman GA, Koziol J, Sanders D: Intravitreal injection of vancomycin in experimental staphylococcal endophthalmitis. Acta Ophthalmol 53:311–320, 1975.
58. Ling CH, Peyman GA, Raichand M: Electron microscopic study of toxicity of intravitreal injections of gentamicin in primates. Can J Ophthalmol 20:179–183, 1985.
59. Smith MA, Sorenson JA, Lowy FD, et al: Treatment of experimental methicillin-resistant *Staphylococcus epidermidis* endophthalmitis with intravitreal vancomycin. Ophthalmology 93:1328–1335, 1986.
60. Talamo JH, D'Amico DJ, Kenyon KR: Intravitreal amikacin in the treatment of bacterial endophthalmitis. Arch Ophthalmol 104:1483–1485, 1986.
61. Zachary IG, Forster RK: Experimental intravitreal gentamicin. Am J Ophthalmol 82:604–611, 1976.
62. Lambert SR, Stern WH: Methicillin- and gentamicin-resistant *Staphylococcus epidermidis* endophthalmitis after intraocular surgery. Am J Ophthalmol 99:725–726, 1985.
63. Kervick GN, Flynn HW, Alfonso E, Miller D: Antibiotic therapy for *Bacillus* species infections. Am J Ophthalmol 110:683–687, 1990.
64. Pflugfelder SC, Hernandez E, Fliesler SJ, et al: Intravitreal vancomycin: Retinal toxicity, clearance, and interaction with gentamicin. Arch Ophthalmol 105:831–837, 1987.
65. Schwalbe RS, Stapleton JT, Gilligan PH: Emergence of vancomycin resistance in coagulase negative staphylococci. N Engl J Med 316:927–931, 1987.
66. Bennett TO, Peyman GA: Toxicity of intravitreal aminoglycosides in primates. Can J Ophthalmol 9:475–478, 1974.
67. McDonald HR, Schatz H, Allen AW, et al: Retinal toxicity secondary to intraocular gentamicin injection. Ophthalmology 93:871–877, 1986.
68. Conway BP, Campochiaro PA: Macular infarction after endophthalmitis treated with vitrectomy and intravitreal gentamicin. Arch Ophthalmol 104:367–371, 1986.
69. Brown GC, Eagle RC, Shakin EP, et al: Retinal toxicity of intravitreal gentamicin. Arch Ophthalmol 108:1740–1744, 1990.
70. Insler MS, Cavanaugh HD, Wilson WA: Gentamicin-resistant *Pseudomonas* endophthalmitis after penetrating keratoplasty. Br J Ophthalmol 69:189–191, 1985.
71. Majerovics A, Tanenbaum HL: Endophthalmitis and pars plana vitrectomy. Can J Ophthalmol 19:25–28, 1984.
72. Meredith TA, Aguilar E, Miller MJ, et al: Comparative treatment of experimental *Staphylococcus epidermidis* endophthalmitis. Arch Ophthalmol 108:857–860, 1990.
73. Jacobs DR, Cohen HB: The inflammatory role of endotoxin in rabbit gram-negative bacterial endophthalmitis. Invest Ophthalmol Vis Sci 25:1074–1079, 1984.
74. Ellerhorst B, Golden B, Jarudi N: Ocular penetration of topically applied gentamicin. Arch Ophthalmol 93:371–378, 1975.
75. Furgiuele FP: Ocular penetration and tolerance of gentamicin. Am J Ophthalmol 64:421–426, 1967.
76. Furgiuele FP: Penetration of gentamicin into the aqueous humor of human eyes. Am J Ophthalmol 69:481–483, 1970.
77. Litwack KD, Pettit T, Johnson BL: Penetration of gentamicin: Administered intramuscularly and subconjunctivally into aqueous humor. Arch Ophthalmol 82:687–693, 1969.
78. Yannis RA, Rissing JP, Buxton TB, Shockley RK: Multistrain comparison of three antimicrobial prophylaxis regimens in experimental postoperative *Pseudomonas* endophthalmitis. Am J Ophthalmol 100:404–407, 1985.
79. O'Day DM, Jones DB, Patrinely J, Elliott JH: *Staphylococcus epidermidis* endophthalmitis: Visual outcome following noninvasive therapy. Ophthalmology 89:354–360, 1982.
80. Trope GE, Lawrence JR, Hind VMD, Everden A: Systemic absorption of topical and subconjunctival gentamicin. Br J Ophthalmol 43:692–693, 1979.
81. Stern WH, Tamura E, Jacobs RA, et al: Epidemic postsurgical *Candida parapsilosis* endophthalmitis: Clinical findings and management of 15 consecutive cases. Ophthalmology 92:1701–1709, 1985.

82. Pavan PR, Brinser JH: Exogenous bacterial endophthalmitis treated without systemic antibiotics. Am J Ophthalmol 104:121–126, 1987.
83. Barza M, Kane A, Baum J: Pharmacokinetics of intravitreal carbenicillin, cefazolin, and gentamicin in rhesus monkeys. Invest Ophthalmol Vis Sci 24:1602–1606, 1983.
84. Ficker L, Meredith TA, Gardner S, Wilson LA: Cefazolin levels after intravitreal injection. Invest Ophthalmol Vis Sci 31:502–505, 1990.
85. Talamo JH, D'Amico DJ, Hanninen LA, et al: The influence of aphakia and vitrectomy on experimental retinal toxicity of aminoglycoside antibiotics. Am J Ophthalmol 100:840–847, 1985.
86. Oum BS, D'Amico DJ, Wong KW: Intravitreal antibiotic therapy with vancomycin and aminoglycoside: An experimental study of combination and repetitive injections. Arch Ophthalmol 107:1055–1060, 1989.
87. Stern GA, Engel HM, Driebe WT: The treatment of postoperative endophthalmitis: Results of differing approaches to treatment. Ophthalmology 96:62–67, 1989.
88. Cottingham AJ, Forster RK: Vitrectomy in endophthalmitis. Arch Ophthalmol 94:2078–2081, 1976.
89. McGetrick JJ, Peyman GA: Vitrectomy in experimental endoph-thalmitis. Part II. Bacterial endophthalmitis. Ophthalmic Surg 10:87–92, 1979.
90. Talley AR, D'Amico DJ, Talamo JH, et al: The role of vitrectomy in the treatment of postoperative bacterial endophthalmitis: An experimental study. Arch Ophthalmol 105:1699–1702, 1987.
91. Hopen G, Mondino BJ, Kozy D, Lipkowitz J: Intraocular lenses and experimental bacterial endophthalmitis. Am J Ophthalmol 94:402–407, 1982.
92. Fox GM, Joondeph BC, Flynn HW, et al: Delayed-onset pseudophakic endophthalmitis. Am J Ophthalmol 111:163–173, 1991.
93. Katz LJ, Cantor LB, Spaeth GL: Early and late bacterial endophthalmitis following glaucoma filtering surgery. Ophthalmology 92:959–963, 1985.
94. Kozarsky AM, Stulting RD, Waring GO, et al: Penetrating keratoplasty for exogenous *Paecilomyces* keratitis followed by postoperative endophthalmitis. Am J Ophthalmol 98:552–557, 1984.
95. Weiss I: *Pseudomonas* orbital cellulitis. Am J Ophthalmol 87:368–370, 1979.
96. Pflugfelder SC, Flynn HW Jr, Zwickey TA, et al: Exogenous fungal endophthalmitis. Ophthalmology 95:19–30, 1988.

Chapter 103

■

Intraocular Foreign Bodies

ALEXANDER R. GAUDIO, ANDREW J. PACKER,
and JOHN C. MADIGAN, JR.

Intraocular foreign bodies present a multifaceted challenge. The diagnosis may be delayed or missed because the small, high-speed projectile penetrates the eye with minimal discomfort and little initial damage. Only later will the patient present with persistent inflammation, visual blurring, iris discoloration, or an abnormal pupil. At other times, the damage may be so extensive that the drama attendant upon its treatment tends to obscure good judgment. Precipitous attempts to remove the intraocular foreign body before properly determining its composition, location, or magnetic properties may aggravate the disaster. Dramatic, prolonged surgical attempts to remove a nonvisualized foreign body with a magnet have in the past resulted in embarrassing and legal implications when the foreign body proved to be nonmagnetic and outside the globe. A more elegant approach to the management of intraocular foreign bodies has been made possible by better technology and a clearer understanding of their chemical and physiologic interactions with the ocular tissues.[1, 2]

Gone are the days of the giant magnet, when the dramatic command of "Turn it on," would allow the previously unseen foreign body to suddenly appear at the magnet's tip, often with fragments of lens, uvea, vitreous, and retina, not to mention the instruments and the tug on the operating room personnel's watches and other metallic belongings in the vicinity. Also virtually gone are the sunflower cataract and the Fleischer ring that developed over the course of observation of a copper intraocular foreign body that was left in the eye undisturbed for prolonged periods because of the greater damage caused by attempting to remove it. Experience, pathobiologic insights, improved vitrectomy techniques, and the advancements in bioengineering are responsible for a more logical approach to intraocular foreign bodies and, because of the lack of irreversible initial ocular damage, a better prognosis.

However, even in cases with a better prognosis because of limited initial damage by the foreign body's penetration, favorable results are obtained only by meticulous attention to the history, examination, appropriate ancillary studies, and timely surgical intervention, with staging as indicated. A review of the Massachusetts Eye and Ear Infirmary experience with intraocular foreign bodies from 1966 to 1991, a period encompassing both the previtrectomy and the vitrectomy years, highlights the fact that despite some real advancements, the prognosis remains guarded for any eye with an intraocular foreign body. Only continued efforts at prevention will diminish the tragic impact of these avoidable, devastating injuries.

CLINICAL PRESENTATION

The history, examination, and ancillary studies are dictated by the extent of the injury and the circumstances surrounding the initial contact with the patient.

Evaluating an intraocular foreign body resulting from an accident involving severe head, facial, and ocular trauma—such as motor vehicle accidents, explosions, or gunshot wounds—might involve little more than a careful inspection prior to repairing the wound, postponing attention to the foreign body or bodies until a more propitious time. Not infrequently such a patient, who may be either comatose or anesthetized, is first seen in the operating room in conjunction with the trauma team; ophthalmologic efforts are per force limited by the patient's general condition.

The intraocular foreign body, which is often quite large and associated with extensive disruption of the ocular structures, may require little more than a brief history and confirmatory radiographic studies. Treatment is directed primarily at restoring the ocular integrity and the avoidance of dreaded complications such as endophthalmitis and sympathetic ophthalmia. The foreign body composition, size, and location determine the method and time of removal in such severely traumatized eyes.

Fortunately, the more common clinical presentations do not involve such ocular devastation. The foreign body, which is usually small, may be hidden by media opacities that may be as mild as a faint track through the cornea and lens, with minimal vitreous hemorrhage (Fig. 103–1), or quite dense secondary to corneal haze, hyphema, cataract, dense vitreous hemorrhage (Fig. 103–2), and detached retina. Whether uncomplicated and mild or complicated and severe, the clinical presentation allows for a thorough preoperative evaluation and logical therapeutic plan.

The clinical presentation of occult foreign bodies is rare and challenging.[3,4] A darker or lighter iris, different pupil size, or elevated intraocular pressure on the involved side may go unnoticed by both patient and physician. Visual loss may be attributed to cataractous changes; complications at cataract surgery resulting from weakened zonules remain unexplained until siderosis or chalcosis is diagnosed and an intraocular foreign body is identified.

HISTORY

The successful management of intraocular foreign bodies begins with a detailed history. The date, time, place, and circumstances of injury have legal as well as medical value. Most states have a legal requirement to report firearms-related injuries. The interval from the time of injury to the time that medical attention is sought may be a determinant of treatment and prognosis. Infection, organization of the vitreous, cicatrization, and metallosis are all dependent on time. Each dictates its own diagnostic and therapeutic approach. If the patient is referred from a colleague, information obtained from previous examinations, diagnostic studies, and treatment is of great value in maximizing the prognosis and avoiding unnecessary repetition of studies and duplication of possibly harmful administration of medicines. In cases in which the media opacifies quickly, the examiner who had the "first look" can provide the most valuable information, i.e., appearance, size, location, retinal damage, if any, and perhaps even magnetic property based on a "magnet test," thus obviating the need for extensive research into the composition of the foreign body and the additional manipulation of the eye necessitated by ultrasonography.

In work-related ocular injuries resulting in intraocular foreign bodies, assiduous attempts should be made to determine the material with which the patient was working, as such information will provide the basis for the therapeutic course. Determining whether goggles or glasses were worn at the time of injury may prove valuable in shedding light on the nature of the foreign body. Some metallic foreign bodies (iron, copper, lead, zinc) may be toxic to the ocular tissues; others (aluminum, gold, platinum, silver) are well tolerated. Only foreign bodies containing iron are magnetic. Nonmetallic foreign bodies also fall into the inert and toxic categories: Glass, stone, and plastic can be tolerated for many years, only rarely causing a reaction;[5] conversely, vegetable matter most often induces a severe inflammatory reaction and frequently endophthalmitis.

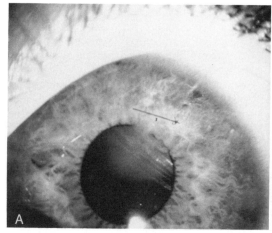
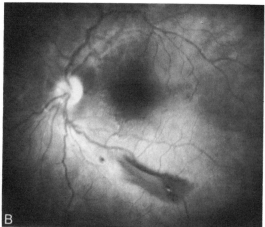

Figure 103–1. A 9-year-old boy with a blasting cap injury of the left eye. A, The anterior tract through the cornea, iris, and lens. B, The foreign body on the retinal surface. Lensectomy, vitrectomy, and forceps removal of the copper-containing foreign body were performed.

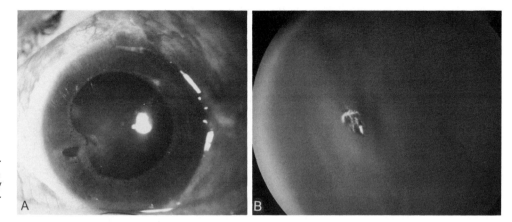

Figure 103–2. *A,* Track of a foreign body through the cornea, iris, and lens. *B,* Foreign body in the vitreous with dense hemorrhage.

Because of the rapidity with which the small metallic projectile penetrates the eye, and the paucity of accompanying symptoms, injuries incurred striking steel on steel may be minimized by the patient and overlooked by the physician initially consulted for the "mild ocular injury." Very rarely do these injuries cause infection, perhaps because of the heat and speed, but unless removed, siderosis is very likely to develop. The use of wire cutters more commonly involves copper foreign bodies. The severity of inflammation and the rapidity with which chalcosis develops is dependent on the location and the size of the piece of copper inside the eye. Small ones located peripherally may cause little if any complication, but that is the exception. Explosives and firearms not infrequently result in binocular damage with multiple foreign bodies, which are usually a combination of copper and lead. Double perforations are common. Trauma involving vegetable matter (lash, thorn, wood, soil) raises the specter of infection in general and fungus infection in particular. Each dictates a specific diagnostic and therapeutic approach. The history of a causative injury resulting in an intraocular foreign body is not always obtainable. Patients with ocular foreign bodies may present with gradual visual loss or intermittent inflammation but with no awareness of the acute event. On occasion, detailed questioning, pursued because of suggestive findings on examination, evokes a vague recollection of a slight ocular injury previously dismissed as a "minor irritation."

EXAMINATION

Examination of the patient with an intraocular foreign body must be tailored to the clinical presentation and the extent of injury. A severely damaged open globe, with uveal prolapse and total hyphema, merits little more than a penlight look. Determining at least the presence of light perception provides a basis for discussion with the patient or family, or both. Radiographic studies, to ascertain the presence and location of the foreign body, and a brief medical history, specifically to rule out allergies and to assess the general medical condition for purposes of general anesthesia, usually suffice.

When faced with a patient who gives a vague history of a possible foreign body and presents with little more than mild localized conjunctival injection, the index of suspicion has to be high and the search detailed. Vision measurement, tonography, adnexal inspection, pupillary responses, iris color, biomicroscopy, gonioscopy, and dilated pupil ophthalmoscopy may each contribute potentially eye-saving information and facilitate the treatment decision. In the case of a suspected long-standing iron-containing intraocular foreign body, anisocoria and abnormal pupillary reaction may be present, along with a different iris color on the involved side (Fig. 103–3). Corneal deposits are usually seen: rust-colored precipitates on the endothelium and "iron lines" at the epithelial level. Cataractous changes may vary from brown

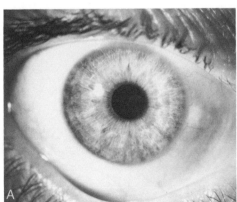
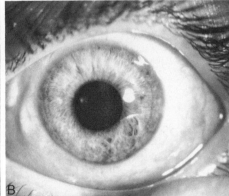

Figure 103–3. Iris color change in an eye harboring an occult ferrous foreign body. *A,* Normal right eye. *B,* Darker iris of the siderotic eye.

dustlike accumulations at the level of the anterior capsule to a mature partially or totally dislocated cataract. When visible, the vitreous fibers may have a rusty appearance, the retinal reflex is altered, the arterioles are narrowed, and the disc is pale.[6]

Studies of the pathologic features of eyes with siderosis have revealed iron deposits accumulated in the regions of ocular pumps—i.e., corneal endothelium and Descemet's membrane, trabecular meshwork, pupillary constrictor muscles, ciliary epithelium, lens epithelium, retinal pigment epithelium, and internal limiting membrane. In chalcosis, marked inflammation has been found around the copper foreign body and in the uvea, along with copper deposits in the peripheral corneal stroma, Descemet's membrane, lens, vitreous, and surface of the retina.[7]

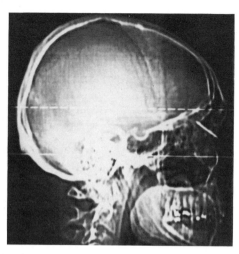

Figure 103–4. Lateral x-ray view demonstrating a large intraocular foreign body.

ANCILLARY STUDIES

What Cogan[48] described as the birth of "a new era in ophthalmic traumatology" took place at Harvard in June 1886 "just six months after Roentgen's epochal discovery," when x-rays were first used to locate an intraocular foreign body. Since then, radiographic image studies have remained the sine qua non of the preoperative evaluation of traumatized eyes. Documentation of the presence, location, and number of intraocular foreign bodies may be achieved with the standard "foreign body x-ray series," including Waters, Caldwell, and lateral views (Fig. 103–4). Computed tomography[8–10] provides much more reliable information as to size, shape, and localization of the foreign body, whether in the anterior or the posterior segment (Fig. 103–5), thus relegating

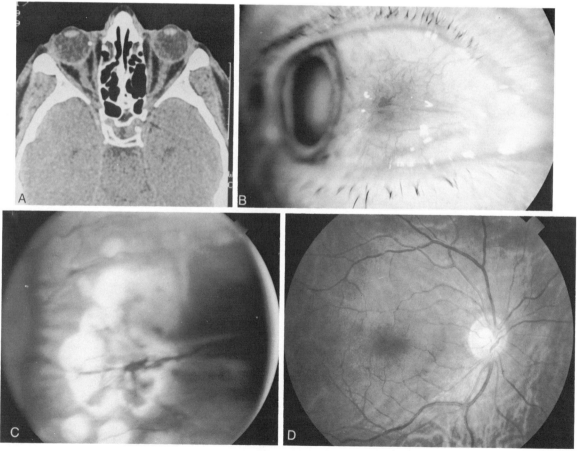

Figure 103–5. A, Computed tomography (CT) scan of a foreign body in the retina at the nasal equator. B, Entry site. C, Scleral buckle at the site of the transscleral posterior extraction. D, Normal posterior pole—20/20 vision.

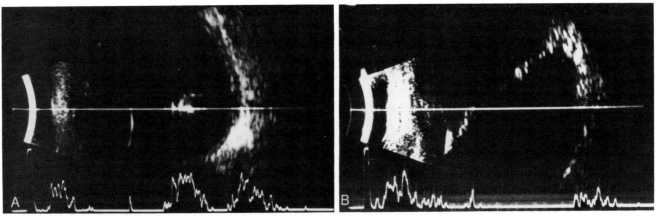

Figure 103–6. *A,* Ultrasonogram of an intraocular foreign body. *B,* Ultrasonogram showing an intraocular foreign body perforating the posterior wall of the globe.

to historical interest previously useful but time-consuming and less accurate localization methods such as soft tissue films to detect foreign bodies in the anterior segment; the Sweet localization technique, which involved no contact with the injured eye but considerable inaccuracy; and the Comberg technique, which was somewhat dangerous because of the need to place a contact lens with a metal marker on the eye; and the various metal locators of Berman, Roper-Hall, and Bronson-Turner. In eyes with opaque media, skillfully performed ultrasonography (Fig. 103–6) has proved of great help in determining the extent of intraocular damage, retinal detachment, and double perforation, as well as in detecting foreign bodies not seen on x-ray studies.[11, 12] The role of magnetic resonance imaging remains peripheral in the evaluation of intraocular foreign bodies.[13-18] Electroretinography (Fig. 103–7) is invaluable in providing information of a diagnostic as well as a prognostic nature. When a difficult decision regarding removal of a long-standing intraocular foreign body is held in abeyance, close follow-up with periodic full-field electroretinograms can provide clear documenta-

tion of the progression of toxic changes and indications for intervention.[19]

TREATMENT

The therapeutic approach to a traumatized eye harboring an intraocular foreign body is predicated on the respected maxim "haste makes waste." The severity and immediacy of the injury determine the treatment course. A patient who has a foreign body in the anterior chamber, iris, or lens, with a self-sealed corneal wound, requires quite different attention from the patient with a large foreign body, corneoscleral rupture, and a prolapsed uvea, lens, and vitreous. In the most extreme case, the ocular treatment has to be coordinated with the plastic surgeon, maxillofacial surgeon, and neurosurgeon, and the most that can be achieved is to identify and close the perforation as cleanly as possible, leaving the foreign body or bodies and additional intraocular surgery for a later time.

Some general therapeutic considerations apply to the

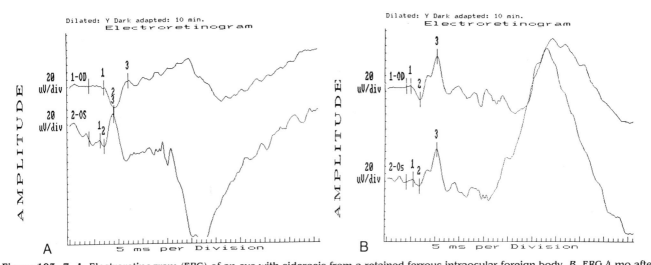

Figure 103–7. *A,* Electroretinogram (ERG) of an eye with siderosis from a retained ferrous intraocular foreign body. *B,* ERG 4 mo after removal of the foreign body. Note the return to normal evidenced by increased b-wave amplitude and decreased implicit time.

entire spectrum of clinical presentations of intraocular foreign bodies. Protection of the perforated globe is of primary importance. A shield, no matter how makeshift, is ideal; care must be taken to avoid any pressure on the lids or globe. Tetanus toxoid booster, 0.5 ml subcutaneously, is advisable if the patient has not had one in 6 mo. Foreign body films and computed tomography are necessary to establish the presence and location of the foreign body. Except in the most extreme case, no intervention is advisable without such information. Broad-spectrum antibiotic prophylaxis is best started as early as feasible. Mannitol or some other hyperosmotic agent is valuable to shrink the vitreous and decrease the likelihood of vitreous loss.

Surgical repair of a perforated globe is best undertaken with general anesthesia that is carefully administered to avoid bucking and postoperative vomiting. Curare-like drugs are less likely to cause contraction of the rectus muscles and the attendant risk of extruding intraocular contents through a perforation of the globe. Preoperative preparation of the globe is limited by the extent of the trauma and the need to minimize the possibility of introducing toxic agents into the open eye. Suturing of the wound should start at its anteriormost extension, followed by gradual posterior exploration and repair as needed. When the sclera is involved, the peritomy is most helpful if it is extensive and starts at a distance of several millimeters from the wound. Disinserting a rectus muscle may be necessary to improve visualization and reduce pressure on the open globe. Prolapsed uveal tissue is reposited if clean and viable; it is excised if necrotic or contaminated. Corneal wounds are sutured with 10–0 nylon and the knot is buried for patient comfort. To close the scleral extension of the wound, 8–0 nylon or a similar nonabsorbable suture is best. When the corneal penetration results in disruption of the anterior chamber, a keratocentesis opposite the wound is useful to re-form the anterior chamber, evacuate blood or debris, introduce a spatula to separate the iris from the wound, or irrigate to test the wound closure. After reestablishing the integrity of the globe, it is safer either to proceed with removal of the foreign body or, if there is any question about proceeding, to wait a few days.

Because the overwhelming majority of intraocular foreign bodies are magnetic, the role of magnets continues to be very important, if not indispensable, in the treatment of intraocular foreign bodies. Myriad magnets have been employed over the years, and new ones continue to appear.[20–24] Those that remain in popular use include the rare earth magnet, the pencil magnet, and the Bronson electromagnet (Fig. 103–8). The first can be introduced into the eye, whereas the second is quite effective when within 1 mm of a magnetic foreign body. Although somewhat unwieldy because of its weight, the last derives its usefulness from the strong magnetic field it can generate, which is maximized by using only short bursts of electrical application to avoid heating the magnet, and thus decreasing its strength, and using the blunt conical tip, which of all the various shapes available generates the strongest magnetic field. Additional important considerations in the magnetic extraction of intraocular foreign bodies follow:

1. The magnetism of a metallic foreign body is directly related to its iron content.

2. A magnetic foreign body orients itself longitudinally to the magnet, a change of orientation that can be damaging if it occurs near the retina.

3. The strength of the magnet decreases as its distance from the foreign body increases, the magnetic force being inversely proportional to the cube of the distance.

When a foreign body is located in the anterior segment, removal is accomplished with either simple forceps or a hand-held magnet via a limbal incision. Occasionally an iridectomy or cataract extraction is made necessary by the location of the foreign body in the lens or posterior chamber (Fig. 103–9). Small, inert foreign bodies causing no corneal or lens problem may require no intervention at all unless dictated by delayed complications (Fig. 103–10). In general, the results of foreign body extraction from the anterior chamber, iris, or lens are excellent.[25]

Posterior segment foreign bodies are most problem-

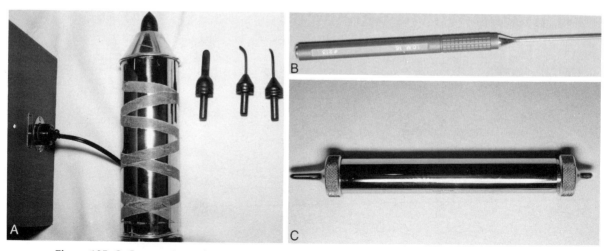

Figure 103–8. Commonly used magnets. A, Electromagnet. B, Rare earth magnet. C, Pencil magnet.

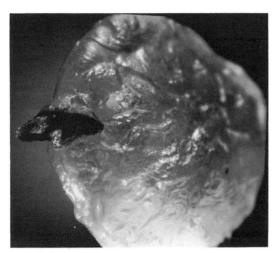

Figure 103–9. Intracapsular cataract extraction performed to remove an intraocular foreign body deeply embedded in a cataractous lens.

atic. Because they are frequently associated with extensive ocular damage, they may be difficult to see, reach, and remove. Pars plana vitrectomy has facilitated the task immensely in those cases in which visualization is poor, and when the foreign body is not magnetic, improved grasping instruments have made a great contribution. The advent of the laser has reduced the incidence of intervention-related bleeding, and more physiologic solutions have decreased the incidence of cataract and corneal decompensation.

The route of removal of a foreign body from the posterior segment is determined by its location, size, magnetic property, and the clarity of the media.[26] Attempts to remove the foreign body blindly or through the entry site are too dangerous and are not recommended. When clearly visible in the vitreous cavity or on the retina, with no encapsulating vitreous organization, a magnetic foreign body can be successfully and safely removed with an electromagnet via a pars plana sclerotomy in a meridian chosen so that the trajectory

of the foreign body will not damage the retina or the lens. Not infrequently, a vitrectomy, with lensectomy as indicated, will be necessary to clear the media prior to removing the foreign body. Retinal tears at the site of impact are treated with laser or cryopexy if the edges are elevated or if early signs of retinal detachment are present (Fig. 103–11). Extraction of an encapsulated foreign body is facilitated by first clearing the condensed vitreous and capsule surrounding it (Fig. 103–12). If the magnetic foreign body is impaled in the retina and possibly the choroid, the removal options are either anteriorly via the pars plana using vitrectomy techniques,[27, 28] or when possible via the posterior transscleral route (Fig. 103–13). In the latter approach, the media is cleared, if necessary, and the foreign body is accurately localized by indirect ophthalmoscopy, marking the sclera. Scleral flaps are dissected, diathermy is applied in the scleral bed in stepping stone fashion, and a sclerotomy is made directly over the foreign body to, but not including, the choroid. After the exposed choroidal knuckle undergoes gentle diathermy to minimize bleeding, placing a small magnet over it will result in a bulging pulsation, thus providing reassurance that it is indeed magnetic and properly localized. A small incision is made in the bulging choroid, and the foreign body is delivered with a hand-held magnet. The trap-door scleral buckle with a small silicone implant is then completed. Failure to remove the foreign body with this technique is attributable either to inaccurate localization or to the erroneous determination of its magnetic property.

Nonmagnetic foreign bodies lying in the vitreous or on the retina are grasped and removed with forceps via the pars plana after a vitrectomy is performed. If such a foreign body is intraretinal, similar methods of extraction are employed, but the retinal penetration site is surrounded by laser treatment prior to grasping and removing the foreign body to reduce the probability of bleeding and detachment. Removal of subretinal nonmagnetic foreign bodies may require a retinotomy or gentle manipulation to move them to a safer location prior to making them accessible to the forceps.[29] Foreign

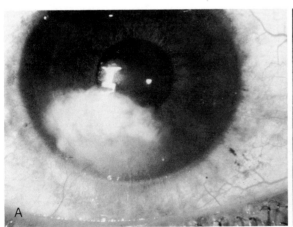
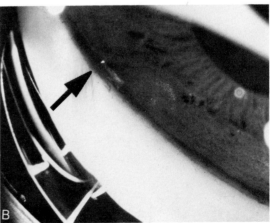

Figure 103–10. A 34-year-old man presented with foreign body sensation in the right eye after an automobile accident involving a shattered windshield. *A,* A pie-shaped area of corneal edema. *B,* Gonioscopy showing a small foreign body *(arrow)* in the angle. Following surgical removal, visual acuity improved from 20/30 to 20/20.

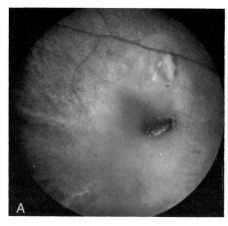
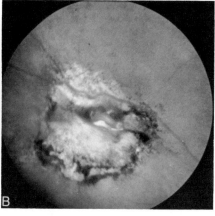

Figure 103–11. *A,* A foreign body lying on the retina amidst vitreous hemorrhage, next to a retinal tear at the site of impact. *B,* After removal of the foreign body and retinopexy.

body forceps, despite several generations of improvements, still leave a number of problems unsolved. Grasping large foreign bodies is often very difficult and occasionally impossible. Holding the foreign body is frequently a challenge, especially when trying to extract it through a pars plana incision belatedly recognized as too small. Therefore, care must be taken to assess the size and shape of the foreign body, choose the appropriate forceps,[30] and properly prepare the pars plana extraction site.

COMPLICATIONS

None of the ocular structures, from orbit and adnexa to the optic nerve, is immune from the potential ravages, direct or indirect, caused by an intraocular foreign body. The extent of the initial injury most often is predictive of the outcome, and the size, number, entry site, and composition are determining factors. Loss of media clarity, hemorrhage, and infection compose the spectrum of complications from visual diminution to loss of the eye. The introduction of vegetable matter with virulent infectious organisms can destroy the eye in a matter of hours. More insidious are the complications in an eye harboring a copper- or iron-containing foreign body. Occult entry or difficulties attendant upon re-

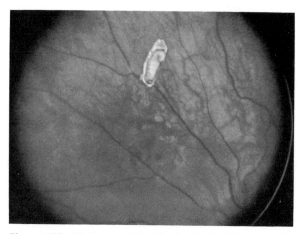

Figure 103–12. Encapsulated foreign body, lying on retina.

moval, which was a problem especially with copper and other nonmagnetic foreign bodies prior to the advent of vitrectomy, most commonly explain the prolonged presence of such a foreign body in the eye. In the case of iron, siderosis may develop within weeks, but the course is variable depending on the iron content in the foreign body and its location. Virtually all ocular structures are involved in the siderotic process—glaucoma, cataract, iris color changes, mydriasis, retinal function destruction, and optic nerve atrophy. The effects of copper are also dependent on size, composition, and location. A small particle near the pars plana quickly and totally encapsulated may cause no reaction, whereas a foreign body of pure copper induces an acutely destructive, violent inflammation.[31] In contrast, the reaction to an alloy is more gradual. Chalcosis develops as copper diffuses from the foreign body and is deposited in the peripheral cornea, iris, vitreous, retinal surface, zonules, and lens, resulting in a classic sunflower cataract.

Appropriate, timely, and successful intervention will minimize but not eliminate complications.[32–34] Endophthalmitis continues to occur, although the incidence has been reduced by antibiotics and prompt intervention. It can be a particularly vexing problem in farming communities.[35] Intraoperative bleeding remains a significant cause of failure, as do the occasional retinal tears and detachments that do not respond to treatment. Sympathetic ophthalmia has been reported as a complication of intraocular foreign bodies and of vitrectomy; however, a review of the 522 cases of intraocular foreign bodies at the Massachusetts Eye and Ear Infirmary between January 1, 1966, and July 1, 1991, revealed not a single case, suggesting that it must be an exceedingly rare occurrence. Similarly rare is the incidence of intraoperative light damage to the macula.[36] The challenge of postoperative visual rehabilitation is increased by the often-present corneal scarring and aphakic status. Delayed vitreous organization, fibrous proliferation, subretinal neovascularization,[37] retinal detachment, and epimacular fibrosis (Fig. 103–14) add to the uncertainty of the prognosis.[38, 39]

The legal ramifications in the field of intraocular foreign bodies, which is surrounded by an aura of emergency and deprived of calm judgment, are not to be overlooked.[40] Difficulties can be minimized by a

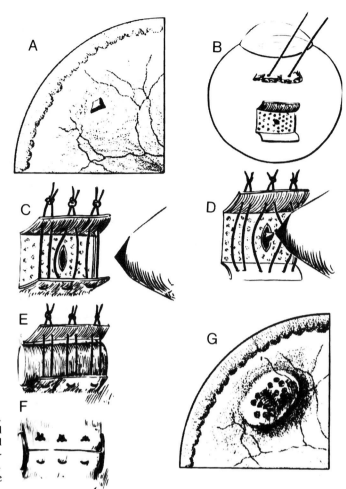

Figure 103–13. *A*, Magnetic foreign body impaled in the retina. *B*, Trap door and diathermy at localization site under disinserted rectus muscle. *C*, Foreign body causing bulge of the choroidal knuckle through sclerotomy, with approach of magnet. *D*, Delivery of foreign body with a pencil magnet. *E*, Silicone implant. *F*, Sutured flaps. *G*, Internal view of the extraction site and buckle effect. (Courtesy of the late Taylor R. Smith, M.D.)

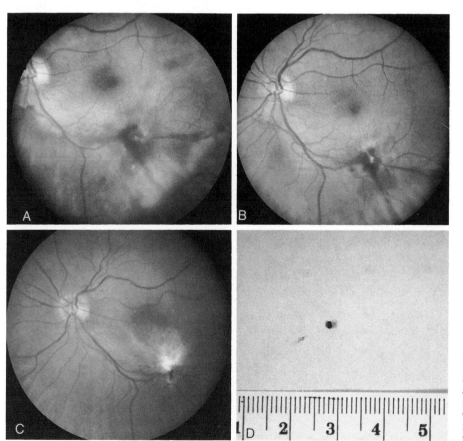

Figure 103–14. Evolution of epimacular fibrosis from a scar at untreated impact site of a foreign body. *A*, Impact site amidst small retinal and vitreous hemorrhage. *B*, Slight clearing 1 mo later. *C*, Cicatrization with epimacular fibrosis 7 mo later. *D*, Causative foreign body. Final vision was 20/200.

complete history, a well-planned preoperative evaluation, and skilled intervention with proper equipment and a support team. Undue haste is counterproductive. An instructive example follows:

CASE HISTORY

RM, a 56-year-old referee at a skeet shoot, was struck in the right eye by what was thought to be a pellet that had ricocheted off the skeet. He noted immediate loss of vision and was taken to a local hospital, where standard localizing foreign body films were taken. The ophthalmologist on call then proceeded with surgery, attempting to remove the foreign body with an electromagnet via the inferonasal corneoscleral entry site. After several attempts, the procedure was terminated because of uncontrollable bleeding. The wound was sutured and a consultation was requested. A period of healing was advised, during which time it was learned that the pellets used at the skeet shoot were of lead and hence nonmagnetic. Additional studies revealed the foreign body to be outside the globe posteriorly. The vitreous hemorrhage subsequently cleared, revealing a scar at the exit site inferotemporal to the macula. After several months, the cataract was removed, a subsequent retinal detachment was repaired, and the patient ultimately recovered 20/60 vision, with slight epimacular fibrosis (Fig. 103–15). The pellet remains in the orbit undisturbed.

Comment: A thorough history, better preoperative studies, and perhaps earlier consultation would have prevented the intraoperative complications and postoperative embarrassment. Removal of an intraocular foreign body blindly is inadvisable; it is better to clear the media or wait for it to clear. Attempted extraction via the entry site, although inviting, is best eschewed. Cataract, retinal detachment, and epimacular fibrosis are not uncommon sequelae. Not all double perforations need to be explored and repaired posteriorly. Orbital foreign bodies that create no problems are best left alone.

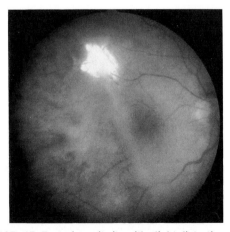

Figure 103–15. Posterior exit site with slight distortion of macula from epimacular fibrosis. Final vision was 20/60.

A careful history and examination are imperative, as sadly shown by the following case:

CASE HISTORY

RT, a 27-year-old mechanic, presented to the emergency room complaining of a scratchy feeling in the left eye. He was found to have a small area of bulbar conjunctival injection inferotemporally and considerable sooty debris on the lids and lashes. Vision was 20/20. Erythromycin ophthalmic ointment was prescribed, and he was advised to see an ophthalmologist if the injury was not better within a week. Shortly thereafter he consulted an ophthalmologist because of redness, tearing, and photophobia. Iritis was diagnosed and local steroid drops and cycloplegics were added to the erythromycin treatment. A cycle of improvement and ingravescence, corresponding to changes in the frequency of medication, eventually ended with abrupt visual loss. He was referred for a retinal evaluation, which revealed a glistening yellow intraocular foreign body lying on the inferior retina, which was detached and gathered into folds (proliferative retinopathy, grade C-2). The foreign body was removed and the retina was reattached, but vision remained at the counting fingers level because of recurrent epimacular fibrosis.

Comment: Nonspecific complaints by a patient whose occupation predisposes him or her to ocular injuries must be thoroughly investigated. A localized spot of conjunctival injection in any patient with a vague complaint cannot be dismissed lightly, unless a detailed history, complete examination, and adequate studies justify doing so. Prior to instituting treatment for iritis, a retinal examination with scleral depression is mandatory. In this case, it most likely would have prevented severe visual loss.

This patient's ocular saga is illustrative of the value of maintaining a high index of suspicion when confronted with unusual findings:

CASE HISTORY

JP, a 40-year-old road worker, consulted an ophthalmologist because of poor vision in his right eye. The vision was at the counting fingers level and was explained by an advanced "unusual" cataract; surgery was undertaken. Early in the procedure, the lens fell into the vitreous. An anterior vitrectomy was performed; a lens implant was placed in the anterior chamber, and the patient was referred for vitreoretinal consultation. After the intraocular pressure was lowered and some corneal clarity was achieved, the iris was noted to be considerably lighter than that of the other eye. Pars plana vitrectomy was performed, followed by Fragmatome extraction of the virtually intact lens lying on the inferior retinal periphery. Prior to terminating the procedure, indirect ophthalmoscopy with scleral depression revealed a small glistening encapsulated foreign body on the pars plana inferiorly. It was removed and scanning electron microscopy and energy-dispersing analysis proved its ferrous nature. Seven months after surgery, the best corrected vision was 20/70, the pupil was frozen at 6 mm, and the macular reflex was suggestive of mild epimacular fibrosis. Electroretinographic studies were compatible with decreased illumination, attributable to the pupil size, and were not felt to be reflective of siderosis. Interestingly, even in retrospect the patient could not recall a specific incident of trauma leading to the intraocular foreign body.

Comment: A monocular "unusual" cataract in a young patient, together with the iris color change, is sufficient to heighten suspicion of an occult intraocular foreign body or at least previous ocular trauma. Approaching surgery on this eye with such concerns, and the knowledge that zonules may be weak in siderosis or ruptured in trauma, may have avoided the complications encountered. Electroretinographic abnormalities in siderosis may disappear within 3 mo after removing the foreign body, thus explaining the findings in this case. Siderosis bulbi respond nicely to treatment.[41]

PREVENTION

Although the incidence of intraocular foreign bodies is small compared with the multitude of problems that affect the eye, their toll (personal and economic) is vastly disproportionate to their number, because those afflicted are overwhelmingly young and often in their most productive years.[42] Further, despite revolutionary therapeutic advances, a significant number of eyes are lost, and of those that are saved, subnormal vision is the most common outcome. The percentage of eyes with excellent vision following intraocular foreign body removal is small.[43] It is obvious, therefore, that in addition to the careful history, examination, ancillary studies, and timely and appropriate intervention, better efforts at preventing such visual catastrophes are necessary. Educating the public to increase the general awareness of the potentially calamitous consequences of seemingly innocuous activities such as hammering a nail is imperative.[44] Equally important is the need to stress the use of protective glasses on the job and in the home when performing tasks involving hammering or other activities that could possibly entail a projectile.[45] Avoiding unnecessary visual loss can best be achieved by pursuing prevention as the paramount goal.[46, 47]

REFERENCES

1. Tawara A: Transformation and cytotoxicity of iron in siderosis bulbi. Invest Ophthalmol Vis Sci 27:226–236, 1986.
2. Burch PG, Albert DM: Transscleral ocular siderosis. Am J Ophthalmol 84:90, 1977.
3. Lebowitz AA, Couch JM, Thompson JT, Shields JA: Occult foreign body simulating melanoma with extrascleral extension. Retina 8:141–144, 1988.
4. Duber JS, Fisher DH: Occult plastic intraocular foreign body. Ophthalmic Surg 20:169–70, 1989.
5. Saar I, Raniel J, Neumann E: Recurrent corneal edema following late migration of intraocular glass. Br J Ophthalmol 75:188–189, 1991.
6. Sneed SR: Ocular siderosis. Arch Ophthalmol 106:997, 1988.
7. Rosenthal AR, Marmor MF, Leuenberger P, Hopkins JL: Chalcosis: A study of natural history. Ophthalmology 86:1956, 1979.
8. Zinreich SJ, Miller NR, Aguayo JB, et al: Computed tomographic three-dimensional localization and compositional evaluation of intraocular and orbital foreign bodies. Arch Ophthalmol 104:1477–1482, 1986.
9. Lindahl S: Computed tomography of intraobital foreign bodies. Acta Radiol 28:235–240, 1987.
10. Etherington RJ, Hourihan MD: Localization of intraocular and intraorbital foreign bodies using computed tomography. Clin Radiol 40:610–614, 1989.
11. Fisher YL: Advances in contact ophthalmic ultrasonography: Ocular trauma and intraocular foreign body patients. Dev Ophthalmol 18:69–74, 1989.
12. Bryden FM, Pyott AA, Bailey M, McGhee CN: Real-time ultrasound in the assessment of intraocular foreign bodies. Eye 4:727–731, 1990.
13. Lagouros PA, Langer BG, Peyman GA, et al: Magnetic resonance imaging and intraocular foreign bodies. Arch Ophthalmol 105:551–553, 1987.
14. Williamson TH, Smith FW, Forrester JV: Magnetic resonance imaging of intraocular foreign bodies. Br J Ophthalmol 73:555–558, 1989.
15. Williams S, Char DH, Dillon WP, et al: Ferrous intraocular foreign bodies and magnetic resonance imaging. Am J Ophthalmol 105:398–401, 1988.
16. LoBue TD, Deutsch TA, Lobick J, Turner DA: Detection and localization of nonmetallic intraocular foreign bodies by magnetic resonance imaging. Arch Ophthalmol 106:260–261, 1988.
17. Kelsey CA, King JN, Keck GM, et al: Ocular hazard of metallic fragments during MR imaging at 0.06 T. Radiology 180:282–283, 1991.
18. Glatt HJ, Custer PL, Barrett L, Sartor K: Magnetic resonance imaging and computed tomography in a model of wooden foreign bodies in the orbit. Ophthalmol Plast Reconstr Surg 6:108–114, 1990.
19. Good P, Gross K: Electrophysiology and metallosis: Support for an oxidative (free radical) mechanism in the human eye. Ophthalmologica 196:204–209, 1988.
20. Crock GW, Janakiraman P, Reddy P: Intraocular magnet of Parel. Br J Ophthalmol 70:879–885, 1986.
21. Nishi O: Magnetic device for removal of intraocular foreign bodies. Ophthalmic Surg 18:232–233, 1987.
22. Mansour AM: New attachment for the ocular magnet. Ann Ophthalmol 20:239, 1988.
23. May DR, Noll FG, Munoz R: A 20-gauge intraocular electromagnetic tip for simplified intraocular foreign-body extraction. Arch Ophthalmol 107:281–282, 1989.
24. McCuen BW II, Hickingbotham D: A new retractable micromagnet for intraocular foreign body removal. Arch Ophthalmol 107:1819–1820, 1989.
25. Hadden OB, Wilson JL: The management of intraocular foreign bodies. Aust NZ J Ophthalmol 18:343–351, 1990.
26. Coleman DJ, Lucas BC, Rondeau MJ, Chang S: Management of intraocular foreign bodies. Ophthalmology 94:1647–1653, 1987.
27. Slusher MM: Intraretinal foreign bodies. Management and observations. Retina 10(Suppl)1:650–654, 1990.
28. Ambler JS, Meyers SM: Management of intraretinal metallic foreign bodies without retinopexy in the absence of retinal detachment. Ophthalmology 98:391–394, 1991.
29. Joondeph BC, Flynn HW Jr: Management of subretinal foreign bodies with a cannulated extrusion needle. Am J Ophthalmol 110:250–253, 1990.
30. McCarthy MJ, Pulido JS, Soukup B: The use of ureter stone forceps to remove a large intraocular foreign body. Am J Ophthalmol 110:208–209, 1990.
31. Micovic V, Milenkovic S, Opric M: Acute aseptic panophthalmitis caused by a copper foreign body. Fortschr Ophthalmol (Germany) 87:362–363, 1990.
32. Armstrong, MF: A review of intraocular foreign body injuries and complications in N. Ireland from 1978–1986. Int Ophthalmol 12:113–117, 1988.
33. Behrens-Baumann W, Praetorious G: Intraocular foreign bodies. 297 consecutive cases. Oftalmologica 198:84–88, 1989.

34. Percival SPB: Late complications from posterior segment intraocular foreign bodies. Br J Ophthalmol 56:462, 1972.

35. Mieler WF, Ellis MK, Williams DF, Han DP: Retained intraocular foreign bodies and endophthalmitis. Ophthalmology 97:1532–1538, 1990.

36. Kingham JD: Photic maculopathy in young males with intraocular foreign body. Milit Med 156:44–47, 1991.

37. Trimble SN, Schatz H: Subretinal neovascularization following metallic intraocular foreign-body trauma. Arch Ophthalmol 104:515–519, 1986.

38. Williams DF, Mieler WF, Abrams GW, Lewis H: Results and prognostic factors in penetrating ocular injuries with retained intraocular foreign bodies. Ophthalmology 95:911–916, 1988.

39. Punnonen E, Laatikainen L: Prognosis of perforating eye injuries with intraocular foreign bodies. Acta Ophthalmol (Copenh) 67:483–491, 1989.

40. Bettman JW: Seven hundred medicolegal cases in ophthalmology. Ophthalmology 97:1379–1384, 1990.

41. Sneed SR, Weingeist TA: Management of siderosis bulbi due to a retained iron-containing intraocular foreign body. Ophthalmology 97:375–379, 1990.

42. Khan MD, Kundi N, Mohammed Z, Nazeer AF: A 6-1/2–years' survey of intraocular and intraorbital foreign bodies in the Northwest Frontier Province, Pakistan. Br J Ophthalmol 71:716–719, 1987.

43. Williams DF, Mieler WF, Abrams GW: Intraocular foreign bodies in young people. Retina 10(Suppl)1:945–949, 1990.

44. Owen P, Keightley SJ, Elkington AR: The hazards of hammers. Injury 18:61–62, 1987.

45. Dunn JP Jr, Berger ST, Mondino BJ, Goodwin LT Jr: Ocular trauma caused by exploding glass bottles containing dry ice and water. Ophthalmic Surg 21:628–631, 1990.

46. Jeffers JB: The role of organized ophthalmology in preventing ocular injuries. Int Ophthalmol Clin 28:255–258, 1988.

47. Pizzarello LD: American Academy of Ophthalmology's commitment to eye safety. [Letter] Arch Ophthalmol 107:1565, 1989.

48. Cogan DG: Williams's ophthalmic connections. [Letter] Harvard Med Alum Bull 64:5, 1990.

SECTION V

Hereditary Retinal Diseases

Edited by
ELIOT L. BERSON

Chapter 104

■

Hereditary Retinal Diseases: An Overview

ELIOT L. BERSON

Hereditary retinal diseases represent a significant cause of visual loss in individuals all over the world. An estimated 100,000 persons are affected in the United States alone. The problem is magnified when we consider that many children are visually impaired and that the majority become legally blind by age 40 yr.

Most of these diseases were originally defined based on the fundus appearance as seen through the ophthalmoscope and, in some cases, through histopathologic examination of autopsied eyes. More recently, visual function assessments, biochemical studies, and molecular genetic analyses have provided new approaches for detecting these diseases and defining pathogenetic mechanisms. Many hereditary retinal diseases can now be diagnosed in early life based on deficits in visual function, biochemical abnormalities, or molecular genetic defects, in some cases many years before symptoms develop and changes are visible with the ophthalmoscope. The capacity to diagnose these conditions at an early stage has provided hope that some of these diseases may be reversed, stabilized, or slowed prior to the death of retinal cells.

This chapter presents an overview for ophthalmologists of some of the current approaches being used for diagnosis of hereditary retinal diseases that involve cone or rod photoreceptor function, or both (Table 104–1). These approaches have not only provided the capability for early detection of these diseases but have also aided in clarifying some pathogenetic mechanisms that lead to photoreceptor cell degeneration.

CONE AND ROD DISTRIBUTION ACROSS THE HUMAN RETINA

An understanding of the normal cone and rod distribution across the human retina is necessary to interpret tests of visual function in patients with hereditary retinal diseases. The normal human retina has about 130 million photoreceptors, and the rods outnumber the cones by about 13:1. Rods are distributed across all of the normal retina except in the foveola (central 1 degree 40 min); rod density is maximal 20 to 40 degrees eccentric to the foveola (Fig. 104–1). Cone density is highest in the fovea or central 5 degrees (Fig. 104–1), but more than 90 percent of the retinal cones are outside the central 5 degrees. Cones and rods are approximately equal in number in the macula (central 18.4 degrees).

Keeping this distribution of the photoreceptors in mind, a patient with advanced macular degeneration with a 10- to 20-degree–diameter central scotoma by definition has lost not only macular cones but also macular rods. A patient with retinitis pigmentosa with a midperipheral scotoma has lost both rods and cones in the midperipheral retinal area corresponding to the scotoma. A patient with advanced cone degeneration by definition has lost cones across all, or nearly all, the retina.

Patients with normal cone function and absent rod function (i.e., stationary night blindness [SNB]) would be expected to have a visual acuity of 20/20 and full kinetic visual fields with white test lights in the Goldmann perimeter. Patients with absent cone function and

Table 104–1. SOME HEREDITARY RETINAL DISEASES*

Autosomal dominant forms of retinitis pigmentosa
Autosomal recessive forms of retinitis pigmentosa
Sex-linked (X chromosome–linked) forms of retinitis pigmentosa
Isolate (simplex) forms of retinitis pigmentosa
Progressive cone-rod degeneration
Sector retinitis pigmentosa
Some syndromes or diseases of which retinitis pigmentosa is a part
  Usher's syndrome, type I and type II
  Laurence-Moon and Bardet-Biedl syndromes
  Bassen-Kornzweig syndrome
  Refsum's disease
  Kearns-Sayre syndrome
  Hereditary cerebroretinal degenerations including Batten's disease
  Olivopontocerebellar atrophy
  Cockayne's syndrome
  Alström's disease
  Mucopolysaccharide disorders
Congenital amaurosis of Leber
Sex-linked choroideremia
Generalized choroidal sclerosis
Gyrate atrophy of the choroid and retina
Retinitis punctata albescens
Cone degenerations
Hereditary macular degenerations including Stargardt's disease, central areolar choroidal dystrophy, Best's vitelliform macular dystrophy, dominant drusen, North Carolina macular dystrophy
Stationary forms of night blindness including dominant (Nougaret) nyctalopia, autosomal recessive and sex-linked nyctalopia, Oguchi's disease, fundus albipunctatus
Congenital rod monochromacy and blue cone monochromacy

*Hereditary retinal diseases that involve rod or cone photoreceptor function.

1183

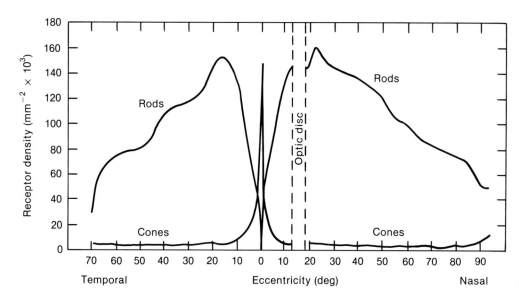

Figure 104–1. Distribution of rods and cones in the normal human retina corresponding to perimetric angles from the fovea at zero degrees as given. (After Østerberg. From Pirenne MH: Vision and the Eye. London, Chapman and Hall, 1967.)

normal rod function (i.e., rod monochromasy) would be expected to have visual acuity of 20/200, a small central scotoma, and an otherwise full kinetic visual field in the Goldmann perimeter. Patients can read fine newspaper print with either their cones or their rods, although patients with only rod function usually require magnifying lenses to read. Patients with macular degeneration and large areas of retained peripheral (i.e., extramacular) cone or rod function can read fine print with either their peripheral cones or their peripheral rods with the appropriate magnification.[1, 2]

DARK–ADAPTATION TESTING

Cone and rod function can be separated by evaluating the course of dark adaptation after exposure to a steady adapting light. Both cones and rods normally can adapt to the dark. The threshold response of a normal subject to an 11-degree white test light presented 7 degrees above the fovea in the dark over 40 min can be described by a biphasic curve with an initial cone limb followed by a rod limb, as illustrated in Figure 104–2. Following

exposure to a standard adapting light, final cone threshold is normally achieved in 5 to 7 min; the final cone threshold is 100- to 1000-fold (i.e., 2 to 3 log units) higher than final rod threshold, which is normally achieved after 40 min of dark adaptation. A patient with SNB with normal cone function and absent rod function has a normal cone limb but no cone-rod break at 5 to 7 min; final threshold even after 40 min is determined by cones and is therefore 2 to 3 log units greater than normal (Fig. 104–2). The patient with SNB can see normally under dim photopic conditions that exist at night near street lights or in dimly lit areas and experiences "night blindness" only under starlight or moonlight (i.e., scotopic) conditions.

Figure 104–2 also shows dark-adaptation curves from two patients with retinitis pigmentosa designated as RP (1) and RP (2). Both report "night blindness" under dim photopic conditions, as they have impairment of the initial cone limb of dark adaptation in contrast to the patient with SNB. Some patients with early macular degeneration may also have difficulty seeing at night, but on further questioning they report that the symptom occurs when they are driving at night and are trying to

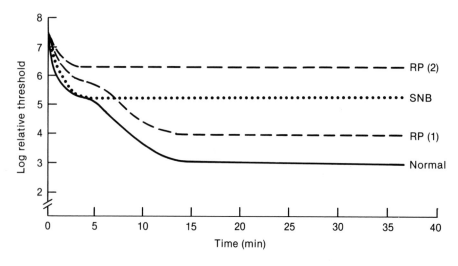

Figure 104–2. Representative dark-adaptation curves for a normal subject; a patient with congenital stationary night blindness (SNB); and two patients with moderately advanced retinitis pigmentosa, *RP(1)* and *RP(2)*. (Reprinted with permission from Berson EL: Night blindness: Some aspects of management. *In* Faye E [ed]: Clinical Low Vision. Boston, Little, Brown and Company, 1976.)

adjust to oncoming headlights; these patients appear to have difficulty at night because of an impairment in dark adaptation of their macular cones.[2-4]

SPECTRAL SENSITIVITY FUNCTIONS

Rod and cone function can also be assessed by measuring the sensitivity of the eye across the visible spectrum under dark-adapted (i.e., scotopic) or light-adapted (i.e., photopic) conditions. The visible spectrum normally extends from the deep blue at 400 nm to the deep red at 700 nm. Under scotopic conditions, the peak sensitivity of the eye, governed by the rod system, is near 500 nm, whereas under photopic conditions, the peak sensitivity, mediated by the cone system, is near 555 nm (Fig. 104–3). The shift from peak sensitivity in the blue-green region under dark-adapted conditions to the orange-yellow region under light-adapted conditions is called the Purkinje shift. Under dark-adapted conditions, a dim blue light presented to a normal subject near threshold will first be reported only as light, as the subject is using the rod system and therefore cannot appreciate color; when the light is made 1000-fold brighter, a normal subject is able to use the cone system to see the test light as blue. Similarly, under dark-adapted conditions, a dim blue light can be used to isolate rod function in the electroretinogram (ERG); a bright blue light can elicit both rod and cone responses if the light is sufficiently bright to be seen by the cones. A dim orange-red light will elicit only a rod response in the ERG, whereas a bright orange-red light (λ >600 nm) will elicit a response from both cones and rods.

The peak ERG sensitivity of the cone system to a 25-Hz white flickering light is near 555 nm under dark-adapted conditions (Fig. 104–4), as rods usually cannot respond to stimuli greater than 20 Hz under these test conditions. We can isolate blue, green, and red cone function, respectively, to a 25-Hz white flickering light in the presence of different colored steady background lights that desensitize one or another cone system by bleaching that system (i.e., dissociating opsin from vitamin A). The blue cone system in the presence of a bright yellow steady background light has a peak sensitivity near 440 nm to the 25-Hz stimulus. In the presence of a purple adapting light that desensitizes the blue and red cone systems, the peak sensitivity is near 540 nm, thereby isolating green cone function. In the presence of a blue-green steady background light that desensitizes the blue cone and green cone systems, the peak sensitivity is near 580 nm, thereby isolating red cone function. The spectral sensitivities of the red, green, and blue cone systems, defined with ERG testing, correspond, respectively, to the absorption characteristics of individual red, green, and blue cones, determined with microspectrophotometry, supporting the conclusion that these three ERG functions are generated by the red (long wavelength–sensitive), green (middle wavelength–sensitive), and blue (short wavelength–sensitive) cones, respectively.[5-8]

Spectral sensitivity testing, whether determined by

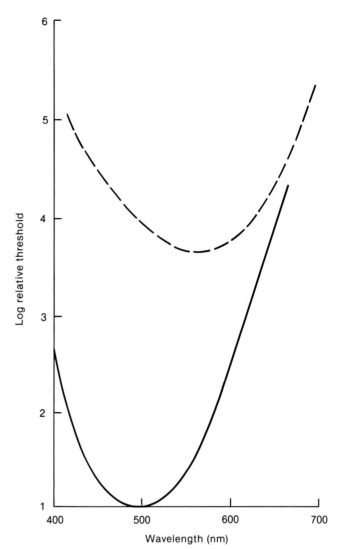

Figure 104–3. *Continuous line* is CIE (Commission International de l'Eclairage) scotopic luminosity curve (rod spectral sensitivity function) derived from psychophysical measurements and placed at a level for normal human subjects; *dashed line* is Wald's photopic luminosity curve (spectral sensitivity function for the cone mechanisms under photopic conditions) derived from psychophysical measurements of peripheral retinal function. Electroretinographic spectral sensitivity curves for normal rod and cone systems also respectively approximate the *solid line* and *dashed line* curves. (From Berson EL: Electrical phenomena in the retina. *In* Hart WM [ed]. Adler's Physiology of the Eye. Clinical Application, 9th ed. St Louis, CV Mosby, 1992.)

psychophysical or ERG measurements, provides a basis for classification of hereditary retinal diseases involving the photoreceptors. For example, patients with autosomal recessive rod monochromasy (i.e., complete monochromatism) with normal rod function and complete loss of cone function have a peak sensitivity near 500 nm under both light- and dark-adapted conditions. Patients with X-linked blue-cone monochromasy are born with no red and green cone function but retain blue cone and rod function; their sensitivity under dark-adapted conditions is governed by rods with peak sensitivity near 500 nm, whereas their sensitivity under light-adapted conditions is governed by blue cones with

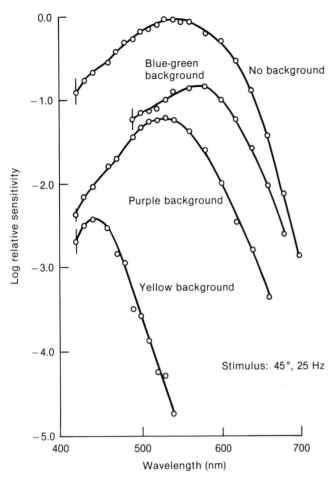

Figure 104–4. Spectral sensitivity curves describing response of monkey cone mechanisms to a 25-Hz stimulus under conditions of dark adaptation or in the presence of intense chromatic backgrounds. Sector disc (50 percent duty cycle) was used to present flickering stimuli (25 Hz). Stimulus subtended a visual angle of 45 degrees and was centrally superimposed on a 68-degree background. Spectral sensitivity data were based on the log relative quantum flux at the retina necessary to elicit a criterion amplitude in the electroretinogram (ERG). The red cone mechanism showed the best separation on a blue-green adapting field, the green cone mechanism on a purple adapting field, and the blue cone mechanism on a yellow adapting field. Data points *(open circles)* are an average of three animals. *Vertical lines* equal ± 1 SD (average). (From Mehaffey L III, Berson EL: Cone mechanisms in the electroretinogram of the cynomolgus monkey. Invest Ophthalmol 13:266, 1974.)

a peak sensitivity near 440 nm. Patients with X-linked cone degeneration, protan type have a partial loss of red and green cone function with predominant loss of red cone function at a time when rod function and blue cone function appear to be normal. Patients with retinitis pigmentosa or other generalized retinal degenerations such as choroideremia or progressive cone-rod degeneration appear to have an abnormality of both rod and cone function across all or nearly all the retina in the early stages.[2, 5]

COLOR VISION TESTING

Cone function can be measured not only by means of dark adaptation and spectral sensitivity testing but also

by evaluating color vision. The Farnsworth panel D15 and the Ishihara plates can be used to screen patients with X-linked red (protan) deficiency or X-linked green (deutan) deficiency. Dominantly inherited blue (tritan) deficiency can also be detected on the Farnsworth panel D15. Blue cone monochromat color plates can be used to distinguish young men with X-linked blue cone monochromasy from young men with autosomal recessive rod monochromasy, as the former individuals pass this test whereas the latter individuals fail it. Color deficiencies can also be monitored with an anomaloscope, which allows color matches; e.g., a patient with choroidal disease and subretinal fluid in the fovea may have cone photoreceptor disorientation with a consequent shift in the Rayleigh color match to a higher red primary ratio (i.e., pseudoprotanomaly).[9–13]

Acquired red-green or blue-yellow color defects, or both, are well known; e.g., a patient with cone dystrophy may report an acquired red-green dyschromatopsia due to loss of cone photoreceptors in the macula, or a patient with retinitis pigmentosa, glaucoma, or diabetic retinopathy with field loss can report acquired blue-yellow deficiency.

When color vision tests are used to assess retinal photoreceptor function, we obtain information about the patches or regions of cones used to perform these tests. A patient with advanced macular degeneration with a central scotoma may fail the Ishihara plates because of loss of central field and yet perform the Farnsworth panel D15 correctly by viewing the color caps eccentrically with extramacular cones.[2]

FULL–FIELD ELECTRORETINOGRAPHIC TESTING

The full-field ERG is a mass response generated by cells across the entire retina in response to flashes of light. The cones account for 20 to 25 percent and the rods account for 75 to 80 percent of the full-field ERG response to single flashes of white light under dark-adapted conditions. The full-field ERG is primarily generated by extramacular (i.e., midperipheral and far peripheral) cones and rods, as patients with a four-disc-diameter central scar and normal extramacular function have normal full-field cone and rod ERG responses. The central macula (central 10 degrees) contains about 450,000 cones or 7 percent of the total retinal cone population, so that abnormalities confined only to the central macula generally do not compromise the full-field ERG. Loss of half the photoreceptors across the entire retina is associated with approximately a 50 percent reduction in full-field ERG amplitude.

The photoreceptors generate the initial cornea-negative component (i.e., negative relative to baseline), or a-wave in the ERG, whereas the Müller cells are responsible for the later cornea-positive component, or b-wave. The full-field ERG, if abnormal, is particularly useful in detecting patients with generalized loss of rod or cone function, or both. Patients with reduced vision due to optic atrophy or cortical disease have preserved outer retinal function and would be expected to have normal ERGs to full-field flashes of light.

Patients with focal loss of cones due to either a large central area of chorioretinal scarring or a large peripheral area of chorioretinal scarring (i.e., greater than 4 disc diameters) have displayed normal b-wave implicit times with reduced amplitudes (Fig. 104–5). In contrast, patients with early retinitis pigmentosa usually display delayed cone b-wave implicit times with or without reductions in amplitude in the early stages (Fig. 104–5). Cone responses to 30-Hz flicker are so delayed that a phase shift occurs between the time of stimulus flash (designated by the vertical hatched lines in the figure) and the corresponding response peaks such that each stimulus elicits the "next-plus-one" response. Similarly, patients with focal loss of patches of rod function due to chorioretinal scarring either in the macula or in the far periphery also show reductions in amplitude with normal b-wave implicit times. In contrast, patients with generalized forms of retinitis pigmentosa display reduced rod amplitudes with delayed rod b-wave implicit times. The full-field ERG therefore can be used as an aid in defining the extent and type of cone and rod involvement, as patients with focal loss of retinal function and self-limited disease have reductions in amplitude with normal implicit times, whereas patients with widespread loss of retinal function and progressive dis-

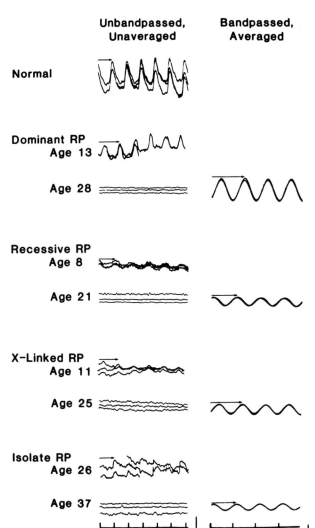

Figure 104–6. Full-field 30-Hz ERGs from a normal subject and four patients with RP tested at an 11- to 15-yr interval. Stimulus onset, vertical markers; calibration symbol *(left column, lower right)* designates 100 μV vertically for the normal subject and the top three patients and 40 μV vertically for the bottom patient and 50 msec horizontally for all traces; calibration *(right column, lower right)* designates 2 μV vertically for the dominant, X-linked, and isolate patients and 0.3 μV for the recessive patient and 20 msec horizontally for all traces. B-wave implicit times are designated with *arrows.* (From Andréasson SOL, Sandberg MA, Berson EL: Narrow-band filtering for monitoring low-amplitude cone electroretinograms in retinitis pigmentosa. Am J Ophthalmol 105:500–503, 1988. Published with permission from The American Journal of Ophthalmology. Copyright by The Ophthalmic Publishing Company.)

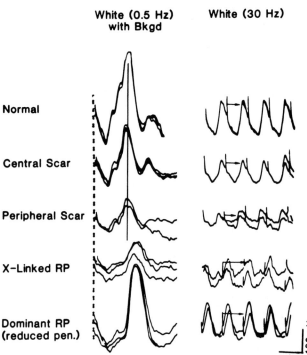

Figure 104–5. Full-field cone ERGs from a normal subject, two patients with large chorioretinal scars, and two patients with retinitis pigmentosa (RP). Responses *(left column)* were obtained to 0.5-Hz white light in presence of steady white 10 ft-L background light sufficient to eliminate rod contribution to full-field ERG. Responses *(right column)* were obtained to 30-Hz white flicker. *Horizontal arrows* designate cone b-wave implicit time. Calibration *(lower right corner)* designates 25 msec horizontally and 40 μV vertically for the left column and 50 msec and 100 μV for the right column.

ease characteristically have reductions in amplitude with delays in b-wave implicit times.

The range of detectability of ERG responses has been extended 100- to 1000-fold with computer averaging and narrow bandpass filtering. Responses that were not detectable without computer averaging or narrow bandpass filtering (i.e., <10 μV) can be monitored down to a level well under 1 μV with these techniques (Fig. 104–6). More than 90 percent of patients aged 6 to 49 yr with retinitis pigmentosa and visual field diameters greater than 8 degrees have detectable ERG responses with computer averaging and narrow bandpass filtering, thereby making it possible to quantify objectively the amount of remaining retinal function and follow the course of the retinal degeneration.[14-18]

FOCAL ELECTRORETINOGRAPHY

Focal cone ERGs can be elicited with a stimulator-ophthalmoscope. With this instrument, a 4-degree, 42-Hz white flickering stimulus is presented within a 10-degree white steady surround; this flickering stimulus allows isolation of cone function, and the steady surround permits the examiner to visualize the fundus. The surround also desensitizes the retina just outside the stimulus, thereby minimizing any possible responses that could be generated by effects of stray light from the stimulus. A patient with a one-disc-diameter central macular scar and visual acuity reduced to 20/200 displays foveal cone ERG responses indistinguishable from noise when the stimulus is centered within the scar but normal responses when the stimulus is centered outside the scar in a parafoveal area that appears normal on fundus examination. A patient with decreased vision due to strabismic amblyopia or optic atrophy displays a normal foveal ERG (Fig. 104-7). Therefore, the focal cone ERG elicited with the stimulator-ophthalmoscope has clinical value in distinguishing patients with hereditary macular degenerations from those with optic atrophy, as the responses are abnormal in the former and normal in the latter.

Responses in the central retina can be elicited not only in response to flashes of light but also in response to a phase-reversing pattern stimulus, usually a grating or checkerboard displayed on a television screen. The pattern elements (checks or bars) periodically reverse position, so that the bright bars become dim and vice versa, although the sum of all bars has a constant brightness at all times. The responses can be reliably measured only when the stimulus is focused on the retina and maintained on the fovea during testing. In contrast to the flash ERG, the pattern ERG is eliminated by transection of the optic nerve (Fig. 104-8), supporting the idea that the pattern response is generated by the inner retina. The pattern ERG may have clinical value in monitoring inner retinal diseases such as glaucoma or optic nerve abnormalities, but an abnormal pattern response should be interpreted as reflecting inner retinal or optic nerve disease only when it is known that the outer retina is functionally intact, as abnormal pattern ERGs have also been reported in macular degenerations involving the photoreceptors.

Visually evoked cortical potentials (VECPs) can be used to assess central foveal cone function in patients with macular disease. It has been estimated that the central 2 degrees generates 65 percent of this response. The problem of stray light can be minimized by use of pattern-reversal stimuli. The VECP has had limited value in measuring macular function behind a lens opacity because smaller than normal responses can result from reduction of stimulus sensitivity and from image blur on the retina produced by the opacity. In contrast to the focal-flash ERG, which is generated by the outer

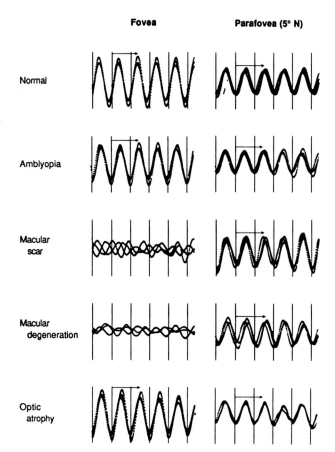

Figure 104-7. Foveal and parafoveal cone ERGs from a normal subject and four patients with visual acuity of 20/200. Two or three consecutive computer summations (n = 128) are shown. *Vertical lines* denote stimulus onset; *arrows* denote b-wave implicit time to corresponding response peak. Calibration symbol in *lower right corner* denotes 20 msec horizontally and 0.25 μV vertically. (From Jacobson SG, Sandberg MA, Effron MH, Berson EL: Foveal cone electroretinograms in strabismic amblyopia: Comparison with juvenile macular degeneration, macular scars, and optic atrophy. Trans Ophthalmol Soc UK 99:353, 1979.)

retina, the VECP can be abnormal in diseases of the outer retina, such as hereditary macular degeneration, as well as in diseases of the optic nerve or visual cortex. Again, abnormalities in the VECP can be more informative in localizing the site of visual loss if the patient is known to have normal photoreceptor function with a normal focal cone ERG.[19-24]

ELECTROOCULOGRAPHY

The electrooculogram (EOG) is recorded with leads placed near the inner and outer canthus and is measured by asking the patient to look straight at a fixation light and then laterally 30 degrees at a second fixation light, alternating between these fixation lights first for 10 to 12 min in the dark and then for an additional 15 to 20 min in the light. The lowest potential, generated per 30 degrees of eye movement in the dark, is compared with the largest potential, generated per 30 degrees of eye movement in the light, and recorded as the light-

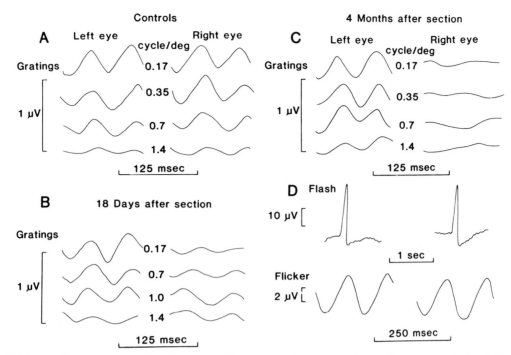

Figure 104–8. Examples of pattern-reversal ERGs recorded from one cat before and after the section of the right optic nerve. *A,* Control records obtained from the two eyes before the section of the optic nerve. *B* and *C,* Records obtained 18 days and 4 mo after the optic nerve section. Each record is the average of 500 responses. Stimulus: vertical sinusoidal grating reversed in contrast 16 times/sec; contrast, 30 percent; mean luminance, 10 cd/sq m. The spatial frequency is indicated next to each record. *D,* ERG in response to 50-msec light flashes (250 trolands) and to light flickering at 8 Hz (mean luminance, 10 cd/sq m; amplitude of square-wave modulation, 40 percent) recorded from the two eyes 4 mo after section of the right optic nerve. (*A–D,* From Maffei L, Fiorentini A: Electroretinographic responses to alternating gratings before and after section of the optic nerve. Science 211:953, 1981. Copyright 1981 by the American Association for the Advancement of Science.)

rise:dark-trough ratio. This ratio is usually greater than or equal to 1.8 for patients aged 50 yr or younger.

The EOG is useful in evaluating patients with known or suspected dominantly inherited Best's vitelliform macular dystrophy. Patients with Best's macular dystrophy have a light-rise:dark-trough ratio of less than 1.5 at a time when the full-field ERG is normal; abnormal EOGs have been observed not only in patients with visible vitelliform macular lesions but also in asymptomatic relatives with normal fundi who nevertheless have this condition. The EOG is normal in patients with dominantly inherited cone degeneration but is abnormal in patients with cone-rod dystrophies, as normal rods are required to generate a normal light-rise in the EOG.[2, 5]

GUIDELINES FOR CLASSIFICATION OF HEREDITARY RETINAL DISEASES BASED ON RETINAL FUNCTION TESTS

In broad outline, hereditary retinal diseases involving the photoreceptors can be subdivided into four groups, as follows: (1) Those diseases that involve cone or rod function alone across all or nearly all the retina (e.g., cone degeneration, SNB); (2) those diseases that involve both cone and rod function but only in localized areas of the retina (e.g., macular degeneration, sector retinitis pigmentosa); (3) those diseases that involve either cone or rod function over all or nearly all the retina with macular degeneration; and (4) those diseases that involve both cone and rod function over all or nearly all the retina (e.g., retinitis pigmentosa, choroideremia). If one photoreceptor system is abnormal and the other is normal in a generalized hereditary retinal disease primarily involving the photoreceptors, as monitored by the full-field ERG, the long-term prognosis for the remaining normal photoreceptor system appears good, as seen in cone degeneration or SNB. Patients who have localized loss of peripheral retinal function due to a hereditary retinal disease such as sector retinitis pigmentosa appear to retain retinal function in those areas that are not involved. Patients with macular degeneration with retention of peripheral rods or cones, or both, at the time of initial examination appear to retain one or both receptor systems outside the macula over the long term; these patients should be distinguished from those with cone-rod degeneration who have abnormal cone and rod function over all or nearly all the retina at an early stage. Patients with impaired cone and rod function over all or nearly all the retina in the early stages of disease have a poor long-term visual prognosis, as seen in cases of retinitis pigmentosa and choroideremia. Therefore, knowledge of the amount and extent of remaining cone and rod function has implications not only with respect to establishing diagnoses but also in estimating long-term visual prognoses.[25]

In performing visual function tests, it is important to understand that different tests provide complementary information; e.g., color vision tests are used to assess patches of cones, either in the macula or in the peripheral retina. A patient can have a normal color vision test and yet have an abnormal full-field cone ERG. Similarly, a patient can have a normal rod threshold on dark-adaptation testing because of retention of a normal region of functioning rods and yet have a subnormal full-field rod ERG because other areas of rod function are compromised. A patient can have an abnormal focal cone ERG and yet have a normal full-field ERG as, for example, in cases of macular degeneration.

In assessing a patient with known or suspected hereditary retinal disease involving the photoreceptors, color vision testing, dark-adaptation testing, full-field ERG testing, and focal-flash ERG testing are particularly useful in defining the extent and type of disease. EOG testing is helpful primarily in patients with Best's vitelliform macular dystrophy. These tests are best performed in patients older than 6 yr of age. ERG testing can be reliably performed in patients younger than 6 yr of age with mild sedation.[2, 5, 25]

BIOCHEMICAL MEASURES

Biochemical abnormalities have been detected in some hereditary retinal diseases involving the photoreceptors. Most notable is the abetalipoproteinemia seen in the Bassen-Kornzweig syndrome,[26-28] the elevated serum phytanic acid seen in Refsum's disease,[29-31] and the elevated serum ornithine levels seen in patients with gyrate atrophy of the choroid and retina.[32-36] In the untreated state, patients with the Bassen-Kornzweig syndrome present with steatorrhea in early life, ataxia in adolescence, and visual symptoms in early adult life. They may compensate for their steatorrhea by reducing fat intake, and they may not be aware of their ataxia. Therefore, they may present initially to an ophthalmologist with the complaint of night deficiency and for that reason serum lipoprotein electrophoresis is recommended for young individuals when this condition is suspected. Similarly, patients with Refsum's disease may not appreciate the initial symptoms of ataxia, loss of smell, or unusual dryness of the skin and present for the first time to an ophthalmologist with the symptom of night deficiency; a serum phytanic acid determination should be considered when this diagnosis is suspected. In early life, peripheral chorioretinal atrophy may be minimal in patients with gyrate atrophy, and a serum ornithine level should be obtained if gyrate atrophy is suspected. Pigmentary retinal degenerations have also been identified in patients with mucopolysaccharidoses[37-41] (e.g., Hunter's, Hurler's, Sanfilippo's, and Scheie's syndromes); these patients are usually identified because of the clinical features and mucopolysacchariduria.

In the case of the Bassen-Kornzweig syndrome, knowledge of a serum deficiency in fat-soluble vitamins led to the recommendation of vitamins A, E, and K administration in the treatment of this condition. In the case of Refsum's disease, knowledge of abnormal storage of phytanic acid in a variety of tissues, including the pigment epithelium, led to the recommendation of a low-phytol, low–phytanic acid diet as a treatment for this condition. In the case of gyrate atrophy, knowledge of an ornithine aminotransferase enzyme deficiency with consequent hyperornithinemia has resulted in trials of vitamin B_6 (a known cofactor for this enzyme) and an arginine-restricted diet (as arginine is the precursor of ornithine) in an effort to lower serum ornithine levels and modify the course of the disease.

MOLECULAR GENETIC ANALYSES

Molecular genetic analyses of leukocyte DNA have provided criteria for early detection of patients with hereditary retinal diseases involving the photoreceptors. By way of background, DNA is configured as a double helix in the nucleus of a cell. Two strands of DNA are schematically represented in Figure 104–9 as two intertwined ribbons; each sugar phosphate strand has nucleotide bases arranged toward the middle. The four nucleo-

Structure of DNA

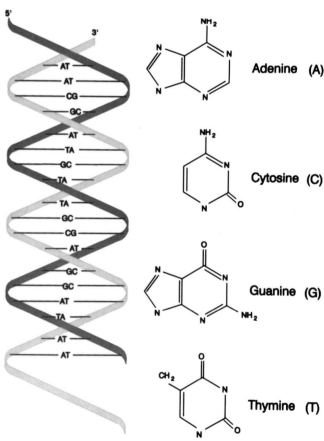

Figure 104–9. Schematic representation of two strands of DNA configured as a double helix with a sugar-phosphate backbone and the bases arranged toward the middle. *Adenine (A)* always pairs with *thymine (T)*, and *cytosine (C)* always pairs with *guanine (G)*.

tide bases of DNA are adenine, cytosine, guanine, and thymine designated by the letters A, C, G, and T; adenine always pairs with thymine, and cytosine pairs with guanine. The two strands of DNA can split apart, with the nucleotide bases serving as the template for synthesizing messenger RNA by which DNA sends its coded instructions to the cytoplasm for protein synthesis.

The genetic code was deciphered by the mid-1960s. A three-base sequence, or codon, was needed to specify each of the 20 amino acids known to compose our proteins (Fig. 104–10); e.g., a three-base codon with cytosines in positions 1, 2, and 3—i.e., CCC—encodes the amino acid proline. The codon cytosine-adenine-cytosine, or CAC, encodes the amino acid histidine. Some redundancy exists in the code, as several codons can designate the same amino acid. Three codons do not encode amino acids but result in a termination of translation and are, therefore, called stop codons (Fig. 104–10). The human genome has about 3 billion A, C, G, and T bases, which are organized into approximately 100,000 genes on 23 chromosomes.[42–45]

Several strategies exist for finding gene abnormalities in patients with hereditary diseases. A chromosomal aberration in a patient with a disease can provide information about a gene or genes that may be responsible for that disease; e.g., a very small deletion in the short arm of the X-chromosome in the band designated as Xp21.2 was found to be associated with Duchenne's muscular dystrophy and retinitis pigmentosa.[46] A limitation of this approach is that many hereditary ocular diseases are not associated with deletions that can be detected simply by looking at the chromosomes.

Methods in common use to identify genes responsible for diseases include gene linkage analysis and the candidate gene approach. Gene linkage analysis involves mapping a gene based on its proximity to another known locus on the same chromosome. Linkage analyses are performed, in general, when several family members are available, so it becomes important initially to collect a few well-defined large families and evaluate the DNA from both affected and unaffected members. Once the gene locus has been mapped to a chromosome band, DNA is cloned from the band and a search is conducted for a sequence of bases in the DNA that is conserved in evolution and therefore thought to be functionally important. One then determines if the conserved DNA sequence is expressed by identifying its messenger RNA transcript in the cell type affected by the disease under study. Once confirmed, one searches for mutations in the newly identified gene.

Another approach uses the concept of a candidate gene. With this approach, it is important to collect a large number of unrelated patients with the same disease and use cloned genes that encode for proteins that are known to have a role in the normal function and structure of the diseased tissue; e.g., genes that encode for proteins known to be important in the phototransduction cascade (e.g., rhodopsin, transducin, cyclic guanosine monophosphate phosphodiesterase) are candidate genes for one or another hereditary photoreceptor disease. A search is conducted in a candidate gene for mutations that may be present in some patients and not in others with the same phenotype.[47]

Analyses of DNA from peripheral white blood cells have so far revealed specific gene defects in forms of autosomal dominant retinitis pigmentosa,[47–49] as well as autosomal recessive gyrate atrophy of the choroid and retina;[50–53] X-linked blue cone monochromacy;[54] X-linked cone degeneration, protan type;[55] and X-linked choroideremia.[56] The specificity of the gene abnormalities found in these conditions now makes it feasible to consider diagnostic blood tests to detect one or another of these conditions.

Discovery of the precise gene defect in a hereditary retinal disease helps to define its cause, allows new insights into pathogenesis, and provides a framework for considering means of treatment. Antibodies to an abnormal protein produced by a mutant gene can be applied to autopsied eyes from patients with a hereditary retinal disease and that gene defect to determine the amount and distribution of the abnormal protein in remaining retinal cells and thereby help clarify pathogenesis. Mutant human gene constructs can be studied in a variety of in vitro systems and in transgenic animal models of these diseases to define pathogenetic mechanisms and to search for treatments.

The Genetic Code

First Position	Second Position				Third Position
	T	C	A	G	
T	Phe	Ser	Tyr	Cys	T
	Phe	Ser	Tyr	Cys	C
	Leu	Ser	STOP	STOP	A
	Leu	Ser	STOP	Trp	G
C	Leu	Pro	His	Arg	T
	Leu	Pro	His	Arg	C
	Leu	Pro	Gln	Arg	A
	Leu	Pro	Gln	Arg	G
A	Ile	Thr	Asn	Ser	T
	Ile	Thr	Asn	Ser	C
	Ile	Thr	Lys	Arg	A
	Met	Thr	Lys	Arg	G
G	Val	Ala	Asp	Gly	T
	Val	Ala	Asp	Gly	C
	Val	Ala	Glu	Gly	A
	Val	Ala	Glu	Gly	G

Examples: Codon CCC encodes Proline (Pro); Codon CAC encodes Histidine (His)

Figure 104–10. Human genetic code: Three nucleotide bases compose a codon; each codon encodes either an amino acid or a message to stop translation. The code is described in this figure as if referable to DNA; in actuality, during the course of transcription of DNA to mRNA, the pyrimidine base uracil (U) replaces thymine (T). Ala, alanine; Arg, arginine; Asn, asparagine; Asp, aspartic acid; Cys, cysteine; Gln, glutamine; Glu, glutamic acid; Gly, glycine; His, histidine; Ile, isoleucine; Leu, leucine; Lys, lysine; Met, methionine; Phe, phenylalanine; Pro, proline; Ser, serine; Thr, threonine; Trp, tryptophan; Tyr, tyrosine; Val, valine.

REFERENCES

1. Østerberg G: Topography of the layer of rods and cones in the human retina. Acta Ophthalmol 6(Suppl):1, 1935.
2. Berson EL: Visual function testing: Clinical correlations. *In* Tasman W, Jaeger E (eds): Foundations of Clinical Ophthalmology, vol. 2. Philadelphia, JB Lippincott, 1991.
3. Mandelbaum J: Dark adaptation. Some physiological and clinical considerations. Arch Ophthalmol 26:203, 1941.
4. Berson EL: Night blindness: Some aspects of management. *In* Faye E (ed): Clinical Low Vision. Boston, Little, Brown, 1976.

5. Berson EL: Electrical phenomena in the retina. *In* Hart WM (ed): Adler's Physiology of the Eye. Clinical Application, 9th ed. St Louis, CV Mosby, 1992.

6. Mehaffey L III, Berson EL: Cone mechanisms in the electroretinogram of the cynomolgus monkey. Invest Ophthalmol 13:266, 1974.

7. Brown PK, Wald G: Visual pigments in single rods and cones of the human retina. Science 144:45, 1964.

8. Marks WB, Dobelle WH, MacNichol EF Jr: Visual pigments of single primate cones. Science 143:1181, 1964.

9. Pokorny J, Smith V: Color vision and night vision. *In* Ryan SJ (ed): Retina, vol. 1. Basic Science and Inherited Retinal Disease. St Louis, CV Mosby, 1989.

10. Weleber RG, Eisner A: Retinal function and physiological studies. *In* Newsome DA (ed): Retinal Dystrophies and Degenerations. New York, Raven, 1988.

11. Pokorny J, Smith VC: Eye disease and color defects. Vision Res 26:1573, 1986.

12. Berson EL, Sandberg MA, Rosner B, et al: Color plates to help identify patients with blue cone monochromatism. Am J Ophthalmol 95:741, 1983.

13. Wyszechi G, Stiles WS: Color Science. New York, John Wiley & Sons, 1967.

14. Gouras P: Electroretinography: Some basic principles. Invest Ophthalmol 9:557, 1970.

15. Berson EL, Gouras P, Hoff M: Temporal aspects of the electroretinogram. Arch Ophthalmol 81:207, 1969.

16. Berson EL: Retinitis pigmentosa and allied retinal diseases: Electrophysiologic findings. Trans Am Acad Ophthalmol Otolaryngol 81:659, 1976.

17. Berson EL, Sandberg MA, Rosner B, et al: Natural course of retinitis pigmentosa over a three-year interval. Am J Ophthalmol 99:240, 1985.

18. Andréasson SOL, Sandberg MA, Berson EL: Narrow-band filtering for monitoring low-amplitude cone electroretinograms in retinitis pigmentosa. Am J Ophthalmol 105:500, 1988.

19. Sandberg MA, Berson EL, Ariel M: Visually evoked response testing with a stimulator-ophthalmoscope: Macular scars, hereditary macular degeneration, and retinitis pigmentosa. Arch Ophthalmol 95:1805, 1977.

20. Sandberg MA, Jacobson SG, Berson EL: Foveal cone electroretinograms in retinitis pigmentosa and juvenile macular degenerations. Am J Ophthalmol 88:702, 1979.

21. Jacobson SG, Sandberg MA, Effron MH, et al: Foveal cone electroretinograms in strabismic amblyopia: Comparison with juvenile macular degeneration, macular scars, and optic atrophy. Trans Ophthalmol Soc UK 99:353, 1979.

22. Sandberg MA, Hanson AH, Berson EL: Foveal and parafoveal cone electroretinograms in juvenile macular degeneration. Ophthalmic Paediatr Genet 3:83, 1983.

23. Maffei L, Fiorentini A: Electroretinographic responses to alternating gratings before and after section of the optic nerve. Science 211:953, 1981.

24. Lawwill T: The bar-pattern electroretinogram for clinical evaluation of the central retina. Am J Ophthalmol 78:1231, 1979.

25. Berson EL: Hereditary retinal diseases: Classification with the full-field electroretinogram. *In* Lawwill T (ed): ERG, VER and Psychophysics, Documenta Ophthalmologica Proceedings Series, 13—XIV ISCERG Symposium, May 10–14, 1976, Louisville, KY, pp 149–171. The Hague, Dr. W. Junk, 1977.

26. Bassen FA, Kornzweig AL: Malformation of the erythrocytes in a case of atypical retinitis pigmentosa. Blood 5:381, 1950.

27. Salt HB, Wolff OH, Lloyd JK, et al: On having no betalipoprotein. A syndrome comprising a-beta-lipoproteinemia, acanthocytosis and steatorrhea. Lancet 2:325, 1960.

28. Gouras P, Carr RE, Gunkel RD: Retinitis pigmentosa in abetalipoproteinemia: Effects of vitamin A. Invest Ophthalmol Vis Sci 10:784, 1971.

29. Refsum S: Heredopathia atactica polyneuritiformis: A familial syndrome not hitherto described. Acta Psychiatr Neurol Scand 38(Suppl):1, 1946.

30. Klenk E, Kahlke W: Über das Vorkommen der 3,7,11,15-tetramethylhexadecansäure (Phytansäure) in den Cholesterinestern und anderen Lipoidfraktionen der Organe bei einem Krankheitsfall unbekannter Genese: Verdacht auf Heredopathia atactica polyneuritiformis (Refsum syndrome). Hoppe Seylers Z Physiol Chem 333:133, 1963.

31. Refsum S: Heredopathia atactica polyneuritiformis, phytanic acid storage disease Refsum's disease: A biochemically well-defined disease with a specific dietary treatment. Arch Neurol 38:605, 1981.

32. Cutler CW: Drei ungewöhnliche Fälle von retino-choroideal Degeneration. Arch Augenheilkd 30:117, 1895.

33. Fuchs E: Über zwei der retinitis pigmentosa verwandte Krankheiten (retinitis pigmentosa albescens und atrophia gyrata choriodieae et retinae). Arch Augenheilkd 32:111, 1896.

34. Simell O, Takki K: Raised plasma ornithine in gyrate atrophy of the choroid and retina. Lancet 1:1031, 1973.

35. Berson EL, Schmidt SY, Shih VE: Ocular and biochemical abnormalities in gyrate atrophy of the choroid and retina. Ophthalmology 85:1018, 1978.

36. Kaiser-Kupfer MI, Caruso RC, Valle D: Gyrate atrophy of the choroid and retina, long-term reduction of ornithine slows retinal degeneration. Arch Ophthalmol 109:1539, 1991.

37. Gills JP, Hobsin R, Harley WB, et al: Electroretinography and fundus oculi findings in Hurler's disease and allied mucopolysaccharidoses. Arch Ophthalmol 74:596, 1965.

38. Bach G, Eisenberg F, Cantz M, et al: The defect in Hunter's disease: Deficiency of sulfoiduronate sulfatase. Proc Natl Acad Sci USA 70:21334, 1973.

39. Bach G, Friedman R, Weissman B, et al: The defect in the Hurler and Scheie syndromes: Deficiency of α-L-iduronidase. Proc Natl Acad Sci USA 69:2048, 1972.

40. Kresse H: Mucopolysaccharidosis III A (Sanfilippo A disease): Deficiency of a heparin sulfamidase in skin fibroblasts and leukocytes. Biochem Biophys Res Commun 54:1111, 1973.

41. Von Figura K, Logering M, Mersmann G, et al: Sanfilippo B disease: Serum assays for detection of homozygous and heterozygous individuals in three families. J Pediatr 83:607, 1973.

42. Drlica K: Understanding DNA and Gene Cloning, A Guide for the Curious. New York, John Wiley & Sons, 1984.

43. Gelehrter TD, Collins FS: Principles of Medical Genetics. Baltimore, Williams & Wilkins, 1990.

44. Watson JD, Tooze J, Kurtz DT: Recombinant DNA. A Short Course. New York, WH Freeman, 1983.

45. Watson JD, Hopkins NH, Roberts JW, et al: Molecular Biology of the Gene, 4th ed. Menlo Park, CA, Benjamin/Cummings, 1987.

46. Francke U, Ochs JD, DeMartinville B, et al: Minor Xp21 chromosome deletion in a male associated with expression of Duchenne muscular dystrophy, chronic granulomatous disease, retinitis pigmentosa, and McLeod syndrome. Am J Hum Genet 37:250, 1985.

47. Dryja TP, McGee TL, Reichel E, et al: A point mutation in the rhodopsin gene in one form of retinitis pigmentosa. Nature 343:364, 1990.

48. Dryja TP, McGee TL, Hahn LB, et al: Mutations within the rhodopsin gene in patients with autosomal dominant retinitis pigmentosa. N Engl J Med 323:1302, 1990.

49. Kajiwara K, Mukai S, Travis G, et al: Mutations in the human retinal degeneration slow gene in autosomal dominant retinitis pigmentosa. Nature 354:480, 1991.

50. Mitchell G, Brody L, Looney J, et al: An initiator codon mutation in ornithine delta aminotransferase causing gyrate atrophy of choroid and retina. J Clin Invest 81:630, 1988.

51. Mitchell GA, Brody LC, Sipila I, et al: At least two mutant alleles of ornithine aminotransferase cause gyrate atrophy of the choroid and retina in Finns. Proc Natl Acad Sci USA 86:197, 1989.

52. Ramesh V, McClatchey AI, Ramesh N, et al: Molecular basis of ornithine aminotransferase deficiency in B-6-responsive and -nonresponsive forms of gyrate atrophy. Proc Natl Acad Sci USA 85:3777, 1988.

53. Inana G, Chambers C, Hotta Y, et al: Point mutation affecting processing of the ornithine aminotransferase precursor protein in gyrate atrophy. J Biol Chem 264:17432, 1989.

54. Nathans J, Davenport CM, Maumenee IH, et al: Molecular genetics of human blue cone monochromacy. Science 245:831, 1989.

55. Reichel E, Bruce AM, Sandberg MA, et al: An electroretinographic and molecular genetic study of X-linked cone degeneration. Am J Ophthalmol 108:540, 1989.

56. Cremers FPM, van de Pol DJR, van Kirkoff LPM, et al: Cloning of a gene that is rearranged in patients with choroideraemia. Nature 347:674, 1990.

Chapter 105

■

Objective Assessment of Retinal Function

MICHAEL A. SANDBERG

The purpose of this chapter is to describe the methodology for, application of, and normal variation in some objective measures of retinal function that are used to establish diagnoses in known or suspected hereditary retinal diseases. Objective assessment of retinal function is important for at least three reasons. First, it provides evidence about the site of localization of visual loss (e.g., whether the site of visual loss is within the eye or visual pathways or whether the abnormality is restricted to the macula or involves the entire retina). Second, in most cases it permits a quantitative assessment of the degree of malfunction that can be followed over time for the purpose of projecting long-term prognosis or evaluating a prospective treatment. Third, outcomes from these measures may be shown to the patient as variations in fundus reflectance or as waveforms on photographs or paper so that the patient can appreciate the type and magnitude of his or her visual malfunction and thereby actively participate with the ophthalmologist in the initial and follow-up examinations.

The techniques addressed include fundus reflectometry, early receptor potential recording, electrooculography, full-field and focal flash electroretinography, pattern-reversal electroretinography, and pattern-reversal visually evoked potential recording. Although visually evoked potential recording does not reflect retinal function directly, it is a necessary test to perform when measures of retinal function fail to disclose the site of abnormality and therefore is discussed briefly at the end of the chapter. Guidelines are presented for obtaining reliable and reproducible results and, in some cases, for interpreting variations within a single session and between visits in a given patient, as well as differences that may exist among normal subjects.

FUNDUS REFLECTOMETRY

Fundus reflectometry (also known as retinal densitometry) is a method for estimating the mass optical density, absorption spectra, and regeneration kinetics of the photolabile pigments within photoreceptors. Although still primarily a research tool, it may be used clinically to help identify stationary forms of nyctalopia that have normal rhodopsin densities but a defect in transmission between rod photoreceptors and more proximal retinal cells,[1] diseases of dark adaptation involving slowed pigment regeneration such as fundus albipunctatus (Fig. 105–1),[2] diseases of dark adaptation with normal pigment regeneration such as Oguchi's disease,[3] and pho-

toreceptor mosaicism in carriers of X-linked retinitis pigmentosa.[4, 5] It is also useful in subtyping patients with dominant retinitis pigmentosa based on generalized rod loss versus regionalized rod and cone loss[6] and in monitoring the course of diseases affecting the uvea and retinal pigment epithelium (RPE).[7]

Two types of reflectometers are in use at present, usually in a clinical research setting. The first, and original, type involves collecting and comparing the amount of light reflected by 1 to 2 degrees of the fundus, initially from the dark-adapted eye and afterward following exposure to a light that bleaches most of the available visual pigment.[8–10] The light from a brief test flash, which in itself bleaches little of the visual pigment, is reflected from the fundus and focused on the head of a photomultiplier tube; the difference in the reflected light preceding and following the bleaching episode provides a measure of the amount of visual pigment. The second, and more recent, type of reflectometer involves imaging the fundus over a visual angle of at least 10 degrees and capturing the reflected light either photographically or on videotape. Density differences are then quantified by comparing unbleached with bleached areas captured in a single image[11, 12] or between successive images.[13, 14]

Both systems may be properly used only in patients

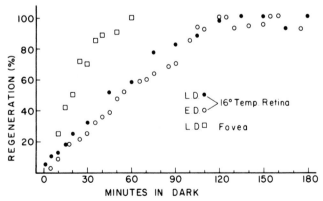

Figure 105–1. Visual pigment regeneration for two brothers (*L.D.* and *E.D.*) with fundus albipunctatus. Recovery times to 50 percent of maximum were about 1 hr for rhodopsin in the peripheral retina and 20 min for cone pigments in the fovea, increases of approximately 20-fold and 16-fold, respectively, compared with normal with this test system. (Modified from Carr RE, Ripps H, Siegel IM: Visual pigment kinetics and adaptation in fundus albipunctatus. Doc Ophthalmol Proc XI International Society for Clinical Electroretinography Symp, 1974, p 193. Reprinted by permission of Kluwer Academic Publishers.)

with clear media and stable fixation. The pupil is maximally dilated and the eye undergoes dark adaptation for at least 30 min, during which time an impression of the patient's bite is made with dental wax. With the patient's head stabilized by the wax impression and the fellow eye fixating on a red lamp or light-emitting diode, the examiner aligns the eye to be tested in dim red or infrared light that causes negligible bleaching. For assessing rhodopsin density, the midperipheral fundus, in which cone photoreceptors are scarce, is generally chosen; for assessing cone pigment density, the fovea, in which rods are fewest, is chosen. A test flash of narrow-band wavelength near the peak of the absorption spectrum (i.e., ~500 nm for rods and ~560 nm for cones) is then presented to quantify reflectance of the dark-adapted eye. After reaffirming alignment in red light, a bright white light is usually presented for many seconds to bleach at least 95 percent of the visual pigment. The test flash is then presented again to quantify reflectance without significant absorption by visual pigment. The logarithmic difference between the two measurements represents the pigment density. This is a "double-density" difference in that the test beam has passed through the photoreceptor layer twice, the second time by reflection from the pigment epithelium and choroid. Additional test flashes may be presented either at other wavelengths in rapid succession to both dark-adapted and bleached eyes to determine the absorption spectrum of the visual pigment or at known intervals after the bleaching episode to assess the time course of pigment regeneration. Figure 105–2 illustrates results from an imaging densitometer. In this case, a midperipheral region of retina was initially bleached for 10 sec over only the right half of the image, the left half remaining adapted to the dark. The figure shows the image pho-

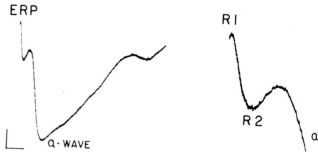

Figure 105–3. Normal human early receptor potential (ERP) followed by an a-wave of electroretinogram (ERG) (*left tracing*) and normal ERP with high sweep speed and amplification (*right tracing*). Both cornea-positive peak (R1) and later cornea-negative peak (R2) of ERP are designated. Stimulus onset is at beginning of each trace. Calibration symbol signifies 2 msec horizontally and 100 μV vertically for the *left tracing*, and 0.5 msec horizontally and 50 μV vertically for the *right tracing*. (From Berson EL, Goldstein EB: The early receptor potential in dominantly inherited retinitis pigmentosa. Arch Ophthalmol 83:412, 1970. Copyright 1970, American Medical Association.)

tographed by a 500-nm test flash and captured on videotape. The bleached half appears brighter than the unbleached half, indicating less remaining visual pigment in the former.

Normal values for rhodopsin double density range from 0.08 to 0.15 log units in different peripheral regions for young adult subjects[15] and from 0.06 to 0.14 log units between regions of a single subject.[16] For cone pigment, the range between subjects is 0.14 to 0.30 within the central 2 degrees, which falls to 0.05 to 0.11 at an average eccentricity of 2.5 degrees.[14] Foveal cone pigment density has been reported to decline linearly with age.[17]

EARLY RECEPTOR POTENTIAL RECORDING

The early receptor potential (ERP) is a very short latency, biphasic response from the eye elicited by a very bright flash of light.[18] It consists of a cornea-positive component (R1) followed by a cornea-negative component (R2), which is then followed by the cornea-negative a-wave of the electroretinogram (ERG) (Fig. 105–3). It derives almost entirely from photoreceptors;[19] R1 reflects the conversion of lumirhodopsin to metarhodopsin I[20] whereas R2 reflects the conversion of metarhodopsin I to metarhodopsin II.[21] As its amplitude is proportional to the amount of pigment bleached by the flash[22] and depends on the orientation of visual pigment molecules within the outer segment,[23] it may be used as a measure of mass outer segment optical density over most of the retina. In humans, 60 to 70 percent of the R2 response is generated by cones and the remainder by rods,[24, 25] so that it may not be possible to specify whether one or both receptor systems are involved if the amplitude reduction is less than 40 percent. The ERP has been used to demonstrate photoreceptor impairment in a variety of retinal diseases, including retinitis pigmentosa.[18, 26, 27]

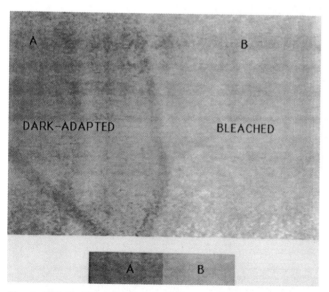

Figure 105–2. Midperipheral regions of a normal human fundus photographed on videotape with 502-nm light immediately following a greater than 95 percent rhodopsin bleach over the right half performed with an imaging reflectometer. Squares at bottom were copied from areas designated with letters to facilitate comparison of double-density gray values, which differ by approximately 0.2 log unit.

The ERP must be elicited with a light flash approximately 10 million times brighter than that required to elicit the b-wave of the ERG (Fig. 105–4).[28] This can be achieved, e.g., with a flashgun focused in the plane of the pupil in maxwellian view. Care must be taken to avoid a photovoltaic artifact superimposed on R1. Investigators have developed custom monopolar contact lenses with either nonmetallic electrodes or metallic electrodes shielded from incident light[29–31] to record an ERP uncontaminated by photovoltaic artifact. Since the light flash must bleach a considerable amount of visual pigment to generate a detectable response, time for pigment regeneration must be allowed before presenting successive flashes to illustrate reproducibility. Intraindividual and interindividual variations in ERP amplitude may be as much as 3:1.[32]

ELECTROOCULOGRAPHY

The light-rise of the electrooculogram (EOG) is a measure of the integrity of the RPE and overlying photoreceptors. It arises from a depolarization of the basal (i.e., choroidal side) membrane of the RPE.[33] The EOG is a measure of the slowly changing voltage difference between the front (positive) and the rear (negative) surfaces of the globe recorded over time under different conditions of illumination (Fig. 105–5). The light-rise represents the largest difference measured in illumination divided by the smallest difference measured in darkness.[34] In clinical practice its important use is to help diagnose Best's vitelliform macular degeneration, a dominantly inherited condition. In this disease, the EOG light-rise is reduced or lacking.[35–38] Asymptomatic carriers of Best's disease may also have abnormal

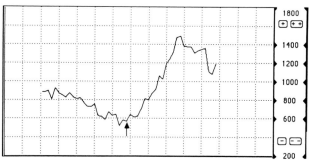

Figure 105–5. Electrooculogram (EOG) recorded from a normal subject. Eye movements were made twice each minute by alternately viewing fixation points separated by 30 degrees in a Ganzfeld dome, differentially amplified at a gain of 200 (−3 db at 0.1 and 100 Hz), digitized, and peak-to-peak amplitudes for each saccade quantified by computer. *Vertical dotted lines* are separated by 2.5 min intervals; *horizontal dotted lines* are separated by 200 μV. *Arrow* designates onset of background illumination.

EOGs.[37] The EOG also differentiates Best's disease from pseudovitelliform macular degeneration, in which there is generally a normal ratio.[38] In other retinal diseases, EOG testing does not add to whatever diagnosis may have been made with the ERG alone.[39] Fast oscillations of the EOG have also been recorded[40] but have not yet been found useful for diagnosis.

The EOG may be measured in cooperative patients with stable fixation who have a visual field diameter of at least 60 degrees. Following exposure to ambient room illumination for 30 min or longer, during which time the pupils are dilated, cup electrodes filled with electrode cream are attached with tape just lateral to the inner and outer canthus of each eye (i.e., two electrodes per eye) and to the forehead as ground. Upon verbal instruction from the examiner, the subject alternately fixates red light–emitting diodes in a Ganzfeld dome placed at 0 and 30 degrees with respect to forward gaze, first in the dark for approximately 12 min and then in the presence of a full-field 10 ft-L white background for about 12 min. A Ganzfeld dome, rather than an x-ray viewing box (or equivalent), should be used so that the entire retina will be illuminated as evenly as possible; otherwise the EOG will reflect primarily only posterior pole function.[41] Intervals of about 12 min of darkness and 12 min of illumination are said to reduce the normal variation.[42] The maximal voltage in the light is compared with the minimal voltage in the dark to derive the light-rise:dark-trough ratio, which is normally greater than 1.8 in patients younger than 50 yr. Care should be taken that the onset of illumination is not too abrupt or else the tested eye might begin to tear, which could alter electrode resistance. Responses from each eye should be differentially amplified at a gain of approximately 200 (d.c. − 100 Hz) and displayed on an x-y plotter or digitized and displayed by computer. Repeat recordings on a given patient should be done at approximately the same time of day because of the presence of an underlying circadian rhythm (see further on).

Intraindividual variability in the light-rise:dark-trough ratio of the EOG generally does not exceed 60 per-

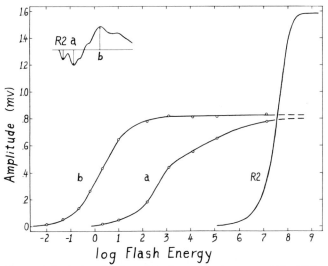

Figure 105–4. Amplitudes of the b-wave and a-wave of the ERG, and the R2 component of the ERP for the dark-adapted albino rat as a function of the log of the flash energy. Responses were obtained with 0.7 msec full-field white flashes. Log flash energy of zero corresponds to 1 quantum absorbed/rod. Amplitudes were measured from baseline. (From Cone RA: The early receptor potential of the vertebrate eye. Cold Spring Harbor Symp Quant Biol 30:483, 1965.)

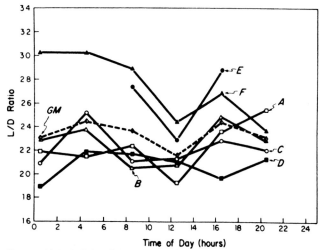

Figure 105–6. EOG light : dark ratios for 6 normal subjects (A–F) and their grand mean at different times of day. (From Anderson ML, Purple RL: Circadian rhythms and variability of the clinical electrooculogram. Invest Ophthalmol Vis Sci 19:278, 1980.)

cent.[43–45] The normal range for the light-rise:dark-trough ratio has been placed at 1.9 to 2.8,[46] although values of 1.5 to 3.4 have been reported.[47] It should be noted that the ratio increases with luminance.[48] The ratio also appears to decline with age, at least among women.[46, 47, 49] Significant differences in the ratio between sexes have been reported, with larger values for females.[45, 47] Between 20 and 50 percent of the variation in the EOG light-rise may be due to circadian rhythmicity.[50] Recordings done at 2-hr intervals for six normal subjects and their means show a sinusoidal temporal pattern in which the ratio was highest in the early morning and late afternoon and lowest around midday (Fig. 105–6).

FULL-FIELD ELECTRORETINOGRAPHY

The normal human ERG elicited by a moderate-intensity white flash from the dark-adapted eye consists of a cornea-negative deflection, called the *a-wave*, followed by a cornea-positive deflection, called the *b-wave* (Fig. 105–7). The a-wave is known to reflect photoreceptor function,[51, 52] and the b-wave is generated by Müller cells reflecting activity in the inner nuclear layer of the retina.[53, 54] In actuality, the recorded b-wave is a summation of photoreceptor and more proximal retinal function, since the photoreceptor component continues beyond the onset of the b-wave.[52] Several wavelets, known as "oscillatory potentials" (see Fig. 105–7), may normally be seen superimposed on the ascending portion of the b-wave. These wavelets reflect bipolar cell responses generated by feedback from amacrine cells.[55, 56] Separation of the ERG into a-wave, b-wave, and oscillatory potentials has important application for objectively diagnosing, classifying, and staging retinal diseases; e.g., in response to a moderate-intensity white light presented to the dark-adapted eye, loss of the a-wave with a slowing of the b-wave in patients with clear

media may signify a photoreceptor degeneration in which photoreceptors have lost optical density. This follows from the fact that in normal eyes reducing stimulus intensity affects a-wave amplitude before b-wave amplitude (see Fig. 105–7). Conversely, loss of the b-wave with preservation of the a-wave may signify retinoschisis[57] or congenital nyctalopia with myopia (Fig. 105–8).[1] In both of these conditions, synaptic transmission from photoreceptors to more proximal elements is disturbed. Selective loss of oscillatory potentials, in contrast, is usually interpreted as specifically reflecting inner retinal ischemia, as occurs in diabetic retinopathy[58] and central retinal vein occlusion (Fig. 105–9).[59]

Careful inspection of the a-wave reveals an inflection (see Fig. 105–7, *arrow*), which reflects a summation of cone and rod components of differing time course. Although not apparent, the same is true of the b-wave. The fact that the normal dark-adapted ERG is a sum-

FULL-FIELD ERGS FROM A NORMAL SUBJECT

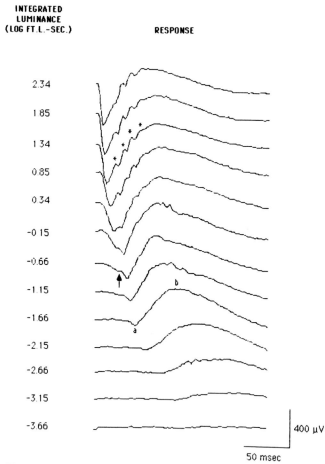

Figure 105–7. Dark-adapted ERGs recorded from a normal subject in response to full-field white flashes of varying integrated luminance. Traces begin at flash onset. Cornea-negative a-wave and cornea-positive b-wave are designated by *letters*; oscillatory potentials designated by *asterisks*. *Arrow* points to inflection in the a-wave, representing combination of cone and rod components. (Modified from Sandberg MA, Lee H, Gaudio AR, et al: Relationship of oscillatory potential amplitudes to a-wave slope over a range of flash luminances in normal subjects. Invest Ophthalmol Vis Sci 32:1508, 1991.)

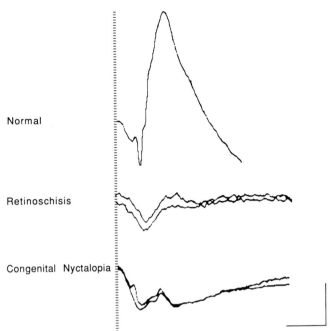

Normal

Retinoschisis

Congenital Nyctalopia

Figure 105–8. Dark-adapted ERGs recorded from a normal subject, a patient with juvenile X-linked retinoschisis, and a patient with congenital nyctalopia with myopia in response to a full-field white flash. Calibration (lower right) designates 100 μV vertically and 50 msec horizontally.

mation of rod and cone components may be demonstrated in two ways. First, placing, in turn, a blue filter or a red filter, scotopically matched to the blue filter (i.e., matched in brightness for the rods), in front of the eye and then flashing a white light results in different waveforms (Fig. 105–10). The waveform with the blue filter in front of the eye consists of a late-onset, bell-shaped b-wave, whereas that with the red filter in front of the eye consists of an early-onset a-wave and b-wave (with oscillations) followed by the same late-onset b-wave. The early components seen to red but not blue light represent cone activity, whereas the late b-wave represents rod activity. When the cone and rod components are well separated in time, they appear to summate linearly.[60–62] However, when the two b-waves occur at the same time with near-maximal amplitudes, as for the conventional white flash, the summation appears to be nonlinear, as may be seen by using a method of digital subtraction.[63] Linear subtraction of a cone-isolated response to red light from a mixed cone and rod response to a bright blue light, photopically matched to the red light, yields a rod-isolated waveform in which the b-wave is "scalloped" (Fig. 105–11). This implies that the b-wave to the bright blue light represents a sublinear summation of rod and cone components. Conversely, even for these bright lights, the two a-waves appear to summate linearly. The presence of a steady white background that desensitizes rods and eliminates their contribution to the ERG reveals a "photopic" a-wave and b-wave from the cone system (Fig. 105–12).[64] In addition to background illumination, a flash rate of 30 Hz may be used to isolate cone function to white light (see Fig. 105–10).[61] This is true because the rod

system is normally incapable of responding to these rates of flicker. Lights of different wavelength and background adaptation have been used to demonstrate both a rod and a cone contribution to oscillatory potentials.[65]

Isolation of rod and cone contributions to the ERG, like comparative analysis of the a-wave and b-wave components, is also important for classifying retinal diseases; e.g., selective loss of cone function may signify congenital rod monochromatism or advanced cone degeneration, whereas loss of a rod contribution may signify an early stage of dominant retinitis pigmentosa. In the cone-isolated response to flicker, the high rate of presentation and sinusoidal nature of the waveform in cases of advanced retinitis pigmentosa make it possible to resolve amplitudes as small as 0.05 μV with signal averaging and electronic filtering (see further on), which can be used to follow the course of this condition.[66]

The full-field ERG may also be used to quantify the amount of remaining function for each of the three cone mechanisms. The middle-wavelength or green cone system and the long-wavelength or red cone system may be evaluated by comparing cone ERGs elicited by a short-wavelength flash or a photopically matched long-wavelength flash superimposed on a photopic background (see Fig. 105–10)[61] or flickering at 30 Hz.[67] If the responses are equivalent in amplitude, the patient is considered to have comparable numbers of cones of

BRIGHT-FLASH FULL-FIELD ERGS

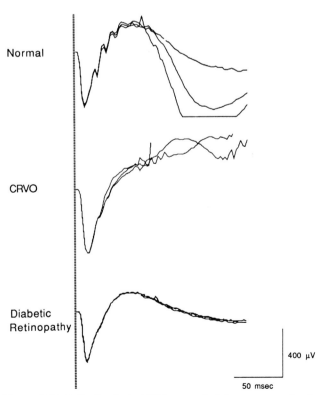

Normal

CRVO

Diabetic Retinopathy

400 μV

50 msec

Figure 105–9. Dark-adapted ERGs recorded from a normal subject, a patient with central retinal vein occlusion (CRVO), and a patient with diabetic retinopathy, in response to a full-field bright white flash.

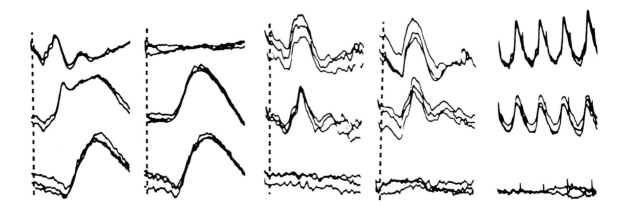

Figure 105–10. Full-field ERGs to scotopically matched red (*column 1*) and blue (*column 2*) flashes, to photopically matched orange (*column 3*) and blue-green (*column 4*) flashes in presence of 5 to 10 ft-L background light, and to 30-Hz white flashes (*column 5*) are shown successively from top to bottom for a patient with Nougaret-type night blindness, a normal subject, and a patient with advanced cone degeneration. Two or three responses to same stimulus are superimposed; calibration symbol signifies 60 msec horizontally and 50 µV vertically for columns 1 and 2, 30 msec horizontally and 50 µV vertically for columns 3 and 4, and 60 msec horizontally and 100 µV vertically for column 5; corneal positivity is an upward deflection; stimulus onset, *vertical hatched line* for columns 1 to 4 and shock artifacts for column 5. (From Berson EL, Gouras P, Hoff M: Temporal aspects of the electroretinogram. Arch Ophthalmol 81:207–214, 1969.)

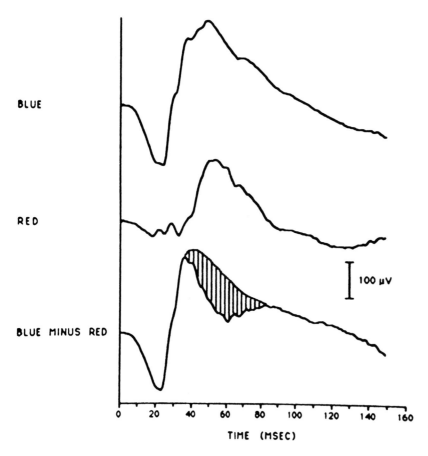

Figure 105–11. Computer-averaged dark-adapted full-field ERGs from a normal subject to photopically matched blue (*top*) and red (*middle*) flashes and the result of subtracting the second response from the first to derive a rod ERG in isolation (*bottom*). The rod component elicited by the red flash had already been eliminated by subtracting the response to a scotopically matched blue flash. In the bottom waveform, the *lower solid line* represents the result of subtraction and the *hatched area* illustrates the suggested rod b-wave correction for nonlinear summation of the cone and rod components to blue light. (From Sandberg MA, Miller S, Berson EL: Rod electroretinograms in an elevated cyclic guanosine monophosphate–type human retinal degeneration. Comparison with retinitis pigmentosa. Invest Ophthalmol Vis Sci 31:2283, 1990.)

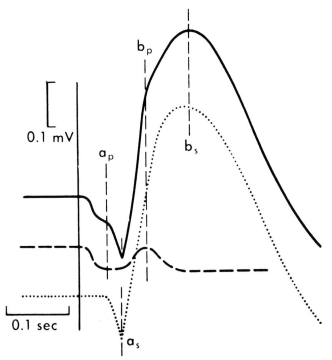

Figure 105–12. Analysis of ERG in dark-adapted human eye as the resultant of photopic (*dashed line*) and scotopic (*dotted line*) components. The a-wave is composed of photopic (a_p) and scotopic (a_s) components, and the b-wave is similarly composed of photopic (b_p) and scotopic (b_s) components. (From Armington JC, Johnson EP, Riggs LA: The scotopic a-wave in the electrical response of the human retina. J Physiol [Lond] 118:289, 1952.)

each type, as has been observed in carriers of blue cone monochromatism.[68] However, if the two responses are unequal in amplitude or differ by a factor of two or greater, then one of the two cone systems is considered to be reduced in number relative to the other or lacking, respectively.[67] Use of a short-wavelength flash superimposed on a bright white background has been shown to isolate in time the short-wavelength or blue cone system from the other systems (Fig. 105–13).[69]

Interest has developed in clinical recording of b-wave amplitude versus flash intensity functions under conditions of dark adaptation in patients with retinal disease. The intent of this approach is to distinguish changes in maximal amplitude (V max), which are thought to reflect cell number and response gain, from changes in sensitivity (k), which are thought to reflect outer-segment optical density and media clarity. Some studies have used white flashes to elicit these functions,[70–72] which complicates interpretation because of the variable summation of cone and rod contributions in diseases that may affect these two systems unequally. One study used digital subtraction to isolate rod function in patients with retinitis pigmentosa or cone-rod degeneration and showed that reductions in sensitivity, irrespective of changes in maximal amplitude, may be used to infer losses of rod photoreceptor optical density.[73] Another study showed that patients with an apparently rare form of retinal degeneration could have increased maximal amplitude with reduced sensitivity, as well as implicit

times that were more delayed for dim flashes than for bright flashes (Fig. 105–14), a combination that could best be explained by an elevation of retinal cyclic guanosine monophosphate rather than in terms of cell and optical density loss.[63]

Full-field ERGs, like EOGs, are conventionally elicited with a Ganzfeld dome (Fig. 105–15) that provides a nearly homogeneous distribution of light over the central 120 degrees of the retina.[74] Although retinal illuminance falls as a consequence of decreasing apparent pupillary area for retinal eccentricities greater than 60 degrees, this is compensated in large part by the curvature of the retina and by reduced light absorption in the ocular media with eccentricity.[75] With virtually uniform retinal illumination, the faster cone and slower rod components of the ERG across the retina respond with a minimal variation in latency and therefore may be separated in time and quantified. In addition, this retinal light distribution is altered little by small changes in eye position, which fosters reproducibility between successive responses.[74, 76]

The eye or eyes to be tested should be initially dilated and adapted to the dark for at least 45 min. Dilatation maximizes amplitudes and generally minimizes implicit times.[77, 78] Complete dark adaptation, which may require 45 min or longer depending on the level of prior exposure, also maximizes amplitudes (Fig. 105–16)[79] while also tending to maximize implicit times. Recordings are best done with a bipolar contact lens electrode, with the positive electrode being a ring around the contact lens and the negative or reference electrode a conductive coating on a lid speculum (Fig. 105–17). The bipolar configuration, in which the lid versus ground response is subtracted from the cornea versus ground response, localizes the response to the eye and provides the best elimination of surrounding 60-Hz noise and any photovoltaic artifact that may be generated by the flashlamp. The lid speculum also prevents the upper and lower eyelids from partially covering the cornea and thereby obstructing the passage of light into the eye; a reduction in retinal illuminance could artifactually reduce ERG amplitudes and increase implicit times.

With the patient fixating on a red light–emitting diode, 0.5-Hz dim, short-wavelength flashes may be given first to isolate the rod ERG; next, 0.5-Hz scotopically matched long-wavelength flashes can be given to obtain a mixed response consisting of a faster cone component and a slower rod component of amplitude comparable with that elicited by the short-wavelength flash. After that, 0.5-Hz dim white flashes may be given to elicit an a-wave and maximal b-wave consisting of a summation of both cone and rod components, and finally 30-Hz dim white flashes or 0.5-Hz dim white flashes superimposed on a background to isolate a cone response may be given.[76] For cases of generalized cone degeneration or when abnormal color vision is found, the spectral lights described earlier may be presented to assess the different cone systems across the retina. When isolating the cone response with flicker or background illumination, the retina may need to be illuminated for several minutes before a maximal response is obtained (Fig. 105–18).[80–82]

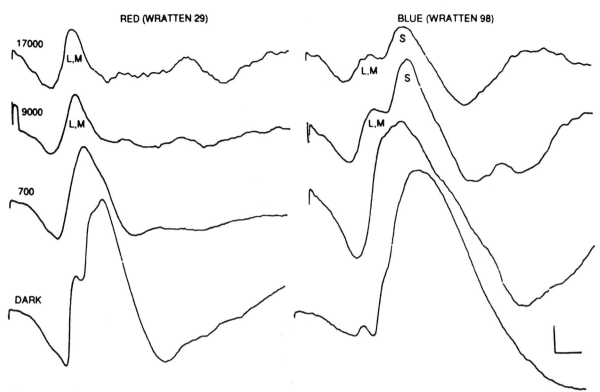

Figure 105–13. Full-field ERGs elicited by red and blue flashes at different levels of background illumination indicated by the photopic troland values on the left above each trace. L, M, and S signify, respectively, the responses of the long-wavelength, middle-wavelength, and short-wavelength sensitive cone systems. The calibration, *lower right*, signifies vertically 4 μV for the upper four and 40 μV for the lower four traces and 9 msec horizontally. (From Gouras P, MacKay CJ: Electroretinographic responses of the short-wavelength-sensitive cones. Invest Ophthalmol Vis Sci 31:1203, 1990.)

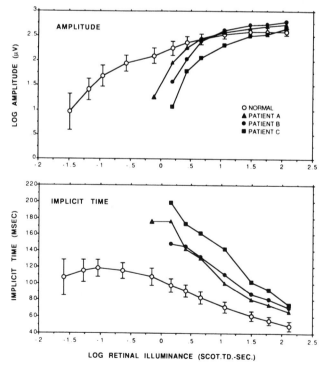

Figure 105–14. Rod b-wave amplitude and implicit time (i.e., time to peak) versus retinal illuminance functions for 17 normal subjects (mean ± S.D.) and 3 patients with a cGMP-type retinal degeneration. Rod ERGs were elicited with full-field blue flashes at low retinal illuminances and by a method of digital subtraction involving photopically matched blue and red flashes at high retinal illuminances. (Redrawn from Sandberg MA, Miller S, Berson EL: Rod electroretinograms in an elevated cyclic guanosine monophosphate–type human retinal degeneration. Comparison with retinitis pigmentosa. Invest Ophthalmol Vis Sci 31:2283, 1990.)

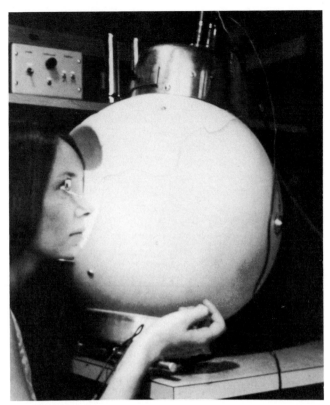

Figure 105–15. Ganzfeld stimulator. Flashlamp enclosed in case and attached to top of diffusing sphere illuminates inner white surface of this dome (40 cm in diameter), providing a full-field stimulus. Lights are recessed in top of dome so that patient can be tested in presence of steady full-field background light. (From Rabin AR, Berson EL: A full-field system for clinical electroretinography. Arch Ophthalmol 92:59, 1974. Copyright 1974, American Medical Association.)

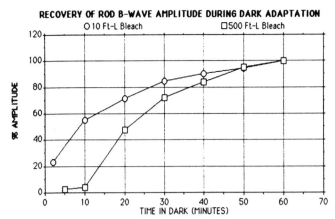

Figure 105–16. Computer-averaged full-field rod ERG percent amplitudes to a 0.5-Hz 10 μsec blue flash (λmax = 440 nm) of 16 ft-L recorded over time in the dark from a normal observer after a 10-min full-field white light bleach of 10 ft-L or 500 ft-L presented to the dilated pupil. Amplitudes for 60 min dark adaptation were arbitrarily designated 100 percent. All the data appear to reflect rod function, except for the low-amplitude 5-min value after the stronger bleach, which probably represents residual cone function. Each set of data represents a single run. (From Sandberg MA: Technical issues in electroretinography. *In* Heckenlively J, Arden G [eds]: Principles and Practice of Clinical Electrophysiology of Vision. St Louis, Mosby–Year Book, 1991.)

nation), with each flash separated from the next by an interval of about 1 min to minimize light adaptation from the preceding flash.

Full-field ERG responses may be photographed in real time from an oscilloscope or digitized and stored for subsequent analysis and hard copy. Digitization may be used to eliminate baseline variation and to isolate

Patients with small dilated pupils or those whose pupils cannot be dilated or, in some cases, who have media opacities that obscure visualization of the fundus may have ERGs that are smaller in amplitude than expected or are nondetectable with single flashes because of reduced stimulus retinal illuminance. An electronic photoflash, with approximately 1000 times the energy of the conventional full-field flash when illuminating a Ganzfeld dome, can be used to elicit larger responses from such eyes.[83] In order to separate the optical density effect of the media obstruction from any change that may be due to a retinal abnormality, responses to a series of stimulus intensities should be compared with those obtained with conventional full-field flashes in normal eyes. If a-wave and b-wave amplitudes and implicit times to the brighter flashes in eyes with opaque media can be matched to those obtained to the dimmer flashes in normal eyes with clear media, large areas of the retina can be considered to be functioning normally.[84] In eyes with large pupils and relatively clear media, these bright flashes may be used to elicit a maximal a-wave with oscillatory potentials superimposed on the ascending limb of the b-wave.[83] Bright flash stimulation should be presented to the dark-adapted eye (i.e., before flicker or background illumi-

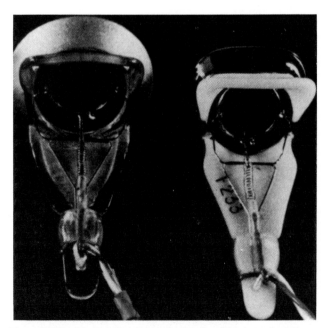

Figure 105–17. Double-electrode (Burian-Allen) contact lenses used to obtain ERG responses. (From Rabin AR, Berson EL: A full-field system for clinical electroretinography. Arch Ophthalmol 92:59, 1974. Copyright 1974, American Medical Association.)

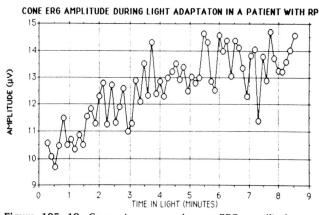

Figure 105–18. Computer-averaged cone ERG amplitudes recorded at different times during presentation of 30-Hz white full-field 10-μsec flashes of 6300 ft-L luminance through the dilated pupil of a previously dark-adapted patient with dominant retinitis pigmentosa (RP) with reduced penetrance. (From Sandberg MA: Technical issues in electroretinography. In Heckenlively J, Arden G [eds]: Principles and Practice of Clinical Electrophysiology of Vision. St Louis, Mosby–Year Book, 1991.)

oscillatory potentials, whose frequency content (50 to 180 Hz) exceeds that of the a-wave (less than 50 Hz) and b-wave (less than 25 Hz).[83, 85–87] Oscillatory potentials may then be quantified either in conventional time domain or, by Fourier analysis, in frequency domain (Fig. 105–19). Consecutive digitized responses may also be summed and averaged and, for 30-Hz flicker, smoothed with narrow bandpass filtering to resolve very small amplitudes (Fig. 105–20).[66, 88] Signal averaging may also be used to reduce large voltages due to eye movements, as, e.g., in cases of nystagmus.

The variation in full-field ERG amplitude for a given stimulus condition across normal subjects is as much as 2.5:1.[89, 90] Age, sex, refraction, ocular pigmentation, and time of day may all contribute to this variation, as follows: With increasing age among adults, a-wave am-

plitude declines,[89] b-wave amplitude declines,[89, 91–93] oscillatory potential amplitude declines (Fig. 105–21), and b-wave implicit time increases with increasing age.[89, 93] These decreases in ERG amplitudes and increases in ERG implicit times with increasing age probably reflect decreasing retinal illuminance with increasing age caused by reduced light transmissivity by the lens[94] and, possibly, to a smaller dilated pupillary diameter with increasing age. Similarly, increased uveal pigmentation lowers amplitude, and decreased uveal pigmentation raises it.[95, 96] The ERG b-wave is also larger in hyperopic eyes than in myopic eyes (Fig. 105–22)[91, 97, 98] and is slightly larger in women than in men.[89, 91, 97, 99, 100]

Intrasubject variation in amplitude in normal subjects across days can be as much as plus or minus 25 percent for large responses. Normal subjects, unentrained to a cyclic pattern of illumination, have shown no significant variations in rod ERG amplitude over daylight hours.[101] However, in normal subjects entrained to cyclic illumination for at least 3 days, rod ERG amplitudes follow a regular pattern, being on average 10 to 15 percent smaller 1.5 hr after light onset than at other times of day (Fig. 105–23).[101] The physiological basis for this ERG diurnal rhythm appears to be an alteration in photoreceptor function associated with rod outer segment disc shedding, since recordings in normal light-entrained rats have demonstrated an ERG variation similar to that seen in humans and that is significantly correlated with the number of phagosomes appearing in the RPE.[102]

FOCAL ELECTRORETINOGRAPHY

Since only some 7 percent of cone photoreceptors are in the central macula, patients with macular degeneration typically retain normal full-field ERGs and must be assessed with a focal stimulus in order to reveal and quantify malfunction.[39] Foveal cone ERGs have been

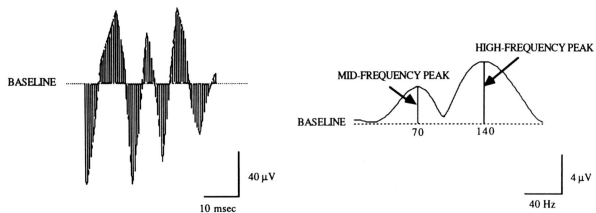

Figure 105–19. Quantification of mean oscillatory potential amplitude in the time domain between the a-wave and the b-wave peaks after 62-Hz high-pass filtering for a normal subject in response to a bright full-field flash white flash. *Vertical lines* represent some of the amplitudes whose absolute values with respect to baseline were summed prior to calculation of the mean (*left*). Quantification of mid- and high-frequency amplitudes for oscillatory potentials by the magnitude fast Fourier transform for a normal subject in response to the same flash (*right*). (Modified from Sandberg MA, Lee H, Gaudio AR, et al: Relationship of oscillatory potential amplitudes to a-wave slope over a range of flash luminances in normal subjects. Invest Ophthalmol Vis Sci 32:1508, 1991.)

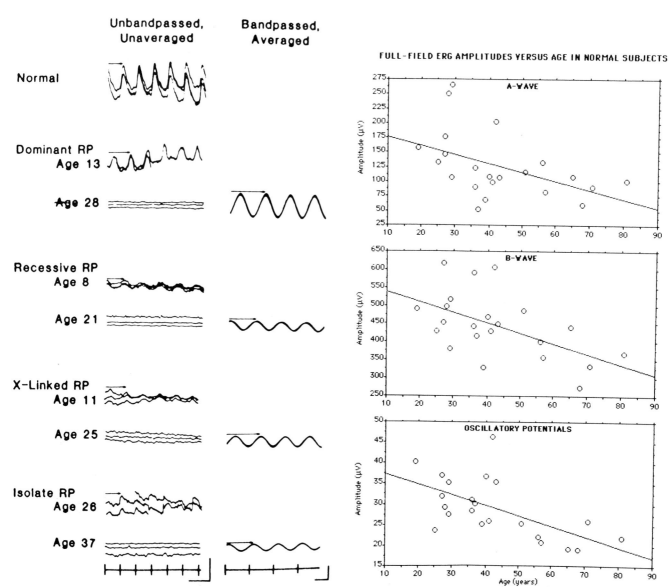

Figure 105–20. ERGs elicited with full-field white 30-Hz flashes from a normal subject and 4 patients with different genetic types of RP at ages spanning intervals of 11 to 15 years. Responses were recorded without (*left column*) or with (*right column*) computer averaging and bandpass filtering. Stimulus onset, *vertical markers*; calibration symbol (*left column, lower right*) designates 100 μV vertically for the normal subject and top three patients and 40 μV vertically for the bottom patient and 50 msec horizontally for all traces; calibration (*right column, lower right*) designates 2 μV vertically for the dominant, X-linked, and isolate patients and 0.3 μV for the recessive patient and 20 msec horizontally for all traces. b-Wave implicit times are designated with *arrows*. (From Andréasson SOL, Sandberg MA, Berson EL: Narrow-band filtering for monitoring low-amplitude cone electroretinograms in retinitis pigmentosa. Am J Ophthalmol 105:500–503, 1988. Published with permission from The American Journal of Ophthalmology. Copyright by The Ophthalmic Publishing Company.)

Figure 105–21. a-Wave, b-wave, and oscillatory potential amplitude versus age in normal subjects. Responses were elicited from dark-adapted eyes with full-field dim white flashes for the *upper* and *middle graphs* or bright white flashes for the *lower graph*. Oscillatory potential amplitudes are calculated as described for Figure 105–19.

EFFECT OF REFRACTION ON B-WAVE AMPLITUDE

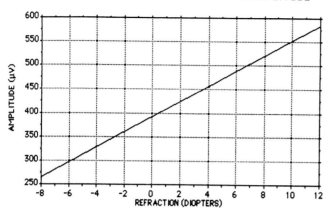

Figure 105–22. Linear regression of b-wave amplitude on refraction based on average of regression equations for men and women from measurements on 86 normal subjects. Maximal b-waves were elicited from the semi–dark-adapted eye with white light flashes derived from a lamp at different distances from the subject and presented through the dilated pupil. (From Sandberg MA: Technical issues in electroretinography. *In* Heckenlively J, Arden G [eds]: Principles and Practice of Clinical Electrophysiology of Vision. St Louis, Mosby–Year Book, 1991; based on the data of Pallin E: The influence of the axial size of the eye on the size of the recorded b-potential in the clinical single-flash electroretinogram. Acta Ophthalmol 101[Suppl]:1, 1969.)

used by various centers over the last 25 yr to detect macular malfunction.[103–110] Abnormal foveal cone responses have been found in patients with Stargardt's disease,[106, 111] in which amplitude varied directly with visual acuity, and with age-related macular degeneration (Fig. 105–24).[107, 112] In patients with macular holes, foveal amplitude varied inversely with hole diameter, and subnormal responses appeared to predict impending holes in the fellow eye.[113] Foveal ERGs may be abnor-

mal in symptomatic patients even when no diagnostic abnormalities can by seen by ophthalmoscopy and fluorescein angiography,[114, 115] and thus they provide an aid in early detection of macular malfunction. Conversely, foveal cone ERGs are normal in patients with strabismic amblyopia[116] or optic neuropathy,[117, 118] indicating that the test provides a differential diagnosis for diseases of the macula versus diseases of the optic nerve or visual cortex (Fig. 105–25). Focal cone ERGs should, in gen-

FULL-FIELD ROD ERGS (WITH ENTRAINMENT)

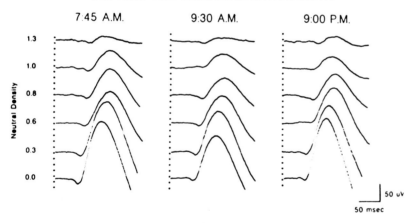

FULL-FIELD ROD ERGS (WITHOUT ENTRAINMENT)

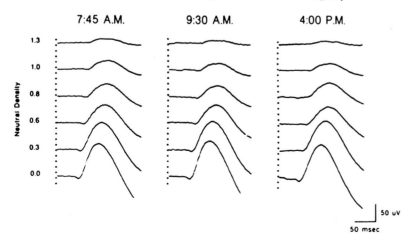

Figure 105–23. Computer-averaged rod ERG responses on one day of testing obtained from a normal subject with or without entrainment to a 14-hr light: 10-hr dark cycle with light onset at 8 AM. The stimulus flash was attenuated by neutral density filters as shown on left. Stimulus onset is indicated with *vertical broken lines.* (From Birch DG, Berson EL, Sandberg MA: Diurnal rhythm in the human rod ERG. Invest Ophthalmol Vis Sci 25:236, 1984.)

FOVEAL CONE ERGs

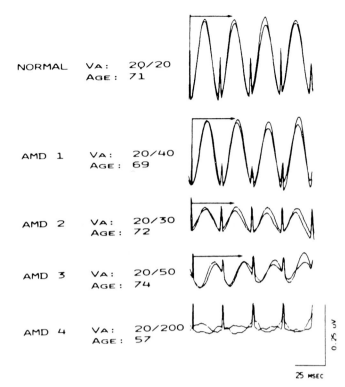

Figure 105–24. Representative foveal cone ERGs from a normal subject and 4 patients with age-related macular degeneration (AMD). Responses were recorded with a stimulator-ophthalmoscope. Each 100-msec trace contains 4 responses to the 42-Hz stimulus. Two consecutive traces (each the average of 200 sweeps) are shown for each patient. *Arrows* indicate b-wave implicit time (time between light flash and response). (From Fish GE, Birch DG, Fuller DG, et al: A comparison of visual function tests in eyes with maculopathy. Published courtesy of Ophthalmology [1986; 93:1177–1182].)

eral, be used in conjunction with full-field recording in order to rule out generalized cone degeneration, which also may not have visible signs of disease.

Focal cone ERGs may now be elicited with a commercially available instrument, the maculoscope. With this instrument, the examiner can visualize the fundus through a short-stalk Burian-Allen bipolar contact lens electrode over the dilated pupil. A 42-Hz, white, 4-degree-diameter stimulus is placed on the fovea and centered within a steady white 10-degree surround. This high rate of flicker not only isolates cone function but also renders the response sinusoidal (Fig. 105–26) so that amplitudes less than 1 μV, which occur normally, can be resolved with the help of electronic filtering, computer averaging, and Fourier analysis. White flashes, rather than red, are used to avoid eliciting subnormal

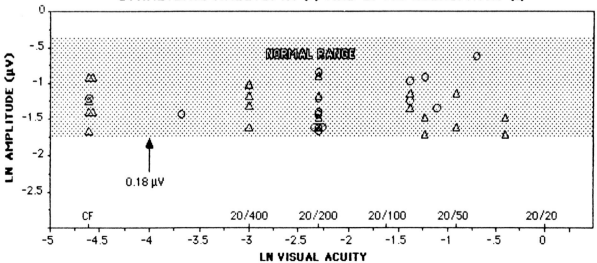

Figure 105–25. Foveal cone ERG amplitude versus acuity in patients with strabismic amblyopia or optic neuropathy. Responses were recorded with a stimulator-ophthalmoscope.

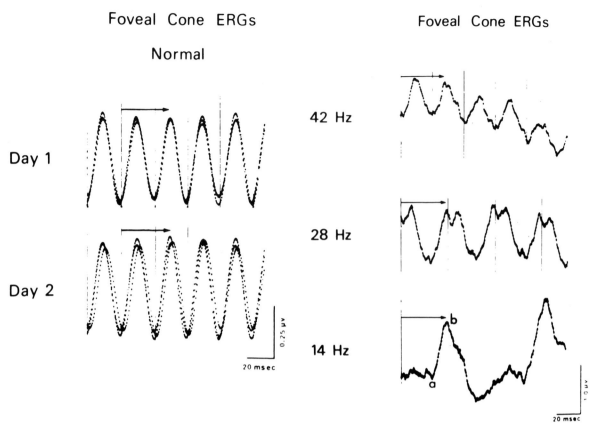

Figure 105–26. Foveal cone ERGs from a normal subject at three stimulus frequencies (*right*) elicited with a hand-held dual-beam stimulator-ophthalmoscope. A single computer summation (n = 512) is shown for each frequency. a-Wave and b-wave peaks are indicated for 14-Hz condition. Responses to 42-Hz stimulation appear sinusoidal and may be bandpass filtered to enhance signal : noise for better reproducibility on the same day and between days (*left*). *Vertical lines* designate stimulus onset; *arrows*, b-wave implicit times. (From Sandberg MA, Jacobson SG, Berson EL: Foveal cone electroretinograms in retinitis pigmentosa and juvenile macular degeneration. Am J Ophthalmol 88:702, 1979. Published with permission from The American Journal of Ophthalmology. Copyright by The Ophthalmic Publishing Company.)

amplitudes from patients with congenital protanopia. Focal cone ERGs may be performed in an unshielded room in dim ambient room illumination. Since foveal cone ERG amplitudes are very small and tend to increase during continued light adaptation,[119] consecutive response averages should be recorded over a period of a few minutes to prove reproducibility.

Foveal cone ERG amplitude has been reported to be inversely correlated with age for 100 normal eyes of subjects between the ages of 5 and 75 yr.[112] A fourfold range for normal foveal cone ERG amplitude has been reported.[111] Although the reason for this large normal range is unclear, it can be effectively reduced by 30 percent on average by adopting a ratio of foveal amplitude divided by parafoveal amplitude.[120] This approach should be used with caution, as some regional variation in the parafoveal cone ERG has been reported.[121] Normal intervisit variability in foveal cone ERG amplitude has not been reported.

PATTERN ELECTRORETINOGRAPHY

Pattern electroretinography uses a spatiotemporal exchange of stripes or checks in which mean luminance is

held fixed to elicit a focal ERG.[122] The theory is that local, time-varying changes in luminance responses generated by photoreceptors cancel at the cornea (or at least make a minimal contribution to the response), whereas cells with center-surround receptive fields (i.e., retinal ganglion cells) are strongly stimulated. One defense of this idea is that the pattern ERG (PERG) shows spatial tuning under some situations; i.e., amplitude is larger for stimulus elements of medium size and smaller for stimulus elements of smaller or larger sizes (Fig. 105–27).[123–128] In other instances, however, a high-pass relationship occurs in which amplitude increases monotonically with the size of the stimulus element.[129] In these cases, primarily resulting from high-luminance, high-contrast targets, a significant luminance component is thought to contaminate the responses to large stimulus elements.[123, 128] Luminance components presumably arise from nonlinear summation of opposite sign responses to "on" and "off" stimulation.[130, 131]

Unlike the focal luminance–evoked ERG (usually referred to as the focal ERG or FERG), the PERG has been found to be predominantly abnormal in patients with glaucoma,[132–135] optic neuritis,[136, 137] or optic atrophy (Fig. 105–28),[138, 139] which further supports the idea that it derives from ganglion cell activity. It has been reported to be both more sensitive[140] and less sensitive[141]

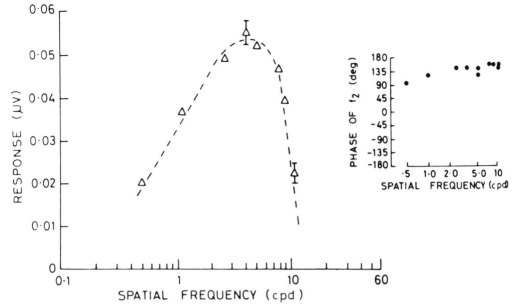

Figure 105–27. Pattern ERG amplitude and phase versus spatial frequency for a normal subject. Responses were elicited with a 1.6 × 1.7 degree, 100 percent contrast sinusoidal grating reversing sinusoidally at 8 Hz. Responses were recorded with a gold-foil electrode. (From Hess RF, Baker CL Jr: Human pattern-evoked electroretinogram. J Neurophysiol 51:939, 1984.)

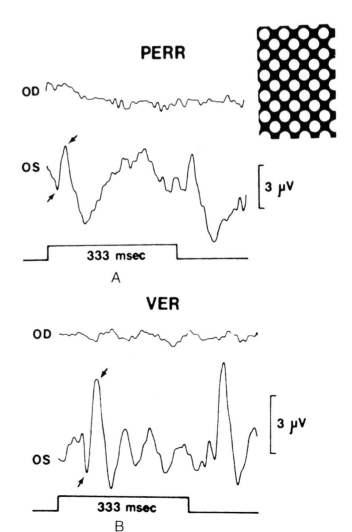

Figure 105–28. Pattern reversal ERGs *(A)* and visual-evoked responses (VERs) *(B)* from the right and left eyes of a patient with a traumatic unilateral (right) optic nerve section. Responses were elicited by a matrix of 40' of arc dots, as illustrated at *upper right*. *Arrows* designate major negative and positive components, respectively. The pattern ERGs were recorded simultaneously from both eyes with DTL electrodes; the pattern VERs were recorded sequentially with the positive electrode 2 cm above the inion referenced to an earlobe. (From Dawson WW, Maida TM, Rubin ML: Human pattern-evoked retinal responses are altered by optic atrophy. Invest Ophthalmol Vis Sci 22:796, 1982.)

than full-field oscillatory potentials in detecting inner retinal malfunction in patients with early stages of diabetic retinopathy. It remains controversial whether the PERG tends to be abnormal in ocular hypertension, as some studies have found many abnormal responses,[142, 143] whereas others have found mostly normal responses.[144] It also remains controversial whether the PERG is abnormal in amblyopia, as some studies have found mainly abnormal responses,[145–147] whereas others have found normal responses.[126, 148]

Based on the preceding normative and clinical studies, studies in mammals involving section of the optic nerve,[149, 150] and current source density analysis,[151] it is now fairly certain that the PERG derives, at least in part, from the ganglion cells. However, the PERG should not be used alone to diagnose the site of retinal malfunction, since it necessarily depends on photoreceptor function and has been shown to be abnormal in macular disease involving the photoreceptors.[152] If the PERG is abnormal, it would also be advisable to obtain a focal flash ERG to evaluate photoreceptor function before assuming that the inner retina is abnormal.

PERGs are usually elicited by phase-reversing square-wave stripes or checks presented on a television monitor or modulated by a moving mirror within an optical system. The temporal modulation may be at a low frequency, (i.e., less than 8 Hz) to elicit transient responses (see Fig. 105–28) or at a high frequency (i.e., ≥8 Hz) to elicit a steady-state, sinusoidal response. The transient response consists of a cornea-negative deflection followed by a cornea-positive deflection (see Fig. 105–28), much like the luminance ERG. The temporal modulation is usually squarewave but may be sinusoidal. Contrast (i.e., the luminance difference between light and dark elements relative to the mean luminance) may be 100 percent or less. Field size is typically 20 degrees or less, but must contain an even number of spatial elements in order to minimize any luminance component, particularly if low spatial frequencies are used.

The patient's pupil may or may not be dilated; in either case, care must be taken that the patient is properly refracted for or can focus on the pattern, which is usually placed between 0.5 and 1 m distant. A pattern that is not focused will have reduced retinal contrast and result in a reduction in amplitude.[123, 126] Two diopters of blur may reduce amplitude 50 percent.[126] The probability that patterns will be out of focus for patients with reduced acuity must be considered when interpreting responses, an issue that has been raised with respect to evaluating strabismic amblyopia.[126]

Signals may be monitored with a silver cup skin electrode on the lower lid,[153] a corneal gold foil or DTL electrode placed in the lower conjunctival sac,[153–155] or a Burian-Allen bipolar contact lens electrode.[156] With the gold foil electrode, but apparently not with the DTL electrode,[157] pattern stimulation of one eye can by volume conduction lead to an artifactual response from the fellow eye.[158–160] With the DTL electrode, the ratio of signal:noise was said to be best if the reference electrode was placed by the outer canthus of the stimulated eye.[157] If a contact lens is used, the eye must be refracted with it in place. PERG signals are typically less than 5 μV in amplitude and must be averaged, preferably with an artifact reject buffer. The skin electrode is reported to be little affected by blinking but yields smaller amplitudes than does a corneal electrode.[153] The contact lens electrode alone prevents reduction of stimulus luminance by closure of the lids.

Although the stimulus fields for eliciting PERGs are usually large relative to those used for eliciting FERGs, fixation near the center of the pattern is still important because the major contribution to the response for a midfrequency check size comes from the fovea. It has been shown that PERG amplitude can fall twofold for an eccentricity of 4 degrees[126] and threefold for an eccentricity of 12 degrees.[161] Eccentric fixation may also help to generate a luminance component, which may be conveniently checked by quantifying the fundamental component of the response by Fourier analysis.[127]

Interocular differences in PERG amplitude among normal subjects have been estimated to be as much as 100 percent.[126] The PERG does not appear to be significantly different between males and females,[156] but a small decline in amplitude[156, 162] and an increase in latency[156] with increasing age have been reported.

VISUAL–EVOKED RESPONSE TESTING

Pattern-reversal visual-evoked responses (VERs) are now preferred over flash VERs for the evaluation of the visual pathways, owing in large part to their smaller range of variation in normal subjects and, undoubtedly related to this, their enhanced sensitivity in detecting axonal conduction defects. The pattern VER is a multiphasic response that, when detectable, contains an inion-positive component with a latency of about 100 msec, called *P100* (see Fig. 105–28). The primary use of the pattern-reversal VER is to identify visual loss secondary to diseases of the optic nerve and anterior visual pathways versus those of psychogenic origin. Demyelination and compressive lesions of the optic nerve, e.g., produce reliable slowing of the pattern response (Fig. 105–29), whereas flash responses in these cases often have normal latencies.[163] As many as 96 percent of patients with multiple sclerosis might be expected to have delayed pattern VERs.[164] Although P100 remains delayed, its amplitude varies monotonically with visual acuity during recovery from optic neuritis.[165] Determining contrast thresholds for a range of spatial frequencies permits the objective assessment of visual acuity (at 100 percent contrast),[166] which can be used to detect malingering.

The stimulus for the pattern VER may be essentially the same as for the PERG, allowing for both measures to be recorded simultaneously, as is becoming increasingly the custom.[124, 145, 156, 161, 162] It is essential that the checkerboard pattern be in proper focus, since lack of focus leads to decreases in VER amplitude[167, 168] and increases in VER latency.[169] Recordings are generally

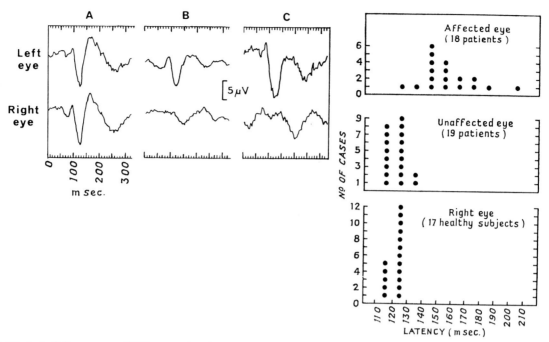

Figure 105–29. *Left,* Pattern reversal VERs recorded from a midline occipital electrode from the left and right eye of a normal subject (A) and two patients who were recovering from acute attacks of optic neuritis in the right eye with onset 4 wk (B) and 3 wk (C) previously. Pattern reversal is at 20 msec; positivity downward. *Right,* Distribution of the peak latencies of the major positive component of the pattern reversal VER from the affected eye of 18 patients with optic neuritis (*upper histogram*), from the unaffected eye of 19 patients with optic neuritis (*middle histogram*), and from the right eye of 17 normal subjects (*lower histogram*). (From Halliday AM, McDonald WI, Mushin J: Delayed visual evoked response in optic neuritis. Lancet 1:982, 1972.)

made from the midline, either using a bipolar configuration with the positive electrode above the inion and the negative electrode on the vertex or using monopolar configurations with positive electrodes above the inion and over the parietal lobe. Earlobes may serve as reference and ground. The electrodes may be conventional electroencephalographic cup electrodes and should be filled with electrode cream and applied to the scalp after reducing scalp resistance with an abrasive. The intent is to obtain a resistance less than 5000 ohms. The electrodes may be held in place with colloidin. Responses must be averaged by computer because amplitudes are generally less than 10 µV.

Unlike retinal responses, scalp responses to pattern reversal show marked interindividual variation in waveform among normal subjects (Fig. 105–30).[170] Nevertheless, remarkable agreement exists for the normal latency for the P100 component across studies. Upper limits for latency differences between left and right eyes of normal subjects have been estimated at 8 to 10 msec.[171] Repeat testing of the same subjects on separate days showed a substantial variation in latency with values that still mostly fell within normal limits obtained on the same patients at a single session.[171] P100 latency increases with age in normal subjects, at a rate of about 2 msec/decade depending on spatial frequency (Fig. 105–

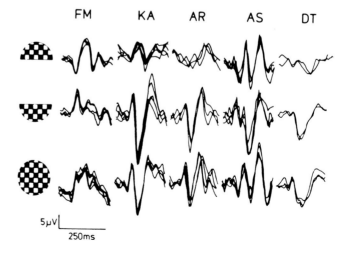

Figure 105–30. VERs from 5 normal subjects to different distributions of pattern reversal stimulation as noted on *left.* Two or more consecutive response averages are superimposed to illustrate intrasubject reproducibility. Check size 50′ of arc, reversal rate 1/sec, field diameter 16 degrees. The positive electrode was 6 cm above the inion, the negative electrode was placed midfrontally, and the ground electrode was on the earlobe (positivity upward). (From Airas KA: Interindividual variation and additivity of the visual evoked potentials to the local checkerboard stimulation of the central and paracentral retina. Acta Ophthalmol 64:557, 1986.)

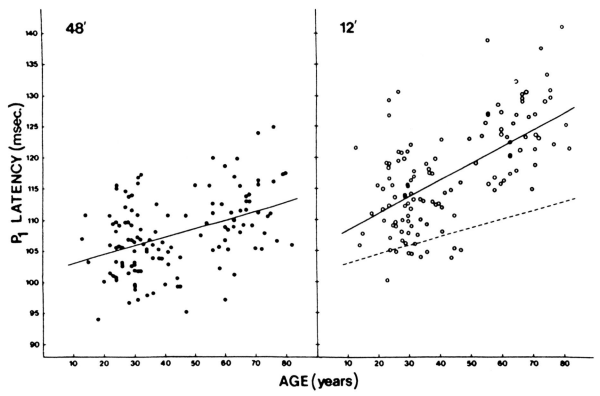

Figure 105–31. P100 (*P1*) latency for 48 min (*closed circles*) and 12 min (*open circles*) checks as a function of age. Each data point is the mean latency of the right and left eye of each subject. For 48-min checks, y = 0.14x + 101.8; for 12-min checks, y = 0.26x + 105.6. For ease of comparison the regression line for 48-min checks has also been plotted as a *dashed line* on the 12-min graph. (From Sokol S, Moskowitz A, Towle VL: Age-related changes in the latency of the visual evoked potential: Influence of check size. Electroencephalogr Clin Neurophysiol 51:559, 1981.)

31).[172] P100 latency also is greater for small pupils than for large pupils;[173] some (but not all) of the increase with age may be due to age-related miosis.

OBJECTIVE EVALUATION OF FUNCTION

When a patient presents with reduced visual acuity, blur, or metamorphopsia or with difficulty seeing at night, increased sensitivity to bright lights, or an impairment in discriminating colors (or any combination of these symptoms), the ophthalmologist must decide if objective tests of visual function are required in addition to a routine examination. It has been our preference to first rule out photoreceptor malfunction by performing full-field and focal flash electroretinography. If results from these tests are abnormal, no additional measurements of function are necessary, and the patient can be advised that the problem is within the eye in the outer retina. If results from flash electroretinography are normal, it would be appropriate to consider the PERG to rule out ganglion cell and optic nerve dysfunction, and then the pattern VER to rule out visual pathway and cortical dysfunction.

REFERENCES

1. Carr RE, Ripps H, Siegel IM, et al: Rhodopsin and the electrical activity of the retina in congenital night blindness. Invest Ophthalmol Vis Sci 5:497, 1966.
2. Carr RE, Ripps H, Siegel IM: Visual pigment kinetics and adaptation in fundus albipunctatus. Doc Ophthalmol Proc XI International Society for Clinical Electroretinography Symp, p 193, 1974.
3. Carr RE, Ripps H: Rhodopsin kinetics and rod adaptation in Oguchi's disease. Invest Ophthalmol 6:426, 1967.
4. Bird AC, Hyman V: Detection of heterozygotes in families with X-linked pigmentary retinopathy by measurements of retinal rhodopsin concentration. Trans Ophthalmol Soc UK 93:221, 1972.
5. Bird AC: X-linked retinitis pigmentosa. Br J Ophthalmol 59:175, 1975.
6. Kemp CM, Jacobson SG, Faulkner DJ: Two types of visual dysfunction in autosomal dominant retinitis pigmentosa. Invest Ophthalmol Vis Sci 29:1235, 1988.
7. Alpern M, Krantz D: Visual pigment kinetics in abnormalities of the uvea-retinal epithelium in man. Invest Ophthalmol Vis Sci 20:183, 1981.
8. Campbell FW, Rushton WAH: Measurement of the scotopic pigment in the living human eye. J Physiol 130:131, 1955.
9. Weale RA: Photo-sensitive reactions in foveae of normal and cone monochromatic observers. Optica Acta 6:158, 1959.
10. Alpern M: Rhodopsin kinetics in the human eye. J Physiol 217:447, 1971.
11. Highman VN, Weale RA: Rhodopsin density and visual threshold in retinitis pigmentosa. Am J Ophthalmol 75:822, 1973.
12. Sheorey UB: Clinical assessment of rhodopsin in the eye. Br J Ophthalmol 60:135, 1976.
13. Kemp CM, Faulkner DJ: Rhodopsin measurement in human disease: Fundus reflectometry using television. Dev Ophthalmol 2:130, 1981.
14. Kilbride PE, Fishman M, Fishman GA, et al: Foveal cone pigment density difference and reflectance in retinitis pigmentosa. Arch Ophthalmol 104:220, 1986.
15. Ripps H, Brin KP, Weale RA: Rhodopsin and visual threshold in retinitis pigmentosa. Invest Ophthalmol Vis Sci 17:735, 1978.

16. Faulkner DJ, Kemp CM: Human rhodopsin measurement using a T.V.-based imaging fundus reflectometer. Vision Res 24:221, 1984.
17. Kilbride PE, Hutman LP, Fishman M, et al: Foveal cone pigment density difference in the aging human eye. Vision Res 26:321, 1986.
18. Berson EL, Goldstein EB: The early receptor potential in dominantly inherited retinitis pigmentosa. Arch Ophthalmol 83:412, 1970.
19. Brown KT, Crawford JM: Melanin and the rapid light-evoked responses from pigment epithelial cells of the frog eye. Vision Res 7:165, 1967.
20. Pak WL: Some properties of the early electrical response in the vertebrate retina. Cold Spring Harbor Symp Quant Biol 30:493, 1965.
21. Cone RA: Early receptor potential: Photoreversible charge displacement in rhodopsin. Science 155:1128, 1967.
22. Cone RA: Early receptor potential of the vertebrate retina. Nature 204:736, 1964.
23. Cone RA, Brown PK: Dependence of the early receptor potential on the orientation of rhodopsin. Science 156:536, 1967.
24. Goldstein EB, Berson EL: Cone dominance of the human early receptor potential. Nature 222:1272, 1969.
25. Carr RE, Siegel IM: Action spectrum of the early receptor potential. Nature 225:88, 1970.
26. Galloway NR: Early receptor potential in the human eye. Br J Ophthalmol 51:261, 1967.
27. Tamai A: Studies on the early receptor potential in the human eye. III. ERP in primary retinitis pigmentosa. Yonago Acta Med 18:18, 1974.
28. Cone RA: The early receptor potential of the vertebrate eye. Cold Spring Harbor Symp Quant Biol 30:483, 1965.
29. Berson EL, Goldstein EB: The early receptor potential in dominantly inherited retinitis pigmentosa. Arch Ophthalmol 83:412, 1970.
30. Barber C, Cotterill DJ, Larke JR: A new contact lens electrode. Doc Ophthalmol Proc Ser 13:385, 1977.
31. Sieving PA, Fishman GA, Maggiano JM: Corneal wick electrode for recording bright flash electroretinograms and early receptor potentials. Arch Ophthalmol 96:899, 1978.
32. Muller W, Topke H: The early receptor potential (ERP). Doc Ophthalmol 66:35, 1987.
33. Steinberg RH, Linsenmeier RA, Griff ER: Three light-evoked responses of the retinal pigment epithelium. Vision Res 23:1315, 1983.
34. Arden GB, Barrada A, Kelsey JH: New clinical test of retinal function based upon the standing potential of the eye. Br J Ophthalmol 46:449, 1962.
35. Krill AE, Morse PA, Potts AM, et al: Hereditary vitelliruptive macular degeneration. Am J Ophthalmol 61:1405, 1966.
36. François J, De Rouck A, Fernandez-Sasso D: Electro-oculography in vitelliform degeneration of the macula. Arch Ophthalmol 77:726, 1967.
37. Deutman AF: Electro-oculography in families with vitelliform dystrophy of the fovea. Detection of the carrier state. Arch Ophthalmol 81:305, 1969.
38. Sabates R, Pruett RC, Hirose T: The electrooculogram in "vitelliform" macular lesions. Doc Ophthalmol Proc Ser 37:93, 1983.
39. Berson EL: Electrical phenomena in the retina. In Hart WM (ed): Adler's Physiology of the Eye. Clinical Application, 9th ed. St Louis, CV Mosby, 1992.
40. Kolder H, Brecher GA: Fast oscillations of the corneoretinal potential in man. Arch Ophthalmol 75:232, 1966.
41. Fishman GA, Young RSL, Schall SP, et al: Electro-oculogram testing in fundus flavimaculatus. Arch Ophthalmol 97:1896, 1979.
42. Kolder HE, Hochgesand P: Empirical model of electro-oculogram. Doc Ophthalmol 34:229, 1973.
43. Kelsey JH: Variations in the normal electro-oculogram. Br J Ophthalmol 51:44, 1967.
44. Lith GHM, Balik J: Variability of the electro-oculogram (EOG). Acta Ophthalmol 48:1091, 1970.
45. Jones RM, Stevens TS, Gould S: Normal EOG values of young subjects. Doc Ophthalmol Proc Ser 13:93, 1976.
46. Arden GB, Barrada A: Analysis of the electro-oculogram of a series of normal subjects. Br J Ophthalmol 46:468, 1962.
47. Adams A: The normal electro-oculogram (E.O.G.). Acta Ophthalmol 51:551, 1973.
48. Jackson SA: The optimum illuminance level for clinical electro-oculography. Acta Ophthalmol 57:665, 1979.
49. Krogh E: Normal values in clinical electrooculography. IV. Analysis of two dimensionless EOG parameters and their relation to other variables. Acta Ophthalmol 55:739, 1977.
50. Anderson ML, Purple RL: Circadian rhythms and variability of the clinical electro-oculogram. Invest Ophthalmol Vis Sci 19:278, 1980.
51. Brown KT, Wiesel TN: Localization of origins of electroretinogram components by intraretinal recording in the intact cat eye. J Physiol (Lond) 158:257, 1961.
52. Brown KT, Watanabe K: Isolation and identification of a receptor potential from the pure cone fovea of the monkey retina. Nature 193:958, 1962.
53. Miller RF, Dowling JE: Intracellular responses of the Müller (glial) cells of mudpuppy retina: Their relation to b-wave of the electreoretinogram. J Neurophysiol 33:323, 1970.
54. Newman EA: Current source density analysis of the b-wave of the frog retina. Am J Neurophysiol 43:1335, 1980.
55. Ogden TE: The oscillatory waves of the primate electroretinogram. Vision Res 13:1059, 1973.
56. Heynen H, Wachtmeister L, van Norren D: Origin of the oscillatory potentials in the primate retina. Vision Res 25:1365, 1985.
57. Hirose T, Wolf E, Hara A: Electrophysiological and psychophysical studies in congenital retinoschisis of X-linked recessive inheritance. Doc Ophthalmol Proc Ser 13:173, 1976.
58. Yonemura D, Aoki T, Tsuzuki K: Electroretinogram in diabetic retinopathy. Arch Ophthalmol 68:19, 1962.
59. Gaudio AR, Lee H, Kini M, et al: Oscillatory potentials in central retinal vein occlusion. Invest Ophthalmol Vis Sci 30(Suppl):477, 1989.
60. Gouras P: Rod and cone independence in the electroretinogram of the dark-adapted monkey's perifovea. J Physiol 187:455, 1966.
61. Berson EL, Gouras P, Hoff M: Temporal aspects of the electro-retinogram. Arch Ophthalmol 81:207, 1969.
62. Chatrian GE, Nelson PL, Lettich E, et al: Computer-assisted quantitative electroretinography. II. Separation of rod and cone components of the electroretinogram in congenital achromatopsia and congenital nyctalopia. Am J EEG Technol 20:79, 1980.
63. Sandberg MA, Miller S, Berson EL: Rod electroretinograms in an elevated cyclic guanosine monophosphate–type human retinal degeneration. Comparison with retinitis pigmentosa. Invest Ophthalmol Vis Sci 31: 2283, 1990.
64. Armington JC, Johnson EP, Riggs LA: The scotopic a-wave in the electrical response of the human retina. J Physiol (Lond) 118:289, 1952.
65. King-Smith PE, Loffing DA, Jones R: Rod and cone ERGs and their oscillatory potentials. Invest Ophthalmol Vis Sci 27:270, 1986.
66. Berson EL, Sandberg MA, Rosner B, et al: Natural course of retinitis pigmentosa over a three-year interval. Am J Ophthalmol 99:240, 1985.
67. Reichel E, Bruce AM, Sandberg MA, et al: An electroretinographic and molecular genetic study of X-linked cone degeneration. Am J Ophthalmol 108:540, 1989.
68. Berson EL, Sandberg MA, Maguire A, et al: Electroretinograms in carriers of blue cone monochromatism. Am J Ophthalmol 102:254, 1986.
69. Gouras P, MacKay CJ: Electroretinographic responses of the short-wavelength–sensitive cones. Invest Ophthalmol Vis Sci 31:1203, 1990.
70. Arden GB, Carter RM, Hogg CR, et al: A modified ERG technique and the results obtained in X-linked retinitis pigmentosa. Br J Ophthalmol 67:419, 1982.
71. Moloney JB, Mooney DJ, O'Connor MA: Retinal function in Stargardt's disease and fundus flavimaculatus. Am J Ophthalmol 96:57, 1983.
72. Massof RW, Wu L, Finkelstein D, et al: Properties of electroretinographic intensity response functions in retinitis pigmentosa. Doc Ophthalmol 57:279, 1984.
73. Birch DG, Fish GE: Rod ERGs in retinitis pigmentosa and cone-rod degeneration. Invest Ophthalmol Vis Sci 28:140, 1987.

74. Berson EL, Gouras PL, Gunkel R: Rod responses in retinitis pigmentosa, dominantly inherited. Arch Ophthalmol 80:58, 1968.

75. Le Grand Y: Form and Space Vision. Bloomington, Indiana University Press, 1967.

76. Rabin AR, Berson EL: A full-field system for clinical electroretinography. Arch Ophthalmol 92:59, 1974.

77. Karpe G, Wulfing B: Importance of pupil size in clinical ERG. Acta Ophthalmol 70(Suppl):53, 1961.

78. Brunette JR, Olivier P, Lafond G: Decreased ocular light penetration and electroretinographic response time. Can J Ophthalmol 15:24, 1980.

79. Sandberg MA: Technical issues in electroretinography. In Heckenlively J, Arden G (eds): Principles and Practice of Clinical Electrophysiology of Vision. St Louis, Mosby–Year Book, 1991.

80. Miyake Y, Horiguchi M, Ota I, et al: Characteristic ERG flicker anomaly in incomplete congenital stationary night blindness. Invest Ophthalmol Vis Sci 28:1816, 1987.

81. Gouras P, MacKay CJ: Growth in amplitude of the human cone electroretinogram with light adaptation. Invest Ophthalmol Vis Sci 30:625, 1989.

82. Miller S, Sandberg MA: Cone electroretinographic change during light adaptation in retinitis pigmentosa. Invest Ophthalmol Vis Sci 25:2536, 1991.

83. Sandberg MA, Lee H, Gaudio AR, et al: Relationship of oscillatory potential amplitudes to a-wave slope over a range of flash luminances in normal subjects. Invest Ophthalmol Vis Sci 32:1508, 1991.

84. Fuller DG, Knighton RW, Machemer R: Bright-flash electroretinography for the evaluation of eyes with opaque vitreous. Am J Ophthalmol 80:214, 1975.

85. Algvere P, Westbeck S: Human ERG in response to double flashes of light during the course of dark adaptation: A Fourier analysis of the oscillatory potentials. Vision Res 12:195, 1972.

86. Gur M, Zeevi Y: Frequency-domain analysis of the human electroretinogram. J Opt Soc Am 70:53, 1980.

87. Van der Torren K, Groenweg G, Van Lith G: Measuring oscillatory potentials: Fourier analysis. Doc Ophthalmol 69:153, 1988.

88. Andréasson SOL, Sandberg MA, Berson EL: Narrow-band filtering for monitoring low-amplitude cone electroretinograms in retinitis pigmentosa. Am J Ophthalmol 105:500, 1988.

89. Martin DA, Heckenlively JR: The normal electroretinogram. Doc Ophthalmol Proc Ser 31:135, 1982.

90. Berson EL: Electroretinographic findings in retinitis pigmentosa. Jap J Ophthalmol 31:327, 1987.

91. Peterson H: The normal b-potential in the single-flash clinical electroretinogram: A computer technique study of the influence of sex and age. Acta Ophthalmol 99(Suppl):5, 1968.

92. Weleber RG: The effect of age on human cone and rod Ganzfeld electroretinograms. Invest Ophthalmol Vis Sci 20:392, 1981.

93. Wright CE, Williams DE, Drasdo N, et al: The influence of age on the electroretinogram and visual evoked potential. Doc Ophthalmol 59:365, 1985.

94. Said FS, Weale RA: The variation with age of the spectral transmissivity of the living human crystalline lens. Gerontologia 3:213, 1959.

95. Dodt E, Copenhaver RM, Gunkel RD: Electroretinographic measurement of the spectral sensitivity in albinos, caucasians, and negroes. Arch Ophthalmol 62:795, 1959.

96. Krill AE, Lee GB: The electroretinogram in albinos and carriers of the ocular albino trait. Arch Ophthalmol 69:32, 1963.

97. Pallin E: The influence of the axial size of the eye on the size of the recorded b-potential in the clinical single-flash electroretinogram. Acta Ophthalmol 101(Suppl):1, 1969.

98. Perlman I, Meyer E, Haim T, et al: Retinal function in high refractive error assessed electroretinographically. Br J Ophthalmol 68:79, 1984.

99. Karpe G, Rickenbach K, Thomasson S: The clinical electroretinogram. I. The normal electroretinogram above fifty years of age. Acta Ophthalmol 28:301, 1950.

100. Zeidler I: The clinical electroretinogram. IX. The normal electroretinogram. Value of the b-potential in different age groups and its difference in men and women. Acta Ophthalmol 37:294, 1959.

101. Birch DG, Berson EL, Sandberg MA: Diurnal rhythm in the human rod ERG. Invest Ophthalmol Vis Sci 25:236, 1984.

102. Sandberg MA, Pawlyk BS, Berson EL: Electroretinogram (ERG) sensitivity and phagosome frequency in the normal pigmented rat. Exp Eye Res 43:781, 1986.

103. Arden GB, Bankes JLK: Foveal electroretinogram as a clinical test. Br J Ophthalmol 50:740, 1966.

104. Biersdorf WR, Diller DA: Local electroretinogram in macular degeneration. Am J Ophthalmol 68:296, 1969.

105. Hirose T, Miyake Y, Hara A: Simultaneous recording of electroretinogram and visually evoked response: Focal stimulation under direct observation. Arch Ophthalmol 95:1205, 1977.

106. Sandberg MA, Jacobson SG, Berson EL: Foveal cone electroretinograms in retinitis pigmentosa and juvenile macular degeneration. Am J Ophthalmol 88:702, 1979.

107. Fish GE, Birch DG, Fuller DG, et al: A comparison of visual function tests in eyes with maculopathy. Ophthalmology 93:1177, 1986.

108. Seiple WH, Siegel IM, Carr RE, et al: Evaluating macular function using the focal electroretinogram. Invest Ophthalmol Vis Sci 27:1123, 1986.

109. Miyake Y, Shiroyama N, Ota I, et al: Local macular electroretinographic responses in idiopathic central serous chorioretinopathy. Am J Ophthalmol 106:546, 1988.

110. Brodie SE, Naidu EM: Combined amplitude and phase criteria for evaluation of macular electroretinograms. Invest Ophthalmol Vis Sci 31(Suppl):425, 1990.

111. Sandberg MA, Hanson AH, Berson EL: Foveal and parafoveal cone electroretinograms in juvenile macular degeneration. Ophthalmic Paediatr Genet 3:83, 1983.

112. Birch DG, Fish GE: Focal cone electroretinograms: Aging and macular disease. Doc Ophthalmol 69:211, 1988.

113. Birch DG, Jost BF, Fish GE: The focal electroretinogram in fellow eyes of patients with idiopathic macular holes. Arch Ophthalmol 106:1558, 1988.

114. Miyake Y, Ichikawa K, Shiose Y, et al: Hereditary macular dystrophy without visible fundus abnormality. Am J Ophthalmol 108:292, 1989.

115. Matthews GP, Sandberg MA, Berson EL: Foveal cone electroretinograms in patients with central visual loss of unexplained etiology. Arch Ophthalmol 110:1568, 1992.

116. Jacobson SG, Sandberg MA, Effron MH, et al: Foveal cone electroretinograms in strabismic amblyopia. Comparison with juvenile macular degeneration, macular scars and optic atrophy. Trans Ophthalmol Soc UK 99:353, 1979.

117. Biersdorf WR: The foveal electroretinogram is normal in optic atrophy. Doc Ophthalmol Proc Ser 40:127, 1984.

118. Sandberg MA, Baruzzi CM, Berson EL: Foveal cone ERGs in optic neuropathy. Invest Ophthalmol Vis Sci 27(Suppl):104, 1986.

119. Weiner A, Sandberg MA: Normal change in the foveal cone ERG with increasing duration of light exposure. Invest Ophthalmol Vis Sci 32:2842, 1991.

120. Weiner A, Sandberg MA, Berson EL: Abnormal foveal to parafoveal cone ERG amplitude ratios in patients with reduced visual acuity and suspected foveal disease. Invest Ophthalmol Vis Sci 31(Suppl):426, 1990.

121. Miyake Y, Shiroyama N, Horiguchi M, et al: Asymmetry of focal ERG in human macular region. Invest Ophthalmol Vis Sci 30:1743, 1989.

122. Riggs LA, Johnson EP, Schick AML: Electrical responses of the human eye to moving stimulus pattern. Science 144:567, 1964.

123. Odom JV, Maida TM, Dawson WW: Pattern evoked retinal response (PERR) in human: Effects of spatial frequency, temporal frequency, luminance and defocus. Curr Eye Res 2:99, 1982/1983.

124. Sokol S, Jones K, Nadler D: Comparison of the spatial response properties of the human retina and cortex as measured by simultaneously recorded pattern ERGs and VEPs. Vision Res 23:723, 1983.

125. Hess RF, Baker CL Jr: Human pattern-evoked electroretinogram. J Neurophysiol 51:939, 1984.

126. Hess RF, Baker CL Jr, Verhoeve JN, et al: The pattern evoked electroretinogram: Its variability in normals and its relationship to amblyopia. Invest Ophthalmol Vis Sci 26:1610, 1985.

127. Plant GT, Hess RF, Thomas SJ: The pattern evoked electroretinogram in optic neuritis. Brain 109:469, 1986.

128. Drasdo N, Thompson DA, Thompson CM, et al: Complemen-

tary components and local variations of the pattern electroretinogram. Invest Ophthalmol Vis Sci 28:158, 1987.

129. Trick GL, Wintermeyer DH: Spatial and temporal frequency tuning of pattern-reversal retinal potentials. Invest Ophthalmol Vis Sci 23:774, 1982.

130. Spekreijse H, Estevez O, Van der Tweel LH: Luminance responses to pattern reversal. Doc Ophthalmol Proc Ser 2:205, 1973.

131. Baker CL, Hess RF: Linear and nonlinear components of human electroretinogram. J Neurophysiol 51:952, 1984.

132. Arden GB, Vaegan, Hogg CR: Clinical and experimental evidence that the pattern electroretinogram (PERG) is generated in more proximal retinal layers than the focal electroretinogram (FERG). Ann NY Acad Sci 388:580, 1982.

133. May JG, Ralston JV, Reed JL, et al: Loss in pattern-elicited electroretinograms in optic nerve dysfunction. Am J Ophthalmol 93:418, 1982.

134. Wanger P, Persson HE: Pattern-reversal electroretinograms in unilateral glaucoma. Invest Ophthalmol Vis Sci 24:749, 1983.

135. Boback P, Bodis-Wollner I, Harnois C, et al: Pattern electroretinograms and visual evoked potentials in glaucoma and multiple sclerosis. Am J Ophthalmol 96:72, 1983.

136. Kirkham TH, Coupland SG: The pattern electroretinogram in optic nerve demyelination. Can J Neurol Sci 10:256, 1983.

137. Mashima Y, Oguchi Y: Clinical study of the pattern electroretinogram in patients with optic nerve damage. Doc Ophthalmol 61:91, 1985.

138. Fiorentini A, Maffei L, Pirchio M, et al: The ERG in response to alternating gratings in patients with diseases of the peripheral visual pathway. Invest Ophthalmol Vis Sci 21:490, 1981.

139. Dawson WW, Maida TM, Rubin ML: Human pattern-evoked retinal responses are altered by optic atrophy. Invest Ophthalmol Vis Sci 22:796, 1982.

140. Arden GB, Hamilton AMP, Wilson-Holt J, et al: Pattern electroretinograms become abnormal when background diabetic retinopathy deteriorates to a preproliferative stage: Possible use as a screening test. Br J Ophthalmol 70:330, 1986.

141. Coupland SG: A comparison of oscillatory potential and pattern electroretinogram measures in diabetic retinopathy. Doc Ophthalmol 66:207, 1987.

142. Weinstein GW, Arden GB, Hitchings RA, et al: The pattern electroretinogram (PERG) in ocular hypertension and glaucoma. Arch Ophthalmol 106:923, 1988.

143. Trick GL, Bickler-Bluth M, Cooper DG, et al: Pattern reversal electroretinogram (PERG) abnormalities in ocular hypertension: Correlation with glaucoma risk factors. Curr Eye Res 7:201, 1988.

144. Wanger P, Persson HE: Pattern-reversal electroretinograms from normotensive, hypertensive and glaucomatous eyes. Ophthalmologica 195:205, 1987.

145. Sokol S, Nadler D: Simultaneous electroretinograms and visual evoked potentials from adult amblyopes in response to pattern stimuli. Invest Ophthalmol Vis Sci 18:848, 1979.

146. Arden GB, Vaegan, Hogg CG, et al: Pattern ERGs are abnormal in many amblyopes. Trans Ophthalmol Soc UK 100:453, 1980.

147. Arden GB, Wooding SL: Pattern ERGs in amblyopia. Invest Ophthalmol Vis Sci 26:88, 1985.

148. Gottlob I, Welge-Lussen L: Normal pattern electroretinograms in amblyopia. Invest Ophthalmol Vis Sci 28:187, 1987.

149. Maffei L, Fiorentini A: Electroretinographic responses to alternating gratings before and after section of the optic nerve. Science 211:953, 1981.

150. Maffei L, Fiorentini A, Bisti S, et al: Pattern ERG in the monkey after section of the optic nerve. Exp Brain Res 59:423, 1985.

151. Sieving PA, Steinberg RH: Proximal retinal contribution to the intraretinal 8-Hz pattern ERG of cat. J Neurophysiol 57:104, 1987.

152. Vaegan, Billson FA: Macular electroretinograms and contrast sensitivity as sensitive detectors of early maculopathy. Doc Ophthalmol 63:399, 1986.

153. Kakisu Y, Mizota A, Adachi E: Clinical application of the pattern electroretinogram with lid skin electrode. Doc Ophthalmol 63:187, 1986.

154. Arden GB, Carter RM, Hogg C, et al: A gold foil electrode: Extending the horizons for clinical electroretinography. Invest Ophthalmol Vis Sci 18:421, 1979.

155. Dawson WW, Trick GL, Litzkow CA: Improved electrode for electroretinography. Invest Ophthalmol Vis Sci 18:988, 1979.

156. Celesia GG, Kaufman D, Cone S: Effects of age and sex on pattern electroretinograms and visual evoked potentials. Electroencephalogr Clin Neurophysiol 68:161, 1987.

157. Odom JV, Maida TM, Dawson WW, et al: Pattern electroretinogram: Effects of reference electrode position. Doc Ophthalmol 65:297, 1987.

158. Seiple WH, Siegel IM: Recording the pattern electroretinogram: A cautionary note. Invest Ophthalmol Vis Sci 24:796, 1983.

159. Peachey NS, Sokol S, Moskowitz A: Recording the contralateral PERG: Effect of different electrodes. Invest Ophthalmol Vis Sci 24:1514, 1983.

160. Arden GB, Carter RM, Hogg C: Uniocular recording of pattern ERG. Vision Res 26:281, 1986.

161. Rover J, Bach M: Pattern electroretinogram plus visual evoked potential: A decisive test in patients suspected of malingering. Doc Ophthalmol 66:245, 1987.

162. Trick GL, Trick LR, Haywood KM: Altered pattern evoked retinal and cortical potentials associated with human senescence. Curr Eye Res 10:717, 1986.

163. Halliday AM, McDonald WI, Mushin J: Delayed visual evoked response in optic neuritis. Lancet 1:982, 1972.

164. Halliday AM, McDonald WI, Mushin J: Visual evoked responses in the diagnosis of multiple sclerosis. Br Med J 4:661, 1973.

165. Halliday AM, McDonald WI, Mushin J: Delayed pattern evoked responses in optic neuritis in relation to visual acuity. Trans Ophthalmol Soc UK 93:315, 1973.

166. Howe JW, Mitchell KW, Robson C: Some clinical experiences using contrast evoked potential techniques in organic and nonorganic visual dysfunction. Doc Ophthalmol Proc Ser 31:353, 1982.

167. Harter MR, White CT: Evoked cortical responses to checkerboard patterns: Effect of check size as a function of visual acuity. Electroencephalogr Clin Neurophysiol 28:48, 1970.

168. Millodot M, Riggs LA: Refraction determined electrophysiologically: Responses to alternation of visual contours. Arch Ophthalmol 84:272, 1970.

169. Sokol S, Moskowitz A: Effect of retinal blur on the peak latency of the pattern evoked potential. Vision Res 21:1279, 1981.

170. Airas KA: Interindividual variation and additivity of the visual evoked potentials to the local checkerboard stimulation of the central and paracentral retina. Acta Ophthalmol 64:557, 1986.

171. Meienberg O, Kutak L, Smolenski C, et al: Pattern reversal evoked cortical responses in normals. A study of different methods of stimulation and potential reproducibility. J Neurol 222:81, 1979.

172. Sokol S, Moskowitz A, Towle VL: Age-related changes in the latency of the visual evoked potential: Influence of check size. Electroencephalogr Clin Neurophysiol 51:559, 1981.

173. Hawkes CH, Stow B: Pupil size and the pattern evoked visual response. J Neurol Neurosurg Psychiatry 44:90, 1981.

Chapter 106

■

Retinitis Pigmentosa and Allied Diseases

ELIOT L. BERSON

Retinitis pigmentosa is a progressive retinal degeneration that usually leads to blindness in later life. The prevalence of this disease is about 1 in 4000 worldwide.[1-6] In a study conducted in the state of Maine in the United States, retinitis pigmentosa was divided into genetic types by families and the percentages were as follows: 19 percent autosomal dominant, 19 percent autosomal recessive, 8 percent X chromosome–linked, 8 percent undetermined, and 46 percent isolates with only one affected member in a given family.[5] In England, the X-linked type has been reported in 16 percent of families and the autosomal recessive type in 7 percent of families.[4]

Genetic heterogeneity is known to exist within a given hereditary pattern.[7-14] Genetic loci have been found respectively on chromosomes 3, 6, and 8 for dominantly inherited retinitis pigmentosa. At least two genetic loci exist for X-linked retinitis pigmentosa on the short arm of the X chromosome. Therefore, retinitis pigmentosa is a group of diseases caused by abnormal genes at various loci within the human genome.

The rapid expansion of knowledge about retinitis pigmentosa and allied night-blinding diseases precludes a comprehensive review in a single chapter. This chapter provides a framework for evaluating patients with these diseases (Table 106–1) and a summary of some recent advances.

SYMPTOMS AND SIGNS

Patients with retinitis pigmentosa characteristically experience night blindness and difficulty with the midperipheral visual field in adolescence. As their condition progresses, they acquire a tendency toward blue blindness, lose the far-peripheral field of vision, and eventually lose central vision as well. Signs on ocular examination include narrowed retinal vessels, depigmentation of the retinal pigment epithelium, intraretinal bone spicule pigmentation, waxy pallor of the optic discs, and vitreous abnormalities.[15-27] Posterior subcapsular cataracts develop in many cases,[28] and some patients show cystoid macular edema.[29, 30] Refractive errors, including astigmatism and myopia, are common.[31, 32] The characteristic bone spicule pigment is typically distributed around the midperipheral fundus (Fig. 106–1A) in the zone in which rods are normally in maximal concentration. Histopathologic studies of autopsy eyes have shown loss of photoreceptors, as well as photoreceptors with shortened or absent outer segments.[33-41]

ELECTRORETINOGRAMS

In 1945, Karpe discovered that patients with advanced retinitis pigmentosa had very small or nondetectable (<10 μV) electroretinograms (ERGs).[42] Subsequently, it was shown that patients with early retinitis pigmentosa could have subnormal but easily detectable ERG a-wave and b-wave responses.[43-46] Responses were not only reduced in amplitude but also delayed in b-wave implicit times,[45-49] and these ERG changes could be detected in some instances many years before diagnostic abnormalities were visible on fundus examination.[48] Figure 106–2 illustrates representative full-field ERGs from a normal subject and four children aged 9 to 14 yr with early retinitis pigmentosa. Rod responses to dim blue light under dark-adapted conditions (left column) are reduced in all genetic types and when detectable are delayed in b-wave implicit times, as designated by *horizontal arrows* in the figure. Cone responses to 30-cycle-per-sec

Table 106–1. RETINITIS PIGMENTOSA AND SOME ALLIED DISEASES

Autosomal dominant forms of retinitis pigmentosa
Autosomal recessive forms of retinitis pigmentosa
Sex-linked (X chromosome–linked) forms of retinitis pigmentosa
Isolate (simplex) forms of retinitis pigmentosa
Progressive cone-rod degeneration
Atypical retinitis pigmentosa including sector, unilateral, and paravenous forms
Some syndromes or diseases of which retinitis pigmentosa is a part:
  Bassen-Kornzweig syndrome
  Refsum's disease
  Usher's syndrome, type I and type II
  Laurence-Moon and Bardet-Biedl syndromes
  Kearns-Sayre syndrome
  Hereditary cerebroretinal degenerations including Batten's disease
  Olivopontocerebellar atrophy
  Cockayne's syndrome
  Alström's disease
Congenital amaurosis of Leber
Sex-linked choroideremia
Gyrate atrophy of the choroid and retina
Retinitis punctata albescens
Stationary forms of night blindness:
  Autosomal dominant nyctalopia (Nougaret type)
  Autosomal recessive nyctalopia (Riggs type)
  Autosomal recessive and sex-linked nyctalopia (Schubert-Bornschein type)
  Oguchi's disease
  Fundus albipunctatus

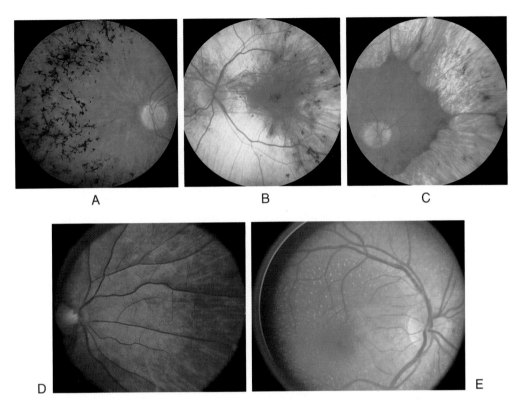

Figure 106–1. Fundus photographs of moderately advanced retinitis pigmentosa (*A*), moderately advanced choroideremia (*B*), gyrate atrophy of the choroid and retina (*C*), Oguchi's disease without dark adaptation (*D*), and fundus albipunctatus (*E*).

(c.p.s. i.e., 30 Hz) white flickering light (Fig. 106–2, right column) are normal or reduced in amplitude and normal or delayed in b-wave implicit times. In most cases, cone b-wave implicit times (Fig. 106–2, right column, *arrows*) are so delayed that a phase shift occurs between the stimulus artifacts (designated by the *vertical lines* in figure) and the corresponding response peaks; each stimulus flash elicits the next-plus-one response, in

contrast to the normal response. In the mixed cone-rod responses to single flashes of white light under dark-adapted conditions (Fig. 106–2, middle column), the cornea-negative a-wave generated by the photoreceptors is reduced in amplitude in all genetic types, pointing to the involvement of the photoreceptors in these early stages.[48]

The subnormal responses with delayed b-wave implicit

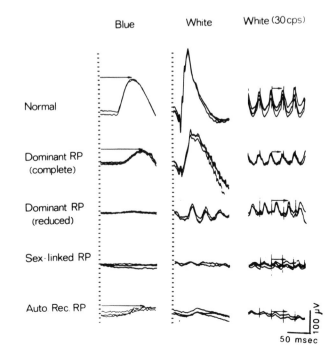

Figure 106–2. Electroretinogram (ERG) responses for a normal subject and four patients with retinitis pigmentosa (ages 13, 14, 14, and 9 yr). Responses were obtained after 45 min of dark adaptation to single flashes of blue light (left column) and white light (middle column). Responses (right column) were obtained to 30 c.p.s. (or 30 Hz) white flickering light. Calibration symbol (lower right corner) signifies 50 msec horizontally and 100 μV vertically. Rod b-wave implicit times in column 1 and cone implicit times in column 3 are designated with *arrows*. (From Berson EL: Retinitis pigmentosa and allied diseases: Electrophysiologic findings. Published courtesy of Trans Am Acad Ophthalmol Otolaryngol 81:OP659–666, 1976.)

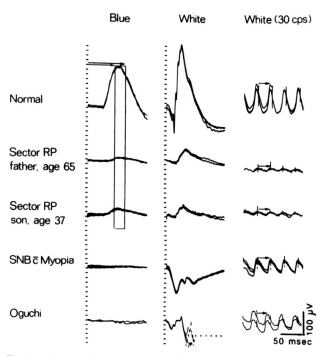

Figure 106–3. ERG responses of a normal subject and four patients with sector or stationary retinal disease. *Horizontal arrows* (column 1) designate range of normal rod b-wave implicit times, and *vertical bar* defining this range (mean ± S.D.) has been extended through responses of patients with sector retinitis pigmentosa. Responses (middle column) from patient with Oguchi's disease are interrupted by reflex blinking, so latter part cannot be illustrated. Cone implicit times in column 3 are designated with *arrows*. (From Berson EL: Retinitis pigmentosa and allied diseases: Electrophysiologic findings. Published courtesy of Trans Am Acad Ophthalmol Otolaryngol 81:OP659–666, 1976.)

times seen in widespread progressive forms of retinitis pigmentosa contrast with the subnormal responses with normal b-wave implicit times seen in self-limited sector retinitis pigmentosa (Fig. 106–3). For example, a father and son with dominantly inherited sector retinitis pigmentosa, separated in age by almost 30 yr, have comparably reduced amplitudes and normal b-wave implicit times. These patients usually have an area of intraretinal pigment confined to one or two quadrants of the periphery of each eye, with loss of peripheral rods and cones and consequent reductions in both rod and cone amplitudes. Rod b-wave implicit times are within the normal range (Fig. 106–3, *vertical bars*). Cone b-wave implicit times are also within the normal range, and each stimulus elicits the succeeding response, as seen in the normal ERG. The ERGs recorded from patients with sector retinitis pigmentosa are comparable to those recorded from patients with large peripheral chorioretinal scars.[48]

Studies of patients with widespread progressive forms of retinitis pigmentosa with detectable rod ERGs and delayed cone b-wave implicit times have demonstrated that cone b-wave implicit time to white flicker is inversely proportional to the log amplitude of the dark-adapted rod b-wave to blue light. In these patients, cone b-wave implicit time did not vary with the amplitudes of the dark-adapted cone b-waves. A tenfold reduction

in rod amplitude was associated with about 5.5 msec slowing in cone b-wave implicit times.[50] These results would suggest that it is the loss of rod photoreceptors among remaining cones that apparently leads to abnormal rod-cone interaction,[51] which can account in large part for the delays in cone b-wave implicit times seen in these forms of retinitis pigmentosa.

The ERG can be used to identify not only which patients have progressive forms of retinitis pigmentosa but also which patients are normal. Relatives of patients with retinitis pigmentosa, aged 6 yr or older, with normal rod and cone ERG amplitudes and implicit times have not been observed to develop this disease at a later time.[48, 49, 52]

CARRIERS OF X-LINKED RETINITIS PIGMENTOSA

Female carriers of X-linked retinitis pigmentosa can show a patch of bone spicule pigmentation in the periphery or an abnormal tapetal reflex in the macula; among carriers of child-bearing age, less than half showed diagnostic findings on fundus examination. ERG testing can be used as an aid in detecting female carriers of X-linked retinitis pigmentosa.[53, 54] ERG testing of obligate carriers has shown that more than 90 percent have abnormal responses that are reduced in amplitude to single flashes of blue or white light under dark-adapted conditions or are delayed in cone b-wave implicit times, or both, in one or both eyes. A few older obligate carriers with visual symptoms have had very small or even nondetectable full-field ERGs (Fig. 106–4).[53] Daughters of obligate carriers have had either normal ERGs or abnormal ERGs similar to those recorded from obligate carriers.

The abnormal ERGs of carriers of X-linked retinitis pigmentosa contrast with the normal full-field ERG amplitudes and normal fundi observed in obligate female carriers of autosomal recessive disease.[53] Once carrier females of X-linked retinitis pigmentosa have been detected by ophthalmoscopy or full-field ERG testing, or both, they would know that they would have a 50 percent chance of having an affected son and a 50 percent chance of having a carrier daughter with each childbirth.

Female carriers can have a slowly progressive retinal degeneration, although the natural course remains to be defined. Some female carriers have had considerable loss of visual field and substantial reductions in ERG amplitudes by age 70 yr.

NATURAL COURSE OF RETINITIS PIGMENTOSA

The ERG provides a quantitative measure of remaining retinal function and therefore can aid in defining the natural course of retinitis pigmentosa. For example, full-field ERGs have been recorded over a 20-yr interval in young patients in a family with a dominant form of disease. Amplitudes decreased over this period, and

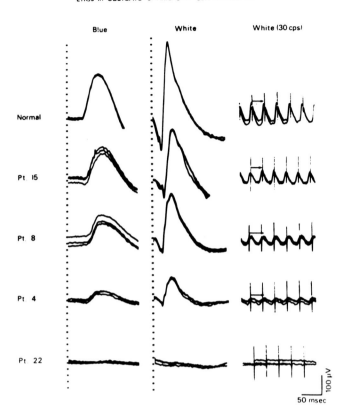

ERGs in OBLIGATE CARRIERS of SEX–LINKED RP

Figure 106–4. ERG responses from a normal subject and four obligate carriers of sex-linked retinitis pigmentosa. Pt (patient) 15, age 39; Pt 8, age 41; Pt 4, age 51; Pt 22, age 70. Stimulus onset is designated by *vertical hatched lines* for columns 1 and 2 and *vertical shock artifacts* for column 3. Cornea-positivity is upward deflection. *Arrows* in column 3 designate cone b-wave implicit times. (From Berson EL, Rosen JB, Simonoff EA: Electroretinographic testing as an aid in detection of carriers of X-chromosome–linked retinitis pigmentosa. Am J Ophthalmol 87:460–468, 1979. Published with permission from The American Journal of Ophthalmology. Copyright by The Ophthalmic Publishing Company.)

patients aged 13 yr or younger with normal fundi and abnormal ERGs in 1967 showed fundus changes of retinitis pigmentosa and further reductions in their ERG amplitudes in 1977 (Fig. 106–5);[55] examination of some members of this family showed further loss in 1987.[49]

Signal averaging with a bipolar artifact reject buffer and bandpass filtering have extended the range of detectability of responses from affected patients. ERGs can now be recorded that are as low as 1 μV to 0.5-Hz flashes of white light with signal averaging alone, and with bandpass filtering and signal averaging, that are as low as 0.05 μV to 30-Hz white flicker. Full-field ERG function could be monitored with at least one test criterion in 90 percent of an outpatient population with a visual field diameter greater than 8 degrees, thereby making this technique useful in defining the natural course of the disease. ERGs in an adult man with X-linked retinitis pigmentosa are illustrated in Figure 106–6 to show changes in ERG function over a 2-yr period.[56, 57]

Among 94 patients, aged 6 to 49 yr, with the common forms of retinitis pigmentosa, full-field ERGs declined significantly over a 3-yr interval in 66 of 86 patients (77 percent), with detectable responses at baseline. Patients lost on average 16 percent of remaining full-field ERG amplitude per year to single flashes of white light (95 percent confidence limits, 13.1 to 18.6 percent) and 18.5 percent of remaining amplitude per year, to 30-Hz white flicker (95 percent confidence limits, 15.1 to 21.5 percent). Patients lost on average 5.2 percent of remaining foveal cone ERG amplitude per year, indicating that

loss of retinal function was primarily extrafoveal in these patients. They lost on average 4.6 percent of remaining visual field area per year in the Goldmann perimeter with a V-4$_e$ white test light, whereas visual acuity and dark-adaptation thresholds remained relatively stable. Bone spicule pigment increased in 54 percent of patients in whom comparisons could be made over a 3-yr interval, suggesting that observation of increased pigmentation as a means of following this condition was not as sensitive as full-field ERG testing.[56]

Caution must be exercised in applying these population ERG results to predict longitudinal patterns in individual patients because standard deviations derived from standard errors indicated considerable variation around the mean for these patients.[56] However, these results, describing the natural course on a quantitative basis, provide a frame of reference for planning interventions in similar populations to stabilize or slow the course of retinitis pigmentosa, particularly if monitored with full-field ERG testing.

ABNORMAL ROD ERG DIURNAL RHYTHM IN RETINITIS PIGMENTOSA

The changes that occur in retinitis pigmentosa can be considered not only in terms of the course over years but also in terms of abnormalities in rod function that can occur over the course of a day. Abnormal rod ERG diurnal rhythms have been observed in light-entrained

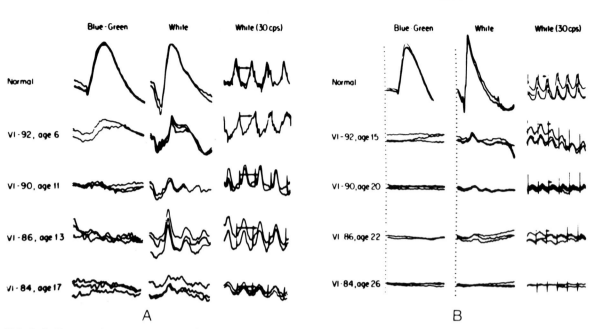

Figure 106–5. *A,* Electroretinograms recorded in 1967 for a normal subject and four affected members from a family with a dominant form of retinitis pigmentosa. One to three responses to the same stimulus are represented. Stimulus onset is designated by *vertical hatched lines* in columns 1 and 2 and *vertical shock artifacts* in column 3; cornea positivity is upward deflection; *arrows* in column 3 designate cone implicit times. Calibration symbol, lower right, designates 50 msec horizontally for columns 1 and 2 and 25 msec for column 3 and 50 μV vertically for column 1 and 100 μV vertically for columns 2 and 3. *B,* Electroretinograms recorded in 1977 for a normal subject and four affected members from the same family as in (*A*) for comparison with ERGs recorded in 1967. Calibration symbol (lower right corner) designates 60 msec horizontally and 100 μV vertically for all tracings. (From Berson EL, Simonoff EA: Dominant retinitis pigmentosa with reduced penetrance: Further studies of the electroretinogram. Arch Ophthalmol 97:1286, 1979. Copyright 1979, American Medical Association.)

patients with dominant retinitis pigmentosa; these patients had abnormal reductions in rod b-wave sensitivity 1.5 and 8 hr after light onset (Fig. 106–7). The abnormal reductions in rod b-wave sensitivity at 9:30 A.M. and 4:00 P.M. raised as one possibility that these patients with dominant retinitis pigmentosa shed abnormally large fractions of rod outer segments throughout the light period and that their rods were slow to renew their pre–light onset outer-segment length. Abnormal diurnal rhythms have also been reported in patients with autosomal recessive and isolate forms of retinitis pigmen-

tosa. The pathogenetic mechanism that leads to these abnormal rod ERG diurnal rhythms remains to be defined.[58–63]

MOLECULAR GENETIC STUDIES OF RETINITIS PIGMENTOSA

Molecular genetic techniques have provided a new approach to finding biochemical abnormalities in retinitis pigmentosa, as well as in other hereditary diseases.

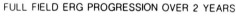

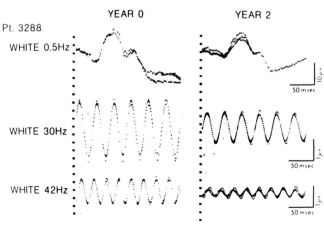

Figure 106–6. Computer-averaged full-field electroretinograms from a 26-year-old man with X-linked retinitis pigmentosa obtained in response to 10-μsec flashes of white light at 16,000 ft-L presented at 0.5 Hz (n = 64), 30 Hz (n = 256), and 42 Hz (n = 256) at base line (year 0) and at 2-year follow-up (year 2). Three consecutive response averages are superimposed in each case. *Vertical broken lines* denote flash onset for 0.5 Hz condition and onset of one of the train of flashes for 30-Hz and 42-Hz conditions. (From Berson EL, Sandberg MA, Rosner B, et al: Natural course of retinitis pigmentosa over a three-year interval. Am J Ophthalmol 99:240–251, 1985. Published with permission from The American Journal of Ophthalmology. Copyright by The Ophthalmic Publishing Company.)

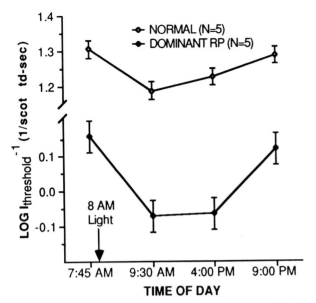

Figure 106–7. Mean log $I_{threshold}^{-1}$ of rod b-wave $V = kI^n$ function versus time of day for five light-entrained normal subjects and five light-entrained patients with dominant retinitis pigmentosa. Subjects were dark-adapted for 1 hr prior to 9:30 A.M., 4 P.M., and 9 P.M. test sessions. Log $I_{thresholds}^{-1}$ were based on criterion amplitudes averaging 28.8 μV for normal subjects and 10.6 μV for patients with retinitis pigmentosa. Error bars designate ± S.E.M. derived from pooled estimates of population variances obtained from analyses of variance. (From Sandberg MA, Baruzzi CM, Hanson AH III, Berson EL: Rod ERG diurnal rhythm in some patients with dominant retinitis pigmentosa. Invest Ophthalmol Vis Sci 29:494, 1988.)

A series of DNA probes linked to various regions of the human genome, if found to cosegregate with a form of retinitis pigmentosa, can be used to localize the region of the chromosome in which the gene for that form is located.

Gene-linkage analyses have localized Usher's syndrome, type II (retinitis pigmentosa with partial deafness) to the long arm of chromosome 1[64, 65] and two forms of X-linked retinitis pigmentosa have been localized to the short arm of the X chromosome, one near the L1.28 locus and one more distal near the OTC locus.[9, 10] Linkage analyses have revealed separate loci for Usher's syndrome, type I on the short arm (R Smith et al, Personal communication) and long arm (W Kimberling et al, Personal communication) of chromosome 11. These linkage analyses are undoubtedly initial steps in the search for the precise gene abnormalities in these conditions.

Linkage analyses revealed that an anonymous polymorphic sequence named CR1–C17 within the long arm of human chromosome 3 was linked to a gene responsible for dominant retinitis pigmentosa in a family in Ireland.[7] Since the rhodopsin gene also mapped to the long arm of chromosome 3,[66, 67] and since rhodopsin is expressed in rod photoreceptors, which are affected early in this disease, a search was conducted for an abnormality in the rhodopsin gene in the leukocyte DNA of patients with dominant retinitis pigmentosa in the United States.

The search initially revealed an abnormal nucleotide sequence in the gene coding for rhodopsin in 17 of 148 unrelated patients with autosomal dominant retinitis pigmentosa and in none of 102 unaffected individuals (Fig. 106–8). The nucleotide base change was a cytosine-to-adenine transversion (i.e., CCC to CAC) in codon 23, corresponding to a substitution of histidine for proline in the 23rd amino acid of rhodopsin. Only clinically affected relatives showed this gene defect in the families studied. These results, coupled with the fact that proline-23 is highly conserved among normal opsins, suggested that this point mutation affected a critical amino acid in rhodopsin and that this mutation could be the cause of one form of autosomal dominant retinitis pigmentosa. This mutation was designated as *rhodopsin, proline-23-histidine* (i.e., Pro23His).[68]

Subsequent studies have revealed many more mutations in the rhodopsin gene (Table 106–2).[68–90] Again, only one mutation has been found in a given family, and each mutation has segregated perfectly with the disease in the families studied so far. All patients with rhodopsin gene mutations tested so far by the author have had abnormal rod ERGs. None of these mutations has been found in unrelated normal subjects. When the incidence of these mutations is added to that of the Pro23His mutation, about 25 to 30 percent of families with autosomal dominant retinitis pigmentosa in the United States have a mutation of the rhodopsin gene.

Some data have been obtained to show that the site of the mutation has implications with respect to the clinical severity of the disease. A group of 17 patients from separate families with Pro23His (mean age 37 yr) retained a mean visual acuity of 20/26, compared with 20/37 for the group of 8 patients from separate families with Pro347Leu (mean age 32 yr). Visual field area was on average 3463 square degrees in the Pro23His group to a V-4$_e$ white test light (normal, >11,399 square degrees) and 1224 square degrees in the Pro347Leu group. ERG responses to single 0.5-Hz flashes of white light were on average 14.4 μV in the Pro23His group, which is almost tenfold larger than the mean amplitude of 1.7 μV in the Pro347Leu group. Cone responses to 30-Hz flicker were also tenfold larger on average for the Pro23His group (i.e., 5.5 μV) compared with the Pro347Leu group (i.e., 0.5 μV). The ERG and other clinical findings taken together would support the idea that patients with Pro23His have, on average, less severe disease than those with rhodopsin, Pro347Leu. Available data would suggest that patients with rhodopsin, Pro23His would be expected to retain vision on average 17 yr longer than would patients with rhodopsin, Pro347Leu, although these estimates are based on small numbers and remain to be confirmed by a prospective longitudinal study.[70–72]

Although patients with the Pro23His mutation retained more retinal function on average than did patients with the Pro347Leu mutation, some variability in clinical expression exists at a given age among patients with these mutations, particularly among the group with Pro23His. This variability in clinical expression among patients with the same gene defect has raised the possibility that some factor or factors other than the gene

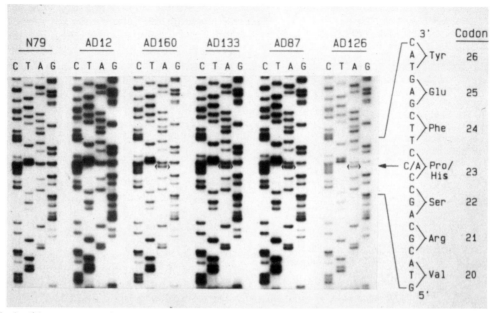

Figure 106-8. Nucleotide sequence of codons 20 to 26 of the human rhodopsin gene derived from leukocyte DNA of a normal individual (N79) and of five representative patients with autosomal dominant retinitis pigmentosa included in this study and identified by their molecular genetic numbers AD12, AD160, AD133, AD87, and AD126. The normal subject and patient AD12 show the normal sequence, whereas the other four patients are heterozygous for the cytosine-to-adenine transversion within codon 23 (CCC to CAC). In these four patients with this mutation, the single base change can be seen as a band marked in brackets. (From Berson EL, Rosner B, Sandberg MA, et al: Ocular findings in patients with autosomal dominant retinitis pigmentosa and a rhodopsin gene defect (Pro23His). Arch Ophthalmol 109:92, 1991. Copyright 1991, American Medical Association.)

Table 106-2. MUTATIONS FOUND IN THE RHODOPSIN GENE IN PATIENTS WITH AUTOSOMAL DOMINANT RETINITIS PIGMENTOSA*

Number	Mutation		Normal Sequence†	References
1	Thr17Met	C→T	GCG ACG GGT	75, 82, 85, 88, 89, 90
2	Pro23His	C→A	AGC CCC TTC	68–71, 75, 80, 85–89
3	Pro23Leu	C→T	AGC CCC TTC	75
4	Phe45Leu	T→C	ATG TTT CTG	88, 89
5	Gly51Val	G→T	CTG GGC TTC	75
6	Thr58Arg	C→G	CTC ACG CTC	69, 75, 77, 82, 84, 85, 88, 89
7	Del68–71	12 bp del	CTG CGC ACG CCT	83
8	Val87Asp	T→A	ATG GTC CTA	88, 89
9	Gly89Asp	G→A	CTA GGT GGC	75, 88, 89
10	Gly106Trp	G→T	TTC GGG CCC	88, 89
11	Leu125Arg	T→G	GCC CTG TGG	75
12	Arg135Leu	GG→TT	GAG CGG TAC	82, 88, 89
13	Arg135Trp	C→T	GAG CGG TAC	82, 88, 89
14	Cys167Arg	T→C	CGG TGC GCC	75
15	Pro171Leu	C→T	CCC CCA CTC	75
16	Tyr178Cys	A→G	AGG TAC ATC	76, 88
17	Glu181Lys	G→A	CCC GAG GGC	75
18	Gly182Ser	G→A	GAG GGC CTG	85, 90
19	Ser186Pro	T→C	TGC TCG TGT	75
20	Gly188Arg	G→A	TGT GGA ATC	75
21	Asp190Asn	G→A	ATC GAC TAC	75, 83
22	Asp190Gly	A→G	ATC GAC TAC	75, 88, 89
23	His211Pro	A→C	GTC CAC TTC	83
24	Ile255Del	3 bp del	GTC ATC ATC ATG	74, 81
25	Pro267Leu	C→T	GTG CCC TAC	85
26	Lys296Glu	A→G	GCC AAG AGC	83
27	Gln344Ter	C→T	AGC CAG GTG	82, 88, 89
28	Val345Met	G→A	CAG GTG GCC	73, 75
29	Pro347Arg	C→G	GCC CCG GCC	79
30	Pro347Leu	C→T	GCC CCG GCC	69, 72, 74, 75, 78, 88, 89
31	Pro347Ser	C→T	GCC CCG GCC	69, 75

*Mutations reported through January 1992.
†Affected base or bases are underlined.

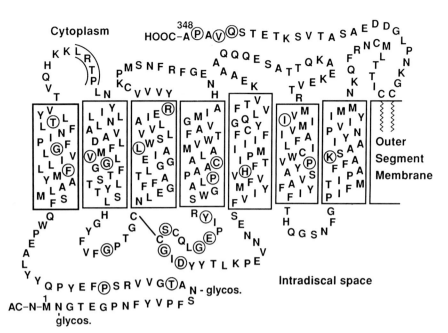

Figure 106–9. This is a model of the rhodopsin protein in a rod outer segment disc membrane. Each letter signifies an amino acid residue, using the standard one-letter code. The protein, which contains 348 amino acids, traverses the outer segment disc membrane seven times, so that different portions of the molecule are in the cytoplasm, within the outer segment membrane, or in the intradiscal space. The amino acids that are affected by point mutations so far reported in patients with autosomal dominant retinitis pigmentosa are circled (see also Table 106–2). The lysine residue [K] highlighted with a circle in the seventh transmembrane domain is covalently bound to the vitamin A aldehyde (i.e., 11-*cis*-retinal). Glycosylation sites are labeled near the N-terminal of the protein. The *solid line* designates a disulfide bond between two cysteines in separate intradiscal loops.

defect itself are responsible for the expression of this condition. Risk factor analyses of patients with this mutation and varying severity of disease may help to determine ameliorating or aggravating factors that may be affecting the course of this condition, with possible implications for therapy.[70–72]

The rhodopsin gene is about 7 kilobases in length with five exons; the gene normally encodes 348 amino acids in the rhodopsin protein. Normal rhodopsin molecules are thought to traverse the rod outer-segment membrane seven times (Fig. 106–9) and are folded in three dimensions, with the first and seventh transmembrane segments in close proximity. Loops on the intradiscal side near the amino terminal tail are thought to be involved in the folding of the molecule, whereas some loops on the cytoplasmic side appear to interact with transducin as the first step in the phototransduction cascade. The normally folded rhodopsin molecule forms a pocket for vitamin A, which is bound to a lysine residue at position 296, designated by the letter *K* in the seventh transmembrane segment (Fig. 106–10). The Pro23His mutation may interfere with the overall folding of rhodopsin and thereby modify the capacity of the pocket to hold vitamin A. It has also been speculated that some of these mutations may affect assembly or transport of molecules through the inner segment, with consequent accumulation of these molecules in the rough endoplasmic reticulum or in the Golgi of the inner segments; this accumulation may compromise the function and viability of rod photoreceptors. The reason why mutations in the rod system eventually also lead to cone photoreceptor cell death is not known. Studies of transgenic mice with these mutations, as well as evaluation of cultured cell systems with these mutations, may help to define the mechanisms by which they lead to photoreceptor cell death.[91, 92]

Mutations in the human retinal degeneration slow (*RDS*) gene on the short arm of chromosome 6 have

been reported in other families with autosomal dominant retinitis pigmentosa.[13, 14] All patients so far studied have had abnormal rod and cone ERGs. This gene encodes for the protein peripherin, a protein thought to help maintain normal outer segment structure. An abnormality in this gene is also known to be responsible for a retinal degeneration in a mouse model called *rds*.

A homozygous nonsense mutation (Glu 249 → Stop) within exon 4 of the rhodopsin gene has been detected in a patient with autosomal recessive retinitis pigmen-

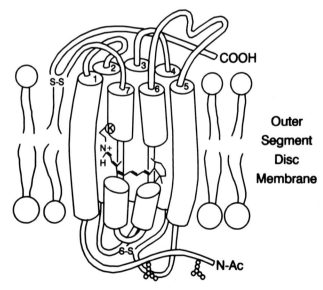

Figure 106–10. Schematic representation of a normal rhodopsin molecule folded in three dimensions to form a pocket to hold the vitamin A–derived chromophore (11-*cis*-retinal), which is covalently attached to a lysine residue, designated by the letter K in the seventh transmembrane segment. (Modified from Applebury ML: Molecular genetics. Insight into blindness. Reprinted by permission from Nature vol. 343, pp 316–317; Copyright © 1990 Macmillan Magazines Limited.)

tosa; this patient had deficient night vision early in life, and had no detectable rod function, a small residual cone ERG, and typical fundus findings of retinitis pigmentosa at age 29 yr. Both parents and some of her siblings had normal-appearing fundi but were heterozygous carriers for this mutation. As a group, these carriers had the same maximal rod ERG responses as did normal controls, but they required a brighter stimulus to achieve a half-maximal response, suggesting that they have less rhodopsin in their rod photoreceptors. This nonsense mutation would be expected to result in a truncated rhodopsin protein that is missing the sixth and seventh transmembrane domains and the 11-cis-retinal attachment site. This mutation is the first report of a gene abnormality responsible for a form of autosomal recessive retinitis pigmentosa and was found in 1 of 132 unrelated patients studied.[93]

TREATMENT TRIALS FOR RETINITIS PIGMENTOSA

Many treatments have been attempted for the common forms of retinitis pigmentosa without proven benefit.[94–100] They include various vitamins and minerals, vasodilators, tissue therapy with placental extract, cortisone, cervical sympathectomy, injections of a hydrolysate of yeast RNA, ultrasound, transfer factor, dimethyl sulfoxide, ozone, and muscle transplants. None of these attempts at treatment was conducted with a randomized, double-masked, controlled protocol, which is necessary to avoid possible patient or examiner biases. Most of these studies were conducted without electroretinography as an end point for evaluating efficacy, so the amount of remaining retinal function was not quantitated in an objective manner.

Claims of success with one or another treatment by patients with retinitis pigmentosa that are based solely on subjective reporting of improved visual function are

to be interpreted with caution. Spontaneous fluctuations in acuity and field are well known in this condition. Given the slow course of the disease without treatment, it will usually require several years to assess whether or not a proposed treatment has any effect on stabilizing or slowing the course of the disease. The problem of assessing treatments may be further complicated by the genetic heterogeneity of this condition and the stage of disease at which treatment is initiated.

RETINITIS PIGMENTOSA ASSOCIATED WITH HEREDITARY ABETALIPOPROTEINEMIA

In hereditary abetalipoproteinemia (Bassen-Kornzweig syndrome),[101–103] patients have fat malabsorption, a form of retinitis pigmentosa, diffuse neuromuscular disease with ataxia, acanthocytosis, and low serum cholesterol and triglyceride levels (<50 mg/dl). Without treatment, these patients usually present with steatorrhea in early life, ataxia in adolescence, and night vision deficiency in early adult life. About 50 cases have been reported around the world. The diagnosis is based on an inability to detect apolipoprotein B in plasma. In this recessively inherited disease, patients appear to have an inability to secrete apolipoprotein B-100, which is a major protein of very low density lipoproteins and low density lipoproteins, and also show an inability to secrete apolipoprotein B-48, which is a major protein of intestinal chylomicrons. Since they do not make chylomicrons, they cannot efficiently absorb fat and fat-soluble vitamins. Patients have a deficiency of vitamins A and E in serum, with consequent effects on retinal function, and vitamin K deficiency, which results in excessive bleeding at surgery.[103]

Large doses of vitamin A have resulted in return of dark-adaptation thresholds and ERG responses to normal in the early stages. Figure 106–11 illustrates full-

ERGs in Hereditary Abetalipoproteinemia

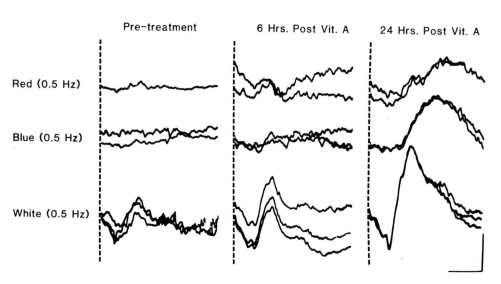

Pre-treatment   6 Hrs. Post Vit. A   24 Hrs. Post Vit. A

Red (0.5 Hz)

Blue (0.5 Hz)

White (0.5 Hz)

Figure 106–11. Full-field ERGs to red (*top*) and blue (*middle*) light, equal for rod vision, and brighter white stimulus (*bottom*) from patient with hereditary abetalipoproteinemia (dark-adapted). Responses in left column were obtained before vitamin A therapy, those in middle column at 6 hr, and those on right at 24 hr after vitamin A therapy. Two to three responses to the same stimulus are superimposed. Light stimulus begins with each trace. Calibration (lower right) signifies 0.06 mV vertically and 60 msec horizontally. (From Gouras P, Carr RE, Gunkel RD: Retinitis pigmentosa in abetalipoproteinemia: Effects of vitamin A. Invest Ophthalmol Vis Sci 10:784, 1971.)

field ERGs to red, blue, and white light prior to treatment (Fig. 106–11, left column), 6 hr after vitamin A therapy (Fig. 106–11, middle column), and 24 hr after vitamin A therapy (Fig. 106–11, right column) to show that the ERG can be reversed to normal in a patient in the early stages of this condition.[104] More advanced stages have not responded to therapy, but in two such cases in which the retinas were examined after the death of the patient considerable loss of photoreceptor cells was observed.[105] Vitamin E has also been advocated to prevent the progression of this retinal degeneration.[106] The recommended treatment is fat restriction sufficient to minimize diarrhea and 300 units/kg/day of vitamin A in water-soluble form, 100 units/kg/day of vitamin E, and 0.15 mg/kg/day of vitamin K.[103] Because these patients have a deficiency of essential fatty acids in serum, omega-3 fatty acids (eicosapentaenoic acid and docosahexaenoic acid) in fish oil have been recommended up to an amount of 0.10 g/kg/day.[103] Some physicians give vitamin K supplementation to normalize clotting parameters only prior to surgery. The long-term effects of vitamins A and E and essential fatty acids in preserving retinal function in this condition remain to be clearly established.[49]

RETINITIS PIGMENTOSA ASSOCIATED WITH REFSUM'S DISEASE

Refsum's disease is an inborn error of metabolism in which the patient accumulates exogenous phytanic acid.[107, 108] Findings include a peripheral neuropathy, ataxia, an increase in cerebrospinal fluid protein with a normal cell count, and retinitis pigmentosa. All patients have elevated serum phytanic acid levels. Some patients have anosmia, neurogenic impairment of hearing, electrocardiographic abnormalities, and skin changes resembling ichthyosis. The fundus can be granular, with areas of depigmentation around the periphery with a subnormal ERG in the early stages or more typical retinitis pigmentosa with a nondetectable ERG in more advanced stages.[109]

A defect exists in the conversion of phytanic acid to α-hydroxy phytanic acid, specifically in the introduction of a hydroxyl group on the α carbon of phytanic acid (Fig. 106–12).[110] The pathogenesis appears to involve accumulation of phytanic acid in a variety of tissues, including the retinal pigment epithelium.[111]

Treatment consists of restricting not only animal fats and milk products (i.e., foods that contain phytanic acid) but also green leafy vegetables containing phytol.[112] Success of treatment depends on the patient's maintaining body weight; if body weight becomes reduced, phytanic acid is released from tissue stores, resulting in an increase of phytanic acid in serum and exacerbation of symptoms. Refsum has reported two patients whose serum phytanic acid levels were lowered to normal and who showed improvement in motor nerve conduction velocity, some relief of ataxia, and return of the cerebrospinal fluid protein to normal. Moreover, the retinitis

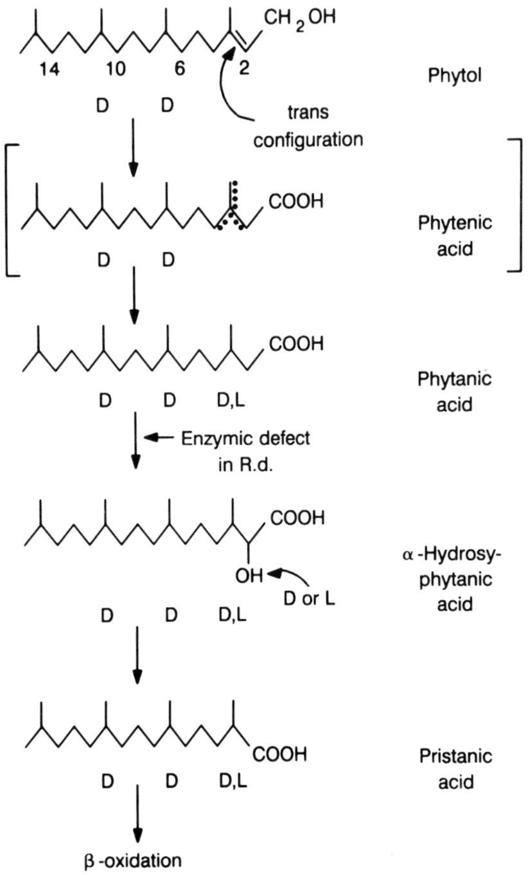

Figure 106–12. Phytanic acid, its immediate precursors and metabolites, and site of enzyme defect in Refsum's disease (R.d.). (From Eldjarn L, Stokke O, Try K: Biochemical aspects of Refsum's disease and principles for the dietary treatment. *In* Vinken PJ, Bruyn GW [eds]: Handbook of Clinical Neurology, Amsterdam, North-Holland, 1976.)

pigmentosa and hearing impairment did not progress; one of these patients was followed for 10 yr and the other for many years.[113] One young adult with a mild form of this disorder has been followed on a low-phytol, low-phytanic acid diet for 4 yr; full-field ERGs, reduced 75 percent below normal prior to commencement of this diet, have remained about the same over this period (Fig. 106–13). Long-term effects of this diet on retinal function continue to be studied.[49]

OTHER FORMS OF RETINITIS PIGMENTOSA

Some 15 to 20 percent of affected individuals with retinitis pigmentosa have associated hearing loss, sometimes referred to as Usher's syndrome in recognition of the British ophthalmologist Usher, who emphasized that this condition was recessively inherited.[114] Patients with Usher's syndrome, type I typically have night blindness in the first or second decade of life, profound congenital deafness (i.e., >70 db loss of all frequencies) with unintelligible speech, and vestibular ataxia, whereas those with Usher's syndrome, type II usually report

Refsum's Disease: Effects of Low Phytanic Acid Diet

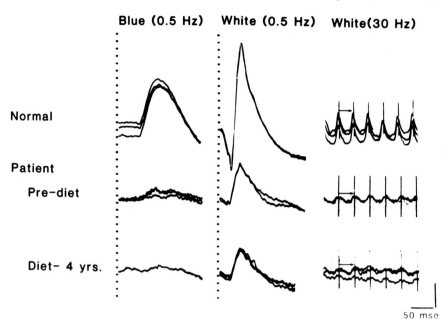

Figure 106–13. Full-field ERGs from a normal subject and a patient with a mild form of Refsum's disease prior to and 4 yr after treatment with low-phytol, low–phytanic acid diet. Pretreatment responses were recorded at age 31 yr. (From Berson EL: Electroretinographic findings in retinitis pigmentosa. Jpn J Ophthalmol 31:327, 1987.)

night blindness in the second to fourth decade of life, have a partial high-tone hearing loss with intelligible speech, and do not show ataxia.[115] Patients with Usher's syndrome, type II have been shown to have abnormalities in the cilia of sperm and abnormalities in the connecting cilia in many remaining photoreceptors in autopsied eyes.[116–119]

Some 2 to 6 percent of congenitally deaf children have Usher's syndrome, type I. If a child presents with profound deafness and a balance disorder manifested by late onset of walking usually after 15 mo of age, the possibility of Usher's syndrome, type I should be considered.[119] The diagnosis of retinitis pigmentosa as part of Usher's syndrome, type I or type II can be made in early life with electroretinographic testing. Once a child is identified, the parents would know that with each succeeding childbirth they have a 25 percent chance of having a child with this condition. No tests are yet available to identify the carrier of Usher's syndrome, type I or type II.

The Laurence-Moon-Bardet-Biedl syndrome includes retinitis pigmentosa, mental retardation, polydactyly, truncal obesity, and hypogonadism as the most frequent features.[120–127] Some authors have noted that there are retinal and other abnormalities common to the two disorders but that polydactyly is found primarily in patients with the Bardet-Biedl form, whereas neurologic findings are found primarily in patients with the Laurence-Moon form.[128, 129] However, some patients have been described with both polydactyly and neurologic abnormalities and therefore would seem to qualify for inclusion in both syndromes.[130, 131] Variability of clinical expression is well known, and some patients may have this condition without mental retardation or without the polydactyly.[132–136] Renal disease can be a part of this syndrome,[137] and therefore patients should have their blood pressure and urine checked periodically.

Retinal degeneration is the most common feature of the Laurence-Moon-Bardet-Biedl syndrome, occurring in about 90 percent of cases.[137] The macula is often involved early, leading to the suggestion that these patients have an inverse form of retinitis pigmentosa. The fundus in early life may be granular without pigment formation so that the diagnosis is established only after electroretinographic testing.[138] A child born with polydactyly to normal parents should be suspected of having this syndrome. Once this syndrome is identified in one individual, parents would know that they have a 25 percent chance with each succeeding childbirth of having another child with this condition.

Leber's congenital amaurosis is an autosomal recessive disorder associated with severe reduction in vision near birth and very reduced ERGs.[139–144] Patients characteristically have hyperopia and nystagmus, and fundus examination reveals granularity, white flecks, or intraretinal bone spicule pigment, or some combination. Again, once this diagnosis is established based on the fundus appearance and an abnormal ERG, parents would know that they have a 25 percent chance with each succeeding childbirth of having a child with this condition. Retardation of mental development has been reported in some patients, possibly secondary to visual impairment.[143] Leber's congenital amaurosis involving the retina and pigment epithelium should not be confused with Leber's optic atrophy, a maternally inherited condition involving the optic nerve associated in some families with an abnormality in mitochondrial DNA.[145, 146] The gene abnormality and biochemical basis of Leber's congenital amaurosis are not yet known.

Retinitis punctata albescens can be associated with some signs and symptoms characteristic of retinitis pigmentosa.[147] Patients usually present with profound adaptational problems and gradual loss of peripheral vision. Examination with a direct ophthalmoscope will reveal multiple punctate white deposits around the mid-periphery at the level of the pigment epithelium for which this condition was named. Patients have retinal arteriolar attenuation and some have intraretinal bone spicule pigment in the midperiphery in one or two quadrants. This raises the possibility that this condition is a variant of retinitis pigmentosa[21, 148, 149] This form of retinal degeneration may affect the eyes of a patient asymmetrically; often these patients receive a neurologic evaluation in search of an intracranial abnormality before it is realized that the visual loss is due to a widespread retinal degeneration. Full-field ERGs in such patients are invariably abnormal, with reductions in amplitude and delays in implicit times. The condition is usually slowly progressive, although the course appears to vary from one individual to another. This condition has been thought to be inherited in an autosomal recessive mode, but a dominant mode of transmission can occur; therefore, ERG testing of relatives of affected patients is recommended to help establish the mode of transmission.

Atypical rare forms of retinitis pigmentosa include those designated as paravenous or unilateral. The paravenous form is usually characterized by slightly reduced full-field ERGs with normal implicit times and intraretinal pigment and atrophy of the pigment epithelium confined to the distribution of the retinal veins in each eye. Unilateral retinitis pigmentosa is characterized by fundus changes of retinitis pigmentosa in one eye with no evidence of retinal degeneration in the other eye. Full-field ERGs are substantially reduced in the affected eye and normal in the other eye. Patients with unilateral retinitis pigmentosa would not be expected to develop retinitis pigmentosa in the fellow eye at a later time. In the author's experience, patients with either paravenous or unilateral disease have presented with a negative family history for retinal degeneration, suggesting that these forms of retinitis pigmentosa are not inherited.

CHOROIDEREMIA

Young men with choroideremia characteristically have normal visual acuities, minimally increased dark-adaptation thresholds, and full visual fields to large test lights at a time when granularity and depigmentation of the retinal pigment epithelium are seen around the fundus periphery. ERGs are reduced in amplitude, with delays in b-wave implicit time (Fig. 106–14). In more advanced stages in adulthood, dark-adaptation thresholds are further increased, and the visual fields become constricted at a time when ERGs are undetectable and extensive choroidal atrophy and clumped pigment are visible around the peripheral fundus (see Fig. 106–1B). Men usually retain little, if any, central vision beyond the age of 60 yr.[150–154]

Obligate female carriers of this X-linked disease[155, 156] may demonstrate fundus changes that include patchy depigmentation of the retinal pigment epithelium and coarse pigment granularity or even pigment clumps in the periphery. However, carriers typically retain normal visual acuity and normal final dark-adapted rod

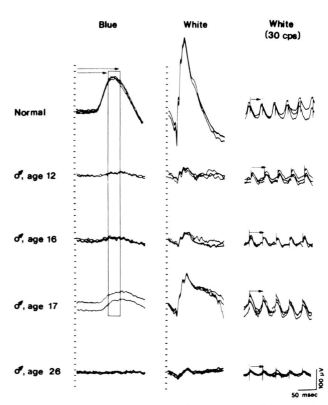

Figure 106–14. Electroretinographic responses of four males with choroideremia. Cone flicker responses to white 30-c.p.s. flicker remained detectable in the oldest male when rod responses to blue light were not detectable. Normal responses are shown for comparison. Time of stimulus onset is designated by *vertical hatched lines* in columns 1 and 2 and *vertical shock artifacts* in column 3. *Arrows* and *vertical bar* on rod responses to blue light show range of normal b-wave implicit times. Responses to single flashes of white light show reduced a- and b-wave amplitudes in all males. *Arrows* on white flicker responses show delayed implicit times in the affected males. (From Sieving PA, Niffenegger JH, Berson EL: Electroretinographic findings in selected pedigrees with choroideremia. Am J Ophthalmol 101:361–367, 1986. Published with permission from The American Journal of Ophthalmology. Copyright by The Ophthalmic Publishing Company.)

thresholds.[156, 157] Generally carriers have been thought to have a nonprogressive course,[158] but carriers with severe disease have been described.[159, 160] In contrast to the carrier state of X-linked retinitis pigmentosa, ERGs of carriers of choroideremia usually have been described as normal,[153, 154, 159] although reduced amplitudes have been reported in some cases.[152, 154, 161]

Study of a patient with choroideremia with a large deletion helped to assign the choroideremia gene to a small segment of the long arm of the X chromosome, specifically in the Xq21 band.[162, 163] By making use of gene linkage analyses and study of additional patients with microdeletions, eight overlapping complementary DNA (cDNA) clones were isolated from this chromosomal region.[164] The corresponding gene is expressed in retina, choroid, and retinal pigment epithelium. The cDNAs encompassed an open reading frame of 948 base pairs that was structurally altered in all eight patients studied.[164] The gene product and its role in the retina and pigment epithelium remain to be clarified.

Interfamilial and intrafamilial variability of clinical expression is known to exist in this disease. The natural course of choroideremia on a year-to-year basis is being investigated. Correlations, if any, between specific deletions and clinical expression of the disease remain to be evaluated. No treatment is yet known.

GYRATE ATROPHY OF THE CHOROID AND RETINA

Patients with gyrate atrophy of the choroid and retina have myopia, constricted visual fields, elevated dark-adaptation thresholds, small or nondetectable full-field ERGs, and characteristic chorioretinal atrophy distributed around the peripheral fundus and sometimes near the optic disc (see Fig. 106–1C).[165–167] The chorioretinal atrophy can differ in extent among young patients of comparable age. Patients develop cataracts and usually become virtually blind between the ages of 40 and 55 yr, with extensive chorioretinal atrophy.[167] Biochemical abnormalities include a 10- to 20-fold elevation of plasma ornithine levels,[168, 169] hypolysinemia,[170] hyperornithinuria,[170] and virtual lack of ornithine keto-acid aminotransferase (OAT) in extracts of cultured skin fibroblasts and in cultured lymphocytes.[170–172] Some patients have been reported to have seizures,[169] although neurologic examinations have been normal.[173] Electron microscopy has revealed morphologic changes in muscle fibers and hair shafts.[173, 174] Swollen mitochondria have been described in the retina.[175]

Genetic heterogeneity appears to exist, as some patients have shown a 30 to 50 percent fall in plasma ornithine levels within a week when given orally administered vitamin B$_6$ (300 to 500 mg/day), whereas other patients have not responded.[170, 176] All patients studied so far have had a decline in plasma ornithine levels of 50 percent or more when placed on a low-protein (15 g/day), low-arginine diet. Some young adults have shown increased areas of atrophy despite lowering of plasma ornithine levels with diet or a vitamin B$_6$ supplement to a plasma level of 300 to 400 nmol/ml (normal range 50 to 100 nmol/ml).[177] When plasma ornithine levels were lowered to less than 200 nmol/ml with diet for 5 to 7 yr in two pairs of siblings younger than 10 yr of age, the two younger affected siblings were virtually free of chorioretinal atrophy at an age when their older siblings were known to have atrophy.[178] The possible long-term beneficial effect of lowering plasma ornithine levels remains under investigation.

OAT is a mitochondrial matrix enzyme that catalyzes the intraconversion of ornithine and α-ketoglutarate to pyrroline-5-carboxylate and glutamate (Fig. 106–15).[179] The OAT structural gene has been assigned to chromosome 10 on the basis of expression of the human enzyme in somatic cell hybrid lines.[180] The OAT structural gene spans 21 kilobases of DNA, encoding a transcript of 2.2 kilobases in 11 exons.[181] Exon 1 appears to be part of the regulatory region of the gene. Exon 2, whose existence was indicated by its presence in a pseudogene from the X chromosome, has been lacking from cDNA, implying that it is spliced out of the mature OAT transcript.[181] Translation of OAT begins with exon 3. More than 20 point mutations in the OAT gene have been detected in gyrate atrophy patients.[182–186] A 9-base-pair deletion covering the splice acceptor region of exon 5 has also been reported, adding to the allelic heterogeneity observed in this disease.[187]

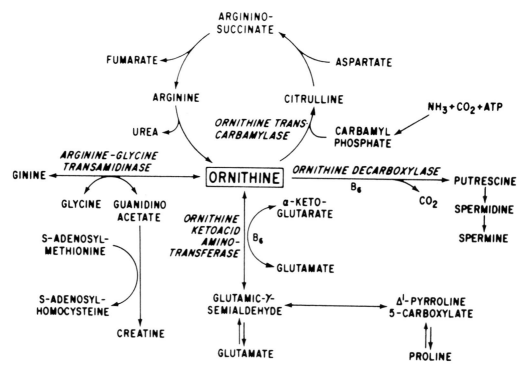

Figure 106–15. Pathways of ornithine metabolism. (From Weleber RG, Kennaway NG, Buist NR: Gyrate atrophy of the choroid and retina. Int Ophthalmol 4:26, 1981. Reprinted by permission of Kluwer Academic Publishers.)

OTHER RETINAL DEGENERATIONS

Retinal degenerations involving the photoreceptors across the retina can exist in association with other systemic findings. If a patient presents with ophthalmoplegia, the Kearns-Sayre syndrome should be considered. Abnormalities include ptosis, chronic progressive external ophthalmoplegia, a disturbance of the retinal pigment epithelium, ERGs that are usually reduced in amplitude, and respiratory distress. Some patients experience heart block and may require a pacemaker.[188–191] The diagnosis is confirmed by the observation of ragged red fibers on muscle biopsy specimens. This syndrome has been associated with mitochondrial DNA mutations; treatment of one patient with coenzyme Q10 and succinate resulted in clinical improvement of respiratory distress.[191] The value, if any, of this treatment for retinal malfunction remains to be established.

Patients who present with a widespread loss of photoreceptor function with abnormal ERGs and symptoms of cerebral deterioration may have a cerebroretinal degeneration, grouped under the overall heading of neuronal ceroid lipofuscinosis, or Batten's disease. Batten's disease can be subdivided into an infantile form (psychomotor deterioration by age 2 yr, ataxia, microcephaly, granular inclusions on conjunctival biopsy), a late-infantile form (seizures, rapid mental deterioration in early childhood, curvilinear inclusions on biopsy specimens), a juvenile form (mental deterioration beginning around age 6 yr, bull's-eye maculopathy, fingerprint inclusions on conjunctival biopsy), and an adult-onset form (seizures, slow dementia, abnormal inclusions best seen on muscle biopsy specimens). No proven treatment exists for these diseases.[192, 193]

Patients with olivopontocerebellar atrophy can present with a history of tremors, ataxia, and dysarthria and can show findings of oculomotor impairment and retinal degeneration. This condition is inherited in a dominant mode with variable penetrance. Some patients have retinal arteriolar attenuation, a diffuse disturbance of the retinal pigment epithelium, and very reduced ERGs. Some patients may show only neurologic findings and have normal fundi and normal retinal function, whereas others have abnormal ERGs with no diagnostic findings on fundus examination and no history of neurologic disease.[194–196] The cause of this condition and the basis for variable clinical expression remain to be defined.

Other rare syndromes associated with retinal degeneration include Alström's disease and Cockayne's syndrome. Patients with Alström's disease have retinitis pigmentosa with profound loss of vision in the first decade of life and very reduced ERGs. Systemic findings include diabetes mellitus, obesity, deafness, renal failure, baldness, and hypogenitalism.[197, 198] Patients with Cockayne's syndrome show extensive loss of vision by the second decade of life and have retinitis pigmentosa, dwarfism, deafness, mental deterioration, and premature aging. No treatments are known for these conditions.[199, 200]

STATIONARY FORMS OF NIGHT BLINDNESS

Five forms of stationary night blindness have been described as follows: (1) dominantly inherited congenital nyctalopia (Nougaret type), (2) recessively inherited stationary night blindness without myopia (Riggs type), (3) recessive or X-linked congenital nyctalopia with myopia (Schubert-Bornschein type), (4) recessively inherited Oguchi's disease, and (5) recessively inherited fundus albipunctatus.[201–210] It is the normality or near-normality of the cone system in the full-field ERGs that allows separation of most stationary forms of night blindness from practically all forms of night blindness associated with the early stages of retinitis pigmentosa (see Fig. 106–3).

Patients with dominantly inherited nyctalopia (Nougaret type) have a normal fundus appearance, normal or nearly normal cone ERGs, and absent rod ERG function. Fundus reflectometry studies have indicated that even though these patients have night blindness and a nondetectable rod ERG, they still have normal rhodopsin kinetics[211] and cone pigment kinetics that are normal or nearly normal.[212] The lack of a rod a-wave and the electrooculogram light-rise have led to the supposition that this condition involves the rod photoreceptors.[211, 213]

Recessively inherited stationary night blindness without myopia (Riggs type) is a rare form of stationary night blindness.[207, 214] In this type, the patient retains a normal cone ERG, has a normal fundus appearance, and after prolonged dark adaptation attains only normal dark-adapted cone threshold on psychophysical testing. The cone responses in patients with recessively inherited stationary night blindness without myopia are similar to those recorded from the dominantly inherited Nougaret type of nyctalopia. Rod ERG responses are lacking.

Patients with congenital nyctalopia with myopia (Schubert-Bornschein type) inherit their condition in either a sex-linked or an autosomal recessive mode.[206, 208, 214] The extent of the myopia is characteristically -3.5 to -14.5 D. Patients cannot attain normal dark-adapted rod thresholds and have fundus findings of myopia; rod ERG b-wave responses to dim blue light are undetectable, and the patients have a characteristic cornea-negative response to white light in the dark-adapted state and normal or nearly normal cone responses to 30-Hz white flicker (see Fig. 106–3). The defect appears to be some abnormality in intraretinal transmission of the response from the rod photoreceptors to proximal retinal cells. Rhodopsin kinetics measured by fundus reflectometry are normal and the light-rise of the EOG is preserved, so this condition is thought to involve a defect that is more proximal in the retina than is the defect in the Nougaret type of nyctalopia.[211] ERG amplitudes are reduced in congenital nyctalopia with myopia compared with those in normal emmetropia; this probably occurs because of the known reductions of ERG amplitude seen in patients with moderate axial myopia as the only finding.[215]

The ERG abnormality in congenital nyctalopia with

myopia has been reported as an acquired defect in patients with cutaneous malignant melanoma, who reported an acquired acute onset of night blindness with selective reduction in the rod b-wave response (Fig. 106–16).[216] Development of an antibody to the melanoma that also reacts to retinal cells with an interruption in rod signal transmission has been considered as a possible mechanism to account for the sudden onset of night blindness in these patients.

Patients with congenital nyctalopia (Schubert-Bornschein type) can be further subdivided into two groups designated as a "complete" or an "incomplete" form of the condition based on dark-adaptation measures and ERG amplitudes. In the complete form, responses are mediated by the cone system. In the incomplete form, rod ERG responses, although reduced in amplitude, are still measurable to dim blue light, and the cone ERG is also subnormal. Although patients with the complete form have moderate or high myopia, those with the incomplete form are thought to have mild myopia or slight hyperopia.[217] The long-term course of patients with the incomplete form remains to be established.

Patients with autosomal recessive Oguchi's disease usually require 2 to 12 hr to attain normal dark-adapted rod thresholds and show a characteristic change from a golden-brown fundus in the light-adapted state (see Fig. 106–1D) to a fundus of normal color in the dark-adapted state (the Mizuo phenomenon).[204] Following 1 hr of dark adaptation, patients with Oguchi's disease have no rod b-wave in response to dim blue light flashes, a cornea-negative response to white light, and a normal cone response to 30-Hz white flicker. Following complete dark adaptation after 12 hr, some patients have a normal rod b-wave amplitude and normal rod b-wave implicit time but only in response to one or two flashes of light.[218] Apparently the test flash used to elicit the ERG, although relatively dim, can be intense enough to cause the rod system to adapt to light. Rhodopsin kinetics are normal, and the light-rise of the EOG is preserved; therefore the defect in Oguchi's disease, like that in congenital nyctalopia with myopia, appears to be located more proximal in the retina than is the defect in the Nougaret type of nyctalopia.

Fundus albipunctatus is another form of recessively inherited stationary night blindness.[209, 219] Patients have yellow-white deposits in the deep retina outside the macula (see Fig. 106–1E). In contrast to the findings in Oguchi's disease, patients with fundus albipunctatus have a delay in rod visual pigment and foveal cone pigment regeneration, as monitored with fundus reflectometry.[209, 210] Changes in visual pigment levels parallel the prolonged cone and rod limbs of the dark-adaptation curve. Full-field ERGs have been found to be normal with respect to both cone and rod amplitudes and b-wave implicit times after full dark adaptation.[219] The findings in fundus albipunctatus suggest an abnormality in visual pigment regeneration secondary to some

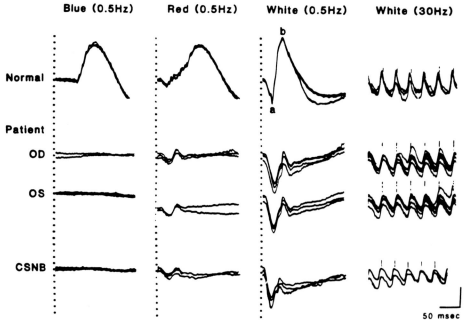

Figure 106–16. Full-field electroretinographic responses from a normal subject, from the right (O.D.) and left (O.S.) eyes of a patient with malignant melanoma, and from a patient with congenital stationary night blindness with myopia (*CSNB*). Stimulus onset is designated by the *vertical hatched lines* in columns 1, 2, and 3 and the *vertical lines* superimposed on the responses in column 4. Two or three consecutive responses are illustrated and cornea positivity is an upward deflection. The peak of the cornea-negative a-wave, generated by photoreceptors, and the peak of the cornea-positive b-wave, generated by activity of cells proximal to the photoreceptors, are designated in the response of the normal subject to single flashes of white light. Lower right, Calibration symbol designates 50 msec horizontally, 200 μV vertically for the top recording in column 3, and 100 μV vertically for all other tracings. Both patients lack the cornea-positive b-wave from the rod system in columns 1, 2, and 3 in contrast to the normal while retaining normal cone amplitudes (≥50 μV) in their responses to 30-Hz white flickering light in column 4. (From Berson EL, Lessell S: Paraneoplastic night blindness with malignant melanoma. Am J Ophthalmol 106:307–311, 1988. Published with permission from The American Journal of Ophthalmology. Copyright by The Ophthalmic Publishing Company.)

abnormality in the relationship between the photoreceptors and the pigment epithelium. The composition of the yellow-white lesions and their relationship to the abnormality in visual pigment regeneration are not known.

The defect in adaptation in Oguchi's disease differs from that in fundus albipunctatus. First, in Oguchi's disease the rod mechanism is affected at a time when psychophysical cone dark adaptation proceeds at a normal rate. Second, the defect appears to be proximal to the photoreceptors in Oguchi's disease, since the rate of rhodopsin regeneration, as measured by fundus reflectometry, is normal in contrast to that seen in fundus albipunctatus. Third, relatively weak illumination will delay the appearance of the rod branch of the dark-adaptation curve, as measured by psychophysical testing, by more than 30 min in Oguchi's disease, whereas exposure to a similar light produces a smaller effect in fundus albipunctatus. Oguchi's disease therefore appears to be a defect in rod neural adaptation, whereas fundus albipunctatus appears to represent a defect in visual pigment regeneration.[220, 221]

Molecular genetic defects for different forms of stationary night blindness remain to be defined. It will be of interest to see if those forms of stationary night blindness with abnormalities proximal to the photoreceptors involving intraretinal rod transmission are associated with a specific abnormality in neuroretinal transmitters. It is of interest that these diseases involving the rod photoreceptor or cells proximal to the rod photoreceptor are not associated with pigment migration or attenuation of the retinal vessels, whereas these latter findings are characteristically seen in patients with rod photoreceptor cell degeneration and retinitis pigmentosa.[221] Although the stationary forms of night blindness are rare, it is important to identify these conditions when patients present with night blindness on a retinal basis, as the long-term prognosis in these patients is good, in contrast to the progressive disease seen in patients with night blindness associated with retinitis pigmentosa.

APPROACH TO THE PATIENT

Patients with known or suspected retinitis pigmentosa or an allied disease should be asked to provide a history of the age of onset of night blindness, visual field loss, and loss of visual acuity. Symptoms of night blindness often reflect problems in adaptation under dim photopic conditions and therefore suggest cone malfunction. Patients with a sudden onset of night blindness, particularly after the age of 50 yr, should be considered candidates for a paraneoplastic process (i.e., nonocular malignancy with associated retinal malfunction) or so-called cancer-associated retinopathy.[216, 222, 223] Difficulties in reading may reflect a generalized loss of cone function or loss of cone function confined to the macula.

The medical history should include information on operations and illnesses as well as current medications and nutritional supplements. Intestinal surgery or liver disease may have affected the absorption or metabolism of vitamin A. Chronic intake of some medications (e.g., hydroxychloroquine, phenothiazines) may have compromised retinal function. The medical history should include information on the status of hearing, as some 15 percent of patients with retinitis pigmentosa have a high-tone partial hearing loss, and some 5 percent have profound congenital deafness. A history of polydactyly, mental retardation, or renal disease, if elicited, should raise the possibility of an association of these abnormalities with a retinal degeneration. A detailed family history is always warranted to determine if other members of the family are affected with retinal degeneration and to determine whether or not consanguinity exists in the parents, as this raises the likelihood of a hereditary disease.

The ocular examination should include a refraction; some 50 percent of patients with retinitis pigmentosa have 1 D or more of astigmatism in the less astigmatic eye.[32] Uncorrected myopia can be a cause of night blindness, and therefore it is important to establish that the patient has the correct prescription. Reading vision should be tested and lenses prescribed as needed to ensure that the patient can read at least 8-point print. Following an assessment of acuity and refractive error, a visual field determination should be performed with small and large test lights. Color vision testing should then be performed, preferably without dilatation and under standard lighting conditions. In our experience, the Farnsworth panel D15 and the Ishihara plates are adequate for initial screening for red and green color deficiencies; a tritan axis of confusion can occur in patients with retinitis pigmentosa.

Pupils are then maximally dilated with phenylephrine hydrochloride and cyclopentolate hydrochloride and the patient is patched. After 30 to 45 min of dark adaptation, final dark-adaptation thresholds are measured to establish whether or not the patient has impaired rod function. After dark-adaptation testing, full-field electroretinography is performed. If the responses are easily detected without computer averaging, the test can be accomplished within 10 to 15 min per eye; if computer averaging is required, the testing may take 20 to 30 min per eye. This sequence of evaluations helps to ensure that the patients have their dark-adaptation and ERG testing prior to more extensive light exposure associated with ophthalmoscopy that might cause light adaptation to occur and thereby affect the dark-adaptation and ERG measurements.

After the results of dark-adaptation and ERG testing are obtained, patients are examined with pupils fully dilated, at which time the refractive error can be confirmed by retinoscopy, and eyeglass prescriptions can be modified if necessary. A slit-lamp examination and direct and indirect ophthalmoscopy are performed; fine retinal deposits (e.g., as those seen in retinitis punctata albescens) and slight retinal arteriolar attenuation may be appreciated best with direct ophthalmoscopy. In patients with cataracts, retinal acuity can be obtained with a retinal potential acuity meter or equivalent instrument to compare retinal acuity with distance acuity.

In the case of isolate males with retinitis pigmentosa in whom X-linked disease must be suspected, the patient's mother should be evaluated if possible with both a fundus examination and ERG testing to determine whether or not she shows signs of a carrier state of X-linked disease and, if affected, how much retinal function remains. Carriers of X-linked retinitis pigmentosa have abnormal full-field ERGs in one or both eyes in more than 90 percent of cases, whereas carriers of autosomal recessive disease have normal fundi and normal ERG amplitudes. Establishment of a diagnosis of X-linked disease can be helpful in determining visual prognosis in a male patient with retinitis pigmentosa, since males with X-linked disease characteristically become legally blind by age 30 to 45 yr, whereas males with autosomal recessive disease usually become legally blind by age 45 to 60 yr.

At the initial examination, every effort should be made to establish the diagnosis, consider the best possible optical devices to maximize remaining vision, explain the genetic implications when indicated, and offer referral to appropriate psychologic, social, and community resources. Follow-up examinations are usually conducted every 2 yr to help determine the course of the disease as monitored by visual acuity, visual fields, and ERGs (computer-averaged in most cases); to adjust eyeglasses and provide low-vision aids if required; and to consider whether or not cataract surgery is indicated. Cataract surgery is usually deferred in the case of retinitis pigmentosa until a time when the patient cannot read with either eye. A trial with dilating drops (e.g., homatropine 2 percent taken at dusk) may be attempted to see if the patient can meet her or his visual needs without surgery. Cataract extraction has the greatest potential for improving vision among those patients who have cataracts large enough to impair visualization of the fundus with the ophthalmoscope as well as detectable ERGs with computer averaging as a measure of some remaining retinal function and evidence of retinal acuity that is better than distance acuity.

Acetazolamide has been advocated for patients with retinitis pigmentosa with cystoid macular edema; some individuals given this drug have shown an improvement in acuity and others have claimed subjective improvement without measurable change in acuity. The value of this treatment for such patients remains to be established.[224–226]

For patients less than 40 yr of age with autosomal recessive retinitis pigmentosa, serum lipoprotein electrophoresis and serum phytanic acid levels can be assessed after fasting for 12 hr if Bassen-Kornzweig syndrome or Refsum's disease are suspected. A plasma ornithine level can be obtained to confirm gyrate atrophy. A fasting serum vitamin A level can be obtained if nutritional deficiency or intestinal malabsorption is suspected. A serologic test for syphilis should be performed if this diagnosis is suspected, as retinitis pigmentosa has been associated with this disease.

Discussion of results of the ocular examination with the patient, and with the patient's family if indicated, must be individualized for each case, but in any event, every effort should be made to answer the patient's questions faithfully and provide a clear description not only of what abnormalities exist but also of how much function remains. In this regard, the measurement of any ERG function (with computer averaging if necessary) is of advantage, as the patient can be shown in positive terms what function remains. It is important to impress upon the patient that these conditions in general progress at a very slow rate. Remarks such as "Your vision may last for 2 yr or 30 yr" should be avoided, as the patient hears only the more severe prognosis and does not understand that in most instances she or he may well retain vision for 20 to 40 yr or more after the initial evaluation, particularly in the case of retinitis pigmentosa or choroideremia. It is often useful to hear what the patient believes she or he was told previously and to try to address any misconceptions. For example, some patients believe that retinal dystrophy and degeneration are "different diseases" and erroneously conclude that none of the physicians agree on the diagnosis.

Literature provided to the patient at the time of the visit is extremely important, as most patients cannot assimilate all the information given to them verbally. Printed information describing their condition, patterns of inheritance, reasons why they should be followed over time by their ophthalmologist, the significance of molecular genetic studies, and so on should be available for distribution in the office. Patients may wish to receive a copy of the results of the ocular examination; a visual display of their ERG responses as part of this report can be helpful in demonstrating to the patient the amount of retinal function remaining.

When a child is detected with retinitis pigmentosa or an allied retinal degeneration, parents must be provided with a full written report. If the parents agree, the child should be provided with sufficient verbal information at the time of the examination to allow the child to understand her or his own symptoms. For example, if the child has night vision deficiency, she or he should be advised to be careful when engaging in activities under conditions of dim illumination. If the child has a deficiency in side vision, she or he should be advised that it may be difficult if not unsafe to play certain sports (e.g., baseball or hockey). A child may well be legally blind because of loss of acuity and still be able to read with magnifying lenses; if this child has sufficient visual field, she or he may well be able to continue functioning in a regular school. In the author's experience, it is psychologically helpful to both the child and the parents to emphasize how much visual function remains rather than how much has been lost and to defer conclusions about long-term visual prognosis until the child has been examined several times over 2-yr intervals.

NIGHT VISION POCKETSCOPE

Advances in electrooptical technology have resulted in night vision devices that allow patients with retinitis pigmentosa, choroideremia, stationary night blindness, and allied diseases to use their cones to function under scotopic conditions (starlight or moonlight conditions) or, if necessary, under dim photopic conditions that exist at night near street lights or in a slightly darkened room.[227, 228] These light-amplifying devices have been incorporated into a monocular pocketscope or binocular goggles that can be used as an aid to alleviate the symptom of night blindness. The instruments contain bright point source protection so that a patient can view a dimly illuminated scene in the presence of automobile headlights or street lights. The monocular pocketscope (Fig. 106–17) is hand-held, with a 40-degree field of view. It provides patients with their best daylight vision at night for one eye. Candidates for this device are patients with best corrected vision of better than 20/200 in at least one eye, a field diameter of greater than 20

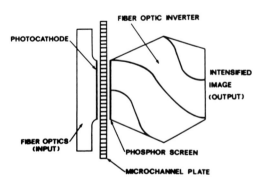

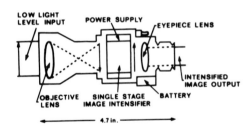

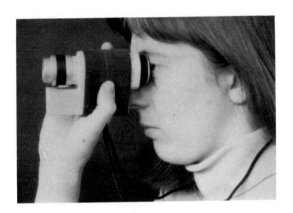

Figure 106–17: *Top,* Generation II night vision pocketscope adapted for patients with night blindness; patient holds to her eye. *Middle,* Diagram of a generation II night vision pocketscope. Instrument is 11.8 cm in length and 0.35 kg in weight and contains a single-stage image intensifier tube. The model is produced by International Telephone and Telegraph Corporation (ITT) and contains rechargeable batteries that are periodically recharged in a portable carrying case that is plugged into an ordinary wall receptacle. *Bottom,* Single-stage image intensifier tube, 3 cm in length, contained in the night vision pocketscope. (Reprinted with permission from Berson EL: Night blindness: Some aspects of management. *In:* Faye EE [ed]: Clinical Low Vision, Boston, Little, Brown and Company, 1976.)

degrees in that eye, and mobility in daylight with one eye patched. Patients who depend heavily on a far-temporal crescent for mobility are not good candidates, nor are patients who, because of a central scotoma, cannot view the output screen in the pocketscope. It is best that the patient be allowed to use the pocketscope in the field before making a decision on whether to obtain it. More than 200 pocketscopes have been prescribed in the United States, and the majority of patients have found the instrument helpful for mobility under conditions of dim illumination.

OTHER OPTICAL AIDS

Some patients with retinitis pigmentosa have reduced acuity. A closed circuit television for magnification is helpful in many instances, particularly because the patient can view the reading material as white on a black background, thereby reducing glare. For those who have difficulty tracking a line, a ruler or cutout window may be of value. Patients with night vision deficiency should be encouraged to carry a small penlight. Magnifying lenses put into an eyeglass frame are also helpful. Bifocals are to be avoided in patients with very constricted visual fields, as the lower segment may cut the visual field, so that the patient finds them less than useful. In the author's experience, field wideners have had limited, if any, value for patients with retinitis pigmentosa and allied conditions.

GENETIC COUNSELING

If retinitis pigmentosa is dominantly inherited (i.e., three consecutive generations with father-to-son transmission), each affected patient has a 1 in 2 chance with each childbirth of having a child of either sex with this condition. If retinitis pigmentosa is inherited by an autosomal recessive mode (i.e., at least two comparably affected female siblings or a male and female sibling comparably affected with normal parents or an isolate case with a family history of consanguinity), an affected patient has a 1 in 80 chance of marrying a carrier with this condition and the carrier has a 1 in 2 chance of passing on the abnormal gene; therefore, the chance of a patient with an autosomal recessive form of retinitis pigmentosa having an affected child is about 1 in 160 with each childbirth ($\frac{1}{80} \times \frac{1}{2}$). If a male has X-linked retinitis pigmentosa or choroideremia, all of his sons will be normal and all of his daughter will be carriers. If a woman is a carrier of X-linked retinitis pigmentosa or choroideremia, she has a 50 percent chance of having an affected son and a 50 percent chance of having a carrier daughter with each childbirth. Patients with isolate (simplex) retinitis pigmentosa (i.e., no known affected family members) can be considered to have recessive disease, although exceptions exist. All offspring of males or females with autosomal recessive retinitis pigmentosa are carriers of this condition; carriers enjoy normal vision but have about a 1 in 320 chance of having an affected child with each childbirth (i.e., 1 in 80 chance of marrying a carrier and, if married to a carrier, a 1 in 4 chance of having an affected child; $\frac{1}{80} \times \frac{1}{4} = \frac{1}{320}$). In the case of Usher's syndrome, type I, Usher's syndrome, type II, Leber's congenital amaurosis, or other autosomal recessive diseases, once a couple has one affected child they have a 1 in 4 chance with each succeeding childbirth of having another affected child.

In families with only one affected male, retinitis pigmentosa can be inherited in an autosomal recessive or X-linked mode; ERG testing and fundus examination of the mother can help determine whether or not she is a carrier of X-linked disease. A careful family history and examination of relatives of an affected patient with ERG testing can aid in establishing this mode of transmission. It is important to recognize that retinitis pigmentosa may skip generations and yet be transmitted in a dominant mode; the dominant mode with variable penetrance should be suspected in patients younger than 20 yr of age who have large cone ERGs (i.e., >40 μV) with substantial delays in implicit time.[55]

Patients often state that their children have had normal routine eye examinations and therefore must not have retinitis pigmentosa or an allied disease. In the author's experience, some young persons may have these diseases and yet appear normal on routine ocular examination. By age 30 yr, more than 90 percent of patients can be diagnosed with the ophthalmoscope, but in individuals less than 30 yr, ERG testing is indicated if the patient wants to be certain whether or not any relatives are affected. The ERG identifies those who are affected and those who are normal; in families with retinitis pigmentosa, patients aged 6 yr and older with normal ERGs would not be expected to develop the condition at a later time.

Advances with molecular genetic techniques undoubtedly will facilitate genetic counseling; e.g., some 25 to 30 percent of patients with autosomal dominant retinitis pigmentosa in the United States have rhodopsin gene mutations detectable through analysis of leukocyte DNA. Patients identified through analysis of DNA would have an ocular examination including ERG testing to confirm the diagnosis and to determine the amount of remaining retinal function, as variable clinical expression at a given age is known to exist among patients with the same rhodopsin gene mutation. Leukocyte DNA analysis should be considered not only for families with a known dominant mode of transmission over three consecutive generations but also for families with transmission over two consecutive generations or for isolate cases with presumably normal parents, as some of these patients may have a rhodopsin gene mutation described in dominant pedigrees, thereby helping to establish that the mode of inheritance is dominant. It is important to establish the correct genetic type in families with retinitis pigmentosa, not only for the sake of providing accurate genetic counseling but also as a guideline in establishing long-term visual prognoses of affected patients, as patients with dominantly inherited disease generally retain vision longer than those with recessive or X-linked disease.

PSYCHOLOGIC AND VOCATIONAL COUNSELING

Patients identified with progressive retinal degenerations for which no treatment is known often need psychologic counseling to help adjust to the knowledge that they are expected to lose their vision over time. Initial expressions of anger, frustration, despair, or depression are normal reactions in such patients, and they may need counseling in order to come to terms with their disease. Similarly, parents of affected patients may feel profound guilt when they learn about the genetic implications of the disease and may need psychologic counseling. Patients and their family members frequently benefit from a support group in which they can talk to others who have similar problems. Patients may also need guidance in selecting an appropriate vocation that they can pursue with their present vision and can continue to pursue in the event their vision fails. To this end, guidance provided by a trained specialist can be extremely helpful. It is very important that the patient be advised to return to an ophthalmologist every 1 to 2 yr. Patients with these diseases need periodic contact with their ophthalmologist to receive information on the course of their disease, to obtain whenever possible optical aids to maximize use of remaining vision, and in some cases to receive psychologic support.

SUNGLASSES

General agreement exists that patients with hereditary degenerations of the retina should avoid excessive exposure to bright sunlight outdoors until more is known about whether light stress will modify the course of this condition.[229] Two patients with retinitis pigmentosa who wore an opaque scleral contact lens over one eye for 8 to 10 hr/day for 5 yr showed comparable degeneration in both eyes, suggesting that this type of protection from light did not alter the course of disease.[230] Some patients have expressed a preference for orange photochromic sunglasses (e.g., Corning CPF 550) with tinted side shields or dark amber sunglasses (e.g., NoIR brand worn over an existing prescription) with tinted side shields. However, no particular type of sunglasses has been shown to alter the course of retinal degeneration. Until more is known, patients should be advised to select sunglasses for outdoor use that provide maximal comfort without compromising vision.

FUTURE DIRECTIONS

Analyses of leukocyte DNA provide an opportunity to determine the biochemical causes of different forms of retinitis pigmentosa and allied diseases. In all families studied so far with rhodopsin gene mutations, the mutations have segregated perfectly with the disease. The potential therefore exists to detect asymptomatic affected patients through analysis of DNA and study the functional consequences of gene abnormalities in the early stages of disease. Preliminary data have already revealed that a mutation near one end of the rhodopsin gene (i.e., Pro23His) is associated, on average, with less severe retinal disease at a given age than is a mutation near the other end (i.e., Pro347Leu). Additional research is needed to determine to what extent genotypes can be related to phenotypes.

It is now possible to inject mutant human gene constructs into mouse eggs to create transgenic models of human retinal degenerations. For example, transgenic mice with the rhodopsin, Pro23His mutation have been produced;[231] they show abnormal ERGs and photoreceptor cell degeneration and transmit the condition to about 50 percent of their offspring. Other transgenic animal models of human hereditary retinal degenerations will undoubtedly be described in the near future; these models can be used not only to define pathogenesis but also to search for treatments. Furthermore, mutant genes may be synthesized in the laboratory and their expression studied in a variety of in vitro systems.[232, 233] Antibodies produced to abnormal gene products may be applied to autopsied eyes of animal models as well as to patients with retinal degenerations to reveal the amount and distribution of the mutant gene product in remaining photoreceptor cells and thereby help clarify pathogenesis.

Electroretinographic testing, using computer averaging and narrow bandpass filtering, provides a basis for objectively monitoring the course of retinal degeneration in most patients with retinitis pigmentosa and allied diseases. Variability of clinical severity at a given age among patients with the same gene defects suggests that some factor or factors other than the gene defects themselves may be involved in the clinical expression of some forms of these diseases. Risk factor analyses of well-defined populations of patients with retinitis pigmentosa over time may reveal ameliorating or aggravating factors associated with the course of degeneration with possible implications for therapies.[234]

REFERENCES

1. Ammann F, Klein D, Franceschetti A: Genetic and epidemiological investigation of pigmentary degeneration of the retina and allied disorders in Switzerland. J Neurol Sci 2:183, 1965.
2. Boughman JA, Conneally PM, Nance WE: Population genetic studies of retinitis pigmentosa. Am J Hum Genet 32:223, 1980.
3. Hu DN: Genetic aspects of retinitis pigmentosa in China. Am J Med Genet 12:51, 1982.
4. Jay M: On the heredity of retinitis pigmentosa. Br J Ophthalmol 66:405, 1982.
5. Bundy S, Crews SJ: Wishes of patients with retinitis pigmentosa concerning genetic counseling. J Med Genet 19:317, 1982.
6. Bunker CH, Berson EL, Bromley WC, et al: Prevalence of retinitis pigmentosa in Maine. Am J Ophthalmol 97:357, 1984.
7. McWilliam P, Farrar GJ, Kenna P, et al: Autosomal dominant retinitis pigmentosa (ADRP): Localization of an ADRP gene to the long arm of chromosome 3. Genomics 5:619, 1989.
8. Inglehearn CF, Jay M, Lester DH, et al: The evidence for linkage between late onset autosomal dominant retinitis pigmentosa and chromosome 3 locus D3547 (C17): Evidence for genetic heterogeneity. Genomics 6:168, 1990.
9. Bhattacharya SS, Wright AF, Clayton JF, et al: Close genetic linkage between X-linked retinitis pigmentosa and a restriction fragment length polymorphism identified by recombinant DNA probe L1.28. Nature 309:253, 1984.
10. Musarella MA, Burghes A, Anson-Cartwright L, et al: Localization of the gene for X-linked recessive type of retinitis pigmentosa (XLRP) to Xp21 by linkage analysis. Am J Hum Genet 43:484, 1988.
11. Chen JD, Halliday F, Keith G, et al: Linkage heterogeneity between X-linked retinitis pigmentosa and a map of 10 RFLP loci. Am J Hum Genet 45:401, 1989.
12. Blanton SH, Heckenlively JR, Cottingham AW, et al: Linkage mapping of autosomal dominant retinitis pigmentosa (RP1) to the pericentric region of human chromosome 8. Genomics 11:857, 1991.
13. Farrar GJ, Kenna P, Jordan S, et al: A three-base-pair deletion in the peripherin-RDS gene in one form of retinitis pigmentosa. Nature 354:478, 1991.
14. Kajiwara K, Hahn L, Mukai S, et al: Mutations in the human retinal degeneration slow gene in autosomal dominant retinitis pigmentosa. Nature 354:480, 1991.
15. Donders FC: Beiträge zur pathologischen Anatomie des Auges. Graefes Arch Clin Exp Ophthalmol 2:106, 1857; 1:139, 1855.
16. Leber T: Die Pigmentdegeneration der Netzhaut und mit ihr verwandte Erkrankungen. In Graefe Saemisch-Hess, Handbuch der Gesamten Augenheilkunde, 2nd ed, vol. 7. Leipzig, Germany, W Engelmann, 1916, p 1076.
17. Bell J: Retinitis pigmentosa and allied diseases of the eye. In Pearson K (ed): Treasury of Human Inheritance, vol. 2. London, Cambridge University, 1922.
18. Franceschetti A, François J, Babel J: Les Héredodégenerescences Choriorétiniennes. Paris, Masson, 1963.
19. Duke-Elder S, Dobrie JH: Diseases of the Retina. In Duke-Elder S (ed): System of Ophthalmology, vol. 10. St Louis, CV Mosby, 1967.
20. Merin S, Auerbach E: Retinitis pigmentosa. Surv Ophthalmol 20:203, 1976.
21. Deutman AF: Rod cone dystrophy: Primary hereditary, pigmentary retinopathy, retinitis pigmentosa. In Krill AE, Archer DB (eds): Krill's Hereditary Retinal and Choroidal Disease, vol 2. Clinical Characteristics. New York, Harper & Row, 1977.
22. Marmor MF, Aguirre G, Arden G, et al: Retinitis pigmentosa, a symposium on terminology and methods of examination. Ophthalmology 90:126, 1983.
23. Pruett RC: Retinitis pigmentosa: Clinical observations and correlations. Trans Am Ophthalmol Soc 81:693, 1983.
24. Heckenlively JR: RP cone-rod degeneration. Trans Am Ophthalmol Soc 85:438, 1987.
25. Pagon RA: Retinitis pigmentosa. Surv Ophthalmol 33:137, 1988.
26. Heckenlively JR: Retinitis Pigmentosa. Philadelphia, JB Lippincott, 1988.
27. Newsome DA: Retinitis pigmentosa, Usher's syndrome, and other pigmentary retinopathies. In Newsome DA (ed): Retinal Dystrophies and Degenerations. New York, Raven, 1988.
28. Heckenlively JR: The frequency of posterior subcapsular cataract in the hereditary retinal degenerations. Am J Ophthalmol 93:733, 1982.
29. Fetkenhour CL, Choromokos E, Weinstein J, et al: Cystoid macular edema in retinitis pigmentosa. Trans Am Acad Ophthalmol Otolaryngol 83:515, 1977.
30. Fishman GA, Maggiero JM, Fishman M: Foveal lesions seen in retinitis pigmentosa. Arch Ophthalmol 95:1993, 1977.
31. Sieving PA, Fishman GA: Refractive errors of retinitis pigmentosa patients. Br J Ophthalmol 52:625, 1978.
32. Berson EL, Rosner B, Simonoff EA: Risk factors for genetic typing and detection in retinitis pigmentosa. Am J Ophthalmol 89:763, 1980.
33. Kolb H, Gouras P: Electron microscopic observations of human retinitis pigmentosa dominantly inherited. Invest Ophthalmol Vis Sci 13:487, 1974.
34. Szamier RB, Berson EL: Retinal ultrastructure in advanced retinitis pigmentosa. Invest Ophthalmol Vis Sci 16:947, 1977.
35. Szamier RB, Berson EL, Klein R, et al: Sex-linked retinitis pigmentosa: Ultrastructure of photoreceptors and pigment epithelium. Invest Ophthalmol Vis Sci 18:145, 1979.

36. Meyer KT, Heckenlively JR, Spitznas M, et al: Dominant retinitis pigmentosa: A clinicopathologic correlation. Ophthalmology 89:1414, 1982.
37. Santos-Anderson RM, Tso MOM, Fishman GA: A histopathologic study of retinitis pigmentosa. Ophthalmic Paediatr Genet 1:151, 1982.
38. Gartner S, Henkind P: Pathology of retinitis pigmentosa. Ophthalmology 89:1425, 1982.
39. Bunt-Milam AH, Kalina RE, Pagon RA: Clinical-ultrastructural study of a retinal dystrophy. Invest Ophthalmol Vis Sci 24:458, 1983.
40. Rodrigues MM, Wiggert B, Hackett J, et al: Dominantly inherited retinitis pigmentosa. Ultrastructure and biochemical analysis. Ophthalmology 92:1165, 1985.
41. Flannery JG, Farber DB, Bird AC, et al: Degenerative changes in a retina affected with autosomal dominant retinitis pigmentosa. Invest Ophthalmol Vis Sci 30:191, 1989.
42. Karpe G: The basis of clinical electroretinography. Acta Ophthalmol 23(Suppl):84, 1945.
43. Goodman G, Gunkel RD: Familial electroretinographic and adaptometric studies in retinitis pigmentosa. Am J Ophthalmol 46:142, 1958.
44. Gouras P, Carr RE: Electrophysiological studies in early retinitis pigmentosa. Arch Ophthalmol 72:104, 1964.
45. Berson EL, Gouras P, Gunkel RD: Rod responses in retinitis pigmentosa, dominantly inherited. Arch Ophthalmol 80:58, 1968.
46. Berson EL, Gouras P, Gunkel RD, et al: Dominant retinitis pigmentosa with reduced penetrance. Arch Ophthalmol 81:226, 1969.
47. Berson EL, Gouras P, Hoff M: Temporal aspects of the electroretinogram. Arch Ophthalmol 81:207, 1969.
48. Berson EL: Retinitis pigmentosa and allied diseases: Electrophysiologic findings. Trans Am Acad Ophthalmol Otolaryngol 81:659, 1976.
49. Berson EL: Electroretinographic findings in retinitis pigmentosa. Jpn J Ophthalmol 31:327, 1987.
50. Birch DG, Sandberg MA: Dependence of cone b-wave implicit time on rod amplitude in retinitis pigmentosa. Vision Res 27:1105, 1987.
51. Sandberg MA, Berson EL, Effron MH: Rod-cone interaction in the distal human retina. Science 212:829, 1981.
52. Berson EL: Retinitis pigmentosa, the electroretinogram, and Mendel's laws. Trans Pa Acad Ophthalmol Otolaryngol 26:109, 1973.
53. Berson EL, Rosen JB, Simonoff EA: Electroretinographic testing as an aid in detection of carriers of X-chromosome–linked retinitis pigmentosa. Am J Ophthalmol 87:460, 1979.
54. Fishman GA, Weinberg AB, McMahon TT: X-linked recessive retinitis pigmentosa: Clinical characteristics of carriers. Arch Ophthalmol 104:1329, 1986.
55. Berson EL, Simonoff EA: Dominant retinitis pigmentosa with reduced penetrance: Further studies of the electroretinogram. Arch Ophthalmol 97:1286, 1979.
56. Berson EL, Sandberg MA, Rosner B, et al: Natural course of retinitis pigmentosa over a three-year interval. Am J Ophthalmol 99:240, 1985.
57. Andréasson SOL, Sandberg MA, Berson EL: Narrow-band filtering for monitoring low-amplitude cone electroretinograms in retinitis pigmentosa. Am J Ophthalmol 105:500, 1988.
58. Birch DG, Berson EL, Sandberg MA: Diurnal rhythm in the human rod ERG. Invest Ophthalmol Vis Sci 25:236, 1984.
59. Birch DG, Sandberg MA, Berson EL: Diurnal rhythm in the human rod ERG: Relationship to cyclic lighting. Invest Ophthalmol Vis Sci 27:268, 1986.
60. Sandberg MA, Pawlyk BS, Berson EL: Electroretinogram (ERG) sensitivity and phagosome frequency in the normal pigmented rat. Exp Eye Res 43:781, 1986.
61. Birch DG: Diurnal rhythm in the human rod ERG—Normal subjects vs. retinitis pigmentosa. Invest Ophthalmol Vis Sci 28:235, 1987.
62. Sandberg MA, Pawlyk BS, Crane WG, et al: Diurnal rhythm in the ERG of the RCS pigmented rat. Invest Ophthalmol Vis Sci 28:111, 1987.
63. Sandberg MA, Baruzzi CM, Hanson AH III, Berson EL: Rod ERG diurnal rhythm in some patients with dominant retinitis pigmentosa. Invest Ophthalmol Vis Sci 29:494, 1988.
64. Kimberling WJ, Weston MD, Möller C, et al: Localization of Usher syndrome type II to chromosome 1q. Genomics 7:245, 1990.
65. Lewis RA, Otterud B, Stauffer D, et al: Mapping recessive ophthalmic diseases: Linkage of the locus for Usher syndrome type II to a DNA marker on chromosome 1q. Genomics 7:250, 1990.
66. Nathans J, Piantanida TP, Eddy RL, et al: Molecular genetics of inherited variation in human color vision. Science 232:203, 1986.
67. Sparkes RS, Klisak I, Kaufman D, et al: Assignment of the rhodopsin gene to human chromosome three, region 3q21–3q24 by in situ hybridization studies. Curr Eye Res 5:797, 1986.
68. Dryja TP, McGee TL, Reichel E, et al: A point mutation of the rhodopsin gene in one form of retinitis pigmentosa. Nature 343:364, 1990.
69. Dryja TP, McGee TL, Hahn LB, et al: Mutations within the rhodopsin gene in patients with autosomal dominant retinitis pigmentosa. N Engl J Med 323:1302, 1990.
70. Berson EL: Ocular findings in a form of retinitis pigmentosa with a rhodopsin gene defect. Trans Am Ophthalmol Soc 88:355, 1990.
71. Berson EL, Rosner B, Sandberg MA, et al: Ocular findings in patients with autosomal dominant retinitis pigmentosa and a rhodopsin gene defect (Pro23His). Arch Ophthalmol 109:92, 1991.
72. Berson EL, Rosner B, Sandberg MA, et al: Ocular findings in patients with autosomal dominant retinitis pigmentosa and rhodopsin, proline-347-leucine. Am J Ophthalmol 111:614, 1991.
73. Berson EL, Sandberg MA, Dryja TP: Autosomal dominant retinitis pigmentosa with rhodopsin, valine-345-methionine. Trans Am Ophthalmol Soc 89:117, 1991.
74. Bhattacharya S, Lester D, Keen TJ, et al: Retinitis pigmentosa and mutations in rhodopsin. Lancet 337:185, 1991.
75. Dryja TP, Hahn LB, Cowley GS, et al: Mutation spectrum of the rhodopsin gene among patients with autosomal dominant retinitis pigmentosa. Proc Natl Acad Sci USA 88:9370, 1991.
76. Farrar GJ, Kenna P, Redmond R, et al: Autosomal dominant retinitis pigmentosa: A mutation in codon 178 of the rhodopsin gene in two families of Celtic origin. Genomics 11:1170, 1991.
77. Fishman GA, Stone EM, Gilbert LD, et al: Ocular findings associated with a rhodopsin gene codon 58 transversion mutation in autosomal dominant retinitis pigmentosa. Arch Ophthalmol 109:1387, 1991.
78. Fujiki K, Hotta Y, Shiono T, et al: Codon 347 mutation of the rhodopsin gene in a Japanese family with autosomal dominant retinitis pigmentosa. Am J Hum Genet 49(Suppl):187, 1991.
79. Gal A, Artlich A, Ludwig M, et al: Pro347Arg mutation of the rhodopsin gene in autosomal dominant retinitis pigmentosa. Genomics 11:468, 1991.
80. Heckenlively JR, Rodriguez JA, Daiger SP: Autosomal dominant sectoral retinitis pigmentosa. Two families with transversion mutation in codon 23 of rhodopsin. Arch Ophthalmol 109:84, 1991.
81. Inglehearn CF, Bashir R, Lester DH, et al: A 3-bp deletion in the rhodopsin gene in a family with autosomal dominant retinitis pigmentosa. Am J Hum Genet 48:26, 1991.
82. Jacobson SG, Kemp CM, Sung CH, et al: Retinal function and rhodopsin levels in autosomal dominant retinitis pigmentosa with rhodopsin mutations. Am J Ophthalmol 112:256, 1991.
83. Keen TJ, Inglehearn CF, Lester DH, et al: Autosomal dominant retinitis pigmentosa: Four new mutations in rhodopsin, one of them in the retinal attachment site. Genomics 11:199, 1991.
84. Richards JE, Kuo CY, Boehnke M, et al: Rhodopsin Thr58Arg mutation in a family with autosomal dominant retinitis pigmentosa. Ophthalmology 98:1797, 1991.
85. Sheffield VC, Fishman GA, Beck JS, et al: Identification of novel rhodopsin mutations associated with retinitis pigmentosa by GC-clamped denaturing gradient gel electrophoresis. Am J Hum Genet 49:699, 1991.
86. Sorscher EJ, Huang Z: Diagnosis of genetic disease by primer-specified restriction map modification, with application to cystic fibrosis and retinitis pigmentosa. Lancet 337:1115, 1991.

87. Stone EM, Kimura AE, Nichols BE, et al: Regional distribution of retinal degeneration in patients with the proline to histidine mutation in codon 23 of the rhodopsin gene. Ophthalmology 98:1806, 1991.
88. Sung CH, Davenport CM, Hennessey JC, et al: Rhodopsin mutations in autosomal dominant retinitis pigmentosa. Proc Natl Acad Sci USA 88:6481, 1991.
89. Sung CH, Schneider BG, Agarwal N, et al: Functional heterogeneity of mutant rhodopsins responsible for autosomal dominant retinitis pigmentosa. Proc Natl Acad Sci USA 88:8840, 1991.
90. Fishman GA, Stone EM, Sheffield VC, et al: Ocular findings associated with rhodopsin gene codon 17 and codon 182 transition mutations in dominant retinitis pigmentosa. Arch Ophthalmol 110:54, 1992.
91. Hargrave PA, O'Brien PJ: Speculations on the molecular basis of retinal degeneration in retinitis pigmentosa. In Anderson RE, Hollyfield JG, La Vail MM (eds): Retinal Degenerations. Boca Raton, FL, CRC Press, 1991.
92. Khorana HG: Rhodopsin, photoreceptor of the rod cell. An emerging pattern for structure and function. J Biol Chem 267:1, 1992.
93. Rosenfeld PH, Cowley GS, McGee TL, et al: Null mutations within the rhodopsin gene as a cause of rod photoreceptor dysfunction and autosomal recessive retinitis pigmentosa. Nature Genet 1:209, 1992.
94. Biro I: Therapeutic experiments in cases of retinitis pigmentosa. Br J Ophthalmol 23:332, 1939.
95. Gordon DM: The treatment of retinitis pigmentosa with special reference to the Filatov method. Am J Ophthalmol 30:565, 1947.
96. Campbell DA, Harrison R, Tonks EL: Retinitis pigmentosa: Vitamin A serum levels in relation to clinical findings. Exp Eye Res 3:412, 1964.
97. Chatzinoff A, Nelson E, Stahl N, et al: Eleven-cis vitamin A in the treatment of retinitis pigmentosa: A negative study. Arch Ophthalmol 80:417, 1968.
98. Bergsma DR, Wolf ML: A therapeutic trial of vitamin A in patients with pigmentary retinal degeneration: A negative study. In Landers MA, Wolbarsht ML, Laties AM, et al (eds): Retinitis Pigmentosa. New York, Plenum, 1976.
99. Katznelson LA, Khoroshilova-Maslova IP, Eliseyeva RF: A new method of treatment of retinitis pigmentosa/pigmentary abiotrophy. Ann Ophthalmol 22:167, 1990.
100. Duke-Elder S, Dobrie JH: System of ophthalmology. In Duke-Elder S (ed): Diseases of the Retina, vol. 10. St Louis, CV Mosby, 1967.
101. Bassen FA, Kornzweig AL: Malformation of the erythrocytes in a case of atypical retinitis pigmentosa. Blood 5:381, 1950.
102. Salt HB, Wolff OH, Lloyd JK, et al: On having no betalipoprotein. A syndrome comprising A-beta-lipoproteinemia, acanthocytosis and steatorrhea. Lancet 2:325, 1960.
103. Schaefer EJ: Diagnosis and management of ocular abnormalities in abetalipoproteinemia. In Zrenner E, Krastel H, Goebel HH (eds): Research in Retinitis Pigmentosa, Advances in Biosciences, vol. 62. Oxford, England, Pergamon Journals, 1987.
104. Gouras P, Carr RE, Gunkel RD: Retinitis pigmentosa in abetalipoproteinemia: Effects of vitamin A. Invest Ophthalmol Vis Sci 10:784, 1971.
105. von Sallmann L, Gelderman AH, Laster L: Ocular histopathologic changes in a case of a-beta-lipoproteinemia (Bassen-Kornzweig syndrome). Doc Ophthalmol 26:451, 1969.
106. Bishara S, Merin S, Cooper M, et al: Combined vitamin A and E therapy prevents retinal electrophysiological deterioration in abetalipoproteinemia. Br J Ophthalmol 66:767, 1982.
107. Refsum S: Heredopathia atactica polyneuritiformis: A familial syndrome not hitherto described. Acta Psychiatr Neurol Scand (Suppl) 38:1, 1946.
108. Klenk E, Kahlke W: Über das Vorkommen der 3,7,11,15-tetramethylhexadecansäure (Phytansäure) in den Cholesterinestern und anderen Lipoidfraktionen der Organe bei einem Krankheitsfall unbekannter Genese: Verdacht auf Heredopathia atactica polyneuritiformis (Refsum syndrome). Hoppe Seylers Z Physiol Chem 333:133, 1963.
109. Berson EL: Nutrition and retinal degenerations: Vitamin A, taurine, ornithine and phytanic acid. Retina 2:236, 1982.
110. Eldjarn L, Stokke O, Try K: α-Oxidation of branched chain fatty acids in man and its failure in patients with Refsum's disease showing phytanic acid accumulation. Scand J Clin Lab Invest 18:694, 1966.
111. Toussaint D, Danis P: An ocular pathologic study of Refsum's syndrome. Am J Ophthalmol 72:342, 1971.
112. Eldjarn L, Stokke O, Try K: Biochemical aspects of Refsum's disease and principles for the dietary treatment. In Vinken PJ, Bruyn GW (eds): Handbook of Clinical Neurology. Amsterdam, North-Holland, 1976.
113. Refsum S: Heredopathia atactica polyneuritiformis, phytanic acid storage disease Refsum's disease: A biochemically well-defined disease with a specific dietary treatment. Arch Neurol 38:605, 1981.
114. Usher CH: The Bowman lecture: On a few hereditary eye affections. Trans Ophthalmol Soc UK 55:164, 1935.
115. Fishman GA, Kumar A, Joseph ME, et al: Usher's syndrome: Ophthalmic and neuro-otologic findings suggesting genetic heterogeneity. Arch Ophthalmol 101:1367, 1983.
116. Hunter DG, Fishman GA, Mehta RS, et al: Abnormal sperm and photoreceptor axonemes in Usher's syndrome. Am J Ophthalmol 104:385, 1986.
117. Barrong SD, Chaitin MH, Fliesler SJ, et al: Ultrastructure of connecting cilia in different forms of retinitis pigmentosa. Arch Ophthalmol 110:706, 1992.
118. Berson EL, Adamian M: Ultrastructural findings in an autopsy eye from a patient with Usher's syndrome, type II. Am J Ophthalmol, in press.
119. Vernon M: Usher's syndrome—Deafness and progressive blindness. Clinical cases, prevention, theory and literature survey. J Chronic Dis 22:133, 1969.
120. Laurence JZ, Moon RC: Four cases of "retinitis pigmentosa," occurring in the same family, and accompanied by general imperfections of development. Ophthalmic Rev (Old Series) 2:32, 1866.
121. Hutchinson J: Slowly progressive paraplegia and disease of the choroids with defective intellect and arrested sexual development in several brothers and a sister. Arch Surg (Lond) 11:118, 1900.
122. Bardet G: Sur un syndrome d'obésité congénitale avec polydactylie et rétinite pigmentaire (contribution à l'étude des formes cliniques de l'obésité hypophysaire). These de Paris: Amédée Legrand, 1920.
123. Biedl A: Ein Geschwisterpaar mit adiposo-genitaler Dystrophie. Dtsch Med Wochenschr 48:1630, 1922.
124. Luz MF, Marques MNT, Jorge E, et al: The Laurence-Moon-Bardet-Biedl syndrome. Metab Pediatr Syst Ophthalmol 8:15, 1985.
125. Ehrenfeld EN, Rowe H, Auerbach E: Laurence-Moon-Bardet-Biedl syndrome in Israel. Am J Ophthalmol 70:524, 1970.
126. Sorsby A, Avery H, Cockayne EA: Obesity, hypogenitalism, mental retardation, polydactyly, and retinal pigmentation; the Laurence-Moon-Bardet-Biedl syndrome. QJ Med (New Series) 8:51, 1939.
127. Stiggelbout W: The Bardet-Biedl syndrome: Including Hutchinson-Laurence-Moon syndrome. In Vinken PJ, Bruyn GW (eds): Handbook of Clinical Neurology, vol. 13. Neuroretinal Degenerations. Amsterdam, North-Holland, 1972.
128. Schachat AP, Maumenee IH: Bardet-Biedl syndrome and related disorders. Arch Ophthalmol 100:285, 1982.
129. Campo RV, Aaberg TM: Ocular and systemic manifestations of the Bardet-Biedl syndrome. Am J Ophthalmol 94:750, 1982.
130. Björk A, Lindblom U, Wadensten L: Retinal degeneration in hereditary ataxia. J Neurol Neurosurg Psychiatry 19:186, 1956.
131. Rizzo J, Berson EL, Lessell S: Retinal and neurological findings in the Laurence-Moon-Bardet-Biedl phenotype. Ophthalmology 93:1452, 1986.
132. Ammann F: Investigations cliniques et génétiques sur le syndrome de Bardet-Biedl en Suisse. J Genet Hum 18(Suppl):287, 1970.
133. Stanescu B, Evrard P, Michiels J, et al: Electroretinographic changes in a case of spino-cerebellar degeneration (SCD). Metab Pediatr Ophthalmol 4:221, 1980.
134. Klein D, Ammann F: The syndrome of Laurence-Moon-Bardet-Biedl and allied diseases in Switzerland: Clinical, genetic, and epidemiological studies. J Neurol Sci 9:479, 1969.
135. Froment J, Bonnet P, Colrat A: Hérédo-dégénérations réti-

nienne et spino-cérébelleuse. Variantes ophthalmoscopiques et neurologiques présentées par trois générations successives. J Med Lyon 18:153, 1937.

136. Berson EL, Gouras P, Gunkel RD: Progressive cone-rod degeneration. Arch Ophthalmol 80:68, 1968.

137. Bell J: The Laurence-Moon Syndrome. In Penrose LS (ed): The Treasury of Human Inheritance, vol. 5, part III. Cambridge, England, Cambridge University Press, 1958.

138. Krill AE, Folk E, Rosenthal IM: Electroretinography in the Laurence-Moon-Biedl syndrome: An aid in diagnosis of the atypical case. Am J Dis Child 102:205, 1961.

139. Leber T: Ueber Retinitis pigmentosa und angeborene Amaurose. Graefes Arch Clin Exp Ophthalmol 15:1, 1869.

140. Franceschetti A, Dieterlé P: Importance diagnostique et prognostique de l'électrorétinogramme (ERG) dans les dégénérescenses tapéto-rétiniennes avec rétrécissement du champ visuel et héméralopie. Confinia Neurologica 14:184, 1954.

141. François J: Leber's congenital tapetoretinal degeneration. Int Ophthalmol Clin 8:929, 1968.

142. Noble KG, Carr RE: Leber's congenital amaurosis. A retrospective study of 33 cases and a histopathological study of one case. Arch Ophthalmol 96:818, 1978.

143. Nickel B, Hoyt CS: Leber's congenital amaurosis: Is mental retardation a frequent associated defect? Arch Ophthalmol 100:1089, 1982.

144. Heher KL, Traboulsi EI, Maumenee IH: The natural history of Leber's congenital amaurosis: Age-related findings in 35 patients. Ophthalmology 99:241, 1992.

145. Wallace DC, Singh G, Lott MT, et al: Mitochondrial DNA mutation associated with Leber's hereditary optic neuropathy. Science 242:1427, 1988.

146. Neumann NJ, Lott MT, Hallare DC: The clinical characteristics of pedigrees of Leber's hereditary optic neuropathy with the 11778 mutation. Am J Ophthalmol 111:750, 1991.

147. Mooren A: Fünf Lustren ophthalmologischer Wirksamkeit. Wiesbaden, Bergmann, 1882.

148. Kurozumi I, Ohara M, Yasui T, et al: Case of retinitis punctata albescens in a boy and degeneratio pigmentosa retinae sine pigmento in his sister. J Clin Ophthalmol (Tokyo) 17:177, 1963.

149. Krill AE: Incomplete rod-cone degenerations. In Krill AD (ed), with special assistance of Archer DB: Krill's Hereditary Retinal and Choroidal Diseases, vol. 2. Clinical Characteristics. New York, Harper & Row, 1977.

150. Mauthner L: Ein Fall von Choroideremia. Ber Natur Med Ver Innsbruch 2:191, 1872.

151. McCulloch C: Choroideremia. A clinical and pathologic review. Trans Am Ophthalmol Soc 67:142, 1969.

152. Pameyer JK, Waardenburgh PJ, Henkes HE: Choroideremia. Br J Ophthalmol 44:724, 1960.

153. Bounds GW Jr, Johnston TL: The electroretinogram in choroideremia. Am J Ophthalmol 39:166, 1955.

154. Sieving PA, Niffenegger JH, Berson EL: Electroretinographic findings in selected pedigrees with choroideremia. Am J Ophthalmol 101:361, 1986.

155. Goedbloed J: Mode of inheritance of choroideremia. Ophthalmologica 104:308, 1942.

156. McCulloch C, McCulloch RJP: A hereditary and clinical study of choroideremia. Trans Am Acad Ophthalmol 52:160, 1948.

157. Sorsby A: Ophthalmic Genetics, 2nd ed. New York, Appleton-Century-Crofts, 1970.

158. Kurstjens JH: Choroideremia and gyrate atrophy of the retina and choroid. Doc Ophthalmol 19:1, 1965.

159. Fraser GR, Friedmann AI: Choroideremia in a female. Br Med J 2:732, 1968.

160. Jacobson J, Stephens G: Hereditary choroidoretinal degeneration. Study of a family including electroretinography and adaptometry. Arch Ophthalmol 67:321, 1962.

161. Harris GS, Miller JR: Choroideremia. Arch Ophthalmol 80:423, 1968.

162. Cremers FPM, Sankila E-M, Brunsmann F, et al: Deletions in patients with classical choroideremia vary in size from 45 kb to several megabases. Am J Hum Genet 47:622, 1990.

163. Cremers FPM, van de Pol DJR, Wieringa B, et al: Chromosomal jumping from the DXS165 locus allows molecular characterization of four microdeletions and a de novo chromosome X/13

164. Cremers FPM, van de Pol DJR, van Kerkhoff LPM, et al: Cloning of a gene that is rearranged in patients with choroideraemia. Nature 347:674, 1990.

165. Cutler CW: Drei ungewöhnliche Fälle von Retino-Choroideal-Degeneration. Arch Augenheilkd 30:117, 1895.

166. Fuchs E: Über zwei der Retinitis pigmentosa verwandte Krankheiten (Retinitis punctata albescens und atrophia gyrata choroideae et retinae). Arch Augenheilkd 32:111, 1896.

167. Takki KK, Milton RC: The natural history of gyrate atrophy of the choroid and retina. Ophthalmology 88:292, 1981.

168. Simmel O, Takki K: Raised plasma-ornithine and gyrate atrophy of the choroid and retina. Lancet 2:1031, 1973.

169. Takki K: Gyrate atrophy of the choroid and retina associated with hyperornithinaemia. Br J Ophthalmol 58:3, 1974.

170. Berson EL, Schmidt SY, Shih VE: Ocular and biochemical abnormalities in gyrate atrophy of the choroid and retina. Ophthalmology 85:1018, 1978.

171. Trijbels JMF, Sengers RCA, Bakkeren JAJM, et al: L-Ornithine-ketoacid-transaminase deficiency in cultured fibroblasts of a patient with hyperornithemia and gyrate atrophy. Clin Chem Acta 79:371, 1977.

172. Valle D, Kaiser-Kupfer MI, Del Valle LA: Gyrate atrophy of the choroid and retina: Deficiency of ornithine amino-transferase in transformed lymphocytes. Proc Natl Acad Sci USA 74:5159, 1977.

173. Kaiser-Kupfer MI, Kuwabara T, Askanas V, et al: Systemic manifestations of gyrate atrophy of the choroid and retina. Ophthalmology 88:302, 1981.

174. Vannas-Sulonen K, Sipila I, Vanna A, et al: Gyrate atrophy of the choroid and retina: A five-year follow-up of creatine supplementation. Ophthalmology 92:1719, 1985.

175. Wilson DJ, Weleber RG, Green WR: Gyrate atrophy of the choroid and retina: A clinicopathologic correlation. Am J Ophthalmol 11:24, 1991.

176. Weleber RG, Kennaway NG: Clinical trial of vitamin B$_6$ for gyrate atrophy of the choroid and retina. Ophthalmology 88:316, 1981.

177. Berson EL, Hanson AH, Rosner B, et al: A two-year trial of low-protein, low-arginine diets of vitamin B$_6$ for patients with gyrate atrophy. In Cotlier E, Maumenee I, Berman E (eds): Birth Defects: Original Article Series. New York, AR Liss, 1982.

178. Kaiser-Kupfer MI, Caruso RC, Valle D: Gyrate atrophy of the choroid and retina, long-term reduction of ornithine slows retinal degeneration. Arch Ophthalmol 109:1539, 1991.

179. Weleber RG, Kennaway NG, Buist NR: Gyrate atrophy of the choroid and retina. Int Ophthalmol 4:23, 1981.

180. O'Donnell JQ, Vannas-Sulonen K, Shaw TB, et al: Gyrate atrophy of the choroid and retina: Assignment of the ornithine aminotransferase structural gene to human chromosome 10 and mouse chromosome 7. Am J Hum Genet 43:922, 1988.

181. Mitchell GA, Looney JE, Brody LC, et al: Human ornithine aminotransferase cDNA cloning and analysis of the structural gene. J Biol Chem 263:14288, 1988.

182. Mitchell G, Brody L, Looney J, et al: An initiator codon mutation in ornithine delta aminotransferase causing gyrate atrophy of choroid and retina. J Clin Invest 81:630, 1988.

183. Ramesh V, McClatchey AI, Ramesh N, et al: Molecular basis of ornithine aminotransferase deficiency in B-6-responsive and -nonresponsive forms of gyrate atrophy. Proc Natl Acad Sci USA 85:3777, 1988.

184. Mitchell GA, Brody LC, Sipila I, et al: At least two mutant alleles of ornithine aminotransferase cause gyrate atrophy of the choroid and retina in Finns. Proc Natl Acad Sci USA 86:197, 1989.

185. Inana G, Chambers C, Hotta Y, et al: Point mutation affecting processing of the ornithine aminotransferase precursor protein in gyrate atrophy. J Biol Chem 264:17432, 1989.

186. Brody LC, Mitchell GA, Obie C, et al: Ornithine δ-aminotransferase mutations in gyrate atrophy. J Biol Chem 267:3302, 1992.

187. McClatchey AI, Kaufman DL, Berson EL, et al: Splicing defect at the ornithine aminotransferase (OAT) locus in gyrate atrophy. Am J Hum Genet 47:790, 1990.

188. Kearns TP, Sayre GP: Retinitis pigmentosa, external ophthal-

moplegia, and complete heart block: Unusual syndrome with histologic study in one of two cases. Arch Ophthalmol 60:280, 1958.

189. Kearns TP: External ophthalmoplegia, pigmentary degeneration of the retina, and cardiomyopathy: A newly recognized syndrome. Trans Am Ophthalmol Soc 63:559, 1965.
190. Eagle RC, Hedges TR, Yanoff M: The atypical pigmentary retinopathy of Kearns-Sayre syndrome: A light and electron microscopic study. Ophthalmology 89:1433, 1982.
191. Shoffner JM, Lott MT, Voljavec AS, et al: Spontaneous Kearns-Sayre/chronic external ophthalmoplegia plus syndrome associated with a mitochondrial DNA deletion: A slip-replication model and metabolic therapy. Proc Natl Acad Sci USA 86:7952, 1989.
192. Batten FE: Cerebral degeneration with macular change (so-called juvenile form of family amaurotic idiocy). Q J Med 7:444, 1914.
193. Weleber RG: Retinitis pigmentosa and allied disorders. In Ryan SJ (ed): Retina, vol. 1. St Louis, CV Mosby, 1989.
194. Hamilton SR, Chatrian GE, Mills RP, et al: Cone dysfunction in a subgroup of patients with autosomal dominant cerebellar ataxia. Arch Ophthalmol 108:551, 1990.
195. Traboulsi EI, Maumenee IH, Green WR, et al: Olivopontocerebellar atrophy with retinal degeneration: A clinical and ocular histopathologic study. Arch Ophthalmol 106:801, 1988.
196. To KW, Adamian M, Jakobiec FA, et al: Olivopontocerebellar atrophy with retinal degeneration: An electroretinographic and histopathologic investigation. Ophthalmology, in press.
197. Alström CH, Hallgren B, Nilsson LB: Retinal degeneration combined with obesity, diabetes mellitus and neurogenous deafness: A specific syndrome (not hitherto described) distinct from the Laurence-Moon-Bardet-Biedl syndrome—Clinical, endocrinological, and genetic examination based on a large pedigree. Acta Psychiatr Neurol Scand 34(Suppl 129):1, 1959.
198. Millay RH, Weleber RG, Heckenlively JR: Ophthalmologic and systemic manifestations of Alström's disease. Am J Ophthalmol 102:482, 1986.
199. Cockayne EA: Dwarfism with retinal atrophy and deafness. Arch Dis Child 11:1, 1936.
200. Pearce WG: Ocular and genetic features of Cockayne's syndrome. Can J Ophthalmol 7:435, 1972.
201. Cunier R: Histoire d'une hémérolopie, héréditaire depuis siecles dans un famille do la commune de Vendemian, pres Montpellier. Ann Soc Med de Gand 4:385, 1838.
202. Nettleship E: A history of congenital stationary night blindness in nine consecutive generations. Trans Ophthalmol Soc UK 27:269, 1907.
203. Oguchi C: Über die eigenartige Hemeralopie mit diffuser weissgraulicher Verfärbung des Augenhintergrundes. Graefes Arch Clin Ophthalmol 81:109, 1912.
204. Mizuo G: On a new discovery in the dark adaptation on Oguchi's disease. Acta Soc Ophthalmol Jpn 17:1148, 1913.
205. Lauber H: Die sogenannte Retinitis punctata albescens. Klin Monatsbl Augenheilkd 48:133, 1910.
206. Schubert G, Bornschein H: Beitrag zur Analyse des Menschlichen Elektroretinogramms. Ophthalmologica 123:396, 1952.
207. Riggs LA, Wooten BR: Electrical measures and psychophysical data on human vision. In Jameson D, Hurvich LM (eds): Handbook of Sensory Physiology, vol. 7/4. New York, Springer-Verlag, 1972.
208. Carr RE: Congenital stationary night blindness. Trans Am Ophthalmol Soc 72:448, 1974.
209. Carr RE, Ripps H, Siegel IM: Visual pigment kinetics and adaptation in fundus albipunctatus. In Documenta Ophthalmologica proceedings series. Eleventh International Society for Clinical Electroretinography Symposium, Bad Nauheim, West Germany. The Hague, Dr W Junk BV, 1974.
210. Ripps H: Night blindness revisited: From man to molecules. Invest Ophthalmol Vis Sci 23:588, 1982.
211. Carr RE, Ripps H, Siegel IM, et al: Rhodopsin and the electrical activity of the retina in congenital night blindness. Invest Ophthalmol 5:497, 1966.
212. Alpern M, Holland MG, Ohba N: Rhodopsin bleaching signals in essential night blindness. J Physiol (Lond) 225:457, 1972.
213. Gouras P: Relationships of the electro-oculogram to the electroretinogram. In The clinical value of electroretinography. International Society for Clinical Electroretinography Symposium, Ghent, Belgium, 1966. Basel, Switzerland, S Karger AG, 1968.
214. Goodman G, Bornschein H: Comparative electroretinographic studies in congenital night blindness and total color blindness. Arch Ophthalmol 58:174, 1957.
215. Hill DA, Arbel KF, Berson EL: Cone electroretinograms in congenital nyctalopia with myopia. Am J Ophthalmol 78:127, 1974.
216. Berson EL, Lessell S: Paraneoplastic night blindness with malignant melanoma. Am J Ophthalmol 106:307, 1988.
217. Miyake Y, Yagasaki K, Horiguchi M, et al: Congenital stationary night blindness with negative electroretinogram: A new classification. Arch Ophthalmol 104:1013, 1986.
218. Gouras P: Electroretinography: Some basic principles. Invest Ophthalmol 9:557, 1970.
219. Marmor MF: Defining fundus albipunctatus. In Lawwill T (ed): Documenta Ophthalmologica proceeding series, No. 13. Fourteenth International Society for Clinical Electroretinography Symposium, Louisville, Kentucky, May 10–14, 1976. The Hague, Dr W Junk BV, 1976.
220. Ripps H: Night blindness and the retinal mechanisms of visual adaptation. Ann R Coll Surg Engl 58:2, 1976.
221. Berson EL: Electrical phenomena in the retina. In Hart WM Jr (ed): Adler's Physiology of the Eye, 9th ed. St Louis, CV Mosby, 1992.
222. Thirkill CE, FitzGerald P, Sergott RC, et al: Cancer-associated retinopathy (CAR syndrome) with antibodies reacting with retinal, optic-nerve and cancer cells. N Engl J Med 321:1589, 1989.
223. Keltner JL, Thirkill CE, Tyler NK, et al: Management and monitoring of cancer-associated retinopathy. Arch Ophthalmol 110:48, 1992.
224. Cox SN, Hay E, Bird AC: Treatment of chronic macular edema with acetazolamide. Arch Ophthalmol 106:1190, 1988.
225. Fishman GA, Gilbert LD, Fiscella RG, et al: Acetazolamide for treatment of chronic macular edema in retinitis pigmentosa. Arch Ophthalmol 107:1445, 1989.
226. Chen JC, Fitzke FW, Bird AC: Long-term effect of acetazolamide in a patient with retinitis pigmentosa. Invest Ophthalmol Vis Sci 31:1914, 1990.
227. Berson EL, Rabin AR, Mehaffey L: Advances in night vision technology: A pocketscope for patients with retinitis pigmentosa. Arch Ophthalmol 90:427, 1973.
228. Berson EL: Retinitis pigmentosa and allied diseases: Some aspects of diagnosis, pathogenesis, and management. In Committee on Vision, National Research Council: Night Vision: Current Research and Future Directions. Washington, DC, National Academy Press, 1987.
229. Newsome DA, Berson EL, Bonner R, et al: Possible role of optical radiation in retinal degenerations. In Waxler M, Hitchins VM (eds): Optical Radiation and Visual Health. Boca Raton, FL, CRC Press, 1986.
230. Berson EL: Light deprivation and retinitis pigmentosa. Vision Res 20:1179, 1980.
231. Olsson JE, Gordon JW, Pawlyk BS, et al: Transgenic mice with a rhodopsin mutation (Pro23His): A mouse model of autosomal dominant retinitis pigmentosa. Neuron 9:815, 1992.
232. Oprian DD, Molday RS, Kaufman RJ, et al: Expression of a synthetic bovine rhodopsin gene in monkey kidney cells. Proc Natl Acad Sci USA 84:8874, 1987.
233. Khorana HG, Knox BE, Nasi E, et al: Expression of a bovine rhodopsin in Xenopus oocytes: Demonstration of light dependent ionic currents. Proc Natl Acad Sci USA 85:7917, 1988.
234. Berson EL: Retinitis pigmentosa. The Friedenwald Lecture. Invest Ophthalmol Vis Sci, in press.

Chapter 107

■

Hereditary Cone Dysfunction Syndromes

ELIAS REICHEL

The physiologic basis of color vision has occupied the interest of some preeminent scientists over the past 300 yr.[1] Newton established that when sunlight passed through a prism, the sunlight was broken down into its constituent rays and formed a spectrum of colors. Young in 1802 proposed that trichromasy was a consequence of humans having three independent light-sensitive mechanisms.[2] von Kries in 1897 arbitrarily defined congenital color vision defects using Greek words.[3] Protan (first) was used for red blindness, deutan (second) was used for green blindness, and tritan (third) was used for blue blindness. There is an additional category called tetartan (fourth), which is a combined blue-yellow defect. To date no congenital tetartan defects have been found. Today, of all the genetic conditions that affect the eye, the most information is known about the abnormalities of the cone pigment genes and how they affect color vision. The spectrum of disease that is seen varies from the trivial to the most devastating.

"NORMAL" COLOR VISION

Human color vision is mediated by cone photoreceptors. There are three different classes of cones, one being maximally sensitive to light near 560 nm (long wavelength or red cones), a second that is maximally sensitive to light near 535 nm (middle wavelength or green cones), and a third that is maximally sensitive to light near 440 nm (short wavelength or blue cones).[4–6] The human retina contains a total of about 6 million red and green cones in approximately equal numbers and about 1 million blue cones.

Normal observers require a combination of three different lights to match the appearance of a given colored light. The matching range is the range of ratio of red:green light that is acceptable as a match of a standard yellow light. The mid-matchpoint of the matching range is the red:green ratio chosen by normal subjects when they are free to adjust both the brightness of the yellow light and the relative intensity of the red and green lights. In any set of normal individuals there are considerable differences in the matching range and in the range in the value of the mid-matchpoint.[7, 8] Differences in mid-matchpoints can vary because of prereceptorial or receptorial differences among individuals.[9, 10]

ABNORMAL COLOR VISION

Functional Observations

Anomalous trichromasy occurs when an individual has an anomalous (deviant) cone photopigment that replaces a normal cone photopigment of one type of cone photoreceptor; therefore, three wavelengths are required to match another wavelength and these persons do not accept the color matches made by normal individuals (Fig. 107–1). Deuteranomaly occurs when the normal middle-wavelength cone photopigment is replaced by one that has a peak sensitivity that is at a longer wavelength. Conversely, protanomaly occurs when the normal long-wavelength photopigment is replaced by one that has a peak sensitivity that is shorter than usual (i.e., middle-wavelength cone photopigment). Protanomaly and deuteranomaly can be defined using the Rayleigh match anomaloscope. An individual with protanomaly requires too much red in the red-green mixture to match the yellow field. Conversely, a person with deuteranomaly requires too much green in the red-green mixture to match the yellow field. Matching ranges of individual persons with anomalous trichromasy can vary, as has been found in normal individuals. Not all red:green ratios are acceptable to the individual with anomalous trichromasy, and it is this feature that separates an individual with anomalous trichromasy from one with dichromasy.

Protanopia and deuteranopia are thought to be caused by a lack of a red cone photopigment and a green cone photopigment, respectively. Protanopes and deuteranopes can match any red-green mixture to the yellow match field by manipulating the brightness function only. When the red-green mixture is all red, protanopes require less illumination of the yellow half-field than normal individuals do; deuteranopes require about the same brightness setting as do normal individuals to make a color match.

Congenital tritanomaly has not been determined to exist, because the diagnosis of this type of defect using psychophysical testing involves the use of short-wavelength lights (blue and blue-green) that are selectively absorbed by the macular yellow pigment (xanthophyll).[12] Since the concentration of this pigment in the macula differs markedly from observer to observer, it is difficult to know whether differences in magnitude of response function are being measured or whether the results that

1238

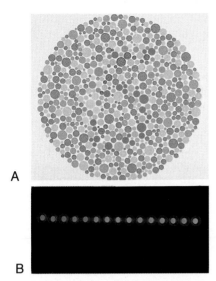

A

B

Figure 107–1. *A,* Ishihara plate test for screening and classifying red-green defects. The Macbeth easel lamp should be used for illumination during color vision testing. *B,* The Farnsworth Dichotomous Test for Color Blindness, or D-15 test, is an arrangement test used to detect congenital color defects. Protan, deutan, or tritan defects can be determined. The Macbeth easel lamp should be used for illumination. The photographic reproductions are not suitable for testing color vision.

are obtained result from differences in macular pigment absorption. In addition, the lens absorbs short-wavelength light, and this absorption increases with age. Therefore, older individuals have a decreased ability for blue color discrimination, and assessment of tritan defects in this group of patients can be particularly difficult.[13]

Incidence

Red and green color vision deficiencies are inherited by an X-linked mode of transmission. Approximately 6 percent of males of European ancestry have anomalous color vision—5 percent being deuteranomalous and 1 percent being protanomalous. Approximately 0.25 percent of females are deuteranomalous and 0.01 percent of females are protanomalous. Carriers of an anomalous gene constitute about 12 percent of the female population. Both protanopia and deuteranopia occur in approximately 1 percent of males of European ancestry. One in 10,000 females has either protanopia or deuteranopia.[14] Female carriers for protanopia and deuteranopia may test similarly to normal individuals, male protanopes or deuteranopes, respectively, or somewhere in between, depending on the degree of lyonization of the X chromosome.[11] Female carriers for protanopia or deuteranopia each compose about 2 percent of the female population.

The incidence of color vision deficiencies among non-Europeans is lower when compared with individuals of European ancestry. Asian males have a 4.9 percent incidence of color deficiency; in females, the incidence is 0.64 percent. Individuals of African, Native Ameri-

can, or Mexican ancestry have an even lower incidence; in males, the incidence is 3.1 percent, and among females, it is 0.7 percent. One study of individuals of European ancestry detected a 15.7 percent incidence of cone pigment gene rearrangements that were consistent with color deficiencies.[15] This result appeared to be significantly different from psychophysical data obtained from a similar population. Even more intriguing is the high frequency of molecular variation at the X-linked color vision loci in individuals of African descent, although they have a much lower incidence of psychophysically proven color deficiencies.[16]

Congenital tritanopia is rare.[17, 18] The incidence is probably one in every several tens of thousands of people. Congenital tritanopia exists as a dominant trait with variable expression, and patients with this condition must be distinguished from those who are affected with dominantly inherited optic atrophy (Kjer's optic atrophy) who can also present with near-normal or normal visual acuity and with a mild to moderate tritan color defect.[19, 20]

Molecular Genetics

The genes for the red and green cone opsins lie on the long arm of the X chromosome.[21] The cone pigment genes lie in a tandem array. A normal trichromat male has one copy of a red gene; however, there can be anywhere from one to five green pigment genes.[15] Furthermore, a normal trichromat can have a normal red and a normal green pigment gene, and in addition, a hybrid red and green pigment gene. Duplication of the green pigment gene most likely results from homologous but unequal recombination or crossover during meiosis. This occurs because of the close similarity of the genes and their intragenic sequences.[22] By this same mechanism of intragenic recombination, hybrid genes can be produced by rearrangement of genetic material for the red and green cone pigment genes.

Deuteranopes can have one red pigment gene and an anomalous hybrid red-green gene with a spectral absorbance that is close to that of the red pigment gene. Protanopes lack a normal red pigment gene, but they can have anywhere from one to three normal green cone pigment genes.[15, 22] A hybrid red-green gene can be found in each of these patients, and its encoded opsin functions as a midspectral wavelength pigment. Deuteranomalous individuals have one normal red pigment gene, at least one normal green pigment gene, and at least one hybrid gene. Protanomalous individuals lack a normal red gene, have one hybrid gene, and can have between one and four normal green genes. Subsequent analysis of the red and green pigment gene cluster in individuals with color deficiencies and in normal individuals will undoubtedly lead to more descriptions of the genetic variation that exists at these gene loci. Ultimately, correlation of these genotypes to their functional alterations and deficiencies will provide for a better understanding of the variation in human color vision.

Neitz and coworkers have determined that the spectral

differences between the middle- (530 nm) and the long- (562 nm) wavelength cone pigments are determined by the additive effects of substitutions at three amino acid positions. These amino acids correspond to positions 180, 277, and 285. A substitution at amino acid site 180 by either an alanine or a serine accounts for a 5-nm difference observed in the long-wavelength cone pigment that was originally observed microspectrophotometrically.[10]

The gene for the blue cone pigment has been localized to chromosome 7.[21] A single amino acid substitution at amino acid position 264 of blue cone opsin has been identified in a Dutch pedigree with tritanopia: A highly conserved proline at position 264 is changed to serine. It is hypothesized that this defect causes the tritan defect in this family.[23]

ABNORMAL COLOR VISION ASSOCIATED WITH SUBNORMAL VISUAL ACUITY

Dominantly Inherited Cone Dysfunction Syndrome

Hereditary progressive cone degenerations have largely been thought to be autosomal dominant conditions. Many sporadic cases have been described.[34] At present, it would be difficult to subdivide progressive cone degenerations that are inherited as autosomal dominant, X-linked, autosomal recessive, or sporadic on clinical grounds alone. Patients with cone degeneration present with complaints of declining central vision and photophobia or light sensitivity. In addition, these patients may complain of difficulty adjusting from a light environment to a dark environment, which is related to a defective mechanism of cone dark adaptation. Color vision may initially be normal or may become defective.[35-39]

In general, cone degenerations present within the first 2 decades of life. Typically, vision can fall to the 20/200 level by age 30 yr. Variability exists in the age of onset of decreased vision among different individuals, even among affected members of the same family. Color vision is moderately to severely affected by the time the patient presents with visual acuity in the 20/40 to 20/60 range.[39] One interesting feature of cone degenerations, especially those that present with a bull's-eye maculopathy, is that in some individuals, central acuity may be excellent (20/20), although there is a pericentral scotoma around the small central area of remaining field. In early cone degenerations, the color defect is usually of the red-green type. As the condition becomes more advanced, patients show variable axes of confusion in the Farnsworth D15 panel and the Rayleigh anomaloscope match widens first toward the red end (pseudoprotanomaly) and then toward both ends. This phenomenon may be due to a misalignment of photoreceptor outer segments.[40] Visual field testing shows central or pericentral scotomas. Individuals who lose central visual acuity and who have large central scotomas experience eccen-

tric viewing. Although the peripheral field remains normal to a I-4$_e$ white test light in pure cone degenerations, in cone-rod degenerations there can be loss of the peripheral field as well.

Full-field electroretinographic (ERG) testing of individuals with cone degenerations shows abnormalities in the components of the ERG that are cone-mediated, including the dark-adapted cone-mediated x-wave (the first cornea-positive wave elicited with red light), 30-Hz flicker, and photopic responses. The cone b-wave implicit time is usually abnormal. Photopically matched long-wavelength and middle-wavelength lights can be used as stimuli in determining whether one of these types of photoreceptors is preferentially involved. Dark-adaptation testing characteristically discloses monophasic curves with a normal final rod threshold (Fig. 107-2).

Typically, patients with cone degenerations can present with several different types of fundus findings. Initially, these patients may have an entirely normal fundus appearance. Later on, they may show some central retinal pigment epithelial changes. Eventually, these patients may show a bull's-eye lesion in each macula (Fig. 107-3).

A pedigree has been described of autosomal dominant macular dystrophy with preferential involvement of the short-wavelength–sensitive cones. This defect was associated with mild macular pigmentary changes, poor foveolar reflexes, and slightly reduced visual acuity. There appeared to be preferential loss of blue cone function with sparing of red and green cone function as

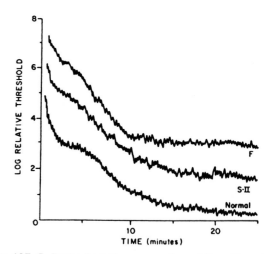

Figure 107–2. Dark-adaptation curves for a father (F) and a son (S-II) with autosomal dominant cone degeneration and a normal subject who were followed for 45 min after light adaptation. Ordinate scales apply to the lowest curve; other curves are shifted upward to avoid overlap. The father and the son show a monophasic curve with no rod-cone break compared with the normal subject. This is typical for cone degenerations. All subjects reached normal final thresholds at similar times. The rate of recovery in the initial phase of adaptation for the affected patients is slower than the rate of recovery at the corresponding time during the cone limb of the normal curve. (From Berson EL, Gouras P, Gunkel RD: Progressive cone degeneration, dominantly inherited. Arch Ophthalmol 80:77, 1968. Copyright 1968, American Medical Association.)

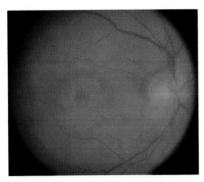

Figure 107–3. A 79-year-old man with autosomal dominant cone degeneration. Visual acuity was 20/400 O.U. Characteristic bull's-eye maculopathy is observed in the fundus photograph. His 35-year-old son had 20/30 visual acuity O.U. and minimal changes on fundus examination.

determined by anomaloscope testing. ERG revealed that there was an abnormality of blue cones that extended beyond the central macula. The reduction in visual acuity and abnormal macular findings helped to distinguish this condition from congenital tritanopia. These individuals also had normal optic discs.[41]

Autosomal Recessive Cone Dysfunction Syndrome

The recessively inherited cone dysfunction syndromes are a group of rare disorders in which color vision is either entirely lacking (complete monochromatism) or severely limited (incomplete monochromatism). Visual acuity, in general, is reduced. Often there is a history of consanguinity.[42–44] In one study, the incidence of complete monochromatism was approximately 0.003 percent. Visual acuity is at the 20/200 level in complete monochromatism but can be as good as 20/50 in incomplete forms. These patients usually have an aversion to bright lights. The fundus may show a lack of the foveal reflex and an irregular distribution of the macular pigment. The ERG shows profoundly reduced or no full-field cone ERGs and normal rod ERG responses.

The complete monochromat can match any two wavelengths by adjusting the brightness of one light only (i.e., only one primary is required to produce a color mixture). All colors can be matched to shades of gray. These individuals arrange the Farnsworth D15 with a nonspecific axis of confusion. It is thought that complete monochromats have some residual cone photoreceptors that can be seen in computer-averaged ERGs. Histopathologic study of eyes with complete monochromatism has revealed 5 to 10 percent of the normal number of extrafoveal cones in all cases studied so far. Foveal cones can be present but are abnormal morphologically.[45, 46]

Incomplete monochromats generally have nystagmus and photophobia, as do complete monochromats. Psychophysical testing is necessary to define the differences between complete monochromatism and incomplete monochromatism and is helpful in distinguishing the

different types of incomplete monochromatisms from one another.[44, 47–49] The ability of an individual with incomplete monochromatism to distinguish among different colors can differ, and this information can be used to define the different types of incomplete monochromatism. Fundus reflectometry has shown both red and green cones, suggesting that these are postreceptorial disorders.[50, 51] Table 107–1 provides a summary of the clinical features of hereditary cone dysfunction syndromes.

X-linked Cone Dysfunction Syndromes

BLUE CONE MONOCHROMATISM

Blue cone monochromatism, also known as π_1 cone monochromatism, X-linked atypical monochromatism, or X-linked recessive incomplete monochromatism, occurs in approximately 1 in every 1 million males.[24] Males with this condition have a peak sensitivity near 504 nm under dark-adapted conditions because of normal rod function and a peak sensitivity near 440 nm under light-adapted conditions because of normal blue cone function in contrast to males with peak sensitivity under light-adapted conditions near 555 nm. Young males with blue cone monochromatism typically have nystagmus, photophobia, reduced visual acuity, and myopia.[25] Visual acuity ranges from 20/60 to 20/400. Fundus examination shows a granular macula in young males and atrophy in the macula in some older males. The full-field cone ERG to 30-Hz white flicker is reduced to less than 3 μV (as blue cones normally contribute less than 3 μV to the 350-μV full-field cone ERG to 30-Hz white flicker). Obligate female carriers have diminished cone ERGs, mildly delayed cone implicit times, loss of the a_1 oscillation to white light under dark-adapted conditions, or some combination of these ERG findings (Fig. 107–4).[26] Carriers may also show a red-green deficiency on psychophysical testing. A series of color vision test plates, called blue monochromat plates, can be used to distinguish young males with X-linked blue cone monochromatism from young males with autosomal recessive rod monochromatism (Fig. 107–5).[27] The blue cone monochromat can perform this test, whereas the rod monochromat fails it.

Given that blue cone monochromatism is an X-linked condition that is characterized by the lack of both red and green cone sensitivities, Nathans and associates postulated that a mutation could occur in the red-green pigment gene array that could explain such a functional defect.[28] Twelve families who had the diagnosis of blue cone monochromatism were studied. Each one of these families fell into one of two classes of genetic alterations that could explain the mutant phenotype. One genotype occurred via a two-step pathway. Unequal homologous recombination reduced the number of pigment genes to only one in affected males (the average normal complement is three per X chromosome). A point mutation caused a functional inactivation of the only remaining opsin gene. The second class of genetic alterations

Table 107–1. SUMMARY OF THE CLINICAL FEATURES OF HEREDITARY CONE DYSFUNCTION SYNDROMES*

Disorder	Inheritance	Visual Acuity	Fundus	Color Testing	ERG	Other
Protanomaly, deuteranomaly	XR	Normal	Normal	Ishihara extremely sensitive for identifying red-green defects. AO-HRR can detect red-green and blue-yellow defects; mild red-green defects can be missed. Farnsworth D-15, protan or deutan axis of confusion can be detected in severe anomalous trichromats or dichromats. Nagel anomaloscope is exceptionally sensitive to quantify the anomaly quotient (red-green).	Mismatch of photopically matched long-wavelength or middle-wavelength responses in protanopia or deuteranopia. Cone ERG to white light is normal. Early cornea-negative oscillations to red light reduced in protanopia.	
Protanopia, deuteranopia	XR	Normal	Normal			
Tritanopia	AD	Normal	Normal	AO-HRR is a good test for screening Farnsworth D-15 tritan axis of confusion.	Normal	
Cone degeneration	AD, AR, XR	20/20–20/200	Bull's-eye maculopathy; tapetal sheen; temporal pallor of optic nerve; RPE changes in macula.	Protan and deutan axes of confusion can be observed in Farnsworth D-15 in early cone degenerations. Pseudoprotanomaly can be observed in cone degenerations as well. Eventual scotopization of axis of confusion in cone degenerations; scotopic axis of confusion in rod monochromatism and blue cone monochromatism.	Full-field cone ERGs are subnormal in cone degenerations (nondetectable to 40 μV responses). Mismatches to long-wavelength and middle-wavelength photopically matched lights can be observed.	Monophasic dark-adaptation profile. Mizuo-Nakamura phenomenon occasionally seen.
Blue cone monochromat	XR	20/60–20/200	RPE changes in macula.	Scotopic axis of confusion (Farnsworth D-15). Matches along rod line of Rayleigh equation. Blue cone monochromat plates useful in distinguishing rod monochromatism from blue cone monochromatism.	Cone ERGs are reduced to less than 3 μV. Full-field rod ERGs are normal. Long-wavelength and middle-wavelength photopically matched lights are reduced but matched in carrier females.	Nystagmus frequently seen. Monophasic dark-adaptation profile.
Rod monochromat	AR	20/200–20/400	RPE changes in macula.	Scotopic axis of confusion (Farnsworth D-15). Matches along rod line of Rayleigh equation.	Cone ERGs are reduced to less than 3 μV. Full-field rod ERGs are normal.	Nystagmus frequently seen. Monophasic dark-adaptation profile.
Cone monochromat with normal acuity	?	Normal	Normal	Abnormal responses to red-green and blue-yellow screening plates.	Full-field ERGs are normal.	

*XR, X-linked recessive; AD, autosomal dominant; AR, autosomal recessive; RPE, retinal pigment epithelium; AO-HRR, American Optical–Hardy–Rand–Rittler.

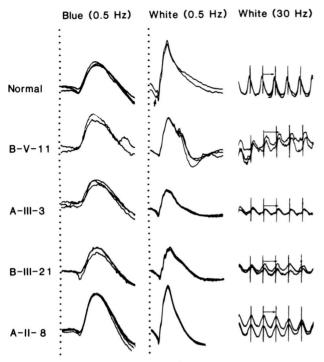

Blue (0.5 Hz)   White (0.5 Hz)   White (30 Hz)

Normal

B-V-11

A-III-3

B-III-21

A-II-8

Figure 107–4. Full-field electroretinograms (ERGs) from a normal subject and obligate carriers of blue cone monochromatism from two families (A and B). Two or three consecutive responses are illustrated for each stimulus condition. Time of stimulus onset is designated by *vertical lines* in columns 1 and 2 and *vertical shock artifacts* in column 3. *Short arrow* designates the a1 oscillation in the normal response; *long arrows* designate cone b-wave implicit times; calibration symbol (lower right) designates 100 μV vertically for columns 1 and 3, 200 μV vertically for column 2, and 50 msec horizontally for all tracings. (From Berson EL, Sandberg MA, Maguire A, et al: Electroretinograms in carriers of blue cone monochromatism. Am J Ophthalmol 102:254–261, 1986. Published with permission from The American Journal of Ophthalmology. Copyright by The Ophthalmic Publishing Company.)

consisted of nonhomologous deletions of genomic DNA that was adjacent to the red and green pigment gene cluster. These deletions defined a 579-base-pair region that is located 4 kilobases upstream from the red pigment gene (Fig. 107–6). It is possible that the 579-base-pair region is essential for the normal expression of the pigment gene array.

X-LINKED CONE DEGENERATION

X-linked cone degeneration is a rare disorder in which affected males can present with slightly reduced visual acuity, no evidence of nystagmus, and no diagnostic abnormalities on fundus examination. A family with this disorder has recently been identified, and the molecular genetic and ERG features of this entity have been defined.[29] In this family, the 15-year-old propositus had near-normal visual acuity, a protan deficiency, and a full-field cone ERG to 30-Hz white flicker that was reduced by 50 percent in amplitude. His maternal grandfather and great uncle had visual acuity of 20/200, a deficiency in color vision, and signs of macular retinal pigment epithelial changes (Fig. 107–7). Both of these

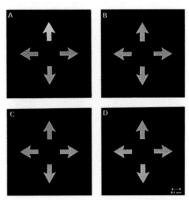

Figure 107–5. Reproductions of color plates that help distinguish patients with blue cone monochromatism from those with rod monochromatism. *A* and *B* are the two instructional plates, and *C* and *D* are two of the four test plates. These reproductions should not be used to test patients, because the printed colors may not be the same as those of our original plates. The plates should be viewed under a Macbeth lamp.

affected males had markedly diminished cone ERGs. History taking revealed that the older affected males had normal vision earlier in life. The carrier females, the mother and maternal aunt of the propositus, had normal visual acuity and diminished cone ERGs with predominant loss of red cone function (Figs. 107–8 to 107–10). Their cone responses to 30-Hz white flicker, although abnormal, were larger than those from the three affected males. Genomic DNA isolated from these patients was analyzed with a red cone pigment gene

Gene Defects in Blue Cone Monochromacy

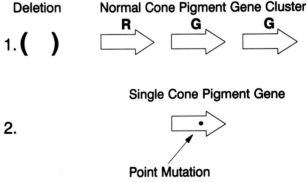

Figure 107–6. Schematic diagram of defects in blue cone monochromasy. One type of defect is characterized by deletions *(parentheses)* that occur downstream of the tandem gene array of the X-linked cone visual pigment genes *(arrows)*. (*R*, red; *G*, green.) Such a deletion always includes a sequence that is 4 kilobases from the beginning of the coding sequence of the first pigment gene. The second type of mutation is characterized by reduction to one pigment gene by homologous cross-overs and the occurrence of a point mutation in the single pigment gene with alteration in the nucleotide sequence that leads to dysfunction of the cone pigment.

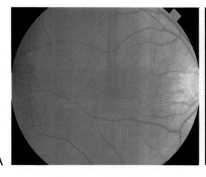
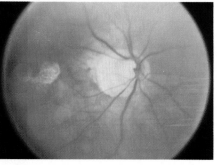

A

B

Figure 107–7. *A,* Fundus photographs from the right eye of a 15-year-old boy with X-linked cone degeneration. The patient displayed mild retinal pigment epithelium (RPE) changes in the foveas. Visual acuity was 20/30 O.U. *B,* The maternal grandfather at age 71 yr had 20/200 acuity and had signs of atrophic RPE changes in both eyes.

complementary DNA probe that disclosed a 6.5-kilobase deletion in the red cone pigment gene. The findings substantiate that a defect in a gene encoding for a cone photoreceptor protein can lead to a cone photoreceptor degeneration. This finding adds to the spectrum of genetic defects of the red-green cone pigment gene family.

Another entity that has been described is X-linked progressive cone dystrophy.[30–32] In pedigrees with this condition, there is also evidence of visual acuity deteri-

oration in older males. The visual acuity changes were associated with bull's-eye lesions and central geographic atrophy of the retinal pigment epithelium in older subjects. Some of the patients displayed a tapetum-like sheen. Cone ERGs were subnormal, and dark adaptation revealed elevated cone thresholds. The Mizuo-Nakamura phenomenon was observed in two different families with this condition.[31] Preliminary linkage studies of one of these families indicated that the gene for this condition was on the short arm of the X chromosome and is therefore distinct from X-linked cone degeneration.[33]

OTHER HEREDITARY DISORDERS ASSOCIATED WITH CONE DYSFUNCTION

Fenestrated sheen macular dystrophy is a rare autosomal dominant macular dystrophy seen in young individuals. A refractile sheen with small red spots is seen in the foveal area. Retinal pigment epithelial hyperpigmentation can be seen in the juxtafoveal area, and an annular zone of depigmentation can follow. Mild changes in the cone ERG and the electrooculogram were observed in patients with this condition.[52] Some have reported reductions in both the cone and rod ERGs.[53]

Several investigators have identified individuals who appear to have typical symptoms of cone dysfunction (loss of visual acuity, decreased color vision, photophobia, profoundly abnormal cone-mediated ERGs) but who have supernormal rod ERGs to high-intensity white light. The rod stimulus response curve (Naka-Rushton equation) of these individuals is steeper than that found in normal individuals. This defect could possibly represent a defect in cyclic nucleotide phosphodiesterase. A deficiency of this enzyme can cause increased intracellular levels of cyclic guanosine monophosphate and thus a supernormal ERG (Fig. 107–11).[54] This form has been designated as an elevated cyclic guanosine monophosphate type of retinal degeneration.[55]

Autosomal dominant olivopontocerebellar degeneration has been found to be associated with cone degeneration as well. These patients present with reduced acuity and macular abnormality. Full-field ERGs suggest that this syndrome is associated with a cone-rod type of retinal degeneration involving both macular and extra-

FULL-FIELD ERGs IN X-LINKED CONE DEGENERATION –PROTAN TYPE

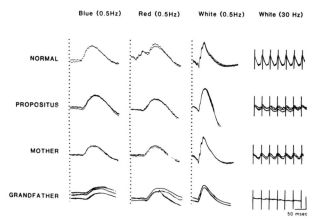

Figure 107–8. Dark-adapted full-field ERGs from a normal subject and three members of a family with X-linked cone degeneration. Calibration symbol *(lower right)* designated 50 msec for all patients and 100 μV vertically for columns 1, 2, and 4 and 200 μV for column 3. Suprathreshold blue and red lights, matched in brightness for rods near threshold in normal subjects, elicited matched responses in the affected patients (in contrast to normals) that is consistent with normal rod function and diminished red and green cone function in these patients. Mixed cone-rod responses to white light were reduced about 40 percent below normal in the propositus's grandfather, which is also consistent with reduced cone function and normal rod function. Cone isolated responses to 30-Hz white flicker showed reduced responses in the propositus and his mother and nondetectable (< 10 μV) responses in the maternal grandfather and maternal great uncle. The propositus had smaller cone responses than those of his mother; his cone responses to 30-Hz flicker were comparable to the amplitude and implicit time recorded from him at age 3 yr under anesthesia and at age 10 yr without anesthesia. (From Reichel E, Bruce AM, Sandberg MA, et al: An electroretinographic and molecular genetic study of X-linked cone degeneration. Am J Ophthalmol 108:540–547, 1989. Published with permission from the American Journal of Ophthalmology. Copyright by The Ophthalmic Publishing Company.)

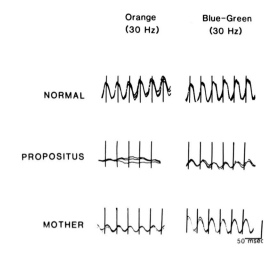

Orange
(30 Hz)

Blue–Green
(30 Hz)

NORMAL

PROPOSITUS

MOTHER

50 msec

Figure 107–9. Full-field ERGs from a normal subject, the propositus, and his mother from a family with X-linked cone degeneration with predominant loss of red cone function obtained in response to 30-Hz orange and blue-green stimuli. Runs were computer-averaged (N = 256 per sweep), and three sweeps are illustrated. Stimulus onset is designated by *vertical lines.* Calibration symbol (lower right) designates 50 msec horizontally and 25 µV vertically for all tracings. Both patients showed mismatched responses in contrast to the normal subject, with predominant loss of amplitude in the responses to the long-wavelength stimulus. The maternal aunt of the propositus also showed the same mismatch consistent with predominant loss of red cone function. (From Reichel E, Bruce AM, Sandberg MA, et al: An electroretinographic and molecular genetic study of X-linked cone degeneration. Am J Ophthalmol 108:540–547, 1989. Published with permission from the American Journal of Ophthalmology. Copyright by The Ophthalmic Publishing Company.)

macular cones and rods.[56, 57] Some affected individuals may show only an abnormal full-field cone ERG.

X-linked adrenoleukodystrophy has been associated with a higher than expected incidence of congenital redgreen defects. It is thought that the gene defect for adrenoleukodystrophy is in close proximity to the redgreen pigment gene cluster and that these two clinical findings are linked in some way.[58]

One other form of cone dysfunction is monochromatism associated with normal visual acuity. This form of atypical monochromatism could be considered to be tritanopia combined with either protanopia or deuteranopia. It should be distinguished from incomplete monochromatism with reduced visual acuity. This condition is thought to affect 1 in every 100 million people. Visual function is otherwise normal, and the ERG to white stimuli has been reported to be normal. The inheritance pattern is unknown, although it is associated with otherwise typical congenital color blindness.[13, 60]

HEREDITARY VERSUS ACQUIRED COLOR DEFECTS

The first distinction that should be made in the examination of any patient with a color deficiency is whether the color deficiency is based on a hereditary or congenital defect or whether it is acquired. This distinction is important in that the underlying cause of an

acquired color vision deficiency may be a potentially reversible ocular or systemic disease that affects the eye. There are several general features that can help distinguish an acquired defect from a congenital defect. In acquired defects, the two eyes are frequently affected to different degrees. An acquired defect may show progression or regression with time and may not appear to be stationary, as most congenital color deficiencies are. The patient with an acquired color defect may remember having normal color vision at one time. Patients who have an acquired color vision deficiency will name colors incorrectly using terminology that is based on their previous experience of normal color vision. Some individuals with acquired defects may have loss of visual field and associated neurologic abnormalities. There may be a history of ingestion or use of drugs or other agents that can cause either cone dysfunction or alterations in color vision (e.g., digitalis retinal toxicity, ethambutol optic neuropathy, tobacco-alcohol amblyopia). Finally, one can usually elicit a history of either an ocular or a systemic disease that can often lead to color vision deficits. These conditions include diabetes, glaucoma, age-related macular degeneration, optic

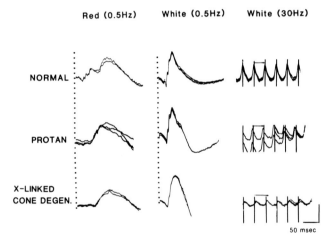

Red (0.5Hz)

White (0.5Hz)

White (30Hz)

NORMAL

PROTAN

X-LINKED
CONE DEGEN.

50 msec

Figure 107–10. Full-field ERG responses from a normal subject, a male with protan deficiency, and the propositus with X-linked cone degeneration. Stimulus onset is indicated by *vertical hatched lines* in columns 1 and 2 and *vertical lines* in column 3. *Horizontal arrows* in column 3 designate 50 msec horizontally for all tracings, and 100 µV vertically for columns 1 and 3 and 200 µV vertically for column 2. The ERGs of the propositus are contrasted with those from a man with a protan deficiency, normal visual acuity, and normal fundi. Both the protan-deficient subject and the propositus with X-linked cone degeneration had diminished early cornea-positive oscillations to red light. However, the individual with protan deficiency retained normal amplitudes in mixed cone-rod responses to 0.5-Hz white light and cone-isolated responses to 30-Hz white flicker, whereas the propositus had borderline normal responses to 0.5-Hz white light and reduced responses to 30-Hz white flicker. Furthermore, the boy with cone degeneration showed a delay (> 32 msec) in cone implicit time to 30-Hz flicker, resulting in a phase shift between stimulus flash onset, which is designated by the *vertical lines,* and the corresponding response peaks. (From Reichel E, Bruce AM, Sandberg MA, et al: An electroretinographic and molecular genetic study of X-linked cone degeneration. Am J Ophthalmol 108:540–547, 1989. Published with permission from the American Journal of Ophthalmology. Copyright by The Ophthalmic Publishing Company.)

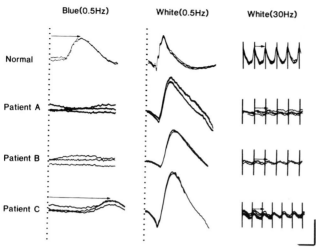

Figure 107–11. Full-field ERGs from a normal subject and three patients with an unusual form of retinal degeneration (Patient A, age 10 yr; Patient B, age 39 yr; and Patient C, age 39 yr) in response to 10-μsec duration, 0.5-Hz blue flashes that isolate rod function, 0.5-Hz white flashes that normally elicit a mixed cone and rod response, and 30-Hz white flashes that isolate cone function. Two or more consecutive sweeps are shown superimposed. *Vertical hatched lines* (left and middle columns) or *vertical lines* (right column) denote flash onset. *Arrows* (left and right columns) designate b-wave implicit times (i.e., time interval between stimulus flash and major cornea-positive response peak) for detectable responses. Calibration (lower right) denotes 100 μV (left and right columns) or 200 μV (middle column) vertically and 50 msec horizontally. These patients have subnormal and delayed or nondetectable rod responses to 0.5-Hz flashes of dim blue light, responses to 0.5-Hz flashes of white light that are normal or supernormal in amplitude, and subnormal and delayed cone responses to 30-Hz flashes of the same white light. (From Sandberg MA, Miller S, Berson EL: Rod electroretinograms in an elevated cyclic guanosine monophosphate–type human retinal degeneration. Invest Ophthalmol Vis Sci 31:2283, 1990.)

neuropathies, cataracts, and chorioretinal degenerative or inflammatory processes. After establishing that an acquired loss of color vision does not exist, the exact nature of the hereditary or congenital loss of color vision should be defined.

The following features should be assessed in any individual in whom a hereditary condition is being considered. It should be determined whether there is a family history that defines the heredity of the color deficiency as being X-linked, autosomal dominant, or autosomal recessive. It is especially important to determine whether the condition is stationary or progressive (i.e., is the visual acuity or color deficit getting worse?). Is there nystagmus or a history of nystagmus, and is there photophobia? On fundus examination, one should determine whether there is any evidence of a maculopathy (i.e., bull's-eye configuration) that would suggest a cone degeneration. An individual who has subnormal visual acuity, photophobia, nystagmus, or signs of a maculopathy and an acquired retinal abnormality warrants further psychophysical and ERG testing to determine if cone dysfunction exists.

In this setting, the full-field ERG, focal ERG testing, and specialized tests of color vision can prove very useful. The cones generate 20 to 25 percent of the dark-adapted response and the rods generate 75 to 80 percent;

a reduction in the dark-adapted response to white light would be expected if the patient has lost cone function. Macular and extramacular cone responses can be isolated with 30-Hz white flicker. Abnormal full-field cone ERGs to 30-Hz white stimulus (indicated by a subnormal amplitude with or without a delay in implicit timing) in this circumstance will help prove the existence of a cone dysfunction syndrome. It must be remembered that the cone ERG elicited by a white light is normal in dichromatism and anomalous trichromatism. Rod function should also be assessed to determine whether the condition is a cone-rod degeneration or primarily a rod degeneration with degeneration of the cones occurring in association (retinitis pigmentosa). Other useful tests are the full-field 0.5-Hz cone ERG in the presence of white background light sufficient to eliminate the rod contribution to the ERG and full-field 30-Hz cone ERGs using photopically matched orange and photopically matched blue-green lights.[29, 61] These two lights elicit ERG responses that are matched in amplitude in normal subjects and are mismatched in amplitude in individuals with protanopia, deuteranopia, or cone degenerations that predominantly affect either the red or the green cone systems. Recently, a technique for determining the ERG response of the blue cone system has been established that may prove to be useful in detecting degenerations of the blue cone system.[62] The focal ERG is a useful adjunct to full-field ERG testing in that it can be used to identify abnormalities of the foveal cones. Finally, color vision testing is of paramount importance in classifying the color defect psychophysically. All color vision tests are concerned with a small area of the retina (less than 10 degrees) and therefore are representative of function in that small area of retina and should be contrasted to the summed response of the full-field cone ERG that measures cone function throughout the entire retina. The systematic approach that was presented earlier will allow one to determine whether a color defect is acquired or is either a hereditary degenerative or a stationary condition.

ACQUIRED COLOR DEFICIENCY CAUSED BY RETINAL DEFECTS

Kollner in 1912 concluded that lesions in the outer retinal layers gave rise to blue-yellow defects, whereas damage to the inner retinal layers and the optic nerve resulted in red-green defects (the so-called Kollner rule).[63] We now know that red-green defects can occur in diseases of the outer retina, and conversely, blue-yellow defects can occur in diseases that affect the optic nerve and inner layers of the retina. A classification scheme of acquired color vision defects was first proposed by François and Verriest.[64] This classification is based on the axis of major chromatic discrimination loss (i.e., the ability to judge redness-greenness and the separate ability to judge blueness-yellowness). There are now three well-recognized patterns of discrimination loss in acquired color vision defects.[13, 40, 65, 66]

Type I acquired red-green defects are characterized

by a progressive deterioration in chromatic discrimination on the red-green axis. There is often a concomitant reduction in visual acuity that is roughly proportional to the severity of the color defect. Eventually, total loss of color discrimination occurs in the affected visual field. A type I defect is usually seen in retinal diseases that primarily involve the photoreceptors of the macula. This defect is thought to reflect the destruction of macular cones. Type II acquired red-green defects show a progressive, moderate to severe, loss of discrimination along the red-green axis and a concomitant milder blue-yellow loss of discrimination. Type II defects are typically seen in conditions that affect the optic nerve: optic neuritis, optic atrophy, tumors of the optic nerve or chiasm, and toxins that affect the optic nerve. Generalizations regarding visual acuity and how it relates to color deficiency cannot be made with this type of acquired color defect. The type III acquired blue-yellow defect is the most frequently observed acquired color vision defect. There is usually a mild to moderate loss of blue-yellow discrimination and the visual acuity deficit is usually mild to moderate. The type III defect can be seen in the following conditions: vascular disorders (diabetes in particular), chorioretinal degenerations and inflammations, age-related macular degeneration, papilledema, glaucoma, autosomal dominant optic atrophy, and optic neuritis. When an acquired color vision defect is diagnosed, one must be wary of a concomitant congenital color deficiency given the high incidence of these conditions in any population.

ACQUIRED COLOR DEFICIENCY CAUSED BY CORTICAL DEFECTS

Acquired disorders of color vision caused by lesions of the central nervous system can be divided into two main groups.[67–69] In one group, the color sense is normal but naming or recognition of colors is impaired. In the other group, there is an actual inability to see colors (dyschromatopsia or monochromatism). For instance, in patients with Wernicke's aphasia, the patient may be unable to name the color of an object because he or she does not comprehend the task and because there is a deficiency in language. Individuals with anomic aphasias may also fail to name colors, but given a choice they can correctly name the color of an object. It is important to note that naming performance is not limited to color naming only in aphasia. There is also a separate group of patients having a specific inability to name colors and no other problem with the naming of other objects. These patients usually also have alexia without agraphia (pure word blindness). They are not aphasic but are unable to match an observed color to its spoken name. Their color sense is normal when tested with color plates and matching tasks.

The second category of cortical defects are those that are described as cerebral dyschromatopsia. This condition can resemble X-linked color blindness. The patient cannot perform the pseudoisochromatic test plate test but can correctly name the colors of brightly colored objects. The color loss does not resemble a protan or deutan defect. Central nervous system dyschromatopsia is frequently associated with prosopagnosia (the inability to recognize faces) and loss of the superior portions of the visual field. The defect is thought to be consistent with bilateral lesions that involve the inferior portions of the visual cortex of the optic radiations.

Chromatopsia occurs when white objects appear to be colored.[13] Chromatopsia has been described after drug ingestions, after the quick absorption of a substance, or when there is an imbalance in retinal physiologic mechanisms. Chromatopsia is temporary because color perception can adapt to a new equilibrium and white can again be perceived as white. Coloropsia is chromatopsia caused by a cortical defect.

OTHER CONSIDERATIONS IN THE DIAGNOSIS OF CONE DEGENERATIONS

Without a doubt, there are several different genetic disorders that can be called cone dysfunction syndromes. Autosomal dominant inheritance appears to be the most common inheritance pattern seen in family studies of progressive hereditary cone degenerations. Autosomal recessive and X-linked pedigrees have also been described. For the simplification of diagnosis, it is best to consider that patients with cone dysfunction syndromes have significant abnormalities in full-field cone-mediated ERGs. There are descriptions of patients who have regional cone disease that may be either central or peripheral.[39, 70] On our clinical service, an individual who displays only features of a central cone degeneration is classified as having either a macular degeneration or dystrophy or an acquired macular disorder.

In patients with suspected cone dysfunction, it is urgent to establish whether the loss is due to cone dysfunction alone, to macular dysfunction, or to cone-rod dysfunction.[71, 72] A progressive cone-rod degeneration can present with macular dysfunction, and peripheral retinal malfunction is revealed with the full-field ERG. Patients with cone-rod degeneration have diminished visual acuity, abnormal color vision, monophasic dark-adaptation curves with slightly elevated rod thresholds, markedly reduced cone ERGs, and reduced rod components of the full-field ERG, whereas patients with cone degenerations have reduced cone ERGs and normal rod function. In cone-rod degeneration, there can be bone spicule pigmentation or clumped pigmentation and retinal arteriolar narrowing as is seen in retinitis pigmentosa. The distinction between cone degenerations and cone-rod degeneration is important in that the prognosis for retaining useful peripheral vision is, as expected, worse in the group of patients with a cone-rod degeneration.

In considering any cone degeneration, chloroquine retinopathy can present with a bull's-eye lesion or with retinal pigment epithelial atrophy that is almost identical to that seen in a hereditary form of cone degeneration (Table 107–2). Hydroxychloroquine toxicity has also

Table 107–2. DIFFERENTIAL DIAGNOSIS OF BULL'S-EYE MACULOPATHY

Cone degeneration
Chloroquine or hydroxychloroquine maculopathy
Cone-rod degeneration
Lipofuscinosis
Bull's-eye maculopathy associated with Stargardt's disease and fundus flavimaculatus
Fenestrated sheen macular dystrophy
Parafoveal atrophy of the retinal pigment epithelium secondary to drusen
Central areolar choroidal dystrophy
Juvenile Batten's disease
Fucosidosis
Clofazimine maculopathy

been associated with atrophy of the pigment epithelium with a bull's-eye lesion in the macula.[73] In general, the full-field ERG and the electrooculogram are usually normal in the early stages unless the condition is very far advanced. Digoxin has been reported to cause toxicity with a subnormal cone ERG amplitude and delayed implicit time that was reversible after cessation of the medication.[74] It is imperative to exclude drug toxicity in any patient who presents with a bull's-eye maculopathy before making the diagnosis of a cone degeneration.

ASSESSMENT AND FOLLOW-UP EXAMINATIONS

In assessing any patient with a cone dysfunction syndrome, visual acuity, color vision, visual field, full-field ERG, and focal ERG testing should be performed in order to classify the condition. Patients should be encouraged to wear tinted glasses to help reduce photophobia. In patients with diminished visual acuity, magnifiers, closed-circuit televisions and specialized software for enlargement of text displayed on computer screens are useful for helping the patient to read and for the performance of tasks at close distances. Telescopes are also useful for patients to pick out objects at a distance (e.g., to watch sporting events or to read street signs). Follow-up examinations are important in establishing decline of visual function by psychophysical and ERG testing.

REFERENCES

1. Daw NW, Hart WMJ: Color vision. In Moses RA, Hart WMJ (eds): Adler's Physiology of the Eye. St Louis, CV Mosby, 1987.
2. Young T: On the theory of light and colours. Philos Trans R Soc Lond (Biol) 92:12, 1802.
3. von Kreis J: Über Farbensysteme. Z Psychol Physiol Sinnesorg 13:241, 1897.
4. Brown PK, Wald G: Visual pigments in human and monkey retinas. Nature 200:37, 1963.
5. Wald G: The receptors of human color vision. Science 145:1007, 1964.
6. Brown PK, Wald G: Visual pigments in single rods and cones of the human retina. Science 144:45, 1964.
7. Weleber RG, Eisner A: Retinal function and physiological studies. In Newsome DA (ed): Retinal Dystrophies and Degenerations. New York, Raven Press, 1988.
8. Pokorny J, Smith V: Color vision and night vision. In Ogden TE, Schachat AP (eds): Retina. St Louis, CV Mosby, 1989.
9. Lutze M, Cox WJ, Smith VC: Genetic studies of variation in Rayleigh and photometric matches in normal trichromats. Vision Res 30:149, 1990.
10. Neitz J, Jacobs GH: Polymorphism of the long-wavelength cone in normal human colour vision. Nature 323:623, 1986.
11. Lyon MF: Gene action in the X-chromosome of the mouse (Mus musculus, L.). Nature 190:372, 1961.
12. Wald G: Human vision and the spectrum. Science 101:653, 1943.
13. Pokorny J, Smith VC, Verriest G, et al: Congenital and Acquired Color Vision Defects. New York, Grune & Stratton, 1979.
14. Hurvich LM: Color Vision. Sunderland, MA, Sinauer Associates, 1981.
15. Drummond-Borg M, Deeb SS, Motulsky AG: Molecular patterns of X-chromosome–linked color vision genes among 134 men of European ancestry. Proc Natl Acad Sci USA 86:983, 1989.
16. Jorgensen AL, Deeb SS, Motulsky AG: Molecular genetics of X-chromosome–linked color vision among populations of African and Japanese ancestry: High frequency of a shortened red pigment gene among Afro-Americans. Proc Natl Acad Sci USA 87:6512, 1990.
17. Wright WD: The characteristics of tritanopia. J Opt Soc Am 42:509, 1952.
18. Went LN, Pronk N: The genetics of tritan disturbances. Hum Genet 69:255, 1985.
19. Krill AE, Smith VC, Pokorny J: Similarities between congenital tritan defects and dominant optic-nerve atrophy: Coincidence or identity? J Opt Soc Am 60:1132, 1970.
20. Krill AE, Smith VC, Pokorny J: Further studies supporting the identity of congenital tritanopia and hereditary dominant optic atrophy. Invest Ophthalmol 10:457, 1971.
21. Nathans J, Piantanida JP, Hogness DS: Molecular genetics of human color vision. The genes encoding blue, green and red pigment. Science 232:193, 1986.
22. Nathans J, Piantanida JP, Eddy RL: Molecular genetics of inherited variation in human color vision. Science 232:203, 1986.
23. Li T, Zierath P, Went L, et al: Substitution of a highly conserved amino acid residue in the S-cone (blue) photopigment may be the cause of tritan defect in a Dutch pedigree. Invest Ophthalmol Vis Sci 32(Suppl):783, 1991.
24. Lewis RA, Holcomb JD, Bromley WC: Mapping X-linked ophthalmic disease. III. Provisional assignment of the locus for blue cone monochromacy to Xq28. Arch Ophthalmol 105:1055, 1987.
25. Spivey BE: The X-linked recessive inheritance of atypical monochromatism. Arch Ophthalmol 95:741, 1983.
26. Berson EL, Sandberg MA, Maguire A: Electroretinograms in carriers of blue cone monochromatism. Am J Ophthalmol 102:254, 1986.
27. Berson EL, Sandberg MA, Rosner B: Color plates to help identify patients with blue cone monochromatism. Am J Ophthalmol 95:741, 1983.
28. Nathans J, Davenport CM, Maumenee IH, et al: Molecular genetics of human blue cone monochromacy. Science 245:831, 1989.
29. Reichel E, Bruce AM, Sandberg MA, et al: An electroretinographic and molecular genetic study of X-linked cone degeneration. Am J Ophthalmol 108:540, 1989.
30. Jacobson DM, Thompson HS, Bartley JA: X-linked progressive cone dystrophy. Clinical characteristics of affected males and female carriers. Ophthalmology 96:885, 1989.
31. Heckenlively JR, Weleber RG: X-linked recessive cone dystrophy with tapetal-like sheen. Arch Ophthalmol 104:1322, 1986.
32. Keunen JEE, van Everdingen JAM, Went LN, et al: Color matching and foveal densitometry in patients and carriers of an X-linked progressive cone dystrophy. Arch Ophthalmol 108:1713, 1990.
33. Bartley J, Gies C, Jacobson D: Progressive cone dystrophy maps between DXS7 (11.28) and DXS206 (XJ1.1) and is linked to DXS84 (754). Cytogenet Cell Genet 51:959, 1989.
34. Ripps H, Noble KG, Greenstein VC, et al: Progressive cone dystrophy. Ophthalmology 94:1401, 1987.
35. Carr RE, Siegel IM: Cone dysfunctions in man. Trans Am Acad Ophthalmol Otolaryngol 81:613, 1976.

36. Goodman G, Ripps H, Siegel IM: Cone dysfunction syndromes. Arch Ophthalmol 70:214, 1963.

37. Krill AE, Deutman AF: Dominant macular degenerations: The cone dystrophies. Am J Ophthalmol 73:352, 1972.

38. Weleber RG, Eisner A: Cone degeneration ("bull's eye dystrophies") and color vision defects. *In* Newsome DA (ed): Retinal Dystrophies and Degenerations. New York, Raven Press, 1988.

39. Krill AE, Deutman AF, Fishman M: The cone degenerations. Doc Ophthalmol 35:1, 1973.

40. Pokorny J, Smith VC, Ernest JT: Macular color vision defects: Specialized psychophysical testing in acquired and hereditary chorioretinal diseases. Int Ophthalmol Clin 20:54, 1980.

41. Bresnick GH, Smith VC, Pokorny J: Autosomal dominantly inherited macular dystrophy with preferential short-wavelength–sensitive cone involvement. Am J Ophthalmol 108:265, 1989.

42. Weale RA: Some aspects of total color blindness. Trans Ophthalmol Soc UK 73:241, 1975.

43. Ikeda H, Ripps H: The electroretinogram of a cone monochromat. Arch Ophthalmol 75:513, 1966.

44. Pokorny J, Smith VC, Pinkers AJLG: Classification of complete and incomplete autosomal recessive achromatopsias. Graefes Arch Clin Exp Ophthalmol 219:121, 1981.

45. Falls HF, Woter JR, Alpern M: Typical total monochromacy. A histological and psychophysical study. Arch Ophthalmol 74:610, 1965.

46. Glickstein M, Heath GG: Receptors in the monochromat eye. Vision Res 15:633, 1975.

47. Smith VC, Pokorny J, Newell FW: Autosomal recessive incomplete achromatopsia with deutan luminosity. Am J Ophthalmol 87:393, 1979.

48. Smith VC, Pokorny J, Newell FW: Autosomal recessive incomplete achromatopsia with protan luminosity function. Ophthalmologica 177:197, 1978.

49. Neuhann T, Krastel K, Jacques W: Differential diagnosis of typical and atypical congenital achromatopsia. Graefes Arch Clin Exp Ophthalmol 209:19, 1978.

50. Weale RA: Photosensitive reactions in foveae of normal and cone-monochromatic observers. Optica Acta 6:158, 1959.

51. Gibson IM: Visual mechanisms in a cone monochromat. J Physiol (Lond) 161:10, 1962.

52. O'Donnell FE, Welch RB: Fenestrated sheen macular dystrophy: A new autosomal dominant maculopathy. Arch Ophthalmol 97:1292, 1979.

53. Sneed SR, Sieving PA: Fenestrated sheen macular dystrophy. Am J Ophthalmol 112:1, 1991.

54. Gouras P, Eggers HM, Mackay CJ: Cone dystrophy, nyctalopia and supernormal rod responses: A new retinal degeneration. Arch Ophthalmol 101:718, 1983.

55. Sandberg MA, Miller S, Berson EL: Rod electroretinograms in an elevated cyclic guanosine monophosphate–type human retinal degeneration. Invest Ophthalmol Vis Sci 31:2283, 1990.

56. Hamilton SR, Chatrian GE, Mills RP: Cone dysfunction in a subgroup of patients with autosomal dominant cerebellar ataxia. Arch Ophthalmol 108:55, 1990.

57. To KW, Adamian M, Jakobiec FA, et al: Olivopontocerebellar atrophy with retinal degeneration: An electroretinographic and histopathologic investigation. Ophthalmology, in press.

58. Chen WW, Webster TD, Moser HW, et al: Alterations of visual pigment genes in adrenoleukodystrophy. Am J Hum Genet 43(Suppl):A140, 1988.

59. Marmor MF, Jacobson SG, Foerster MH, et al: Diagnostic clinical findings of a new syndrome with night blindness and enhanced S cone sensitivity. Am J Ophthalmol 110:124, 1990.

60. Went LN, Pronk N: Achromatopsia and combination defects of protan, deutan and tritan genes. Colour vision deficiencies. VII. Doc Ophthalmol 39:319, 1984.

61. Gouras P: Electroretinography. Some basic principles. Invest Ophthalmol Vis Sci 9:557, 1970.

62. Gouras P, Mackay CJ: Electroretinographic responses of the short-wavelength–sensitive cones. Invest Ophthalmol Vis Sci 31:1203, 1990.

63. Kollner H: Die Störungen des Farbensinnes. Ihre klinische Bedeutung und ihre Diagnose. Berlin, S Karger, 1912.

64. François J, Verriest G: Ib acquired deficiency of color vision with special reference to its detection and classification by means of the tests of Farnsworth. Vision Res 1:201, 1961.

65. Hart WMJ: Acquired dyschromatopsias. Surv Ophthalmol 32:10, 1987.

66. Verriest G: Further studies on acquired deficiency of color discrimination. J Opt Soc Am 185:195, 1983.

67. Meadows JC: Disturbed perception of colours associated with localized cerebral lesions. Brain 97:615, 1974.

68. Green GJ, Lessell S: Acquired cerebral dyschromatopsia. Arch Ophthalmol 95:121, 1977.

69. Pearlman AL, Birch J, Meadows JC: Cerebral color blindness: An acquired defect in hue discrimination. Ann Neurol 5:253, 1979.

70. Pinckers A, Deutman AF: Peripheral cone disease. Ophthalmologica 174:145, 1977.

71. Berson EL, Gouras P, Gunkel RD: Progressive cone degeneration, dominantly inherited. Arch Ophthalmol 80:77, 1968.

72. Berson EL, Gouras P, Gunkel RD: Progressive cone-rod degeneration. Arch Ophthalmol 80:68, 1968.

73. Weiner A, Sandberg MA, Gaudio AR: Hydroxychloroquine retinopathy. Am J Ophthalmol 112:528, 1991.

74. Weleber RG, Shults WT: Digoxin retinal toxicity. Arch Ophthalmol 99:1568, 1981.

Chapter 108

▪

Hereditary Macular Degenerations

ELIAS REICHEL and MICHAEL A. SANDBERG

As a group, hereditary macular disorders constitute a significant cause of visual loss in children and young adults. These conditions usually progress to legal blindness. Symptoms frequently begin in childhood or early adolescence and may hamper learning in school because affected children must sit as close to the blackboard as possible or use telescopic aids. Young adults may fail vision tests for driving and thereby be forced to adjust not only their vocational aspirations but also their lifestyle in general around public conveyance or the assistance of family and friends. Loss of visual acuity may prevent performance in occupations that depend on fine distance vision. Many of these patients are extremely sensitive to bright lights or outdoor illumination, for reasons that are not yet clear, and find it necessary to wear sunglasses in many situations. In addition, the knowledge that these conditions may be passed on to children and future generations can lead to emotional problems with long-term consequences.

This chapter presents these disorders according to their pattern of inheritance, first considering autosomal dominant and then autosomal recessive forms. X-linked retinoschisis and X-linked cone dysfunction syndromes that can affect the macula are discussed in Chapters 106 and 107. For each condition, funduscopic appearance, electrophysiologic description, prognosis for retaining central vision, and histopathologic descriptions are reviewed. The chapter then concludes with some comments on our approach to patients with these diseases.

Until recently, all of the heredomacular degenerations have been thought to have normal full-field electroretinograms (ERGs), consistent with loss of only macular function and the basis of their original grouping. As will be shown further on, patients with a subtype of Stargardt's disease exhibit abnormal full-field cone ERGs. Many patients referred with conditional diagnoses of macular degeneration, based on funduscopic abnormalities that are limited to the posterior pole (e.g., central geographic atrophy or bull's-eye maculopathy) are found to have generalized cone or cone-rod degeneration based on abnormal full-field cone or cone and rod ERGs, respectively. In fact, one can make the generalization that most macular dystrophies without the pathognomonic fundus features that are described in this chapter (e.g., flecks, drusen, or myopia on fundus examination or a widespread blocked choroidal fluorescence on fluorescein angiography) are cone or cone-rod degenerations until proved otherwise by full-field ERG testing.

DOMINANTLY INHERITED MACULAR DEGENERATIONS

Cystoid Macular Edema

An autosomal dominant form of cystoid macular edema has been described.[1-3] These patients show cystoid macular edema at a young age and invariably are hyperopic because of elevation of the macula. They have no findings or underlying features that predispose to cystoid macular edema (e.g., uveitis). Ophthalmoscopically, these patients show typical cystoid macular edema, which is characterized by thickening of the macula with multiple cystic macular changes; later, they may experience macular atrophy and pigmentary changes. Fluorescein angiography shows cystoid macular edema with leaking perifoveal capillaries and retinal pigment epithelial (RPE) window defects. Full-field ERGs are normal; however, there appears to be a subnormal ratio of the light-peak:dark-trough voltage in the electrooculogram (EOG),[3] suggesting a defect at the

level of the RPE. Affected patients show a gradual progressive decrease of visual acuity starting anywhere from the first to the fourth decades of life. Visual acuity declines to less than the 20/100 level in more than 50 percent of patients by the fourth decade of life. An acquired red-green dyschromatopsia can be seen as well. No histopathologic studies of this condition have yet been reported.

Progressive Foveal Dystrophy

Several pedigrees have been described with a dominant pattern of inheritance in which affected patients have macular dystrophy with white flecks (Fig. 108–1).[4-6] Fundus findings include flecks similar to those seen in fundus flavimaculatus, as well as atrophy of the pigment epithelium in the macula. The flecks block choroidal fluorescence, whereas the choroidal circulation is otherwise visible.

In one large pedigree, some individuals showed marked diminution of visual acuity (20/200 or 20/400) in the first or second decade of life, whereas others did not show onset of visual loss until the fourth or fifth decade of life, typical of the variable expressivity seen in many autosomal dominant conditions.[5] An acquired color defect was also present later in life. Electrophysiologic testing showed normal full-field cone and rod ERG responses and a normal EOG. There is one report of a histopathologic study of eyes from an individual affected by a dominant form of Stargardt's disease.[6] This study revealed aggregates of enlarged RPE cells with apices distended with lipofuscin and melanolipofuscin. These results are similar to those found in individuals with the recessive form of the condition (see further on).

Best's Disease

Best's disease (vitelliform macular dystrophy) is seen in individuals of European, African, and Hispanic ancestry and is variably expressed.[7] Patients can present with blurred vision, diminished visual acuity, and me-

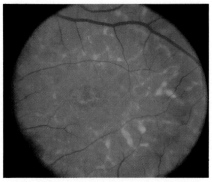

Figure 108–1. Fundus photograph of a 10-year-old girl with dominant Stargardt's disease. Visual acuity was 20/200 O.U. (Courtesy of PF Lopez, M.D, IH Maumenee, M.D., and WR Green, M.D.)

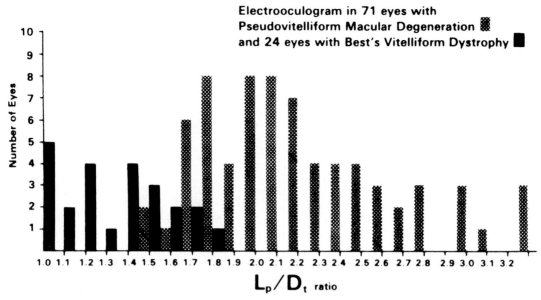

Figure 108–2. Frequency histogram of electrooculogram (EOG) light peak (L_p): dark trough (D_t) ratios in 24 eyes with Best's vitelliform macular degeneration and 71 eyes with pseudovitelliform macular degeneration. (From Sabates R, Pruett RC, Hirose T: Pseudovitelliform macular degeneration. Retina 2:197, 1982.)

tamorphopsia. Best's disease has been described as going through four phases based on fundus examination.[8, 9] The first, called the previtelliform stage, is characterized by a normal fundus appearance. The second stage, the vitelliform stage, usually occurs in early childhood and is characterized by a well-circumscribed 0.5- to 2-disc-diameter yellow lesion that looks like the yolk of an egg and appears to be located under the pigment epithelium. This is usually 0.5 to 2 optic disc diameters in size. Acuity is usually normal or slightly reduced. The lesion may be unilateral, and a yellowish change may be noted in the RPE throughout the fundus. During the teenage years, or thereafter, the yellow lesion can break through the RPE into the subretinal space, and the yellow material can accumulate inferiorly in the macula in the subretinal space to form pseudo-hypopyon (the third stage). A scrambled egg appearance to the fundus then follows, with yellow deposits scattered throughout the posterior pole (the fourth stage). Usually patients are hypermetropic, and visual acuity is in the 20/40 range at this point in the evolution of the disease. Atrophy, choroidal neovascularization, serous detachment of the retina, and disciform scarring can occur in patients with Best's disease.[10, 11] A case of a patient with Best's disease has been described in which a macular hole and rhegmatogenous retinal detachment occurred.[12] Fluorescein angiography in patients with Best's disease reveals blockage of choroidal fluorescein by the vitelliform lesion.[13] After breakup of the vitelliform lesion, there may be depigmentation and staining of atrophic RPE.

The EOG is diagnostic for this dominantly inherited condition (Fig. 108–2). It generally shows a markedly reduced or nondetectable light-peak:dark-trough ratio in affected patients.[14–16] In a minority of cases, however, the EOG is only slightly reduced (see Fig. 108–2).[17] The diagnosis of Best's disease can be made when one sees

any of the four characteristic fundus stages associated with an EOG ratio less than or equal to 1.5 (normal ≥1.8) (Fig. 108–3). Obligate carriers of this condition, who may be asymptomatic and lack visible fundus abnormalities, will also have an abnormal EOG.[16, 18] Full-field ERGs are typically normal,[14, 15] whereas foveal ERGs may be abnormal, even when visual acuity is preserved (Fig. 108–4). The prognosis is good for retaining useful vision in at least one eye throughout life in patients with Best's disease.[19] Eighty-eight percent of patients will have better than 20/40 vision in their better eye. Only 4 percent of patients will have vision less than 20/200 in their better eye.

A variant of Best's disease has multifocal lesions

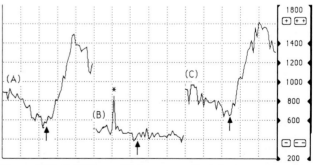

Figure 108–3. EOG amplitudes versus time for a normal subject (A), a 19-year-old patient with Best's vitelliform macular degeneration and visual acuity of 20/25 (B), and a 38-year-old patient with pseudovitelliform macular degeneration and visual acuity of 20/30 (C) tested with a Ganzfeld dome. *Vertical dotted lines* designate 5-min intervals; *horizontal dotted lines* designate 200-µV intervals; *arrows* designate onset of background illumination; *asterisk* denotes transient change in resistance between electrodes. The patient with Best's disease showed no increase in amplitude in the light, whereas the patient with pseudovitelliform macular degeneration showed a normal increase.

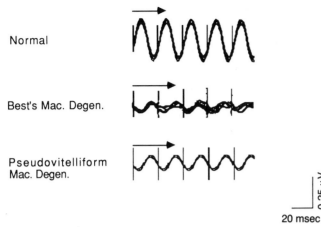

Normal

Best's Mac. Degen.

Pseudovitelliform
Mac. Degen.

0.25 μV

20 msec

Figure 108–4. Foveal cone electroretinograms (ERGs) from a normal subject, a 27-year-old patient with Best's disease and visual acuity of 20/25, and a 50-year-old patient with pseudovitelliform macular degeneration and visual acuity of 20/30 obtained with a stimulator-ophthalmoscope. Two or more consecutive computer summations are superimposed. *Arrows* designate b-wave implicit times. Both patients had subnormal and delayed responses.

throughout the posterior pole (Fig. 108–5).[20] The patients whom we have observed with this condition tend to be older than those with the unifocal form of Best's disease. It is important, therefore, to consider the possibility that this variant represents multifocal pigment epithelial detachments that are filled with chronic serous exudates.[21, 22]

Studies of eyes from patients with Best's disease show RPE cells with excessive amounts of lipofuscin-like material, particularly in the fovea.[23–25] Material derived from deteriorating RPE cells located between Bruch's

membrane and the pigment epithelium in the fovea was considered to represent a previtelliform lesion. There appears to be a secondary loss of photoreceptor cells as well as collections of outer segment debris.

Adult Vitelliform (Pseudovitelliform) Macular Dystrophy

Affected individuals have a small (less than 1 disc diameter), slightly elevated, yellow subretinal lesion, and there may be small yellow flecks in the paracentral region (Fig. 108–6). The lesion can easily be confused with small serous detachments that can be seen in central serous retinopathy or solar retinopathy. Fluorescein angiography shows a lesion that is nonfluorescent sometimes surrounded by a ring of hyperfluorescence.[26, 27]

As in Best's disease, full-field ERGs are normal, whereas foveal ERGs may be abnormal in pseudovitelliform macular degeneration (see Fig. 108–4). The EOG has been observed to be between 1.5 and 1.8 (see Fig. 108–2) and may be well within the normal range (see Fig. 108–3). These patients may present with mild loss of acuity and metamorphopsia in one or both eyes, usually between the ages of 30 and 50 yr.[17, 28–31] The prognosis for retaining good central vision in one eye is usually good, even until late adulthood.[17, 32] According to one study, pseudovitelliform macular degeneration can be differentiated from Best's disease based on its late age of onset, typically normal EOG reading, negative family history for dominant inheritance, slow course, and final atrophic scar.[17]

Gass studied one eye with adult-onset vitelliform macular dystrophy using histopathologic techniques.[33]

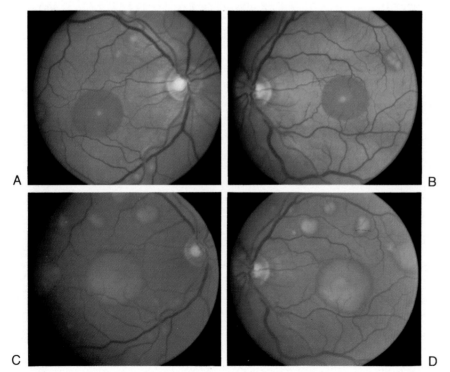

A B C D

Figure 108–5. *A* and *B*, Fundus photographs of a 62-year-old man with Best's disease showing multifocal lesions. He presented with what appeared to be a serous elevation of the macula in both eyes. Follow-up examination revealed multiple small foci of yellowish material throughout the posterior pole. EOG showed a light-peak:dark-trough of 1.0 in both eyes. Visual acuity was 20/20 at this time. *C* and *D*, Examination 8 mo later revealed a typical vitelliform lesion in both eyes associated with multiple deposits of lipofuscin throughout the posterior pole and best corrected visual acuity was 20/20 O.U. (Courtesy of Albert R. Frederick, Jr., M.D.)

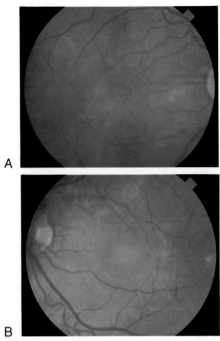

Figure 108–6. Fundus photographs of a 30-year-old man with adult-onset foveomacular dystrophy. Visual acuity was 20/15 O.D. and 20/40 O.S. (A and B). Left eye shows typical pseudovitelliform lesion. EOG testing showed a light-peak:dark-trough of 2.1 O.D. and 2.4 O.S. Full-field ERGs were normal.

suggesting a continuum between vitelliform macular dystrophy and butterfly-shaped dystrophy at least in some pedigrees.[41, 42] In one family, four different types of patterns were observed on fundus examination.[43] Fluorescein angiography shows a darkly pigmented lesion surrounded by hyperfluorescence. Functional testing is, in general, normal. Color vision may be slightly affected when visual acuity is subnormal. These findings suggest that this condition is limited to the RPE. Changes that simulate what is seen in the pattern dystrophies of the RPE can be observed in older individuals with signs of age-related macular degeneration (AMD; i.e., drusen). No histopathologic studies of this condition have been done.

Central Areolar Dystrophies

Central areolar choroidal dystrophy is an autosomal dominant dystrophy with variable expression, characterized by the gradual development of symmetric, well-defined areas of geographic atrophy of the RPE not associated with drusen, myopia, serous or hemorrhagic disciform detachment of the RPE, or inflammation of the choroid (Fig. 108–7).[44–48] Another condition called central areolar pigment epithelial dystrophy is probably the same disease.[49] Examination of the fundus may show RPE granularity in the fovea. Full-field ERGs can be

This eye showed focal loss of photoreceptors and atrophy and partial loss of the RPE in the fovea of both eyes. Pigment-laden cells and extracellular melanin appeared to be the causative feature of the central pigmentation. This pigmented material was found to lie between the retina and Bruch's membrane. Eosinophilic, PAS-positive material was seen surrounding the central pigment clumps. Gass observed no abnormal amount of lipofuscin present in the RPE-containing cells in his study. Another study showed a high concentration of lipofuscin that may be responsible for the foveal lesion.[34]

Pattern Dystrophies of the RPE

This group of conditions is named for the patterns of deposits of pigment that can be seen in the macular area. In some individuals, pigmentation in the macula has been described as displaying a butterfly shape; other patterns have been described as well.[35–39] These patients usually have normal to slightly subnormal visual acuity. Patients with these conditions have mild disturbances of central vision. Color vision may be abnormal. Full-field ERGs are normal, whereas the EOG can be subnormal in some patients. This is a very slowly progressive condition. Visual prognosis is good for retaining vision in at least one eye until late adulthood. Choroidal neovascularization can occur in any of the pattern dystrophies, particularly in those with the butterfly pattern.[40] In some individuals, a vitelliform lesion has also been seen; these patients have subnormal EOGs as well,

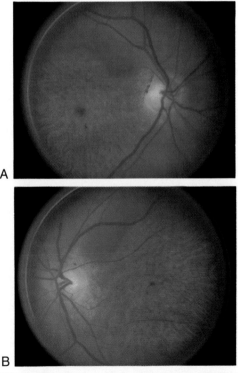

Figure 108–7. Right fundus (A) and left fundus (B) of a 59-year-old woman with central areolar choroidal dystrophy O.U. Visual acuity was 20/50 O.D. and at the counting fingers level O.S. Full-field cone and rod ERGs were reduced 60 percent below normal in both eyes. Cone implicit time was slightly delayed. Dark adaptation was normal. The patient was hypermetropic and had no signs of drusen or other stigmata of age-related macular degeneration.

subnormal.[49, 50] We have observed in patients who have symmetric geographic atrophy without evidence of drusen or myopia that the full-field cone ERG and rod ERG are reduced, suggesting that this is a condition that affects more than just the posterior pole.[51] Young patients with this condition present with macular granularity and normal visual acuities and visual fields. Individuals with this condition have a slow decline of visual acuity starting at approximately age 40 to 50 yr that is associated with the geographic depigmentation of the RPE. One can readily see choroidal vessels within the area of RPE atrophy. The area of atrophy expands slowly, and visual acuity can eventually fall to the "counting fingers" range. Fluorescein angiography shows hyperfluorescence corresponding to the areas of pigment epithelial atrophy. Choroidal vessels can be observed to be outlined by fluorescein. Hyperfluorescence can be detected at the edges of the lesions, indicating leakage of dye from intact choriocapillaris.

Histologic studies have shown a well-demarcated avascular zone that is atrophic and fibrotic.[52] The vessels, including the posterior ciliary arteries, have been found to be normal. The outer retinal layers, including the RPE, were not found to be present in the areas with underlying choroidal atrophy. Bruch's membrane appeared to be normal.

Some individuals characterize benign concentric annular macular dystrophy[53] and fenestrated sheen macular dystrophy[54] as forms of geographic atrophy or bull's-eye maculopathy that primarily affect the macula. Both are autosomal dominant conditions. Benign concentric annular macular dystrophy is characterized by a bull's-eye pattern of geographic atrophy of the RPE around the fovea. It is important to point out that in a long-term follow-up of individuals with benign concentric macular dystrophy, most showed worsening of ERGs (both cone and rod systems), and there was the appearance of bone spicule pigment in some of these patients.[55] Fenestrated sheen macular dystrophy is characterized by small red fenestrations in the macula associated with a golden sheen. The macula in this condition typically has a tapetal reflex. Prognosis for retaining visual acuity is good in both of these conditions. No long-term follow-up is available for fenestrated sheen macular dystrophy. In addition, some patients with fenestrated sheen macular dystrophy have widespread abnormalities of the cone and rod systems.[56] Therefore, we prefer to classify benign concentric annular macular dystrophy and fenestrated sheen macular dystrophy as degenerations involving the cone and rod photoreceptors. We would reserve comment regarding prognosis for retaining peripheral vision in either of these conditions until more follow-up data are available.

Dominantly Inherited Drusen

The spectrum of disease caused by dominantly inherited drusen has been given a wide variety of names: Doyne's honeycomb dystrophy, Hutchinson-Tay choroiditis, malattia léventinese, Holthouse-Batten superficial chorioretinitis, and guttate choroiditis. These different names may represent variants of the same condition. Doyne described the occurrence of colloid bodies (drusen) observed to lie on Bruch's membrane in certain families who lived in Oxford, England. These drusen tended to merge together and eventually become confluent, resembling a honeycomb, hence the name Doyne's honeycomb choroiditis (Fig. 108–8). Vogt and Klainguti described a family with a macular dystrophy similar to Doyne's that lived in the Valley of the Leventine in the Canton of Tessin in Switzerland.[57]

Dominant drusen is difficult to separate from AMD. Some authors believe that many individuals who are affected with AMD have a form of dominant drusen.[58] Although dominant drusen may represent a subset of AMD, it would be unlikely that all types of AMD represent the varied expression of a single gene defect that would cause a disease as prevalent as AMD (upward of 15 percent of individuals older than the age of 75 yr have signs of this condition).[59] However, a case control study of patients with AMD found that there was a statistically significant association between AMD and family history of the disease.[60] Another study attempted to distinguish dominant drusen from age-related (acquired) drusen using histopathologic methods.[61] Only two eyes were examined in this study. The individual thought to have familial drusen showed a widespread disturbance of the RPE throughout the retina characterized by an irregularity of the pigment granule content of the retinal pigment epithelial cells. In addition, some of the pigment epithelial cells contained a granular basophilic material. In contrast, the individual with AMD showed focal RPE changes that were confined to

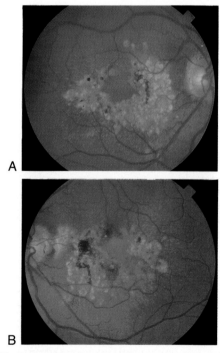

Figure 108–8. Fundus photographs of a 37-year-old man who has the diagnosis of Doyne's honeycomb macular dystrophy with visual acuity of 20/20 O.D. and 20/100 O.S. *A,* Right eye. *B,* Left eye. Fundus examination revealed the typical honeycomb appearance of multiple, confluent drusen with associated pigmentary changes. Full-field and focal ERG testing was normal.

the site of the drusen. The pigment epithelium between the drusen appeared to be normal. Ultrastructurally, drusen from both patients showed an abnormal distribution of pigment granules throughout the cytoplasm of the RPE. The mitochondria showed marked degeneration, and there was an increase in lysosomes. A fibrillar material was found in the plasma membrane's infoldings, and there were also deposits of this material on Bruch's membrane. Histochemically, there was no difference in the composition of the drusen, with both containing sialic acid and cerebrosides.

We reserve the diagnosis of dominant drusen for individuals who present with drusen at an early age (second to third decade of life) and when there is a clear family history of the condition affecting several generations (Fig. 108–9). Usually there is a halo of drusen surrounding the foveola and symmetric changes in both eyes. These drusen are distributed mainly in the macula and around the optic nerve head, often with a nasal predominance. Some have suggested that the location of drusen nasal to the disc is pathognomonic of familial drusen.[62, 63]

Individuals with dominant drusen have been noted as early as childhood and usually present with normal to near-normal acuity.[64] These patients are in general asymptomatic; however, if there are symptoms, they usually consist of difficulty with central vision, particularly under dim lighting conditions or when driving at night. Fluorescein angiography shows well-defined hyperfluorescent areas beginning in the early arterial phase that correspond to the drusen. The hyperfluorescence is due to RPE window defects that overlie the drusen. If subretinal neovascularization occurs, there can be a sudden reduction in visual acuity or new or worsening metamorphopsia. Fluorescein angiography is a necessity

in the management of these patients when a choroidal neovascular membrane is suspected. Full-field ERGs and EOGs, in our experience, have been normal in patients with dominant drusen (and AMD). When performing such studies, it is important to compare these results to those of normal age-matched controls.

Sorsby's pseudoinflammatory macular dystrophy or autosomal dominant hemorrhagic macular dystrophy was studied initially in five families showing a dominantly inherited condition that is characterized by the development of choroidal neovascular membranes, subretinal hemorrhages, and changes consistent with disciform degeneration (Fig. 108–10).[65–68] Loss of central vision occurs in the fifth decade of life because of these exudative changes, and there is a progressive loss of peripheral vision due to chorioretinal atrophy. Patients with Sorsby's pseudoinflammatory macular dystrophy have been identified who have abnormal rhodopsin kinetics.[69, 70] When areas with the abnormal yellow subretinal material were tested, there were delays in both psychophysical dark adaptation and rhodopsin regeneration. In areas without the subretinal material, dark adaptation and rhodopsin regeneration were normal. It was proposed that the abnormal rhodopsin kinetics represented a reduced metabolic exchange across an altered Bruch's membrane. Full-field ERGs and EOGs are normal in patients with this condition.

Histopathologic data are available on two sisters. Findings were consistent with both AMD and angioid streaks in patients with pseudoxanthoma elasticum. In addition, thick, lipid-rich deposits have been seen within Bruch's membrane.[71] The fundus changes observed in Sorsby's macular degeneration are also common in AMD. To add further confusion, a follow-up study of Sorsby's original five families showed that there were

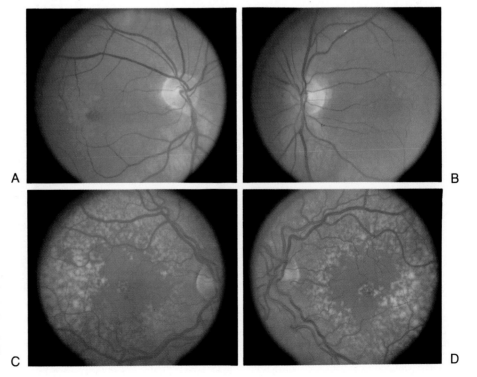

Figure 108–9. A and B, Fundus photographs of a 21-year-old woman with dominant drusen of both eyes. Visual acuity was 20/50 O.D. and 20/40 O.S. Her 57-year-old mother had 20/20 vision O.U. There were drusen in the posterior poles of both eyes (C and D). Her 81-year-old maternal grandfather's vision was at the counting fingers level in the right eye and 20/40 in the left eye. Drusen and depigmentation of the retinal pigment epithelium were observed on funduscopic examination.

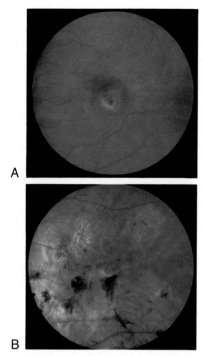

Figure 108–10. Fundus photograph of a 40-year-old man with autosomal dominant hemorrhagic macular dystrophy (Sorsby's pseudoinflammatory dystrophy). A choroidal neovascular membrane (CNVM) is seen in the left eye (A). Twelve months later a CNVM developed in the right eye. His 63-year-old mother currently shows extensive retinal scarring and loss of retinal pigment epithelium and choriocapillaris (B). She suffered an acute loss of vision in her left eye at the age of 50 yr, and laser surgery at that time failed to stem the choroidal neovascular membrane. (Courtesy of Steven A. Boskovich, M.D., and Paul A. Sieving, M.D.)

funduscopic features that were typical of angioid streaks with multiple, fine, drusen-like deposits that were identical to the peau d'orange changes occurring in patients with pseudoxanthoma elasticum.[72] Another interesting feature of this condition is that the diagnosis is rarely made in the United States, with most people considering this a form of AMD.

A large pedigree from North Carolina has been described, consisting of 545 family members affected by a dominantly inherited macular dystrophy characterized by a slowly progressive loss of central vision.[73, 74] The earliest fundus changes that can be seen occur in childhood and the early teenage years (Fig. 108–11). Drusenlike deposits are seen in the macula with associated pigmentary changes. Visual acuity may remain normal; however, acuity can drop to the 20/200 level with development of atrophy of the choroid, RPE, and retina. This condition is, in general, thought to be very slowly progressive.[75] Choroidal neovascular membranes can also occur in these patients. Staphylomas with outpouching of the area of atrophy have also been observed in patients with this condition. Visual function testing, aside from acuity and field, is normal in these patients. Systemic evaluation of these individuals revealed aminoaciduria that segregates independently of the foveal dystrophy but is also dominantly inherited. The wide variety of lesions that are seen in the condition probably reflect the variable expressivity of this dominant trait.

AUTOSOMAL RECESSIVE MACULAR DEGENERATIONS

Familial Foveal Retinoschisis

This condition resembles X-linked retinoschisis; the peripheral fundus appears normal, however, and the full-field ERG is also normal.[76]

Stargardt's Disease (Fundus Flavimaculatus)

Stargardt's disease is perhaps the most common heredomacular degeneration. A history of parental consanguinity can often be obtained from patients who are thought to have a recessive form of Stargardt's disease. The definition of Stargardt's disease is confusing in that it is also known by another name (fundus flavimaculatus) and has been subdivided into several categories that may represent the same genetic condition. It is likely

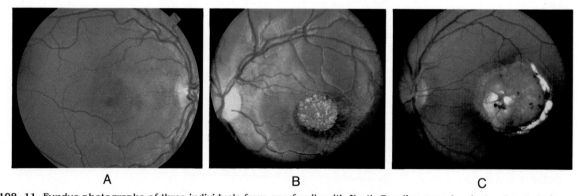

Figure 108–11. Fundus photographs of three individuals from one family with North Carolina macular dystrophy. A, Left eye of a 22-year-old woman with 20/20 vision (grade I fundus). B, Right eye of a 7-year-old girl with 20/30 visual acuity (grade II fundus. C, Right eye of a 29-year-old man with 20/40 visual acuity and grade III fundus. Seventeen affected members of this family were observed over a 10-yr period, and only one patient showed a progressive loss of vision with development of a disciform lesion. (From Small KW, Killian J, McLean WC: North Carolina's dominant progressive foveal dystrophy: How progressive is it? Br J Ophthalmol 75:401, 1991.)

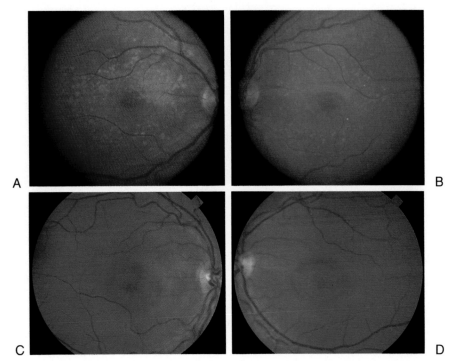

Figure 108–12. Fundus photographs of two sisters with Stargardt's disease. The older sister (A and B), aged 17 yr, had 20/200 visual acuity O.U. and shows white flecks at the level of the retinal pigment epithelium. The fovea showed granular retinal pigment epithelium changes. Her 10-year-old sister (C and D) had 20/200 visual acuity O.U. with granular retinal pigment epithelium changes in the fovea. No white deposits were seen, illustrating intrafamilial variability.

that Stargardt's disease and fundus flavimaculatus are a continuum of the same condition[77] and that the varied fundus appearances may represent a progression of a particular genetic form of the disease, although multiple genetic forms of this condition cannot be excluded.[78–82] Franceschetti was the first to use the term *fundus flavimaculatus* when describing the appearance of yellow-white, irregularly shaped flecks in the fundus at the level of the RPE (Figs. 108–12 to 108–14).[82] The flecks are always present in the posterior pole and can extend as far as the equator of the eye. Stargardt's disease is also characterized by flecks in the posterior pole of the eye, and early on patients with this condition may show normal maculas, with atrophy occurring later as the disease progresses.

The fundus appearance of the yellow flecks can appear similar to drusen. These lesions have also been described as having a pisiform (fishlike) shape. Fluorescein angiography is useful in distinguishing drusen from the presence of the yellow flecks in that drusen hyperfluoresce or block fluorescein in correspondence to their location and size in the posterior pole, whereas the flecks of Stargardt's disease either do not fluoresce or

show an irregular pattern of fluorescence.[83] Some authors have described a heavily pigmented RPE ("vermilion fundus") that shows a "silent" choroid (obscured choroidal fluorescence).[84] In the central macula, the RPE may be observed to have areas of geographic atrophy, a beaten-metal appearance, or a bull's-eye pattern of dystrophy.[81]

Some authors have classified the fundus appearance of Stargardt's disease into many different stages, ranging from a normal-appearing fundus to atrophy of the macula with or without flecks to flecks with or without atrophy of the macula, and in addition, flecks that may be peripheral to the macula.[79, 81] Using such a categorization is arbitrary, especially in a disease in which any individual may go through more than one of these stages of fundus appearance. More importantly, it is difficult to stage fundus appearance to the level of visual acuity.[85] Initially, the fundus may appear to be normal. Lack of the foveolar reflex may precede any changes in the RPE before flecks are seen. Fluorescein angiography can show choroidal silence because of the filtering action of the RPE. With the appearance of RPE atrophy, hyperfluorescence of the atrophic spots can occur.

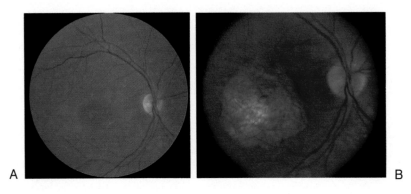

Figure 108–13. Progression of macular changes in a patient with Stargardt's disease. Flecks can be seen throughout the posterior pole with retinal pigment epithelium changes noted in the fovea and parafovea at age 16 yr (A). Visual acuity was 20/200 at this time. Eleven years later, the visual acuity is unchanged; however, there is a large area of retinal pigment epithelium and choriocapillaris drop-out in the posterior pole (B).

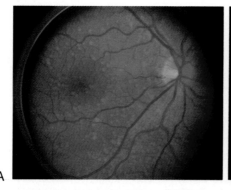
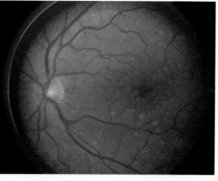

Figure 108–14. Fundus photographs of a 29-year-old woman with fundus flavimaculatus. Visual acuity was 20/20 O.U. Multiple white, round, and pisiform flecks are seen throughout the posterior pole spanning a 30-degree radius throughout the fundus. Full-field ERGs were normal. Patient was seen 5 yr later with no change in acuity or funduscopic examination. Focal ERG testing at that time was normal.

Patients with Stargardt's disease usually present by their teenage years with bilateral diminution of vision.[80, 86] Visual acuity can often be ascertained to be normal by previous history. Visual acuity usually falls to less than the 20/100 level after approximately 5 yr in patients who initially present with 20/40 vision or better. Retinal function testing shows visual acuity declining to the 20/200 level or slightly worse by the early 20s. Visual field testing can show a relative central scotoma that later progresses to an absolute central scotoma. An acquired red-green dyschromatopsia may occur. Dark adaptation is normal. Full-field ERGs are typically normal, whereas foveal ERGs are often abnormal, even in patients with nearly normal visual acuity.[87] Foveal ERGs may be subnormal in amplitude or delayed in peak time, or both (Fig. 108–15).[88] Both changes were correlated with visual acuity (e.g., Fig. 108–16). The EOG has been reported to be subnormal in most patients who have been examined, although normal values were found using a diffusing sphere (as is standard in ERG) in patients with early stages of disease.[89] The test is difficult to perform in patients who have diminished

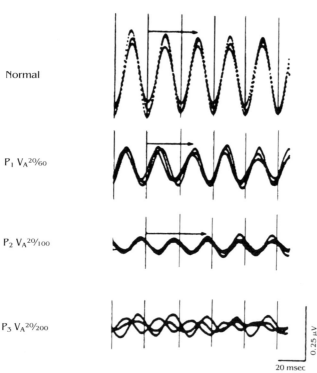

Figure 108–15. Foveal cone ERGs from a normal subject and three patients with Stargardt's disease obtained with a stimulator-ophthalmoscope. Three consecutive computer summations are shown. *Arrows* designate b-wave implicit times for detectable responses. Responses for the patients are subnormal (P_1), subnormal and delayed (P_2), and nondetectable (P_3). (From Sandberg MA, Jacobson S, Berson E: Focal cone electroretinograms in retinitis pigmentosa and juvenile macular degenerations. Am J Ophthalmol 88:702–707, 1979. Published with permission from The American Journal of Ophthalmology. Copyright by The Ophthalmic Publishing Company.)

FOVEAL CONE ERG AMPLITUDES IN
JUVENILE MACULAR DEGENERATION

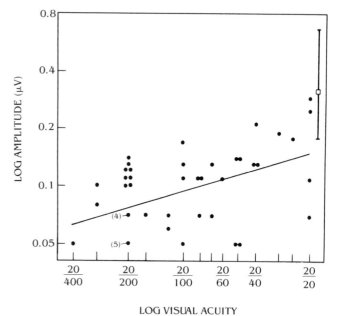

LOG VISUAL ACUITY

Figure 108–16. A double logarithmic plot of foveal cone ERG amplitude versus Snellen visual acuity based on one eye of each of 46 patients with Stargardt's disease *(filled circles)*. Numbers in parentheses denote multiple values. For statistical purposes, nondetectable responses (<0.05 μV) were set equal to 0.05 μV. The solid line is the best-fitting linear regression line, $\log_e y = 0.29 \log_e x - 1.89$, where y is ERG amplitude in microvolts and x is decimal visual acuity; the correlation coefficient (r) is 0.51, $p < 0.001$. The median *(open square)* and range *(vertical bars)* for foveal ERG amplitudes elicited from 67 normal observers are shown for an average normal visual acuity of 20/18. (From Sandberg MA, Hanson AH, Berson EL: Foveal and parafoveal cone electroretinogram in juvenile macular degeneration. Ophthalmic Paediatr Genet 3:83, 1983. Published with permission from the journal Ophthalmic Paediatrics and Genetics. Copyright by Aeolus Press.)

visual acuity (less than 20/200); in fact, many of the previous studies that have been done indicate that subnormal EOGs may reflect the poor visual acuity rather than actually provide evidence for the occurrence of a disturbance of the RPE as the primary problem.

When 55 individuals between the ages of 6 and 34 yr with a diagnosis of Stargardt's disease were reviewed, peripheral cone malfunction was determined to occur in 40 percent of these patients, as evidenced by delayed full-field cone ERG b-wave implicit times and diminished full-field cone ERG b-wave amplitudes.[90] Peripheral rod function was determined to be normal in these patients. Follow-up was available for approximately half of the patients with cone malfunction. These patients lost 13 percent of remaining full-field cone function per year in comparison to those with normal cone function who lost only 5 percent function per year. Therefore, full-field cone ERGs can be helpful in prognosticating the preservation of peripheral cone function. It is interesting to speculate that the group that shows peripheral cone malfunction may actually have a form of cone or cone-rod degeneration.

Histopathologic study of Stargardt's disease has indicated that there is an accumulation of material in the apex of the RPE cell that is identified as an acid mucopolysaccharide.[81] The defects in the photoreceptors may be secondary to the RPE abnormality. More recently, some investigators determined that the intercel-lular accumulation of material was of a lipofuscin-like substance.[91] Scanning electron microscopy revealed RPE cells that were engorged to ten times their normal size with this material. Subretinal neovascularization has been seen in cases of fundus flavimaculatus, and this complication must be watched for in patients with this condition.[92]

Sjögren's Reticular Dystrophy of the RPE

This is a rare, usually autosomal recessive, condition characterized by an accumulation of dark pigment in a meshwork or fishnet-like pattern.[93–95] The network starts centrally and then extends toward the periphery in later stages of the disease. Eventually, the pigment disappears. This pigment is thought to reside at the level of the RPE. As one might expect, there is hyperfluorescence between the hyperpigmented meshwork. The pigmented network blocks the choroidal fluorescence (Fig. 108–17). Visual acuity is minimally affected in this condition. Tests of retinal function are normal. We recorded from one patient with this condition who showed both normal full-field and foveal ERGs (e.g., Fig. 108–18). No histopathologic information is available for this condition.

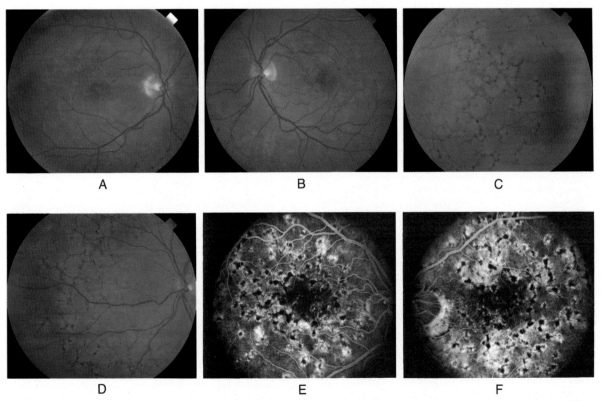

Figure 108–17. Fundus photographs and fluorescein angiograms of a 32-year-old man with Sjögren's reticular dystrophy of the retinal pigment epithelium. Visual acuity was 20/20 in both eyes. Fundus photography shows a netlike pattern of pigmentation in the posterior pole and the midperiphery (A–D). Fluorescein angiography shows blockage of dye in the areas of hyperpigmentation and hyperfluorescence along the reticulated pattern corresponding to retinal pigment epithelium loss (E and F). Full-field and foveal ERGs were normal.

Normal

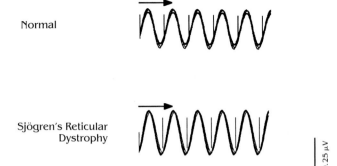

Sjögren's Reticular
Dystrophy

0.25 μV

20 msec

Figure 108–18. Foveal cone ERGs from a normal subject and a 32-year-old patient with Sjögren's reticular dystrophy and visual acuity 20/20 obtained with a stimulator-ophthalmoscope. Three consecutive computer summations are superimposed. *Arrows* designate b-wave implicit times. The patient with Sjögren's reticular dystrophy had normal responses.

APPROACH TO THE PATIENT

Patients, especially children and young adults, who present with subnormal visual acuity with or without associated macular changes should receive a careful evaluation regarding the possibility of their having a hereditary macular condition. Exclusion of optic nerve disorders (e.g., optic neuritis) and acquired conditions (e.g., solar maculopathy) by careful examination and history taking is crucial in establishing the diagnosis of a hereditary macular condition. Many of these conditions have typical fundus features that make diagnosis easy. Conversely, many conditions that have a similar fundus appearance may display different functional (ERG) abnormalities. Full-field ERG testing is therefore useful in evaluating whether the cone or both the cone and the rod systems are involved. Not only is this useful for diagnostic purposes but it also can be used for determining whether peripheral visual loss may occur in a patient who seemingly has only macular changes on ophthalmoscopic examination. Focal ERG testing is useful for establishing the course of malfunction of the foveal photoreceptors and can be helpful in distinguishing amblyopia and optic nerve disorders from macular malfunction. EOG testing is useful in evaluating patients who are thought to have Best's disease. Fluorescein angiography is useful for diagnostic purposes and for determining the evaluation and treatment of choroidal neovascular membranes that can be seen in dominant drusen, Best's disease, and the pattern dystrophies.

After making the diagnosis of a hereditary macular degeneration, the patient's needs for visual aids should be assessed. Magnifiers and high add glasses for near use have been found to be useful for reading. Devices for enlarging reading material have also been helpful. Since many of these patients present at a young age, they can be helped by receiving vocational counseling that is geared to their visual deficit. Patients with disease that solely affects the macula should be encouraged that they will maintain the use of their peripheral vision for the rest of their lives. Many patients benefit from the use of a hand-held pocket telescope for use at ball games or the theater and for other activities that require fine distance acuity. We encourage our patients who are sensitive to bright light to wear sunglasses. Patients are followed every several years to assess their visual function and reassess their need for visual aids.

If a hereditary condition is thought to exist, the individual is counseled regarding the possibility of having other affected family members, and if a mode of inheritance is established, he or she is told about the possibility of having children affected with the same condition.

REFERENCES

1. Deutman AF, Pinckers AJLG, Van de Kerk AL: Dominantly inherited cystoid macular edema. Am J Ophthalmol 82:540, 1976.
2. Notting JGA, Pinckers AJLG: Dominant cystoid macular dystrophy. Am J Ophthalmol 83:234, 1977.
3. Pinckers A, Deutman AF, Notting JG: Retinal function in dominant cystoid macular dystrophy. Arch Ophthalmol 94:579, 1976.
4. Cavender JC: Fundus flavimaculatus: Variable fundus findings in a dominant pedigree. Invest Ophthalmol Vis Sci 17(Suppl):204, 1978.
5. Cibis GW, Morey M, Harris DG: Dominantly inherited macular dystrophy with flecks (Stargardt). Arch Ophthalmol 98:1785, 1980.
6. Lopez PF, Maumenee IH, de la Cruz Z, et al: Autosomal-dominant fundus flavimaculatus. Ophthalmology 97:798, 1990.
7. Maloney W, Robertson D, Duboff S: Hereditary vitelliform macular degeneration. Arch Ophthalmol 95:979, 1977.
8. Barricks M: Vitelliform lesions developing in normal fundi. Am J Ophthalmol 83:324, 1977.
9. Kraushar M, Margolis S, Morse P, et al: Pseudohypopyon in Best's vitelliform macular dystrophy. Am J Ophthalmol 94:30, 1982.
10. Miller SA, Bresnick GH, Chandra SR: Choroidal neovascular membrane in Best's vitelliform macular dystrophy. Am J Ophthalmol 82:252, 1976.
11. Benson WE, Kilker AE, Enoch JM, et al: Best's vitelliform macular dystrophy. Am J Ophthalmol 79:59, 1975.
12. Schachat AP, de la Cruz Z, Green WR: Macular hole and retinal detachment in Best's disease. Retina 5:22, 1985.
13. Curry H Jr, Moorman L: Fluorescein photography of vitelliform macular degeneration. Arch Ophthalmol 79:705, 1968.
14. Krill AE, Morse PA, Potts AM, et al: Hereditary vitelliruptive macular degeneration. Am J Ophthalmol 61:1405, 1966.
15. François J, De Rouck A, Fernandez-Sasso D: Electro-oculography in vitelliform degeneration of the macula. Arch Ophthalmol 77:726, 1967.
16. Deutman AF: Electro-oculography in families with vitelliform dystrophy of the fovea: Detection of the carrier state. Arch Ophthalmol 81:305, 1969.
17. Sabates R, Pruett RC, Hirose T: Pseudovitelliform macular degeneration. Retina 2:197, 1982.
18. Thorborn W, Nordstrom S: EOG in a large family with hereditary macular degeneration. Acta Ophthalmol 56:455, 1976.
19. Mohler CW, Fine SL: Long-term evaluation of patients with Best's vitelliform dystrophy. Ophthalmology 88:688, 1981.
20. Miller SA: Multifocal Best's vitelliform dystrophy. Arch Ophthalmol 95:984, 1977.
21. Noble K, Levitzky M, Carr R: Detachments of the retinal pigment epithelium at the posterior pole. Am J Ophthalmol 82:296, 1976.
22. Burgess D, Olk R, Uniat L: Macular disease resembling adult foveomacular dystrophy in older adults. Ophthalmology 94:1987, 1987.
23. Frangieh GT, Green WR, Fine SL: A histopathologic study of Best's vitelliform dystrophy. Arch Ophthalmol 100:1115, 1982.
24. O'Gorman S, Flaherty WA, Fishman GA, et al: Histopathologic findings in Best's vitelliform macular dystrophy. Arch Ophthalmol 106:1261, 1988.
25. Weingeist TA, Kobrin JL, Watzke RC: Histopathology of Best's macular dystrophy. Arch Ophthalmol 100:1108 1982.

26. Gass JDM: A clinicopathologic study of a peculiar foveomacular dystrophy. Trans Am Ophthalmol Soc 72:139, 1974.
27. Vine AK, Schatz H: Adult-onset foveomacular pigment epithelial dystrophy. Am J Ophthalmol 89:680, 1980.
28. Bloom LH, Swanson DE, Bird AC: Adult vitelliform macular degeneration. Br J Ophthalmol 65:800, 1981.
29. Fishman GA, Trimble S, Rabb MF, et al: Pseudovitelliform macular degeneration. Arch Ophthalmol 95:73, 1977.
30. Wiznia R, Perina B, Noble K: Vitelliform macular dystrophy of late onset. Br J Ophthalmol 65:866, 1981.
31. Hodes B, Feiner L, Sherman S, et al: Progression of pseudovitelliform macular dystrophy. Arch Ophthalmol 102:381, 1984.
32. Epstein G, Rabb M: Adult vitelliform macular degeneration: Diagnosis and natural history. Br J Ophthalmol 64:733, 1980.
33. Gass JDM: A clinicopathologic study of a peculiar foveomacular dystrophy. Trans Am Ophthalmol Soc 72:139, 1974.
34. Patrinely JR, Lewis RA, Font R: Foveomacular vitelliform dystrophy, adult type: A clinicopathologic study including electron microscopic observations. Ophthalmology 92:1712, 1985.
35. Deutman AF, van Blommestein JDA, Henkes HE, et al: Butterfly-shaped pigment dystrophy of the fovea. Arch Ophthalmol 83:558, 1970.
36. Hsieh RC, Fine BS, Lyons JS: Patterned dystrophies of the retinal pigment epithelium. Arch Ophthalmol 95:429, 1977.
37. Marmor M, Byers B: Pattern dystrophy of the pigment epithelium. Am J Ophthalmol 84:32, 1977.
38. O'Donnell FE, Schatz H, Reid P, et al: Autosomal dominant dystrophy of the retinal pigment epithelium. Arch Ophthalmol 97:680, 1979.
39. Prensky JG, Bresnick GH: Butterfly-shaped macular dystrophy in four generations. Arch Ophthalmol 101:1198, 1983.
40. Burgess D: Subretinal neovascularization in a pattern dystrophy of the retinal pigment epithelium. Retina 1:151, 1981.
41. Gutman I, Walsh JB, Henkind P: Vitelliform macular dystrophy and butterfly-shaped epithelial dystrophy: A continuum? Br J Ophthalmol 66:170, 1982.
42. Giuffre G: Autosomal dominant pattern dystrophy of the retinal pigment epithelium: Intrafamilial variability. Retina 8:169, 1988.
43. Jong PD, Delleman J: Pigment epithelial pattern dystrophy: Four different manifestations in a family. Arch Ophthalmol 100:1416, 1982.
44. Ferry AP, Llovera I, Shafer DM: Central areolar choroidal dystrophy. Arch Ophthalmol 88:39, 1972.
45. Nettleship E: Central senile areolar choroidal atrophy. Trans Ophthalmol Soc UK 4:165, 1884.
46. Sandvig K: Familial, central, areolar, choroidal atrophy of autosomal dominant inheritance. Acta Ophthalmol 33:1, 1955.
47. Sorsby A: Choroidal angio-sclerosis with special reference to its hereditary character. Br J Ophthalmol 23:433, 1939.
48. Sorsby A, Crick RP: Central areolar choroidal sclerosis. Br J Ophthalmol 37:129, 1953.
49. Noble K: Central areolar choroidal dystrophy. Am J Ophthalmol 84:310, 1977.
50. Carr R: Central areolar choroidal dystrophy. Arch Ophthalmol 73:32, 1965.
51. Reichel E, Berson EL: Abnormal full-field cone electroretinograms in central areolar choroidal dystrophy. Invest Ophthalmol Vis Sci 31(Suppl):496, 1990.
52. Ashton N: Central areolar choroidal sclerosis: A histo-pathological study. Br J Ophthalmol 37:140, 1953.
53. Deutman A: Benign concentric annular macular dystrophy. Am J Ophthalmol 78:384, 1974.
54. O'Donnell FE Jr, Welch RB: Fenestrated sheen macular dystrophy: A new autosomal dominant maculopathy. Arch Ophthalmol 97:1292, 1979.
55. Biesen P, Deutman A, Pinckers A: Evolution of benign concentric annular macular dystrophy. Am J Ophthalmol 100:73, 1985.
56. Sneed SR, Sieving PA: Fenestrated sheen macular dystrophy. Am J Ophthalmol 112:1, 1991.
57. Duke-Elder S: The tapeto-retinal dystrophies. In Duke-Elder S (ed): System of Ophthalmology, vol. 10. St Louis, CV Mosby, 1967.
58. Gass JDM: Drusen and disciform macular detachment and degeneration. Arch Ophthalmol 90:206, 1973.
59. Leibowitz HM, Krueger DE, Maunder LR, et al: The Framingham Eye Study monograph. Surv Ophthalmol 24(Suppl):434, 1980.
60. Hyman LA, Lilienfeld A, Ferris F III: Senile macular degeneration: A case-control study. Am J Epidemiol 118:213, 1983.
61. Farkas TG, Krill AE: Familial and secondary drusen: Histologic and functional correlations. Trans Am Acad Ophthalmol Otolaryngol 75:333, 1971.
62. Deutman A, Jansen LMAA: Dominant drusen of Bruch's membrane. In Deutman A (ed): The Hereditary Dystrophies of the Posterior Pole of the Eye. Assen, The Netherlands, van Gorcum, 1971.
63. Pearce WG: Doyne's honeycomb retinal degeneration: Clinical and genetic features. Br J Ophthalmol 52:73, 1968.
64. Deutman AF, Jansen LMAA: Dominantly inherited drusen of Bruch's membrane. Br J Ophthalmol 54:373, 1970.
65. Fraser HB, Wallace DC: Sorsby's familial pseudoinflammatory macular dystrophy. Am J Ophthalmol 71:1216, 1971.
66. Sorsby A, Mason MEJ, Gardener N: A fundus dystrophy with unusual features. Br J Ophthalmol 33:67, 1949.
67. Carr RE, Noble KG, Nasaduke I: Hereditary hemorrhagic macular dystrophy. Am J Ophthalmol 85:318, 1978.
68. Carr RE, Noble KG: Pseudoinflammatory macular dystrophy. Trans Am Ophthalmol Soc 75:255, 1977.
69. Steinmetz RD, Polkinghorne D, Fitzke F, et al: Abnormal dark adaptation and rhodopsin kinetics in Sorsby's fundus dystrophy. Invest Ophthalmol Vis Sci 31(Suppl):413, 1990.
70. Boskovich S, Sieving P: Autosomal dominant hemorrhagic macular dystrophy. Ophthalmology, in press.
71. Ashton N, Sorsby A: A fundus dystrophy with unusual features: A histological study. Br J Ophthalmol 35:751, 1951.
72. Hoskin A, Sehmi K, Bird AC: Sorsby's pseudoinflammatory macular dystrophy. Br J Ophthalmol 64:859, 1981.
73. Frank HR, Landers MB Jr, Williams RJ, et al: A new dominant progressive foveal dystrophy. Am J Ophthalmol 78:903, 1974.
74. Lefler WH, Wadsworth JAC, Sidbury J Jr: Hereditary macular degeneration and amino-aciduria. Am J Ophthalmol 71:224, 1971.
75. Small KW, Killian J, McLean WC: North Carolina's dominant progressive foveal dystrophy: How progressive is it? Br J Ophthalmol 75:401, 1991.
76. Lewis RA, Lee GB, Martonyi CL, et al: Familial foveal retinoschisis. Arch Ophthalmol 95:1190, 1977.
77. Hadden OB, Gass JDM: Fundus flavimaculatus and Stargardt's disease. Am J Ophthalmol 82:527, 1976.
78. Carr RE: Fundus flavimaculatus. Arch Ophthalmol 74:163, 1965.
79. Fishman GA: Fundus flavimaculatus: A clinical classification. Arch Ophthalmol 94:2061, 1976.
80. Klien BA, Krill AE: Fundus flavimaculatus: Clinical, functional and histopathologic observations. Am J Ophthalmol 64:3, 1967.
81. Noble KG, Carr RE: Stargardt's disease and fundus flavimaculatus. Arch Ophthalmol 97:1281, 1979.
82. Franceschetti A, François J: Fundus flavimaculatus. Arch Ophthal (Paris) 25:505, 1965.
83. Ernest JT, Krill AE: Fluorescein studies in fundus flavimaculatus and drusen. Am J Ophthalmol 62:1, 1966.
84. Gass JDM: Stereoscopic Atlas of Macular Diseases. St Louis, CV Mosby, 1987.
85. Aaberg T: Stargardt's disease and fundus flavimaculatus: Evaluation of morphologic progression of intrafamilial co-existence. Trans Am Ophthalmol Soc 84:453, 1986.
86. Moloney JBM, Mooney DJ, O'Connor MA: Retinal function in Stargardt's disease and fundus flavimaculatus. Am J Ophthalmol 96:57, 1983.
87. Sandberg MA, Jacobson SG, Berson EL: Focal cone electroretinograms in retinitis pigmentosa and juvenile macular degenerations. Am J Ophthalmol 88:702, 1979.
88. Sandberg MA, Hanson AH, Berson EL: Foveal and parafoveal cone electroretinogram in juvenile macular degeneration. Ophthalmic Paediatr Genet 3:83, 1983.
89. Fishman GA, Young RSL, Schall SP, et al: Electro-oculogram testing in fundus flavimaculatus. Arch Ophthalmol 97:1896, 1979.
90. Berson EL, Jin J: Full-field electroretinograms in patients with juvenile macular degeneration without or with peripheral cone involvement. Invest Ophthalmol Vis Sci 28:236, 1987.
91. Eagle RC, Lucier AC, Bernardino VB Jr, et al: Retinal pigment epithelial abnormalities in fundus flavimaculatus: A light and electron microscope study. Ophthalmology 87:1189, 1980.
92. Klein RR, Lewis R, Meyers S, et al: Subretinal neovascularization

associated with fundus flavimaculatus. Arch Ophthalmol 96:2054, 1978.

93. Chopdar A: Reticular dystrophy of the retina. Br J Ophthalmol 60:342, 1976.

94. Fishman GA, Woolf MB, Goldberg MF, et al: Reticular tapeto-retinal dystrophy: A possible late stage of Sjögren's reticular dystrophy. Br J Ophthalmol 60:35, 1976.

95. Kingham JD, Fenzi RE, Willerson D, Aaberg TM: Reticular dystrophy of the retinal pigment epithelium. Arch Ophthalmol 96:1177, 1978.

SECTION VI

Retinal Detachment: Historical Perspectives

Edited by
CHARLES L. SCHEPENS

Chapter 109

Retinal Detachment: Historical Perspectives

CHARLES L. SCHEPENS and NABIL G. CHEDID

OVERVIEW

Great inventions are seldom the result of a totally new concept. They are nearly always based on previous thinking that somehow did not mature to its full potential. This was true for ophthalmoscopy and for the discovery of the treatment of retinal detachment. Because of this observation, each of the three sections of this chapter—methods of examination, pathogenesis, and treatment—has been subdivided into an early and a modern period. The early period was characterized by "fishing expeditions" in various directions without real continuity in thinking. The modern period describes the gradual progress that was made once solid fundamental facts were established. It is interesting to note that in every section, the early period already contained the embryonic ideas that were developed in the modern period, but these ideas were not pursued to their logical conclusions until later years.

METHODS OF EXAMINATION

Early Period

The early period of examination techniques precedes the discovery of ophthalmoscopy and extends over 159 years, from 1691 to 1850. During that period, a number of observations were made about retinal detachment. In 1691, the anatomic description of a retinal detachment was first recorded by Maitre-Jan, who reported it in his book, first published in 1707. Since this was the first modern textbook on ophthalmology, it became popular and several editions were published. The author noted a dislocated lens, total retinal detachment, and retraction of the vitreous body in the eye of a dead cow.[1] He also observed that many eyes that had suffered a contusion or perforation of the globe also showed retinal detachment or retinal edema at autopsy. Morgagni[2] and later Wardrop[3] published pathologic observations of retinal detachment in human eyes.

In 1722, De Saint Yves[4] described clinical symptoms of retinal detachment that he called a "separation of the retina from the choroid." He reported "kind of shadows" in the visual field that corresponded to the detached area. However, he did not make a distinction between the visual effects of retinal detachment and those of dense vitreous opacities. In 1765, Morgagni described a retinal detachment with shriveled retina in a case of intraocular tumor.[5] Beer,[6] Sichel,[7] Desmarres,[8] and others described clinical signs of retinal detachment. Their reports originated mostly in their interpretation of the light reflection seen in the dilated pupil of the abnormal eye.

Details of the fundus of the living eye were accidentally seen by Méry[9] while he was holding a cat under water to study its pupillary reaction (Fig. 109–1). He failed to provide the correct explanation for what he observed. Five years later, de la Hire[10] correctly explained Mery's observation. He proposed that when the cat was placed under water, the water neutralized the refractive power of the cornea. In addition, he supplied a diagram that showed the optical effect of using what in fact amounted to a contact lens with a flat anterior surface.

In subsequent years, advantage was not taken of the observations of the authors described previously, but in a number of cases it was noted that under special circumstances, the fundus reflection (but limited fundus detail) was visible. One of the first such observations in humans was by Purkinje in 1823.[11] Cumming[12] made more elaborate observations about the fundus reflex and came close to discovering ophthalmoscopy. Similar observations were made by Brücke in 1847.[13]

Modern Period

Examination of the living ocular fundus, known as ophthalmoscopy, was not possible before Helmholtz's invention of the ophthalmoscope. The word *ophthalmoscope* derives from two Greek words—*ophthalmos,* which means eye and *skopeo,* which means to observe.

MONOCULAR OPHTHALMOSCOPY

Helmholtz described the principles of ophthalmoscopy in his famous monograph in 1851.[14] He named his instrument *Augenspiegel* (Fig. 109–2). Helmholtz's ophthalmoscope consisted of two essential parts. The first part was made of three or four thin plates of glass acting as a semitransparent mirror, which reflected light into the examined eye and also allowed an observer to see

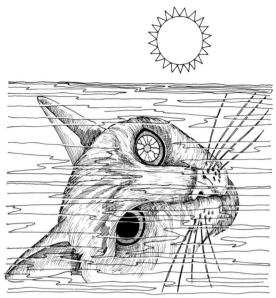

Figure 109–1. When a cat's head is under water, its pupils dilate and the fundus becomes clearly visible because the refractive power of the cornea is neutralized.

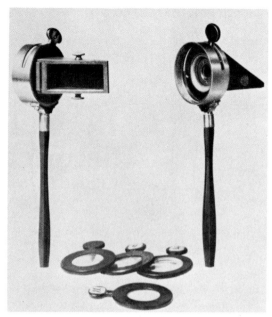

Figure 109–3. Helmholtz direct ophthalmoscope (1850). Light was reflected into the patient's pupil by multiple layers of thin glass. The observer could see the fundus by looking through glass layers. Helmholtz used corrective lenses as necessary. (From Engelking E: Dokumente zur Erfindung des Augenspiegels durch Hermann von Helmotz im Jahre 1850. München, Verlag von JF Bergmann, 1950.)

through the glass plates. The second part consisted of a lens inserted between the glass plates and the observer's eye to bring the fundus image of the examined eye in focus onto the retina of the observer (Fig. 109–3). There is no doubt that Helmholtz is the true inventor of ophthalmoscopy because he not only made an ophthalmoscope but also was able to detail its optical functioning. It should be noted, however, that Jones[15] described the model of an instrument contrived by Babbage in 1847, "for the purpose of looking into the interior of the eye." Jones did not think much of the invention because he felt that it had not increased the efficacy of his treatments!

Barely 2 mo after Helmholtz's publication, a Dutch instrument maker named Epkens built a similar direct ophthalmoscope in which the glass plates were replaced by a mirror without silvering in its center.[16] The observer

could see the fundus through the unsilvered part of the mirror.

Helmholtz also described indirect ophthalmoscopy but did not make the instrument because he thought that this technique would offer no advantage over the direct method. Initially, not every ophthalmologist was enthused by Helmholtz's invention. One ophthalmologist told him the instrument should never be used: "It would be too dangerous to admit the naked light into a diseased eye." Another stated that "The mirror might be of service to oculists with defective eyesight—he himself had good eyes and wanted none of it."[17] However, many diseases causing blindness that had until that time been called *black cataract* could now be studied and became gradually treatable in the course of the next century, including glaucoma and retinal, choroidal, and optic nerve diseases.

Ruete[18] made the first indirect ophthalmoscope (Fig. 109–4), a practical system using a concave mirror with an observation hole in its center and one or two mobile convex lenses set between the mirror and the patient's eye. His introduction of a concave mirror to reflect light into the patient's eye improved fundus illumination. Indirect ophthalmoscopy provided a larger field of view, a smaller magnification, and an inverted image of the observed fundus.

Many technical modifications rapidly followed Helmholtz's invention and Ruete's innovation. To reflect the light into the patient's eye, other reflectors were used in addition to glass plates and a concave mirror, such as plain glass mirrors, silvered lenses, prisms, and polished metal mirrors. For observation with a direct ophthalmoscope, lenses were mounted on a Rekoss disc, sliding

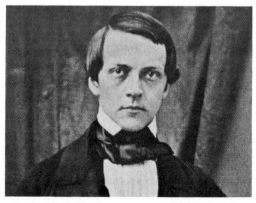

Figure 109–2. Herrmann Helmholtz in 1848 at age 27 yr, 2 yr prior to his discovery of the ophthalmoscope. (From Engelking E: Dokumente zur Erfindung des Augenspiegels durch Hermann von Helmotz im Jahre 1850. München, Verlag von JF Bergmann, 1850, p 7.)

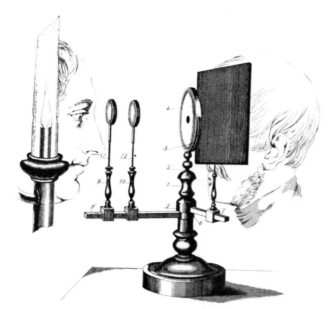

Figure 109–4. Ruete's indirect ophthalmoscope (1852). The light source was placed next to the patient's head. Light was reflected into the patient's eye through the concave mirror. Reflected light passed through two lenses that formed an image of the light source onto the patient's dilated pupil. Light from the patient's retina emerged through the dilated pupil and was condensed into an inverted fundus image located between the observer and the condensing lenses. The observer watched this image through the central hole in the concave mirror. (From Ruete CGT: Bildliche Darstellung der Krankheiten des menschlichen Auges. Leipzig, BG Teubner, 1854–1866.)

bars, or revolving chains. The light sources for all these reflecting ophthalmoscopes were sunlight, candlelight, oil lamps, or coal gas lamps. Models with numerous changes in design were seen in the first 3 decades that followed the discovery of monocular ophthalmoscopy. From 1851 to 1880, no less than 78 different models were described.[19] By 1902, 50 yr after the ophthalmoscope's invention, 140 models of the instrument were on exhibit at a special meeting of the American Medical Association.[20] Many models combined optical principles of direct and indirect ophthalmoscopy, but only a few survived.

A significant change was the introduction by Dennett of the first electrical ophthalmoscope in 1885.[21] Soon after, a number of electrical modifications were described. Notable was the introduction by Juler in 1885 of batteries with nonspillable liquid (Fig. 109–5).[22] Dry batteries were first introduced by Marple in 1906.[23] In the 20th century, many improvements were made to electrically powered direct ophthalmoscopes. However, all these instruments (May, Welch Allyn, Giantscope, Friedenwald, Keeler) were based on the same principles and differed only in details. They are described in Rucker's monograph.[24] Indirect ophthalmoscopes did not change much until the middle of the 20th century.

BINOCULAR OPHTHALMOSCOPY

In 1861, Giraud-Teulon[25] devised the first binocular ophthalmoscope (Fig. 109–6). He was inspired by two

types of technical developments: (1) the reflecting concave mirror and the technique of indirect ophthalmoscopy used by Ruete, and (2) the prism system used by Nachet in the construction of the first binocular microscope. Movable prisms permitted binocular observation of the patient's fundus while the examiner used a handheld condensing lens.

In 1911, Gullstrand[26, 27] carefully studied the parameters affecting indirect ophthalmoscopy. Basing his work on a simplified mathematical model of the optics of the human eye, he developed an instrument that avoided reflections from the patient's cornea and lens. This instrument could be used monocularly or binocularly. It provided a clear image with excellent magnification and illumination. This fundamental progress is the basis on which all current fundus cameras are constructed. In fact, they are nothing more than carefully designed indirect ophthalmoscopes.

Schepens described the binocular indirect headband ophthalmoscope in 1945.[28] It was originally designed to facilitate examination of retinal detachments. This instrument had two components: a headband to hold the stereoscopic viewing system and a powerful light source fixed on a flexible balanced arm. In addition, the observer held a condensing lens in front of the patient's eye to see the aerial image of the fundus (Fig. 109–7).[29] The magnification obtained was inversely proportional

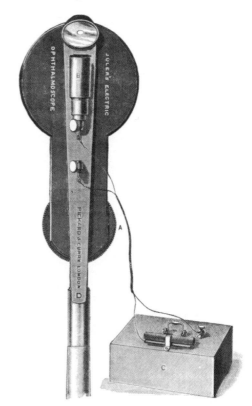

Figure 109–5. Juler's electric ophthalmoscope (1886). Direct ophthalmoscope whose light was supplied by a small bulb that was lit by battery with nonspillable liquid. (From Juler H: Refraction ophthalmoscope, with a special arrangement for the electric light. Trans Ophthalmol Soc UK 6:503, 1886.)

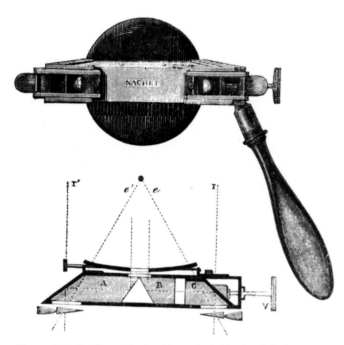

Figure 109–6. Giraud-Teulon binocular indirect ophthalmoscope (1861). The light source and reflecting concave mirror were like those of Ruete's instrument (see Fig. 109–4). A set of prisms allowed binocular vision. The instrument was made by Nachet, constructor of the first binocular microscope (From Zander A: The Ophthalmoscope: Its Varities and its Use. [Translated from the German by RB Carter] London, R Hartwicke, 1864. *A,* p 60; *B,* p 59.)

to the dioptric power of the condensing lens, and the depth of field varied inversely with magnification.[30] In 1951, Schepens modified his instrument by incorporating the viewing system and the light source into the headband. He also described a scleral depressor mounted on a thimble. Its use rendered details of the fundus periphery much more readily visible. He reported a series of 400 consecutive cases of idiopathic retinal detachment and found one or more breaks in 99 percent of the cases.[31]

Trantas was the first to describe scleral depression.[32] When he indented the overlying sclera with his thumbnail he could see the peripheral fundus with a direct ophthalmoscope. Trantas' technique was difficult to use, and as a result he was unable to accurately describe many changes in the fundus periphery. It soon fell into oblivion.

Combined with the binocular indirect ophthalmoscope, the Schepens technique of scleral depression[33] became widely used and recognized as a method of choice for evaluation and treatment of peripheral vitreoretinal pathologic conditions. An articulated scleral depressor of improved design offers more flexibility for the examiner and less discomfort to the patient.[34]

Pomerantzeff in 1968[35] optimized the Schepens ophthalmoscope by applying Gullstrand's principle,[27] which avoids reflections from the patient's cornea and crystalline lens. The Schepens-Pomerantzeff ophthalmoscope is most useful for seeing through a small patient's pupil

or through opacities of the media and for optimizing the view and maximizing stereopsis when looking at the fundus periphery.[36]

Gonin and, later, Weve, Amsler, and Arruga emphasized the importance of making an accurate fundus sketch in every case of retinal detachment. Weve's color code has been adopted for these sketches and is now used by most retina surgeons around the world.[37]

Both direct and indirect ophthalmoscopes had their advocates through the years. Gonin, the distinguished pioneer of modern retinal detachment surgery, used monocular indirect ophthalmoscopy. Although electric hand-held ophthalmoscopes were especially popular in English-speaking countries in the 1930s and are still widely used at present, since the 1950s, binocular indirect ophthalmoscopy has been increasingly perceived as the most effective clinical method of vitreoretinal evaluation. None of the models of binocular indirect headband ophthalmoscopes is fundamentally different from the Schepens and the Schepens-Pomerantzeff original models. The modern indirect ophthalmoscope and scleral depressor are most important for the correct evaluation of the retina and vitreoretinal relationships preoperatively, intraoperatively, and postoperatively.[38]

FUNDUS PHOTOGRAPHY

Howe[39] managed to photograph a fundus of a living human for the first time. He used an Auerbach gas burner placed in the focus of a perforated concave mirror that reflected light into the eye through a planoconvex lens. Fick[40] proposed to use the indirect method of Ruete with a camera on a footstand and a water chamber to eliminate the corneal reflex. Guilloz[41] produced the first usable photos of the human ocular

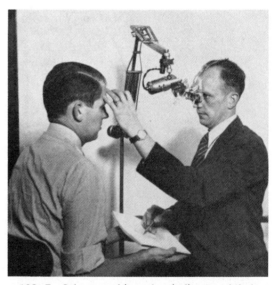

Figure 109–7. Schepens binocular indirect ophthalmoscope (1945). The illumination system was attached to a flexible arm. The observation device was worn on the observer's head. (From Schepens CL: A new ophthalmoscope demonstration. Trans Am Acad Ophthalmol Otolaryngol 51:298–301, 1947.)

fundus. He used the principle of the "mirror reflex camera" in conjunction with a photographic plate. When the oblique mirror plate of his camera was flipped out of the way, he could synchronously blow magnesium powder from a rubber ball into the observation flame to produce a flashlight (Fig. 109–8).

At the turn of the century, pioneers of fundus photography still faced three serious technical difficulties: (1) light sources were inadequate, (2) light reflections from the refractive media of the patient's eye partially obscured the fundus view, and (3) it was impossible to keep the photographed eye motionless for the long exposure needed. Around 1905, Dimmer[42–44] and the Zeiss Company designed and constructed a complicated machine that produced acceptable quality fundus photographs (Fig. 109–9). These photographs were published later by Dimmer and Pillat[45] in the first atlas of fundus photography. Bedell's atlas followed 2 yr later.[46]

Based on the principles of Gullstrand's reflex-free ophthalmoscopy,[26, 47] Nordenson (Fig. 109–10) developed a new and relatively compact fundus camera.[48] It was equipped with a carbon arc light but still produced an annoying central reflection that adversely affected the quality of the photographs. The reflection was later blotted out with a small black dot on the objective lens.[49] The Nordenson-improved camera worked according to the same basic optical principles as did the Gullstrand indirect ophthalmoscope. It consisted of a table-mounted indirect ophthalmoscope with a single-lens reflex camera. In the late 1930s, films replaced photographic glass plates, and the electronic flash appeared.[50]

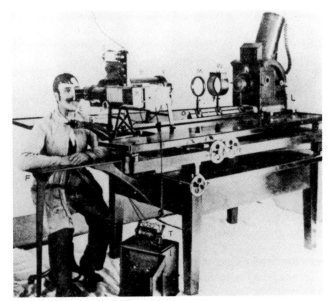

Figure 109–9. The fundus camera of Dimmer, constructed by Zeiss (1907). It produced the first acceptable fundus photographs. (From Haugwitz TV: The history of optical instruments for the examination of the eye. *In* Hirschberg J [ed]: The History of Ophthalmology, vol 11, part 2. Bonn, JP Wayenborgh, 1986.)

Numerous improvements were introduced in the fundus camera in later years[51, 52] but without a basic change in its design.

The development of all optical instruments for ex-

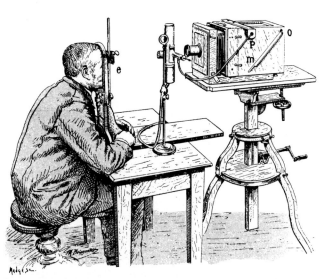

Figure 109–8. Guilloz fundus camera (1893). It contains an ophthalmoscopic condensing lens and a gas light that is flashed by a system that automatically blows magnesium powder into the flame at the appropriate moment. The camera contains a 45-degree mirror that projects the fundus image vertically on frosted glass. When the fundus picture is in focus, the mirror is rotated out of the way and at the same instant magnesium powder is automatically blown into the gas flame to create a flash. The fundus picture is recorded on a glass plate. (From Guilloz Th: La photographie instantanée du fond d'oeil humain. Arch d'Ophtalmol 13:472, 1893.)

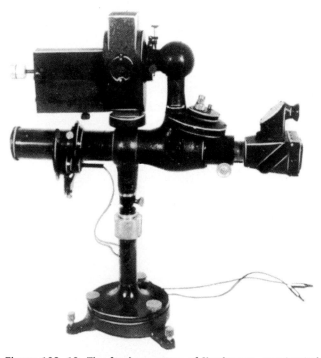

Figure 109–10. The fundus camera of Nordenson, constructed by Zeiss (1925), used a carbon arc lamp. (From Haugwitz TV: The history of optical instruments for the examination of the eye. *In* Hirschberg J [ed]: The History of Ophthalmology, vol 11, part 2. Bonn, JP Wayenborgh, 1986.)

amination and photography of the retina was based on Gullstrand's simplified optical model of the eye.[27] In this model, three restrictive assumptions were made: (1) Optical elements of the eye (cornea and lens) are infinitely thin, (2) light rays considered are exclusively those that form an infinitely small angle with the axis of the optical system, and (3) the portion of the retina that is imaged by the optical system is infinitely small (punctual).

Pomerantzeff and associates (Fig. 109–11) made a gigantic step forward when they constructed the most realistic optical model of the eye in existence in 1972.[53] The greatest obstacle was the crystalline lens with its many layers of different refractive indices and aspherical surfaces. It is thanks to this epoch-making work that modern optical instruments to examine and photograph the eye could be optimized; several of these instruments are described in the following section.

Equator-plus Instrumentation. The solid angle visible by ophthalmoscopy varies with the instrumentation used: It is 15 degrees with a direct ophthalmoscope and 30 to 60 degrees with an indirect ophthalmoscope, depending on the strength and diameter of the condensing lens. In order to obtain the maximal solid angle of view, three conditions must be realized: (1) A large solid angle of retina must be illuminated, (2) the illuminated solid angle must be made visible to the observer, and (3) disturbing reflections from the cornea and lens must be avoided. Pomerantzeff and Govignon fulfilled these conditions in their Equator-plus ophthalmoscope and camera.[54, 55] It requires the use of a specially designed contact lens and covers an angle that ranges between 175 and 203 degrees, depending on the method of illumination.

Ninety-degree Noncontact Camera. A 90-degree noncontact fundus camera was designed and built.[56] It avoids disturbing corneal and lens reflections by using a special system of illumination from a crown of fibers around the objective lens (Fig. 109–12A and B).

High-magnification Contact Camera. Any detail in the retina that the fundus camera can record must necessarily be present in the aerial image made by the objective lens. Magnifying this aerial image photographically cannot reveal details not already recorded in this image.

A system was designed and constructed by Pomerantzeff in 1980 called the Macula-Disc camera.[56] It uses optic fibers for illumination through a contact lens and records the aerial image of the fundus directly on film. It has better contrast, more resolution, and better illumination than does any regular fundus camera. Its field is 18 degrees measured from the nodal point of the eye (Fig. 109–13).

SCANNING LASER OPHTHALMOSCOPE

In Gullstrand's reflex-free ophthalmoscopy, several conditions must be fulfilled: (1) A sharp image of the light source must be projected on the patient's pupil, (2) a sharp image of the observer's pupils (or the camera's diaphragm in fundus photography) must also be projected on the patient's pupil (these pupillary images are small and all the light that reaches the observer's retina—or the camera's film—must pass through them), and (3) the image of the light source and that of the pupils must be separated in the pupil to prevent scattered light from blurring the fundus image.

Scanning laser ophthalmoscopy is based on a new principle proposed by Pomerantzeff and coworkers.[57] Fundus illumination is produced by a narrow flying beam of weak laser light, which is a well-known process.[58] This makes it possible to use the major portion of the pupillary area to collect light reflected from the fundus. The apparatus itself was developed and constructed by Webb and colleagues (Fig. 109–14).[59]

The advantages of this system are multiple. Because a major portion of the pupillary area is used to collect light from the fundus, 1000 to 10,000 times less light is needed to illuminate the fundus than in regular ophthalmoscopy or fundus photography. As a result, the pupil does not need to be dilated for ophthalmoscopy. Since laser light is monochromatic and illuminates only one point at a time, it causes less light scattering and permits a sharper image to be obtained than when a polychromatic light source is used.

The light emerging from the pupil is collected by a lens system and photomultiplied. The photomultiplier tube drives a television monitor. Each picture element (pixel) on the monitor corresponds directly to a picture element in the fundus. As the illuminating spot flies across the fundus, the electron beam flies synchronously across the television screen and a television picture is built up. There is no other ophthalmoscopic image in the system, the only visible image being on the television screen. The picture is monochromatic, being produced by a single-wavelength laser beam. It can reveal details not visible by any other means, and it can make a visible picture with infrared rays. Finally a videocassette can be made for later frame-by-frame study of the dynamic pictures on the television screen. Hard copies can also be made of selected views.

The scanning laser ophthalmoscope is manufactured by Rodenstock and has many applications unrelated or

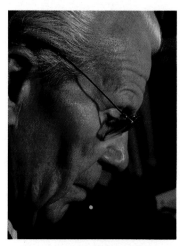

Figure 109–11. Oleg Pomerantzeff, physicist, is probably the greatest contributor to ophthalmic physics in this century.

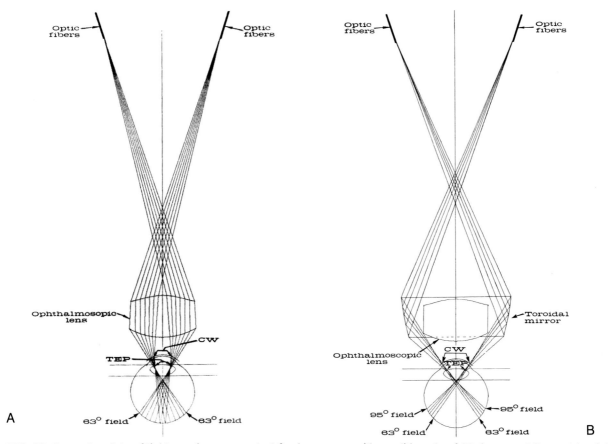

Figure 109–12. Computer plots of light rays in a noncontact fundus camera with a solid angle of 90 degrees at the nodal point. *A,* Light provided by annulus of optic fibers illuminates a 63-degree field. Sufficient size corneal window (*CW*) and entrance pupil (*TEP*) are free of light in order to give a reflexless view of the fundus. *B,* In order to illuminate 95-degree field, second annulus of fibers provides light that is reflected into the patient's eye by a circular toroidal mirror attached to a condensing lens. (From Schepens CL: Retinal Detachment and Allied Diseases, vol 2. Philadelphia, WB Saunders, 1983, pp 1115–1116.)

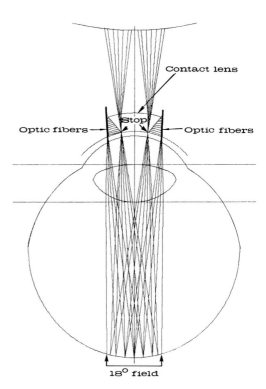

Figure 109–13. A computer plot of light rays in a high-definition contact fundus camera. Illuminating rays come from optic fibers forming a circle around the corneal periphery. The retinal image is recorded directly on film. (From Schepens CL: Retinal Detachment and Allied Diseases, vol 2. Philadelphia, WB Saunders, 1983, p 1117.)

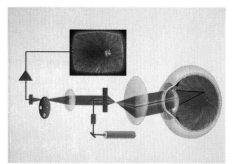

Figure 109–14. Sketch of a scanning laser ophthalmoscope. Weak laser tube (*below*) projects thin pencil of light, which flies over the fundus illuminating successively a large area. Light reflected from the fundus passes practically through the whole pupil, is collected by the condensing lens, and then photomultiplied. The light collected may be diaphragmed and is then transmitted to a television apparatus.

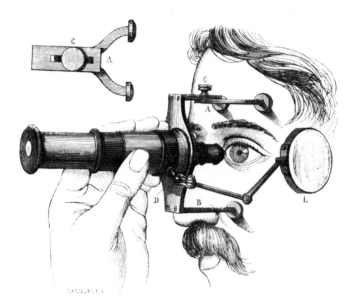

Figure 109–15. The de Wecker monocular ophthalmomicroscope (1863) used oblique illumination supplied by a light source not shown on the picture. The whole instrument was portable. (From de Wecker L: Traité théorique et pratique des maladies des yeux. Paris, Baillière, 1863, p 272.)

related only distantly to retinal detachment. The field of view with the scanning laser ophthalmoscope depends on the power of the condensing lens that is placed in front of the patient's eye. The system has a great depth of focus and therefore is ideal to reproduce, in a single picture, the details of a retinal detachment, even with ballooning retinal elevation.[60] This is accomplished by using a strong condensing lens (+28 D) in front of the patient's dilated pupil.

SLIT–LAMP MICROSCOPY

For years, the development of slit-lamp microscopy was essentially aimed at the study of the anterior segment. For vitreous and fundus examination, three components are needed: an observation microscope, a slit lamp, and an optical device with which the retina and posterior vitreous can be imaged into the focal plane of the microscope. Each of these components evolved separately.

The modern observation microscope is derived from the Czapski binocular corneal microscope.[61] At that time, an oblique light[62] and a monocular microscope[63] to examine the eye were already in use (Fig. 109–15). The main deficiency of the Czapski microscope was the lack of an adequate illumination system to produce a clear-cut optical section of the transparent eye tissues (Fig. 109–16).

Focal illumination of the retina was first introduced by Wolff in 1901,[64] but his technique had two major limitations: (1) The illumination beam was relatively weak and (2) the angle formed between illumination and observation beams could not be varied. The first problem was solved by Gullstrand and the second by Koeppe.

In 1911, Gullstrand introduced the slit lamp and called his illumination system *Nernstspaltlampe*.[65] This instrument consisted essentially of a closed tube with a "Nernst" electrical bulb at one end and an optical system designed to produce a strong and clear-cut beam of light, emanating from an adjustable slit, at the other end.[66] The same year Gullstrand won a Nobel Prize for his contribution related to the dioptric system of the eye,[27] but his slit lamp was ignored at the time because

it initially appeared to be nothing more than a modification of available oblique illumination methods.[67]

The preliminary steps that were to make slit-lamp examination of the fundus possible in humans had already been taken by Mery in 1704[9] and by de la Hire

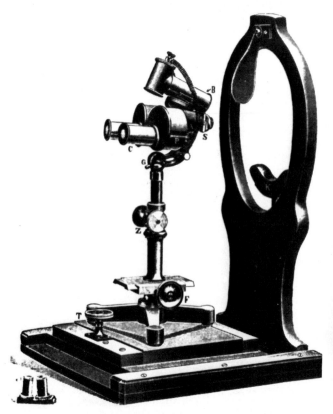

Figure 109–16. Czapski binocular corneal microscope (1899). (From Czapski S: Binoculares Cornealmikroskop. Arch Ophthalmol [Berlin] 48:231, 1899.)

in 1709.[10] However, it was not until Helmholtz's discovery of the ophthalmoscope that Czermak[68, 69] and Coccius[70] designed two devices called *Orthoscope*, with which to neutralize the refractive power of the ocular media. Czermak used a small tub that he pressed against the orbital margin and filled with water while the patient was in a supine position. Observation was conducted with an ophthalmoscope. Coccius designed a different type of water bath that resembled small diver's goggles.

Koeppe[71] realized the importance of Gullstrand's invention of slit-lamp illumination. He postulated that for an observer to see optical sections of the fundus, two prerequisites are indispensable: (1) The angle formed between the axis of illumination and that of observation has to be adjustable and small and (2) the fundus image ought to be brought into the focusing range of the microscope. The first prerequisite was met by using a front-silvered mirror that reflected the illumination beam at an acute angle into the eye. For the second, Koeppe designed a flat contact lens[71] with a dioptric power of −69.4 D and a diameter of 17 mm. Using this lens was not easy, but for the first time examination of the posterior segment of the eye with a flat contact lens and a slit beam of light became possible. At that time, a monocular microscope was used.

The prototype of the modern slit-lamp microscope was built by Zeiss, combining the slit illumination of Gullstrand and the corneal microscope of Czapski. Gallemaerts and Kleefeld[72] fitted the slit lamp vertically and improved the illumination, magnification, and stereopsis. Schmidt[73] developed the most modern type of slit-lamp microscope, built with a vertical illumination arm (Haag-Streit 900). Other recent models are not substantially different.

Instead of nullifying the refractive power of the eye with a contact lens, a negative precorneal lens has been used. This was first suggested by Stilling in 1879.[74] The technique was improved by Lemoine and Valois in 1923.[75] In 1940, Hruby[76] improved and later popularized[77] this method by using a precorneal lens of about −55 D.

A different technique for examination of optical sections of the inner eye was introduced by El Bayadi in 1953.[78] He proposed using a planoconvex lens of about +60 D with the slit-lamp microscope. This lens is held in front of the examined eye and provides an inverted ophthalmoscopic slit-lamp image of the vitreous and fundus. This image is observed with a microscope.

A flat three-mirror contact lens for slit-lamp examination of the fundus was developed by Goldmann in 1948.[79] Widely used today, this lens provides an excellent view of fundus details around the macula and at the periphery. The three-mirror lens can be replaced by a lens with a single mirror, the angle of which can be appropriately varied.[80, 81]

Photography of retinal slit images is relatively easy, but photography of vitreous details is difficult for two reasons: (1) The contrast of vitreous structures is very low and (2) the image to be photographed is seen on the reddish and fairly brilliant background of the fundus. An apparatus was built for this purpose and consisted of a special aspherical condensing lens of +58.6 D mounted in front of a photographic slit lamp that supplies illumination of exceptional luminance.[82, 83] This arrangement also permits cinematography of moving vitreous structures. Its disadvantage is that its use makes it difficult to examine the peripheral vitreous. More recently,[84] a +90-D double-aspherical lens was tried for the same purpose, with certain advantages.

OTHER METHODS OF EXAMINATION

Other techniques, which are used extensively to study other ophthalmic diseases, are very useful in certain specific cases of retinal detachment. Some of these techniques are relatively recent and have a short history. We shall limit ourselves to a brief discussion of ultrasonic evaluation, electrophysiologic measurements, and Doppler measurement of retinal blood flow.

A- and B-scan ultrasonic examination of unusual cases of retinal detachment has been used since the early 1960s.[85, 86] Its obvious indication is to study an eye with opaque media that is suspected of harboring a retinal detachment. This examination will determine the presence, extent, and mobility of a retinal detachment, the existence of vitreous and retinal organization, the density of vitreous opacities, the thickness of the choroid (a thick choroid makes the surgical prognosis poorer), and the size of the eye. An especially valuable application of B-scan ultrasound is for the preoperative evaluation of retinal detachment in stage 5 retinopathy of prematurity.[87] In such cases, the surgical prognosis depends, to a high degree, on the ultrasound findings.

Electrophysiologic examination of an eye with diagnosed or suspected retinal detachment is very important in special cases.[88, 89] The use of this technique is indicated particularly when the media are too opaque to examine the retina by ophthalmoscopy and when there is reason to wonder whether reattaching the retina will bring about functional improvement. A typical example is retinal detachment of long duration with opaque media. In a total retinal detachment, the electroretinographic signal is extinguished. A partial retinal detachment exhibiting an electroretinogram in which the b-wave is smaller than the a-wave (b/a < 1) is characteristic of impairment of the retinal circulation. The visual-evoked response and especially the pattern visual-evoked response are helpful in evaluating the integrity of the optic fibers and visual pathways.[90] For instance, a pattern visual-evoked response that is very abnormal or unrecordable in the presence of a normal electroretinogram generally indicates a severely damaged optic nerve.

The velocity of blood through retinal blood vessels has been determined by high-speed cinematography.[91] This technique requires intracarotid injection of fluorescein. Laser Doppler velocimetry is based on Doppler's original studies in which he demonstrated theoretically that if a beam of light is reflected by moving particles, the wavelength of the reflected radiation is shifted away from the wavelength of the incident radiation.[92] The shift is proportional to the velocity of the moving particles. Because the frequency shift caused by the moving blood cells in the retinal vessels is incredibly small, an extremely high resolution technique is required to detect it.[93] The minute frequency shift causes an electrical current that can be recorded. The laser beam used for this purpose is very weak. It is kept on a retinal vessel by an optical tracking system.[94] The exposure time needed to make a recording is of the order of a fraction of a second so that the variation in blood velocity with each heartbeat can be recorded. By measuring the retinal vessel's diameter, it is easy to calculate the retinal blood flow.[95, 96]

It has been demonstrated that certain retinal detachments that are reattached by an uncomplicated scleral buckling operation gradually lose visual field and central vision postoperatively. Their retinal artery blood speed and blood flow are reduced when measured by laser Doppler. After removal of the scleral buckling the vision improves, as does the retinal blood flow.[97] Successful retinal detachment procedures often impose circulatory changes upon the operated eyes. Some of these changes are permanent in eyes with an encircling band.[98]

CONCEPTS OF PATHOGENESIS

The concepts of pathogenesis of retinal detachment have a most instructive history. No meaningful work could be done in this field before the advent of ophthalmoscopy.

Early Period

The early period lasted 66 yr (1853 to 1919) and was characterized by groping in an attempt to find a logical cause for idiopathic retinal detachment. It ended when the all-important role of the retinal break was established by Gonin in 1919. Coccius in 1853[70] first described retinal breaks, but their full importance went unrecognized until Gonin discovered that they were actually the cause of retinal detachment.[99]

During this period, opinions as to the pathogenesis of idiopathic retinal detachment varied widely. In the early days,[100] von Graefe thought that retinal detachment was due to either choroidal effusion or hemorrhage. Later,[101] he expressed the opinion that in highly myopic eyes, the distention of the globe stretched the retina to the point that it followed the chord of the ocular sphere rather than the arc. He further thought that retinal breaks were part of the healing process. Arlt[102] felt that the main cause was choroidal exudation.

The possible role played by the vitreous was first recognized by Müller in 1858.[103] He observed that in rare cases of traumatic origin, tractional vitreous bands caused retinal detachment. Iwanoff noted that a vitreous detachment often preceded detachment of the retina and was probably a precipitating factor.[104]

It was generally accepted that retinal breaks were not the cause of retinal detachment but one of its results. De Wecker and de Jaeger[105] were probably the first to suspect that retinal breaks were essential in the causation of retinal detachment. They postulated two different mechanisms: (1) Hypersecretion of fluid between the vitreous gel and the retina pushed the gel forward and caused traction on the retina, a mechanism most frequent in eyes with staphyloma. (2) In cases of perforating trauma or inflammation, vitreoretinal traction bands tore the retina and caused retinal detachment. These two theories accounted only for relatively rare instances and did not explain the pathogenesis of retinal detachment in the majority of cases.

Leber in 1882[106] rejected the ideas advanced by de Wecker and de Jaeger. Instead he ascribed a fundamental importance to alterations of the vitreous that were so tenuous as to be clinically undetectable at the time. He insisted that retinal breaks always cause an increase in the extent of the retinal detachment. De Wecker observed the frequent presence of retinal breaks in cases of retinal detachment, even when the clinician failed to recognize them. In subsequent years, Leber experienced difficulty in producing microscopic evidence to support his thesis. In consequence, his concepts were bitterly criticized and he gradually changed his mind. By 1888, de Wecker made very pertinent observations.[107] First he understood, as we do today, the vitreoretinal process that gives rise to retinal tears. Consequently, he thought that a retinal tear always precedes the appearance of a retinal detachment. He concluded by stating that all the surgical procedures recommended at that time were totally ineffective.

In 1908, Leber held that retinal breaks were secondary events caused by extensive preretinal organization (which today we call *proliferative vitreoretinopathy* [PVR]).[108] He observed these changes in eyes with long-standing retinal detachment. In 1906, Dufour and Gonin[109] revived Leber's original theory and that of de Wecker, which ascribed retinal tears to isolated vitreoretinal adhesions occurring in a vitreous that, at the time, appeared clinically normal.

Modern Period

Gonin in 1920[110] confirmed the relationship between vitreous detachment and vitreous traction upon the retina, which, in turn, produced retinal tears and retinal detachment. His confirming evidence resulted mostly from the study of pathologic eye specimens and secondarily from clinical observations in vivo. He thought that the preretinal cellular proliferation reported by Leber as the cause of retinal breaks and retinal detachment was a secondary phenomenon, resulting mostly from the proliferation of the ciliary epithelium.[111] Contrary to Leber's thinking, he ascribed no role to the proliferation of the retinal pigment epithelium. He thought the latter only caused the formation of subretinal membranes.

Gonin's ideas about the pathogenesis of retinal detachment were soon reinforced by Vogt in 1936.[112] He began to study detailed vitreoretinal pathologic features in clinical cases using focal illumination. Further clinical demonstration of the role played by the vitreous in the pathogenesis of retinal detachment was described by Hruby in 1950.[113] He used the slit lamp and a precorneal minus lens. Busacca and associates[114] described more details of the vitreoretinal relationships and gave excellent demonstrations of the existence of vitreoretinal newly formed membranes in cases of retinal detachment. The relationship between preretinal organization and fixed retinal folds was also clearly described.[115]

With the development of techniques to examine the fundus periphery by slit-lamp microscopy, changes leading to certain types of retinal detachment were further studied in vivo by Eisner in 1973.[116] Improved techniques of vitreous examination made it possible to evaluate more clearly the relationship between vitreous traction and retinal breaks.

For nearly 50 yr after Gonin's publication in 1920, retinal breaks were considered the pivotal event in the pathogenesis of retinal detachment. There were, however, some unexplained observations. First, even Gonin observed cases in which retinal holes were produced by retinal thinning, without detectable vitreous traction. Second, it gradually became apparent that a number of retinal tears existed in subjects who did not experience retinal detachment.[117, 118] Such retinal tears are generally small but may occasionally be large; they heal spontaneously by forming a pigmented scar around their periphery. It remains accepted, however, that in the presence of a retinal detachment, a retinal break always needs to be closed (either by an artificial chorioretinal reaction or by the physiologic chorioretinal adhesion) if permanent reattachment of the retina is to be assured.

The strength and nature of the physiologic chorioretinal adhesion has been studied. In 1969, Zauberman and coworkers[119, 120] established that this adhesion was due to two factors: one, which was rather weak, was located in the interphotoreceptor matrix and the other, which was much stronger, disappeared with the animal's death. The matrix was studied in detail,[121] and it was established that the cone matrix sheath is the element that firmly attaches the cones to the apices of the retinal pigment cells. Rods have a similar but less conspicuous attachment. The stronger retinal adhesion is produced by fluid transport from the retina across the pigment epithelium. It does not seem to result from an Na-K pump but primarily from the active absorption of bicarbonate.[122, 123] This mechanism appears to be the same in the mammalian eye as it is in the frog eye.[124]

A more realistic view of the pathogenesis of retinal detachment has emerged from the preceding observations. It is based on the following cardinal ideas:

1. A rhegmatogenous retinal detachment necessarily involves the existence of a retinal break. Most retinal breaks are tears, i.e., they result from vitreous traction. A few are holes and are produced by extreme atrophy of retinal tissue.

2. Retinal tears result from an abnormal vitreoretinal adhesion, combined with shrinkage of the vitreous gel. This has two consequences: It creates a traction on the retina that is limited to the area of abnormal adhesion and it produces liquefied vitreous.

3. Once a retinal tear is produced, the liquid vitreous can gradually enter the subretinal space. The speed of growth of the retinal detachment depends on the strength and the extent of the retinochoroidal adhesion,[120, 125] on the amount of fluid vitreous available, and

on the degree of vitreoretinal traction. Fluid vitreous not only makes liquid available to detach the retina from the pigment epithelium but also acts by inertial movement, pushing more fluid under the retina each time the eye is rotated.[126, 127]

4. Retinal holes can give rise to a retinal detachment, depending on the equilibrium between the vitreoretinal traction, the amount of liquid vitreous available, and the strength of the retinochoroidal adhesion.

5. Retinal tears that do not lead to retinal detachment are those that are accompanied by relatively weak vitreoretinal traction or relatively strong retinochoroidal adhesion, or both.

6. Repair of an existing retinal detachment can involve three possible steps: (a) closure of retinal breaks, (b) release of vitreoretinal traction, and (c) approximation of the retina with the choroid. There are no known means at this time to reinforce the natural retinochoroidal adhesion. The therapeutic retinochoroidal adhesions that are used are of variable strength.

7. Membrane formation by cells that proliferate on the anterior surface of the retina, on the detached posterior hyaloid, on the posterior surface of the detached retina, and finally, in the vitreous gel itself is a secondary phenomenon that often prevents retinal reattachment. These cells originate mostly from the retinal pigment epithelium and from the retina itself.[111, 128, 129]

8. In order to understand more deeply the processes that cause retinal detachment, we will need to learn more about the molecular events that lead to this disease. These events occur in the matrix that attaches the photoreceptors to the retinal pigment epithelium, in the retina itself, and in the vitreous. This study was started by Balazs in 1968[130] and is being continued by a number of other investigators.[131]

TREATMENT

The techniques of treatment for rhegmatogenous retinal detachment have followed closely our understanding of the pathogenesis of the disease. In the early period, before Gonin published his cardinal observations, treatment was somewhat haphazard and uniformly followed by unfavorable results. Starting with Gonin's publications, the results of treatment have steadily improved to reach their present high level.

Early Period

It was quite natural that the earliest attempts at treating retinal detachment consisted of releasing the subretinal fluid. In 1814, Ware perforated the sclera in an eye with presumptive "effusion of fluid between the choroid coat and retina" to relieve the patient's excruciating pain. His presumption was confirmed by the immediate escape of a "yellow coloured fluid."[132] This procedure was used in early surgical treatments of retinal detachment and was modified by draining the subretinal fluid with a needle and syringe.[107]

As we have mentioned in the discussion on pathogenesis, von Graefe thought that idiopathic retinal detachment was caused by a choroidal exudation that was pushing the retina forward, thereby compressing the vitreous gel into a retracted mass. Based on this concept, he thought that the retinal breaks resulted from nature's effort to equalize the pressure between the subretinal and the vitreous cavities. He therefore perforated the retina with one or two discission needles.[133] When this treatment failed, more conservative attempts were made, consisting of prolonged bedrest[134] and bilateral compressive bandages. This was often supplemented by rubbings with mercury ointment and pilocarpine injections, which were supposed to hasten resorption of the subretinal fluid. Some surgeons thought that there was a pathogenic relationship between retinal detachment and glaucoma. For this reason, they recommended iridectomy as a curative and even a preventive measure in cases of retinal detachment.[135, 140] De Wecker explained the failure of all these treatments because Leber's theory was correct.[107, 136, 137] This theory hypothesized that the disease was caused by adhesions of the retracting vitreous to the retina. Efforts were then made to either cause an adhesive chorioretinitis or push the retina against the choroid. The adhesive chorioretinitis was not aimed at closing the retinal breaks. Various methods were proposed to accomplish these aims such as galvanocautery,[138] electrolysis,[139] retinal sutures,[140] and injections of tincture of iodine into the subretinal space[140] or vitreous.[141] Vitreous injections of several substances were also attempted, such as subretinal fluid,[142] and later saline solution,[143] cerebrospinal fluid,[144] and aqueous humor.[145]

In 1895, Deutschmann[146] used multiple discissions to cut the vitreoretinal adhesions; he then refilled the vitreous cavity with rabbit vitreous diluted in saline solution, thinking that the injected material tended to dissolve the traction bands. He reported successes that could not be duplicated by others.

The pathogenic theory of Leber,[108] that vitreous traction was the cause of retinal detachment, led to the idea of reducing the volume of the globe. Excision of a full-thickness strip of sclera was first performed by Alaimo in 1893.[147] A similar operation based on a different pathogenic concept was proposed later by Müller.[148] He maintained that retinal detachment resulted from stretching of the choroid and transudation between the retina and the choroid. He suggested an extensive full-thickness scleral resection to reduce the size of the eye and to bring the choroid closer to the retina. A lamellar scleral resection with tucking of the scleral flap was first performed by Blaskowics in 1911.[149] These scleral operations were recommended exclusively in cases of retinal detachment with high myopia.

Since all these techniques were unconcerned with the localization of the retinal breaks, the surgical success rate was estimated to be between less than 1 percent[150] and 6 percent,[151] in spite of the fact that many cases were considered inoperable, and thus only favorable cases were operated upon.

Modern Period

The modern period is characterized by two major efforts to reattach a detached retina. Following the theory of de Wecker and Gonin, a technique was developed by Gonin to close the retinal breaks by extraocular surgery. Another class of operations later was aimed at neutralizing or eliminating the vitreous traction on the retina by intraocular manipulations. It should be remembered that in two sentences Gonin summarized everything that can be done, even today, in order to repair a retinal detachment: "Retinal reattachment to be durable requires that traction exerted on the retina by the vitreous be eliminated or be counterbalanced by an appropriate chorioretinal adhesion. The possibility of such a reattachment is conceivable only after closure of the retinal break(s)."[99]

CLOSURE OF RETINAL BREAKS BY EXTRAOCULAR SURGERY

Extraocular surgery to close retinal breaks started after Gonin recognized the key role played by retinal breaks in retinal detachment. Inspired by Leber, Gonin proposed transscleral thermocauterization[152] to close retinal breaks, known as *Gonin's ignipuncture technique*. This method followed two essential steps. The first was to find the retinal breaks, determine the meridian, and estimate the distance—in disc diameters—between the extreme fundus periphery and the breaks. This distance was translated into millimeters, and from this measurement, the distance between the limbus and the break was then computed. The second step was to seal the retinal break by introducing a hot thermocautery into the subretinal space through a small scleral incision.

Gonin was the first to accomplish systematic reattachment of rhegmatogenous retinal detachments by causing a localized chorioretinal reaction in the area of the breaks (Fig. 109–17).[153] This procedure improved results drastically from less than 6 percent to more than 50 percent. In 1931, he published his first series of 221 eyes operated on with a success rate of 53 percent.[154] In using an actual cautery, he deliberately perforated the eye wall, and as a result, subretinal fluid escaped (Fig. 109–18).

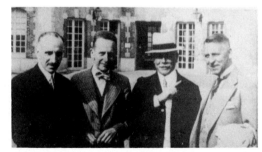

Figure 109–17. Jules Gonin (with hat) photographed in 1934 with his first followers: Arruga (*left*), Amsler (*middle*), and Weve (*right*).

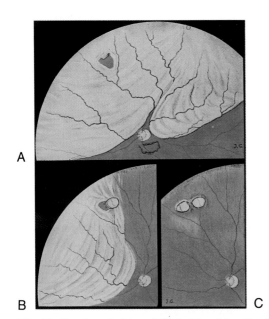

Figure 109–18. Fundus sketches initialed by Jules Gonin. *A,* Superior retinal detachment with an equatorial horseshoe break. *B,* Following first ignipuncture, the break is only partially closed and residual detachment persists. *C,* After second ignipuncture, the break is occluded and the detachment cured. (From Gonin J: Le Décollement de la Rétine: Pathogénie-Traitment. Lausanne, Payot, 1934, pp 112–117.)

In the absence of binocular indirect ophthalmoscopy combined with scleral depression, accurate localization of retinal breaks was often a complicated task. Methods to localize retinal breaks were based on estimation by ophthalmoscopy, on combined ophthalmoscopic-perimetric calculations,[155, 156] or on transillumination.[157] Gonin's method to localize retinal breaks was similar to the original method suggested by von Graefe in 1882.[158] In addition, the documentation and recording of retinal breaks used by Gonin resembled the representation commonly used today in the patient preoperative fundus chart. This chart was initially designed by Amsler and Dubois in 1928.[159]

A less traumatic and more easily controlled technique than Gonin's single ignipuncture was the use of diathermy, introduced independently by Heim[160] and Weve.[161] With surface diathermy, it was easier to treat an extensive area of the eye wall and to regulate the intensity of the reaction.

Techniques that had been used in the last quarter of the 19th century to cause a chorioretinal reaction without concern for the location of the retinal breaks were now revived and applied over the areas of the retinal breaks and chorioretinal degeneration. Thus Vogt in 1936[162] modified electrolysis, first used in 1895,[139] and called it *catholysis*. Guist in 1931[163] revived the use of chemical irritation, first tried in 1889,[141] by placing the irritant in the subchoroidal space rather than in the vitreous or in the subretinal space, and by using potassium hydroxide rather than tincture of iodine.

Gonin had already observed that sharpshooting at multiple retinal breaks and areas of degeneration was difficult and could be ineffective. Treatment, in such cases, was modified by building a barrage of chorioretinal reaction to wall off weak retinal areas. This was described separately by Gonin[154] and Lindner[164] in 1931. In addition, various methods of diathermy applications to cover large areas with chorioretinal reaction and compensate minor localization errors were used.[165–167]

In the 2 decades that followed Gonin's discovery, it became evident that attempts at closing the retinal breaks by inducing a chorioretinal reaction and releasing subretinal fluid were not always successful. Therefore, reattachment techniques were sometimes combined with procedures aimed at reducing the volume of the globe. Reviving and modifying a technique devised in 1893,[147] Lindner[168] and Hildesheimer[169] used full-thickness scleral resection in addition to closure of the retinal breaks. A similar technique was first reported in the United States in 1939 by Pischel and Miller.[170]

The lamellar scleral resection of Blaskowics[149] was revived in 1951 independently by three surgeons.[171–173] In addition, a variety of eye wall shortening operations without scleral resection were described: Inward folding of the sclera was introduced by Weve in 1949,[174] outward full-thickness scleral folding was described by Everett in 1955[175] and by Castroviejo in 1956,[176] and partial-thickness scleral imbrication was proposed by Lemoine and coworkers in 1958.[177] Each of these techniques created a ridgelike buckling that had little effect on walling off retinal breaks and in reducing vitreoretinal traction.

Temporary reduction of the vitreous volume by introduction of subchoridal material was suggested by several authors. Strampelli injected subchoroidal blood plasma in 1933[178] and later inserted a subchoroidal gelatin sponge.[179] Smith injected air under the choroid in 1952.[180] As procedures to reduce the ocular volume multiplied, less attention was paid to closing the retinal breaks, and the percentage of favorable surgical results declined. For instance, lamellar scleral resections were generally performed just posterior to the insertions of the rectus muscles, rather than at the equator, at which point most of the retinal tears were located.

In the English-speaking countries, interest in modern treatment of retinal detachment was not aroused until the early 1930s. An important factor that decreased the rate of success in retinal detachment surgery in these countries was the great popularity of the electric direct ophthalmoscope. With this instrument, retinal breaks were often difficult to find, and frequently their closure was not carried out adequately.

Two elements made retinal detachment surgery substantially more successful in the 1950s: a revival of binocular indirect ophthalmoscopy[29] with scleral depression[33] and surgical procedures that paid strict attention to closure of the retinal breaks.

Scleral operations, aimed at indenting the sclera in the area of the retinal breaks, were probably initiated by Jess in 1937.[181] He temporarily placed a gauze pad on the sclera overlying the retinal break. This type of operation accomplished two purposes: First, it indented the choroid in the area of the retinal break after a chorioretinal reaction had been induced. Second, it tended to relax vitreoretinal traction in the area of the retinal break. Custodis used polyviol—a mixture of polyvinyl alcohol and Congo red—as buckling material.[182, 183] The procedure was abandoned because it led to complications. Schepens and associates used polyethylene tubing as indenting material and introduced the practice of using a tube that encircled the equatorial area of the globe to treat complex cases.[184] They coined the term *scleral buckling*. Later, in 1960,[185] soft silicone rubber was substituted for polyethylene tubing, and this material is still used extensively today. Silicone sponge was introduced as an episcleral implant by Lincoff and colleagues in 1965[186] and is still quite popular today mainly because it enables the surgeon to perform the operation more quickly. The latest implant material is a hydrogel called MAI (copolymer of 2-hydroxyethyl acrylate with methyl acrylate and ethylene diacrylate).[187] It has nearly all of the properties that are desirable in an implant, and in addition, it can absorb water-soluble antibiotics or other medication for sustained release.

Implants whose buckling effect could be adjusted intra- and postoperatively were designed. One was an inflatable silicone rubber implant that was sutured to the sclera.[188] Another was a silicone balloon that was inserted episclerally over the retinal breaks and removed as soon as choroidal adhesion was achieved.[189, 190] Finally, an absorbing implant was recommended for favorable-looking cases. Gelatin, which had been used as a subchoroidal implant in 1954,[179] was inserted intrasclerally under scleral flaps at which point it was absorbed within approximately 6 mo.[191]

Until the 1950s, bedrest was used extensively before and after operation. Prior to surgery, the patient's head was turned and immobilized to place the retinal breaks in the most dependent position with the purpose of flattening the ballooning retina. After operation, the patient was kept in the same position in the hope of keeping retina and choroid in apposition, thus accelerating the development of a retinochoroidal adhesion in the area of the retinal breaks. The advent of the scleral buckling operation changed all that and permitted the shortening or complete elimination of pre- and postoperative bedrest. It also made it possible to obtain better results in unfavorable cases.

There is one instance in which positioning of the patient is still very helpful: giant retinal tears with an inverted retinal flap. Gravity, with well-thought-out exercises, frequently helps to demonstrate how mobile the flap of a giant tear is. This has great prognostic value. Gravity also helps considerably during certain surgical steps.[192] For this purpose, a multipositional power-driven operating table was devised.[193, 194] It allows the surgeon to take advantage of the gravitational force and considerably facilitates the injection of air over the optic disc. Such an injection often repositions the retina against the choroid, thus making it easier to perform the balance of the reattachment operation.

One of the main reasons that bedrest was practically eliminated with the advent of scleral buckling operations was that this operation was accompanied by thorough drainage of subretinal fluid. This either brought about a complete retinal reattachment on the operating table or made fixed retinal folds easily visible and easier to deal with.

Scleral indentation in the area of the retinal break was used in two types of procedures that are simple and effective in favorable cases of retinal detachment. The first consisted of treating the sclera in the area of the retinal break and then indenting it without releasing subretinal fluid. It often brought about the immediate reapplication of retina against choroid in the area of the retinal break. The subretinal fluid could then be left in the eye for spontaneous absorption by the choroid.[183, 186, 195] This concept was originally introduced by Custodis and later popularized by Lincoff. It should be noted, however, that a nondrainage technique had already been used by Gonin (Fig. 109–19), and the scleral indentation simply allowed a widening of the possible indications of nondrainage, but the procedure was still limited to favorable cases. Absence of drainage avoided the complications that could result from release of subretinal fluid. However, when a correct technique of perforation is used, such complications are nearly always avoidable.[196] The disadvantage of the nondrainage technique is that the surgical result may be in doubt at the end of the operation because the retina is still detached.[197]

The second procedure that was a simplification of the original scleral indentation procedures was the athermal buckle. It consisted of scleral buckling as originally described, with thorough release of subretinal fluid but without using any type of cryoapplication, diathermy, or photocoagulation; hence, its name *athermal*. It was originally described by Zauberman in 1975[198, 199] and promptly used by others.[200, 201] Its main advantages were that it was a less traumatic procedure and it was less likely to precipitate PVR. It is very effective in relatively favorable cases of retinal detachment. A disadvantage is that the buckling has to be located somewhat more posteriorly than with regular scleral buckling.[202]

Along with improvements in techniques of scleral indentation and scleral buckling came new and better

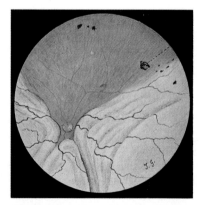

Figure 109–19. Fundus sketch initialed by Jules Gonin. There is a retinal detachment affecting the lower two thirds of fundus, apparently caused by a small break in a practically attached retina, at the 2 o'clock position. Complete reattachment followed ignipuncture over break, found to be located 15 mm from the limbus. Subretinal fluid was not released. (From Gonin J: Le Décollement de la Rétine: Pathogénie-Traitment. Lausanne, Payot, 1934, pp 112–117.)

methods of inducing a chorioretinal reaction. Diathermy was improved by using high-frequency crystal-controlled machines, electrodes with a much smaller active area at the tip, and applications made over thinned sclera.[184] It also gradually became evident that sparse diathermy applications were often most effective.[203]

Diathermy applications have been made more reliable and usable through thick sclera or even through conjunctiva with only minimal damage to these surface structures.[204] This result was obtained with an electrode whose active tip is very small (0.5 to 0.75 mm) and round. When using a return path rather than employing ground as a return, the applications were more consistent and allowed current settings that were 20 to 40 percent lower.[205]

Another modality used to produce chorioretinal reaction is cryoapplication. It was originally accomplished by applying carbonic snow over the sclera[206, 207] or over the choroid through scleral trephinations.[208] These techniques were not practical and were forgotten until the procedure was revived by Cooper, who used liquid nitrogen.[209] Later, carbon dioxide or nitrous oxide was used by releasing the gas in a silver envelope. By these means, well-controlled areas of freezing were obtained.[210, 211] At the present time, the latest types of diathermy and cryotherapy machines can be used over undissected conjunctiva or on bare sclera. Controversy still exists over the contention that since cryoapplications destroy a larger area of choroid and retinal pigment epithelium than do diathermy applications or photocoagulation, they tend to cause more cases of PVR.[212] This danger is likely to be greater when the retinal breaks are large.

In 1959, Meyer-Schwickerath developed photocoagulation.[213] This technique became popular with the advent of lasers.[214] The ruby laser, which was used first, was found to be clinically unreliable because the exposure time was fixed and very short (0.5 msec).[215] It was soon replaced by argon and krypton lasers.[216] The blue wavelength of argon (488 nm) was demonstrated to be potentially dangerous, especially in the macula, whereas the argon green (514.5 nm), krypton yellow (582.6 nm), and red (647.1 nm) were all found to have their useful applications.[217, 218] More recently, the use of an infrared diode laser (810 nm) was studied.[219, 220] The instrument is small and highly portable. It does not require a special electrical outlet or water cooling and has an output power of up to 1 watt. It may be hand-held or used in conjunction with a standard slit-lamp microscope.[221]

CLOSURE OF RETINAL BREAKS BY INTRAOCULAR SURGERY

Since Gonin, it has been recognized that two main elements can prevent retinal reattachment: (1) traction on the retina by a degenerated and partly organized vitreous body and (2) the proliferation of preretinal and subretinal newly formed membranes. The latter may cause severe PVR. Three intraocular surgical techniques have been recommended to combat these retinal breaks: vitreous injections, vitreous manipulations without tissue removal, and vitrectomy.

Vitreous Injections. Injections of various substances into the vitreous, in the hope of pushing the retina back into place, date back to 1874.[142] After Gonin, they were performed following release of subretinal fluid in order to appose the retina with the choroid and obtain a normal ocular tonus. Aside from saline solution, which had been used for a long time, Cibis revived the tapping and reinjection of subretinal fluid into the vitreous cavity.[222] Air was first injected by Ohm in 1911[223] and was popularized by Arruga,[224] Rosengren,[225–227] Schepens and Freeman,[228] and Norton.[229] Air had the advantage of being buoyant and not water-miscible. Consequently, it was less likely than was saline solution to escape into the subretinal space. Because of these advantages, a search was made for a more permanent gas, because air in the vitreous was absorbed in 2 to 5 days.

Many other gases were evaluated, such as oxygen, carbon dioxide, nitrogen, xenon, argon, krypton, and radon. Several gaseous complex molecules that absorb slowly in the vitreous cavity were also tried, most prominently sulfur hexafluoride (SF_6), which has been used since 1973.[229] An SF_6 bubble in the vitreous expands because gases in solution in the blood diffuse into the bubble. As a result, it doubles its original size within 24 hr and lasts twice as long as air in a monkey eye.[230]

Straight-chain perfluorocarbon gases[231] are inert, and the more complex molecules tend to stay in the eye for a long time after injection. The slowness of their absorption is related to their poor solubility in water. As is the case for SF_6, the injected bubble increases in size until it is in equilibrium with blood gases. These expansile gases are useful in treating complicated retinal detachments. The clinically preferred perfluorocarbon for vitreous injection is perfluoropropane (C_3F_8), which expands four times and stays in the vitreous for several weeks. The intraocular inflammatory reaction these gases cause[232] seems to increase with their longevity in the vitreous cavity.

Recently, a technique was introduced that combines internal tamponade with gas-induced chorioretinal reaction and postoperative positioning without release of subretinal fluid.[233, 234] Hilton and Grizzard coined the term *pneumatic retinopexy* to describe this procedure.[234] It is an outpatient operation that consists of treating the area of the retinal break with transconjunctival cryoapplications or photocoagulation. This is followed by injection of an expanding gas into the vitreous and patient positioning that orients the bubble such that it closes the retinal break. Several reports recommended primary use of this procedure in selected, uncomplicated retinal detachments involving the upper 240 degrees of the ocular fundus.[235–238] This method gave good results in carefully selected patients and reduced costs of surgery. However, associated complications were reported,[239–242] especially in aphakic or pseudophakic eyes.[243]

Intraocular expanding gas and episcleral inflatable balloons for temporary tamponade of retinal breaks were compared.[244] Both techniques are nondrainage methods and do not permanently address the vitreoretinal traction component of many rhegmatogenous retinal detachments. It was difficult to produce a valid comparison between the two techniques because of a number of unmatched variables in the groups of patients used. It appears, however, that pneumatic retinopexy, which requires an intraocular injection, offers little advantage and leads to more complications than does the Lincoff balloon, which is an extraocular procedure. Experimentally, expanding intravitreous gas has a morbid effect on the vitreous: In monkey eyes it caused shrinking and tearing of the cortical vitreous lamellae and membrane formation at the edge of the torn lamellae.[245] Cortical vitreous that covers a retinal break plugs the break, thus preventing further escape of fluid vitreous into the subretinal space. Consequently, it has a favorable effect on healing of rhegmatogenous retinal detachment. In a series of 116 patients treated with scleral buckling, the condition of the vitreous body was assessed photographically. Primary surgery was successful in all instances in which the cortical vitreous covered the horseshoe-shaped retinal tear.[246]

Perfluorocarbons with a high boiling point have been used as liquids for temporary injection into the vitreous cavity.[247] Perfluorooctane (C_8F_{18}) has been found useful because it has a low viscosity, a specific gravity of 1.76, and a high vapor pressure. It is employed to flatten the posterior retina and to displace the subretinal fluid anteriorly. It is easily removed at the end of the operation, although problems can occur if the heavy perfluorocarbon should enter the subretinal space through a retinal break.

Attempts were also made to use more physiologic and longer-lasting substances. Rabbit vitreous was tried,[146] and Lenz suggested the possibility of injecting human vitreous,[248] but it was Cutler who first used this substance to correct retinal detachment.[249, 250] It was popularized by Shafer,[251] and further improved by lyophilization,[252] which made the preparation more viscous. Because injection of vitreous preparations presented no curative advantage, this practice was abandoned. Efforts toward producing a better vitreous constituent that could be injected led to trials with hyaluronic acid by Hruby[253] and Pruett and colleagues.[254] It is a viscous material that is well tolerated and can be injected through a small needle. However, it liquefies in the vitreous cavity within a short period. Attempts to use a collagen vitreous substitute produced an inflammatory reaction in the vitreous.[255]

It was clear that a more permanent and nonreactive viscous material would be very useful in severe cases of retinal detachment. Silicone oil (polydimethyl siloxane) is viscous, immiscible with water, and has a high surface tension. It was first used to correct severe retinal detachments, with encouraging results.[256] Subsequent trials revealed that it can penetrate all eye tissues.[257] Long-term studies in monkeys[258] showed spaces between Müller's fibers that contained spherical bodies, presumed to be silicone oil, encircled by homogeneous electron-opaque phospholipid material. Ganglion cells were degenerated. The inner segments of the photoreceptors had lost their phospholipids. Adenosine triphosphatase activity was abnormally high in the plexiform layers. In another study, monkeys showed severe atrophy of the retinal ganglion cells, loss of axons, and degeneration of the corresponding cells in the lateral geniculate

body.[259, 260] The macular elements were affected least, which may explain why a silicone oil injection in humans causes little or no loss of visual acuity.[260] Being a lipid, silicone oil dissolves other lipids such as cholesterol and retinol.[260, 261] Animal and human eyes show the presence of retinol and its derivatives and of cholesterol in silicone oil or fluorosilicone oil that has been present in the eye from a few days to many weeks.[262] Because of these findings, silicone oil injected into the vitreous is generally removed from the vitreous cavity as soon as is deemed clinically practical.

Fluorosilicone was also studied.[263] Its advantage is that its specific gravity (1.28) is higher than that of silicone (0.97) and of water (1.00). Therefore it can be used in a manner analogous to C_8F_{18} (see preceding discussion). Several other substances were tried, among them polygeline, polyacrylamide, polyglyceryl methacrylate, and particularly, hydroxypropyl methylcellulose,[264] but in general only animal experiments were performed with them.

Vitreous Manipulations. Transcleral vitreous surgery is not new. In 1863, von Graefe attempted to cut a dense posterior vitreous membrane by introducing a knife needle into the vitreous cavity through the pars plana ciliaris.[265] Systematic and safe vitreous manipulations had to wait for the development of adequate instruments, which began in 1952.[266] At first, these instruments were forceps or scissors that fitted into a needle 1.4 mm in diameter. Capsular forceps and scissors of a similar model had already been built in 1863 (Fig. 109–20). In many cases, a single instrument was used, although forceps and scissors could be employed simultaneously. Observation was made either by headband indirect ophthalmoscopy or through a microscope with axial illumination and a flat contact lens. These instruments were subsequently improved.[267] They were made watertight and provided with an infusion system,[268] and their closure was automated.[269] Other instruments were devised for vitreous surgery, such as an intraocular balloon to gently reposition the detached retina[270] and

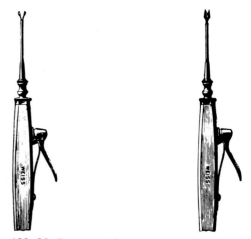

Figure 109–20. Forceps (*left*) and scissors (*right*) built in 1863 according to the principle used at present for vitreous surgery instruments. (From Schepens CL: Retinal Detachment and Allied Diseases, vol 2. Philadelphia, WB Saunders, 1983, p 745.)

an underwater diathermy electrode.[271] This armamentarium was very helpful for cutting vitreoretinal bands and membranes, removing small vitreous foreign bodies, and closing blood vessels prior to cutting. Such steps helped to substantially improve the surgical prognosis of complex retinal detachments.

Vitrectomy. Two basic types of vitrectomy were developed: closed technique and open-sky vitrectomy.

Closed Vitrectomy. Before the advent of vitrectomy, opaque vitreous had been removed.[272] Later, surgeons replaced the liquid removed with saline solution[273] or air.[274] By 1928, Zur Nedden reported on 300 such cases.[275]

Inspired by an invention to perform kidney or liver biopsies atraumatically, a vitreous nibbler was devised in 1970 (Fig. 109–21).[276] Working independently, Machemer and associates devised a vitreous infusion suction cutter and were the first to report results in humans (Fig. 109–22).[277] Initially, vitrectomy instruments were used to remove vitreous opacities. Later, they were also used to remove clear vitreous in order to eliminate vitreoretinal traction and facilitate retinal reattachment. In attempts to improve the versatility and safety of the instruments, several models were built with different cutting devices, suction and infusion, and various kinds of automation. Safety devices were particularly important when the retina was floating in the vitreous and could easily be damaged by the instruments. At first, the vitrectomy instrument contained all the functions: tissue removal, infusion, illumination, and automation.[278] At least a dozen different, but somewhat similar, instruments were described by a number of authors between 1968 and 1974.

Machemer demonstrated that lateral illumination with fiberoptics was more useful than was axial light.[279] O'Malley and Heintz[280] used a third opening in the pars plana ciliaris for infusion of fluid to maintain a constant ocular pressure. This allowed the vitrectomy instrument to be of the same diameter as a second instrument used simultaneously in the vitreous cavity, thus making them freely interchangeable. It also corrected another frequent defect of vitrectomy instruments: The suction of material was often faster than its replacement by saline solution, leading to possibly dangerous hypotony.

Not only did closed vitrectomy make it possible to remove opacities from the eye, even the lens when necessary, but it also made formerly incurable cases accessible to effective treatment. This included instances complicated by severe trauma or by proliferative diabetic retinopathy. Such complex surgery often necessitated the use of different types of second instruments: fiberoptics light equipped with a fine pick, various types of forceps and scissors, and underwater diathermy or other form of cauterization. Other intravitreous techniques became available such as intraocular laser pho-

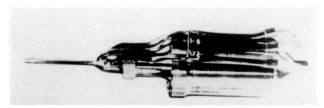

Figure 109–21. Vitreous nibbler (1970) developed by Banko and Tolentino. (From Schepens CL: Vitreous surgery. II. Tissue removal. *In* Pruett RC, Regan CDJ (eds): Retina Congress. New York, Appleton-Century-Crofts, 1974, p 677.)

tocoagulation or cryoprobe to treat posterior retinal breaks from within. Similarly, subretinal fluid could be gently sucked out through a retinal break, and air-fluid exchange could be performed to secure a retinal reattachment on the operating table. The new instrumentation has also made it possible to peel preretinal membranes and to correct macular pucker.[281] Severe degrees of PVR (grades D1, D2, or D3)[232] have yielded to this technique, even when the PVR was mostly or exclusively located in the anterior portion of the fundus.[283] This type of case may be easier to attack via open-sky vitrectomy (see further on).

Another procedure that is occasionally performed during a closed vitrectomy is a retinotomy that liberates viable retina from retina that is excessively adherent to other eye tissue.[284] Similarly, retinectomy has occasionally been performed successfully to eliminate shrunken retina that could not be unfolded.[285]

Thanks to closed vitrectomy, the progress made in the management of severe or formerly desperate cases of retinal detachment has been spectacular. This has occasionally led to excessive surgical enthusiasm, either by using this technique for cases that could be operated on successfully with less risky methods or by operating on eyes with no chance of functional improvement, regardless of the surgical procedure used. An example is traction detachment caused by diabetic retinopathy. Many patients with this condition maintain visual acuity without operation or even improve over a period of observation longer than 4 yr.[286] Other cases were successfully operated on by simply performing a lamellar scleral resection around the equator.[287]

An odd result of the enthusiasm for retinal detachment surgery is the abandonment of painstaking examination of the retina and vitreous. Many vitreoretinal surgeons have totally given up the practice of sketching the details of the fundus preoperatively—using scleral depression on a patient lying down—and of studying the vitreous changes with a three-mirror contact lens. There is no doubt that such negligence occasionally leads to unnecessary reoperations, often involving an

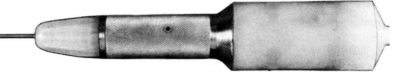

Figure 109–22. Vitreous infusion suction cutter (VISC) developed by Machemer and coworkers in 1971. (From Schepens CL: Retinal Detachment and Allied Diseases, vol 2. Philadelphia, WB Saunders, 1983, p 807.)

unneeded and potentially dangerous vitrectomy procedure.

Open-sky Vitrectomy. In this operation, the anterior route is used by making a large incision in the cornea and removing the lens. It seems to have been first attempted in 1960.[288] Kasner and coworkers were the first to publish cases successfully operated on by this technique.[289] Later, the technique was pioneered by Schepens and Constable[290, 291] and Schepens and Hirose.[292] For this operation, a long focal length (125-mm) microscope is used to avoid interference with instrument manipulations. Initially, a 300-degree corneal incision was made and the cornea was housed in a latex protector and bathed in tissue culture solution and hyaluronic acid.[293] Another approach was to use a 170-degree pars plana incision,[294] which gave better protection to the cornea and better access to the peripheral vitreous. Later, it was found that use of a corneal trephine (7.5- to 8.5-mm) was the most practical technique.[295] After two iridotomies, intracapsular lens removal is practiced. The vitreous gel and liquid is removed with a vitrectomy instrument. Scar tissue and preretinal membranes are dissected with miniaturized scissors, forceps, and spatulas. Subretinal fluid is almost routinely sucked out through existing retinal breaks.

The lack of intraocular pressure tends to cover the exposed tissues, especially the iris and ciliary process, with fibrin. This tendency is combated by a technique used in other fields of medicine, consisting of refrigerating the tissues that are manipulated surgically.[296] The irrigating solution used in animal vitreous surgery was cooled to 7°C. The result was a decrease in intraocular bleeding volume, fibrin production, and postoperative inflammation. Since 1987, Hirose[297] has been irrigating the vitreous cavity with a physiologic solution that is cooled with ice, lowering the temperature of irrigation fluid as mentioned previously.

Hyaluronic acid is used to cover the iris and prevent its adhesion to the corneal wound. It is also used to fill the emptied vitreous cavity, which facilitates posterior dissection.[298] When the eye is filled with hyaluronic acid, a flat contact lens can be temporarily fitted over the corneal trephine opening, which helps further with posterior dissection. Bleeding is controlled with underwater diathermy, which also serves to treat retinal breaks. Iridotomies and the corneal button are sutured, and the eye is refilled with hyaluronic acid to increase its tonus.

The main indications of open-sky vitrectomy are for cases in which the pathologic condition is located mostly in the anterior portion of the vitreous cavity (with the retina often adherent to the ciliary body or another part of the anterior segment) and for removal of large foreign bodies and dense or hard cicatricial tissue. Cases of severe anterior PVR are easier to correct with this technique than with the closed technique. Giant tears complicated by severe PVR may be helped with an open-sky technique in which the retina is sutured to the choroid.[298, 299]

Suturing the retina to the wall of the eye is not new. Galezowski[140] had already used this technique on a closed eye before systematic attempts to close the retinal breaks were carried out. Rubbrecht[300] described his experience with a similar procedure. Later, it was per-

Table 109–1. THE GREAT LANDMARKS: RETINAL EXAMINATION

Landmark	Year	Author (Ref)
Retina first seen in living eye	1704	Méry[9]
First ophthalmoscope	1851	Helmholtz[14]
First binocular ophthalmoscope	1861	Giraud-Teulon[25]
Reflex-free ophthalmoscopy	1911	Gullstrand[27]
Comprehensive optical model of the eye	1972	Pomerantzeff et al[53]
Scanning laser ophthalmoscope	1980	Pomerantzeff and Webb[57]

formed as part of various techniques,[301, 302] some of which were performed at the end of a closed vitrectomy procedure.[303–305] When suturing a giant tear to the choroid, the retinal pigment epithelium that is not covered by the retina was surgically removed to decrease the risk of postoperative recurrence of PVR.[299, 306]

Grade V retinopathy of prematurity causes a total fixed retinal detachment without retinal breaks. It is one of the best indications for the open-sky procedure,[307] which is more effective than closed vitrectomy.[308] In 46 percent of surgically reattached retinas, otherwise totally blind children acquired ambulatory vision.[309] The operation permits the removal of the cicatricial tissue in the vitreous cavity en bloc.

Open-sky vitrectomy is a last-resort operation that has allowed the repair of a variety of desperate cases of detached retina caused either by retinal breaks or by vitreous traction.

WHAT HISTORY TEACHES US
(Tables 109–1 and 109–2)

The aim of all the work related to retinal detachment was to cure and prevent the disease. Clearly, the first step was to be able to see the retina in detail. The landmark discovery in this respect was ophthalmoscopy.[14] Once a retinal detachment could be seen, which happened in 1851, it was 70 yr before its pathogenesis was understood. Repair of rhegmatogenous retinal detachment then became immediately possible because the central role played by the retinal break came to light.[152]

Ophthalmoscopy could have been discovered 147 yr earlier, but in 1704, the observer was in fact looking for

Table 109–2. THE GREAT LANDMARKS: PATHOGENESIS AND TREATMENT

Landmark	Year	Author (Ref)
Retinal break first seen	1853	Coccius[70]
Vitreous as cause of retinal detachment	1882	Leber,[106] de Wecker[107]
Closing break cures detachment	1919	Gonin[99]
Thorough retinal examination	1951	Schepens[31]
Modern buckling	1957	Schepens et al[184]
Photocoagulation	1959	Meyer-Schwickerath[213]
Modern vitrectomy	1971	Machemer et al[277]
Athermal buckling	1975	Zauberman and Garcia Rosell[198]

something else, and his view of the fundus did not raise questions in his mind.[9] Ophthalmoscopy was probably discovered in 1847,[15] but at this time some clinicians did not feel it improved the efficacy of their treatments! Similarly, binocular ophthalmoscopy was known a century before it was popularized,[25] and scleral pressure was described half a century before its use was generalized.[32] This illustrates the slowness of clinicians in realizing the importance of new findings from researchers. Such delays can only be corrected by having more clinicians genuinely interested in clinically applicable eye research.

The way pathogenesis of retinal detachment was unraveled is of great interest. Leber[106] could not convince his colleagues that he was right in 1882 because he lacked enough evidence to demonstrate the importance of vitreoretinal traction. It was only 40 yr later that indispensable evidence was brought forward by Gonin.[152] Even then, it took 30 yr more for the bulk of ophthalmologists to accept the fact that closure of retinal breaks was key to successful reattachment. This slow development is ascribable to slow acceptance of modern techniques for performing ophthalmoscopy (including ophthalmoscopy of the extreme fundus periphery) and slit-lamp microscopy of the vitreous cavity.

In the second half of this century a synthesis was gradually developed concerning the various elements of the pathogenesis of rhegmatogenous retinal detachment: the roles of retinal breaks, PVR, and the physiologic elements that normally keep the retina attached to the retinal pigment epithelium. This led to more effective and less traumatic techniques of surgical reattachment, allowing retinal break closure with better control of the forces that pull the retina off. Today, techniques to accomplish the latter are either extraocular (buckling) or intraocular vitreous manipulations and vitrectomy. Now we can reattach more than 90 percent of all retinal detachments.

The treatment of choice for simple cases seems to be a scleral buckling, using modern diathermy in preference to cryoapplication. The best alternative appears to be the use of a temporary balloon rather than pneumatic retinopexy. Photocoagulation is preferred to close retinal breaks with little or no detachment of the retina. In difficult cases, the vitreous approach has been a key element. However, this surgical progress is unwittingly delaying rational efforts to prevent retinal detachment. Such efforts require a detailed study of the molecular biology of the vitreous. By spreading the ill-conceived idea that the vitreous is an embryonic appendage without useful function in the adult, vitreous surgeons are popularizing an erroneous concept and delaying, perhaps for many years, the day when research in molecular biology of the vitreous becomes adequately funded, thus getting us closer to the day when retinal breaks can be effectively prevented.

References

1. Maitre-Jan A: Traité des maladies de l'oeil et des remèdes propres pour leur guérison enrichi de plusieurs expériences de physique. Paris, Veuve D'Houry, 1740, pp 199–201.
2. Morgagni JB: De Sedibus et Causis Morborum per Anatomen Indagatis Libri Quinque, vol. 1, letter 13. Ebroduni, Switzerland, 1779, p 203.
3. Wardrop J: Essays on Morbid Anatomy of the Human Eye, vol. 2, plate XIV. London, Constable, 1818, pp 270–272.
4. de Saint-Yves C: Nouveau Traité des Maladies des Yeux. Paris, Pierre-Augustin Le Mercier, 1722. (Stockton J. [trans.]: A New Treatise of the Diseases of the Eyes. London, J Crokatt, 1741, pp 285–287.)
5. Morgagni JB: De Sedibus, et Causis Morborum per Anatomen Indagatis, vol. 1. Louvain, Belgium, Typographia Academica, 1765, 182.
6. Beer GJ: Lehre von den Augenkrankheiten, als Leitfaden zu seinen offentlichen Vorlesungen entworfen, vol. 2. Vienna, Camesina, Huebner und Volke, 1817, p 496.
7. Sichel J: Mémoire sur le glaucome, deuxième partie. Ann d'Ocul 5:225–250, 1841.
8. Desmarres LA: Traité Théorique et Pratique des Maladies des Yeux. Paris, Germer Baillière, 1847, pp 710–712.
9. Méry M: Des mouvemens de l'iris et par occasion de la partie principale de la vue. Hist Acad R Sci 1704, pp 261–271.
10. de la Hire M: Explication de quelques faits d'optique, et de la manière dont se fait la vision. Hist Acad R Sci 1709, pp 95–106.
11. Thau W: Purkyne: A pioneer in ophthalmoscopy. Arch Ophthalmol 27:299–316, 1942.
12. Cumming W: On a luminous appearance of the human eye, and its application to the detection of disease of the retina and posterior part of the eye. R Med Chir Soc Lond 29:283–296, 1846.
13. Brücke E: Ueber das Leuchten der menschlichen Augen. Arch Anat Physiol Wissensch Med 1847, pp 225–227.
14. Helmholtz H: Beschreibung eines Augenspiegels zur Untersuchung der Netzhaut im lebenden Auge. Berlin, A. Forstner, 1851.
15. Jones TW: Report on the ophthalmoscope. Med Clin Rev 14:425–432, 1854.
16. Wetenschappelijke Mededeelingen, Ophthalmoskopie. Nederlandsch Weekblad Voor Geneeskundigen. 1:526–528, 1851.
17. Koenigsberger L: Hermann von Helmholtz. (Welby FA, trans.) London, Henry Frowde, 1906, pp 74–81.
18. Ruete CGT: Der Augenspiegel und das Optometer fur practische Aerzte. Gottingen, Dieterichschen Buchhandlung, 1852, pp 1–27.
19. Schepens CL: Retinal Detachment and Allied Diseases, vol. 1. Philadelphia, WB Saunders, 1983, p 6.
20. Friedenwald H: The history of the invention and of the development of the ophthalmoscope. JAMA 38:549–569, 1902.
21. Dennett WS: The electric light ophthalmoscope. Trans Am Ophthalmol Soc 4:156–157, 1885.
22. Juler H: Refraction ophthalmoscope, with a special arrangement for the electric light. Trans Ophthalmol Soc UK 6:502–504, 1886.
23. Marple WB: An improved electric ophthalmoscope. Trans Am Ophthalmol Soc 11:225–229, 1906.
24. Rucker CW: A History of the Ophthalmoscope. Rochester, MN, Whiting Printers, 1971, pp 100–113.
25. Giraud-Teulon M: Ophthalmoscopie binoculaire ou s'exerçant par le concours des deux yeux associés. Ann d'Ocul 45:233–250, 1861.
26. Gullstrand A: Neue Methoden der reflexlosen Ophthalmoskopie. Ber Dtsch Ophthalmol Ges 36:75–80, 1910.
27. Gullstrand A: Einführung in die Methoden der Dioptrik des Auges des Menschen. Leipzig, S Hirzel, 1911.
28. Schepens CL: Un nouvel ophtalmoscope binoculaire pour l'examen du décollement de la rétine (avec la projection d'un film sonore). Bull Soc Belge Ophtalmol 82:9–13, 1945.
29. Schepens CL: A new ophthalmoscope demonstration. Trans Am Acad Ophthalmol Otolaryngol 51:298–301, 1947.
30. Schepens CL: Retinal Detachment and Allied Diseases, vol. 1. Philadelphia, WB Saunders, 1983, p 103.
31. Schepens CL: Examination of the ora serrata region: Its clinical significance. Acta XVI Concilium Ophthalmologicum (Britannia, 1950) 2:1384–1393, 1951.
32. Trantas A: Moyens d'explorer par l'ophtalmoscope—et par translucidité—la partie antérieure du fond oculaire, le cercle ciliaire y compris. Arch d'Ophtalmol 20:314–326, 1900.
33. Brockhurst RJ: Modern indirect ophthalmoscopy. Am J Ophthalmol 41:265–272, 1956.

34. Hovland KR, Tanenbaum HL, Schepens CL: New scleral depressor. Am J Ophthalmol 66:117–118, 1968.
35. Pomerantzeff O: A new stereoscopic indirect ophthalmoscope. In McPherson A (ed): New and Controversial Aspects of Retinal Detachment. New York, Hoeber Medical Division, Harper & Row, 1968, pp 137–146.
36. Hovland KR, Elzeneiny IH, Schepens CL: Clinical evaluation of the small-pupil binocular indirect ophthalmoscope. Arch Ophthalmol 82:466–474, 1969.
37. Schepens CL: Retinal Detachment and Allied Diseases, vol. 1. Philadelphia, WB Saunders, 1983, pp 116–118.
38. Michels RG, Wilkinson CP, Rice TA: Retinal Detachment. St Louis, CV Mosby, 1990, p 250.
39. Howe L: Photography of the interior of the eye. Trans Am Ophthalmol Soc 4:568–571, 1887.
40. Fick EA: Einige Bemerkungen über das photographiren des Augenhintergrundes. Ber Ophthalmol Ges Heidelberg, 1891, pp 197–201.
41. Guilloz Th: La photographie instantanée du fond d'oeil humain. Arch d'Ophtalmol 13:465–481, 1893.
42. Dimmer F: Ueber die Photographie des Augenhintergrundes. Ber Dtsch Ophthalmol Ges 29:162–169, 1901.
43. Dimmer F: Die Photographie des Augenhintergrundes. Ein Wort zur Aufklärung und zur Abwehr. Klin Monatsbl Augenheilkd 45:256–283, 1907.
44. Dimmer F: Die Photographie der Augenhintergrundes. Wiesbaden, Bergmann, 1907, pp 1–28.
45. Dimmer F, Pillat A: Atlas photographischer Bilder des menschlichen Augenhintergrundes. Leipzig, Deuticke, 1927.
46. Bedell AJ: Photographs of the Fundus Oculi. Philadelphia, FA Davis, 1929.
47. Gullstrand A: Die reflexlose Ophthalmoskopie. Arch Augenheilkd 68:101–144, 1911.
48. Nordenson JW: Augenkamera zum stationären Ophthalmoskop von Gullstrand. Ber Dtsch Ophthalmol Ges 45:278, 1925.
49. Hartinger H: Die vollkommen reflexfreie Zeiss-Nordensonsche Netzhautkammer. XIII Concil Ophthalmol Acta (Hollandia, 1929) 1:40–42, 1930.
50. Ogle KN, Rucker CW: Fundus photographs in color using a high-speed flash tube in the Zeiss retinal camera. Arch Ophthalmol 49:435–437, 1953.
51. Littmann H: Die Zeiss-Funduskamera. Ber Dtsch Ophthalmol Ges 59:318–321, 1955.
52. Mann WA: History of photography of the eye. Surv Ophthalmol 15:179–189, 1970.
53. Pomerantzeff O, Fish H, Govignon J, Schepens CL: Wide-angle optical model of the eye. Optica Acta 19:387–388, 1972.
54. Pomerantzeff O, Govignon J: Design of a wide-angle ophthalmoscope. Arch Ophthalmol 86:420–424, 1971.
55. Pomerantzeff O: Equator-plus camera. Invest Ophthalmol 14:401–406, 1975.
56. Pomerantzeff O: Wide-angle noncontact and small angle contact cameras. Invest Ophthalmol Vis Sci 19:973–979, 1980.
57. Pomerantzeff O, Webb R: Scanning Ophthalmoscope for Examining the Fundus of the Eye. US Patent No. 4, 213, 678, 1980.
58. Zworykin VK, Morton GA: Television: The Electronics of Image Transmission in Color and Monochrome, 2nd ed. New York, John Wiley & Sons, 1954, pp 238–244, 946–952.
59. Webb RH, Hughes GW, Pomerantzeff O: Flying spot TV ophthalmoscope. Appl Opt 19:2991–2997, 1980.
60. Acosta F: Personal communication.
61. Czapski S: Binoculares Cornealmikroskop. Arch Ophthalmol (Berlin) 48:229–235, 1899.
62. Von Graefe A: Notiz über die im Glaskörper vorkommenden Opacitäten. Arch Ophthalmol (Berlin) 1:351–361, 1854.
63. Wecker L: Traité Théorique et Pratique des Maladies des Yeux, vol. 1. Paris, JB Baillière. 1863, p 272.
64. Wolff H: I. Ophthalmoskopische Beobachtungen mit dem elektrischen Augenspiegel. II. Anhang: Ueber die fokale Beleuchtung der Netzhaut und des Glaskorpers. Z Augenheilkd 5:101–109, 1901.
65. Gullstrand A: Demonstration der Nernstspaltlampe. Ber Dtsch Ophthalmol Ges 37:374–376, 1911.
66. Gullstrand A: Die Nernstspaltlampe in der ophthalmologischen Praxis. Klin Monatsbl Augenheilkd 50:483–485, 1912.
67. Haugwitz TV: The history of optical instruments for the examination of the eye. In Hirschberg J: The History of Ophthalmology, vol. 11, part 2. (Blodi FC, trans.) Bonn, JP Wayenborgh, 1986, p A117.
68. Czermak J: Ueber eine neue Methode zur genaueren Untersuchung des gesunden und kranken Auges. Vierteljahrschrift Praktische Heilkd 31:154–165, 1851.
69. Czermak J: Beiträge zur Ophthalmoskopie. Vierteljahrschrift Praktische Heilkd 37:137–141, 1853.
70. Coccius A: Ueber die Anwendung des Augenspiegels nebst Angabe eines neuen Instruments. Leipzig, Immanuel Muller, 1853, pp 130–131, 150–156.
71. Koeppe L: Die Mikroskopie des lebenden Augenhintergrundes mit starken Vergrösserungen im fokalen Lichte der Gullstrandschen Nernstspaltlampe. 1. Die Theorie, Apparatur und Anwendungstechnik der Spaltlampenuntersuchung des Augenhintergrundes im fokalen Licht. Graefes Arch Ophthalmol 95:282–306, 1918. 2. Die Histologie des lebenden normalen Augenhintergrundes und einiger seiner angeborenen Anomalien im Bilde der Nernstspaltlampe. Graefes Arch Ophthalmol 97:346–381, 1918.
72. Gallemaerts E, Kleefeld G: Etude microscopique du fond d'oeil vivant. Ann d'Ocul 159:264–274, 1922.
73. Schmidt T: Zur Theorie und Praxis der Spaltlampe. Acta XVIII Concilium Ophthalmologicum, Belgica, 1958. 2:1818–1823, 1959.
74. Stilling J: Notiz über Orthoskopie des Augengrundes. Klin Monatsbl Augenheilkd 17:52–55, 1879.
75. Lemoine P, Valois G: Ophtalmoscopie microscopique (sans verre de contact). Clin Ophthalmol 12:423–428, 1923.
76. Hruby K: Spaltlampenmikroskopie des hinteren Augenabschnittes ohne Kontaktglas. Klin Monatsbl Augenheilkd 108:195–200, 1942.
77. Hruby K: Slit-lamp microscopy of the posterior section of the eye with the new preset lens. Arch Ophthalmol 43:330–336, 1950.
78. El Bayadi G: New method of slit-lamp micro-ophthalmoscopy. Br J Ophthalmol 37:625–628, 1953.
79. Goldmann H: Slit-lamp examination of the vitreous and the fundus. Br J Ophthalmol 33:242–247, 1949.
80. Tolentino FI, Rietzler X, Pomerantzeff O, et al: Adjustable mirror contact lens for fundus and vitreous examinations. Ann Ophthalmol 4:95–98, 1972.
81. Frisen L: An adjustable biomicroscopy contact glass with erect imagery. Arch Ophthalmol 87:202–205, 1972.
82. Takahashi M, Trempe CL, Schepens CL: Biomicroscopic evaluation and photography of posterior vitreous detachment. Arch Ophthalmol 98:665–668, 1980.
83. Schepens CL: Retinal Detachment and Allied Diseases, vol. 2. Philadelphia, WB Saunders, 1983, pp 1127–1130.
84. Kakehashi A, Akiba J, Trempe CL: Vitreous photography with a +90-diopter double aspheric preset lens vs. the El Bayadi-Kajiura preset lens. Arch Ophthalmol 109:962–965, 1991.
85. Oksala A: Experimental and clinical observations on the echograms in vitreous hemorrages. Br J Ophthalmol 47:65–70, 1963.
86. Coleman DJ: Ultrasound in vitreous surgery. Trans Am Acad Ophthalmol Otolaryngol 76:467–479, 1972.
87. Jabbour NM, Eller AE, Hirose T, et al: Stage 5 retinopathy of prematurity. Prognostic value of morphologic findings. Ophthalmology 94:1640–1646, 1987.
88. Hirose T: Evaluation of retinal function in the presence of vitreous opacities. In Freeman HM, Hirose T, Schepens CL (eds): Vitreous Surgery and Advances in Fundus Diagnosis and Treatment. New York, Appleton-Century-Crofts, 1977, pp 79–97.
89. Fuller DG, Knighton RW, Machemer R: Bright-flash electroretinography for the evaluation of eyes with opaque vitreous. Am J Ophthalmol 80:214–223, 1975.
90. Sakaue H, Katsumi O, Mehta M, Hirose T: Simultaneous pattern reversal ERG and VER recordings. Invest Ophthalmol Vis Sci 31:506–511, 1990.
91. Delori FC, Airey RW, Dollery CT, et al: Image intensifier cineangiography. Adv Electronics Electron Phys 33B:1089–1099, 1972.
92. Drain LE: The Laser Doppler Technique. New York, John Wiley & Sons, 1980, p 1.

93. Tanaka T, Riva C, Ben Sira I: Blood velocity measurements in human retinal vessels. Science 186:830–831, 1974.
94. Milbocker MT, Pflibsen KP, Feke GT, et al: A modular eye fundus tracker and image stabilizer. Noninvasive Assessment of the Visual System, Technical Digest Series, vol. 7. Washington, DC, Optical Society of America, 1989, pp 50–53.
95. Feke GT: Human retinal blood flow and laser velocimetry. [Abstract] J Opt Soc Am 65:1171, 1975.
96. Feke GT, Goger DG, Tagawa H, Delori FC: Laser Doppler technique for absolute measurement of blood speed in retinal vessels. IEEE Trans Biomed Eng 34:673–680, 1987.
97. Yoshida A, Feke GT, Green GT, et al: Retinal circulation changes after scleral buckling procedures. Am J Ophthalmol 95:182–188, 1983.
98. Dobbie GJ: Circulatory changes in the eye associated with retinal detachment and its repair. Trans Am Ophthalmol Soc 78:503–566, 1980.
99. Gonin J: Le diagnostic clinique et le traitement des différentes formes de décollement rétinien. Korrespondenzblatt fuer Schweizer Aerzte 49:1675–1678, 1919.
100. von Graefe A: Notiz über die Ablösungen der Netzhaut von der Chorioidea. Arch Ophthalmol (Berlin) 1:362–371, 1854.
101. von Graefe A: Zur Prognose der Netzhautablösung. Arch Ophthalmol (Berlin) 3:394–396, 1857.
102. Arlt F: Die Krankheiten des Auges, für pratische Aerzte geschildert. Prague, FA Credner, 1858, pp 158–184 (vol. 2); 1859, pp 116–129 (vol. 3).
103. Müller H: Anatomische Beitrage zur Ophthalmologie. 7. Beschreibung einiger von Prof. v. Graefe exstirpirter Augapfel. Arch Ophthalmol (Berlin) 4:363–388, 1858.
104. Iwanoff: Beiträge zur normalen und pathologischen Anatomie des Auges. 1. Beiträge zur Abloösung des Glaskörpers. Arch Ophthalmol (Berlin) 15:1–69, 1869.
105. de Wecker L, de Jaeger E: Traité des maladies du fond de l'oeil et atlas d'ophthalmoscopie. Paris, Adrien Delahaye, 1870, pp 151–158.
106. Leber T: Ueber die Entstehung der Netzhautablösung. Ber Dtsch Ophthalmol Ges 14:18–45, 1882.
107. de Wecker L: Quel but doit poursuivre le traitement du décollement de la rétine? Reprinted by Arruga H: Un document historique relatif au décollement de la rétine. Ophthalmologica 98:1–6, 1939.
108. Leber T: Ueber die Entstehung der Netzhautablösung. Ber Dtsch Ophthalmol Ges 35:120–134, 1908.
109. Dufour M, Gonin J: Maladies de la rétine. XXI. Décollement rétinien. In Lagrange F, Valude E. (eds): Encyclopédie Française d'Ophtalmologie, vol. 6. Paris, Octave Doin, 1906, pp 975–1025.
110. Gonin J: Pathogénie et anatomie pathologique des décollements rétiniens (à l'exclusion des décollements traumatiques, néoplasiques et parasitaires). Bull Mem Soc Fr Ophtalmol 33:1–120, 1920.
111. Gonin J: Le Décollement de la Rétine: Pathogénie-Traitement. Payot, Lausanne, 1934, pp 112–117.
112. Vogt A: Die Operative Therapie und die Pathogenese der Netzhautablösung. Stuttgart, F Enke, 1936, pp 64–82.
113. Hruby K: Spaltlampenmikroskopie des Hinteren Augenabschnittes. Vienna, Urban & Schwarzenberg, 1950.
114. Busacca A, Goldmann H, Schiff-Wertheimer S: Biomicroscopie du Corps Vitré et du Fond de l'Oeil. Paris, Masson, 1957, pp 285–324.
115. Tolentino FI, Schepens CL, Freeman HM: Massive preretinal retraction. A biomicroscopic study. Arch Ophthalmol 78:16–22, 1967.
116. Eisner G: Biomicroscopy of the Peripheral Fundus. An Atlas and Textbook. New York, Springer, 1973, pp 60–81.
117. Rutnin U, Schepens CL: Fundus appearance in normal eyes. IV. Retinal breaks and other findings. Am J Ophthalmol 64:1063–1078, 1967.
118. Byer NE: Prognosis of asymptomatic retinal breaks. Arch Ophthalmol 92:208–210, 1974.
119. Zauberman H, Berman ER: Measurement of adhesive forces between the sensory retina and the pigment epithelium. Exp Eye Res 8:276–283, 1969.
120. Zauberman H, de Guillebon H: Retinal traction in vivo and post mortem. Arch Ophthalmol 87:549–554, 1972.
121. Hageman GS, Johnson LV: Structure, composition and function of the retinal interphotoreceptor matrix. Prog Retinal Res 10:207–249, 1991.
122. Miller SS, Steinberg RH: Active transport of ions across frog retinal pigment epithelium. Exp Eye Res 25:235–248, 1977.
123. Hughes BA, Miller SS, Machen TE: Effects of cyclic AMP on fluid absorption and ion transport across frog retinal pigment epithelium. Measurements in the open-circuit states. J Gen Physiol 83:875–899, 1984.
124. Steinberg RH, Miller SS, Stern WH: Initial observations on the isolated retinal pigment epithelium–choroid of the cat. Invest Ophthalmol Vis Sci 17:675–678, 1978.
125. de Guillebon H, de la Tribonnière MM, Pomerantzeff O: Adhesion between retina and pigment epithelium: Measurement by peeling. Arch Ophthalmol 86:679–684, 1971.
126. Lindner K: Über die Herstellung von Modellen zu Modellversuchen der Netzhautabhebung. Klin Monatsbl Augenheilkd 90:289–300, 1933.
127. Machemer R: The importance of fluid absorption, traction, intraocular currents, and chorioretinal scars in the therapy of rhegmatogenous retinal detachments. Am J Ophthalmol 98:681–693, 1984.
128. Machemer R, Van Horn D, Aaberg TM: Pigment epithelial proliferation in human retinal detachment with massive periretinal proliferation. Am J Ophthalmol 85:181–191, 1978.
129. Zinn KM, Constable IJ, Schepens CL: The fine structure of human vitreous membranes. In Freeman HM, Hirose T, Schepens CL (eds): Vitreous Surgery and Advances in Fundus Diagnosis and Treatment. New York, Appleton-Century-Crofts, 1977, pp 39–49.
130. Balazs EA: The molecular biology of the vitreous. In McPherson A (ed): New and Controversial Aspects of Retinal Detachment. New York, Hoeber Medical Division, Harper & Row, 1968, pp 3–15.
131. Seery CM, Davison PF: Collagens of the bovine vitreous. Invest Ophthalmol Vis Sci 32:1540–1550, 1991.
132. Ware J: Remarks on the Ophthalmy, Psorophthalmy, and Purulent Eyes of the New Born Children, case XXIV. London, Underwood & Mawman, 1814, pp 233–238.
133. von Graefe A: Perforation von abgelöst Netzhauten. Arch Ophthalmol 2:85–104, 1863.
134. Samelsohn: Ueber mekanische Behandlung der Netzhaut-ablösung. Med Centr Blatt 49:833–836, 1875.
135. Coppez H: Traitement du décollement par l'iridectomie. Bull Mém Soc Fr Ophtalmol 5:78–99, 1887.
136. de Wecker L: Pourquoi le décollement de la rétine guérit—Il si difficilement. Arch d'Ophtalmol 8:271–274, 1888.
137. de Wecker L, Landolt E: Traité Complet d'Ophthalmologie, vol. 4. Paris, Lecrosnier & Babé, 1889, pp 140–168.
138. de Wecker L, Masselon J: Emploi de la galvano-caustique (galvano-poncture) en chirurgie oculaire. Ann d'Ocul 87:39–44, 1882.
139. Terson: Quelques considérations sur l'application de l'électrolyse à douze cas de décollement de la rétine. Ann d'Ocul 114:22–39, 1895.
140. Galezowski X: Du décollement de la rétine et de son traitement par ophtalmotomie postérieure. Recueil Ophtalmol 17:385–390, 1895.
141. Schoeler HL: Zur operativen Behandlung und Heilung der Netzhautablösung. Berlin, Hermann Peters, 1889, p 41.
142. Weber A: Quoted by Arlt F. In von Graefe A, Saemisch T (eds): Handbuch der gesammten Augenheilkunde, vol. 3, part 1. Leipzig, Wilhelm Engelmann, 1874, p 372.
143. Andrews TA: On the injection of a weak sterile solution of sodium chloride into collapsed eyes. Arch Ophthalmol 29:50–53, 1883.
144. Hegner CA: Ueber Glaskörperersatz. Ber Deutsch Ophthalmol 47:391–394, 1928.
145. Kurachi Y: Aqueous humor as a substitute for cloudy vitreous. Opthal Lit Lon 4:402, 1950.
146. Deutschmann R: Über ein neues Heilverfahren bei Netzhautablosung. Beitr Augenheilkd 2:849–928, 1895.
147. Alaimo: Cura chirurgica del distacco retinico. Ann Ottal 22:542–543, 1893.

148. Müller L: Eine neue operative Behandlung der Netzhautabhebung. Klin Monatsbl Augenheilkd 41:459–462, 1903.
149. Blaskowics L, Szemeszet No. 2, 1911. Cited by Torok E In The treatment of detachment of the retina, with special reference to Müller's resection of the sclera. Arch Ophthalmol 46:466–474, 1917.
150. Vail DT: An inquiry into results of the established treatment of detachment of the retina and a new theory. Trans Am Acad Ophthalmol Otolaryngol 17:29–70, 1912.
151. Binkhorst PG: Resultaten der Diathermische Behandeling van Netvliesloslating over de Jaren 1935 tot 1939 in het Nederlandsch Gasthuis voor Ooglijders te Utrecht. Amsterdam, JK Smit, 1940.
152. Gonin J: Le traitement du décollement rétinien. Ann d'Ocul 158:175–194, 1921.
153. Gonin J: Guérisons opératoires de décollements rétiniens. Rev Génér Ophthalmol 37:337–340, 1923.
154. Gonin J: Les résultats de la thermo-ponction oblitérante des déchirures rétiniennes. Ann d'Ocul 168:689–736, 1931.
155. Lindner R: Ein Weg zur Lagebestimmung von Netzhautstellen. Klin Monatsbl Augenheilkd 82:119–120, 1929.
156. Guist G: Ein Lokalisationsophthalmoskop. Ber Dtsch Ophthalmol Ges 48:343–348, 1930.
157. Majewski KW: Essai d'un repérage diascléral des lésions ophtalmoscopiques. Arch d'Ophtalmol 47:440, 1930.
158. von Graefe A: Epikritische Bemerkungen über Cysticercusoperationen und Beschreibung eines Lokalisierungsophthalmoskops. Arch Ophthalmol 28:187–202, 1882.
159. Amsler M Dubois H: Topographie ophtalmoscopique et décollement rétinien. Ann d'Ocul 165:667–675, 1928.
160. Heim H: Quoted by Gonin J: In Le Décollement de la Rétine: Pathogénie-Traitement. Lausanne, Payot, 1934, p 171.
161. Weve HJM: Over netvliesloslating en den gloeiprik van Gonin. Ned Tijdschr Geneeskd 74:2354–2365, 1930.
162. Vogt A: Die operative Therapie und die Pathogenese der Netzhautablösung. Stuttgart, Ferdinand Enke, 1936, p 38.
163. Guist G: Eine neue Ablatiooperation. Z Augenheilkd 74:232–242, 1931.
164. Lindner K: Ein Beitrag zur Entstehung und Behandlung der idiopathischen und der traumatischen Netzhautabhebung. Graefes Arch Ophthalmol 127:177–295, 1931.
165. Safar K: Behandlung der Netzhautabhebung mit Elektroden für multiple diathermische Stichelung. Ber Dtsch Ophthalmol Ges 49:119–124, 1932.
166. Larsson S: Electro-diathermy in detachment of the retina. Arch Ophthalmol 7:661–680, 1932.
167. Walker CB: Retinal detachment. Technical observations and new devices for treatment with a specially arranged diathermy unit for general ophthalmic service. Am J Ophthalmol 17:1–17, 1934.
168. Lindner K: Heilungsversuche bei prognotisch ungünstigen Fällen von Netzhautabhebung. Z Augenheilkd 81:277–299, 1933.
169. Hildesheimer S: Ablatio-Operation mit streifenförmiger Elektroexcision der Sklera und chemischer Aetzung, vol. 2, part 2. Acta XIV Concilium Ophthalmologicum, Hispania, 1933 Blass, Madrid, pp 52–54.
170. Pischel DK and Miller M: Retinal detachment cured by an eyeball-shortening operation: Report of a case. Arch Ophthalmol 22:974–979, 1939.
171. Dellaporta A: Die Verkürzung des Bulbus mittels Skleralfaltung. Klin Monatsbl Augenheilkd 119:135–140, 1951.
172. Paufique L, Hugonnier R: Traitement du décollement de la rétine par la résection sclérale: Technique personnelle, indications et résultats. Bull Mém Soc Fr Ophtalmol 64:435–456, 1951.
173. Shapland CD: Scleral resection—Lamellar. Trans Ophthalmol Soc UK 71:29–51, 1952.
174. Weve H: Bulbusverkürzung durch Reffung der Sclera. Ophthalmologica 118:660–665, 1949.
175. Everett WG: A new scleral shortening operation. Arch Ophthalmol 53:865–869, 1955.
176. Castroviejo R: New clips and clip-applying forceps for scleral shortening procedure. Trans Am Acad Ophthalmol Otolaryngol 60:483–485, 1956.
177. Lemoine AN Jr, Robinson JT Jr, Calkins LL: Scleral imbrication technique. Arch Ophthalmol 60:237–238, 1958.
178. Strampelli B: Trattamento del distaco di retina con iniezioni sottoretiniche di plasma sanguigno. Boll Ocul 12:629–632, 1933.
179. Strampelli B: Introduzione di spugna di gelatina nello spazio sopracoroideale nella operazione del distacco di retina non riducibile con il riposo. Ann Ottal Clin Ocul 80:275–281, 1954.
180. Smith R: Suprachoroidal air injection for detached retina: Preliminary report. Br J Ophthalmol 36:385–388, 1952.
181. Jess A: Temporäre Skleraleindellung als Hilfsmittel bei der Operation der Netzhautablösung. Klin Monatsbl Augenheilkd 99:318–319, 1937.
182. Custodis E: Beobachtungen bei der diathermischen Behandlung der Netzhautablösung und ein Hinweis zur Therapie der Amotio Retinae. Ber Dtsch Ophthalmol Ges 57:227–230, 1952.
183. Custodis E: Bedeutet die Plombenaufnahung auf die Sklera einen Fortschritt in der operativen Behandlung der Netzhautablösung? Ber Dtsch Ophthalmol Ges 58:102–105, 1953.
184. Schepens CL, Okamura ID, Brockhurst RJ: The scleral buckling procedures. I. Surgical techniques and management. Arch Ophthalmol 58:797–811, 1957.
185. Schepens CL, Okamura ID, Brockhurst RJ, Reagan CDJ: Scleral buckling procedures. V. Synthetic sutures and silicone implants. Arch Ophthalmol 64:868–881, 1960.
186. Lincoff HA, Baras I, McLean J: Modifications to the Custodis procedure for retinal detachment. Arch Ophthalmol 73:160–163, 1965.
187. Refojo MF, Leong FL: Poly (methylacrylate-co-hydroxyethyl acrylate) hydrogel implant material of strength and softness. J Biomed Material Res 15:497–509, 1981.
188. Banuelos A, Refojo MF, Schepens CL: Expandable silicone implants for scleral buckling. I. Introduction of a new concept. Arch Ophthalmol 89:500–502, 1973.
189. Hopping W: Die Ballonplombe: Bericht über die ersten Ergebnisse mit einem neuen Operationsverfahren bei Netzhautablösung. Mod Probl Ophthalmol 5:289–292, 1967.
190. Lincoff HA, Kreissig I, Hahn YS: A temporary buckle for the treatment of small retinal detachments. Ophthalmology 86:586–592, 1979.
191. Borras A: Inclusion of absorbable gelatin film between the scleral lamellae in the treatment of retinal detachment. Am J Ophthalmol 52:561–565, 1961.
192. Schepens CL: Retinal Detachment and Allied Diseases, vol. 1. Philadelphia, WB Saunders, 1983, pp 526–535.
193. Snow JC: Positioning of anesthetized patients for repair of giant retinal breaks: Prone, head down and flexed position. Anesth Analg 43:140–143, 1964.
194. Schepens CL, Freeman HM, Thompson RF: A power-driven multipositional operating table. Arch Ophthalmol 73:671–673, 1965.
195. Chignell AH: Retinal detachment surgery without drainage of subretinal fluid. Am J Ophthalmol 77:1–5, 1974.
196. Schepens CL: Retinal Detachment and Allied Diseases, vol. 1. Philadelphia, WB Saunders, 1983, pp 409–416.
197. Schepens CL: Current management of retinal detachment: Progress or chaos? Ann Ophthalmol 3:21–41, 1971.
198. Zauberman H, Garcia Rosell F: Treatment of retinal detachment without inducing chorioretinal lesions. Trans Am Acad Ophthalmol Otolaryng 79:835–844, 1975.
199. Zauberman H, Berson D: Treatment of retinal detachment without chorioretinal scars. In Shimizu K, Oosterhuis JO (eds): XXIII Concil Ophthalmol Kyoto, 1978, part I. Acta Amsterdam-Oxford, Excerpta Medica, 1979, pp 715–718.
200. Chignell AH: Retinal detachment surgery without cryotherapy. Trans Ophthalmol Soc UK 97:30–32, 1977.
201. Fetkenhour CL, Hanch TL: Scleral buckling without thermal adhesion. Am J Ophthalmol 89:662–666, 1980.
202. Schepens CL: Retinal Detachment and Allied Diseases, vol. 1. Philadelphia, WB Saunders, 1983, pp 1146–1147.
203. Schepens CL: Methods of producing a chorioretinal scar. I. Diathermy. In Retinal Detachment and Allied Diseases, vol. 1. Philadelphia, WB Saunders, 1983, pp 289–299.
204. Jabbour NM, McCormick SA, Gong H: Transcleral and transconjunctival diathermy. Retina 9:127–130, 1989.
205. Budd R, Jabbour NM, Furlong M, et al: Consistent monopolar diathermy delivery using a return path. Invest Ophthalmol Vis. Sci 31(ARVO Suppl):26, 1990.
206. Schoeler F: Experimentelle Erzeugung von Aderhaut-Netzhaut-Entzündung durch Kohlensäureschnee. Monatsbl Augenheilkd 60:1–2, 1918.

207. Bietti GB: Criocausticazioni episclerali come mezzo di terapia nel distacco retinico. Boll Ocul 13:576–617, 1934.
208. Deutschmann R: Ueber zwei Verfahren bei Behandlung der Netzhautablösung (eines davon der Diathermie scheinbar entgegengesetz) nebst Bemerkungen zur Genese des Netzhautrisses und seines Verhältnisses zur Enstehung der Ablösung. Klin Monatsbl Augenheilkd 91:450–456, 1933.
209. Cooper IS: Principles and rationale of cryogenic surgery. St Barnabas Hosp Med Bull 1:5–10, 1962.
210. Amoils SP, Walker AJ: The thermal and mechanical factors involved in ocular cryosurgery. Proc R Soc Med 59:1056–1064, 1966.
211. Amoils SP: The Joule Thomson retinal cryopencils. Arch Ophthalmol 80:128–131, 1968.
212. Campochiaro PA, Kaden IH, Vidauri Leal J, Glaser BM: Cryotherapy enhances intravitreal dispersion of viable retinal pigment epithelial cells. Arch Ophthalmol 103:434–436, 1985.
213. Meyer-Schwickerath G: Lichtkoagulation. Klin Monatsbl Augenheilkd 33(Beihefte):1–96, 1959.
214. Koester CJ, Snitzer E, Campbell CJ, Rittler MC: Experimental laser retina coagulator. [Abstract] J Opt Soc Am 52:607, 1962.
215. Pomerantzeff O, Delori F: Physical aspects of ruby-laser and xenon-arc photocoagulation. In McPherson A (ed): New and Controversial Aspects of Retinal Detachment. New York, Hoeber Medical Division, Harper & Row, 1968, pp 247–260.
216. Bloom AL: Gas lasers. Appl Optics 5:1500–1514, 1966.
217. Pomerantzeff O, Kaneko H, Donovan RH, et al: Effect of the ocular media on the main wavelengths of argon laser emission. Invest Ophthalmol 15:70–77, 1976.
218. Delori FC, Pomerantzeff O: Monochromatic light for treatment and diagnosis: Physical principles. In Freeman HM, Hirose T, Schepens CL (eds): Vitreous Surgery and Advances in Fundus Diagnosis and Treatment. New York, Appleton-Century-Crofts, 1977, pp 587–597.
219. Brancato R, Pratesi R: Applications of diode lasers in ophthalmology. Lasers Light Ophthalmol 1:119–129, 1987.
220. McHugh JDA, Marshall J, Capon M, et al: Transpupillary retinal photocoagulation in the eyes of rabbit and human using a diode laser. Lasers Light Ophthalmol 2:125–143, 1988.
221. McHugh JDA, Marshall J, Ffytche TJ, et al: Initial clinical experience using a diode laser in the treatment of retinal vascular disease. Eye 3:516–527, 1989.
222. Cibis PA: Vitreous transfer and silicone injections. Trans Amer Acad Ophthalmol Otolaryngol 68:983–997, 1964.
223. Ohm J: Ueber die Behandlung der Netzhautablösung durch operative Entleerung der Subretinal-Flüssigkeit und Einspritzung von Luft in den Glaskörper. Graefes Arch Ophthalmol 79:442–450, 1911.
224. Arruga H: Décollement rétinien, l'urgence opératoire, l'injection d'air, les grandes désinsertions. Bull Mém Soc Fr Ophthalmol 49:288–303, 1936.
225. Rosengren B: Ueber die Behandlung der Netzhautablösung mittels Diathermie und Luftinjektion in den Glaskörper. Acta Ophthalmol 16:3–42, 1938.
226. Rosengren B: Air injection in retinal detachment. Acta XVI Concil Ophthalmol (Britannia), 1950, pp 1212–1217.
227. Rosengren B: 300 cases operated upon for retinal detachment, methods and results. Acta Ophthalmol 30:117–122, 1952.
228. Schepens CL, Freeman HM: Current management of giant retinal breaks. Trans Am Acad Ophthalmol Otolaryngol 71:474–487, 1967.
229. Norton E: Intraocular gas in the management of selected retinal detachments. Trans Am Acad Ophthalmol Otolaryngol 77:OP85–98, 1973.
230. Fineberg E, Machemer R, Sullivan P, et al: Sulfur hexafluoride in owl monkey vitreous cavity. Am J Ophthalmol 79:67–76, 1975.
231. Lincoff H, Coleman J, Kreissig I, et al: The perfluorocarbon gases in the treatment of retinal detachment. Ophthalmology 90:546–551, 1983.
232. Constable I: Effect of vitreous replacement with gases: Preliminary note on perfluoropentane. In Freeman HM, Hirose T, Schepens CL (eds): Vitreous Surgery and Advances in Fundus Diagnosis and Treatment. New York, Appleton-Century-Crofts, 1977, pp 427–431.
233. Dominguez DA: Cirurgica precoz y ambulatoria del disprendimiento de retina. Arch Soc Esp Oftal 48:47–54, 1985.
234. Hilton GF, Grizzard WS: Pneumatic retinopexy. A two-step outpatient operation without conjunctival incision. Ophthalmology 93:626–640, 1986.
235. Hilton G, Kelly N, Salzano T, et al: Pneumatic retinopexy, a collaborative report of the first 100 cases. Ophthalmology 94:307–314, 1987.
236. Tornambe P, Hilton G, Kelly N, et al: Expanded indications for pneumatic retinopexy. Ophthalmology 95:597–600, 1988.
237. Tornambe P, Hilton G, The Retinal Detachment Study Group: Pneumatic retinopexy, a multicenter randomized controlled clinical trial comparing pneumatic retinopexy with scleral buckling. Ophthalmology 96:772–784, 1989.
238. Tornambe P, Hilton G, Brinton D, et al: Pneumatic retinopexy, a two-year follow-up study of the multicenter clinical trial comparing pneumatic retinopexy with scleral buckling. Ophthalmology 98:1115–1123, 1991.
239. Dreyer R: Sequential retinal tears attributed to intraocular gas. Am J Ophthalmol 102:276–278, 1986.
240. Poliner L, Grand G, Schoch L, et al: New retinal detachment after pneumatic retinopexy. Ophthalmology 94:315–318, 1987.
241. Freeman W, Lipson B, Morgan C, Liggett P: New posteriorly located retinal breaks after pneumatic retinopexy. Ophthalmology 95:14–18, 1988.
242. Chen J, Robertson J, Coonan P, et al: Results and complications of pneumatic retinopexy. Ophthalmology 95:601–608, 1988.
243. McDonald R, Abrams G, Irvine A, et al: The management of subretinal gas following attempted pneumatic retinal reattachment. Ophthalmology 94:319–326, 1987.
244. Kreissig I, Failer J, Lincoff H, Ferrari F: Results of a balloon buckle in the treatment of 500 retinal detachments and a comparison with pneumatic retinopexy. Am J Ophthalmol 107:381–389, 1989.
245. Lincoff H, Horowitz J, Kreissig I, Jakobiec F: Morphological effects of gas compression on the cortical vitreous. Arch Ophthalmol 104:1212–1215, 1986.
246. Okubo A, Okubo Y, Ohara K, Shimizu H: Vitreous as tamponade in healing of rhegmatogenous retinal detachment. Jpn J Ophthalmol 34:36–43, 1990.
247. Chang S, Repucci V, Zimmerman NJ, et al: Perfluorocarbon liquids in the management of traumatic retinal detachments. Ophthalmology 96:785–792, 1989.
248. Lenz G: Die Behandlung der Netzhautablösung. In Axenfeld T, Elschnig A (eds): Handbuch der gesamten Augenheilkunde, 3rd ed. Elsching A (ed): Augenärtzliche Operationslehre, vol. 2. Berlin, Julius Springer, 1922, pp 1289–1362.
249. Cutler NL: Transplantation of human vitreous. A preliminary report. Arch Ophthalmol 35:615–623, 1946.
250. Cutler NL: Vitreous transplantation. Trans Am Acad Ophthalmol Otolaryngol 51:253–259, 1947.
251. Shafer DM: Vitreous implants in retina surgery. In Schepens CL (ed): Importance of the Vitreous Body in Retina Surgery with Special Emphasis on Reoperations. St Louis, CV Mosby, 1960, pp 131–160.
252. Paufique L, Moreau PG: Les greffes de vitré lyophilisé. Ann d'Ocul 186:873–875, 1953.
253. Hruby K: Weitere Erfahrungen mit Hyaluronasäure als Glaskörperersatz bei Netzhautablösung. In Streiff EB (ed): Modern Problems in Ophthalmology. New York, Karger, 1966, pp 228–229.
254. Pruett RC, Schepens CL Swann DA: Hyaluronic acid vitreous substitute. A six-year clinical evaluation. Arch Ophthalmol 97:2325–2330, 1979.
255. Pruett RC, Schepens CL, Freeman HM: Collagen vitreous substitute. II. Preliminary clinical trials. Arch Ophthalmol 91:29–32, 1974.
256. Cibis PA, Becker B, Okun E, Canaan S: The use of liquid silicone in retinal detachment surgery. Arch Ophthalmol 68:590–599, 1962.
257. Mukai N, Lee PF, Schepens CL: Intravitreous injection of silicone. An experimental study. II. Histochemistry and electron-microscopy. Ann Ophthalmol 4:273–287, 1972.
258. Mukai N, Lee PF, Oguri M, Schepens CL: A long-term evaluation of silicone retinopathy in monkeys. Can J Ophthalmol 10:391–402, 1975.

259. Rockland K, Pankratov MM, Sebag J, et al: Central nervous system changes following intraocular injection of silicone oil. [Abstract] Invest Ophthalmol Vis Sci 29:405, 1988.
260. Zucker CL, Pankratov MM, Sebag J, et al: Topography and time course of retinal effects by intraocular silicone oil. [Abstract] Invest Ophthalmol Vis Sci 30:102, 1989.
261. Nakamura K, Refojo MJ, Crabtree DV, et al: Ocular toxicity of low-molecular-weight components of silicone and fluorosilicone oils. Invest Ophthalmol Vis Sci 32:3007–3020, 1991.
262. Refojo MF, Leong FL, Chung H, et al: Extraction of retinol and cholesterol by intraocular silicone oils. Ophthalmology 95:614–618, 1988.
263. Tolentino FI, Refojo M, Cajita V, et al: Experience with silicone and fluorosilicone oil in ophthalmology. In Caramazza R, Versura P (eds): Biomaterials in Ophthalmology: An Interdisciplinary Approach. Congressi Bologna, Italy, Studio E.R., 1990.
264. Fernandez-Vigo J, Refojo MF, Verstraeten T: Evaluation of a viscoelastic solution of hydroxypropyl methylcellulose as a potential vitreous substitute. Retina 10:148–152, 1990.
265. von Graefe A: Therapeutische Miscellen. Arch Ophthalmol 9:43–152, 1863.
266. Schepens CL: Retinal Detachment and Allied Diseases, vol. 2. Philadelphia, WB Saunders, 1983, pp 770–804.
267. Freeman HM, Schepens CL: Vitreous surgery. Mod Probl Ophthalmol 7:311–316, 1968.
268. Couvillion GC, Freemen HM, Schepens CL: Vitreous surgery. V. Modification of the vitreous scissors. Arch Ophthalmol 83:722–723, 1970.
269. Freeman HM: Vitreous surgery. X. Current status of vitreous surgery in cases of rhegmatogenous retinal detachment. Trans Am Acad Ophthalmol Otolaryngol OP77:202–215, 1973.
270. Couvillion GC, Freeman HM, Schepens CL: Vitreous surgery. III. Intraocular balloon. Instrument report. Arch Ophthalmol 83:713–714, 1970.
271. Schepens CL, Delori F, Rogers FJ, Constable IJ: Optimized underwater diathermy for vitreous surgery. Ophthalmic Surg 6:82–89, 1975.
272. Ford V: Proposed surgical treatment of opaque vitreous. Lancet 1:462–463, 1890.
273. Komoto : Ueber Glaskörperwaschung bei unheilbarer Glaskörperblutung. Klin Monatsbl Augenheilkd 50:265, 1912.
274. Elschnig A: Ueber Glaskorperersatz. Vers Ophthalmol Ges Heidelberg, 1911, pp 11–15.
275. Zur Nedden M: The curative value of aspiration of the vitreous. Arch Ophthalmol 57:109–120, 1928.
276. Schepens CL: Retinal Detachment and Allied Diseases, vol. 2. Philadelphia, WB Saunders, 1983, pp 805–806.
277. Machemer R, Buettner H, Norton EWD, Parel JM: Vitrectomy: A pars plana approach. Trans Am Acad Ophthalmol Otolaryngol 15:813–820, 1971.
278. Tolentino FI, Banko A, Schepens CL, et al: Vitreous surgery. IX. New instrumentation for vitrectomy. Arch Ophthalmol 93:667–672, 1975.
279. Machemer R: A new concept for vitreous surgery. Two instrument techniques in pars plana vitrectomy. Arch Ophthalmol 92:407–412, 1974.
280. O'Malley C, Heintz RM: Vitrectomy via the pars plana. A new instrument system. Trans Pacific Coast Otolophthalmol Soc 53:121–137, 1972.
281. Machemer R: Die chirurgische Entfernung von epiretinalen Makulamembranen (macular puckers). Klin Monatsbl Augenheilkd 172:36–42, 1978.
282. The Retina Society Terminology Committee: The classification of retinal detachment with proliferative vitreoretinopathy. Ophthalmology 90:121–125, 1983.
283. Freeman HM, Elner SG, Tolentino FI, et al: Anterior PVR. Part I: Clinical findings and management. In Freeman HM, Tolentino IF (eds): Proliferative Vitreoretinopathy (PVR). New York, Springer, 1988, pp 22–33.
284. Machemer R: Retinotomy. Am J Ophthalmol 92:768–774, 1981.
285. Machemer R, McCuen BW, de Juan E: Relaxing retinotomies and retinectomies. Am J Ophthalmol 102:7–12, 1986.
286. Cohen HB, McMeel JW, Franks EP: Diabetic traction detachment. Arch Ophthalmol 97:1268–1272, 1979.
287. McMeel JW: Treatment of traction detachment of the retina by scleral resection. In Pruett RC, Reagan CDJ (eds): Retina Congress. New York, Appleton-Century-Crofts, 1974, pp 511–521.
288. Schepens CL: Retinal Detachment and Allied Diseases, vol. 2. Philadelphia, WB Saunders, 1983, p 891.
289. Kasner D, Miller GR, Taylor WH, et al: Surgical treatment of amyloidosis of the vitreous. Trans Am Acad Opthalmol Otolaryngol 72:410–418, 1968.
290. Schepens CL, Constable IJ: Open-sky vitrectomy: Operative technique and instrumentation. In Freeman HM, Hirose T, Schepens CL (eds): Vitreous Surgery and Advances in Fundus Diagnosis and Treatment. New York, Appleton-Century-Crofts, 1977, pp 465–477.
291. Constable IJ, Schepens CL: Open-sky vitrectomy: Indications and preliminary results. In Freeman HM, Hirose T, Schepens CL (eds): Vitreous Surgery and Advances in Fundus Diagnosis and Treatment. New York, Appleton-Century-Crofts, 1977, pp 451–463.
292. Hirose T, Schepens CL: Complications in open-sky vitrectomy. In Freeman HM, Hirose T, Schepens CL (eds): Vitreous Surgery and Advances in Fundus Diagnosis and Treatment. New York, Appleton-Century-Crofts, 1977, pp 479–495.
293. Ashrafzadeh MT, Schepens CL, Lee PF: Vitreous surgery. VII. Corneal protector for subtotal vitrectomy. Arch Ophthalmol 89:138–142, 1973.
294. Liu HS, Tolentino FI, Schepens CL, Freeman HM: Experimental vitreous surgery. XIII. Open-sky partial vitrectomy through pars plana incision. Arch Ophthalmol 91:311–312, 1974.
295. Schepens CL: Clinical and research aspects of subtotal open-sky vitrectomy. Am J Ophthalmol 91:143–171, 1981.
296. Jabbour NM, Schepens CL, Buzney SM: Local ocular hypothermia in experimental intraocular surgery. Ophthalmology 95:1687, 1988.
297. Hirose T: Personal communication.
298. Hirose T, Schepens CL, Lopansri C: Subtotal open-sky vitrectomy for severe retinal detachment occurring as a late complication of ocular trauma. Ophthalmology 88:1–9, 1981.
299. Hirose T: Retino-choroidal suturing in proliferative vitreoretinopathy in giant retinal tear. In Neetens A (ed): Modern Concepts in Vitreoretinal Diseases. Belgium, University of Antwerp, UIA Press, 1985, p 195.
300. Rubbrecht R: La suture dans le traitement du décollement rétinien. Arch d'Ophthalmol 50:608–613, 1933.
301. Scott JD: A new approach to the vitreous base. Mod Probl Ophthalmol 12:407–410, 1974.
302. Heimann K: Zur Behandlung komplizierter Einrisse der Netzhaut. Klin Monatsbl Augenheilkd 176:491–492, 1980.
303. Usui M, Hamazaki S, Takano S, Matsuo H: A new surgical technique for the treatment of the giant tear. Transvitreoretinal fixation. Jpn J Ophthalmol 23:206–215, 1979.
304. Federman JL, Shakin JL, Lanning RG: The microsurgical management of giant retinal tears with trans-scleral sutures. Ophthalmology 89:832–839, 1982.
305. Freeman HM: Management of giant retinal breaks with an inverted retinal flap. In Neetens A (ed): Modern Concepts in Vitreoretinal Diseases. Belgium, University of Antwerp, UIA Press, 1985, pp 183–194.
306. Hirose T: Ablation of retinal pigment epithelium in treatment of giant retinal tears. In Neetens A (ed): Modern Concepts in Vitreoretinal Diseases. Belgium, University of Antwerp, UIA Press, 1985, p 195.
307. Hirose T: Advanced retinopathy of prematurity: Treatment by open-sky vitrectomy. In Neetens A (ed): Modern Concepts in Vitreoretinal Diseases. Belgium, University of Antwerp, UIA Press, 1985, p 199.
308. Machemer R: Closed vitrectomy for severe retrolental fibroplasia in the infant. Ophthalmology 90:436–441, 1983.
309. Hirose T, Lou P: Retinopathy of prematurity. Int Ophthalmol Clin 26:1–23, 1986.

Index

Note: Page numbers in *italics* refer to illustrations; page numbers followed by t refer to tables.

Limbus, incision into, in intracapsular cataract extraction, 614, *615*, 616, *616*

Lime [Ca(OH)₂] injury, emergency treatment of, 3376–3377, 3376t

Limiting membrane, internal, wrinkling of, 919. See also *Epiretinal membranes.*

Lincoff balloon, retinal detachment treatment with, 1101

Lindau tumor, 3311

Linear nevus sebaceous syndrome, *1773*, 1774, 3323

Lipid(s), deposition of, corneal, 61, *62*, 63, 66, *66–67*
　in Terrien's marginal degeneration, 64, *64*
　stromal, 314, *315*
　diabetic retinopathy and, 748t
　in central crystalline dystrophy, 41, *46*
　in sebaceous glands, 101
　metabolic disorders of, ocular manifestations of, 299–303

Lipid-containing granuloma, orbital, 2083, 2085, *2085*

Lipid exudate, in retinal arterial macroaneurysm, 796, *796*

Lipid layer, of tear film, 259

Lipidosis, corneal abnormalities in, 2786
　eye movement disorders in, 2439
　ocular manifestations of, 2781–2783, *2782*

Lipodermoid, *1898*, 1898–1899
　excision of, sequelae of, 1898, *1898*
　pediatric, at lateral canthus, 2792, *2794*

Lipofuscin, in pseudovitelliform macular dystrophy, 1253
　in retinal pigment epithelium, *2245*

Lipofuscinosis, ceroid, neuronal, ocular manifestations of, 2781–2783, *2782*
　retinal findings in, 1227, *2522*

Lipogranuloma, *2095*, 2095–2096

Lipogranulomatosis, ocular manifestations of, 2778
　skeletal/facial changes in, 2783

Lipohyalinosis, in penetrating artery disease, 2666

Lipoid granulomatosis, 1860–1861

Lipoid proteinosis, of eyelid, 1861

Lipoma, orbital, 2331

Lipoprotein, 300, *300*
　familial deficiency of, 302–303, 302t, *303*, 2783, 2786
　metabolic disorders of, ocular manifestations of, 299–303
　particle of, 300, *300*

Liposarcoma, orbital, 2331–2332, *2332*

Liposomes, drug delivery in, 1681

Lisch's nodules, 3205, *3205*, 3259
　histopathology of, 3304
　in neurofibromatosis, 2168, 3304, *3304*

Listeria, 162

Listeria monocytogenes, in endogenous endophthalmitis, 416–417, 3122

Lithium, gaze deviation and, 2502, *2502*
　ophthalmologic effects of, 3738, 3738t

Litigation, malpractice, 3798–3799

Little, James, 611–612

Liver, in candidiasis, 3033, 3036
　in sarcoidosis, 3137

Liver disease, *2979*, 2979–2980
　surgical risk and, 2855
　upper eyelid retraction in, 1836

Loa loa, 3072–3073

Loa loa *(Continued)*
　in diffuse unilateral subacute neuroreti-nopathy, 980

Localized acrodermatitis continua of Hallopeau, 3153

Locked-in syndrome, vs. coma, 2499

Lockwood's ligament, 1691, 1871, *1872*, *1877*

Locus ceruleus, *2448*

Lodoxamide, in allergic conjunctivitis, 82

Loewi's sign, 2945t

Löfgren's syndrome, 3135

Loiasis, 3072–3073
　in diffuse unilateral subacute neuroreti-nopathy, 980

Louis-Bar syndrome, 3320–3322. See also *Ataxia-telangiectasia.*

Low vision. See also *Vision loss.*
　aging and, 3664, 3666
　definitions in, 3664, 3665t
　examination in, 3673–3676, 3673t, 3674t
　　color vision in, 3675
　　components of, 3673t
　　contrast sensitivity in, 3674
　　education in, 3673
　　for severe vision loss, 3690–3691
　　functional history in, 3673, 3674t
　　glare sensitivity in, 3675
　　refraction in, distance, 3675
　　　near, 3675–3676
　　visual acuity in, 3665, 3673–3674
　　visual assessment in, 3673–3675
　　visual fields in, 3674–3675
　functional problems in, 3666–3667
　incidence of, 3663
　macular degeneration and, 3663–3664
　multiple impairments in, 2667
　pediatric, 3665, 3667, 3682–3683
　problems in, 3665–3666
　rehabilitation of, 3663–3695
　　aging and, 3664
　　closed circuit television in, 3681, *3681*
　　contact lenses in, 3678–3679
　　coping and, 3721, 3721t
　　devices for, 3676–3683
　　　approach magnification in, 3681
　　　contrast enhancement in, 3681, *3681*, *3682*
　　　large type in, 3681, *3682*
　　　lighting in, 3681
　　　nonoptical, *3681*, 3681–3683, *3682*, 3682t
　　　optical, 3676–3681
　　　purchase of, 3689
　　educational services in, 3721, 3721t
　　effectiveness of, 3673
　　examination in, 3671
　　failure of, prevention of, 3670
　　families in, 3669–3670
　　follow-up care in, 3683
　　hand-held magnifiers in, 3680, *3680*
　　in choroidal neovascularization, 850
　　library/information services in, 3688–3689, *3689*
　　mobility in, 3689
　　occupational therapy in, 3671–3672, 3683–3686, 3683t
　　　adaptive, 3685
　　　for cooking/eating, 3685, *3685*
　　　for environmental modifications, *3685*, 3685–3686
　　　for vision substitution techniques, 3686

Low vision *(Continued)*
　　　for writing, 3684, 3684–3685, *3685*
　　　multiple impairments and, 3686
　　　treatment plans/sessions in, 3686
　　　with nonoptical devices, *3684*, 3684–3686, *3685*
　　　with optical devices, 3684
　　ophthalmologic residency in, 3672
　　orientation in, 3689
　　patient courtesies in, 3689
　　patient population in, 3672
　　pediatric, 3682–3683
　　program model for, 3671, *3672*
　　psychosocial factors in, 3667–3670, 3687–3688
　　recommendations for, 3683
　　referral criteria in, 3672–3673
　　social worker in, 3672, 3687–3688, 3687t
　　　financial assistance by, 3688
　　　in legal blindness registration, 3687–3688
　　　patient advocacy by, 3688
　　　psychosocial assessment by, 3687–3688
　　　referral responsibilities of, 3688
　　spectacle magnifiers in, 3679, *3679*
　　stand magnifiers in, *3680*, 3680–3681
　　teamwork in, 3672
　　telescopic systems in, 3676–3678, *3677*
　　　aphakia and, 3678
　　　astronomical, 3676–3677, *3677*
　　　bioptic, 3677, *3677*
　　　distance viewing with, 3678
　　　driving with, 3677–3678
　　　Galilean, 3676, *3677*
　　　intermediate viewing with, 3678
　　　investigative, 3678
　　　monocular, 3678
　　　near viewing with, 3678
　　　types of, 3677, *3677*
　　timing of, 3670
　　treatment options in, 3670–3671
　　vocational services in, coping and, 3721, 3721t

Lowe's syndrome, lens pathology in, 2188–2189, *2189*
　ocular manifestations of, 2779, *2779*
　renal rickets in, 2783
　visual system in, 3561

Lubricant preparations, in corneal ulcer, 225

Lumbar peritoneal shunt, in idiopathic intracranial hypertension, 2704

Lumbar puncture, in idiopathic intracranial hypertension, 2701–2702, *2702*, 2704

Lung(s), aspergilloma of, 3038, *3038*, 3039, *3039*
　diagnosis of, 3040
　prognosis for, 3041
　treatment of, 3040
　biopsy of, in sarcoidosis, 3140
　blastomycosis of, 3059
　carcinoid tumor of, 2060
　coccidioidomycosis of, 3055, 3057
　cryptococcosis of, 3047
　in amyloidosis, 2959
　in sarcoidosis, 3135–3136, 3136t
　in scleroderma, 2921
　in Wegener's granulomatosis, 2909, 2909t, 2910, 2910t
　mucormycosis of, 3042
　sporotrichosis of, 3045

Lung cancer, CAR syndrome and, 3353
　metastases from, 3517

Retinal arterial macroaneurysms *(Continued)*
 histopathology of, 797
 natural history of, 797–799, *798*
 pathogenesis of, 797
 treatment of, 799–800, *800*
Retinal artery (arteries), central. See *Central retinal artery* entries.
 embolism of, in transient monocular visual loss, 2654
 in amyloidosis, *2966, 2967*
 macroaneurysms of, 795–801. See also *Retinal arterial macroaneurysms.*
 occlusion of. See *Branch retinal artery occlusion; Central retinal artery occlusion.*
Retinal break(s), 1056–1062. See also *Retinal detachment; Retinal dialysis; Retinal hole(s); Retinal tear(s).*
 after vitreoretinal surgery, 1133–1134
 concussive, 3406
 cystic retinal tuft and, 1065, *1065, 1066*
 horseshoe, retinal detachment and, 1095, *1096*
 in Behçet's disease, 1022, *1024*
 in familial exudative vitreoretinopathy, 815
 in proliferative diabetic retinopathy, 765, *765*
 in retinopathy of prematurity, 788
 localization of, Gonin's method of, 1277
  in scleral buckling surgery, 1097
 pathogenesis of, 1274
 pathologic myopia and, 880
 proliferative vitreoretinopathy treatment and, 1118
 traumatic, 3372, 3406, *3406*
 treatment of, retinal pigment epithelium apposition in, 1129, *1130*
  vitrectomy in, 1128–1130, 1129t
Retinal cells, atrophy of, in neurologic disease, 2520t
Retinal degeneration, cancer and, 3352–3353, *3353*
 cyclic guanosine monophosphate in, 1244
 cystoid, in diabetic retinopathy, *2259,* 2259–2260
  peripheral, 1067–1068
 heparan sulfate storage and, 307
 in Alström's disease, 1227
 in Batten's disease, 1227
 in Cockayne's syndrome, 1227
 in Kearns-Sayre syndrome, 1227
 in Laurence-Moon-Bardet-Biedl syndrome, 1224
 in Leber's congenital amaurosis, 1224
 in neuronal ceroid lipofuscinosis, 1227
 in olivopontocerebellar atrophy, 1227
 inherited metabolic diseases and, 2788t
 neonatal, 2836–2837, *2837*
 pigmentary, in Laurence-Moon-Bardet-Biedl syndrome, *2522*
 progressive. See *Retinitis pigmentosa.*
 siderosis and, 2256, *2257*
 snail track, retinal tears and, 1057, *1057*
 snowflake, 1055
Retinal degeneration slow gene, 1221
Retinal detachment, 1084–1089
 acquired retinoschisis and, 1074–1075, *1075, 1076,* 1076t
 at pigment epithelium, in primary ocular–CNS non-Hodgkin's lymphoma, 527, *529*
  in serpiginous choroiditis, 519

Retinal detachment *(Continued)*
 bullous, with chorioretinopathy, vs. idiopathic uveal effusion, *558, 559*
 congenital retinoschisis and, *1081,* 1081–1082, *1082*
 cystic retinal tuft and, 1064–1065
 definition of, 2248
 degenerative retinoschisis and, 1061
 examination of, 1265–1274
  binocular ophthalmoscopy in, 1267–1268, *1268*
  blood flow study in, 1273–1274
  electrophysiologic, 1273
  fundus photography in, 1268–1270, *1269–1271*
  historical perspectives on, 1265–1274
  monocular ophthalmoscopy in, 1265–1267, *1266, 1267*
  scanning laser ophthalmoscope in, 1270, *1272, 1272*
  slit-lamp microscopy in, *1272,* 1272–1273
  ultrasonography in, 1273
 floaters in, miotic glaucoma therapy and, 1552
 glaucoma in, 1552
 hemorrhagic, 2248, 2250
 historical perspectives on, 1265–1274
 in acute retinal necrosis, 950, 958–960, *959, 960*
 in central retinal vein occlusion, 739
 in cytomegalovirus retinitis, 941, 941t, 942, *942*
 in familial exudative vitreoretinopathy, 815, 816, 817
 in intermediate uveitis, 427, *429*
 in intracapsular cataract extraction, 611
 in morning glory syndrome, 1089
 in primary ocular–CNS non-Hodgkin's lymphoma, 526–527, *527, 528*
 in retinopathy of prematurity, 2802, 2804, *2804*
 in sickle cell disease, 1013–1014, *1014*
 in sympathetic ophthalmia, 498, *499*
 in uveal effusion, 549, *549, 550*
 in Vogt-Koyanagi-Harada syndrome, 482, *482*
 lattice degeneration and, 1052–1054, 1053t, *1054*
 macular hole and, treatment of, 1146–1147
 malpractice and, 3800
 mechanisms of, 2248, *2248, 2249,* 2250
 melanoma and, 3516
 miotic glaucoma therapy and, 1552
 nanophthalmos and, 1532–1533
 neovascular glaucoma and, 1497, 1499
 optic nerve pit and, 1089
 pathogenesis of, 1274–1275, 1283
 pathology of, 2248, *2248–2250,* 2250–2251
 pediatric, after cataract extraction, 2765
 pediatric lensectomy and, 2768
 peripheral, vs. uveitis, 404t
 posterior, pathologic myopia and, 879–880, *880*
 posterior vitreous detachment and, 2246
 postvitrectomy neovascular glaucoma and, 1497
 proliferative vitreoretinopathy risk with, 1118–1119
 radiology of, 3513–3514
 retinal attachment and, 2248
 rhegmatogenous, 1084, *1085,* 1085–1088
  cataract extraction and, 1086

Retinal detachment *(Continued)*
 choroidal coloboma and, 1087
 clinical presentation of, 1094
 Ehlers-Danlos syndrome and, 1088
 epiretinal membranes in, 897
 examination of, 1095–1096
 fluid shifts in, 549–550
 genetic factors in, 1553
 Goldmann-Favre syndrome and, 1087
 homocystinuria and, 1088
 in branch retinal vein occlusion, 742
 in intermediate uveitis, 430–431, *431*
 intraocular infection and, 1087
 intraocular inflammation and, 1087
 lens dislocation in, 2225, *2225*
 Marfan's syndrome and, 1087–1088
 myopia and, 1086
 open-angle glaucoma with, 1561
 pars plana vitrectomy and, 1086–1087
 pathology of, 2248, *2248, 2249*
 penetrating keratoplasty and, 1086–1087
 peripheral fundus lesions and, 1085–1086
 pigmentary dispersion syndrome and, 1555
 posterior vitreous detachment and, 1085
 primary open-angle glaucoma and, 1553
 radiology of, 3513
 retinal coloboma and, 1087
 retinal drawings in, 1095–1096
 scleral perforation and, 1087
 senile retinoschisis and, 1086
 traumatic, 1087
  glaucoma and, 1443
 treatment of, 1094–1107
  cryotherapy in, 1101
  extraocular surgery in, 1276–1279, *1276–1279*
  historical perspectives on, 1275–1282
  intraocular surgery in, 1279–1282, *1280, 1281*
  laser photocoagulation in, 1101
  Lincoff balloon in, 1101
  pneumatic retinopexy in, 1100–1101, 1101t
  scleral buckling surgery in, 1092–1107, 1126
   alternatives to, 1100–1101
   anesthesia for, 1096
   appliance application in, *1098,* 1098–1099, *1099*
   care after, 1100
   chorioretinal adhesion stimulation in, *1097,* 1097–1098
   closure in, 1100
   complications of, 1104–1107, 1105t
    intraoperative, 1104–1105, *1106*
    postoperative, 1105–1107, *1106*
   giant break and, 1102–1103, *1103*
   goals of, 1094–1095, *1095*
   history of, 1092–1093
   incision for, *1096,* 1096–1097, *1097*
   intraocular volume adjustment in, 1099–1100
   macular break and, 1102, *1102*
   prognosis for, 1107
   proliferative vitreoretinopathy and, 1104, *1104, 1105*
   retinal break localization in, 1097
   subretinal fluid drainage in, 1099, 1105, 1107
   unseen retinal breaks and, 1101–1102

Retinal necrosis *(Continued)*
in acquired immunodeficiency syndrome, 940, *940*, 3111
intraretinal hemorrhage in, 948–949, *949*
neural spread of, 955
pathophysiology of, 951–954, *952–954*
pigmentary changes of, 948
progressive, in acquired immunodeficiency syndrome, 951
proliferative vitreoretinopathy in, 960
resolution of, 948
retinal detachment in, 959–960, *960*
rhegmatogenous retinal detachment and, 1087
Swiss cheese appearance of, 947, *948*
treatment of, 956–959, *958, 959*
acute optic neuropathy treatment in, 959
acyclovir in, 950, 952, 956–958, *958*
antiinflammatory agents in, 958
antithrombotic agents in, 958
antiviral agents in, 956–958, *958*
retinal detachment prophylaxis in, 958–959, *959*
retinal reattachment in, 960
types of, 946
variants of, 950–951
varicella-zoster virus in, 945–946
viral etiology in, 951–953, *952, 953*
vs. Behçet's disease, 3129
Retinal neovascularization, central retinal vein occlusion and, 739
fluorescein angiography in, 706, 711, *711, 712*
in branch retinal vein occlusion, 742, *742*
in Eales disease, 793–794, *794*
in hemicentral retinal vein occlusion, 744
in leukemia, 2992
in sarcoidosis, 447, 1002, *1003*
in sickle cell disease, 1012–1013, *1013, 1014*
radiation treatment and, 1039
stages of, *429*
Retinal nerve, 2119
Retinal periphlebitis, acute, diffuse. See *Frosted branch angiitis.*
Retinal pigment epitheliopathy, disseminated, acute, 913–918. See also *Multiple evanescent white dot syndrome.*
Retinal pigment epithelium, 699, *699*
absence of, in normal-tension glaucoma, 1354
adenocarcinoma of, 3256, *3256*
aging of, 2251–2252, *2252*
anatomy of, 699, *699*
angioid streaks of, 2172, *2172*
antiangiogenesis factor of, 1493
atrophy of, choroidal folds and, 896, *897*
extramacular, in central serous chorioretinopathy, 819
geographic, in age-related macular degeneration, 827–828, *828*
in onchocerciasis, 463
nongeographic, in age-related macular degeneration, 828, *828*
central areolar dystrophy of, *1253*, 1253–1254
choriocapillaris atrophy and, 762
contusion of, 1028, 3408, *3408*
cytomegalovirus infection of, 2161
depigmentation of, vs. macular hole, 886
destruction of, choriocapillaris atrophy and, 2253–2254

Retinal pigment epithelium *(Continued)*
detachment of, age-related macular degeneration and, 839–840
drusenoid, 839
fibrovascular, *836*, 839
fluorescein angiography in, 706, *709*
hemorrhagic, 839
in ocular histoplasmosis syndrome, 866
serous, *837*, 839
in central serous chorioretinopathy, 818–819
dystrophic calcification of, in age-related macular degeneration, 828, *828*
fluorescein angiography of, 699, *699*, 704, *704*
focal hyperpigmentation of, in age-related macular degeneration, 828
granulomatous lesions of, 482, *483*
hamartoma of, 3254–3256, *3255, 3256*
hemorrhage of, vs. choroidal melanoma, 3213, *3213*
hyperplasia of, congenital, 3253
in presumed ocular histoplasmosis, 2163, *2163*
in retinal detachment, 2248
reactive, 3253, *3254*
vs. choroidal melanoma, 3213
hypertrophy of, congenital, 3251–3253, *3252, 3253*
classification of, 2978
in familial adenomatous polyposis, 2978
in Gardner's syndrome, 2977–2978, 3351, *3352*
vs. choroidal melanoma, 3213, *3214*
in choroideremia, 2175, *2175*
in cystinosis, 2169, *2169*
in intermediate uveitis, 434
in Kearns-Sayre syndrome, 2492–2493
in Leber's idiopathic stellate neuroretinitis, 811
in leukemia, 537, *538*, 998
in macular degeneration, 828, *828*, 830, *830, 836, 837*, 839, 2251
in placoid pigment epitheliopathy, 2167
in primary ocular–CNS non-Hodgkin's lymphoma, 526–527
in pseudoxanthoma elasticum, 855
in retinitis pigmentosa, 2244, *2245*
in sarcoidosis, 1003
in scleroderma, 2923, *2923*
in systemic lupus erythematosus, 2898–2899
in uveal effusion, 550
in Vogt-Koyanagi-Harada syndrome, 482, *483*
in x-linked ocular albinism, 376–377, *377*
inflammation of, fluorescein angiography in, 916
vs. acute macular neuroretinopathy, 928
vs. central serous chorioretinopathy, 823
vs. multiple evanescent white dot syndrome, 916
inherited metabolic diseases and, 2788t
migration of, in photoreceptor disease, 2521, *2522*
pattern dystrophy of, 1253
vs. age-related macular degeneration, 830, *830*
peau d'orange lesion of, in angioid streaks, 853, *854*
proliferation of, vs. retinoblastoma, 2266

Retinal pigment epithelium *(Continued)*
retinal attachment to, 2248
Sjögren's reticular dystrophy of, *1257, 1258*, 1259
tears of, choroidal neovascularization and, 838, *839*
subretinal neovascularization and, 2254, *2254*
termination of, in optic nerve hypoplasia, 2795, *2797*
tumors of, 3251–3256
malignant, 3256, *3256*
vs. choroidal melanoma, 3213, *3214*
Retinal pigment epithelium cells, age-related degeneration of, 2251, *2251*
collagen fiber accumulation by, 1111–1112
contractility of, 1111–1112
fibronectin of, 1112
in acute posterior multifocal placoid pigment epitheliopathy, 909, 911
in epiretinal macular membranes, 922
in epiretinal membrane, 2247, *2247*
in proliferative vitreoretinopathy, 1111, 2250
Retinal potential, in acute macular neuroretinopathy, 927–928
Retinal reattachment, in acute retinal necrosis, 960
Retinal tear(s), 1056–1060, *1057–1059*
asymptomatic, treatment of, 1059
cystic retinal tufts and, 1057
enclosed ora bays and, 1067
giant, 1058, *1059*
retinal detachment and, 1102–1103, *1103*
treatment of, surgical, perfluorocarbon liquids in, 1146, *1147*
perfluoroethane in, 1150
silicone liquid in, 1152–1153, 1152t
horseshoe (flap), 1057, *1058*
operculation of, 1057, *1058, 1059*
treatment of, 1059
in acute retinal necrosis, 950, *950*
necrotic, 3406
paravascular vitreoretinal adhesions and, 1057
posterior vitreous detachment and, 1056
retinal lattice degeneration and, 1057, *1057*
symptomatic, treatment of, *1058*, 1058–1059
traction, retinal lattice degeneration and, 1051, 1052–1053, 1054, *1054*
traumatic, 1029, 2255, 3372
treatment of, *1058*, 1058–1060
prophylactic, 1059–1060
types of, 1057–1058, *1058, 1059*
vitreoretinal adhesion and, 1056–1057
vitreous base and, 1057
vs. enclosed ora bays, 1067
Retinal telangiectasia, congenital, 801–808. See also *Coats' disease.*
exudative retinal detachment and, 1089
foveal, 806–808. See also *Juxtafoveal retinal telangiectasia.*
primary, 801–808. See also *Coats' disease.*
Retinal threshold profile, in chloroquine-associated retinal toxicity, 1043
Retinal tight junctions, loss of, fluorescein angiography of, 705, *706–708*
Retinal trauma, 1027–1031, 2254–2257, *2255–2257*
retinal detachment and, 1029
retinal dialysis and, 1029

Skull *(Continued)*
    inflammatory, 3558
    neoplastic, 3559–3560, *3560*
    ophthalmic syndromes in, 3560–3561
    osseous, 3559
    physiologic states and, 3560
    radiology of, 3557–3561, *3558–3560*,
        3561–3587. See also specific areas,
        e.g., *Cranial fossa, middle.*
    systemic, 3557
    traumatic, 3557–3558, *3559*
    visual system in, 3556–3560, *3558–3560*
SLACH (soft *lens*-associated *corneal
    hypoxia*) syndrome, hydrogel contact
    lenses and, 3640
Sleep, aqueous production during, 1369,
    1371
    disruption of, in birdshot retinochoroiditis,
        477
Slit-lamp microscopy, 4–6, *5, 6*, 691–696,
    692–695
    aspherical lenses in, *693*, 693–694
    contact methods of, 694–696, *694–696*
    contrast in, adjacent illumination and, *5, 6*
        fundal illumination and, *5, 6*
        limbal scatter and, *5, 6*
        narrow-beam illumination and, 4–5
        narrow sectioning and, 4, *5*
        side illumination and, 4, *5*
        specular reflection and, 5, *5*
    Goldmann's posterior fundus contact lens
        in, 696
    Goldmann's three-mirror lens in, *694*, 694–
        695, *695*
        scleral depression with, *695*, 695–696
    history of, *1272*, 1272–1273
    illumination in, 4
    in corneal edema, *5*, 250
    in cortical cataract, *572*
    in glaucoma, 1296–1298
    in intermediate uveitis, 366
    in posterior subcapsular cataract, *572*
    in pupillary evaluation, 2472
    in senescent noncataractous lens, 565, *565*–
        566
    Mainster lens in, *695*, 696
    noncontact methods of, *693*, 693–694
    observation system in, 5–6
    panfunduscopic lens in, *695*, 696
    photic retinopathy from, 1034
    photography in, 1273
    three-mirror contact lens in, 1273
Sly's syndrome, 310
    pediatric, corneal abnormalities in, 2786
        ocular manifestations of, 2781
Small blue cell tumor, pediatric, 2329–2330
Smallpox. See *Vaccinia.*
Smith, Henry, 609
Smith-Indian expression, in cataract surgery,
    609
Smooth muscle actin, immunohistochemical
    staining with, 2376t
Smooth pursuit system, examination of, 2415
    neural substrate for, 2403–2404
    ocular tracking and, 2404
    palsy of, 2423, *2424*
    performance of, 2403
Snail track degeneration. See *Retinal lattice
    degeneration.*
Snellen chart, in cataract evaluation, 671
    in neuroophthalmology, 2390

Snellen equivalents, in contrast sensitivity
    tests, 674, *674*
Snellen system, in low vision examination,
    3676
Snellen-Donder's sign, 2945t
Snell's law, 3603, *3603, 3604*
    prisms and, 3604
Snell's plaque, in pars plana cysts, 386
Snowflake degeneration, retinal, 1055
Snowmobiling, ocular injury in, 3496t
Soccer, ocular injury in, 3497, 3497t
Social environment, vision loss and, 3181–
    3182
Sodium bicarbonate, in local anesthetic mix,
    2862
Sodium chloride, toxicity of, 270
Sodium fluorescein, 698–699. See also
    Fluorescein angiography.
Sodium hyaluronate (Healon), as vitreous
    substitute, 1143–1144
    postoperative intraocular pressure and,
        1512–1513
Soemmerring's ring cataract, 2208, *2208*
Soemmerring's ring configuration, in Lowe's
    syndrome, 2189
Soft tissue, radiation effects on, 3295–3296
    reconstruction of, 3489
Softball, ocular injury in, 3494–3495
Solar keratosis. See *Actinic keratosis.*
Solar lentigo, of eyelid, 1799, *1799*
Solar retinitis, 1032–1034, *1033*
Solar retinopathy, 1032–1034, *1033*, 3417,
    3417–3418
    fluorescein angiography in, 1033, *1033*
    histopathology of, 1034
    symptoms of, 1033
    visual acuity in, 1033
    vs. macular hole, 885–886
Sole proprietorship, 3790
Somatoform disorders, 3747–3749
    anxiety in, 3747–3748
    body dysmorphic disorder in, 3748–3749,
        3749t
    classification of, 3749t
    conversion reactions in, 3748, 3749t
    differential diagnosis of, 3747
    hypochondriasis in, 3747, 3749t
    pain, 3748–3749, 3749t
    psychologic-physiologic features of, 3750–
        3751
    social-psychologic components of, 3747,
        3748t
    symptoms of, 3747, 3749t
    vs. stress-related physiologic responses,
        3749–3750
Somogyi phenomenon, 2929–2930
Sorbate, ocular toxicity of, 93
Sorbinil, complications of, 758
    in diabetic retinopathy, 757–758, 757t
Sorbitol, accumulation of, cataracts from,
    2212
Sorsby's pseudoinflammatory dystrophy,
    1255–1256, *1256*
Sound, velocity of, average, 605t
Southern blot, in hereditary retinoblastoma
    testing, 3272–3273
Sowda, in onchocerciasis, 3071
Spasm, convergence, abduction palsy and,
    2416–2417, 2425
    near reflex, 2405
Specificity, of visual function tests, 670–671,
    671

Spectacles, in aphakia correction, 3648–3649,
    3649, 3650
    magnifiers with, in low vision rehabilita-
        tion, 3679, *3679*
Spectinomycin, in purulent gonococcal
    conjunctivitis, 164
Spectral sensitivity functions, in hereditary
    retinal disease, *1185*, 1185–1186, *1186*
Specula, in cataract extraction, 614, *614*, 630
Sphenoid bone, greater wing of, *1873, 1878*
    congenital absence of, in neurofibroma-
        tosis, 3305
    in encephalocele, 1899, *1899*
    lesser wing of, *1873, 1878*
    meningioma of, orbital extension of, 2047,
        2047
Sphenoid sinus, *1876*
    mucocele of, treatment of, 1903
Sphere, Inbert-Fick principle of, 1330
Spherophakia, brachymorphism and, 2231
    dominant, lens dislocation in, 2231, *2232*
    isolated, 2188
    pathology of, 2188–2189, *2189*
    zonule-related, 2188
Sphingolipidosis, corneal findings in, 305–
    306, *305–306*
Spielmeyer-Vogt disease, ocular
    manifestations of, 2782, 2783
Spinal cord, hemangioblastoma of, 3311
Spindle cell(s), embryologic migration of,
    788, 789
    in iridic melanoma, 3202, *3202*
    in persistent hyperplastic primary vitreous,
        2197, 2198
    in retinopathy of prematurity, 789
Spindle cell carcinoma, conjunctival, 285
    immunohistochemical staining of, 2377,
        2380t
Spindle cell nevus, of eyelid, 1801
Spindle-epithelioid cell nevus, of eyelid,
    1801, *1801*
Spinothalamic tract, *2446*
Spiradenoma, of eyelid, 1782
Spirochetal disease, conjunctiva in, 168–169
    cornea in, 168–169
Spirochetes, in keratitis, 166t
Spitz nevus, of eyelid, 1801, *1801*
Splenomegaly, pediatric, in inherited
    metabolic disease, 2785t
Spondylitis, ankylosing, anterior uveitis in,
    409
    HLA-B27–positive, uveitis in, 2166
    iridocyclitis in, 471
    iritis in, 471
    pediatric, 2787
    retinal manifestations of, 993
    arthritis and, retinal manifestations of, 993
    cervical, pediatric, 2787–2788
    juvenile, 2877–2878
Spondyloarthropathy, clinical course of, 2788
    juvenile, 2787–2788
        definition of, 2787
        incidence of, 2787
        subtypes of, 2787–2788
Sporothrix schenckii, 3043
    of eyelids, 1707
Sporotrichosis, 3043–3045
    central nervous system, 3045
    clinical manifestations of, *3044*, 3044–3045
    cutaneous, 3044, 3045
    definition of, *3043*, 3044
    diagnosis of, 3045

Trichofolliculoma, of eyelid, 1789, 1791, *1791*
Trichomegaly, 1852, *1852*
Trichomonas vaginalis, 471
Trichophyton rubrum, 3156
Trichotillomania, 1854
Trichromasy, anomalous, 1238. See also *Color vision, abnormal.*
Trifluoperazine, ophthalmologic effects of, 3738t, 3739
Trifluorothymidine, ocular toxicity of, 91–92
Trifluridine, 3028
in ocular viral disease, 118–119, 119t
Trigeminal ganglion, latent herpes simplex virus in, 123
Trigeminal nerve, cornea and, 262
divisions of, distribution of, *124*
in herpes zoster ophthalmicus, 136–137, 143, 415, 458, *459*
maxillary division of, *1874*, 1879
ophthalmic division of, 1873–1874, *1874*
spinal, *2449*
squamous cell carcinoma of, 1738, *1740*, 2679, *2679*
traumatic lesions of, 3467–3468
viral entry to, 123–124, *124*
Trigeminal-vagal reflex, extraocular muscle traction and, 2863–2864
Triglycerides, diabetic retinopathy and, 748t
Triiodothyronine (T3), in Graves' disease, 2947
Trimethoprim, in ocular toxoplasmosis, 933
Trimethoprim-sulfamethoxazole, in *Pneumocystis carinii* infection, 3068
in Wegener's granulomatosis, 2916
Trimetrexate, in *Pneumocystis carinii* infection, 3068
Triparanol, cataracts from, 2216
Triple test, in angle-closure glaucoma testing, 1337
Trisomy 13, cataracts in, 2189, 2762, *2762*
lens abnormalities in, 2787t
Trisomy 18, lens abnormalities in, 2787t
Trisomy 21, iris in, 375, *375*
lens abnormalities in, 2787t
ocular findings in, 375t
Tritanomaly, congenital, 1238. See also *Color vision, abnormal.*
Tritanopia, 1242t
congenital, 1239
Triton tumor, 1994, *1995*, 2063
Trochlear fossa, 1872
Trochlear nerve, *1874*, 1874, *1875*, *1876*, 2444, 2447, *2448*
aberrant regeneration of, upper lid retraction and, 1833
abnormalities of, 2454–2456, *2455*, 2455t, 2456t
anatomy of, 2444, 2447, *2448*
palsy of, acquired, 2454–2456, 2455t
at subarachnoid space, 2455, 2455t
congenital, 2454
elevator-depressor, 2419
evaluation of, 2456, 2456t
fascicular, 2454–2455, 2455t
Harada-Ito procedure for, 2751
hypertropia in, assessment of, *2738*, 2738–2739, *2739*
treatment of, 2739
nuclear, 2454–2455, 2455t
paralytic strabismus in, *2738*, 2738–2739, *2739*

Trochlear nerve *(Continued)*
treatment of, 2456
vertical ocular deviation from, 2454, *2455*
within cavernous sinus, 2455, 2455t
superior, *1875*
trauma to, 3472
traumatic injury to, 3471, 3472
Tropheryma whippelli, 2979
Tropicamide, in angle-closure glaucoma testing, 1336, 1337
in pediatric cycloplegia, 2727
mydriasis with, in cataract extraction, 626, 627t
Trypanosoma cruzi, 3074
Trypanosomiasis, African, 3074
Tryptase, in mast cell secretory granules, 80–81
in vernal conjunctivitis, 84, 84t
Tryptophan, *579*
light-absorptive properties of, 581
N-formylkynurenine conversion from, 581, *582*
photooxidation by, 583
photosensitization by, 581–582, *582*
ultraviolet B radiation absorption by, 576
Tryrosinemia, neonatal, 295
type I, 295
type II, corneal findings in, 295, *296*
dermatologic findings in, 295, *296*
enzymatic deficiencies in, 295, *295*
Tuberculin skin test, 3011
Tuberculoma, choroidal, 2157, *2157*
Tuberculosis, 3011–3016
choroiditis in, 453, *453*
classification of, 3011, 3012t
clinical manifestations of, 3012–3014, *3013*
computed tomography of, 3525
definition of, 3011
diagnosis of, *3014*, 3014–3015
Eales disease and, 795
epidemiology of, 3011
extrapulmonary, 3013–3014, 3013t, *3014*
glaucoma with, 1560
granulomatous anterior uveitis in, 417
in acquired immunodeficiency syndrome, 941, 3106
in interstitial keratitis, 2136
magnetic resonance imaging of, 3525
miliary, 3014, *3014*
ocular, 467, 472, 2157, *2157*, *2158*
vs. serpiginous choroiditis, 522
of eyelids, 1708
optic neuropathy in, 2610
orbital, 2310
pathogenesis of, 3012
prevention of, 3016
primary, 3012
pulmonary, 3013
radiology in, *3013*, *3014*, 3015
reactivation, 3012–3013, *3013*
treatment of, 3015–3016, 3015t
uveitis in, vs. birdshot retinochoroiditis, 478
vs. frosted branch angiitis, 983t, 984
Tuberculum sellae, meningioma of, 2620–2621
Tuberous sclerosis, 3307–3310
astrocytic hamartoma of, vs. retinoblastoma, 3281, *3281*
central nervous system in, 3308–3309
cutaneous involvement in, 3308, *3308*

Tuberous sclerosis *(Continued)*
diagnosis of, 3307
heredity of, 3308
history of, 3299
ophthalmic involvement in, *3309*, 3309–3310
optic nerve drusen in, 3309, *3309*
pathology of, 2270t
prevalence of, 3307
prognosis for, 3310
retinal astrocytic hamartoma in, 3309, *3309*
visceral involvement in, 3309
vitreous hemorrhage in, 3309
Tuberous xanthoma, orbital, *2094*, 2094–2095
Tubingen perimetry, in glaucoma, 1302
Tufts, retinal. See *Retinal tuft(s).*
Tumbu fly, orbital infection with, *1950*, 1951
Tumor(s), 3, 2670. See *Orbital schwannoma; Sebaceous cell carcinoma;* specific structures and types, e.g., *Melanoma.*
frequency of, 1886–1889, 1888t, 1889t
Tumor angiogenesis factor, 1492
Tumor necrosis factor, effects of, 2110t
Tunica media, vascular, hyperplasia of, 2258, *2258*
Tunica vasculosa lentis, 370
persistent, 2145–2146
glaucoma and, 1555
Turcot's syndrome, 2978
Tuton giant cell, of juvenile xanthogranuloma, 3340, *3341*
TWAR agent, 3100
Type A personality, in central serous chorioretinopathy, 818, 821
Tyrosinase, in albinism, 376
Tyrosine, deficiency of, 295
sources of, 295, *295*
ultraviolet B radiation absorption by, 576, *577*
Tyrosinemia, type II, in dendritic keratitis, 2135–2136
Tyrosinosis, pediatric, treatment of, 2788
Tzanck preparation, 3028, *3028*

Ubidecarenone, in Kearns-Sayre syndrome, 2493
UCHL-1, immunohistochemical staining with, 2376t, 2382, *2382*
UGH (*uveitis, glaucoma, and hyphema*) syndrome, 1514
in anterior chamber intraocular lens, 642
Uhthoff's symptom, in multiple sclerosis, 2684
in optic neuritis, 2541–2542, 2541t
Ulcer. See also specific types, e.g., *Mooren's ulcer.*
ameboid, 126
aphthous, in Behçet's disease, 413, 466
corneal. See *Corneal ulcer.*
corneoscleral, after cataract surgery, 206
genital, in Behçet's disease, 413
in Wegener's granulomatosis, 2910, *2911*
rodent. See *Basal cell carcinoma.*
treatment of, 3
von Hippel, in Peters' anomaly, 19
Ulcerative colitis, 2975–2977, 2976t, *2977*
anterior uveitis in, 409, 2788
ocular inflammation in, 400–402, 469
retinal manifestations of, 993